Hung's

MANAGEMENT OF THE DIFFICULT AND FAILED AIRWAY

NOTICE

FOURTH EDITION

Hung's
MANAGEMENT OF THE DIFFICULT AND FAILED AIRWAY

ORLANDO R. HUNG, BSC (PHARMACY), MD, FRCP(C)
Professor, Departments of Anesthesia, Surgery, and Pharmacology
Department of Anesthesia, Pain Management and Perioperative Medicine
Dalhousie University
Queen Elizabeth II Health Sciences Centre
Department of Anesthesia
Halifax, Nova Scotia, Canada

MICHAEL F. MURPHY, MD, FRCP(C)
Professor Emeritus, Department of Anesthesiology and Pain Medicine
University of Alberta
Walter C Mackenzie Health Sciences Centre
Edmonton, Alberta, Canada

Mc Graw Hill

New York Chicago San Francisco Athens London Madrid Mexico City
Milan New Delhi Singapore Sydney Toronto

Hung's Management of the Difficult and Failed Airway, Fourth Edition

1 2 3 4 5 6 7 8 9 LWI 28 27 26 25 24 23

ISBN 978-1-264-27832-9
MHID 1-264-27832-2

This book was set in Adobe Garamond Pro by MPS Limited.
The editors were Tim Hiscock and Christie Naglieri.
The production supervisor was Catherine H. Saggese.
Production management was provided by Poonam Bisht, MPS Limited.

Library of Congress Cataloging-in-Publication Data

Names: Hung, Orlando R., editor. | Murphy, Michael F. (Michael Francis), 1954- editor.
Title: Hung's management of the difficult and failed airway / [edited by] Orlando R. Hung, Michael F. Murphy.
Other titles: management of the difficult and failed airway
Description: Fourth edition. | New York : McGraw Hill, [2023] | Includes bibliographical references and index. | Summary: "A case-based guide that helps prepare physicians for the most demanding airway emergencies. The text is was created out of Dr. Hung's training programs and puts practice into the pages of this very popular textbook. A full-color, case-based guide to effectively managing airway emergencies reflect the latest devices and techniques"—Provided by publisher.
Identifiers: LCCN 2022061520 | ISBN 9781264278329 (hardcover) | ISBN 9781264278336 (ebook)
Subjects: MESH: Airway Management—methods | Airway Obstruction—therapy | Airway Obstruction—prevention & control | Intubation, Intratracheal | Emergency Treatment
Classification: LCC RC732 | NLM WF 145 | DDC 616.2—dc23/eng/20230501
LC record available at https://lccn.loc.gov/2022061520

ASSOCIATE EDITORS

Thomas J. Coonan, MD, FRCP(C)
Professor, Departments of Anesthesia, Pain Management and Perioperative Medicine, and Surgery
Faculty of Medicine
Dalhousie University
Halifax, Nova Scotia, Canada

Narasimhan Jagannathan, MD
Vice Chair & Division Head, General Anesthesia
Director, Pediatric Anesthesia Research
Professor of Anesthesiology
Northwestern University Feinberg School of Medicine
Department of Pediatric Anesthesia
Ann & Robert H. Lurie Children's Hospital of Chicago
Chicago, Illinois

George Kovacs, MD, FRCP(C)
Professor, Emergency Medicine
Dalhousie University
Attending Emergency Physician
Charles V. Keating Emergency & Trauma Centre
Queen Elizabeth II Health Sciences Centre
Nova Scotia Health Authority
Halifax, Nova Scotia, Canada

Matteo Parotto, MD, PhD
Associate Professor
Department of Anesthesiology and Pain Management
Interdepartmental Division of Critical Care Medicine
University of Toronto
Toronto General Hospital
Toronto, Ontario, Canada

Nicholas Sowers, MD, FRCP(C)
Assistant Professor, Department of Emergency Medicine
Dalhousie University
Attending Emergency Physician
Nova Scotia Health Authority
Halifax, Nova Scotia, Canada

Kathryn Sparrow, BSc, MD, FRCP(C), MScHQ
Assistant Professor, Discipline of Anesthesia
Memorial University of Newfoundland
Faculty of Medicine
St. John's, Newfoundland and Labrador, Canada

Ronald D. Stewart, OC, ONS, ECNS (hon), BA, BSc, MD, FACEP, FAEM, DSc (hon), LLD
Professor Emeritus
Departments of Anesthesia, Pain Management and Perioperative Medicine and Emergency Medicine
Faculty of Medicine
Dalhousie University
Queen Elizabeth II Health Science Centre
Halifax, Nova Scotia, Canada

DEDICATION

We would like to thank our families for their unfailing support of our academic and clinical work by dedicating this edition to: Jeanette, Christopher, David, and Ana Hung and to Debbi, Amanda, Ryan, and Teddy Murphy. We also dedicate this edition to all our colleagues whose commitment to developing their expertise in airway management education has impacted our profession by improving patient outcomes.

CONTENTS

SECTION 1

PRINCIPLES OF AIRWAY MANAGEMENT

SECTION 2

AIRWAY TECHNIQUES

SECTION 5

AIRWAY MANAGEMENT IN THE INTENSIVE CARE UNIT (ICU)

SECTION 6

AIRWAY MANAGEMENT IN THE OPERATING ROOM

SECTION 7

AIRWAY MANAGEMENT IN THE PEDIATRIC POPULATION

SECTION 8

AIRWAY MANAGEMENT IN OBSTETRICS

SECTION 9

AIRWAY MANAGEMENT IN UNIQUE ENVIRONMENT

SECTION 10

PRACTICAL CONSIDERATIONS IN AIRWAY MANAGEMENT

CONTRIBUTORS

Mathieu Asselin, MD
Clinical Professor
Département d'anesthésiologie et de soins intensifs
Université Laval
Département d'anesthésiologie du CHU de Québec—Pavillons Hôpital Enfant-Jésus
Québec, Québec, Canada
Chapter 40

Kelly Au, MD, FRCP(C)
Clinical Assistant Professor
Discipline of Anesthesia
Memorial University of Newfoundland
Faculty of Medicine
St. John's, Newfoundland, Canada
Chapter 52

Michael Aziz, MD
Professor and Interim Vice Chair for Clinical Affairs
Anesthesiology and Perioperative Medicine
Oregon Health & Sciences University
Portland, Oregon
Chapter 42

Jonathan G. Bailey, MD, MSc, FRCP(C)
Assistant Professor, Department of Anesthesia, Pain Management and Perioperative Medicine
Dalhousie University
Queen Elizabeth II Health Sciences Centre
Department of Anesthesia
Halifax, Nova Scotia, Canada
Chapter 4

Paul A. Baker, MBChB, MD, FANZCA, FEAMS
Associate Professor, Department of Anaesthesiology
University of Auckland
Specialist Anaesthetist, Starship Children's Hospital
Auckland, New Zealand
Chapter 50

Paulin R. Banguti, MD
Associate Professor
Academic Head of Department of Anesthesia, Critical Care and Emergency Medicine
School of Medicine and Pharmacy
College of Medicine and Health Sciences
University of Rwanda
Kigali, Rwanda
Chapter 60

Lauren F. Becker, MD
Critical Care Medicine Fellow
University of Maryland Medical Center
Baltimore, Maryland
Chapter 24

Kimberly R. Blasius, MD
Scope Anesthesia of North Carolina
University of North Carolina
Wake Forest School of Medicine
Matthews, North Carolina
Chapter 15

Ryan S. Brandt, MD
Medical Education Fellow
Department of Emergency Medicine
University of Florida College of Medicine—Jacksonville
Jacksonville, Florida
Chapter 23

Darren Braude, MD, FACEP
Chief, Division of Prehospital, Austere and Disaster Medicine
Professor of Emergency Medicine and Anesthesiology
University of New Mexico Health Sciences Center
Corrales, New Mexico
Chapter 26

Peter G. Brindley, MD, FRCP(C), FRCP (Edin)
Professor, Critical Care Medicine
University of Alberta
Adjunct Professor, Dosseter Ethics Centre
Adjunct Professor, Anesthesiology and Pain Medicine
University of Alberta Hospital
Edmonton, Alberta, Canada
Chapters 6, 35

Samuel G. Campbell, MB BCh, FRCP (Edin)
Professor, Emergency Medicine
Dalhousie University
Attending Emergency Physician
Charles V. Keating Emergency & Trauma Centre
Queen Elizabeth II Health Sciences Centre
Halifax, Nova Scotia, Canada
Chapter 9

David A. Caro, MD
Professor, Residency Program Director
Associate Chair of Education
Department of Emergency Medicine
University of Florida College of Medicine—Jacksonville
Jacksonville, Florida
Chapters 23, 28

Chris C. Christodoulou, MBChB, Cum Laude DA (UK), FRCP(C)
Head, Department of Anesthesiology, Perioperative and Pain Medicine
Provincial Anesthesia Specialty Lead, Shared Health
Max Rady College of Medicine, Rady Faculty of Health Sciences
University of Manitoba
Winnipeg, Manitoba, Canada
Chapter 12

Thomas J. Coonan, MD, FRCP(C)
Professor, Departments of Anesthesia, Pain Management and Perioperative Medicine, and Surgery
Faculty of Medicine
Dalhousie University
Halifax, Nova Scotia, Canada
Chapters 13, 60

Edward T. Crosby, MD, FRCP(C)
Professor, Department of Anesthesiology
University of Ottawa
Ottawa, Ontario, Canada
Chapter 17

Brandon D'Souza, BHSc, RRT/CCAA, FCSRT
Department of Pediatric Anesthesia & Respiratory Therapy
IWK Health Centre
Halifax, Nova Scotia, Canada
Chapter 47

Dennis Drapeau, BSc, MD, FRCP(C)
Assistant Professor, Department of Anesthesia, Pain Management and Perioperative Medicine
Dalhousie University
Queen Elizabeth II Health Sciences Centre
Halifax, Nova Scotia, Canada
Chapter 38

Tristan Dumbarton, MSc, MD, FRCP(C)
Assistant Professor, Department of Anesthesia, Pain management and Perioperative Medicine.
IWK Health Centre
Pediatric Anesthesia
Halifax, Nova Scotia, Canada
Chapter 47

Louise Ellard, MBBS, FANZCA
Consultant Anaesthetist
Department of Anaesthesia
Austin Health
Melbourne, Victoria, Australia
Chapter 33

Anna K. Engeln, MD, FACEP
Associate Professor
Department of Emergency Medicine
Denver Health Medical Center
Denver, Colorado
Chapter 24

Leo Fares, MD, FRCP(C)
Anesthesia Fellow, Department of Women's & Obstetric Anesthesia
Dalhousie University
IWK Health Centre
Halifax, Nova Scotia, Canada
Chapter 53

Holger Gaessler, MD
Abteilung Anaesthesie und Intensivmedizin
Bundeswehrkrankenhaus Ulm
Ulm, Germany
Chapters 18, 48

Susan Galgay, BSc, BN(Hons), MD, FRCP(C)
Assistant Professor
Department of Anesthesia, Pain Management and Perioperative Medicine
Dalhousie University
Victoria General Hospital
Halifax, Nova Scotia, Canada
Chapter 36

Mallory Garza, MD, FRCP(C)
Assistant Professor, Department of Anesthesia, Pain Management and Perioperative Medicine
Dalhousie University
Staff Anesthesiologist
Queen Elizabeth II Health Sciences Centre
Halifax, Nova Scotia, Canada
Chapter 58

Ronald B. George, MD, FRCP(C)
Chief and Professor of Obstetric Anesthesia, Department of Anesthesia and Perioperative Care
University of California San Francisco
Mission Bay Betty Irene Moore Women's Hospital
San Francisco, California
Chapter 56

Carrie L. Goodine, BScH, MD, FRCP(C)
Assistant Professor
Department of Anesthesia, Pain Management and Perioperative Medicine
Dalhousie University
Queen Elizabeth II Health Sciences Centre
Halifax, Nova Scotia, Canada
Chapter 37

James Gould, MD, FRCP(C)
Assistant Professor
Department of Emergency Medicine
Dalhousie University
Queen Elizabeth II Health Science Centre
Halifax, Nova Scotia, Canada
Chapter 21

Akua Gyambibi, MD, FRCP(C)
Clinical Lecturer
Department of Anesthesiology and Pain Medicine
University of Alberta
Edmonton, Alberta, Canada
Chapter 3

Lucien Hackett, MBBS
Staff Anaesthetist, Department of Anaesthesia and Pain Management
Concord Repatriation General Hospital
Concord, New South Wales, Australia
Chapter 66

John Hajduk
Clinical Research Coordinator
Department of Pediatric Anesthesiology
Northwestern University Feinberg School of Medicine
Chicago, Illinois
Chapter 51

Michele Heath, CCP
Duke University Medical Center and Durham VA Medical Center
Raleigh, North Carolina
Chapter 15

Matthias Helm, MD, Professor
University of Ulm
Bundeswehr Hospital
Blaustein, Germany
Chapter 59

Jacob Heninger, DO
Assistant Professor of Anesthesiology
Northwestern University Feinberg School of Medicine
Department of Pediatric Anesthesia
Ann & Robert H. Lurie Children's Hospital of Chicago
Chicago, Illinois
Chapters 46, 51

Dietrich Henzler, MD, PhD, FRCP(C)
Professor of Anesthesiology
Ruhr University Bochum
Bochum, Germany
Dalhousie University
Halifax, Nova Scotia, Canada
Department of Anesthesia, Surgical Critical Care, Emergency and Pain Medicine
Klinikum Herford
Herford, Germany
Chapter 32

Bjoern Hossfeld, MD, Professor
Abteilung Anaesthesie und Intensivmedizin
Bundeswehrkrankenhaus Ulm
Ulm, Germany
Chapters 18, 48, 59

Johannes M. Huitink, MD, PhD
Anesthesiologist
Airway Management Academy
Amsterdam, The Netherlands
Chapter 1

Christopher Hung, MD
Discipline of Anesthesia, Faculty of Medicine
Memorial University of Newfoundland
St. John's, Newfoundland, Canada
Chapter 59

David Hung, MD
Department of Emergency Medicine
Dalhousie University
Queen Elizabeth II Health Science Centre
Halifax, Nova Scotia, Canada
Chapters 20, 21

Orlando R. Hung, BSc (Pharmacy), MD, FRCP(C)
Professor, Departments of Anesthesia, Pain Management and Perioperative Medicine, Surgery, and Pharmacology
Dalhousie University
Queen Elizabeth II Health Sciences Centre
Department of Anesthesia
Halifax, Nova Scotia, Canada
Chapters 4, 7, 11, 12, 13, 19, 20, 38, 41, 43

Narasimhan Jagannathan, MD, MBA
Vice Chair & Division Head, General Anesthesia
Director, Pediatric Anesthesia Research
Professor of Anesthesiology
Northwestern University Feinberg School of Medicine
Department of Pediatric Anesthesia
Ann & Robert H. Lurie Children's Hospital of Chicago
Chicago, Illinois
Chapters 46, 51

Nicola Jarvis, MBBS
Advanced Airway Management Fellow
Department of Anesthesiology and Pain Management
University of Toronto
Toronto General Hospital
Toronto, Ontario, Canada
Chapters 30, 34

Liane B. Johnson, MDCM, FRCSC, FACS
Associate Professor, Department of Surgery, Division of Pediatric Otolaryngology
Dalhousie University
IWK Health Centre
Halifax, Nova Scotia, Canada
Chapter 47

George W. Kanellakos, MD, FRCP(C)
Assistant Professor
Department of Anesthesia, Pain Management and Perioperative Medicine
Dalhousie University
Queen Elizabeth II Health Sciences Centre
Halifax, Nova Scotia, Canada
Chapter 39

Janny Xue Chen Ke, MD, MSc, FRCP(C)
Assistant Professor, Department of Anesthesiology, Pharmacology and Therapeutics
University of British Columbia
Vancouver, British Columbia, Canada
Chapter 65

Mathew B. Kiberd, MD, FRCP(C)
Assistant Professor, Department of Anesthesia, Pain management and Perioperative Medicine
Pediatric Cardiac Anaesthesiology
Dalhousie University
Halifax, Nova Scotia, Canada
Chapter 47

Chang Kim, MCBhB, FANZCA
Cardiothoracic and ORL Anaesthesia Department
Auckland City Hospital
Auckland, New Zealand
Chapter 45

Rebecca Klinger, MD
Department of Anesthesiology
Duke University Health System
Durham, North Carolina
Chapter 15

Sree Kolli, MD, EDRA
Clinical Assistant Professor
Department of General Anesthesiology and Pain Management
Anesthesiology Institute, Cleveland Clinic
Cleveland, Ohio
Chapter 3

George Kovacs, MD, FRCP(C)
Professor, Emergency Medicine
Dalhousie University
Attending Emergency Physician
Charles V. Keating Emergency & Trauma Centre
Queen Elizabeth II Health Sciences Centre
Nova Scotia Health Authority
Halifax, Nova Scotia, Canada
Chapters 8, 9

Michael S. Kristensen, MD
Professor
Department of Anaesthesia
Rigshospitalet, University Hospital of Copenhagen
Frederiksberg, Denmark
Chapter 64

M. Kwesi Kwofie, MD, FRCP(C)
Associate Professor
Director of Regional Anesthesia and Acute Pain
Department of Anesthesia, Perioperative Medicine and Pain Management
Dalhousie University
Halifax, Nova Scotia, Canada
Chapter 3

J. Adam Law, MD, FRCP(C)
Professor, Department of Anesthesia, Pain Management and Perioperative Medicine
Faculty of Medicine
Dalhousie University
Queen Elizabeth II Health Science Centre
Halifax, Nova Scotia, Canada
Chapter 2

François Lemay, MD
Medical Director
Département d'anesthésiologie et de soins intensifs
Université Laval
Québec, Québec, Canada
Département d'anesthésiologie du CHU de Québec—Pavillon Hôtel-Dieu de Québec
Québec, Québec, Canada
Chapter 40

Laeben Lester, MD
Assistant Professor
Co-Director, Johns Hopkins Airway Program
The Johns Hopkins University, School of Medicine
Department of Anesthesiology and Critical Care Medicine
Division of Cardiothoracic Anesthesia
Affiliate Department of Emergency Medicine
Baltimore, Maryland
Chapter 26

Kar-Soon Lim, MBBS, FANZCA
Staff Anaesthetist, Department of Anaesthesia and Pain Management
Concord Repatriation General Hospital
Concord, New South Wales, Australia
Chapter 66

Konstantin Lorenz, MD
Assistant Professor, Department of Anesthesia, Pain Management and Perioperative Medicine
Dalhousie University
Staff Anesthesiologist, Queen Elizabeth II Health Sciences Centre
Halifax, Nova Scotia, Canada
Chapter 58

Matthew Mackin, MD
Resident, Department of Anesthesia, Pain Management and Perioperative Medicine
Dalhousie University
Queen Elizabeth II Health Sciences Centre
Halifax, Nova Scotia, Canada
Chapter 13

Gemma Malpas, MBChB, FANZCA
Specialist Anaesthetist, Anaesthesia Department
Auckland City Hospital
Auckland, New Zealand
Chapter 45

Katherine Mayer, MD
Assistant Professor, Departments of Emergency Medicine and Pulmonary and Critical Care Medicine
Department of Medicine
The University of Colorado Anschutz Medical Campus
Aurora, Colorado
Chapter 25

James R. McAlpine, BSc, MBChB, FANZCA
Department of Anaesthesia and Pain Management
Capital, Coast and Hutt Valley
Te Whatu Ora—Health New Zealand
Newtown, Wellington, New Zealand
Chapter 11

Dolores M. McKeen, MD, FRCP(C), MSc, CCPE
Professor
Discipline of Anesthesia
Vice Dean, Education & Faculty Affairs
Faculty of Medicine
Memorial University of Newfoundland
St. John's, Newfoundland, Canada
Chapter 52

Genevieve McKinnon, MD, FRCP(C)
Assistant Professor
Department of Anesthesia, Pain Management and Perioperative Medicine
Dalhousie University
Attending Physician Anesthesiology
Capital District Health Authority
Queen Elizabeth II Health Sciences Centre
Halifax, Nova Scotia, Canada
Chapters 27, 67

Franziska Miller, MD
Resident
Department of Anesthesia, Pain Management and Perioperative Medicine
Dalhousie University
Queen Elizabeth II Health Sciences Centre
Halifax, Nova Scotia, Canada
Chapter 62

Andrew D. Milne, B.Eng, MSc, MD, FRCP(C)
Associate Professor, Department of Anesthesia, Pain Management and Perioperative Medicine
Faculty of Medicine
Dalhousie University
Queen Elizabeth II Health Science Centre
Halifax, Nova Scotia, Canada
Chapter 61

Brendan E. Morgan, MD, FRCP(C)
Pediatric Fellow, Department of Anesthesia and Pain Medicine
University of Toronto
The Hospital for Sick Children, Toronto, Ontario, Canada
Chapter 56

Loran T. Morrison, BSc (Physics), BSc (Microbiology/Immunology), MD
Resident (Anesthesiology)
Department of Anesthesia, Pain Management and Perioperative Medicine
Dalhousie University
Queen Elizabeth II Health Sciences Centre
Halifax, Nova Scotia, Canada
Chapter 12

Jarrod M. Mosier, MD
Associate Professor of Emergency Medicine and Medicine
Department of Emergency Medicine
Department of Medicine
Division of Pulmonary, Allergy, Critical Care and Sleep
University of Arizona College of Medicine
Tucson, Arizona
Chapters 25, 35

Holly A. Muir, MD, FRCP(C)
Chair and Professor
Department of Anesthesiology
University of Southern California
Los Angeles, California
Chapters 54, 55

Allana Munro, BSc Pharm, MD, FRCP(C)
Associate Professor, Department of Women's & Obstetric Anesthesia
Dalhousie University
IWK Health Centre
Halifax, Nova Scotia, Canada
Chapter 56

Michael F. Murphy, MD, FRCP(C)
Professor
Departments of Anesthesia, Pain Management and Perioperative Medicine and Emergency Medicine
Faculty of Medicine
Dalhousie University
Queen Elizabeth II Health Science Centre
Halifax, Nova Scotia, Canada
Professor Emeritus
Department of Anesthesiology and Pain Medicine
University of Alberta
Edmonton, Alberta, Canada
Chapters 1, 2, 7, 16, 22, 57, 63, 67

Nate Murray, MD
Resident Physician
Anesthesiology and Perioperative Medicine
Oregon Health & Sciences University
Portland, Oregon
Chapter 42

Sara Najmeh, MD, MSc, FRCS
Division of Thoracic and Upper GI Surgery, Department of Surgery
McGill University
Montreal General Hospital
Montreal, Quebec, Canada
Chapter 15

Batgombo Natsagdorj, MD
Board Member of Mongolian Society of Anesthesiologists
Head of Anesthesia and Intensive Care Department
"Intermed" Hospital
Ulaanbaatar, Mongolia
Chapter 60

James Nielsen, MBBS, FANZCA
Staff Anaesthetist, Department of Anaesthesia and Pain Management
Concord Repatriation General Hospital
Concord, New South Wales, Australia
Chapter 66

Ashley B. Norse, MD
Professor, Clinical Operations Director, Associate Chair of Operations
Department of Emergency Medicine
University of Florida College of Medicine—Jacksonville
Jacksonville, Florida
Chapters 23, 28

Stephanie Pan, MD, FAAP
Clinical Assistant Professor
Department of Anesthesiology, Perioperative and Pain Medicine
Stanford University School of Medicine
Stanford, California
Lucile Packard Children's Hospital
Palo Alto, California
Chapter 49

Jade Panzarasa, MD
Resident, Department of Anesthesia, Pain Management and Perioperative Medicine
Dalhousie University
Halifax, Nova Scotia, Canada
Chapter 31

Matteo Parotto, MD, PhD
Associate Professor
Department of Anesthesiology and Pain Management
Interdepartmental Division of Critical Care Medicine
University of Toronto
Toronto General Hospital
Toronto, Ontario, Canada
Chapters 30, 34

Haydn Perndt, AM, FFARCS, FANZCA, MPH, TM
Clinical Associate Professor
School of Medicine
University of Tasmania
Tasmania, Australia
Chapter 60

David Pescod, AO, MBBS, FANZCA
Associate Deputy Director
The Northern Hospital
Epping, Victoria, Australia
Associate Professor of Anaesthesiology
School of Medicine and Health Sciences
University of Melbourne
Melbourne, Australia
Council Member
World Federation of Societies of Anaesthesiologists
Chapter 60

Rachael Pescod
Bachelor of Medical Science
Australian National University
Medical Student
University of Wollongong
Beveridge, Victoria, Australia
Chapter 60

Alexander Poulton, MD, FRCP(C)
Assistant Professor
Department of Anesthesia, Pain Management and Perioperative Medicine
Dalhousie University
Queen Elizabeth II Health Sciences Centre
Victoria General Hospital
Halifax, Nova Scotia, Canada
Chapters 11, 29

Saul Pytka, MD, FRCP(C)
Associate Professor (Clinical)
Department of Anesthesiology
University of Calgary
Attending Anesthesiologist
Rockyview General Hospital
Flight Physician
STARS Air Ambulance
Calgary, Alberta, Canada
Chapters 5, 63

Yeshith Rai, MD
Anesthesia Resident
Department of Anesthesiology and Pain Medicine
Mount Sinai Hospital
University of Toronto
Toronto, Ontario
Chapter 64

Christina Ratto, MD
Assistant Professor
Department of Anesthesiology
University of Southern California
Los Angeles, California
Chapters 54, 55

Alison Robles, MD
Department of Pediatric Anesthesia
Ann & Robert H. Lurie Children's Hospital of Chicago
Instructor in Anesthesiology
Northwestern University Feinberg School of Medicine
Chicago, Illinois
Chapter 51

Richard D. Roda, B.Eng, MASc, MD, FRCP(C)
Clinical Lecturer, Department of Anesthesiology & Pain Medicine
University of Alberta
Royal Alexandra Hospital
Edmonton, Alberta
Canada
Chapter 61

Matthew Rowland, MD
Fellow in Pediatric Critical Care & Anesthesiology
Northwestern University Feinberg School of Medicine
Department of Pediatric Anesthesia
Ann & Robert H. Lurie Children's Hospital of Chicago
Chicago, Illinois
Chapters 46, 51

Jessica A. Ryder, MD
Operations and Disaster Medicine Fellow
Department of Emergency Medicine
Carolinas Medical Center
Charlotte, North Carolina
Chapter 28

John C. Sakles, MD
Professor, Department of Emergency Medicine
University of Arizona College of Medicine
Tucson, Arizona
Chapter 22

Jeanette Scott, MBChB, FANZCA
Specialist Anaesthetist, Department of Anaesthesia and Pain Medicine
Middlemore Hospital
Auckland, New Zealand
Department of Cardiac and ORL Anaesthesia
Auckland City Hospital
Auckland, New Zealand
Chapter 44

Edwin Seet, MBBS, MMED, FAMS
Senior Consultant and Associate Professor
Department of Anaesthesia
Khoo Teck Puat Hospital
Singapore
Chapter 43

Naveed Siddiqui, MD, MSc
Associate Professor
Department of Anesthesiology and Pain Medicine
Mount Sinai Hospital
University of Toronto
Toronto, Ontario
Chapter 64

Matt hew G. Simms, MSc, MD, FRCP(C)
Assistant Professor
Department of Anesthesia, Pain Management and Perioperative Medicine
Dalhousie University
Queen Elizabeth II Health Sciences Centre
Halifax, Nova Scotia, Canada
Chapter 62

Ana Sjaus, MD, FRCP(C)
Assistant Professor, Department of Women's & Obstetric Anesthesia
Dalhousie University
IWK Health Centre
Halifax, Nova Scotia, Canada
Chapter 53

Jocelyn Slemko, MD, FRCP(C)
Critical Care Fellow
Critical Care Medicine, University of Alberta
University of Alberta Hospital
Edmonton, Alberta, Canada
Chapter 6

Cédric Sottas, MD, FANZCA
Intensive Care Specialist
Starship Children's Hospital
Auckland, New Zealand
Chapter 50

Nicholas Sowers, MD, FRCP(C)
Assistant Professor, Department of Emergency Medicine
Dalhousie University
Attending Emergency Physician
Nova Scotia Health Authority
Halifax, Nova Scotia, Canada
Chapter 8

Kathryn Sparrow, BSc, MD, FRCP(C), MScHQ
Assistant Professor, Discipline of Anesthesia
Memorial University of Newfoundland
Faculty of Medicine
St. John's, Newfoundland and Labrador, Canada
Chapter 41

Mark Stafford-Smith, MD, CM, FRCP(C), MBA
Professor, Department of Anesthesiology
Duke University Medical Center
Durham, North Carolina
Chapter 15

Ronald D. Stewart, OC, ONS, ECNS (hon), BA, BSc, MD, FACEP, FAEM, DSc (hon), LLD
Professor Emeritus
Departments of Anesthesia, Pain Management and Perioperative Medicine and Emergency Medicine
Faculty of Medicine
Dalhousie University
Queen Elizabeth II Health Science Centre
Halifax, Nova Scotia, Canada
Chapter 20

Russell Taylor, PhD
Director, Laboratory for Computational Sensing and Robotics
Engineering Research Center for Computer-Integrated Surgical Systems and Technology
Professor, Department of Computer Science
Whiting School of Engineering
The Johns Hopkins University
Baltimore, Maryland
Chapter 65

Daniel Thomson, MD
Department of Pediatric Anesthesia
Ann & Robert H. Lurie Children's Hospital of Chicago
Fellow in Pediatric Anesthesiology
Northwestern University Feinberg School of Medicine
Chicago, Illinois
Chapter 51

Ban C.H. Tsui, Dip Eng, BSc (Maths), BSc (Pharm), MSc (Pharm), MD, FRCP(C), PG Dip Echo
Professor
Director, Stanford University Pediatric Regional Anesthesia (SUPRA)
Director of Research, Division of Adult Regional Anesthesia
Department of Anesthesiology, Perioperative and Pain Medicine
Stanford University School of Medicine
Stanford, California
Lucile Packard Children's Hospital
Palo Alto, California
Chapter 49

Arnim Vlatten, MD,
Associate Professor
Department of Anesthesia, Pain Management and Perioperative Medicine
Dalhousie University
Queen Elizabeth II Health Sciences Centre
Assistant Professor of Anesthesia
Department of Anesthesia
Dalhousie University
Department of Pediatric Anesthesia
Department of Pediatric Critical Care
IWK Health Centre
Halifax, Nova Scotia, Canada
Chapters 18, 48, 59

David Vokes, MBChB, FRACS
Laryngologist, Head and Neck Surgeon
Department of Otorhinolaryngology
Auckland City Hospital
Auckland, New Zealand
Chapter 44

Mark P. Vu, MD, FRCP(C)
Clinical Assistant Professor
Department of Anesthesia, Pharmacology and Therapeutics
University of British Columbia
Faculty of Medicine
Vancouver, British Columbia, Canada
Chapters 16, 19

Erik N. Vu, CCP, MD, FRCP(C), DAvMed
Assistant Professor, Faculty of Medicine
University of British Columbia
Departments of Emergency and Critical Care Medicine
British Columbia Emergency Health Services
Vancouver, British Columbia, Canada
Chapter 16

Karim Wafa, MD, FRCP(C), PhD
Fellow, Pain Medicine
Department of Anesthesia
McMaster University
Hamilton, Ontario, Canada
Chapter 4

Haotian Wang, MD, FRCP(C)
Lecturer, Department of Anesthesia, Pain Management and Perioperative Medicine
Dalhousie University
Queen Elizabeth II Health Sciences Centre
Halifax, Nova Scotia, Canada
Chapter 39

David T. Wong, MD, FRCP(C)
Professor, Department of Anesthesiology
Department of Anesthesiology and Pain Medicine
University of Toronto
Toronto, Ontario, Canada
Chapters 14, 33

Michael J. Wong, MD, FRCP(C)
Assistant Professor, Department of Anesthesia, Pain Management and Perioperative Medicine
Dalhousie University
Halifax, Nova Scotia, Canada
Chapter 31

Eric You-Ten, MD, PhD, FRCP(C)
Associate Professor, Department of Anesthesiology and Pain Medicine
Mount Sinai Hospital
University of Toronto
Toronto, Ontario, Canada
Chapters 14, 64

Fabricio B. Zasso, MD, MHSc, MBA
Assistant Professor, Department of Anesthesiology and Pain Medicine
Mount Sinai Hospital
University of Toronto
Toronto, Ontario, Canada
Chapters 14, 64

Jinbin Zhang, MBBS, MMED (Anesthesiology)
Senior Consultant, Department of Anaesthesia
Tan Tock Seng Hospital
Singapore
Chapters 10, 43

George Zhong, MBBS, FANZCA
Staff Anaesthetist, Department of Anaesthesia and Pain Management
Concord Repatriation General Hospital
Concord, New South Wales, Australia
Chapter 66

FOREWORD

When the flight attendant calls for a physician, the cabin crew is relieved when an anesthesiologist shows up. We readily manage common events such as nausea and vomiting, but we are equally facile with acute life-threatening events such as heart attacks, loss of consciousness, and anaphylaxis. By far, our most important skill in any emergency is that we can manage an airway.

An hour out of London, I responded to "is there a doctor on board?" A post-ictal passenger was turning dark blue. A simple jaw lift opened the airway. I added a little oxygen. In a minute the passenger became pink. The next minute he awoke from his post-ictal stupor. (A minute later he threw up on me; no good deed goes unpunished.)

By the end of training, newly minted anesthesiologists are highly proficient at managing airways. They have seen thousands of easy airways. They have also seen dozens, or perhaps hundreds, of deeply treacherous airways. Intense residency training appropriately leads to confidence in airway management. However, are they perhaps too confident? Have they seen everything there is to see?

The Nobel prize winning psychologist Daniel Kahneman talks about the cognitive bias "what you see is all there is." It is easy to conclude from our training and experience that we have seen all the airway challenges that exist. That's what I thought. Having practiced anesthesiology for decades, I believed I had seen pretty much everything.

My self-confidence was quickly shattered by the fourth edition of *Hung's Difficult and Failed Airway Management.* In 67 concisely written and well-referenced chapters, the authors introduce aspects of airway management I had never even considered. Chapters on unusual scenarios comprise a little shop of airway horrors: blunt anterior neck trauma, deadly asthma, penetrating facial trauma, deep neck infection, obstructive sleep apnea with goiter. Have you been called to the ICU for a patient in a halo jacket who has bitten his wire-reinforced endotracheal tube? What will you do for an unconscious motorist with a compromised airway trapped in an overturned motor vehicle, or a motorcyclist with a full helmet and severe head injury. When did you last encounter the "cannot intubate/cannot oxygenate" scenario in an infant? The list goes on and on. This is the stuff of anesthesiologists' nightmares.

Nearly all of these are accompanied by case scenarios. The prone airway scenario starts "A 35-year-old intoxicated male 179 cm tall and weighing 110 kg (BMI 34 kg·m^{-2}) presents to the emergency room with a 12-inch hunting knife lodged in his upper thoracic spine after an altercation at a cottage party" What the hell happens in Halifax?

The book is also an endless string of pearls. Using scenarios to capture the reader's interest and harness his or her clinical imagination, the chapters offer practical, evidence-based advice. Consider the patient with the 12-inch hunting knife in his upper thoracic spine. The patient needs to be in the prone position, so you would likely consider face-mask ventilation or the use of an extraglottic device. But, what about tracheal intubation? It would be challenging. Would you have considered positioning two operating room tables side by side? With two tables placed side by side, the patient can be supine with the knife in the gap between the tables, permitting management of a supine patient airway. Alternatively, you might place the patient prone but advance the body caudad until the head is fully supported by an assistant. In this position the table can be placed in full reverse Trendelenburg, elevating the head so you can face the patient directly to facilitate fiberoptic intubation.

I have no way of knowing if reading this book will change clinical outcomes. However, I believe the author's use of case scenario → background information → tips and tricks → case resolution → knowledge assessment questions represents state-of-the-art written didactic teaching. The vivid cases are readily envisioned, such as the patient with the 12-inch hunting knife. The stress of the anesthesiologist is palpable. Wrapping these envisioned cases with strings of clinical pearls commits the tips and tricks to memory. That is why anesthesiologists should read the book now, before they encounter these cases in real life. There is no time to look up a reference in the intensely focused seconds of airway compromise. But, there is time to call for help, of course, which the authors repeatedly identify as the first step in managing a difficult airway.

The authors also present the most recent advances in airway management. For example, I was completely unfamiliar with the rapid deployment of ECMO in anticipated difficult or impossible airways, or the use of ECMO in the ER where a difficult airway might arrive any second by ambulance. This is a huge advance! The authors also discuss the use of artificial intelligence, including the development of new airway management devices that use AI image recognition to facilitate tracheal intubation.

During my residency in the early 1980s, the "best anesthesiologist" at University of Pennsylvania was the one who could shove a 7.0-mm ID endotracheal tube into any trachea using a MAC-3 blade. We were in awe of these masters. However, they had nothing on modern anesthesiologists. We come to the operating room armed with video laryngoscopes, an array of extraglottic devices, novel fiberoptic or chip-guided scopes, and high-flow nasal cannulae. Our everyday skills are far beyond yesteryear's masters of MAC-3 intubation.

Hung's Difficult and Failed Airway Management shows that our everyday airway skills pale in comparison to our potential. It's a masterful textbook, beautifully conceived, well organized, clearly written, extensively referenced, and utterly relevant to our most important task as anesthesiologists.

On a personal note, Dr. Orlando Hung was one of my first fellows at Stanford. Orlando and his family have remained close personal friends. He trained at Stanford in Clinical Pharmacology (and the pharmacology section of the textbook is excellent). What research mentors want for their mentees, and what friends want for their friends, is to make a difference in the world. This book fills me with joy and pride, because my mentee and friend continues to make profound contributions to the well-being, and survival, of the patients we serve.

Steven L. Shafer, MD
Professor Emeritus of Anesthesiology,
Perioperative and Pain Medicine
Stanford University
Editor-in-Chief of Anesthesia & Analgesia (2006–2016)

PREFACE

While earlier guidelines and strategies from the American Society of Anesthesiologists (ASA), the Canadian Airway Focus Group (CAFG), and the Difficult Airway Society (DAS) in the United Kingdom help in managing patients with a difficult or failed airway, there are no specific strategies recommended to manage patients when all four fundamental techniques of oxygenation (face-mask ventilation, use of extraglottic devices, tracheal intubation, and front-of-neck access) are likely to fail; this situation is commonly considered an "impossible" airway.

Recent revisions of the ASA (2022) and CAFG (2021) strategies and guidelines for managing challenging airways recognized the importance of extracorporeal membrane oxygenation (ECMO) in the management of patients with an "impossible" airway. These guidelines have been updated and are reflected in all chapters of this fourth edition. For example, in this edition several chapters (Chapters 15, 21, 31, and 45) discuss the utilization of ECMO in various clinical settings for managing patients with "impossible" airways due to critically obstructive tracheal lesions or upper airway anatomical abnormalities. In other words, while the application of the four basic methods of oxygenation remains the most practical approach in managing a difficult or failed airway, ECMO should be considered in the setting of an impossible airway. However, it takes time to establish ECMO support, which needs specialized equipment and specialized practitioners, and for these reasons, ECMO is impractical in managing an emergency impossible airway or as a rescue airway technique.

Our goal is to provide the practitioner with a single resource with text and videos that provides strategies in managing the full spectrum of airway-related issues. This edition is divided into 10 sections: the first section consists of the foundational information on airway management; the second section reviews airway devices and techniques; the third to the ninth sections discuss context-sensitive airway management in a variety of clinical settings, including prehospital care, in the emergency department, the intensive care unit, the operating room, the post-anesthetic care unit, as well as other parts of the hospital; and the last section highlights practical issues in airway management. A number of new chapters and clinical cases have been added to this edition. As indicated above, four chapters have been added to discuss the role of ECMO in predicted impossible airway management. In addition, chapters discussing the management of patients with COVID infection, patients with opioid overdose, and patients undergoing robotic surgery, and the role of robotics and artificial intelligence in airway management and point-of-care ultrasound (POCUS) of the upper airway in airway management have been included.

In addition to the previous 30 videos on airway techniques, which can be accessed through McGraw Hill AccessAnesthesiology website, three more new videos have been added: Combined Intubation Techniques, Tips and Tricks to Improve Hyperangulated Video-Laryngoscopic Intubation, and the Utility of Extracorporeal Membrane Oxygenation (ECMO) in Airway Management.

ACKNOWLEDGMENTS

We would like to thank all the contributing authors for making this book possible. In addition, we would like to thank all the associate editors (three new associate editors) for their tireless efforts to ensure that the information in this book is clear, concise, and accurate. Several previous associate editors, authors, and coauthors were not able to contribute to this edition of our textbook. These include Aaron Bair, Sebastian Bienia, Kerryann Broderick, Tim Brown, Frances Chung, Richard Cooper, Jo Davies, Laura Duggan, Lorraine Foley, Alison B. Froese, Angelina Guzzo, John Hajduk, Carin Hagberg, Shawn Hicks, Liem Ho, Andrea Huang, Andy Jagoda, Sara Kim, Danae Krahn, Gordon Launcelott, Laeben Lester, Richard Levitan, Anthony Longhini, Kirk MacQuarrie, Kelly McQueen, Ian Morris, David Petrie, Dmitry Portnoy, Brian Ross, Kitt Turney, Narendra Vakharia, and Richard Zane. We would like to thank them for their contributions in previous editions of this textbook and their dedication to education in the narrow field of airway management. In addition, we would like to thank Sara Whynot for her editorial assistance, Christopher Hung and David Hung for the production of the images and videos. We would also like to thank all of the McGraw Hill editorial and production staff for their continuing support.

Orlando R. Hung, MD, FRCPC
Michael F. Murphy, MD, FRCPC

SECTION 1

PRINCIPLES OF AIRWAY MANAGEMENT

CHAPTER 1

Evaluation of the Airway

Michael F. Murphy and Johannes M. Huitink

Failure to evaluate the airway and predict difficulty is the single most important factor leading to a failed airway.[1,2]

The Difficult Airway is something you anticipate; the Failed Airway is something you experience. (*Walls*, 2002)

INTRODUCTION

"Airway management" may be defined as the application of therapeutic interventions that are intended to effect gas exchange, namely oxygenation and the removal of carbon dioxide, and to protect the airway from aspiration in patients who are unable to do it for themselves. *Gas exchange* is fundamental to this definition.[3] A number of devices and techniques are commonly employed in health care settings to achieve this goal. These include the use of face-mask ventilation (FMV), extraglottic airway devices (EGDs), oral or nasal endotracheal intubation (ETI), and invasive or front-of-neck airway (FONA) techniques.

The failure to adequately manage the airway has been identified as a major factor leading to poor outcomes in anesthesia, critical care, emergency medicine, hospital medicine, and emergency medical services (EMS). Adverse respiratory events constituted the largest single cause of injury in the 1991 American Society of Anesthesiologists (ASA) Closed Claims Project.[2] These medical legal actions have persisted over 30 years despite major advances in the identification and management of the difficult airway, the failed airway, inadvertent esophageal intubation, and improvement in airway management devices.[4]

The 4th National Audit Project (NAP4) conducted in the United Kingdom over a 1-year period of time identified major airway management complications in the operating rooms (ORs), intensive care units (ICUs), and emergency departments (EDs) leading to death, brain damage, emergency FONA, or unexpected ICU admission.[5,6] NAP4 reinforced the findings of the National Reporting and Learning System in the United Kingdom that found 18% of 1085 airway management complications in ICU over a 2-year period (2005-2007) were directly related to the act of intubation.[7]

The following narrative will discuss what is new or has changed in the evaluation of the airway prior to airway intervention since the last edition of this textbook.

RECENT INSIGHTS IN ASSESSING THE DIFFICULT AIRWAY

What Are the Dimensions of Difficult Airway?

The Value of Anatomic Predictors Redefined

The first *ASA Guidelines for the Management of the Difficult Airway* was published almost 30 years ago.[1] In the ASA Closed Claims Analysis conducted 12 years later, Peterson et al.[8]

reported that there is evidence to suggest that the incidence of airway management failure could be minimized, or perhaps eliminated, by a prior airway examination to identify anatomic predictors of difficulty.

However, a large Danish study (188,064 patients) evaluated the diagnostic accuracy of predicting difficult airway management in everyday anesthetic practice.[9] The investigators found that when difficult FMV was predicted based on the preoperative evaluation it was actually difficult in only 22% of those cases. Similarly, when difficult intubation was predicted it was difficult in only 25% of those cases. Perhaps more importantly, of the 3391 intubations that were actually difficult, 93% were unanticipated; and difficult bag-mask ventilation was unanticipated in 94%. Their conclusion reiterated the long-held mantra of airway management experts that practitioners should constantly be prepared for unanticipated difficulty or failure. There are limitations to the Danish study because no specific airway assessment tools were disclosed in the preinduction assessment. In fact, only two questions were asked in the preoperative airway assessment: (1) Is difficult direct laryngoscopic (DL) intubation anticipated? (2) Is difficult FMV anticipated? It is difficult to draw any conclusion regarding the value of preanesthesia airway assessment if many of the accepted airway evaluation tools for DL were not used.[10]

The fundamental dilemma facing the airway practitioner is to predict if the airway is "reassuring" or "non-reassuring." The task is to identify nonchallenging versus challenging airways employing tools with poor predictive value alone and in combination. As mentioned above, the ASA guidelines have used the terms "reassuring" and "non-reassuring." Huitink and Bouwman[11] have recently advanced the proposition that a trained practitioner should be able to manage a patient with a reassuring airway (they use the term "basic airway") employing basic airway management techniques (FMV and ETI) after proper training. A basic airway has no complexity factors and it is expected that the airway can be managed without complications with basic airway management techniques by a trained medical professional. In the unlikely event that airway rescue techniques are needed in these patients it is expected to be relatively easy because the anatomy is normal. Conversely, they maintain that the less reassuring the airway, the greater the need to prepare for failure. These airways are defined as advanced airways. Is it advisable to look for complexity factors? Complexity factors can be in six different domains: human factors, equipment, location, patient factors, evaluation of vital signs, and time pressure.[11] For advanced airways, management techniques or a dedicated team with special skills may be needed. If there are multiple complexity factors in various domains the risk of complications increases. The classification into basic or advanced airway can objectively be done with the PHASE and HELPET checklists,[11] a very common sense approach!

Notwithstanding the above, it seems logical to believe that for the rate of airway management failure to diminish, the following factors must all be present at a minimum:

- A thorough airway examination is performed.
- The examination is focused on anatomical and nonanatomical features that reliably foretell failure.
- The practitioner has access to airway management devices and is properly trained in employing them.

Unfortunately, none of these factors are always present for every airway management intervention and lawsuits associated with airway management failure continue to occur.[4,12]

In their 2021 two-part publications the Canadian Airway Focus Group (CAFG)[13,14] identified 14 predictors of difficult tracheal intubation employing direct laryngoscopy (DL), 12 predictors when video laryngoscopy (VL) is used, 13 predictors for difficult FMV, 11 predictors of difficult EGD placement or ventilation, and 6 predictors of performing difficult FONA.

Fortunately, many of the anatomic features overlap. All things being equal, failing specific risk-related conditions such as morbid obesity, the parturient at term, obstructing airway pathologies, and others to be identified below, several of the anatomic features seem to be standing the test of time[14]:

- Neck circumference at the level of the thyroid cartilage >40 to 50 cm[15]
- Mallampati III or IV
- Thyromental distance <6 cm
- Neck radiation
- Obstructing airway pathology

This is not meant to imply that the other myriad of anatomical predictors is not useful, because these predictors are in specific individuals and populations.

Further information on the reliability of anatomic factors was published by Detsky et al.[16] They reviewed studies from 1946 to 2018 to determine which airway examination characteristics were the best predictors of difficult intubation. Sixty-two studies including 33,559 patients found the best predictor was inability of the lower incisors to touch the top lip, followed by shorter hyomental distance, retrognathia, and Wilson score. These all had a higher positive likelihood ratio than the commonly used Mallampati score equal to or greater than III.

The concept of difficulty has been expanded to include:

- The physiologically difficult airway[17]
- Human factors and expertise[18–20]
- Other contextual factors such as time of day, location, expertise of assistance, and others (see Chapter 7)[21]
- Time-pressured emergency situations

The Physiologically Difficult Airway

Mosier et al.[22] identified physiologic factors that enhanced the degree of difficulty in managing the airway in the ICU often contributing to an increase in morbidity and mortality. In 2021, Kornas et al.[17] on behalf of the Society for Airway Management published consensus guidelines for the management of the physiologically difficult airway. They highlighted the importance of hypoxemic respiratory failure and also identified few key factors such as the ability to maintain oxygenation during intubation, manage hypotension and right ventricular dysfunction, and the transition to positive pressure ventilation. These authors have appropriately dubbed these factors as the "physiologically difficult airway." Chapters 4 and 30 elaborate on this important "dimension of difficulty."

The Role of Human Factors in Leading to Adverse Outcomes

Aziz et al.,[19] while focusing on difficult VL, identified the experience and expertise of the practitioner as important factors leading to difficulty and failure. The critically important role of human factors in airway management is well summarized in McClelland's publication.[20] It has become clear that communication is fundamental to managing the difficult and failed airway. The pre-emptive clarification of the plan explains what the sequence of techniques will be, what the triggers are to change gears, and what roles the various team members are expected to perform. It also positions that there is a sense of order: team members know what to expect and when the technique will change and it permits them to prepare in advance for changes to their role. The results of effectively managing human factors are as follows: only those essential to the task are present, the focus of the team is on the patient, idle chat is eliminated, perseveration is managed, cricothyrotomy is now part of the plan and not emblematic of failure, and team members feel free to contribute suggestions. Chapters 6 and 35 elaborate on these human factors.

The Contribution of Context to Difficulty and Failure

Hung and Murphy[21] initially identified that difficult and failed airway management was integrally entwined with the context of when, where, and who were tasked with managing the airway. They proposed that many factors impacted the expertise of those managing the airway, the resources available to them, and the devices they are able to access. Taken together, these contextual factors had the potential to materially affect the outcome. Chapter 7 provides a detailed discussion of this important topic.

So, at the end of the day, there is no recipe, weighted scoring system, or other objective system that will predict success or failure with any certainty. Any evaluation for difficulty must involve an analysis of:

- Anatomic factors
- Physiologic factors
- Human factors (including one's skill set)
- Contextual factors

Taken together, an analysis of these factors will define who requires the airway intervention awake and how to best manage the airway—sedated or anesthetized.

What Are the Newer Techniques and Tools in Airway Management?

Denitrogenation (Often Referred to as Preoxygenation or Perioxygenation)

The functional residual capacity (FRC) is the amount of gas left in the lungs after a normal tidal expiration. It is composed of the residual volume (RV) and the expiratory reserve volume (ERV). Normally this equates to approximately 30 $mL{\cdot}kg^{-1}$. The amount of oxygen storage for an average-size adult is about 1.5 L (approximately 1 L stored in the hemoglobin and myoglobin and 0.5 L in the FRC) [23] With a basal oxygen consumption of 3 to 4 $mL{\cdot}kg^{-1}{\cdot}min^{-1}$ and the FRC filled with air (20% oxygen), a healthy individual would have depleted all oxygen storage after 6 to 8 minutes of apnea.

This replacement of nitrogen in the FRC with oxygen ("denitrogenation") is foundational to airway management. It functions as an "apneic buffer" with an increase in oxygen storage so that a prolonged duration of acceptable oxygen saturation can be maintained during tracheal intubation while the patient is being rendered apneic. The most recent Guidelines from the ASA regarding denitrogenation provide little guidance for the practitioner in this regard.[24] Recent advances, however, have identified that in addition to conventional recommendations (100% oxygen for 3-5 minutes; 5-12 VC breaths; ETO_2 >90%) high-flow nasal oxygen (i.e., high-flow nasal cannula or HFNC) with flows between 10 and 70 $L{\cdot}min^{-1}$ (LPM) administered throughout the preparation and intubation phases, denitrogenation, can significantly increase the "safe" apneic period[25–27] leading to a reduction in mortality.

So, what does this mean to the airway practitioner? It is clear that continuous HFNC during the preparation and execution of intubation administered concurrently with conventional recommendations as above should be employed in all emergency intubations and for all patients judged to be prone to oxygen desaturation (e.g., morbidly obese, underlying lung disease). HFNC should also be considered during awake tracheal intubation (ATI).

Sugammadex in Airway Management

Most literature indicates that the introduction of sugammadex into clinical practice has led to reductions in postoperative respiratory compromise (PORC) and the complications associated with it,[28–30] though there have been contrary publications.[31] The real question regarding sugammadex, as it relates to difficult and failed airway management, is whether a patient with a "Cannot Intubate, Cannot Oxygenate" (CICO) failed airway after receiving a large dose of rocuronium (e.g., 1.2 $mg{\cdot}kg^{-1}$) as part of a rapid sequence intubation (RSI) technique can be rescued (spontaneous ventilation restored) by administering sugammadex. Paton et al. reported a case in 2013[32] where sugammadex was used to reverse rocuronium neuromuscular block in a highly engineered approach to the airway in a patient with subglottic stenosis and known as "impossible" airway. However, this does not answer the question as to whether sugammadex can be relied upon to restore spontaneous ventilation when encountering unanticipated difficulty and/or failed airway. Further information from the study by Bisschops et al.[33] sheds important light on the issues impacting this operation.

The Role of Ultrasound (US) in the Evaluation of the Airway for Difficulty

The use of ultrasound as a diagnostic and procedural assist in acute care medicine (i.e., point-of-care ultrasound [POCUS]) has become ubiquitous.

Three principal applications should be noted:

1. *Locating the cricothyroid membrane (CTM):* It is well known that in an emergency the reliability of skilled airway practitioners to locate the CTM is poor.[5,34–36] This factor, in large

part, has led to the recommendation of open cricothyrotomy (FONA) to supplant Seldinger techniques in CICO situations, but there is evidence that skill in applying ultrasound to this problem rectifies this issue.[37–39] Thus, in a planned approach to the difficult airway, one may employ ultrasound to find and mark the CTM prior to airway intervention.

2. *Evaluating for a difficult airway:* Ultrasound has been used to evaluate the airway for difficulty in both nonpregnant and pregnant patients.[40–46] Investigators have found, having examined 45 potential indicators of difficult airway on ultrasound, that the thicknesses of the anterior neck soft tissues at the level of the hyoid bone and the epiglottis, and the hyomental distance in both supine and ramped positions, were the most reliable at predicting difficult laryngoscopy. While there is further elucidation of the value of ultrasound in evaluating "what cannot be seen" during a naked-eye examination of the airway, this modality bears watching in the literature.
3. *Evaluating gastric contents:* It is feasible to quickly scan the stomach to find out fasting status. Studies have been currently undertaken to find out if this information is useful for the airway strategy (see Chapter 41).

Consequential Publications in the Airway Space in the Last 2 Years

Law JA, Duggan LV, Asselin M, et al. Canadian Airway Focus Group updated consensus-based recommendations for management of the difficult airway: part 1. Difficult airway management encountered in an unconscious patient. *Can J Anesth.* 2021;68:1373-1404. doi: 10.1007/s12630-021-02007-0. Epub 2021 Jun 18.[13]

Law JA, Duggan LV, Asselin M, et al. Canadian Airway Focus Group updated consensus-based recommendations for management of the difficult airway: part 2. Planning and implementing safe management of the patient with an anticipated difficult airway. Can J Anesth. 2021;68:1405-1436.[14] doi: 10.1007/s12630-021-02007-0. Epub 2021 Jun 18.

Cook TM, El-Boghdadly K, McGuire B, McNarry AF, Patel A, Higgs A. Consensus guidelines for managing the airway in patients with COVID-19: guidelines from the Difficult Airway Society, the Association of Anaesthetists, the Intensive Care Society, the Faculty of Intensive Care Medicine and the Royal College of Anaesthetists. *Anaesthesia.* 2020;75:785-799.[47]

Kornas RL, Owyang CG, Sakles JC, Foley LJ, Mosier JM. Evaluation and management of the physiologically difficult airway: consensus recommendations from Society for Airway Management. *Anesth Analg.* 2021;132:395-405.[17] doi: 10.1213/ANE.0000000000005233

Apfelbaum JL, Hagberg CA, Connis RT, et al. 2022 American Society of Anesthesiologists practice guidelines for management of the difficult airway. *Anesthesiology.* 2022;136(1):31-81.[24] https://doi.org/10.1097/ALN.0000000000004002

Ahmad I, El-Boghdadly K, Bhagrath R, et al. Difficult Airway Society guidelines for awake tracheal intubation (ATI) in adults. *Anaesthesia.* 2020;75(4):509-528.[40]

THE STANDARD OF CARE

The growth in knowledge and evidence related to the practice of airway management is relentless. Advances in airway management over the past two decades have significantly improved patient outcome with a reduction in the incidence of death and disability.[4,12,48] The challenge for the practitioner is to keep abreast of new information and techniques to practice within the standard of care.

The "standard of care" is broadly defined as: "The *average* degree of skill, care, and diligence exercised by members of the same profession, practicing in the *same or similar locality* in light of the *present state* of medical and surgical science." This definition incorporates several important features: Average degree of skill; Same or similar locality; Present state of knowledge.

Taking these into consideration, the standard of care is the conduct and skill of an average and prudent practitioner. A bad result due to a failure to meet the standard of care is generally considered to be malpractice. There are two main sources of information as to exactly what is the expected standard of care:

1. The beliefs and opinions of experts in the field
2. The published scientific evidence, standards of care, practice guidelines, and protocols

Driven by the complex nature of this clinical dilemma and the need for successful solutions that are easily learned and maintained (and cost-effective), the standard of care in airway management is exceedingly dynamic. Continuing evolution of new devices and techniques, or ways of thinking, modify the existing standard of care on an ongoing basis. It is incumbent on practitioners to keep abreast of new devices and techniques and remain facile with existing rescue techniques. They can do so by continually perusing the literature and attending educational programs related to airway management.

International, national, regional, and local professional organizations generally address issues relevant to airway management in a variety of ways. Most societies, such as the American Society of Anesthesiologists (ASA), the Difficult Airway Society (DAS-UK), the American College of Emergency Physicians (ACEP), the Canadian Anesthesiologists' Society (CAS), European Airway Management Society (EAMS), and others, engage in crafting practice guidelines.[13,14,17,24,47,49]

Nonetheless, the standard of care remains elusive, particularly when it applies to the management of the difficult and failed airway. Though we know **what it is not**:

- It is neither much better nor much worse care than that delivered on average by one's peers.
- It is not the same as the care provided by *experts* managing difficult and failed airways every day.
- It is not what "ivory-tower" academic experts *think* it *ought to be*.
- It is not a single study published in a reputable journal last week, or a position advocated by *experts* in an editorial in a similarly reputable journal.

We do know that the standard of care is dynamic and our patients expect to receive it at a minimum. Perhaps the best test with respect to difficult and failed airway management is to ask a specific question: "Should the average, reasonable, and prudent practitioner

- Be able to recognize and manage an anticipated difficult airway?
- Be able to manage an unanticipated difficult airway?
- Be able to perform an awake intubation?
- Be able to recognize and manage the failed airway?
- Be facile with one or two rescue airway devices or techniques in the face of a failed airway?
- Be able to work in a team, communicate clearly, and be able to perform under stressful circumstances?
- Be able to perform a FONA?
- Be able to recognize a situation when a call for help or expert advice is needed?"

It is reasonable to expect that most practitioners charged with managing airways would answer yes to all of these questions and thereby define the standard of care. But we should acknowledge the fact that airway skills and experience can be different among and between paramedics, emergency physicians, anesthesiologists, or critical care specialists. Therefore, help should be solicited when the medical practitioner does not have enough experience with the procedure. In patients with highly complex advanced airways, assistance should be called for before the airway management procedure starts—time permitting of course.

MEMORY AIDS TO ASSIST IN THE EVALUATION FOR DIFFICULTY

The most important anatomic predictors were listed at the beginning of this chapter. The reader is referred to the CAFG publications for a complete list of predictors based on the particular operation (e.g., FMV, EGD) being contemplated.[13,14]

It is useful to have a framework for airway evaluation for difficulty. Conceptually, the *difficult airway* has several dimensions:

1. Difficult FMV
2. Difficult placement of an EGD
3. Difficult DL
4. Difficult VL
5. Difficult ATI
6. Difficult emergency FONA (eFONA)

These six dimensions can be reduced to five technical operations:

1. Difficult FMV
2. Difficult EGD
3. Difficult DL intubation
4. Difficult VL intubation
5. Difficult eFONA

Let's look at each one independently.

Difficult Face-Mask Ventilation (FMV): MOANS

The degree of difficulty encountered while performing or attempting to perform FMV has been classified by several authors. The classification scheme of Han[50] and Kheterpal[51] is presented in Tables 1.1 and 1.2, respectively. Research has validated many of those anatomical features that over the years have been implicated in heralding difficult FMV (difficult mask ventilation or DMV).[51,52]

These features can be grouped into five indicators that can be easily recalled by using the mnemonic **MOANS**:

- ***M***ask seal, high ***M***allampati scores, ***M***inimal jaw protrusion, or ***M***ale gender: Bushy beards, crusted blood on the face, or a disruption of lower facial continuity are the commonest examples of conditions that may make an adequate mask seal difficult. Bushy beards can be taped with Tegaderm™. This will improve mask seal and is easy to remove.
- ***O***bese or ***O***bstructing lesions: Patients who are obese defined by Langeron et al.[53] as BMI >26 kg·m^{-2} as opposed to the conventional definition of obese as BMI $= 30$ to 35 kg·m^{-2}; Kheterpal[51] identified a BMI >30 kg·m^{-2} as being associated with difficult FMV. FMV can also be difficult in parturients at term and in patients with upper airway obstruction, angioedema, Ludwig's angina, upper airway abscesses (e.g., peritonsillar), and epiglottitis.
- ***A***ged: Age greater than 55 is associated with a higher risk of difficult BMV, perhaps because of a loss of muscle and tissue tone in the upper airway.[51,53]
- ***N***o teeth or ***N***eck radiation or fixed flexion deformity of the neck: An adequate mask seal may be difficult in the edentulous patient as the face tends to cave in. An option is to leave dentures in situ (if available) for FMV and remove

TABLE 1.1. Han's Mask Ventilation Classification and Description Scale[50]

Classification	Description/Definition
Grade 0	Ventilation by mask not attempted
Grade 1	Ventilated by mask
Grade 2	Ventilated by mask with oral airway or other adjuvant
Grade 3	Difficult mask ventilation (inadequate, unstable, or requiring two practitioners)
Grade 4	Unable to mask ventilate

TABLE 1.2. Mask Ventilation Scale and Incidence[51]

Grade	Description	*N* (%)
1	Ventilated by mask	37,857 (71.3%)
2	Ventilated by mask with oral airway/adjuvant with or without muscle relaxant	13,966 (26.3%)
3	Difficult ventilation (inadequate, unstable, or requiring two providers) with or without muscle relaxant	1,141 (2.2%)
4	Unable to mask ventilate with or without muscle relaxant	77 (0.15%)
	Total Cases	53,041

them for intubation. Radiation therapy in the past to the head and neck[52] and fixed cervical spine deformity[14] may hinder mask ventilation.

- ***S**nores* or ***S**tiff*: For the former, this mnemonic affords one a reminder to check for obstructive sleep apnea (OSA), an increasingly important consideration in anesthetic practice today. FMV may be difficult or impossible in the face of **S**tiff lungs: substantial increases in airways resistance (e.g., severe asthma) or decreases in pulmonary compliance (e.g., pulmonary edema).

Difficult DL Intubation: LEMON

Difficult DL and intubation ordinarily implies that the practitioner had a poor view of the glottis. Cormack and Lehane[54] provided some clarity to the way we think of the *difficult airway* by parsing the act of intubation into its two subcomponents: laryngoscopy and intubation. They also introduced the most widely utilized system of categorizing the degree to which the glottis can be visualized during laryngoscopy (Figure 1.1). Cormack/Lehane view Grades 3 (epiglottis-only visible) and 4 (no glottic structures at all visible) are often used as surrogates to define a difficult laryngoscopy and predict difficult intubation. View Grades 1 (visualization of the entire laryngeal aperture) and 2 (visualization of the posterior cords and arytenoids) are not typically associated with difficult intubation, though some Grade 2s may be difficult or impossible to intubate. Tough Grade 2s and 3s are *tailor-made* for intubating introducers such as the Eschmann Tracheal Introducer and Frova devices (see Chapter 12).

As can be gleaned from the descriptions, the Cormack/Lehane grading system is insensitive to the degree to which the laryngeal aperture is visible during laryngoscopy: a little bit of it (Grade 2) or all of it (Grade 1). The question often asked is: How much of the cords must be viewed to assure intubation success? How much is enough? Some authors have created a 2A view to indicate that some of the cords are visible, and Grade 2B if only the arytenoid cartilages are seen.[55] Likewise, the Grade 3 view has been divided into 3A where the epiglottis is sitting upright and tracheal introducer (commonly known as "bougie") intubation is possible, and 3B where the epiglottis is flipped backward over the glottic aperture and "bougie-guided" intubation is not possible. In attempting to provide a framework or an approach to answering the question "how much of the glottis is visualized?," Levitan et al.[56] devised a scoring system, percentage of glottic opening (POGO), to quantify glottic view. While attractive in many ways, this scale has yet to gain wide acceptance (Figure 1.2).

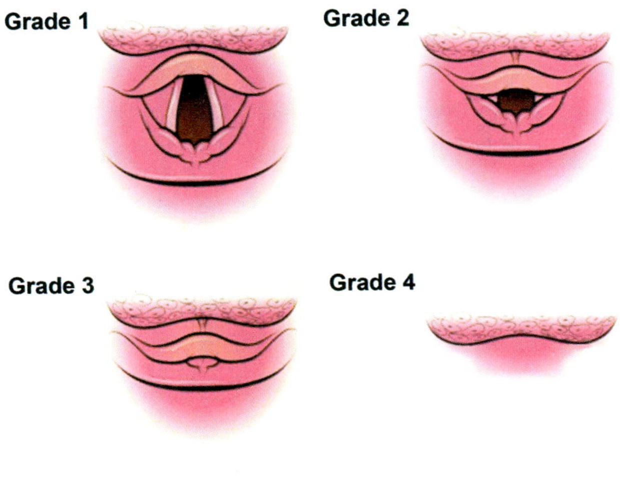

FIGURE 1.1. Cormack/Lehane laryngeal view grading score.

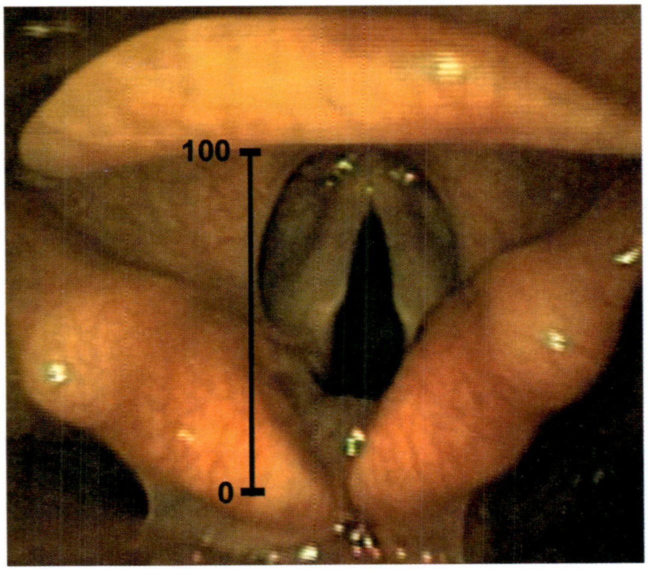

FIGURE 1.2. Levitan's Percent of Glottic Opening (POGO): 100—if the complete glottis can be seen; and 0—if no part of the glottis can be seen.

The Cormack/Lehane grading system is predicated upon grading during the best attempt at conventional DL, and the best attempt in turn requires definition. Benumof[57] defines the best attempt as being composed of six components:

1. Performance by a reasonably experienced practitioner
2. No significant muscle tone
3. The use of the optimal *sniffing* position
4. The use of external laryngeal manipulation (backward upward rightward pressure [BURP] or optimum external laryngeal manipulation [OELM])
5. Length of the blade
6. Type of blade

Most times, intubation demands that the first attempt be the best attempt, particularly in an emergency, although some compromises may be necessary (e.g., residency training). Should an orotracheal intubation attempt fail and an additional attempt be contemplated, it seems reasonable to *change something* on the subsequent attempt to enhance the chances of success. That *something* may be one, some, or all of these factors. Reminding oneself of the components of the optimum or best attempt provides a framework to address "what to change?"

Optimization of all six components may not be in the patient's best interest in an emergency. For example, if difficulty is anticipated, it may not be advisable to paralyze the patient. Additionally, in the event the cervical spine is immobilized, it may not be possible to place them in the *sniffing* position.

Most experts in airway management agree that positioning the head and neck is an important step in optimizing conventional laryngoscopy as a prelude to orotracheal intubation.[58]

If it is possible to consistently and precisely predict direct laryngoscopic intubation failure, the initial selection of direct laryngoscopic oral intubation could be eliminated as a strategy, and alternative techniques entertained (e.g., video-laryngoscopic intubation, flexible bronchoscopic intubation, cricothyrotomy). However, they may be technically more challenging, risky, and time-consuming. During the last several decades, this has not proven to be possible. Lists of anatomical features, radiologic findings, and complex scoring systems have all been explored without consistent success.[13,14]

Therefore, we are left to assemble the known risks, and other contextual issues such as time of day, location, position, availability of devices, and sophistication of assistance coupled with the skill, experience, and judgment of the practitioner, and make a decision: Does this airway meet the threshold of being sufficiently difficult to warrant using a Difficult Airway Algorithm or ask for help, or am I safe to proceed directly to induction of anesthesia, muscle paralysis, laryngoscopy, and intubation.

So, how do we quickly identify as many of the risks associated with DL intubation as possible? The mnemonic ***LEMON*** is a useful guide:

- ***L****ook externally*: If the airway looks difficult, it probably is (Figure 1.3). A litany of physical features has been associated with difficult laryngoscopy and intubation—a small mandible may indicate that the tongue is *retro-fitted* over the larynx; a large mandible elongates the pharyngeal axis serving to extend the distance to the larynx and perhaps move it beyond the horizon of view. Buck teeth block access to the oral cavity and elongate the length of the oral axis. A high, arched palate is often associated with a long, narrow oral cavity making access a problem. A short neck may mean the larynx is positioned higher in the neck relative to the base of the tongue making it more difficult to bring the glottis into view. Lower facial disruption is inconsistent with adequate mask seal and may make the glottis impossible to find. It is often said that when it comes to orotracheal intubation, the "tongue is your enemy" because it gets in your way and the "epiglottis is your friend" because once you find it, you ought to be able to find the glottic opening. However, in the event it is difficult to bypass a large epiglottis with a tracheal introducer or other device, a flexible bronchoscopic-assisted intubation may be indicated. With upper airway disruption, the tongue may actually be a friend as it leads to the epiglottis and the glottic opening.
- ***E****valuate 3-3-2*: Although there is no scientific basis to support the 3-3-2 rule, it serves to ensure that the relevant geometry of the upper airway is assessed adequately. The first *3* assesses the adequacy of oral access (Figure 1.4). One ought to be able to open one's mouth three of one's own finger breadths (approximately 5 cm). The second *3* and the *2* recognize the interplay of the geometric relationships among the various components of the upper airway. A thyromental distance of less than 6 cm was associated with difficult intubation (Figure 1.5). As described earlier, the thyromental distance is the hypotenuse of a triangle (Figure 1.5), the base being the length of the mandible (Figure 1.6) and the third

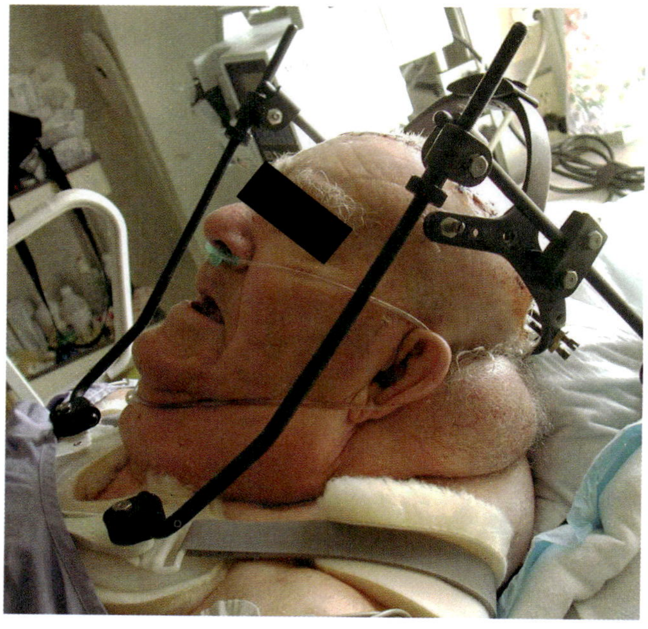

FIGURE 1.3. This patient provides an image recognizable instantly as a difficult airway.

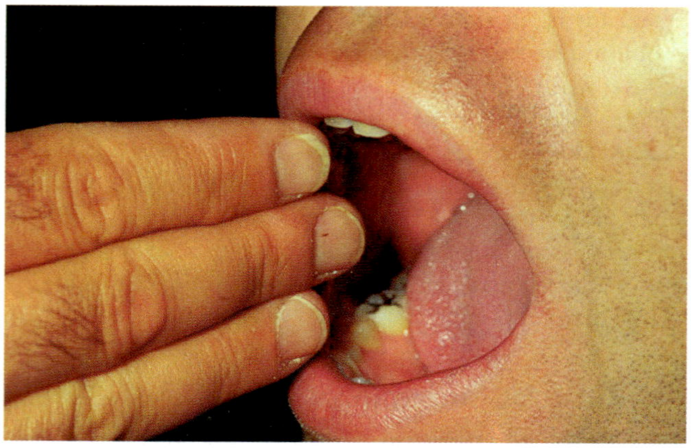

FIGURE 1.4. Airway evaluation: The first 3 of 3-3-2 evaluation indicates the extent of the mouth opening.

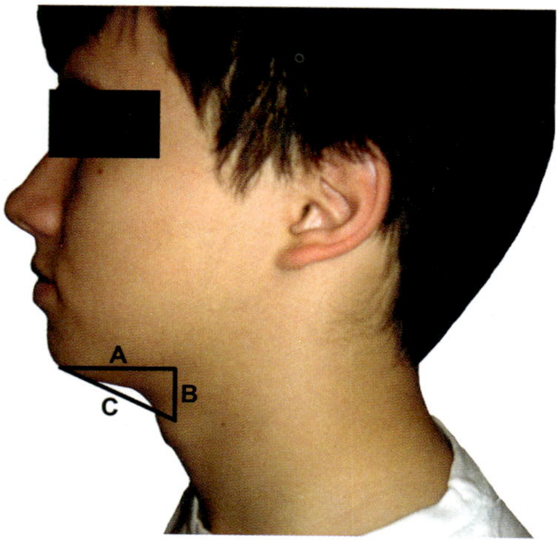

FIGURE 1.5. A thyromental distance of less than 6 cm was associated with difficult intubation.

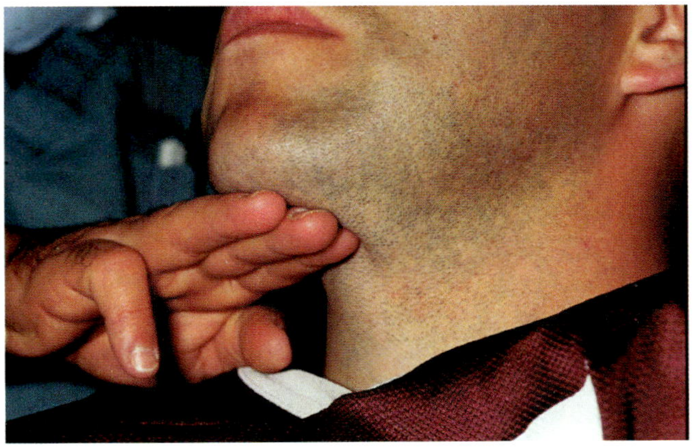

FIGURE 1.6. Airway evaluation: The second 3 of 3-3-2 evaluation indicates the length dimension of the mandibular space.

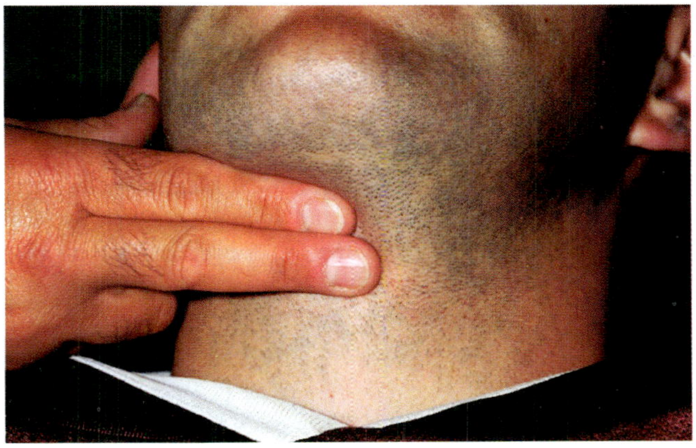

FIGURE 1.7. Airway evaluation: The 2 of 3-3-2 evaluation indicates the position of the larynx relative to the base of the tongue.

leg being the distance between the base of the tongue (neck–mandible junction at the level of the hyoid bone) and the top of the larynx (Figure 1.7). One ought to be able to accommodate three of one's own fingers (approximately 5 cm) between the tip of mentum and the mandible–neck junction (Figure 1.6) and fit two fingers between the mandible–neck junction and the thyroid notch (Figure 1.7). The second *3* steers one in assessing the capacity or volume of the mandibular space to accommodate the tongue on laryngoscopy. More than, or less than, three fingers (approximately 5 cm) are associated with greater degrees of difficulty in visualizing the larynx. The length of the oral axis is elongated if it is longer than three fingers, and the mandibular space may be too small to accommodate the tongue during laryngoscopy if it is shorter than three fingers, leaving it to obscure the view of the glottis. This *mandibular space volume* is determined by three dimensions: its length, its width, and its depth. The *2* identifies the location of the larynx in relation to the base of the tongue. If more than two fingers are accommodated, meaning the larynx is further below the base of the tongue, it may be difficult to visualize the glottis on laryngoscopy because it is too far down the neck and beyond the visual horizon. Fewer than two fingers may mean that the larynx is tucked up under the base of the tongue and may be difficult to expose. This condition is often called "anterior larynx."

- *M*allampati class: Mallampati studied the relationship between the visibility of the posterior oropharyngeal structures and the success rate of laryngoscopic intubation.[59,60] He had patients sit on the side of the bed, open their mouth as widely as possible, and protrude their tongue as far as possible, without phonating. Figure 1.8 depicts how the scale is constructed. Although Class I and II patients are associated

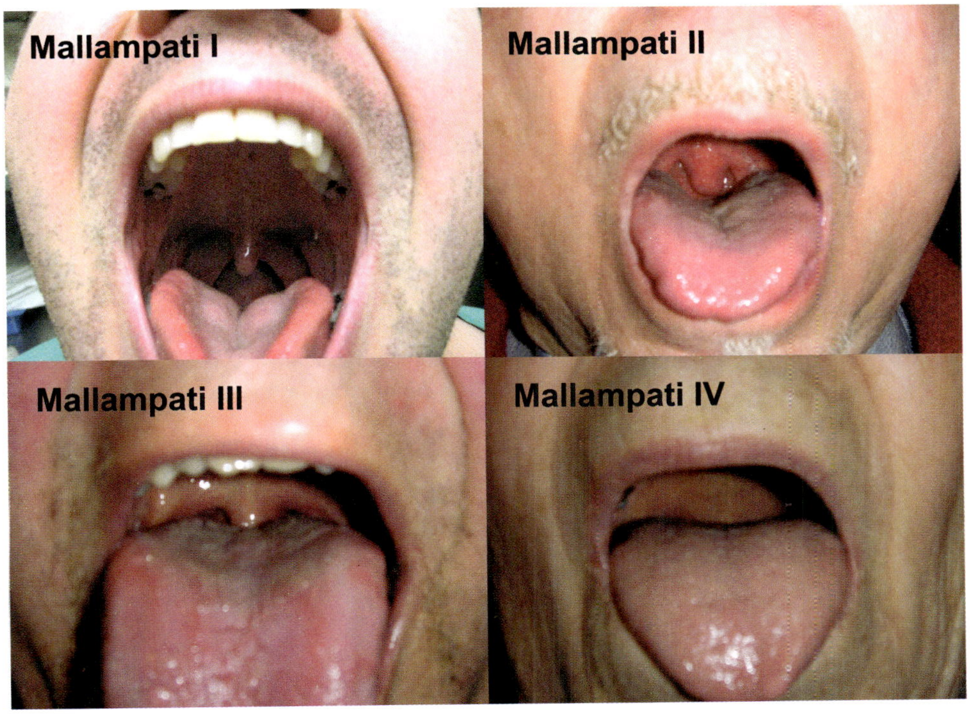

FIGURE 1.8. Mallampati classification.

with low intubation failure rates, circumspection with respect to the wisdom of utilizing neuromuscular blockade to facilitate intubation rests with those in Classes III and IV, particularly Class IV in which intubation failure rates may exceed 10%. This scale, by itself, is neither sensitive nor specific.[61] However, it is commonly used because it is easily performed, particularly in an emergency, and it may reveal important information about access to the oral cavity and potentially difficult glottic visualization.

- ***O***bstruction: There are four cardinal signs of upper airway obstruction: muffled voice (*hot potato voice*); difficulty in swallowing secretions, either because of pain or obstruction; dyspnea and stridor. The first two signs do not ordinarily herald imminent total upper airway obstruction. The presence of dyspnea and/or stridor generally indicates that the diameter of the airway has been reduced to 4.0 mm or less. Upper airway obstruction should always be considered a difficult airway and managed with extreme care. The administration of small doses of opioids and benzodiazepines to manage anxiety may induce total obstruction as the stenting tone of the upper airway musculature relaxes.
- ***N***eck mobility: The ability to position the head and neck is one of the six components of achieving an optimal view of the larynx on oral laryngoscopy. Although there is some dissention,[58] it has long been taught that the "sniffing the morning air," or "sipping English tea" positioning (neck flexion, head extension) of the head and neck, when possible, is at least the best place to start. While cervical spine immobilization alone may not constitute a difficult laryngoscopy, airway practitioners should be cautious in managing patients with limited cervical spine movement.

Difficult VL Intubation: CRANE

VL when compared to DL has been shown to produce better laryngeal views than DL in difficult airways, improve first-pass success rates in difficult and emergency intubations, and reduce the incidence of serious complications associated with laryngoscopic intubation.[13,14,62,63]

This technology has clearly benefited the field of difficult airway management. However, failures do occur and it should not deter a practitioner from performing an awake intubation in a nonemergency patient. Neither should it delay the performance of an open cricothyrotomy in the face of a CICO failed airway.

Predicting difficult VL intubation can be recalled by employing the mnemonic **CRANE**[14]:

C	Contamination and **C**ormack/Lehane 3 or 4 with DL
R	Radiation or **R**estricted mouth opening
A	Abnormal anatomy: mass; previous surgery
N	Neck thick or limited motion
E	Epiglottitis or **E**nlarged tongue

Difficulty with an EGD: RODS

The insertion of an EGD may be a planned backup maneuver (*Plan B*) when faced with a failed conventional orotracheal intubation. It can be used as a conduit for tracheal intubation or it may also serve as a bridging technique to reestablish gas exchange in a CICO setting while one prepares to perform a cricothyrotomy (see Chapter 2). To minimize wasting valuable time, airway practitioners should place the EGD concurrently while setting up to perform a FONA realizing that a perfect seal is not required for rescue oxygenation.

In the former case, when *Plan B* is an EGD, one ought to have performed an evaluation for difficult EGD placement before it is relied on as a primary or backup plan. While there are no prospective studies to evaluate predictors of difficult use of EGDs, there are many clinical reports of difficult use of EGDs, such as the laryngeal mask airway (LMA).

RODS is a mnemonic that is intended to identify problem patients when an EGD is contemplated. Most of these are common sense factors:

- ***R***estricted mouth opening: Depending on the EGD to be employed, more or less oral access may be needed. For instance, at least 2 cm of mouth opening is required to accommodate an LMA-Fastrach™.
- ***O***bstruction: Upper airway obstruction at the level of the larynx or below. An EGD will not bypass this obstruction. The use of an LMA can be potentially difficult in patients with lingual tonsillar hypertrophy.
- ***D***isrupted or ***D****istorted* airway: At least in as much as the *seat and seal* of the EGD may be compromised.
- ***S***tiff lungs or ***S***tiff cervical spine: Ventilation with an EGD may be difficult or impossible in the face of substantial increases in airway resistance (e.g., deadly asthma) or decreases in pulmonary compliance (e.g., pulmonary edema). Seal may be exceedingly difficult or impossible to achieve in the face of a fixed flexion deformity of the neck. In addition, LMA insertion can be difficult in patients with limited neck movement (e.g., ankylosing spondylitis).

Difficult FONA: SHORT

There are no absolute contraindications to performing an emergency FONA or cricothyrotomy. However, some conditions may make FONA difficult or impossible to perform, making it imperative to identify those conditions up front, particularly if one is relying on a rapidly performed cricothyrotomy as a rescue technique. Similarly, while there are no prospective trials to determine predictors of difficult cricothyrotomy, a number of clinical reports have identified situations associated with difficulties in performing a surgical airway. The mnemonic **SHORT** is used to quickly identify features that may indicate a difficult cricothyrotomy:

- ***S***urgery/disrupted airway: The anatomy of the neck may be subtly or obviously distorted due to previous surgery, making the airway difficult to access.
- ***H***ematoma or infection: An infective process or hematoma in the pathway of the cricothyrotomy incision may make the procedure technically difficult but should never be considered a contraindication in a life-threatening situation.
- ***O***bese/access problem: A fixed flexion deformity of the cervical spine, halo traction, and other situations may also make access to the neck difficult.

- *R*adiation: The tissue changes associated with past radiation therapy may alter tissues, making the procedure difficult.
- *T*umor: Tumor either in or around the airway may present difficulty, from both an access perspective and bleeding.

SUMMARY

Failure to evaluate the airway and accurately predict difficulty is the single most important factor leading to a failed airway. Despite decades of study, no system of evaluation is able to discern with certainty (100% reliability) those airways that can be managed with conventional laryngoscopic intubation and those where an alternative method is advisable. For this reason, each and every airway management episode must be approached with a view that some other devices or techniques may be necessary should the primary plan fail. Many factors can make airway management a challenge, such as human factors, location, experience, and clinical situation. The context is very important. Furthermore, the airway practitioner must evaluate the airway for difficulty relative to each of the alternatives contemplated. Once Plan A has failed, it is too late to suddenly realize that Plan B is also impossible because a factor that could have been detected had a prior evaluation for difficulty been conducted.

The PHASE and HELPET checklists can be used to triage airways into basic or advanced and find complexity factors that can increase the risk of complications.

While not exhaustive in covering all of the features of a difficult airway, the mnemonics **MOANS**, **LEMON**, **CRANE**, **RODS**, and **SHORT** provide guidance in evaluating all airways for difficulty, even though they are specifically designed to be employed rapidly in the face of an urgent or emergency clinical circumstance.

Finally, recognizing that one is in the midst of a failed airway is crucial in embarking on maneuvers that may rescue the airway. Persisting with a failing technique and forgetting to ask for help are fundamental contributors to bad outcomes in airway management.

SELF-EVALUATION QUESTIONS

1.1. The most common factor leading to a failed airway is:

A. Morbid obesity

B. Distorted airway anatomy

C. Upper airway obstruction

D. Failure to predict a difficult airway

E. Not knowing enough rescue techniques well

1.2. The standard of care in airway management is related to all of the following **EXCEPT**:

A. The skill of an average practitioner

B. Similar localities

C. Procedures that give the best results

D. The expectations of the reasonable patient

E. Opinions offered by experts

1.3. The standard of care expects that the average, reasonable airway practitioner ought to be able to do all of the following **EXCEPT**:

A. Be able to manage an unanticipated difficult airway

B. Be an expert and be able to use a flexible bronchoscope to intubate immediately in the face of a CICO airway

C. Be facile with one or two rescue devices or techniques in the face of a failed airway

D. Be able to perform a surgical airway

E. Be able to recognize and manage a failed airway

REFERENCES

1. Practice guidelines for management of the difficult airway. A report by the American Society of Anesthesiologists Task Force on management of the difficult airway. *Anesthesiology*. 1993;78:597-602.
2. Cheney FW, Posner KL, Caplan RA. Adverse respiratory events infrequently leading to malpractice suits. A closed claims analysis. *Anesthesiology*. 1991;75:932-939.
3. Hung O, Murphy M. Unanticipated difficult intubation. *Curr Opin Anaesthesiol*. 2004;17:479-481.
4. Crosby ET, Duggan LV, Finestone PJ, Liu R, De Gorter R, Calder LA. Anesthesiology airway-related medicolegal cases from the Canadian Medical Protection Association. *Can J Anaesth*. 2021;68:183-195.
5. Cook TM, Woodall N, Frerk C. Major complications of airway management in the UK: results of the Fourth National Audit Project of the Royal College of Anaesthetists and the Difficult Airway Society. Part 1: Anaesthesia. *Br J Anaesth*. 2011;106:617-631.
6. Cook TM, Woodall N, Harper J, Benger J. Major complications of airway management in the UK: results of the Fourth National Audit Project of the Royal College of Anaesthetists and the Difficult Airway Society. Part 2: Intensive care and emergency departments. *Br J Anaesth*. 2011;106:632-642.
7. Nolan JP, Kelly FE. Airway challenges in critical care. *Anaesthesia*. 2011;66(Suppl 2):81-92.
8. Peterson GN, Domino KB, Caplan RA, Posner KL, Lee LA, Cheney FW. Management of the difficult airway: a closed claims analysis. *Anesthesiology*. 2005;103:33-39.
9. Nørskov AK, Rosenstock CV, Wetterslev J, Astrup G, Afshari A, Lundstrøm LH. Diagnostic accuracy of anaesthesiologists' prediction of difficult airway management in daily clinical practice: a cohort study of 188064 patients registered in the Danish Anaesthesia Database. *Anaesthesia*. 2015;70:272-281.
10. Hung O, Law JA, Morris I, Murphy M. Airway assessment before intervention: what we know and what we do. *Anesth Analg*. 2016;122:1752-1754.
11. Huitink JM, Bouwman RA. The myth of the difficult airway: airway management revisited. *Anaesthesia*. 2015;70:244-249.
12. Joffe AM, Aziz MF, Posner KL, Duggan LV, Mincer SL, Domino KB. Management of difficult tracheal intubation: a closed claims analysis. *Anesthesiology*. 2020:818-829.
13. Law JA, Duggan LV, Asselin M, et al. Canadian Airway Focus Group updated consensus-based recommendations for management of the difficult airway: part 1. Difficult airway management encountered in an unconscious patient. *Can J Anaesth*. 2021;68(9):1373-1404.
14. Law JA, Duggan LV, Asselin M, et al. Canadian Airway Focus Group updated consensus-based recommendations for management of the difficult airway: part 2. Planning and implementing safe management of the patient with an anticipated difficult airway. *Can J Anaesth*. 2021;68(9):1405-1436.
15. Kim JH, Kim H, Jang JS, et al. Development and validation of a difficult laryngoscopy prediction model using machine learning of neck circumference and thyromental height. *BMC Anesthesiol*. 2021;21(1):125.
16. Detsky ME, Jivraj N, Adhikari NK, et al. Will this patient be difficult to intubate? The rational clinical examination systematic review. *JAMA*. 2019;321:493-503.
17. Kornas RL, Owyang CG, Sakles JC, Foley LJ, Mosier JM. Evaluation and management of the physiologically difficult airway: consensus recommendations from Society for Airway Management. *Anesth Analg*. 2021;132(2):395-405.
18. Aziz MF. Advancing patient safety in airway management. *Anesthesiology*. 2018;128:434-436.

19. Aziz MF, Bayman EO, Van Tienderen MM, et al. Predictors of difficult videolaryngoscopy with GlideScope® or C-MAC® with D-blade: secondary analysis from a large comparative videolaryngoscopy trial. *Br J Anaesth.* 2016;117:118-123.
20. McClelland GSM. Just a routine operation: a critical discussion. *J Perioper Pract.* 2016;26:114-117.
21. Hung O, Murphy M. Context-sensitive airway management. *Anesth Analg.* 2010;110:982-983.
22. Mosier JM, Joshi R, Hypes C, Pacheco G, Valenzuela T, Sakles JC. The physiologically difficult airway. *West J Emerg Med.* 2015;16:1109-1117.
23. Lumb AB, Thomas CR. *Nunn and Lumb's Applied Respiratory Physiology*, 9th ed. Elsevier Canada; 2020.
24. Apfelbaum JL, Hagberg CA, Connis RT, et al. 2022 American Society of Anesthesiologists practice guidelines for management of the difficult airway. *Anesthesiology.* 2022;136:31-81.
25. Pavlov I, Medrano S, Weingart S. Apneic oxygenation reduces the incidence of hypoxemia during emergency intubation: a systematic review and meta-analysis. *Am J Emerg Med.* 2017;35:1184-1189.
26. Perera A, Alkhouri H, Fogg T, Vassiliadis J, Mackenzie J, Wimalasena Y. Apnoeic oxygenation was associated with decreased desaturation rates during rapid sequence intubation in multiple Australian and New Zealand emergency departments. *Emerg Med J.* 2021;38:118-124.
27. Sakles JC, Mosier JM, Patanwala AE, Dicken JM. Apneic oxygenation is associated with a reduction in the incidence of hypoxemia during the RSI of patients with intracranial hemorrhage in the emergency department. *Intern Emerg Med.* 2016;11:983-992.
28. Kheterpal S, Vaughn MT, Dubovoy TZ, et al. Sugammadex versus Neostigmine for reversal of neuromuscular blockade and postoperative pulmonary complications (STRONGER): a multicenter matched cohort analysis. *Anesthesiology.* 2020;132:1371-1381.
29. Ledowski T, Szabo-Maak Z, Loh PS, et al. Reversal of residual neuromuscular block with neostigmine or sugammadex and postoperative pulmonary complications: a prospective, randomised, double-blind trial in high-risk older patients. *Br J Anaesth.* 2021;127:316-323.
30. Murphy GS, Avram MJ, Greenberg SB, et al. Neuromuscular and clinical recovery in thoracic surgical patients reversed with neostigmine or sugammadex. *Anesth Analg.* 2021;133:435-444.
31. Li G, Freundlich RE, Gupta RK, et al. Postoperative pulmonary complications' association with sugammadex versus neostigmine: a retrospective registry analysis. *Anesthesiology.* 2021;134:862-873.
32. Paton L, Gupta S, Blacoe D. Successful use of sugammadex in a "can't ventilate" scenario. *Anaesthesia.* 2013;68:861-864.
33. Bisschops MM, Holleman C, Huitink JM. Can sugammadex save a patient in a simulated 'cannot intubate, cannot ventilate' situation? *Anaesthesia.* 2010;65:936-941.
34. Aslani A, Ng SC, Hurley M, McCarthy KF, McNicholas M, McCaul CL. Accuracy of identification of the cricothyroid membrane in female subjects using palpation: an observational study. *Anesth. Analg.* 2012;114:987-992.
35. Elliott DSJ, Baker PA, Scott MR, Birch CW, Thompson JMD. Accuracy of surface landmark identification for cannula cricothyroidotomy. *Anaesthesia.* 2010;65:889-894.
36. Lamb A, Zhang J, Hung O, et al. Exactitude du repérage de la membrane cricothyroïdienne par des stagiaires et des patrons en anesthésie dans un établissement canadien. *Can J Anaesth.* 2015;62:495-503.
37. Ansari U, Malhas L, Mendonca C. Role of ultrasound in emergency front of neck access. *A & A Practice.* 2019;13:382-385.
38. Desai D, You-Ten KE, Arzola C, Friedman Z, Siddiqui N. Improved cricothyrotomy outcomes in human cadavers using ultrasound-guided compared to conventional digital palpation. *J Clin Anesth.* 2014;26:166-167.
39. Siddiqui N, Yu E, Boulis S, You-Ten KE. Ultrasound is superior to palpation in identifying the cricothyroid membrane in subjects with poorly defined neck landmarks a randomized clinical trial. *Anesthesiology* . 2018;129:1132-1139.
40. Adi O, Fong CP, Sum KM, Ahmad AH. Usage of airway ultrasound as an assessment and prediction tool of a difficult airway management. *Am J Emerg Med.* 2021;42:263.e1-e4.
41. Agarwal R, Jain G, Agarwal A, Govil N. Effectiveness of four ultrasonographic parameters as predictors of difficult intubation in patients without anticipated difficult airway. *Korean J Anesthesiol.* 2021;74:134-141.
42. Falcetta S, Cavallo S, Gabbanelli V, et al. Evaluation of two neck ultrasound measurements as predictors of difficult direct laryngoscopy. *Eur J Anaesthesiol.* 2018;35:605-612.
43. Gomes SH, Simões AM, Nunes AM, et al. Useful ultrasonographic parameters to predict difficult laryngoscopy and difficult tracheal intubation—a systematic review and meta-analysis. *Front Med (Lausanne).* 2021;8:671658.
44. Moura ECR, Filho ASM, de Oliveira EJSG, et al. Comparative study of clinical and ultrasound parameters for defining a difficult airway in patients with obesity. *Obes Surg.* 2021;31(9):4118-4124.
45. Sotoodehnia M, Rafiemanesh H, Mirfazaelian H, Safaie A, Baratloo A. Ultrasonography indicators for predicting difficult intubation: a systematic review and meta-analysis. *BMC Emerg Med.* 2021;21(1):76.
46. Zheng BX, Zheng H, Lin XM. Ultrasound for predicting difficult airway in obstetric anesthesia: Protocol and methods for a prospective observational clinical study. *Medicine.* 2019;98:e17846-e.
47. Cook TM, El-Boghdadly K, McGuire B, McNarry AF, Patel A, Higgs A. Consensus guidelines for managing the airway in patients with COVID-19: guidelines from the Difficult Airway Society, the Association of Anaesthetists the Intensive Care Society, the Faculty of Intensive Care Medicine and the Royal College of Anaesthetists. *Anaesthesia.* 2020;75:785-799.
48. Domino KB. Death and brain damage from difficult airway management: a "never event". *Can J Anaesth.* 2021;68(2):169-174.
49. Ahmad I, El-Boghdadly K, Bhagrath R, et al. Difficult Airway Society guidelines for awake tracheal intubation (ATI) in adults. *Anaesthesia.* 2020;75:509-528.
50. Han R, Tremper KK, Kheterpal S, O'Reilly M. Grading scale for mask ventilation. *Anesthesiology.* 2004;101(1):267.
51. Kheterpal S, Martin L, Shanks AM, Tremper KK. Prediction and outcomes of impossible mask ventilation: a review of 50,000 anesthetics. *Anesthesiology.* 2009;110(4):891-897.
52. Kheterpal S, Healy D, Aziz MF, et al. Incidence, predictors, and outcome of difficult mask ventilation combined with difficult laryngoscopy: a report from the multicenter perioperative outcomes group. *Anesthesiology.* 2013;119:1360-1369.
53. Langeron O, Masso E, Huraux C, et al. Prediction of difficult mask ventilation. *Anesthesiology.* 2000;92(5):1229-1236.
54. Cormack RS, Lehane J. Difficult tracheal intubation in obstetrics. *Anaesthesia.* 1984;39:1105-1111.
55. Yentis SM. Predicting difficult intubation—worthwhile exercise or pointless ritual? *Anaesthesia.* 2002;57:105-109.
56. Levitan RM, Ochroch EA, Kush S, Shofer FS, Hollander JE. Assessment of airway visualization: validation of the percentage of glottic opening (POGO) scale. *Acad Emerg Med.* 1998;5:919-923.
57. Benumof JL. Difficult laryngoscopy: obtaining the best view. *Can J Anaesth.* 1994;41(5 Pt 1):361-365.
58. Adnet F, Baillard C, Borron SW, et al. Randomized study comparing the "sniffing position" with simple head extension for laryngoscopic view in elective surgery patients. *Anesthesiology.* 2001;95:836-841.
59. Mallampati SR. Clinical sign to predict difficult tracheal intubation (hypothesis). *Can Anaesth Soc J.* 1983;30:316-317.
60. Samsoon GL, Young JR. Difficult tracheal intubation: a retrospective study. *Anaesthesia.* 1987;42:487-490.
61. Lee A, Fan LTY, Gin T, Karmakar MK, Kee WDN. A systematic review (meta-analysis) of the accuracy of the mallampati tests to predict the difficult airway. *Anesth. Analg.* 2006;102:1867-1878.
62. Carron M, Linassi F, Ieppariello G. Videolaryngoscopy versus direct laryngoscopy for patients with obesity requiring tracheal intubation: a meta-analysis. *Obes Surg.* 2021;31:3327-3329.
63. Law JA, Kovacs G. Videolaryngoscopy 2.0. *Can J Anaesth.* 2021.

CHAPTER 2

The Airway Management Algorithms

J. Adam Law and Michael F. Murphy

INTRODUCTION

What Is the Challenge of Difficult and Failed Airway Management?

Competency in airway management is fundamental to the practice of anesthesia, emergency medicine, emergency medical services (EMS), critical care medicine, hospital medicine, and other acute care specialties. The airway practitioner is faced with two particular challenges: to be able to accurately and expeditiously predict a difficult airway, and to be able to recognize when airway management has failed.[1] No matter the situation, reliably and reproducibly ensuring timely and effective oxygenation and ventilation is imperative. Appropriate planning, selection of the airway devices and techniques, clear communication of that plan, and calm execution based on learned methods and experience enhances success even in the most difficult cases. The need for clearly communicated Plan A (first line or initial plan), B (backup or salvage plan), and C (failed airway plan) cannot be overemphasized.

How Reliably Can We Predict a Difficult Airway?

There are several means through which effective ventilation occurs: spontaneous ventilation by the patient, or positive pressure ventilation provided through face-mask ventilation (FMV), extraglottic device (EGD), tracheal intubation, or surgical (front-of-neck) airway. The latter four of these are *artificial* or non-natural interventions, or methods of active airway management. If a patient is unable to sustain adequate spontaneous gas exchange, or if during therapy the patient's ability to maintain adequate gas exchange is compromised or eliminated (e.g., due to the use of medications), one of these four methods must be employed successfully to assure survival. They constitute the four dimensions of airway management. Hence, before embarking on airway management, the patient should be assessed for predictors of the following:

- Difficult FMV
- Difficult laryngoscopy and tracheal intubation (e.g., using direct laryngoscopy [DL] or video laryngoscopy [VL])
- Difficult EGD use
- Difficult front-of-neck airway (FONA)

Ordinarily, FMV and orotracheal intubation are the usual methods employed in managing the airway of patients unable to adequately breathe for themselves. If a difficult airway is anticipated, and it is not to be managed "awake," EGDs and FONA techniques are usually considered rescue options. Importantly, rescue techniques should not be considered de facto evidence of "failure" when they are part of the airway management plan, a fundamental concept advanced in this text. Techniques under consideration as first-line or rescue depend in large part on the context of the situation, including the indication for airway management, the condition of the patient, the skill of the practitioner, the availability of skilled assistance, the location and equipment available, and the time of day (see Chapter 7).

In elective situations, difficulty with FMV is uncommon. Langeron was the first to address codifying "difficult mask ventilation" (DMV) by prospectively reviewing the management of 1502 patients undergoing elective surgery under general anesthesia.[2] DMV was defined as:

A. An inability to maintain SpO_2 greater than 92% while using 100% O_2 via the bag-mask anesthesia circuit unit
B. Significant gas leak around the face mask
C. A need to increase the fresh gas flow to rates greater than 15 $L{\cdot}min^{-1}$ and to use the flush valve more than twice
D. No perceptible chest wall movement during ventilation
E. The need to perform a two-handed mask technique
F. Changing the practitioner

The anesthesia practitioner was asked to identify ventilation as difficult only if perceived to be clinically relevant, that is, potentially leading to a patient threat. In 5% of the patients, ventilation was considered difficult, and in only one patient was ventilation impossible. Following multivariate analysis, five criteria were recognized as independent factors for DMV: age more than 55 years; body mass index (BMI) greater than 26 $kg{\cdot}m^{-2}$; lack of teeth; presence of a beard; and a history of snoring (see Chapter 1).

Kheterpal et al.[3,4] confirmed that obesity (BMI > 30 $kg{\cdot}m^{-2}$), snoring and sleep apnea, age (>56 years), and Mallampati of Grade III or IV were risk factors for difficult ventilation and in addition, noted that a history of radiation therapy to the neck and severely limited jaw protrusion predicted DMV (see Chapter 8 for a detailed discussion). Han[5] and Kheterpal[4] proposed DMV scales for the purposes of clarity and communication (see Table 2.1).

Difficult FMV in patients under general anesthesia is likely to occur in 2% to 5% of patients and impossible mask ventilation in about one per thousand anesthetics.[2,4,6]

In the emergency situation, other factors may become relevant when considering whether difficulty with FMV is more likely to be encountered. Trauma to the face with resultant edema, bleeding, or debris in the airway, and the need to maintain in-line C-spine immobilization when required may increase the degree of difficulty with FMV. In addition, if used, cricoid pressure is recognized to increase the likelihood of difficult FMV. Petito and Russell[7] evaluated the impact of cricoid pressure on lung ventilation during FMV. Fifty patients were randomized to have cricoid pressure applied or not applied during a 3-minute period of standardized mask-ventilation. Patients who had cricoid pressure applied were considered more difficult to ventilate (36% vs. 12%), and these patients tended to have more air in the stomach than those patients considered easy to ventilate without applied cricoid pressure.

Most studies dealing with the assessment of the airway in anticipation of tracheal intubation using DL have limited applicability to currently available alternative devices (e.g., video laryngoscopes, rigid or flexible bronchoscopic devices, and intubating EGDs).[8–11] Modification of Mallampati's original schema[12] as well as alternative strategies to assess the airway (see Chapter 1) has been proposed. These strategies include using simple anatomical descriptors, ranking and summating anatomical scoring systems, and using logistic regression to create predictive scales to derive performance indices. They share some common characteristics, that is, they have limited sensitivity and positive predictive values with respect to predicting difficult and failed laryngoscopy and intubation. For example, in a meta-analysis by Shiga et al. a score incorporating Mallampati and temporomandibular joint displacement components found a positive association with difficult intubation of only 9.9%.[13] Additionally, many of the tests have only moderate interobserver reliability.[14,15] Such limitations may help to explain why these tests often fail to predict difficult tracheal intubation in the apparently normal population, and why perhaps some practitioners question the ability of preanesthetic airway assessments to predict or rule out difficulty with certainty.[16]

A number of new schemes and techniques used to predict potential airway difficulty have been described; their accuracy and widespread applicability are not yet determined. However, it is likely that they too will have a low positive predictive value, similar to current strategies, because of the low incidence of airway difficulty.[16,17] This will lead to unanticipated difficulty occurring in some instances.[17,18] Therefore, strategies to manage the unanticipated difficult airway should be preformulated for every patient to minimize adverse outcomes resulting from the inevitable occurrence of false-negative predictions.

AIRWAY EMERGENCIES

How Is Airway Management in an Emergency Setting Different?

Airway management in an emergency setting may be complicated by a multitude of factors. Trauma to the face and neck may distort anatomical features or obscure them with blood

TABLE 2.1. Classification of Difficult Bag Mask Ventilation According to Han[5]

Classification	Description/Definition	No. of Selections	% of Cases
Grade 0	Ventilation by mask not attempted	449	24.2
Grade 1	Ventilated by mask	1010	54.4
Grade 2	Ventilated by mask with oral airway or other adjuvant	366	20.0
Grade 3	Difficult mask ventilation (inadequate , unstable, or requiring two practitioners)	22	1.2
Grade 4	Unable to mask ventilate	1	0.05
Comments		6	0.3
Total		1854	

and debris. Additionally, blood in the airway may absorb a significant amount of the light cast by airway devices making recognition of anatomic features more difficult. The requirement for in-line stabilization in patients with known or potential cervical spinal injury may make DL more difficult.[19] Unprepared patients are often associated with a full stomach and are at a higher risk of regurgitation and aspiration of gastric contents. Use of cricoid pressure has been advocated; however, most evidence supporting its use is observational only. There is some evidence that the maneuver imposes an element of obstruction to the passive regurgitation of gastric contents[20] and anecdotal evidence that it has prevented aspiration.[21] On the other hand, it has been shown to be difficult to teach and perform,[22] may not protect against aspiration in all patients at risk,[23–25] hinders FMV and EGD insertion, and may make tracheal intubation more difficult.[26–28] A Cochrane Review was unable to resolve the controversy as to whether cricoid pressure should or should not be abandoned in high-risk patients,[29] and a more recent large, randomized trial indicated that *not* applying cricoid pressure in an at-risk population was noninferior to its application.[30]

Emergency situations and hemodynamically unstable patients may contraindicate the use of drugs to facilitate laryngoscopy, resulting in intubating conditions which may be less than ideal. Finally, a chaotic emergency environment may distract the practitioner, making it more difficult to manage the airway.

DIFFICULT AND FAILED AIRWAY

What Does Experience Tell Us About Rescuing the Difficult Airway?

Airway management guidelines often recommend *default-to* strategies to improve the success of rescue airway interventions and reduce the occurrence of adverse outcomes.[31–33] This follows from published data indicating that persisting with failing techniques rather than defaulting to rescue strategies results in higher rates of morbidity and mortality.[34,35] There is consistent evidence of a significant rise in the rate of airway-related complications in all hospital environments as the number of attempts at laryngoscopy and intubation increases (<2 vs. ≥ 2).[36–50] These complications include esophageal intubation, hypoxemia, regurgitation, aspiration, bradycardia, and cardiac arrest.

Avoiding the morbidity associated with multiple futile attempts at tracheal intubation implies an early move to an alternative technique, as long as the patients' ventilation and oxygenation are nonproblematic. Published studies document the success of a variety of techniques after unsuccessful tracheal intubation by DL, including VL,[51–55] use of a lighted stylet,[56] flexible bronchoscopy,[57] or use of a tracheal tube introducer.[58,59] Connelly et al.[60] noted that alternatives to DL were far more likely to be successful than persistent use of DL in the setting of multiple failed attempts. Exactly which alternative technique is used may be less important than the fact that it is a *practiced alternative* and chosen early in a planned approach when DL has proven to be difficult or has failed.

Is There a Pattern to the Way Airway Practitioners Behave in the Face of a Difficult or Failed Airway?

Although the use of VL is increasing, many tracheal intubations are still performed orally under DL. Difficulties related to tracheal intubation facilitated by DL relate chiefly to difficulty in obtaining a view of the larynx. Multiple patient factors, individually or in combination, may conspire to prevent obtaining an adequate view of the larynx. The ability to predict all patients in whom it will be impossible to establish a line of sight during DL is sufficiently imprecise that sole reliance on the direct laryngoscope to perform tracheal intubation is a precarious strategy. Nevertheless, there is evidence that such behavior has been common among anesthesia practitioners. Rosenblatt surveyed a random sample of the active membership of the American Society of Anesthesiologists (ASA).[61] The survey presented difficult airway scenarios involving cooperative adult patients who required tracheal intubation. Physicians were asked to identify their preferred management technique. In one scenario described as a patient with a history of previous difficult intubation, 60% of practitioners would induce general anesthesia and 59% would proceed with DL. Experienced practitioners tended to use higher risk induction techniques and were more likely to use a laryngeal mask airway in situations commonly agreed to be unconventional or contraindicated. The use of alternative devices was uncommon in the survey, occurring in less than 5% of all scenarios. While this study predated the ready availability of video laryngoscopes, other publications of airway morbidity and closed claims studies continue to indicate risky decision-making in the face of anticipated difficult airway management.[34,35,62,63]

There has also been a substantial change in our thinking with respect to FONA as presented in Chapter 1. In the past, airway practitioners were given the option to perform a needle-guidewire-cannula (Seldinger) technique or an open surgical cricothyrotomy.[64,65] Compared with an open surgical technique, the Seldinger technique was felt to be psychologically more acceptable to the average practitioner. However, reliably identifying the location of the cricothyroid space for initial needle placement in elective surgical patients is difficult, particularly if they are female or obese.[66–69] Subsequently, the Fourth National Audit Project of the Royal College of Anaesthetists and the Difficult Airway Society in the United Kingdom (NAP4)[34,35] and others[70] identified that needle techniques were often unsuccessful and open techniques were more successful; although in many instances, surgeons were more likely than anesthesia practitioners to perform the open techniques. It is currently recommended that an open surgical cricothyrotomy (e.g., scalpel-bougie-tube) be performed in the "cannot intubate, cannot oxygenate" (CICO) situation or that, in the event of problems with needle techniques, conversion to an open technique takes place.[31,32 34]

It is now taught that if the airway practitioner considers a CICO situation even remotely possible then the cricothyroid space be identified (e.g., with the use of ultrasound) and the incision line marked preemptively. Thus, should a cricothyrotomy be needed, it will be part of the plan as opposed to "emblematic of failure." The psychology of this approach is compelling in motivating individuals to move earlier to a cricothyrotomy as soon as a CICO situation is identified. Analysis of NAP4 and closed legal claim databases has identified delay in performing cricothyrotomy as a substantial issue leading to poor outcomes.[34,35,62,63]

What Is the Medical–Legal Experience with Respect to Airway Management Failure?

The largest series of published medical–legal cases involving airway management is that of the ASA Closed Claims Project. Data from the airway cases reviewed in the ASA Closed Claims Project were originally published in 1990, with additional publications in 1991, 2000, 2005, 2011, and 2019.[63,71–74] In the original (1990) report, respiratory adverse event claims accounted for 34% (522/1541) of all claims. Inadequate ventilation was the most common single event overall, accounting for 12.7% of all claims and more than a third of the respiratory claims. Esophageal intubation and difficult intubation claims each occurred at about half the rate of those for inadequate ventilation. In this report, Caplan et al.[71] speculated that improved monitoring would reduce the incidence of inadequate ventilation and esophageal intubation, and enhanced training would reduce the occurrence of difficult intubation and its sequelae.

An updated analysis of closed legal claims relating to the difficult airway was published in 2005.[75] Two-thirds of the documented events took place during induction of anesthesia and the remaining third during surgery, extubation of the trachea, or recovery. Care was judged to be less than appropriate or substandard in nearly half of the difficult airway claims. In the claims with an anticipated difficult airway, the first strategy was more likely to be tracheal intubation after induction of general anesthesia with ventilation ablated (61%) than awake tracheal intubation (ATI) (32%). Awake intubation was attempted but unsuccessful in 12 claims, resulting in death or brain damage in 75% of these claims. In 5 of these 12 claims, airway difficulties arose when general anesthesia was induced after attempts at awake intubation were abandoned. Finally, in claims in which an emergency airway situation developed, the outcome was worse with persistent attempts at intubation before attempting emergency nonsurgical ventilation or emergency surgical airway access.

A more recent ASA closed claims report was published in 2019.[63] As with previous reports, one-third of airway claims originated from intraprocedure, extubation, or recovery phases of operative cases with the remainder at the induction of general anesthesia. Inappropriate management was deemed to have occurred in 73% of cases with sufficient information to assess. The most common management failures included perseveration with a failed technique, failure to use an EGD as a bridge, and the failure to plan appropriately when difficult tracheal intubation was anticipated. Other themes included a delay in initiating surgical airway management, and inadequate preoperative airway evaluation.[63]

Similar themes to the ASA closed claims publications emerged in a 2021 Canadian publication of anesthesiology airway-related medicolegal cases.[62] Originating from Canada's not-for-profit mutual defense union that represents 95% of Canadian physicians, 11% of all reported claims from 2007 to 2016 were airway-related. As with the ASA reports, themes included inadequate or no preoperative airway evaluation, the failure to plan for potentially difficult airway management, and perseveration with failing techniques. There were some cases of failure to recognize esophageal intubation, and others of failure to follow standards for respiratory monitoring.[62]

What Were the Major Messages from the NAP4 Study?

The year-long NAP4 study[34,35] gathered patient cases of major airway complications from all 309 National Health Service (NHS) hospitals in the United Kingdom. It identified cases from the operating room, intensive care unit (ICU), and emergency department (ED). Triggers for inclusion in the database were complications of airway management, defined by the authors as those leading to death, brain damage, need for an emergency surgical airway, unexpected ICU admission, or prolongation of ICU stay. After final review, 184 cases were included: 133 from anesthesia, 36 from ICU, and 15 from the ED. Importantly, when it came to surgical airway, the study identified a high failure rate of percutaneous cricothyrotomy performed by anesthetists. Of 25 attempts, only 9 were successful (36%). An open surgical technique, often performed by a surgeon, was associated with a 100% success rate of tracheal cannulation, although not all patients survived. In the ICU environment, 14 tracheotomies were accidentally dislodged, resulting in a 50% mortality. Other important conclusions could be drawn from this landmark study:

- Poor assessment and poor planning led to poor outcomes.
- If an awake intubation was indicated, it was advisable to use the technique.
- Repeated attempts at orotracheal intubation or EGD use were rarely successful: better to perform a surgical airway early.
- It was good to plan for failure.
- Failure to detect carbon dioxide meant that the endotracheal tube was not in the trachea, even in recently arrested patients.
- Inhalation induction of anesthesia on adult patients with upper airway obstruction was often unsuccessful.

AIRWAY ALGORITHMS

Why Are Algorithms Useful in Airway Management?

Automatic responses are not typical when we are confronted by rare events such as the CICO situation, or other types of airway emergency. Therefore, fundamental to successfully managing the emergency or failed airway is the development of a systematic approach to clinical situations rarely encountered in day-to-day practice. Algorithms, decision trees, and mnemonics feature prominently in these approaches, and they must be evidence-based and quickly and easily applied. It is fair to say that after years of formal medical education and practice, many of us harbor an aversion to *algorithms*. Nevertheless, while it is recognized that rigidity stifles innovation and constrains personal preference, adherence to sensibly constructed decision trees minimizes variation, conserves valuable time, and can provide the greatest chance for success.

James Reason has defined two basic mechanisms whereby practitioners deal with critical incidents.[76] The first is a rule-based solution, whereby upon recognizing the event for what it is, one identifies and applies a solution that experience has shown will likely be useful in solving the problem. Recognizing the event involves a process called "similarity-matching," based on identifying that the characteristics of the events are similar to those of past events (in a sense, *pattern recognition*). The practitioner then decides upon a particular solution that is likely to be effective in resolving the threat. This presupposes that the practitioner has had sufficient experience to both immediately recognize the problem and to know which rule to apply. This ability constitutes what is called "expertise."

The second mechanism for dealing with critical incidents is to apply a knowledge-based solution. This is a ground-up, first-principle strategy whereby without significant past experience with similar situations, the practitioner attempts to find an appropriate solution. Not surprisingly, such strategies often involve multiple decisions, are time-consuming, and when made under the pressure of time, are more likely to fail. For this reason, preformulated airway algorithms are helpful in these situations and deserve to be considered by all airway practitioners.

Coincident with the development of the algorithms (*strategies*) and vital to airway management success is skill in the application of an array of devices and techniques (*tactics*) that can optimize clinical outcomes. As with algorithms, techniques and devices advocated in this chapter are anchored by evidence and expert opinion, rather than personal preference.

Algorithms meant to *guide practice in crisis situations* must exhibit the following design elements:

- Entry and exit points are easily recognized.
- They are based on the best available evidence.
- Branch points are binary.
- There are a limited number of actions at each step.
- They are easy to remember and represent graphically.

Many of the algorithms accompanying airway guidelines are intended as graphic representation of the overall strategy detailed in the narrative, rather than being meant for use as a cognitive aid during an episode of difficulty.

What Are the Features of the American Society of Anesthesiologists' (ASA) Difficult Airway Algorithms and How Has the Most Recent (2022) Version Changed from Previous Ones?

In an attempt to avert airway management disasters, The ASA first produced the *ASA Difficult Airway Algorithm* in 1993.[77] Revisions have been published in 2003,[78] 2013,[65] and most recently, in 2022.[33] All iterations of the ASA Difficult Airway algorithm are derived from the *Practice Guidelines for the Management of the Difficult Airway*, developed by the ASA Task Force on Difficult Airway Management.

The ASA algorithms guide management strategies for patients with anticipated or unanticipated difficult airways (Figure 2.1). They emphasize the importance of possessing expertise in more than one airway management technique and recommend that each time an airway is managed, the practitioner formulates a variety of backup plans to address failure of the primary plan. Rescue tactics are recommended for difficulty with, and the failure of ventilation.

The 2022 ASA algorithms and the accompanying narrative contain a number of substantive changes from previous iterations, as follows:

- A number of infographics have been published to further illustrate the algorithms (Figure 2.2).
- The guidelines are now intended for use by anesthesia practitioners and all others who perform airway management in inpatient and ambulatory settings. Previous iterations were limited to anesthesia practitioners delivering anesthetic care and airway management under the direct supervision of anesthesia practitioners.
- There is additional guidance on when to perform ATI. If a patient anticipated to be a difficult tracheal intubation is also suspected to be difficult to ventilate by face mask or an EGD, is at increased risk of aspiration or apnea intolerance, or if there is expected difficulty with emergency invasive airway rescue, then ATI is recommended. This guidance appears in the narrative, in an expanded section of the accompanying algorithm, and in a separate infographic (Figure 2.3).
- Advice now appears in the algorithms that when a failed attempt at tracheal intubation has occurred, further attempts should be limited, and to remain aware of the passage of time.
- As in previous iterations, when tracheal intubation is unsuccessful, but FMV is adequate, the algorithm's nonemergency pathway recommends considering awakening the patient, use of alternative approaches to tracheal intubation, invasive access to the airway, or other options, including proceeding with the procedure using FMV or EGD ventilation. When FMV is not adequate after failed tracheal intubation, an attempt at EGD ventilation is advised. If unsuccessful, the emergency pathway recommends attempting alternative approaches while preparing for emergency invasive FONA; if still unsuccessful, emergency invasive FONA should proceed.
- A new distinction is made within the category of invasive airway options. Retrograde intubation and percutaneous tracheotomy are now being advised only as elective techniques. Rigid bronchoscopy and extracorporeal membrane oxygenation (ECMO) should also be considered.
- Updated and expanded recommendations are made for the extubation of the difficult airway.

Importantly, the ASA guidelines now include a second version of the difficult airway algorithm that specifically addresses the pediatric patient, along with a similarly dedicated infographic (Figure 2.4). While the structure and messages are similar to the adult patient algorithm, key differences include the following:

- Advice on when to perform an awake or sedated approach to tracheal intubation is predicated only upon suspected concurrent difficulty with ventilation using face mask or an EGD when difficult laryngoscopy is suspected; additional factors are advised for consideration in the adult algorithm.

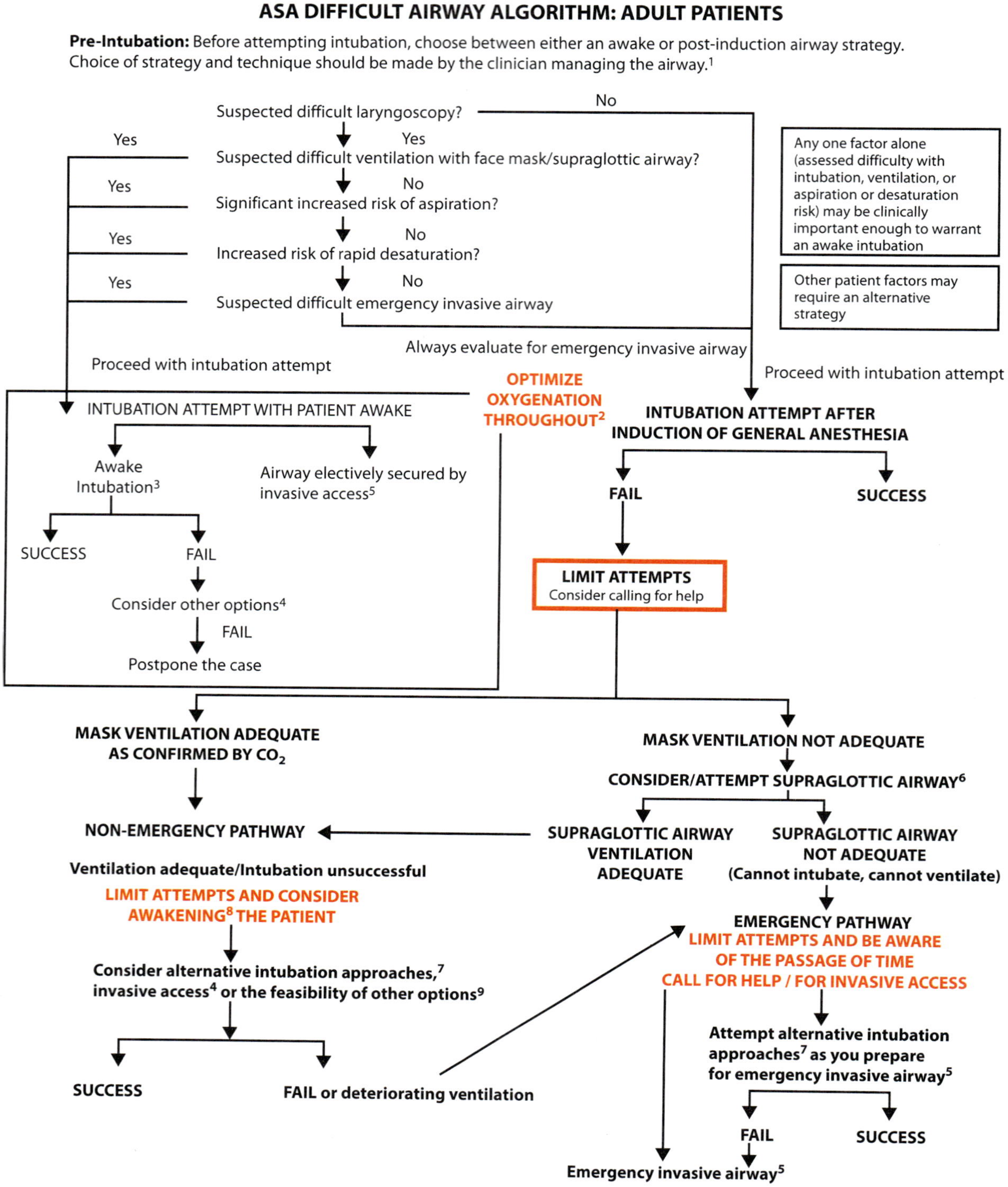

FIGURE 2.1. ASA Difficult Airway Algorithm: adult patients. (Reproduced with permission from Apfelbaum JL, Hagberg CA, Connis RT, et al. 2022 American Society of Anesthesiologists Practice Guidelines for Management of the Difficult Airway. *Anesthesiology*. 2022;136(1):31-81.)

- With a failed attempt at tracheal intubation, when oxygenation/ventilation with face mask or EGD is assessed as being marginal or impossible, the practitioner is advised to exclude/treat anatomical and functional (e.g., adverse airway reflexes) obstruction, and to consider calling for invasive FONA or ECMO.

For both adult and pediatric patients, there is additional information appearing in the infographics and their legends that do not appear in the main article narrative or algorithms. For example, although advice appears in the narrative and main algorithms to "limit attempts," this is clarified in the infographic and accompanying legend as being three attempts at any technique class, with one additional attempt by a practitioner with higher skills. Similarly, other information, including mention of specific techniques is relegated to footnotes or legends, so

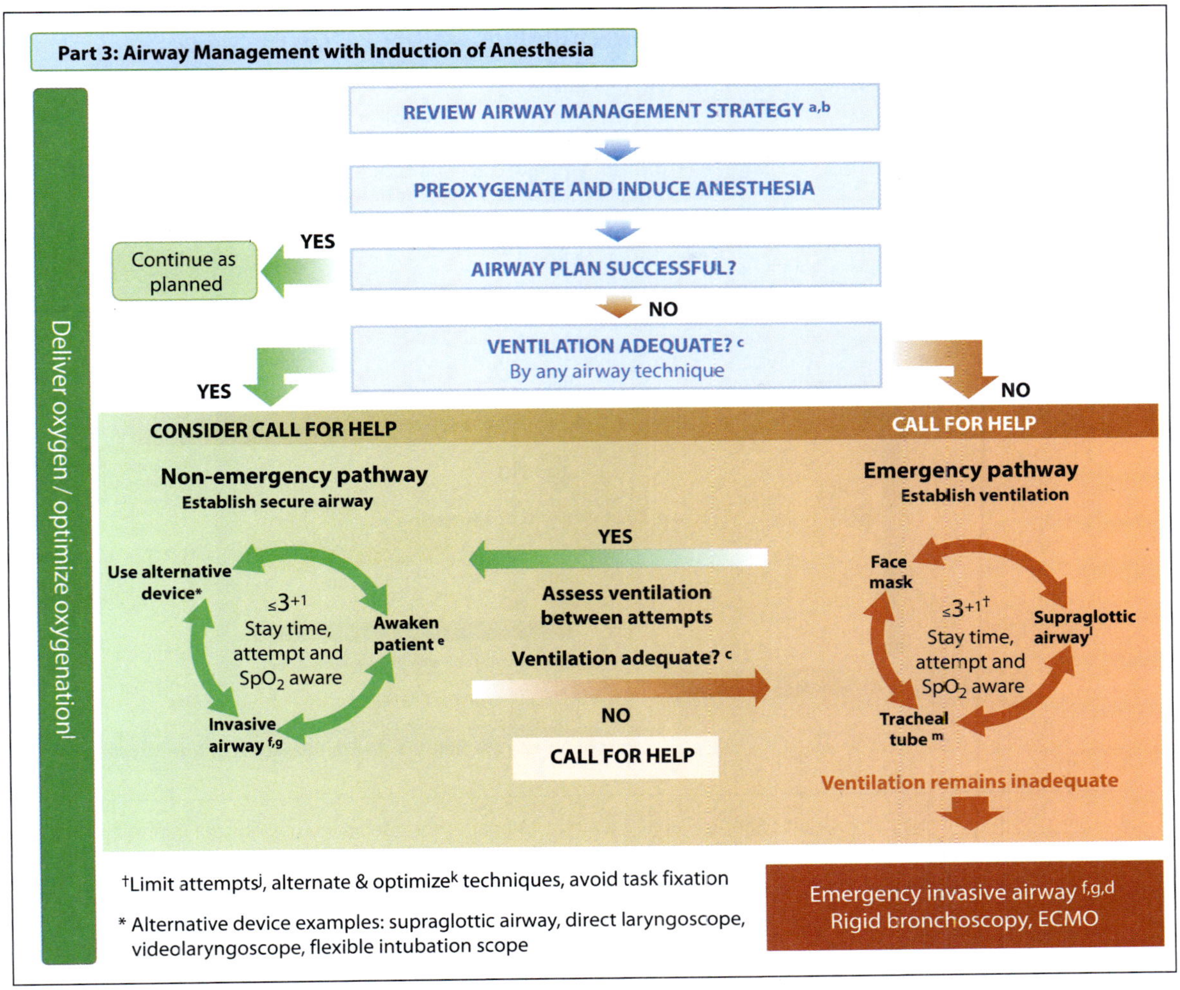

FIGURE 2.2. Difficult airway infographic: adult patients. Part 3: Airway management with induction of anesthesia. For information on superscripts appearing in this infographic, the reader is advised to consult the original publication. (Reproduced with permission from Apfelbaum JL, Hagberg CA, Connis RT, et al. 2022 American Society of Anesthesiologists Practice Guidelines for Management of the Difficult Airway. *Anesthesiology*. 2022;136(1):31-81.)

careful reading of all aspects of the document is required. As always, an early disclaimer states that the ASA guidelines are not intended to replace local institutional policies and that they are not intended as standards or absolute requirements.

What Are the Features of the 2021 Canadian Airway Focus Group Guidelines and Algorithms?

The Canadian Airway Focus Group (CAFG) originally published recommendations for the management of the unanticipated difficult airway in 1998.[79] These were updated in two 2013 publications, the first of which addressed difficult tracheal intubation encountered in an unconscious patient,[64] while the second publication focused on management of the anticipated difficult airway.[80] Both articles have been further updated in 2021.[32,81] With working group representation from Anesthesia, Emergency Medicine and Critical Care, the CAFG has sought to make their recommendations relevant to all three practice environments. The recommendations are based on the best available evidence in the literature; where none exists, consensus opinion is used. Both articles appear with algorithms to illustrate the accompanying narrative.

For the unconscious patient (i.e., general anesthesia has been induced, or an emergency patient was unconscious at presentation) the entry point to the algorithm and discussion is with an unsuccessful first attempt at tracheal intubation (Figure 2.5).

Key points and recommendations include the following:

- After a failed attempt at tracheal intubation, further management will be dictated by the patient's oxygenation status. If the patient's oxygen saturation remains in a safe range for the patient (e.g., by use of successful FMV or EGD ventilation, or due to denitrogenation or use of apneic oxygenation), the left-hand side of the two pathways is selected, allowing the option of proceeding with further attempts at tracheal intubation.
- Additional attempts at tracheal intubation should address the likely cause of the preceding unsuccessful attempt, and not simply repeat the unsuccessful technique. Examples are provided in the narrative and include the use of a tracheal tube introducer to help with a restricted view situation during DL

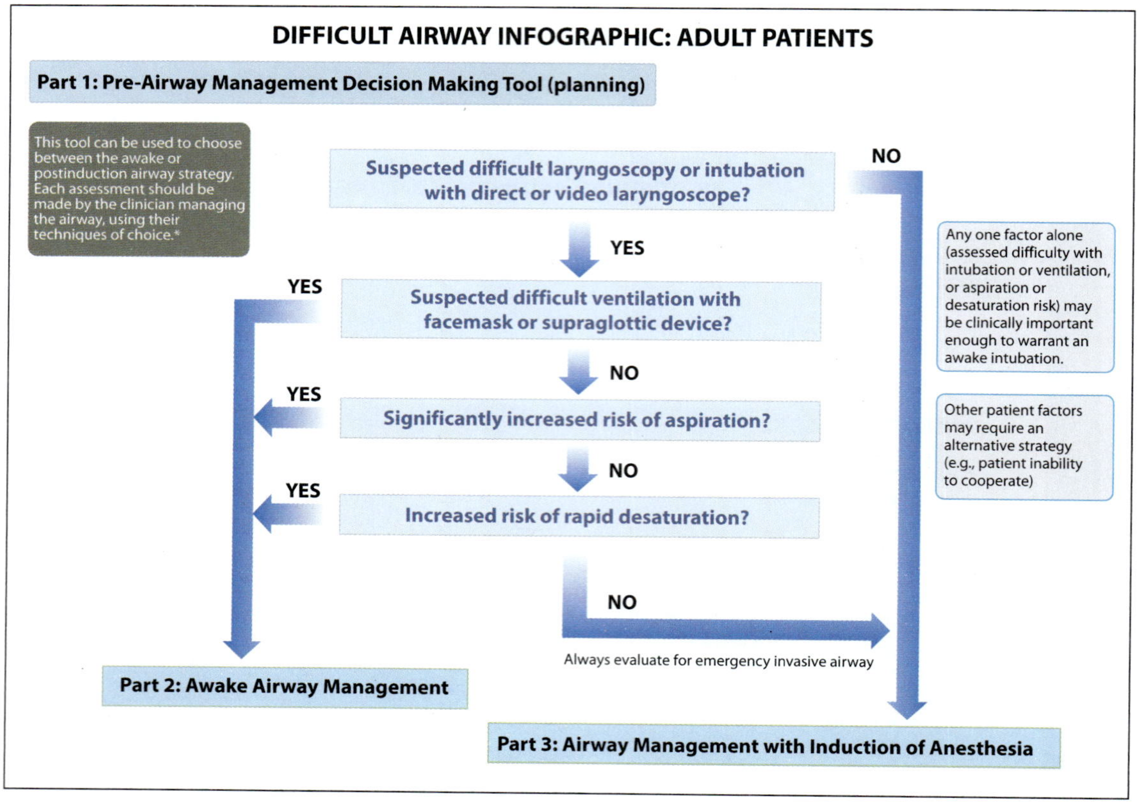

FIGURE 2.3. Difficult airway infographic: adult patients. Part 1: Preairway management decision making tool (planning). For information on superscripts appearing in this infographic, the reader is advised to consult the original publication. (Reproduced with permission from Apfelbaum JL, Hagberg CA, Connis RT, et al. 2022 American Society of Anesthesiologists Practice Guidelines for Management of the Difficult Airway. *Anesthesiology*. 2022;136(1):31-81.)

or Macintosh blade VL, or moving to hyperangulated blade VL. Alternatively, a more experienced practitioner could make a further attempt.

- A maximum of three attempts at tracheal intubation is recommended; if the patient is still not successfully intubated at that point, the algorithm suggests calling for help and pausing to consider *exit strategy* options, provided the patient's oxygen saturation remains nonproblematic. Advice to move to the exit strategy after three failed attempts exists chiefly as a cognitive aid to avoid becoming fixated on multiple futile intubation attempts with a technique already proven to have failed. Exit strategy options include awakening the patient (if feasible and appropriate) or placing an EGD to temporize ventilation and oxygenation pending the arrival of help or additional equipment. An additional intubation attempt can occur as an exit strategy option, although this should be limited to a single attempt by an experienced practitioner, using a technique that is likely to succeed with minimal further trauma to the patient. This will often involve use of a flexible bronchoscope alone or in combination with VL or an EGD unless already tried and failed. A FONA can be considered as an exit strategy option, although this would be rare in the still-oxygenated patient outside the context of an emergency situation.
- The emergency strategy is displayed on the right-hand side of the algorithm and addresses management of the "cannot ventilate, cannot oxygenate (CVCO)" situation. The CVCO term replaces "cannot intubate, cannot ventilate (CICO)" in the publication and is defined as the failure of all three of tracheal intubation, FMV, and EGD use to successfully ventilate the patient (cannot ventilate), resulting in imminent or current patient hypoxemia (cannot oxygenate). The default response becomes emergency FONA.
- While emergency FONA must be undertaken without delay in the CVCO scenario, the 2021 CAFG guidelines suggest concurrent actions while rapidly preparing for emergency FONA. These include ensuring neuromuscular blockade and a single attempt at optimized FMV, EGD placement, and intubation using hyperangulated blade VL, *if not already attempted.*
- A scalpel-bougie-tube technique is the single recommended technique for emergency FONA in adult patients.

The Part 1 CAFG guidelines go on to address difficulty occurring in the obstetrical patient and pediatric patients.

The Part 2 CAFG article[81] addresses how to approach the conscious patient presenting with predictors of difficult airway management. As more airway practitioners become comfortable with intubation techniques such as VL, there is a need to identify when the difficult airway patient can safely be managed after the induction of general anesthesia, or when the airway should be secured in the still conscious, spontaneously breathing patient. Key points and recommendations include the following:

- In the accompanying algorithm (Figure 2.6), to help determine whether airway management of the difficult airway

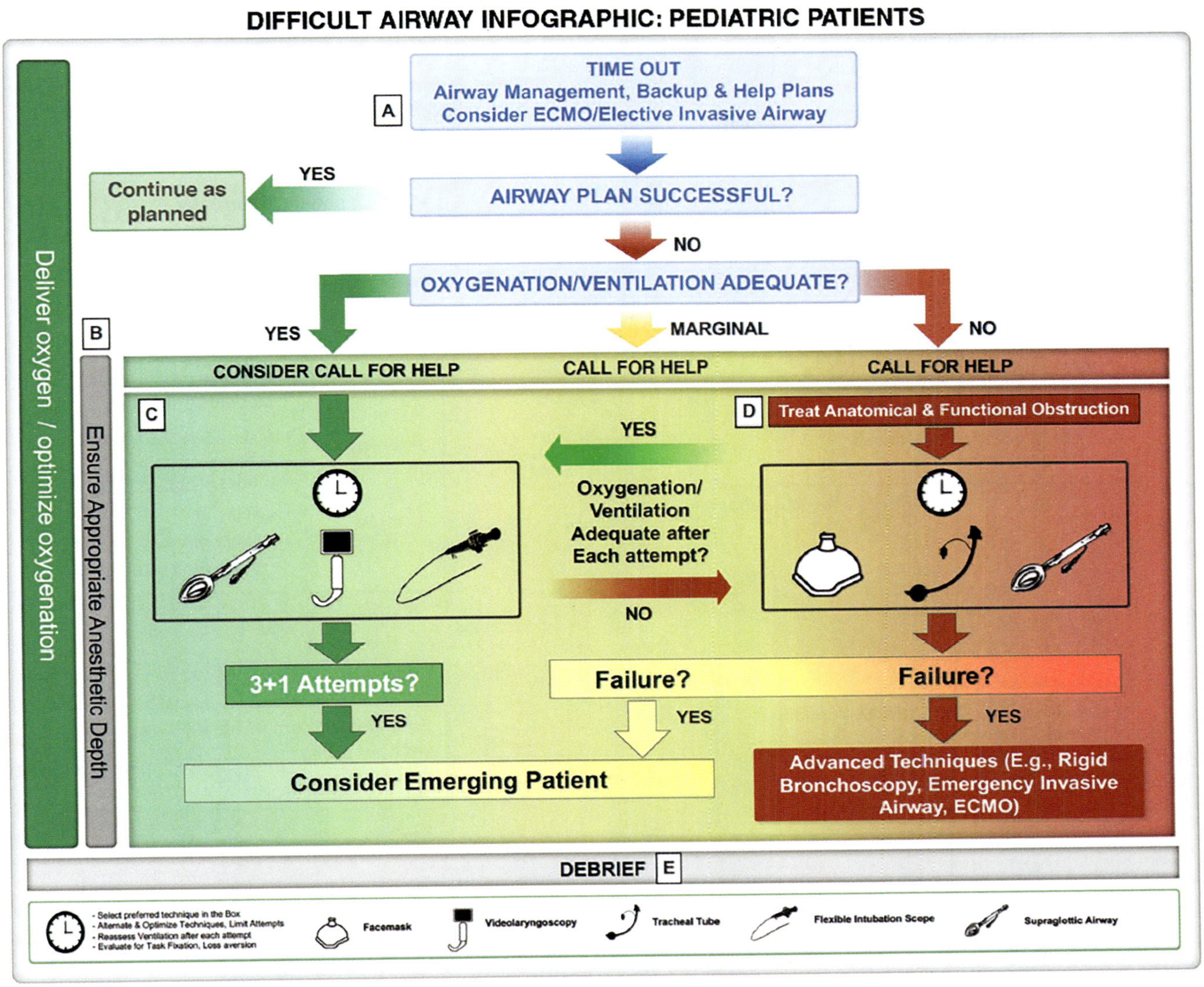

FIGURE 2.4. Difficult airway infographic: pediatric patients. (Reproduced with permission from Apfelbaum JL, Hagberg CA, Connis RT, et al. 2022 American Society of Anesthesiologists Practice Guidelines for Management of the Difficult Airway. *Anesthesiology*. 2022;136(1):31-81.)

patient can safely occur after the induction of general anesthesia, the practitioner is advised to address four key questions. If all four are answered in the negative, then with appropriate preparation, management after the induction of general anesthesia can be considered. Conversely, if the answer is "yes" to any, the practitioner is advised to consider ATI as the safer option.

- The first question is whether ATI is clearly indicated based on profound anatomic anomalies that would render routine techniques such as DL or VL impossible.
- The second is whether difficulty is also predicted with the use of fallback ventilation using one or both of FMV or EGD use.
- The third is whether predicted difficult tracheal intubation coincides with a significant physiologic disturbance such as a high risk of aspiration, predicted apnea intolerance, or hemodynamic instability.
- The fourth asks whether contextual/situational issues exist, such as limited access to additional experienced personnel to help (e.g., due to time of day or a remote location) or availability of necessary equipment to manage the situation.

- Even if one or more of the foregoing questions are answered affirmatively, patient cooperation and time to complete ATI are necessary preconditions. If these are not available yet tracheal intubation must proceed imminently (e.g., for emergency surgery or when tracheal intubation is occurring in the ED or ICU during a resuscitation), the practitioner is advised to perform an airway "double set-up" (i.e., identifying the location of the cricothyroid membrane [CTM], ideally using ultrasound if time permits, together with ensuring that equipment and an individual to perform emergency FONA is present). At that point, management after the induction of general anesthesia may have to proceed, on a "forced-to-act" basis.

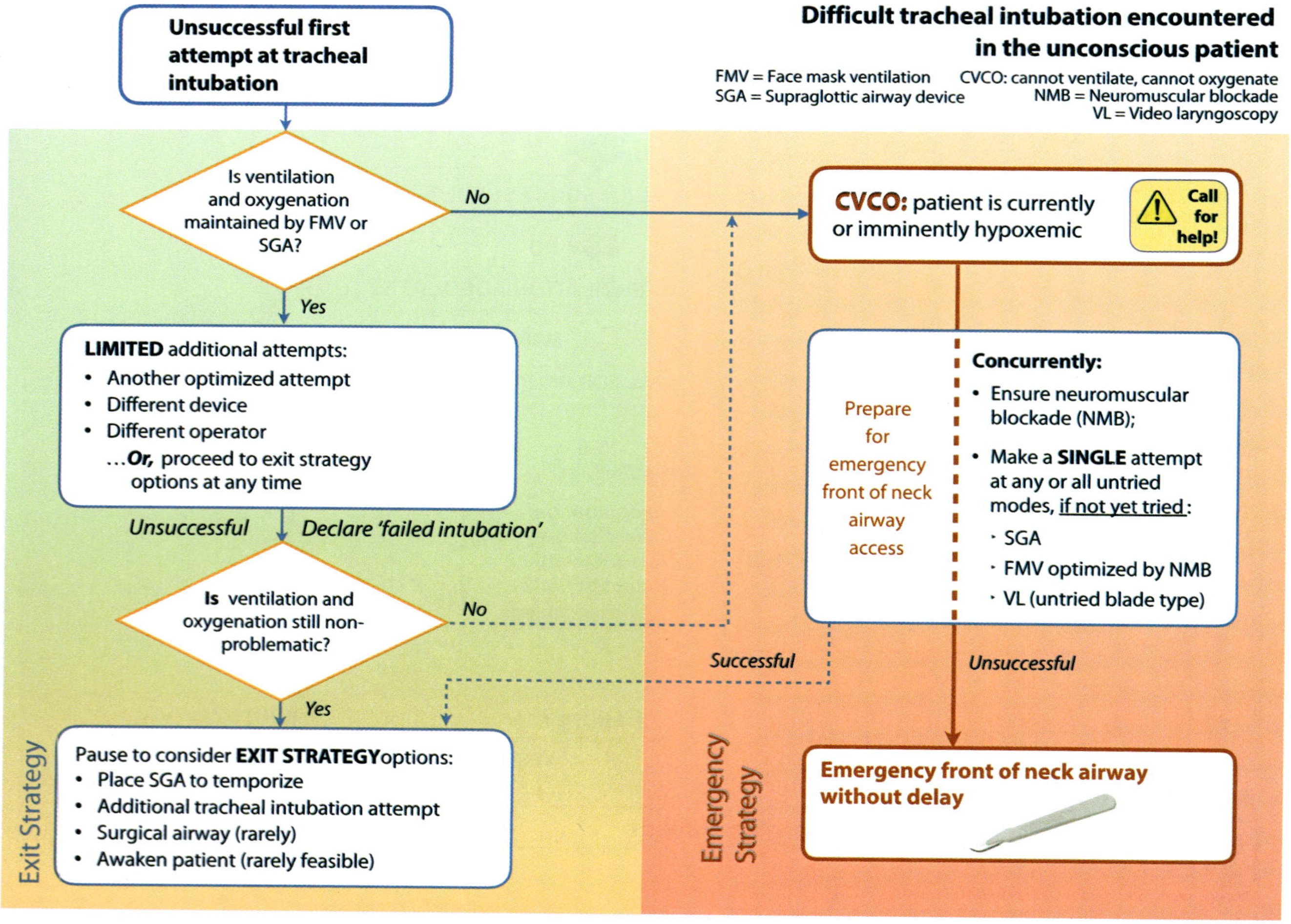

FIGURE 2.5. Canadian Airway Focus Group Algorithm for difficult tracheal intubation encountered in the unconscious patient. (Reproduced with permission from Law JA, Duggan LV, Asselin M, et al. Canadian Airway Focus Group updated consensus-based recommendations for management of the difficult airway: part 1. Difficult airway management encountered in an unconscious patient. *Can J Anaesth.* 2021;68(9):1373-1404.)

A strategy for any encountered difficulty should be predetermined and communicated to all personnel involved.

What Is the Vortex Cognitive Aid?

Developed in Australia by Drs. Nicholas Chrimes and Peter Fritz, the Vortex is a cognitive aid designed to be applied to the unanticipated difficult airway situation.[82] It is meant to be easily recalled by all types of airway practitioners and applicable to all practice environments. Viewed from above, the aid is circular, and is funnel-shaped when viewed from the side (Figures 2.7 and 2.8). The outer green rings represent confirmed alveolar oxygen delivery via a patent airway, while three inner blue segments of the funnel represent the three nonsurgical methods (FMV, EGD ventilation, and tracheal intubation) of establishing a patent airway. The innermost darker blue ring at the bottom of the funnel represents emergency surgical airway. Key points are as follows:

- Difficulty with any of the three nonsurgical airway techniques can be used as an entry point into the aid—for example, tracheal intubation; FMV while awaiting the onset of neuromuscular blockade, or primary use of an EGD in an operating room.
- Failure of an *optimized* attempt at any one technique triggers spiraling forward to the next segment, in any order. For example, failed tracheal intubation may be followed by FMV or EGD ventilation. The narrowing funnel emphasizes that options and time are being used up.
- For each of the three nonsurgical techniques, five optimization maneuvers can be considered, including manipulation of head or neck, use of adjuncts, an alternate size or type of device, suctioning, or addressing pharyngeal muscle tone.
- Recognizing that an optimized performance may not have occurred on the first attempt, a second attempt should be optimized, purposefully trying something different than the previous attempt. A maximum of three attempts can occur with each of the three non-surgical techniques.
- If alveolar oxygen delivery cannot be established with any of the three nonsurgical techniques, the downward spiral into the dark blue zone of the Vortex indicates the need for emergency FONA, regardless of oxygen saturation.

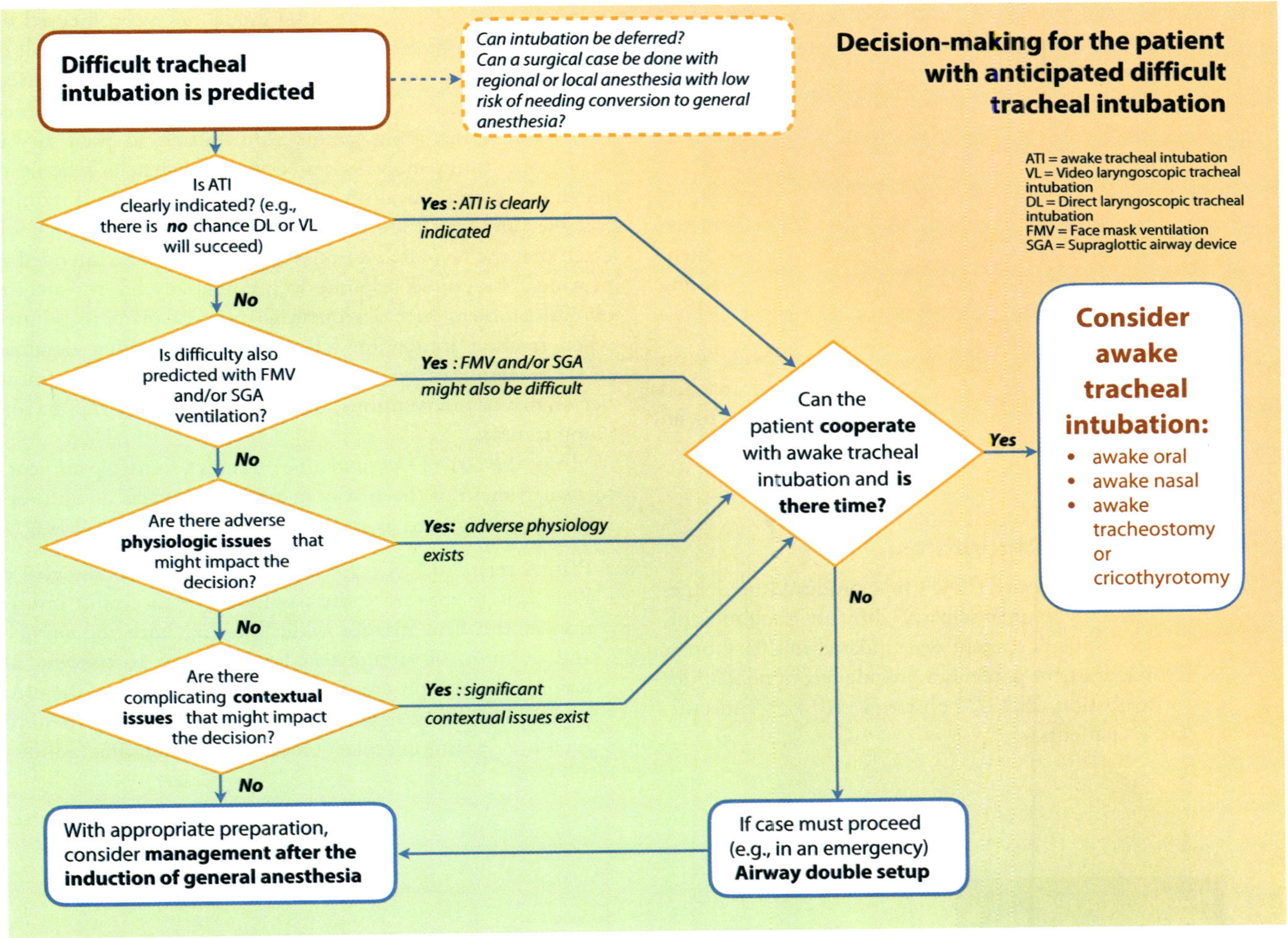

FIGURE 2.6. Canadian Airway Focus Group algorithm for decision-making when difficult tracheal intubation is predicted. (Reproduced with permission from Law JA, Duggan LV, Asselin M, et al. Canadian Airway Focus Group updated consensus-based recommendations for management of the difficult airway: part 2. Planning and implementing safe management of the patient with an anticipated difficult airway. *Can J Anaesth*. 2021;68(9):1405-1436.)

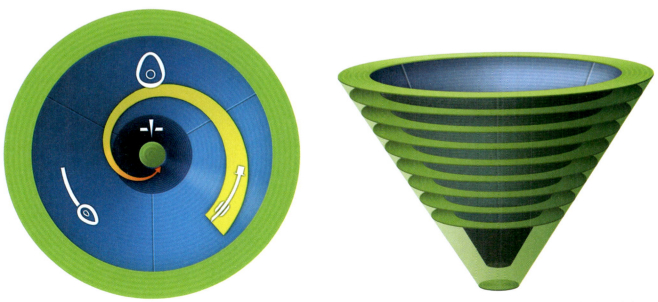

FIGURE 2.7. The Vortex cognitive aid from above. Copyright Nicholas Chrimes 2016. Used with permission.

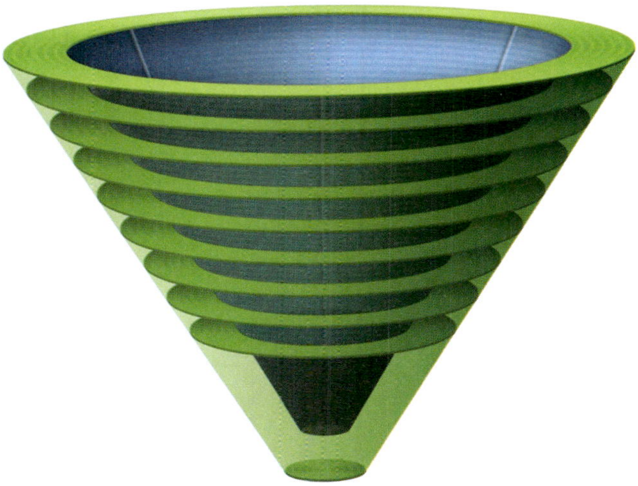

FIGURE 2.8. The Vortex cognitive aid from the side. Copyright Nicholas Chrimes 2016. Used with permission.

- The bottom of the funnel is open to indicate that emergency surgical airway is not necessarily considered definitive, but rather, is simply another way of restoring airway patency and alveolar oxygen delivery.
- Once a patent airway is established and alveolar oxygen delivery is confirmed with any of the nonsurgical or surgical techniques, one moves to the outer horizontal green zone, where time exists to consider options and establish a plan for further management. For example, this might include awakening the patient, calling for additional expertise, or obtaining additional equipment.

The Vortex approach has gained traction worldwide as an effective cognitive aid. More information on the approach is available at www.vortexapproach.com, including links to an e-book and videos on the topic.

What Are the Difficult Airway Society Guidelines and Algorithms?

The Difficult Airway Society (DAS) first produced guidelines for the management of unanticipated difficult tracheal intubation in 2004.[83] This document was updated in 2015; other DAS airway management guidelines provide recommendations for tracheal extubation (2012),[84] obstetric (2015),[85] and critically ill (2018)[86] patients.

The 2015 update to the 2004 guidelines again focused on unanticipated difficult tracheal intubation.[31] In the preamble to the updated guideline, the authors cited a number of influences on the revised recommendations. This included lessons learned from NAP4, including factors contributing to poor airway management outcomes associated with deficiencies relating to judgment, communication, planning, equipment, and training (see the summary findings of NAP4 above). The authors indicated that the revised and updated guidelines were intended to provide a structured response to a potentially life-threatening clinical problem with a sequential series of plans to be used when tracheal intubation failed and, were further designed to place emphasis on oxygenation while limiting the number of airway interventions, in order to minimize trauma and complications.

Thus, the 2015 DAS guideline outlines a four-step approach to management of the airway in anesthetic practice, with each step being designated as a plan (see Figure 2.9), as follows:

- Plan A refers to FMV and tracheal intubation. The goal of Plan A is to maximize the likelihood of successful intubation at the first attempt while limiting both the number and duration of attempts at laryngoscopy, to prevent airway trauma and progression to a CICO situation. The usual recommendations regarding optimal positioning, denitrogenation, neuromuscular block and facilitating adjuncts

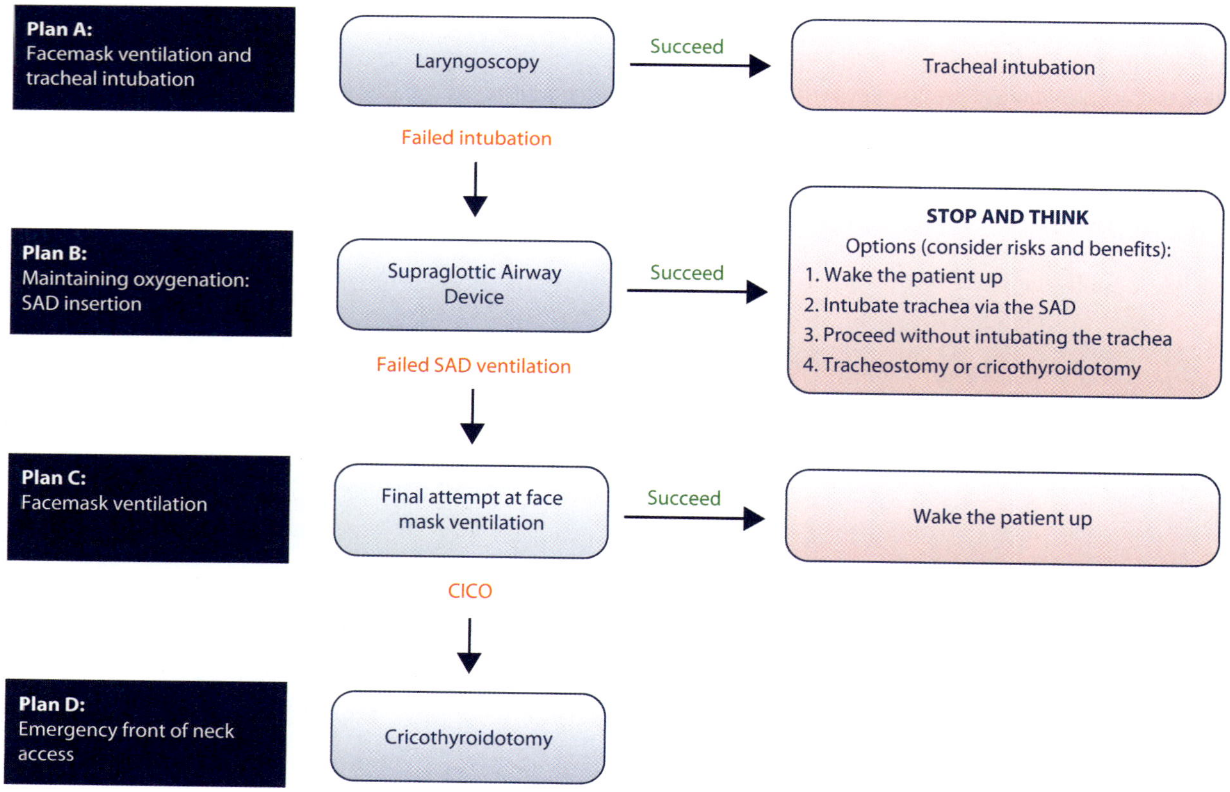

FIGURE 2.9. DAS difficult intubation guidelines—overview algorithm. (Reproduced with permission from Frerk C, Mitchell VS, McNarry AF, et al. Difficult Airway Society 2015 guidelines for management of unanticipated difficult intubation in adults. *Br J Anaesth.* 2015;115(6):827-848.)

(e.g., tracheal introducers or "bougies"), and maneuvers (e.g., laryngeal manipulation) are made. These guidelines recommend a maximum of three attempts at intubation; a fourth attempt by a more experienced colleague is permissible. These attempts include those made with alternative devices such as video laryngoscopes. If intubation has not been achieved after a maximum of four attempts, failed intubation should be declared and Plan B implemented, even if FMV continues to be possible.

- Plan B emphasizes maintaining oxygenation with the insertion of an EGD. The guideline advances the notion that successful placement of an EGD creates the opportunity to "Stop and Think" about whether to wake the patient up, make a further attempt at intubation via the EGD, continue anesthesia without a tracheal tube, or rarely, to proceed directly to a tracheotomy or cricothyrotomy. Patient factors, the urgency of the surgery, and the skill set of the airway practitioner all influence the decision, but the underlying principle is to maintain oxygenation while minimizing the risk of aspiration. There is a discussion about the potential advantages of second-generation EGDs, which are designed to achieve separation of the respiratory and gastrointestinal tracts. If oxygenation through an EGD cannot be achieved after a maximum of three attempts, further attempts should be abandoned and Plan C implemented.
- Plan C relates to final attempts at FMV. If FMV results in adequate oxygenation, the patient should be woken up in all but exceptional circumstances, and this will require a full reversal of neuromuscular block, if feasible. A number of possible scenarios are developing at this stage. During Plans A and B, it will have been determined whether FMV was easy, difficult, or impossible, although the situation may have changed over time as repeated attempts at intubation and EGD placement were made. If it is not possible to maintain oxygenation using a face mask and before critical hypoxemia develops, ensuring full paralysis would offer a final chance of rescuing the airway. The recommendation to ensure full paralysis in a patient who cannot be oxygenated nor intubated will be criticized by some but it can be defended on a number of grounds. If the patient can be neither oxygenated nor intubated using the skill sets and technology available, the situation has become desperate with a good outcome being far from assured. By abolishing laryngeal reflexes, increasing chest wall compliance and facilitating FMV, ensuring full paralysis may permit successful Plan C FMV. As well, if ventilation cannot be established despite the optimized conditions, the FONA becomes necessary and it will be facilitated with paralysis. The decision to not paralyze could only be defended if there was clear evidence of patient recovery and self-correction of a desperate situation, which is unlikely if significant hypoxemia has already developed.
- Plan D—emergency FONA access—is established if Plan C has failed to establish effective ventilation with oxygenation. Likely based on the observations in NAP4 that needle techniques applied by anesthesia practitioners in desperate clinical scenarios were often unsuccessful, the DAS guideline emphasizes scalpel cricothyrotomy with placement of a wide-bore cuffed tube through the CTM, to facilitate normal minute ventilation with a standard breathing system. The authors recommend that all anesthesia practitioners should be trained to perform a FONA and that training should be repeated at regular intervals to ensure skill retention. Although it is possible that the adoption of scalpel cricothyrotomy will reverse the poor outcomes evident in NAP4 arising out of the use of needle cricothyrotomy, it is likely that outcomes will not improve if the scalpel technique continues to be applied late during events, by desperate practitioners who are neither trained nor practiced in the technique.

How Do the 2018 DAS ICU Guidelines Differ from the Foregoing 2015 Publication?

Addressing tracheal intubation of the critically ill patient, the 2018 DAS publication[86] departs somewhat from the sequential Plan A to D approach espoused in the 2015 guidelines on unanticipated tracheal intubation. In the 2018 guidelines, there is additional emphasis in the Plan A recommendations on preparation before proceeding with tracheal intubation, including optimized head-up positioning, pre- and per- (apneic) oxygenation, and availability of VL. The use of a sedative-hypnotic with neuromuscular blockade is recommended to facilitate tracheal intubation in most cases. Failure of a first attempt should trigger a call for help and consideration of VL for further attempts, if not already in use. Failed tracheal intubation should be declared after no more than three attempts; at that point the emphasis shifts to "airway rescue," representing the combination of the 2015 guidelines' sequential Plans B and C into "Plan B/C" efforts at rescue oxygenation using an EGD, interspersed with FMV if needed between attempts (Figure 2.10). Reflecting and acknowledging the Vortex cognitive aid, failure of any technique should be declared if unsuccessful after a maximum of three attempts. Successful Plan B/C oxygenation provides the opportunity to consider "Stop and Think" options, including awakening the patient, awaiting the arrival of additional expertise, a single attempt at flexible endoscopic intubation via the EGD, or proceeding with FONA. Regardless of the patient's oxygenation status, failure of successful patient ventilation after a maximum of three attempts at all three methods of ventilation (tracheal intubation, EGD, and FMV) mandates proceeding with FONA. A scalpel-bougie-tube cricothyrotomy technique is espoused for emergency FONA in this situation.

Both the 2015 and 2018 DAS guidelines emphasize the importance of human factors in dedicated sections, as well as throughout the articles' narrative.[85,86]

Discuss the Project for Universal Management of Airways (PUMA)

Recognizing that the existence of comprehensive airway guidelines from multiple different countries might represent substantial duplication of effort at best or be confusing to the average practitioner at worst, an international group of airway experts is working to arrive at universal airway management principles.[87,88] The PUMA group is planning to publish this work in a series of articles. Their website is www.universalairway.org.

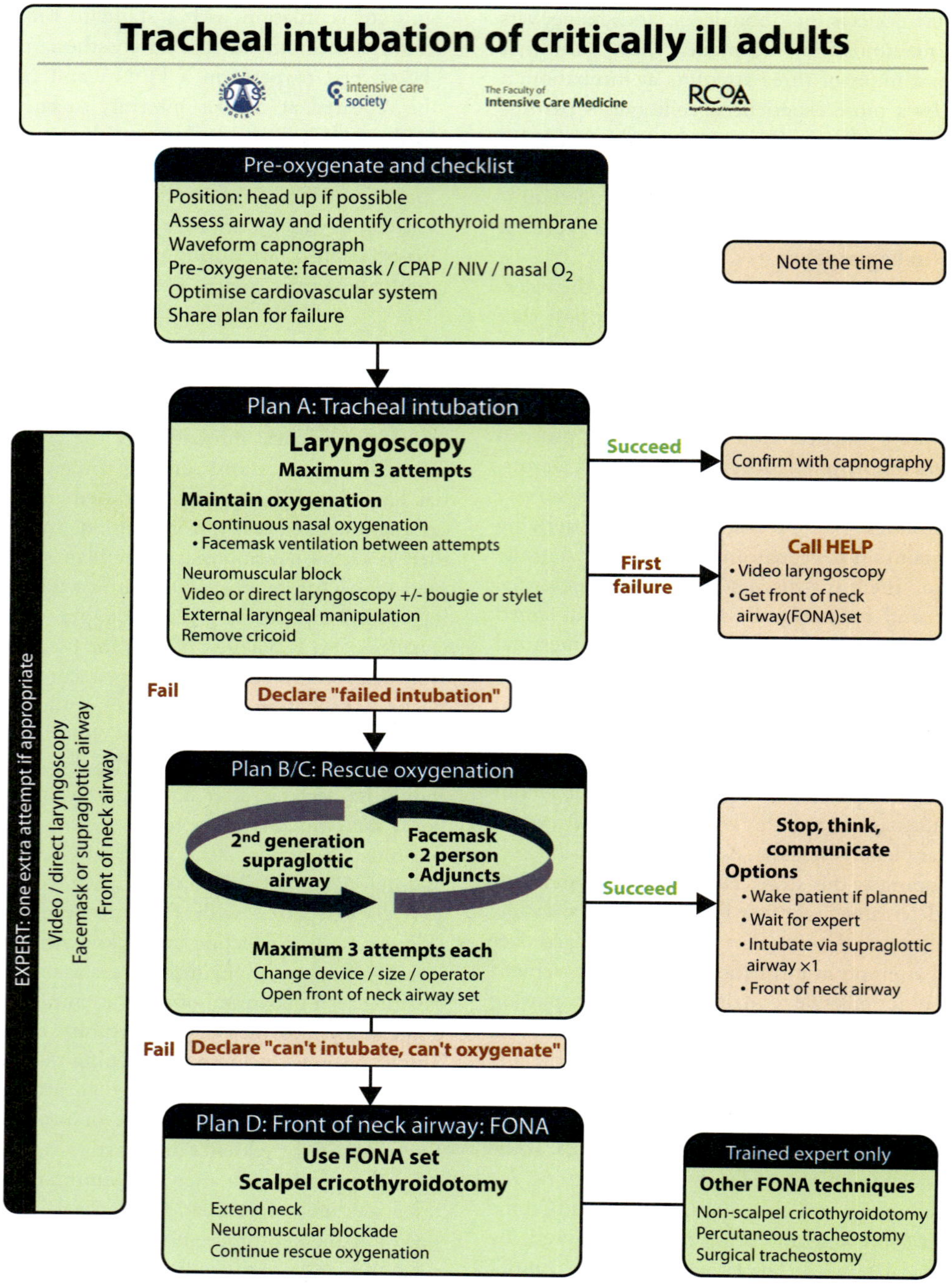

FIGURE 2.10. DAS Tracheal Intubation of Critically Ill Adults Algorithm. For information on superscripts appearing in this algorithm, the reader is advised to consult the original publication. (Reproduced with permission from Higgs A, McGrath BA, Goddard C, et al. Guidelines for the management of tracheal intubation in critically ill adults. *Br J Anaesth*. 2018;120(2):323-352.)

THE DIFFICULT AIRWAY COURSE AIRWAY ALGORITHMS

Why Were These Algorithms Developed?

The airway management algorithms in the next sections are taken from The Difficult Airway Course teachings over the years. They have been crafted in a similar fashion to published national algorithms in that they are substantially based on expert opinion, taking into account the best evidence available. They have been modified over time and adhere to the design elements of effective algorithms articulated above and the content of various national airway guidelines. They describe a logical progression of *thinking* and *doing* when faced with a variety of scenarios, including the *crash* situation, the failed airway, predicted difficult airway management, and extubation of the difficult airway patient. Importantly, the algorithms presented are not meant to be memorized and used as a recipe. Rather, they represent a way of rapidly thinking through difficult clinical situations, helping to make crucial decisions and act effectively. These algorithms appear in Figures 2.11 to 2.15. Please refer to these figures while reading the following text descriptions.

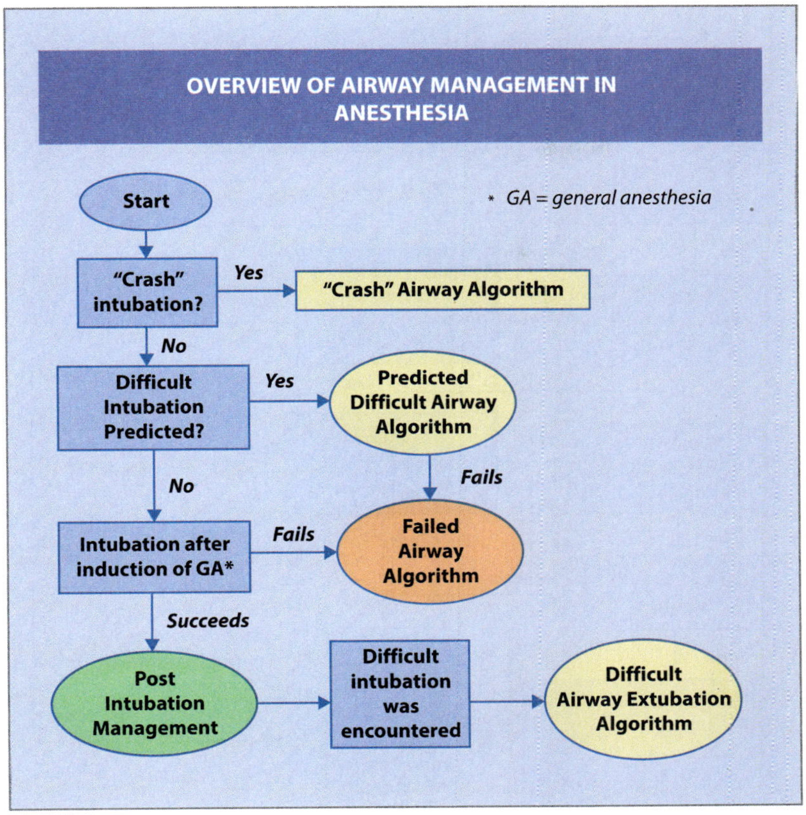

FIGURE 2.11. Airway Management Overview Algorithm. (Reproduced with permission from Airway Management Education Centre (theairwaysite.com) and The Difficult Airway Course : Anesthesia™.)

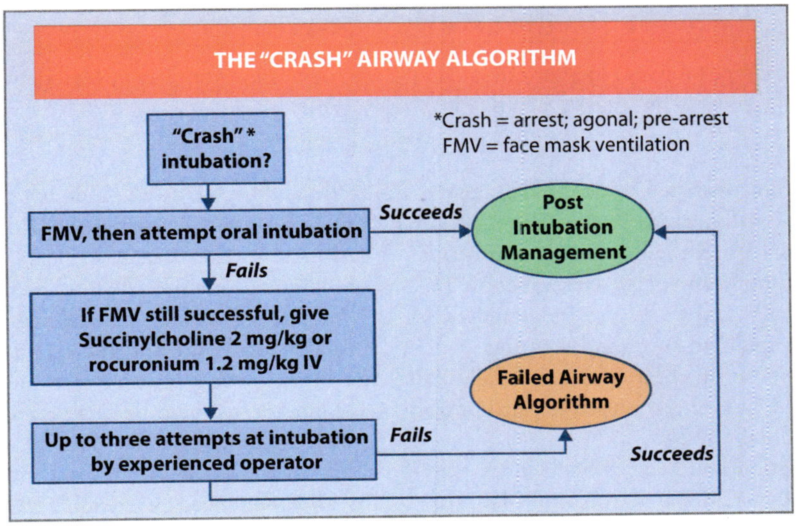

FIGURE 2.12. The Crash Airway Algorithm. (Reproduced with permission from Airway Management Education Centre (theairwaysite.com) and The Difficult Airway Course: Anesthesia™.)

The Overview Algorithm (Figure 2.11)

The Overview Algorithm presents the way most practitioners approach airway management. Essential features are as follows:

- In the event the patient is arrested or near death, a "crash" tracheal intubation is often indicated, and the Crash Airway Algorithm (Figure 2.12) is employed.
- If a "crash" situation does not exist, but airway management is anticipated to be potentially difficult (e.g., based on a nonreassuring airway examination [Table 2.2], adverse patient physiology, or an awkward environment), ATI may be indicated, per the Predicted Difficult Airway Algorithm (Figure 2.13). Chapter 1 presents strategies for assessing the airway for difficulty.

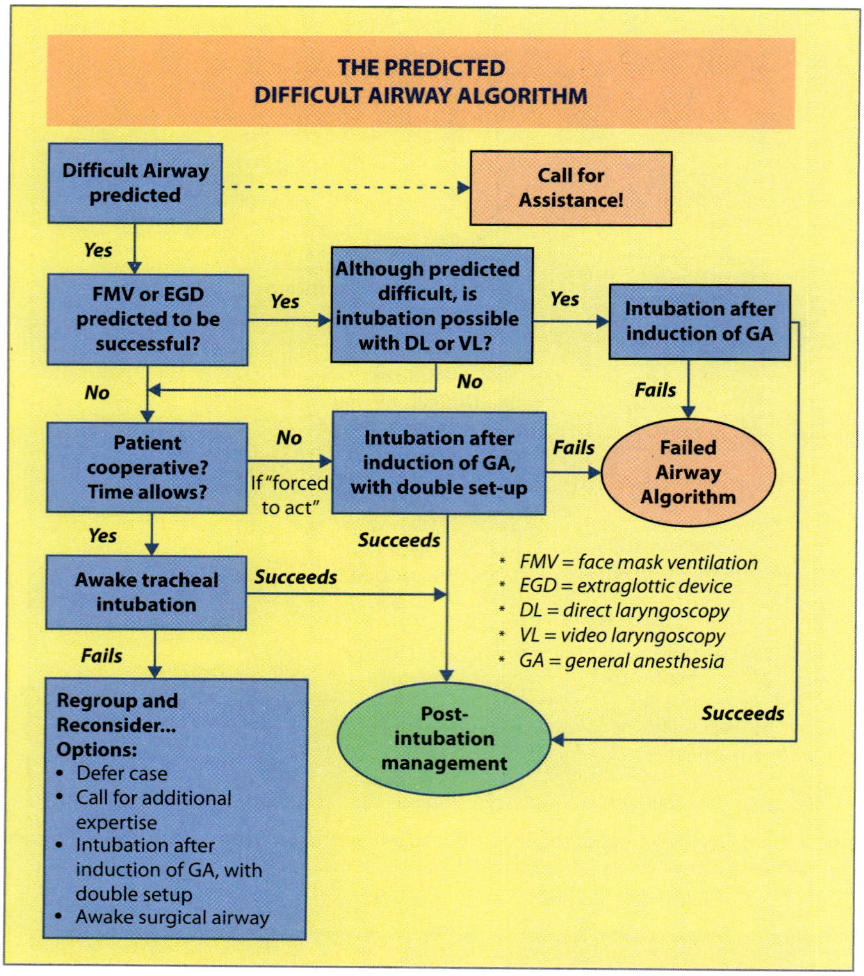

FIGURE 2.13. The Predicted Difficult Airway Algorithm. (Reproduced with permission from Airway Management Education Centre (theairwaysite.com) and The Difficult Airway Course : Anesthesia™.)

- If tracheal intubation is not predicted to be difficult, airway management can generally safely proceed after the induction of general anesthesia (e.g., using rapid-sequence intubation [RSI]). By optimizing conditions for all laryngoscopy, tracheal intubation, and FMV and EGD use, this method is most likely to facilitate rapid and successful securing of the airway.[89] Should attempts at tracheal intubation fail, the Failed Airway Algorithm (Figure 2.14) is used to gain control of the airway rapidly and definitively.
- Finally, if tracheal intubation had been difficult, once extubation is indicated, a Difficult Airway Extubation Algorithm (Figure 2.15) forms the basis of a safe extubation plan.

The Crash Airway Algorithm (Figure 2.12)

Entry into the Crash Airway Algorithm is with an unconscious, unresponsive patient requiring immediate airway management. "Unresponsive" in this context refers to a "newly or nearly dead" patient who is unlikely to respond adversely to oral laryngoscopy (i.e., arrested, agonal or prearrest situations). This algorithm is most likely to apply in out-of-operating room environments. The first step is to immediately perform FMV, quickly followed by oral tracheal intubation facilitated by DL or VL. In many cases, this can proceed without pharmacologic assistance, although this might be inappropriate in the patient with an isolated head injury. If the oral intubation is successful, then the practitioner proceeds with postintubation management. If oral intubation is not initially successful but FMV remains possible, neuromuscular blockade (e.g., succinylcholine 2 $mg{\cdot}kg^{-1}$ or rocuronium 1.2 $mg{\cdot}kg^{-1}$) should be established if not yet done, and additional attempts made at tracheal intubation, with interposed FMV. If the patient is still not intubated after three attempts by an experienced practitioner, the Failed Airway Algorithm (Figure 2.14) is engaged.

The Predicted Difficult Airway Algorithm (Figure 2.13)

This algorithm is specifically designed to guide airway management when difficulty is predicted. Decisions are binary by design. With predicted difficulty, the algorithm seeks to help clarify for the practitioner when tracheal intubation can safely proceed after the induction of general anesthesia, or when ATI is likely to be the safer approach. Algorithm features are as follows:

- Difficulty is predicted chiefly by bedside airway evaluation. The LEMON and CRANE mnemonics (see Chapter 1) can

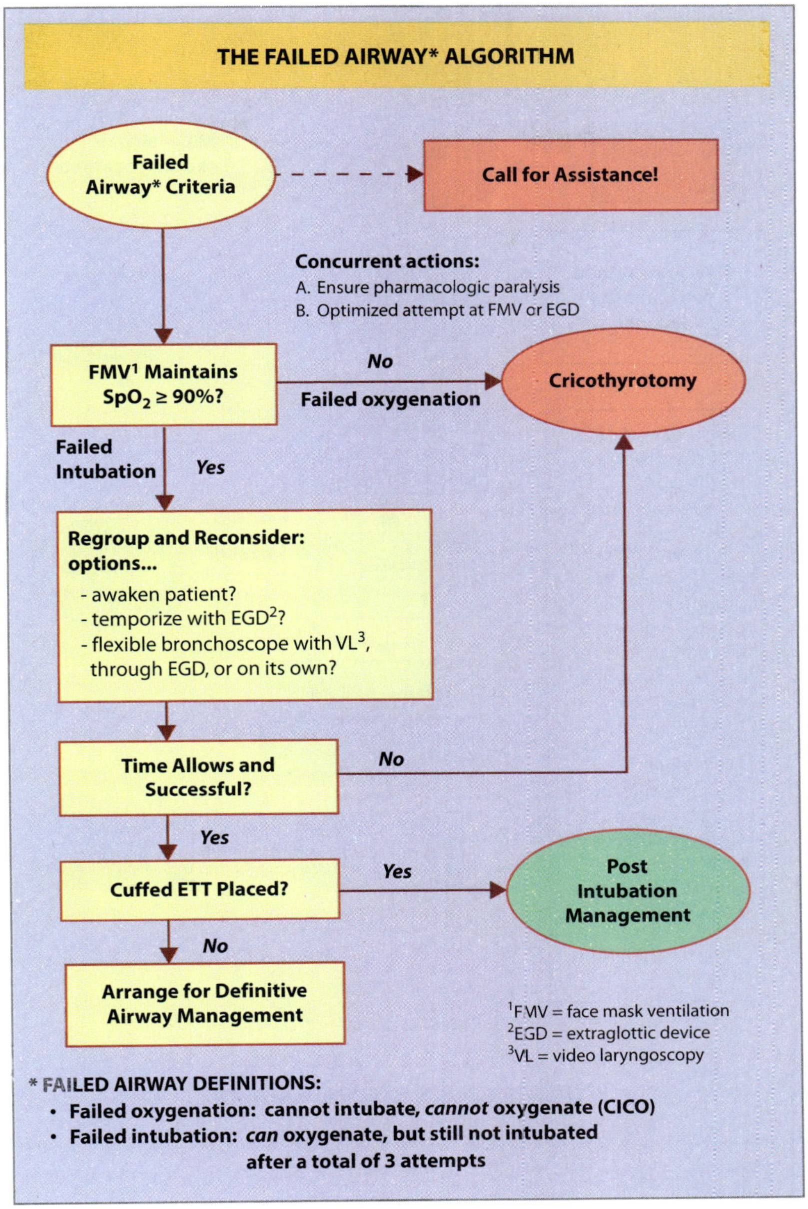

FIGURE 2.14. Failed Airway Algorithm. (Reproduced with permission from Airway Management Education Centre (theairwaysite.com) and The Difficult Airway Course: Anesthesia™.)

be used to help the practitioner recall anatomic predictors of difficult DL and VL, respectively. Additional assessment may sometimes be warranted using awake nasal flexible bronchoscopy[90] or awake oral VL[91] when internal upper airway anatomy might be distorted by obstructing pathology.

- Especially if difficulty is predicted with laryngoscopy and intubation, the practitioner should also evaluate the patient for difficulty with fallback ventilation techniques: FMV (MOANS mnemonic); EGD use (RODS mnemonic), and emergency surgical airway (SHORT mnemonic). See Chapter 1 for further information on these predictors of difficulty.
- When laryngoscopy/intubation is predicted to be difficult but fallback FMV and/or EGD use is predicted to be successful, further assessing the situation is warranted to help determine the safest approach. This includes evaluating whether DL or VL might still succeed even though predicted to be potentially difficult, and whether other factors such as significant physiologic issues (e.g., significant aspiration risk or apnea intolerance) or situational issues (e.g., lack of access to additional expertise for help) exist. A favorable response to this secondary assessment of difficulty might indicate that tracheal intubation can still safely proceed after the induction of general anesthesia.
- Even if ATI is predicted to be the optimal approach, an assessment must first occur of whether time and patient cooperation will allow for an awake approach. If not, then with an "airway double set-up" (preidentification of the location of the CTM and physical presence of equipment

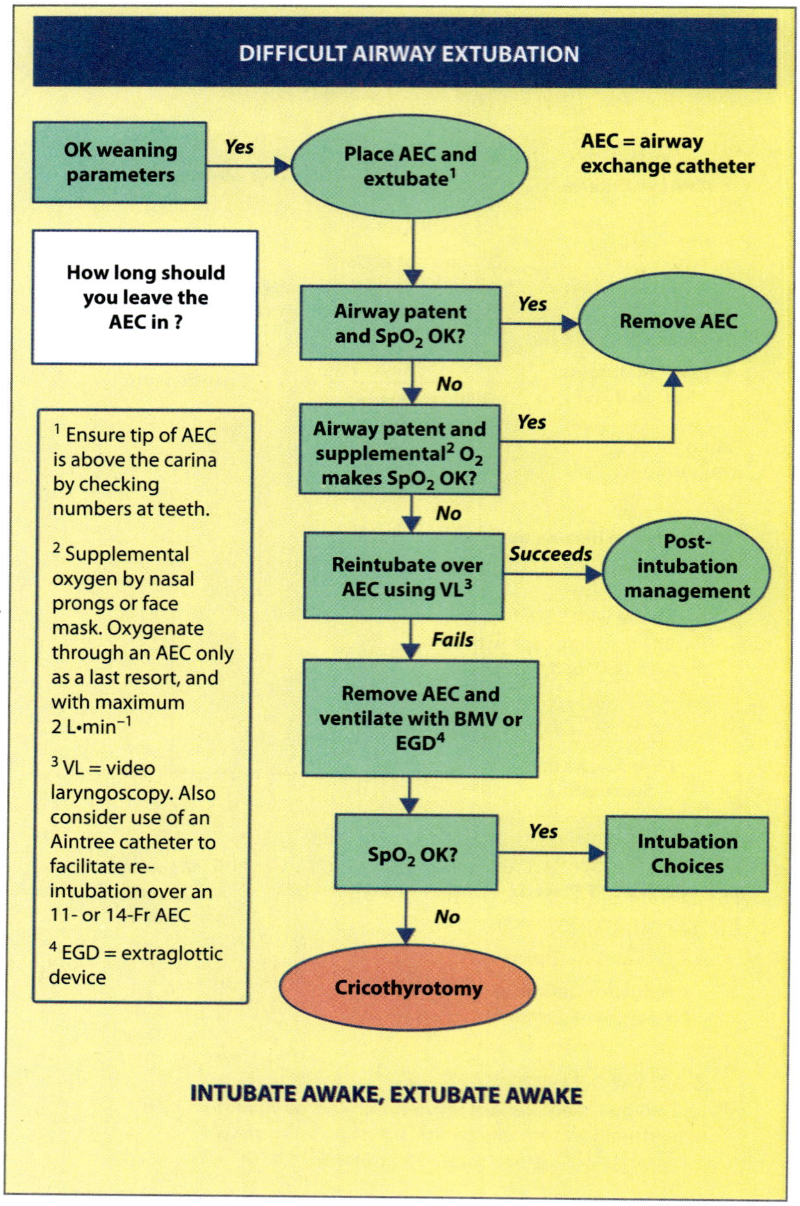

FIGURE 2.15. Difficult Airway Extubation Algorithm. (Reproduced with permission from Airway Management Education Centre (theairwaysite.com) and The Difficult Airway Course: Anesthesia™.)

and an individual to perform emergency FONA), tracheal intubation may need to occur after the induction of general anesthesia on a "forced to act" basis. If tracheal intubation fails in this scenario, the Failed Airway Algorithm is entered.

- When indicated, ATI is most often successful,[92–94] but if it fails, the practitioner is advised to "regroup and reconsider" by considering several options including calling for additional expertise, deferring a surgical case if elective, or proceeding with management after the induction of general anesthesia with an airway "double set-up."

The Failed Airway Algorithm (Figure 2.14)

Early recognition of a failed airway situation is essential to avoiding airway management-related morbidity. For the purposes of this discussion, the term "failed airway" encompasses two related situations, each with different management implications:

A. Tracheal intubation is unsuccessful after a maximum of three attempts, but patient ventilation and oxygenation remain nonproblematic, e.g., using interposed FMV or an EGD (i.e., cannot intubate but CAN oxygenate).
B. Tracheal intubation has failed after one or more attempt(s), and patient ventilation and oxygenation cannot be successfully maintained by fallback use of FMV or EGD ventilation (i.e., cannot intubate, CANNOT oxygenate [CICO]).

Failed Tracheal Intubation, but CAN Oxygenate. *Difficulty* encountered with tracheal intubation should be met with a standard response of transitioning between devices (e.g., from DL to hyperangulated VL), use of adjuncts, or changing to

TABLE 2.2. Components of the Preoperative Airway Physical Examination

Airway Exam Component	Nonreassuring Finding
Length or upper incisors	Relatively long
Relation of maxillary and mandibular incisors during normal jaw closure	Prominent overbite (maxillary incisors anterior)
Relation of incisors during protrusion of mandible	Overbite remains present
Interincisor distance	Less than 3.0 cm
Visibility of uvula (Mallampati Class)	Not visible with tongue protruded, patient sitting (>II)
Shape of palate	High-arched or narrow
Compliance of mandibular space	Stiff and indurated
Thyromental distance	Less than three fingerbreadths (5.0 cm)
Length of neck	Short
Thickness of neck	Thick
Range of motion of head on neck	Limited

Reproduced with permission from American Society of Anesthesiologists Task Force on Management of the Difficult Airway. Practice guidelines for management of the difficult airway: an updated report by the American Society of Anesthesiologists Task Force on Management of the Difficult Airway. *Anesthesiology*. 2003;98(5):1269-1277.

a more experienced practitioner, rather than simply repeating a technique already proven to be unsuccessful. FMV should occur between attempts. Patient morbidity increases with each successive attempt at tracheal intubation, so that a *failed* tracheal intubation situation should be recognized and declared after no more than three unsuccessful attempts. At that point, provided patient ventilation and oxygenation remain adequate (e.g., a waveform capnographic trace is present and SpO_2 is ≥90% with the use of FMV), proceeding vertically down the Failed Airway Algorithm, the practitioner is advised to "regroup and reconsider," with management options as follows:

- *Awakening the patient* may be an option, when feasible. Most often, this will be appropriate chiefly in the elective surgical environment. The state of neuromuscular blockade and sedative agents must be considered and managed, and ventilation supported until the patient is able to maintain gas exchange and airway patency unassisted.
- *An EGD may be placed (if not already attempted).* This can be used to temporize pending the arrival of additional expertise or equipment, or to support the airway until the patient awakens, if this is chosen as an option. Proceeding with surgery using the EGD when the original plan was for tracheal intubation is hazardous and should only occur if the benefit is considered to exceed the risk.
- *A further attempt at tracheal intubation* can be made. However, after the multiple preceding unsuccessful attempts at tracheal intubation, this should be performed by an experienced practitioner, using a technique likely to address why earlier attempts had failed. This might include the use of a flexible bronchoscope, often used in combination with VL or through a compatible EGD.
- If none of the foregoing options have been successful, or when the urgency of other resuscitation priorities precludes their performance in an emergency, FONA might rarely be indicated, despite the still-oxygenated status of the patient.

Failed Tracheal Intubation, CANNOT Ventilate/Oxygenate.

The CICO (failed oxygenation) situation is a clinical emergency of sufficient magnitude that it will lead to neurologic compromise or death if not recognized and rectified rapidly. Decisive action is essential in selecting a technique most likely to lead to a secure airway (i.e., an emergency FONA) in such a situation. In addition:

- The CICO situation can and should be declared as soon as one or more attempts at tracheal intubation have failed when fallback attempts at FMV or EGD ventilation are also unsuccessful. Thus, a CICO situation has occurred when all three modes of ventilation (tracheal intubation, FMV, and EGD ventilation) have been attempted and failed, even after only a single optimized attempt at any one technique.
- When recognized, the CICO situation should be verbally declared to all present, and the default maneuver becomes emergency FONA—most often cricothyrotomy in the adult patient. Even when technically successful, cricothyrotomy has sometimes been done too late to avoid brain damage or death, underscoring the need for early identification of this situation.
- Once the CICO situation is recognized and concurrent with preparations to proceed with cricothyrotomy, pharmacologic paralysis should be established or confirmed, and final attempts at optimized FMV or EGD ventilation can occur.

The Difficult Airway Extubation Algorithm (Figure 2.15)

The Difficult Airway Extubation Algorithm should be employed when reintubation, if needed, might be difficult or impossible. This could arise because the initial tracheal intubation was difficult or, even if originally easy to intubate, reintubation might now be difficult, e.g., due to intervening surgery or suspected development of airway edema. Careful planning for extubation in these cases is imperative.[34,63,81,84] Extubation over an airway exchange catheter is at the core of the algorithm. Properly positioned above the carina, an 11- or 14 French AEC is usually well-tolerated in the awake patient[95] and can provide a guide for early reintubation, if required. Nevertheless, despite the use of the AEC during extubation of the difficult airway patient, it must be emphasized that standard extubation criteria must still be met, including adequate gas exchange and tidal volumes, with a regular pattern of respiration and a level of consciousness sufficient to protect and maintain the airway unassisted. In addition:

- After extubation, if the airway remains patent and patient ventilation and oxygenation are unchallenged, the AEC can be removed once there is little risk of deterioration of the patient's status.
- If the patient requires supplemental oxygen while the AEC is in situ, this should be supplied by standard means, rather than via the AEC. To help avoid the risk of barotrauma, oxygen insufflation should only occur through an AEC in extenuating circumstances, limited to a maximum flow of 2 $L{\cdot}min^{-1}$.[96]
- If tracheal reintubation is required over an AEC, especially if management occurs after the induction of general anesthesia, concomitant VL will facilitate tube passage over the AEC.[97]
- If tracheal reintubation over the AEC fails and fallback FMV or EGD ventilation is required, the AEC should be removed to facilitate those actions. Thereafter, further management should occur according to the previously described principles.

SUMMARY

The failure to adequately manage the airway is a major contributor to poor outcomes in anesthesia, emergency medicine, EMS, and critical care. Adverse respiratory events constitute a significant source of injury in the ASA Closed Claims Project. The single most important factor leading to a failed airway is failure to predict the difficult airway.

Airway management is always stress provoking. Crucial decisions must be made in a timely manner, and the airway practitioner is expected to possess expertise in a variety of primary and rescue maneuvers.

Well-designed algorithms based on the best available evidence are intended to improve the outcome of difficult and failed airway emergencies. Although many airway management guidelines exist with their corresponding algorithms, most espouse very similar management principles. Of these, it is incumbent on the airway practitioner to identify which algorithm to employ, particularly when a *difficult* airway has progressed to a *failed* airway.

SELF-EVALUATION QUESTIONS

2.1 All of the following are features of well-designed, clinically useful algorithms **EXCEPT**:

A. They are designed by reputable organizations.

B. They have clear entry and exit points.

C. Decision points are binary.

D. They are easily remembered in crisis.

E. They are easy to represent graphically.

2.2 All of the following are true of the ASA Difficult Airway Algorithm **EXCEPT**:

A. It is evidence-based.

B. It has likely helped to reduce the rate of airway management failure in anesthesia practice.

C. It is meant to represent the "standard of care" in medicolegal proceedings.

D. It has two sections: one for the difficult airway and one for the failed airway.

E. The use of an extraglottic airway is a discrete step.

2.3 Which of the following is **TRUE** regarding airway guidelines and their accompanying algorithms?

A. If a country has published airway guidelines, the practitioner is legally required to adhere to the recommended actions contained therein.

B. The failure to adhere to the step-wise progression recommended in most national guidelines is responsible for many poor airway-related outcomes.

C. National practice algorithms should be reproduced and displayed for easy reference in all airway management locations.

D. Airway algorithms in national guidelines should be committed to memory for use when difficulty is encountered.

E. Airway guidelines are only applicable to the practice environment of the organization that published them.

REFERENCES

1. Rose DK, Cohen MM. The airway: problems and predictions in 18,500 patients. *Can J Anaesth*. 1994;41(5 Pt 1):372-383.
2. Langeron O, Masso E, Huraux C, et al. Prediction of difficult mask ventilation. *Anesthesiology*. 2000;92(5):1229-1236.
3. Kheterpal S, Han R, Tremper KK, et al. Incidence and predictors of difficult and impossible mask ventilation. *Anesthesiology*. 2006;105(5):885-891. doi:00000542-200611000-00007 [pii].
4. Kheterpal S, Martin L, Shanks AM, Tremper KK. Prediction and outcomes of impossible mask ventilation: a review of 50,000 anesthetics. *Anesthesiology*. 2009;110(4):891-897. doi:10.1097/ALN.0b013e31819b5b87.
5. Han R, Tremper KK, Kheterpal S, O'Reilly M. Grading scale for mask ventilation. *Anesthesiology*. 2004;101(1):267. doi:10.1097/00000542-200407000-00059.
6. Kheterpal S, Healy D, Aziz MF, et al. Incidence, predictors, and outcome of difficult mask ventilation combined with difficult laryngoscopy: a report from the multicenter perioperative outcomes group. *Anesthesiology*. 2013;119(6):1360-1369. doi:10.1097/ALN.0000435832.39353.20.
7. Petito SP, Russell WJ. The prevention of gastric inflation--a neglected benefit of cricoid pressure. *Anaesth Intensive Care*. 1988;16(2):139-143.
8. Mallampati SR. Clinical sign to predict difficult tracheal intubation (hypothesis). *Can Anaesth Soc J*. 1983;30(3 Pt 1):316-317.
9. Mallampati SR, Gatt SP, Gugino LD, et al. A clinical sign to predict difficult tracheal intubation: a prospective study. *Can Anaesth Soc J*. 1985;32(4):429-434.
10. Detsky ME, Jivraj N, Adhikari NK, et al. Will this patient be difficult to intubate? The Rational Clinical Examination systematic review. *JAMA*. 2019;321(5):493-503. doi:10.1001/jama.2018.21413.
11. Roth D, Pace NL, Lee A, et al. Bedside tests for predicting difficult airways: an abridged Cochrane diagnostic test accuracy systematic review. *Anaesthesia*. 2019;74(7):915-928. doi:10.1111/anae.14608.

12. Samsoon GL, Young JR. Difficult tracheal intubation: a retrospective study. *Anaesthesia*. 1987;42(5):487-490.
13. Shiga T, Wajima Z, Inoue T, Sakamoto A. Predicting difficult intubation in apparently normal patients: a meta-analysis of bedside screening test performance. *Anesthesiology*. 2005;103(2):429-437. doi:00000542-200508000-00027 [pii].
14. Karkouti K, Rose DK, Wigglesworth D, Cohen MM. Predicting difficult intubation: a multivariable analysis. *Can J Anaesth*. 2000;47(8):730-739.
15. Karkouti K, Rose K, Cohen M, Wigglesworth D. Models for difficult laryngoscopy. *Can J Anaesth*. 2000;47(1):94-95.
16. Yentis SM. Predicting difficult intubation—worthwhile exercise or pointless ritual? *Anaesthesia*. 2002;57(2):105-109. doi:2515 [pii]
17. Huitink JM, Bouwman RA. The myth of the difficult airway: airway management revisited. *Anaesthesia*. 2015;70(3):244-249. doi:10.1111/anae.12989.
18. Yentis SM. Predicting trouble in airway management. *Anesthesiology*. 2006;105(5):871-872. doi:00000542-200611000-00003 [pii].
19. Thiboutot F, Nicole PC, Trepanier CA, Turgeon AF, Lessard MR. Effect of manual in-line stabilization of the cervical spine in adults on the rate of difficult orotracheal intubation by direct laryngoscopy: a randomized controlled trial. *Can J Anaesth*. 2009;56(6):412-418. doi:10.1007/s12630-009-9089-7.
20. Rice MJ, Mancuso AA, Gibbs C, Morey TE, Gravenstein N, Deitte LA. Cricoid pressure results in compression of the postcricoid hypopharynx: the esophageal position is irrelevant. *Anesth Analg*. 2009;109(5):1546-1552. doi:109/5/1546 [pii]10.1213/ane.0b013e3181b05404.
21. Sellick BA. Cricoid pressure to control regurgitation of stomach contents during induction of anaesthesia. *Lancet*. 1961;2(7199):404-406. doi:10.1016/s0140-6736(61)92485-0.
22. Clark RK, Trethewy CE. Assessment of cricoid pressure application by emergency department staff. *Emerg Med Australas*. 2005;17(4):376-381. doi:10.1111/j.1742-6723.2005.00760.x.
23. Neilipovitz DT, Crosby ET. No evidence for decreased incidence of aspiration after rapid sequence induction. *Can J Anaesth*. 2007;54(9):748-764. doi:54/9/748 [pii].
24. Ellis DY, Harris T, Zideman D. Cricoid pressure in emergency department rapid sequence tracheal intubations: a risk-benefit analysis. *Ann Emerg Med*. 2007;50(6):653-665. doi:10.1016/j.annemergmed.2007.05.006.
25. Brimacombe JR, Berry AM. Cricoid pressure. *Can J Anaesth*. 1997;44(4):414-425.
26. Aoyama K, Takenaka I, Sata T, Shigematsu A. Cricoid pressure impedes positioning and ventilation through the laryngeal mask airway. *Can J Anaesth*. 1996;43(10):1035-1040. doi:10.1007/BF03011906.
27. Asai T, Barclay K, McBeth C, Vaughan RS. Cricoid pressure applied after placement of the laryngeal mask prevents gastric insufflation but inhibits ventilation. *Br J Anaesth*. 1996;76(6):772-776. doi:10.1093/bja/76.6.772.
28. Hartsilver EL, Vanner RG. Airway obstruction with cricoid pressure. *Anaesthesia*. 2000;55(3):208-211. doi:10.1046/j.1365-2044.2000.01205.x.
29. Algie CM, Mahar RK, Tan HB, Wilson G, Mahar PD, Wasiak J. Effectiveness and risks of cricoid pressure during rapid sequence induction for endotracheal intubation. *Cochrane Database Syst Rev*. 2015;(11):CD011656. doi:10.1002/14651858.CD011656.pub2.
30. Birenbaum A, Hajage D, Roche S, et al. Effect of cricoid pressure compared with a sham procedure in the rapid sequence induction of anesthesia: the IRIS Randomized Clinical Trial. *JAMA Surg*. 2019;154(1):9-17. doi:10.1001/jamasurg.2018.3577.
31. Frerk C, Mitchell VS, McNarry AF, et al. Difficult Airway Society 2015 guidelines for management of unanticipated difficult intubation in adults. *Br J Anaesth*. 2015;115(6):827-848. doi:10.1093/bja/aev371.
32. Law JA, Duggan LV, Asselin M, et al. Canadian Airway Focus Group updated consensus-based recommendations for management of the difficult airway: part 1. Difficult airway management encountered in an unconscious patient. *Can J Anaesth*. 2021;68(9):1373-1404.
33. Apfelbaum JL, Hagberg CA, Connis RT, et al. 2022 American Society of Anesthesiologists Practice Guidelines for Management of the Difficult Airway. *Anesthesiology*. 2022;136(1):31-81. doi:10.1097/ALN.0000000000004002.
34. Cook TM, Woodall N, Frerk C, Fourth National Audit P. Major complications of airway management in the UK: results of the Fourth National Audit Project of the Royal College of Anaesthetists and the Difficult Airway Society. Part 1: anaesthesia. *Br J Anaesth*. 2011;106(5):617-631. doi:10.1093/bja/aer058.
35. Cook TM, Woodall N, Harper J, Benger J, Fourth National Audit P. Major complications of airway management in the UK: results of the Fourth National Audit Project of the Royal College of Anaesthetists and the Difficult Airway Society. Part 2: intensive care and emergency departments. *Br J Anaesth*. 2011;106(5):632-642. doi:10.1093/bja/aer059.
36. Galvez JA, Acquah S, Ahumada L, et al. Hypoxemia, bradycardia, and multiple laryngoscopy attempts during anesthetic induction in infants: a single-center, retrospective study. *Anesthesiology*. 2019;131(4):830-839. doi:10.1097/ALN.0000000000002847.
37. Amalric M, Larcher R, Brunot V, et al. Impact of videolaryngoscopy expertise on first-attempt intubation success in critically ill patients. *Crit Care Med*. 2020;doi:10.1097/CCM.0000000000004497.
38. Stinson HR, Srinivasan V, Topjian AA, et al. Failure of invasive airway placement on the first attempt is associated with progression to cardiac arrest in pediatric acute respiratory compromise. *Pediatr Crit Care Med*. 2018;19(1):9-16. doi:10.1097/PCC.0000000000001370.
39. Engelhardt T, Virag K, Veyckemans F, Habre W, Network AGotESoACT. Airway management in paediatric anaesthesia in Europe-insights from APRICOT (Anaesthesia Practice In Children Observational Trial): a prospective multicentre observational study in 261 hospitals in Europe. *Br J Anaesth*. 2018;121(1):66-75. doi:10.1016/j.bja.2018.04.013.
40. Fiadjoe JE, Nishisaki A, Jagannathan N, et al. Airway management complications in children with difficult tracheal intubation from the Pediatric Difficult Intubation (PeDI) registry: a prospective cohort analysis. *Lancet Respir Med*. 2016;4(1):37-48. doi:10.1016/S2213-2600(15)00508-1.
41. Lee JH, Turner DA, Kamat P, et al. The number of tracheal intubation attempts matters! A prospective multi-institutional pediatric observational study. *BMC Pediatr*. 2016;16:58. doi:10.1186/s12887-016-0593-y.
42. Bodily JB, Webb HR, Weiss SJ, Braude DA. Incidence and duration of continuously measured oxygen desaturation during emergency department intubation. *Ann Emerg Med*. 2016;67(3):389-395. doi:10.1016/j.annemergmed.2015.06.006.
43. Kerslake D, Oglesby AJ, Di Rollo N, et al. Tracheal intubation in an urban emergency department in Scotland: a prospective, observational study of 3738 intubations. *Resuscitation*. 2015;89:20-24. doi:10.1016/j.resuscitation.2015.01.005.
44. Goto T, Watase H, Morita H, et al. Repeated attempts at tracheal intubation by a single intubator associated with decreased success rates in emergency departments: an analysis of a multicentre prospective observational study. *Emerg Med J*. 2015;32(10):781-786. doi:10.1136/emermed-2013-203473.
45. Sakles JC, Chiu S, Mosier J, Walker C, Stolz U. The importance of first pass success when performing orotracheal intubation in the emergency department. *Acad Emerg Med*. 2013;20(1):71-78. doi:10.1111/acem.12055.
46. Rognas L, Hansen TM, Kirkegaard H, Tonnesen E. Pre-hospital advanced airway management by experienced anaesthesiologists: a prospective descriptive study. *Scand J Trauma Resusc Emerg Med*. 2013;21:58. doi:10.1186/1757-7241-21-58.
47. Hasegawa K, Shigemitsu K, Hagiwara Y, et al. Association between repeated intubation attempts and adverse events in emergency departments: an analysis of a multicenter prospective observational study. *Ann Emerg Med*. 2012;60(6):749-754 e2. doi:10.1016/j.annemergmed.2012.04.005.
48. Martin LD, Mhyre JM, Shanks AM, Tremper KK, Kheterpal S. 3,423 emergency tracheal intubations at a university hospital: airway outcomes and complications. *Anesthesiology*. 2011;114(1):42-48. doi:10.1097/ALN.0b013e318201c415.
49. Griesdale DE, Bosma TL, Kurth T, Isac G, Chittock DR. Complications of endotracheal intubation in the critically ill. *Intensive Care Med*. 2008;34(10):1835-1842. doi:10.1007/s00134-008-1205-6.
50. Mort TC. Emergency tracheal intubation: complications associated with repeated laryngoscopic attempts. *Anesth Analg*. 2004;99(2):607-613, table of contents. doi:10.1213/01.ANE.0000122825.04923.15.
51. Aziz MF, Brambrink AM, Healy DW, et al. Success of intubation rescue techniques after failed direct laryngoscopy in adults: a retrospective comparative analysis from the multicenter perioperative outcomes group. *Anesthesiology*. 2016;125(4):656-666. doi:10.1097/ALN.0000000000001267.
52. Sakles JC, Mosier JM, Patanwala AE, Dicken JM, Kalin L, Javedani PP. The C-MAC(R) video laryngoscope is superior to the direct laryngoscope for the rescue of failed first-attempt intubations in the emergency department. *J Emerg Med*. 2015;48(3):280-286. doi:10.1016/j.jemermed.2014.10.007.
53. Park R, Peyton JM, Fiadjoe JE, et al. The efficacy of GlideScope(R) videolaryngoscopy compared with direct laryngoscopy in children who are difficult to intubate: an analysis from the paediatric difficult intubation registry. *Br J Anaesth*. 2017;119(5):984-992. doi:10.1093/bja/aex344.
54. Piepho T, Fortmueller K, Heid FM, Schmidtmann I, Werner C, Noppens RR. Performance of the C-MAC video laryngoscope in patients after a limited glottic view using Macintosh laryngoscopy. *Anaesthesia*. 2011;66(12):1101-1105. doi:10.1111/j.1365-2044.2011.06872.x.
55. Amathieu R, Combes X, Abdi W, et al. An algorithm for difficult airway management, modified for modern optical devices (Airtraq laryngoscope; LMA CTrach): a 2-year prospective validation in patients for elective abdominal, gynecologic, and thyroid surgery. *Anesthesiology*. 2011;114(1):25-33. doi:10.1097/ALN.0b013e318201c44f.

56. Hung OR, Pytka S, Morris I, Murphy M, Stewart RD. Lightwand intubation: II—Clinical trial of a new lightwand for tracheal intubation in patients with difficult airways. *Can J Anaesth.* 1995;42(9):826-830.
57. Heidegger T, Gerig HJ, Ulrich B, Kreienbuhl G. Validation of a simple algorithm for tracheal intubation: daily practice is the key to success in emergencies—an analysis of 13,248 intubations. *Anesth Analg.* 2001;92(2):517-522.
58. Combes X, Le Roux B, Suen P, et al. Unanticipated difficult airway in anesthetized patients: prospective validation of a management algorithm. *Anesthesiology.* 2004;100(5):1146-1150. doi:00000542-200405000-00016 [pii].
59. Driver BE, Prekker ME, Klein LR, et al. Effect of use of a bougie vs endotracheal tube and stylet on first-attempt intubation success among patients with difficult airways undergoing emergency intubation: a randomized clinical trial. *JAMA.* 2018;319(21):2179-2189. doi:10.1001/jama.2018.6496.
60. Connelly NR, Ghandour K, Robbins L, Dunn S, Gibson C. Management of unexpected difficult airway at a teaching institution over a 7-year period. *J Clin Anesth.* 2006;18(3):198-204. doi:S0952-8180(05)00340-5 [pii] 10.1016/j.jclinane.2005.08.011.
61. Rosenblatt WH, Wagner PJ, Ovassapian A, Kain ZN. Practice patterns in managing the difficult airway by anesthesiologists in the United States. *Anesth Analg.* 1998;87(1):153-157.
62. Crosby ET, Duggan LV, Finestone PJ, Liu R, De Gorter R, Calder LA. Anesthesiology airway-related medicolegal cases from the Canadian Medical Protection Association. *Can J Anaesth.* Feb 2021;68(2):183-195.
63. Joffe AM, Aziz MF, Posner KL, Duggan LV, Mincer SL, Domino KB. Management of difficult tracheal intubation: a closed claims analysis. *Anesthesiology.* 2019;131(4):818-829. doi:10.1097/ALN.0000000000002815.
64. Law JA, Broemling N, Cooper RM, et al. The difficult airway with recommendations for management—part 1: difficult tracheal intubation encountered in an unconscious/induced patient. *Can J Anaesth.* 2013;60(11):1089-1118. doi:10.1007/s12630-013-0019-3.
65. Apfelbaum JL, Hagberg CA, Caplan RA, et al. Practice guidelines for management of the difficult airway: an updated report by the American Society of Anesthesiologists Task Force on Management of the Difficult Airway. *Anesthesiology.* 2013;118(2):251-270. doi:10.1097/ALN.0b013e31827773b2.
66. Lamb A, Zhang J, Hung O, et al. Accuracy of identifying the cricothyroid membrane by anesthesia trainees and staff in a Canadian institution. *Can J Anaesth.* 2015;62(5):495-503. doi:10.1007/s12630-015-0326-y.
67. Aslani A, Ng SC, Hurley M, McCarthy KF, McNicholas M, McCaul CL. Accuracy of identification of the cricothyroid membrane in female subjects using palpation: an observational study. *Anesth Analg.* 2012;114(5):987-992. doi:10.1213/ANE.0b013e31824970ba.
68. Elliott DS, Baker PA, Scott MR, Birch CW, Thompson JM. Accuracy of surface landmark identification for cannula cricothyroidotomy. *Anaesthesia.* 2010;65(9):889-894. doi:10.1111/j.1365-2044.2010.06425.x.
69. Law JA. Deficiencies in locating the cricothyroid membrane by palpation: we can't and the surgeons can't, so what now for the emergency surgical airway? *Can J Anaesth.* 2016;63(7):791-796.
70. Duggan LV, Ballantyne Scott B, Law JA, Morris IR, Murphy MF, Griesdale DE. Transtracheal jet ventilation in the "can't intubate can't oxygenate" emergency: a systematic review. *Br J Anaesth.* 2016;117(Suppl 1):i28-i38. doi:10.1093/bja/aew192.
71. Caplan RA, Posner KL, Ward RJ, Cheney FW. Adverse respiratory events in anesthesia: a closed claims analysis. *Anesthesiology.* 1990;72(5):828-833.
72. Cheney FW, Posner KL, Caplan RA. Adverse respiratory events infrequently leading to malpractice suits. A closed claims analysis. *Anesthesiology.* 1991;75(6):932-939.
73. Miller CG. *Management of the Difficult Intubation in Closed Malpractice Claims.* 2000. www.asahq.org/Newsletters/2000.
74. Metzner J, Posner KL, Lam MS, Domino KB. Closed claims' analysis. *Best Pract Res Clin Anaesthesiol.* 2011;25(2):263-276. doi:10.1016/j.bpa.2011.02.007.
75. Peterson GN, Domino KB, Caplan RA, Posner KL, Lee LA, Cheney FW. Management of the difficult airway: a closed claims analysis. *Anesthesiology.* 2005;103(1):33-39. doi:00000542-200507000-00009 [pii].
76. Reason J. Human error: models and management. *BMJ.* 2000;320(7237):768-770. doi:10.1136/bmj.320.7237.768.
77. Practice guidelines for management of the difficult airway. A report by the American Society of Anesthesiologists Task Force on Management of the Difficult Airway. *Anesthesiology.* 1993;78(3):597-602.
78. Practice guidelines for management of the difficult airway: an updated report by the American Society of Anesthesiologists Task Force on Management of the Difficult Airway. *Anesthesiology.* 2003;98(5):1269-1277.
79. Crosby ET, Cooper RM, Douglas MJ, et al. The unanticipated difficult airway with recommendations for management. *Can J Anaesth.* 1998;45(8):757-776. doi:10.1007/BF03012147.
80. Law JA, Broemling N, Cooper RM, et al. The difficult airway with recommendations for management—part 2—the anticipated difficult airway. *Can J Anaesth.* 2013;60(11):1119-1138. doi:10.1007/s12630-013-0020-x.
81. Law JA, Duggan LV, Asselin M, et al. Canadian Airway Focus Group updated consensus-based recommendations for management of the difficult airway: part 2. Planning and implementing safe management of the patient with an anticipated difficult airway. *Can J Anaesth.* 2021;68(9):1405-1436.
82. Chrimes N. The vortex: a universal "high-acuity implementation tool" for emergency airway management. *Br J Anaesth.* 2016;117(Suppl 1):i20-i27. doi:10.1093/bja/aew175.
83. Henderson JJ, Popat MT, Latto IP, Pearce AC. Difficult Airway Society guidelines for management of the unanticipated difficult intubation. *Anaesthesia.* 2004;59(7):675-694. doi:10.1111/j.1365-2044.2004.03831.x.
84. Popat M, Mitchell V, Dravid R, Patel A, Swampillai C, Higgs A. Difficult Airway Society guidelines for the management of tracheal extubation. *Anaesthesia.* 2012;67(3):318-340. doi:10.1111/j.1365-2044.2012.07075.x.
85. Mushambi MC, Kinsella SM, Popat M, et al. Obstetric Anaesthetists' Association and Difficult Airway Society guidelines for the management of difficult and failed tracheal intubation in obstetrics. *Anaesthesia.* 2015;70(11):1286-1306. doi:10.1111/anae.13260.
86. Higgs A, McGrath BA, Goddard C, et al. Guidelines for the management of tracheal intubation in critically ill adults. *Br J Anaesth.* 2018;120(2):323-352. doi:10.1016/j.bja.2017.10.021.
87. Chrimes N, Higgs A, Law JA, et al. Project for Universal Management of Airways—part 1: concept and methods. *Anaesthesia.* 2020;75(12):1671-1682. doi:10.1111/anae.15269.
88. Chrimes N, Higgs A, Sakles JC. Welcome to the era of universal airway management. *Anaesthesia.* 2020;75(6):711-715. doi:10.1111/anae.14998.
89. Brown CA 3rd, Bair AE, Pallin DJ, Walls RM, Investigators NI. Techniques, success, and adverse events of emergency department adult intubations. *Ann Emerg Med.* 2015;65(4):363-370 e1. doi:10.1016/j.annemergmed.2014.10.036.
90. Rosenblatt W, Ianus AI, Sukhupragarn W, Fickenscher A, Sasaki C. Preoperative endoscopic airway examination (PEAE) provides superior airway information and may reduce the use of unnecessary awake intubation. *Anesth Analg.* 2011;112(3):602-607. doi:10.1213/ANE.0b013e3181fdfc1c.
91. Jones PM, Harle CC. Avoiding awake intubation by performing awake GlideScope laryngoscopy in the preoperative holding area. *Can J Anaesth.* 2006;53(12):1264-1265. doi:10.1007/BF03021590.
92. Law JA, Morris IR, Brousseau PA, de la Ronde S, Milne AD. The incidence, success rate, and complications of awake tracheal intubation in 1,554 patients over 12 years: an historical cohort study. *Can J Anaesth.* 2015;62(7):736-744. doi:10.1007/s12630-015-0387-y.
93. El-Boghdadly K, Onwochei DN, Cuddihy J, Ahmad I. A prospective cohort study of awake fibreoptic intubation practice at a tertiary centre. *Anaesthesia.* 2017;72(6):694-703. doi:10.1111/anae.13844.
94. Joseph TT, Gal JS, DeMaria S Jr, Lin HM, Levine AI, Hyman JB. A retrospective study of success, failure, and time needed to perform awake intubation. *Anesthesiology.* 2016;125(1):105-114. doi:10.1097/ALN.0000000000001140.
95. Mort TC. Continuous airway access for the difficult extubation: the efficacy of the airway exchange catheter. *Anesth Analg.* 2007;105(5):1357-1362, table of contents. doi:10.1213/01.ane.0000282826.68646.a1.
96. Duggan LV, Law JA, Murphy MF. Brief review: supplementing oxygen through an airway exchange catheter: efficacy, complications, and recommendations. *Can J Anaesth.* 2011;58(6):560-568. doi:10.1007/s12630-011-9488-4.
97. Mort TC, Braffett BH. Conventional versus video laryngoscopy for tracheal tube exchange: glottic visualization, success rates, complications, and rescue alternatives in the high-risk difficult airway patient. *Anesth Analg.* 2015;121(2):440-448. doi:10.1213/ANE.0000000000000825.

CHAPTER 3

Preparation for Awake Intubation

Akua Gyambibi, Sree Kolli, and M. Kwesi Kwofie

INTRODUCTION

Consider the following case: A 54-year-old female with a multinodular goiter is scheduled for thyroidectomy. She has a history of non-insulin-dependent diabetes, obstructive sleep apnea (OSA), and is morbidly obese with a body mass index (BMI) of 54 kg·m^{-2}. She provides a history of difficult airway management at another institution 10 years previously at cholecystectomy, but unfortunately, these records are unavailable. Airway examination reveals a small mouth opening (3 cm or approximately 2 finger-breadths), full dentition with prominent upper incisors, and a receding mandible. When asked to protrude her lower mandible, she is unable to bite her upper lip with her lower incisors. Her neck extension is unremarkable but her neck is notably short and has a circumference of 44 cm. She has a Mallampati score of IV. As expected, her cricothyroid membrane (CTM) is difficult to identify.

This patient presents with multiple predictors of difficult face-mask ventilation, difficult direct laryngoscopy (DL), difficult video laryngoscopy (VL), difficult extraglottic device (EGD) use, and difficult front-of-neck airway (FONA).[1] Additionally, she is scheduled for surgery in which avoiding tracheal intubation is not a practical option. Awake intubation using a flexible bronchoscope is an appropriate initial management plan, and alternative techniques including awake intubation using a video laryngoscope or an optical stylet can also be considered. Regardless of the method used, adequate regional anesthesia of the airway is a prerequisite for safe and successful intubation in the awake, cooperative patient.[2]

What Are the Fundamentals of an "Awake, Bronchoscopically Facilitated" Intubation?

Awake bronchoscopic intubation is a core skill set for awake management of a difficult airway. A practitioner requires a working knowledge of applied airway anatomy to aid in the targeted application of local anesthetics to anesthetize the airway (applied either topically or via nerve blocks of the airway), and adequate dexterity and experience to drive a flexible bronchoscope to successfully use this technique.

APPLIED AIRWAY ANATOMY

The upper airway functionally consists of four regions: the nasal cavities, the pharynx, the larynx, and the trachea (Figure 3.1).[3] The mouth provides an additional route to the pharynx.

The Nose

The nose has several functions including the facilitation of breathing, the humidification and filtering of inspired gases, the housing of the olfactory receptors, and the drainage of the paranasal sinuses and nasolacrimal ducts.[3,4] The skeleton of the external nose is composed of bone superiorly and posteriorly,

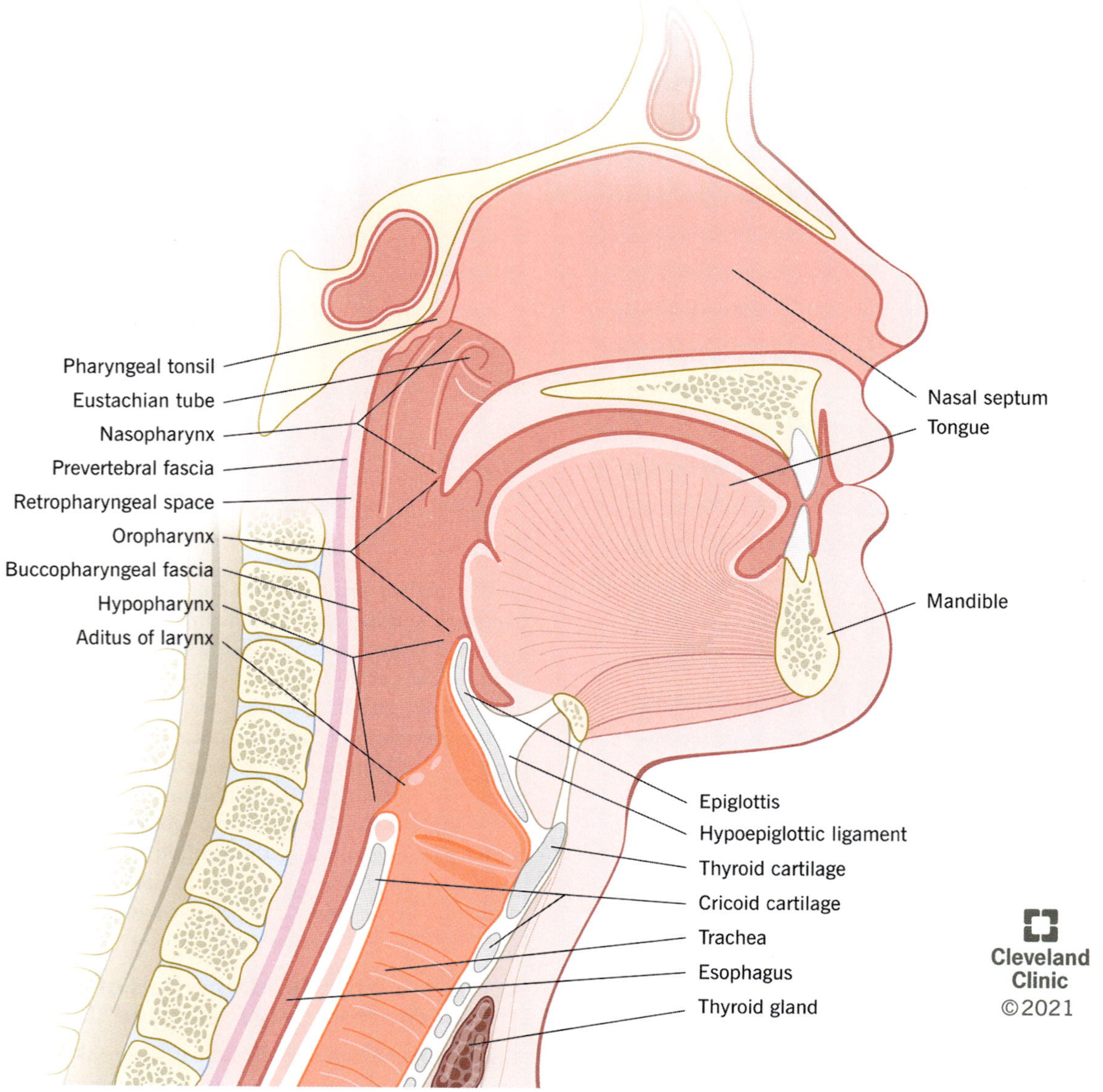

FIGURE 3.1. Sagittal view of the upper airway. (Reprinted with permission Cleveland Clinic Center for Medical Art & Photography ©2021. All Rights Reserved.)

and cartilage inferiorly. The left and right nasal cavities are divided by the nasal septum in the midline and provide a conduit from the nares anteriorly to the posterior nasal aperture (nasal choanae) and nasopharynx posteriorly (Figure 3.2).[4]

The nasal cavities each have a floor, roof, and lateral and medial walls formed by a series of facial bones and cartilages.[4,5] The floor of each nasal cavity is slightly concave and extends in a horizontal plane from the vestibule to the nasopharyngeal opening (Figure 3.2). The floor is formed from the palatine processes of the maxilla and the horizontal process of the palatine bone.[5] The turbinates, or conchae, are three horizontal ridges that project from the lateral walls of each nasal cavity toward the midline and create a superior, middle, and inferior meatus below each respective ridge (Figures 3.2 and 3.3). The superior and middle turbinates are part of the ethmoid bone while the inferior concha is a separate bone altogether.[4] The inferior turbinate and its accompanying meatus is the largest of the three, and as such, is often the route chosen for passing a flexible bronchoscope and nasotracheal tube along the floor of the nose (Figure 3.3).[3,4] Septal deviation may be associated with compensatory hypertrophy of the turbinates, and can produce nasal obstruction.[3] Occasionally, the posterior aspect of the inferior turbinate may be hypertrophied and resistance to the passage of a nasotracheal tube may be encountered at this location.[6] Alternating counterclockwise/clockwise rotation of the tube changes the orientation of the bevel and may facilitate negotiation of the nasal cavity. The paranasal sinuses and the nasolacrimal duct empty

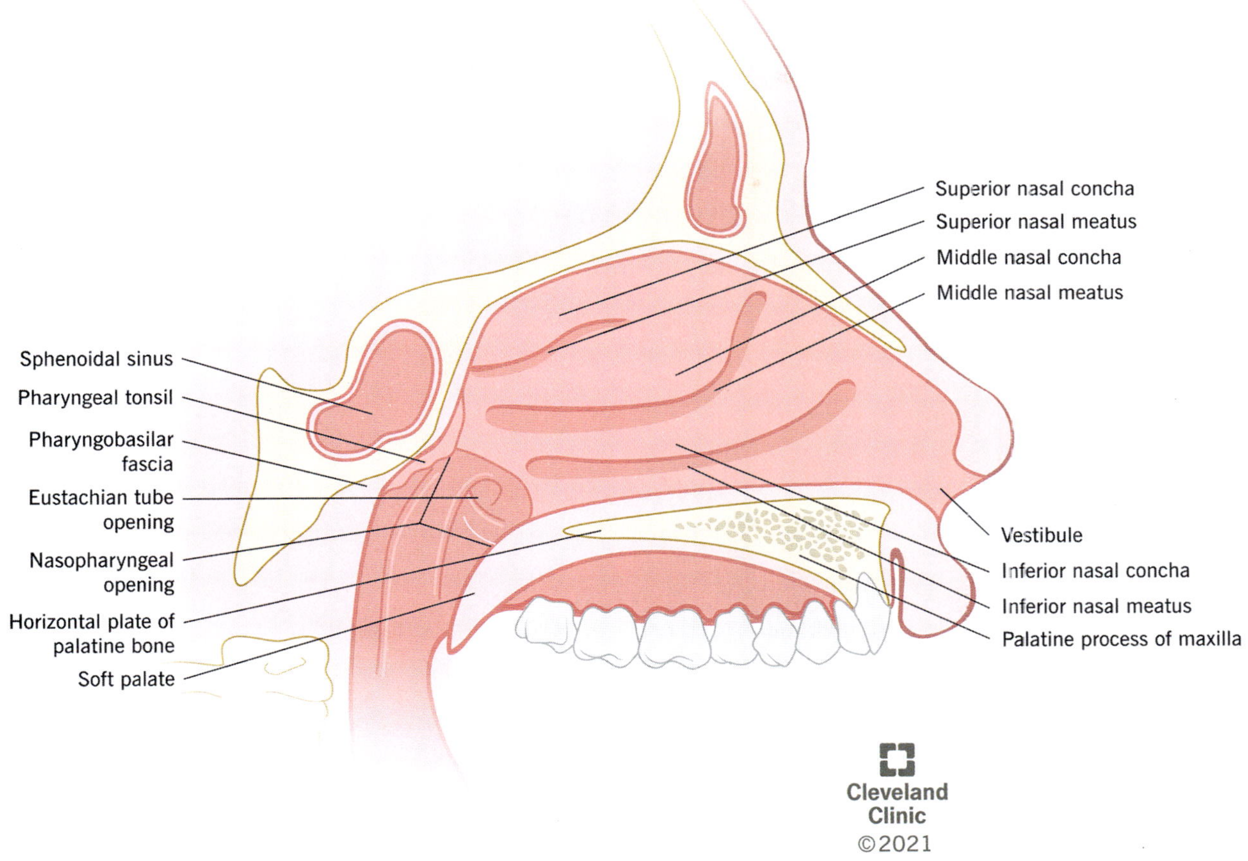

FIGURE 3.2. Lateral nasal wall. (Reprinted with permission Cleveland Clinic Center for Medical Art & Photography ©2021. All Rights Reserved.)

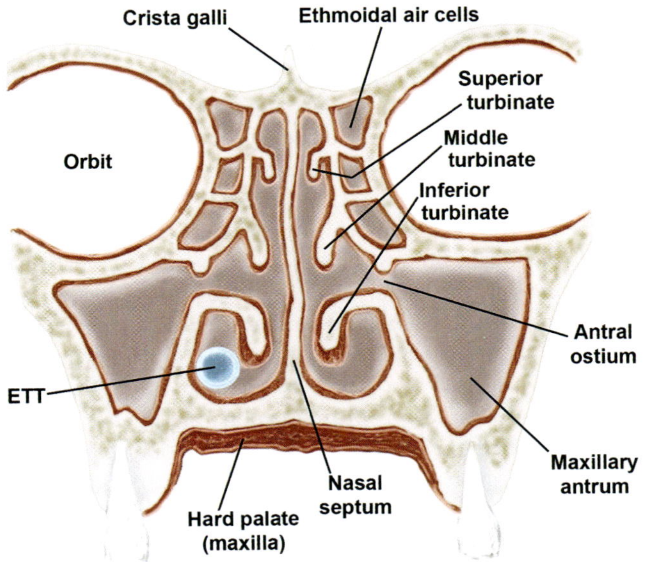

FIGURE 3.3. Coronal section of the maxillary sinus. The position of an endotracheal tube (ETT) is shown in the right nasal cavity.

into the nasal cavity through ostia in the lateral wall.[4,5] Obstruction of these ostia can occur with prolonged nasal intubation and can cause sinusitis, bacteremia, and sepsis.[3,7,8]

The blood supply of the anterior-superior aspect of the nasal cavity comes from the anterior and posterior ethmoidal branches of the ophthalmic artery, which in turn is a branch of the internal carotid.[6] The posterior-inferior portion is supplied by the sphenopalatine artery, branching from the maxillary artery and originating from the external carotid.[3,4,6] While the sphenopalatine artery is the usual culprit in posterior epistaxis, the multiple anastomoses between the anterior ethmoidal, sphenopalatine, and labial branches of the facial artery found at the anterior septum (known as Little's area or Kiesselbach's plexus) is responsible for the majority of epistaxis cases overall (Figure 3.4). Venous drainage occurs through a rich submucosal plexus that joins the sphenopalatine, facial, and ophthalmic veins, the last of which drains into the cavernous sinus.[4–6] Therefore, it comes as no surprise that the most common complication of nasotracheal intubation is epistaxis from abrasion of the mucosa as the tube passes through the nasal cavity.[9] The incidence of epistaxis during nasal intubation varies among studies and with the airway practitioner's level of experience but can range from 9.6% to approximately 73%.[10–14] Tintinalli and Claffey[10] reported mild (blood-tinged mucous) to moderate bleeding in 16% of 71 emergency nasal intubations performed by emergency physicians and nurse anesthetists. Only one case of severe bleeding requiring nasal packing and suctioning of gross blood occurred, and two patients suffered a retropharyngeal laceration. Woodall

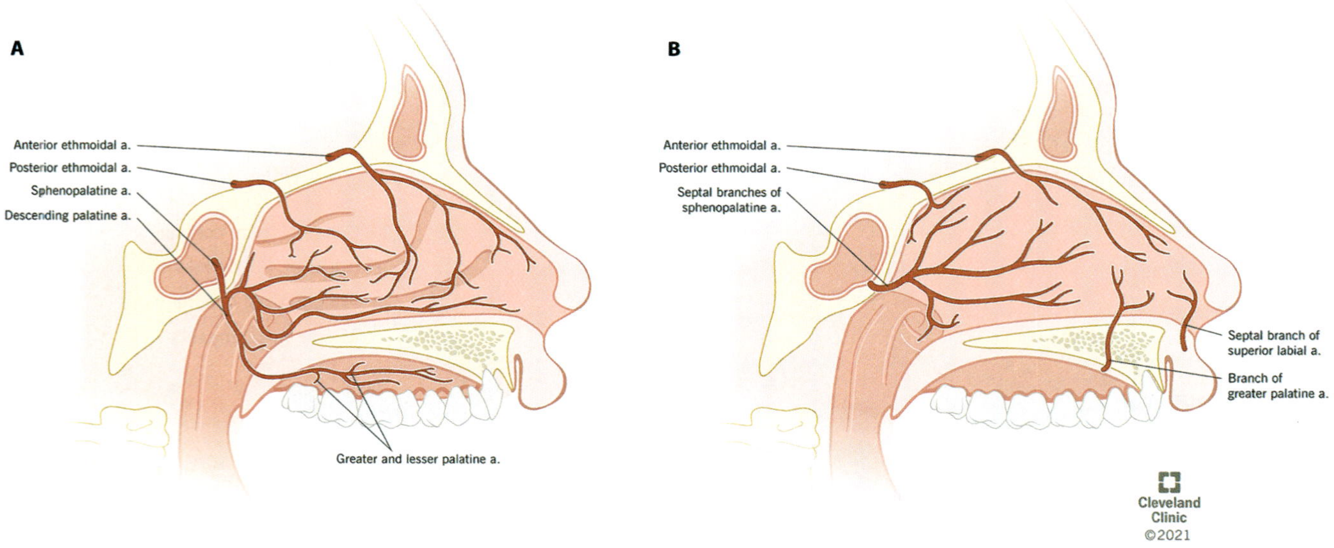

FIGURE 3.4. Blood supply to mucosa of **(A)** lateral nasal wall and **(B)** septum. (Reprinted with permission Cleveland Clinic Center for Medical Art & Photography ©2021. All Rights Reserved.)

et al. published the immediate and late complications at 24 to 48 hours after awake bronchoscopic intubation in 175 anesthesia practitioners who volunteered for a nasotracheal intubation training course.[15] Minor nasal bleeding was seen in 20 subjects during endoscopy or after extubation and none of these subjects required suction to control bleeding or clear the airway. Further, bleeding did not interfere with endoscopy. In a randomized controlled trial comparing nasal intubation in children 4 to 10 years of age using a red-rubber catheter to guide the tube through the nose versus inserting the nasotracheal tube alone, obvious bleeding requiring suctioning was found in 10% versus 29%, respectively.[14]

Passing the tube with the bevel facing the septum during intubation is thought to direct the leading edge away from the vascular septum. However, the optimum orientation of the tube remains controversial.[16] Another common method used to reduce the incidence of epistaxis during nasal intubation is softening the tube with warm sterile saline prior to use. When compared to a room temperature nasotracheal tube, a study of 150 patients found the incidence of both epistaxis and nasal damage (bruising, crusting, and/or tearing of the nasal mucosa) were significantly reduced when using a warmed tube.[13] The softened tip seemingly allowed the tube to slide more easily through the nasal passages, presumably causing less mucosal trauma and bleeding. The Portex North Polar nasotracheal tube is made of a velvet-soft polyvinyl chloride and has been shown to decrease epistaxis when compared to a wire-reinforced tube.[17] Age, sex, anatomic abnormalities of the nose, obesity, tube size, and choice of the left or right nostril did not correlate with epistaxis.[13]

Sensation to the nasal cavities is provided by the ophthalmic and maxillary divisions of the trigeminal nerve (CN V). The anterosuperior aspects of the lateral nasal walls and septum are supplied primarily by the anterior ethmoidal nerve originating from the ophthalmic division, while the posteroinferior portions are supplied by the short, long, and posterolateral branches of the sphenopalatine nerve originating from the maxillary division (Figure 3.5).[3,4] The floor of the nose is supplied by the anterior-superior dental branch of the infraorbital nerve anteriorly, and by the greater palatine nerve posteriorly.[3,6] The special sense of olfaction is provided via rootlets of the olfactory nerve (CN I) located in the roof of the nose adjacent to the cribriform plate.[3,4]

The Mouth

Anatomically, the mouth consists of two parts: the vestibule, which is bounded externally by the lips and cheeks and internally by the gums and teeth, and the mouth cavity proper, bounded by the hard palate and anterior aspect of the soft palate superiorly, the dental arches and teeth anteriorly and laterally, the tongue inferiorly, and the oropharyngeal isthmus posteriorly where it meets the oropharynx.[3,4]

The hard palate, formed by the maxilla anteriorly and the paired palatine bones posteriorly (Figure 3.6), is continuous with the pliable, curtain-like soft palate whose structure is reinforced by a tough, fibrous sheath within it called the palatine aponeurosis.[3,6,18] The lateral edges of the soft palate blend into the pharyngeal walls on each side, and the uvula hangs from the free border of the soft palate in the midline.[6,18] The uvula is a key midline landmark that is often relied upon during bronchoscopic and video-laryngoscopic intubation. The anterior surface of the palate faces the oral cavity and the posterior aspect faces, and is part of, the nasopharynx. In addition, the posterior surface is lined with ciliated columnar epithelial cells that overlay a thick layer of mucous and serous glands, as well as lymphoid tissue.[4] Finally, movement of the soft palate and uvula to seal off the nasopharynx during swallowing and during phonation is controlled by the action of five paired muscles, most notably the palatoglossus and palatopharyngeus, which blend with and insert on the lateral sides of the tongue and side walls of the pharynx, respectively, and approximate the palatoglossal and palatopharyngeal arches (anterior and posterior tonsillar pillars).[6,18] These

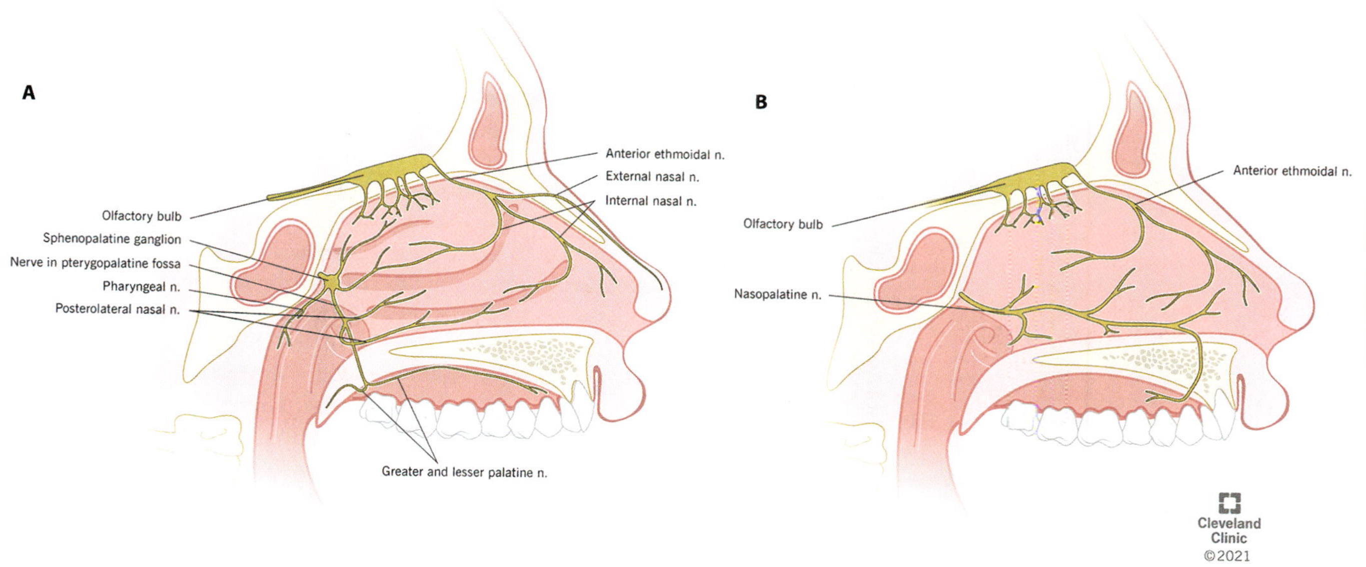

FIGURE 3.5. Nerve supply to mucosa of **(A)** lateral nasal wall and **(B)** septum. (Reprinted with permission Cleveland Clinic Center for Medical Art & Photography ©2021. All Rights Reserved.)

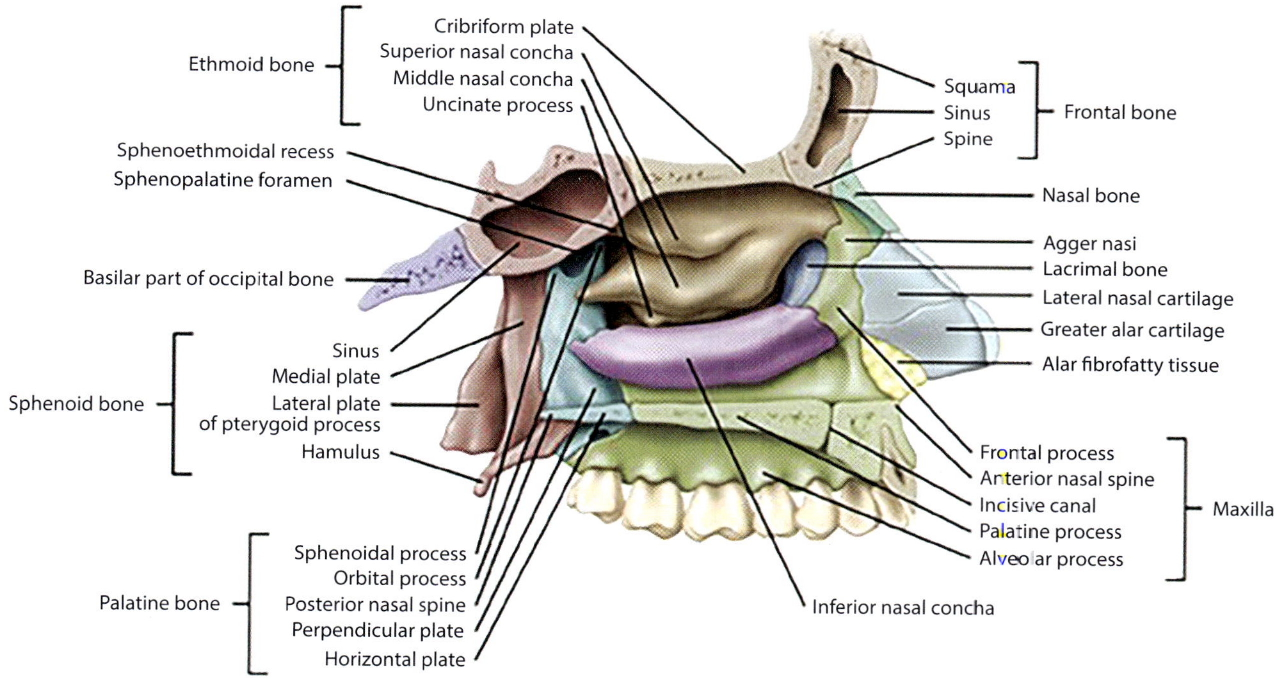

FIGURE 3.6. Bony components of lateral nasal wall.

folds can be used as important landmarks for glossopharyngeal nerve blocks of the airway (*discussed later*). Paralysis of these muscles results in regurgitation of food into the nasal cavity and nasal speech.[6] Sensation to the palate is supplied primarily by the trigeminal nerve. Motor innervation of the various palatine muscles (except the tensor palati) is supplied by the pharyngeal plexus of the vagus nerve, which contains fibers of the accessory nerve (CN XI) (Figure 3.7).[6,18] Backward movement of the tongue against the pharyngeal wall during sedation and anesthesia in a supine position has traditionally been thought to be the primary cause of upper airway obstruction but collapse at the level of the velopharyngeal segment of the upper airway and the soft palate have been found to predominately limit airflow during sleep, sedation, and anesthesia.[18–20]

The anterior two-thirds and posterior one-third of the tongue are separated by a V-shaped groove on its dorsal aspect called the sulcus terminalis.[21] The dorsal surface also often has a shallow groove in the midline that can be a useful landmark during bronchoscopic bronchoscopy for intubation (Figure 3.8). The posterior one-third of the tongue lies within the oropharynx and has a collection of lymphoid tissue called the lingual tonsil, which, together with the palatine, nasopharyngeal, and Eustachian tubal tonsils, form a somewhat continuous "ring" of lymphoid tissue in the pharynx (Waldeyer's

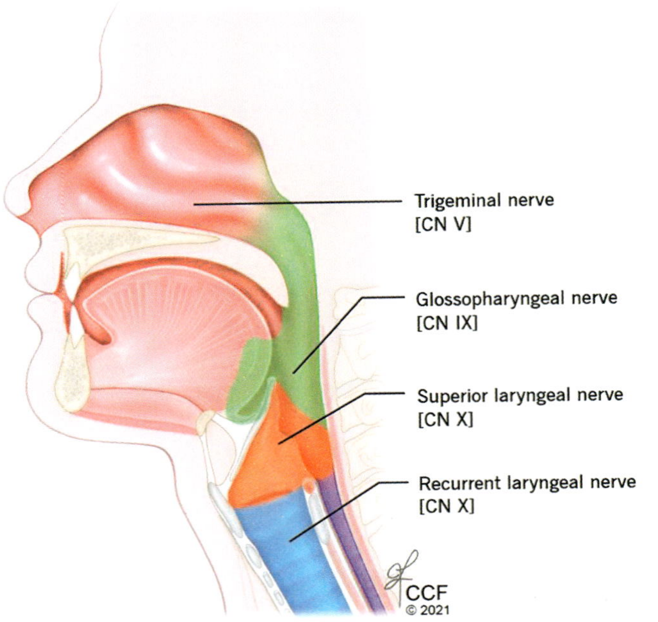

FIGURE 3.7. The sensory distribution of the nerves of the naso, oro, and laryngopharynx. (Reprinted with permission Cleveland Clinic Center for Medical Art & Photography ©2021. All Rights Reserved.)

ring).[18] Lingual tonsil hypertrophy may be a contributor to difficult or impossible DL and face-mask ventilation.[22] General sensation to the anterior two-thirds of the tongue is provided by the lingual branch of the mandibular nerve (CN V), while the special sensation of taste is provided by the chorda tympani, a branch of the facial nerve.[21,23,24] The glossopharyngeal nerve (CN IX) is responsible for both general sensation and taste for the posterior one-third of the tongue (Figure 3.7).[21,25] Stimulation of the posterior third of the tongue (as well as other mucosa innervated by the glossopharyngeal nerve) during awake intubation typically provokes the gag reflex and can be particularly problematic during bronchoscopic intubation. The internal branch of the superior laryngeal nerve (SLN), itself a branch of the vagus nerve (CN X), provides sensation to the base of the tongue in addition to numerous other pharyngeal and laryngeal structures (Figure 3.7).[18,25]

The paired sublingual salivary glands lie just deep to the mucous membranes in the floor of the mouth on either side of the tongue. Deep to these structures lies the mylohyoid muscle which forms a sling to support the floor of the mouth and simultaneously forms the roof of the submandibular space and floor of the sublingual space.[3,6,18,21] The submandibular space lies deep to the mylohyoid muscle—between the mandible and the hyoid bone–and contains fat, lymphatic tissues, and the superficial portion of the submandibular salivary gland, found at the posterior edge of the mylohyoid.[21] Acute cellulitis and swelling within this space, termed Ludwig's angina, forces the tongue and floor of the mouth upward, creating life-threatening airway obstruction and reducing the area into which the tongue can be displaced during DL. Extension to sublingual and hypopharyngeal spaces can produce tongue and pharyngeal swelling, and potential exists for infection to spread down the airway and into the mediastinum, creating significant edema throughout the airway.[26] While awake bronchoscopic intubation can be considered in these patients, many may require awake tracheotomy under local anesthesia.[27,28]

The Pharynx

The pharynx is a 12- to 15-cm long fibromuscular tube that extends from the base of the skull to the lower border of the cricoid cartilage anteriorly and the sixth cervical vertebrae posteriorly where it becomes continuous with the esophagus (Figure 3.1).[18] Posteriorly, it rests against the fascia covering the prevertebral muscles. Anteriorly, it communicates freely with

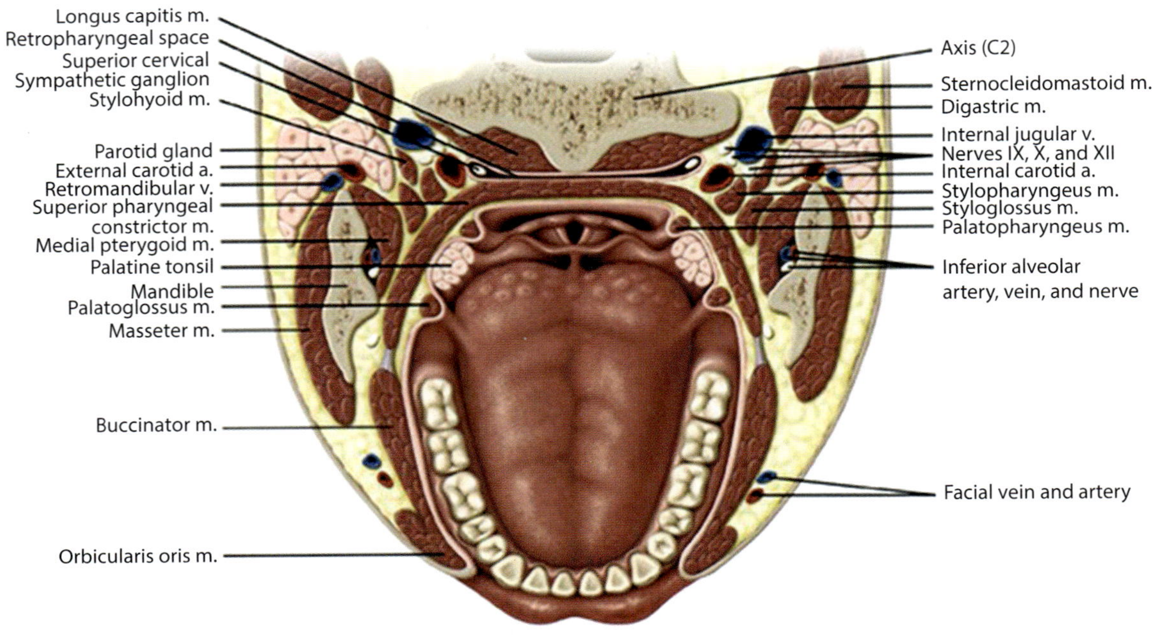

FIGURE 3.8. Horizontal section below lingula of mandible: superior view.

the nasal cavity, mouth, and the larynx at the naso-, oro-, and laryngopharynx, respectively (Figure 3.9). The pharyngeal wall is comprised of a superficial layer of mucosal tissue and a layer of three telescoping constrictor muscles (superior, middle, and inferior) separated by a fibrous layer called the pharyngobasilar fascia.[6,18] The outer surfaces of these muscle are covered in the buccopharyngeal fascia, a thin fibrous capsule that envelopes the pharynx. These muscles work together to coordinate the movement of food from the oropharynx into the esophagus during swallowing (deglutition).[18] The inferior constrictor consists of an upper portion with oblique muscle fibers arising from the thyroid cartilage and a lower transverse portion (the cricopharyngeus) arising from the cricoid that functions as an upper esophageal sphincter. The junction of the pharynx with the esophagus is the narrowest part of the gastrointestinal tract and is a common place for foreign bodies to impact.[3,18,29]

The nasopharynx lies directly behind the nasal cavities, above the soft palate, and communicates with the oropharynx via the pharyngeal isthmus (Figure 3.1). Posterosuperiorly, the sphenoid bone and sphenoid sinus form the roof of the nasopharynx.[4] Sensation to the nasopharynx and oropharynx is supplied primarily by the glossopharyngeal nerve (Figure 3.7).[3,4,6,18] In addition, the maxillary branch of the trigeminal nerve contributes to the sensation of the roof of the nasopharynx, as well as the soft palate and the adjacent part of the tonsil. The nasopharyngeal tonsil (adenoids), a collection of lymphoid tissue, is also located on the roof of the nasopharynx and lies against the superior constrictor muscle.[3,6,18] The opening of the Eustachian tube is found on the lateral wall of each side of the nasopharynx.[6] In some patients, the first cervical vertebra (atlas) has a prominent anterior arch (or tubercle) that projects in the nasopharynx, impeding the passage of the endotracheal tube during nasal intubation.[30] Persistent attempts to push past this obstruction can result in trauma to the nasopharynx and unintentional submucosal placement of the tube. Rotation of the tube may facilitate passage around this prominence. However, on occasion, digital manipulation of the tip of the tube by the index and middle fingers inserted through the mouth may be required.[31] If these maneuvers fail, or as an alternative, a soft nasal trumpet can be passed first through the nose into the pharynx beyond the anterior tubercle of the atlas. A nasogastric (NG) tube cutoff at its proximal end can then be passed into the pharynx through the trumpet and the trumpet removed. A nasal endotracheal tube can then be passed over the NG tube beyond the tubercle of the atlas. The NG tube can then be removed, and the endotracheal tube passed into the trachea. A red-rubber catheter can also be used in place of an NG tube, using a technique described by Elwood et al.[14]

The oropharynx is the space posterior to the mouth cavity, bounded by the palatoglossal arches, soft palate, and the posterior third of the tongue, and extends vertically from the soft palate to the tip of the epiglottis.[6] The palatine tonsils lie within triangular recesses (fauces) formed by the palatoglossal and palatopharyngeal arches and the tongue on each side of the oropharynx (Figure 3.8).[6] The tip of the epiglottis represents the upper border of the laryngopharynx.[3,6] It is tethered to the tongue in the midline by the median glossoepiglottic fold (a fold of mucous membrane that overlies the hyoepiglottic ligament) and to the walls of the pharynx laterally by the lateral glossoepiglottic folds.[3,18,29] The depressions formed on each side of the median glossoepiglottic fold are the valleculae.[6,18,21] During DL, the Macintosh blade is inserted into the base of

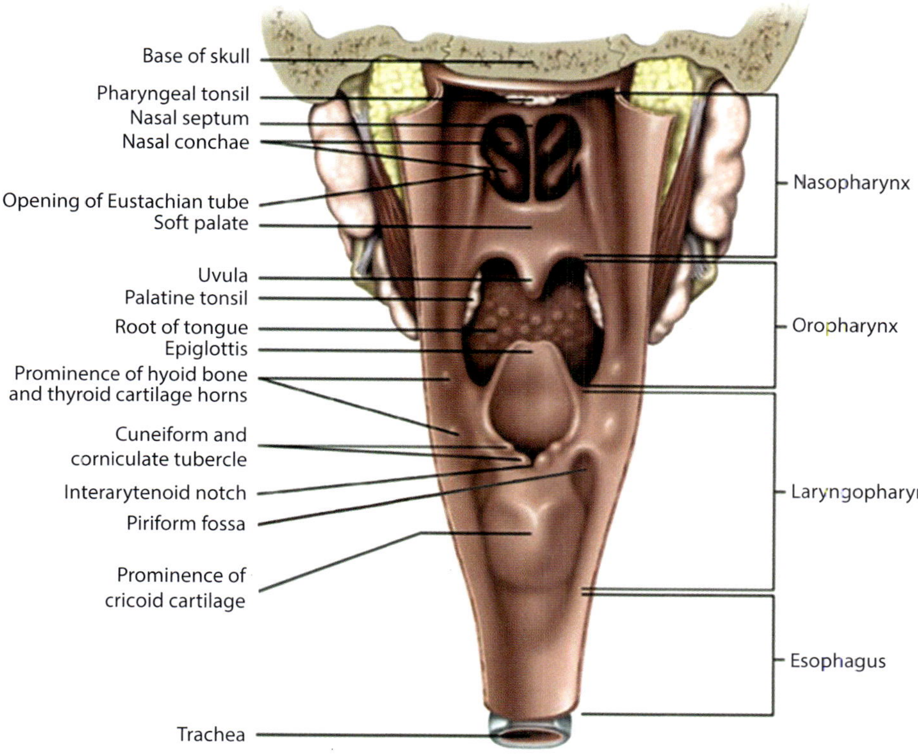

FIGURE 3.9. Opened posterior view of the pharynx.

the vallecula to engage the hyoepiglottic ligament and lift the epiglottis anteriorly to expose the glottis.

The laryngopharynx (hypopharynx) extends from the tip of the epiglottis to the lower border of the cricoid cartilage, and is continuous with the esophagus (Figures 3.9 and 3.10).[3,6] The aditus (inlet) of larynx is bounded anteriorly by the epiglottis, laterally by the aryepiglottic folds, posteriorly by the arytenoid cartilages and a fold of mucous membrane stretch between them.[3,29] The larynx bulges into the center of the laryngopharynx, and the deep recesses found on either side are the piriform fossae (Figure 3.9).[6] As seen during DL, the larynx and pharynx can be conceptualized to be a smaller cylinder placed within and at the anterior aspect of a larger cylinder, respectively. The laryngopharynx receives sensory innervation from the internal branch of the superior laryngeal branch of the vagus nerve, which pierces the thyrohyoid membrane and runs in the submucosa of the piriform fossae. This same nerve supplies some sensation from the base of the tongue (along with the glossopharyngeal nerve) to the level of the vocal cords.[3,18,29,32] The epiglottis is densely innervated, and the true vocal folds are more heavily innervated posteriorly than anteriorly.[18,29,32] Cotton pledgets or balls soaked in local anesthetic can be held against the mucosa of the piriform fossa using Kraus or Jackson forceps to produce a block of the internal branch of the SLN, or the nerve can be approached percutaneously (see the following text). While some authors state that both surfaces of the epiglottis are innervated by the superior laryngeal branch of the vagus,[23] others have stated that the anterior aspect of the epiglottis is innervated by the glossopharyngeal nerve[33] or a combination of the two nerves.[34]

The Larynx

The larynx lies opposite the fourth through sixth cervical vertebrae and is comprised of a framework of articulating cartilages, ligaments, fibrous membranes, and muscles.[3,6,29] It extends from its oblique entrance formed by the aryepiglottic folds, the tip of the epiglottis, and the posterior commissure to the lower border of the cricoid cartilage.[3] Its primary functions are (1) to

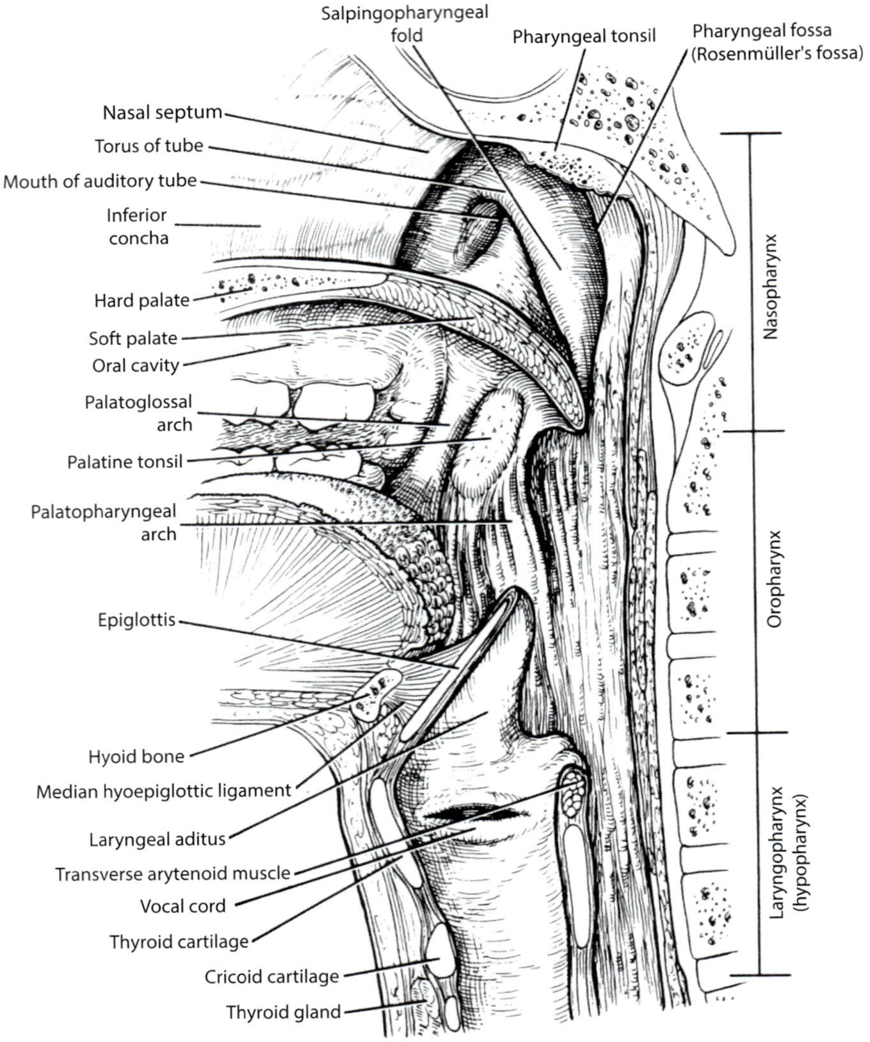

FIGURE 3.10. The medial view of the pharyngeal mucosa. (Reproduced with permission from Cummings CW. *Otolaryngology Head and Neck Surgery*, 3rd ed. St. Louis, MO: Mosby; 1998.)

prevent the inadvertent passage of secretions, food, and foreign bodies into the trachea, and (2) to allow for phonation.[29]

The laryngeal cartilages include the unpaired thyroid, cricoid, and epiglottic cartilages, and the paired arytenoid, corniculate, and cuneiform cartilages.[29] The thyroid cartilage is the largest structure in the larynx and its unique shape is the result of the embryonic fusion of two distinct quadrilateral laminae in the midline, producing a shield-like prominence (also known as the Adam's apple in males) and the thyroid notch (Figure 3.11). The upper edge of the thyroid cartilage is attached to the hyoid bone by the thyrohyoid membrane.[6,29] Posteriorly, the edges of the laminae extend superiorly and inferiorly to form the greater and lesser cornua (horns), respectively. The inferior horn, by means of a facet on its inner surface, articulates with the cricoid cartilage while the superior horn attaches to the hyoid bone via the lateral thyrohyoid ligament.[6,29] The cricoid cartilage is the only complete skeletal ring of the airway. Anteriorly, the thyroid cartilage is attached to the cricoid by the easily palpable CTM, a suitable site for emergency surgical airway access (or FONA) in adults or intratracheal injections.[6,29,34] The pyramid-shaped arytenoid cartilages articulate with the superolateral aspects of the back of the cricoid cartilage (Figure 3.11). These act as true ball-and-socket joints and control the adduction and abduction of the vocal cords. The corniculate cartilages articulate with the apices of the arytenoids, and the posterior commissure is the shallow groove between them. This mucosa-covered

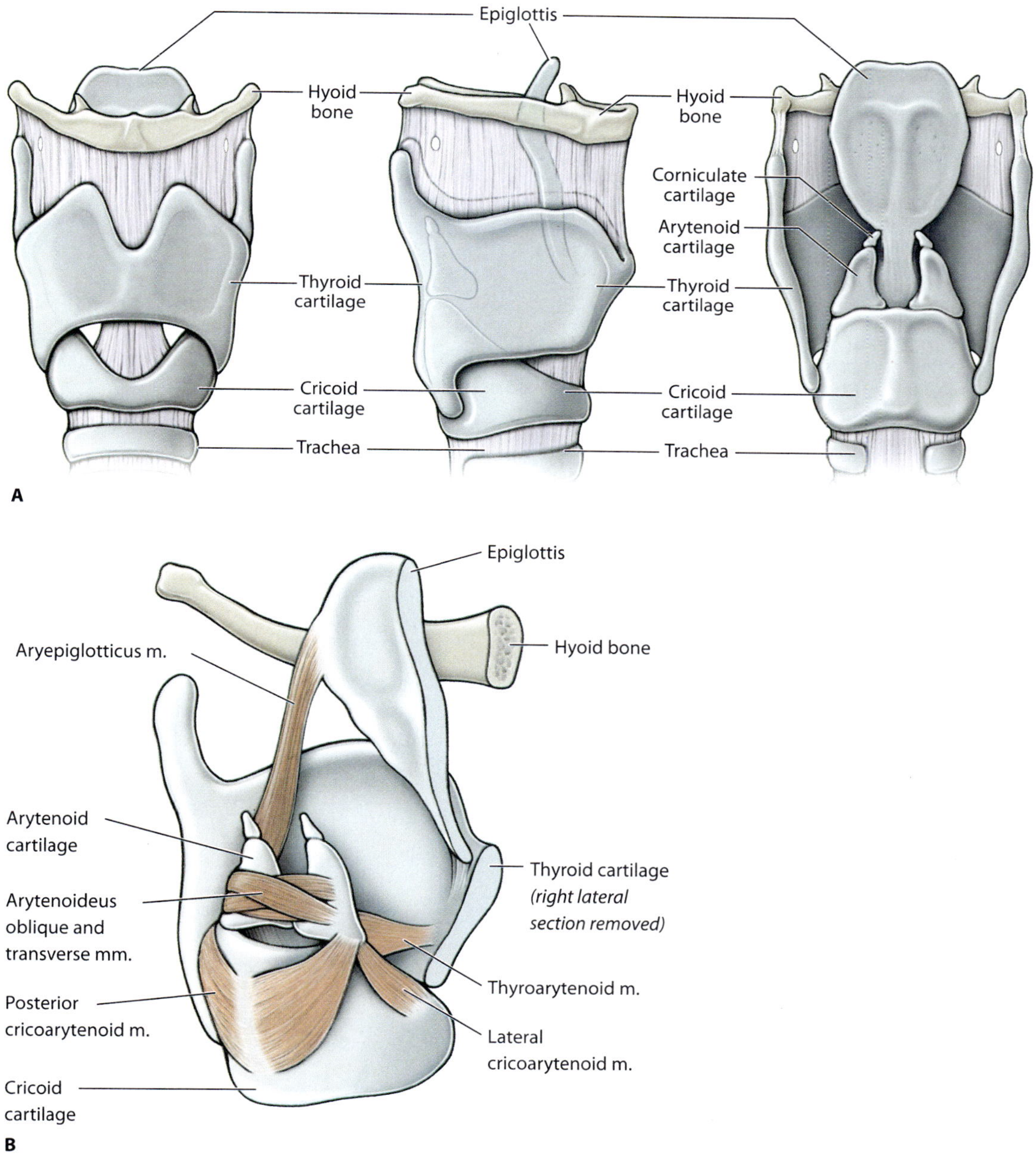

FIGURE 3.11. Cartilages of the larynx. (Reproduced with permission from Lalwani AK. *Current Diagnosis & Treatment Otolaryngology—Head and Neck Surgery*, 4th ed. New York, NY: McGraw Hill; 2020.

depression can be a useful landmark during laryngoscopy.[3] The cuneiforms are tiny cartilages found lateral to the corniculates, but also within the aryepiglottic folds.[6] The epiglottis is leaf-shaped and bears attachments to the thyroid cartilage and hyoid bone through the thyroepiglottic and hyoepiglottic ligaments, respectively.[6,29] The remaining elements that form the structure of the larynx are two paired fibroelastic membranes, the quadrangular and triangular membranes (conus elasticus) (Figure 3.12).[3,29] The quadrangular membrane connects the lateral border of the epiglottis and the arytenoid cartilages.[29] Its free upper edge forms the aryepiglottic ligament, and its thickened lower border, covered in mucosa, forms the vestibular ligament (false vocal cord).[3,29] The cricothyroid ligament or CTM can be identified in the anterior neck as a concavity between the inferior border of the thyroid cartilage and the superior border of the cricoid cartilage (Figures 3.11 and 3.13). It connects

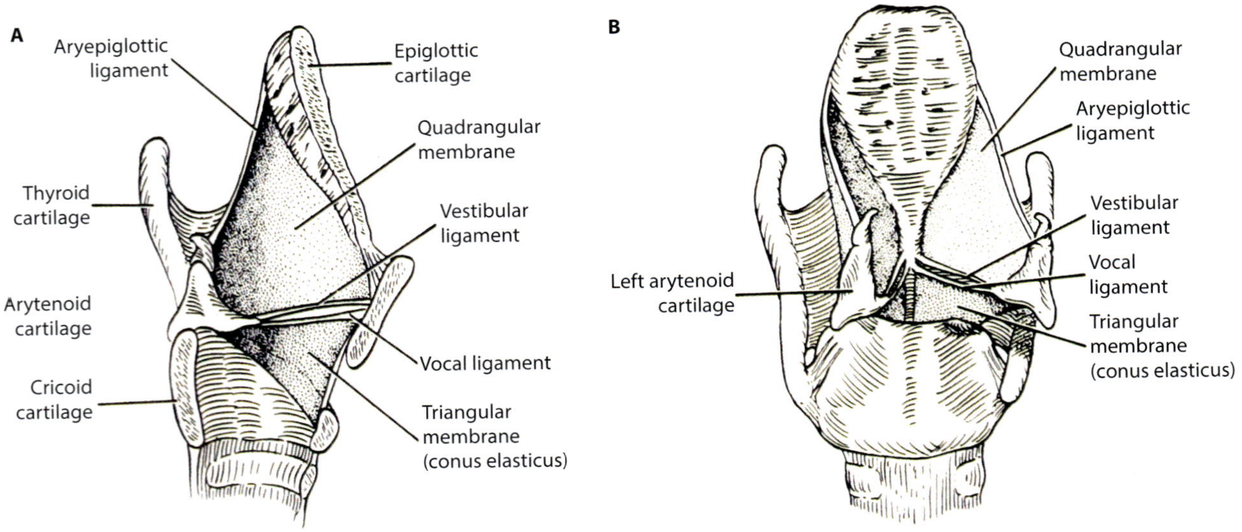

FIGURE 3.12. (A) Sagittal section of laryngeal membranes and **(B)** Posterior view of laryngeal membranes (right arytenoid cartilage moved lateral y). (Reproduced with permission from Cummings CW. *Otolaryngology Head and Neck Surgery,* 3rd ed. St. Louis, MO: Mosby; 1998.)

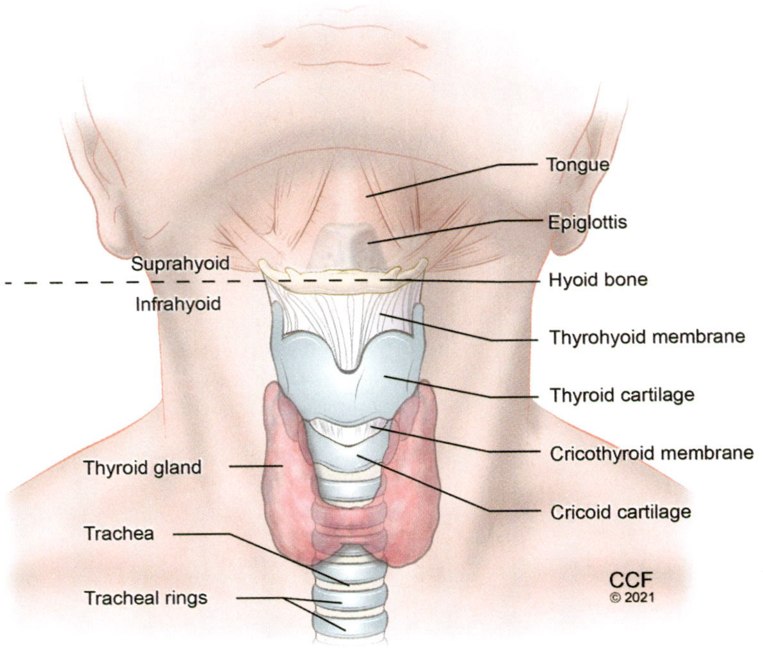

FIGURE 3.13. Anterior view of cricothyroid membrane (ligament). (Reprinted with permission Cleveland Clinic Center for Medical Art & Photography ©2021. All Rights Reserved.)

the thyroid and cricoid cartilages anteriorly in the midline and is continuous with the conus elasticus (cricovocal membrane), which extends posterolaterally from the ligament to attach to the arytenoids on each side. The slightly thickened, free upper edges of the conus elasticus form the true vocal cords.[3,6,29] The CTM is a key landmark for emergency FONA by surgical cricothyrotomy. The width of the membrane ranges from 27 to 32 mm and the reported vertical height of the membrane varies depending on the age (see Chapter 46) and the source but ranges anywhere from 5 to 19 mm in cadavers, with a smaller width and height in females compared to males.[35–39] The CTM can usually be palpated one to one and a half finger breadths below the laryngeal prominence (thyroid cartilage or Adam's apple) and the average vertical distance between the true cords and the midpoint of the CTM is 13 mm in the adult.[36] Vasculature of the anterior neck is considerably variable, but cricothyroid branches of the superior thyroid artery commonly run across the upper portion of the CTM, and branches of the superior and inferior thyroid veins may also cross the membrane. As such, an incision in the lower third of the membrane is recommended.[39] While it is clear these vessels can potentially be injured during cricothyrotomy, bleeding is usually self-limited and of little clinical significance.[39]

In coronal section, the relationship of the true vocal cords to the false vocal cords and the laryngeal ventricle or sinus (between the true and false cords) can be readily appreciated (Figure 3.14). Together, the aryepiglottic, the vestibular (false cords), and the vocal folds (true cords) form a trilevel sphincter mechanism that protects the airway.[3,29] The space between the vestibular and vocal folds is referred to as the glottis, with the laryngeal cavity above the false cords termed the supraglottis and cavity below the vocal cords to the lower border of the cricoid cartilage termed the subglottis.[3,29] The mucosa of the larynx is primarily a ciliated columnar epithelium with mucous-secreting goblet cells scattered throughout, except for the mucosa overlying the anterior aspect of the epiglottis, the upper part of its posterior aspect, and the upper parts of the aryepiglottic folds, where the mucosa becomes stratified squamous epithelium in continuity with the upper gastrointestinal tract.[6,32] Of note, the mucosa covering the vocal folds is devoid of mucus glands and the epithelium adheres directly to the vocal ligaments, limiting swelling of the true cords during edematous states.[40] In

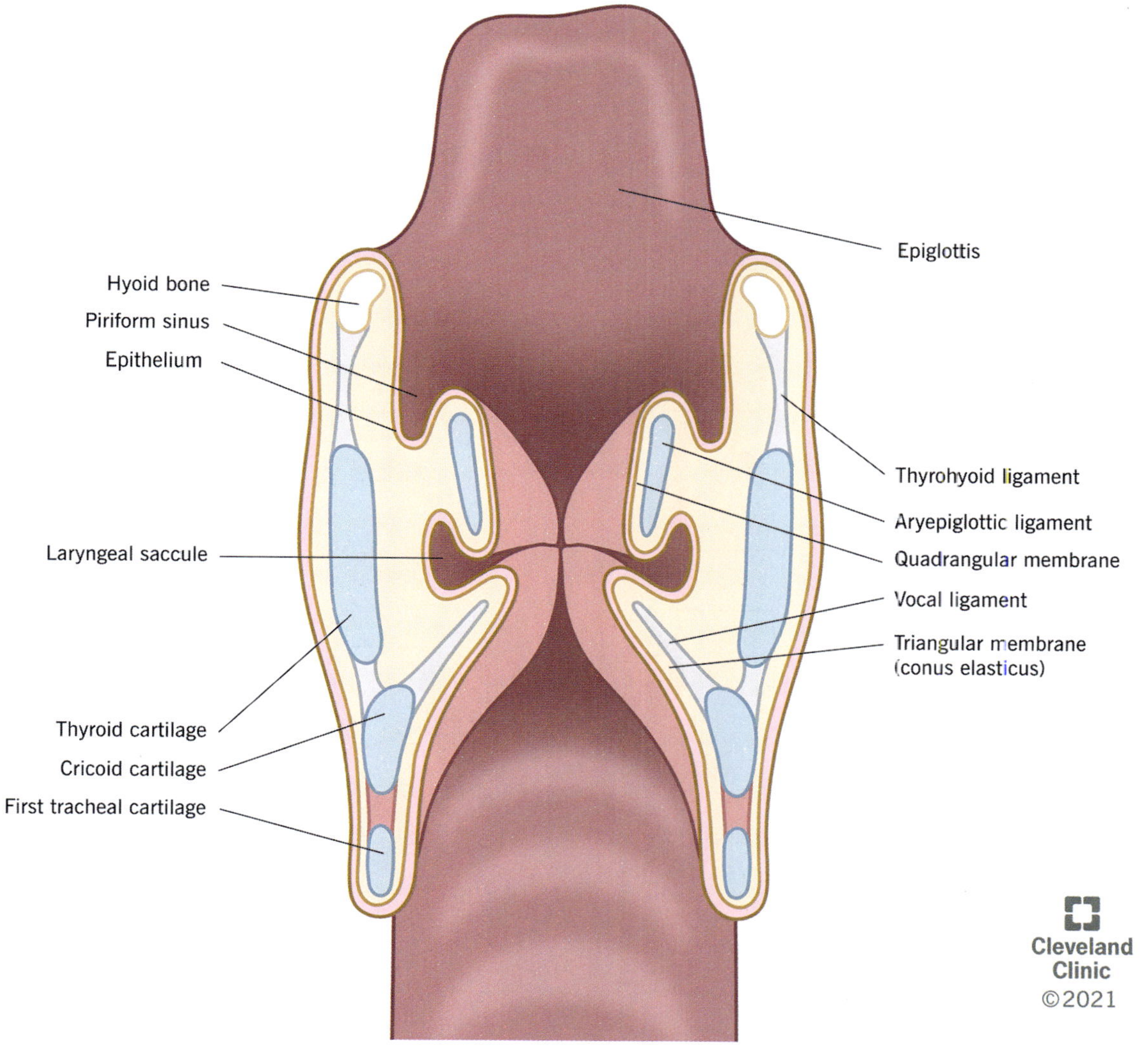

FIGURE 3.14. Coronal section of larynx. (Reprinted with permission Cleveland Clinic Center for Medical Art & Photography ©2021. All Rights Reserved.)

the adult, the vocal cords lie between 12 and 15 cm beyond the teeth.[41] The movement of the laryngeal cartilages and vocal folds is controlled by a complex series of intrinsic muscles, of which the cricothyroid is the sole muscle that lies outside the larynx's cartilaginous skeleton.[6,29] The larynx is innervated by the superior and recurrent laryngeal branches of the vagus (CN X). The SLN arises from the main trunk of CN X just after it exits the jugular foramen and divides into a large sensory internal and a small motor external branch that supplies the cricothyroid muscle (Figure 3.15).[3,29,37] The internal branch travels with the superior laryngeal artery (SLA) and pierces the lateral portion of the thyrohyoid membrane between the greater cornu of the thyroid cartilage and the hyoid bone to provide sensation to the laryngeal mucosa above the level of the vocal cords.[3,29] The left recurrent laryngeal nerve branches from the vagus in the thorax, loops around the aortic arch near the ligamentum arteriosum before traveling superiorly between the trachea and esophagus to innervate the larynx (Figure 3.16). On the right, the recurrent laryngeal nerve leaves the vagus as it crosses the subclavian artery, loops posteriorly under it, and then similarly travels cephalad within the right tracheoesophageal groove.[3,6,23,25,29] The recurrent laryngeal nerves supply all intrinsic muscles of the larynx, except the cricothyroid, and also provides sensation to the mucosa below the vocal cords.[3,6,29] Damage to a single SLN results in hoarseness temporarily, as the contralateral cricothyroid muscle eventually compensates.[6] Unilateral recurrent laryngeal nerve palsy affects the ipsilateral vocal cord, producing hoarseness. Possible causes include malignancies of the neck or thorax, and cardiovascular pathology (i.e., aortic aneurysm or left atrial enlargement). If both nerves are affected, the vocal cords may be held in a partially abducted (complete palsy) or fully adducted (incomplete palsy) position, and stridor and severe airway obstruction may occur.[29]

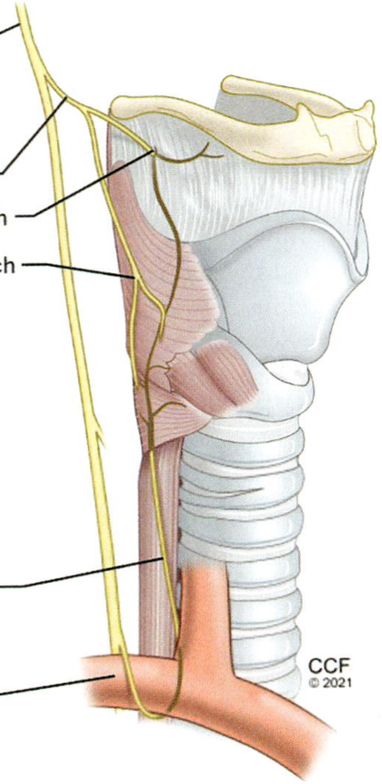

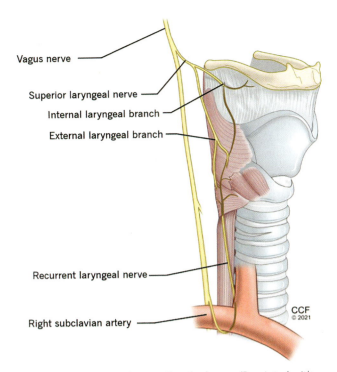

FIGURE 3.15. Nerves innervating the larynx. (Reprinted with permission Cleveland Clinic Center for Medical Art & Photography ©2021. All Rights Reserved.)

The Trachea

The trachea extends inferiorly from the lower border of the cricoid cartilage at approximately the sixth cervical vertebra (in females) or seventh cervical vertebra (in males)[42] to the carina at the fourth[33] or fifth[6,34,43] thoracic vertebra (Figure 3.17). It is 10 to 15 cm long in the adult,[34] and in the sagittal plane

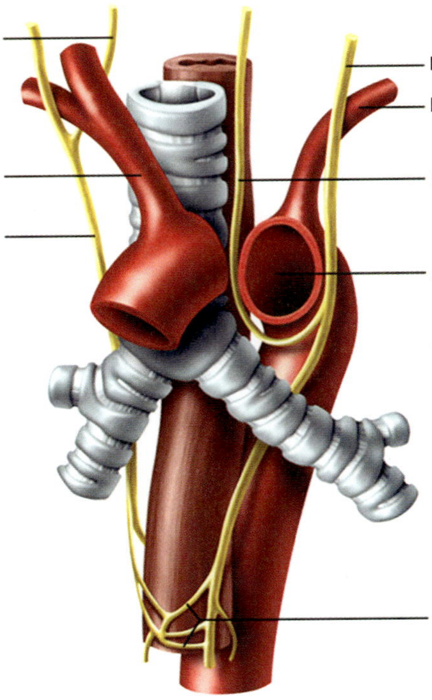

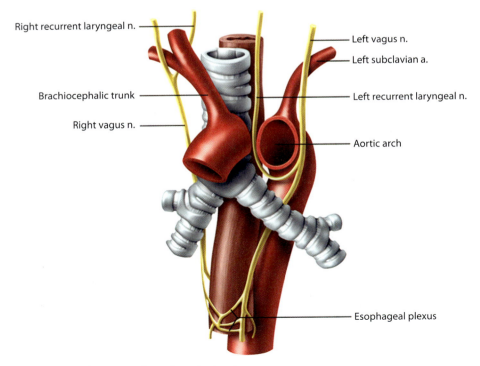

FIGURE 3.16. The distal trachea and mainstem bronchi and related structures.

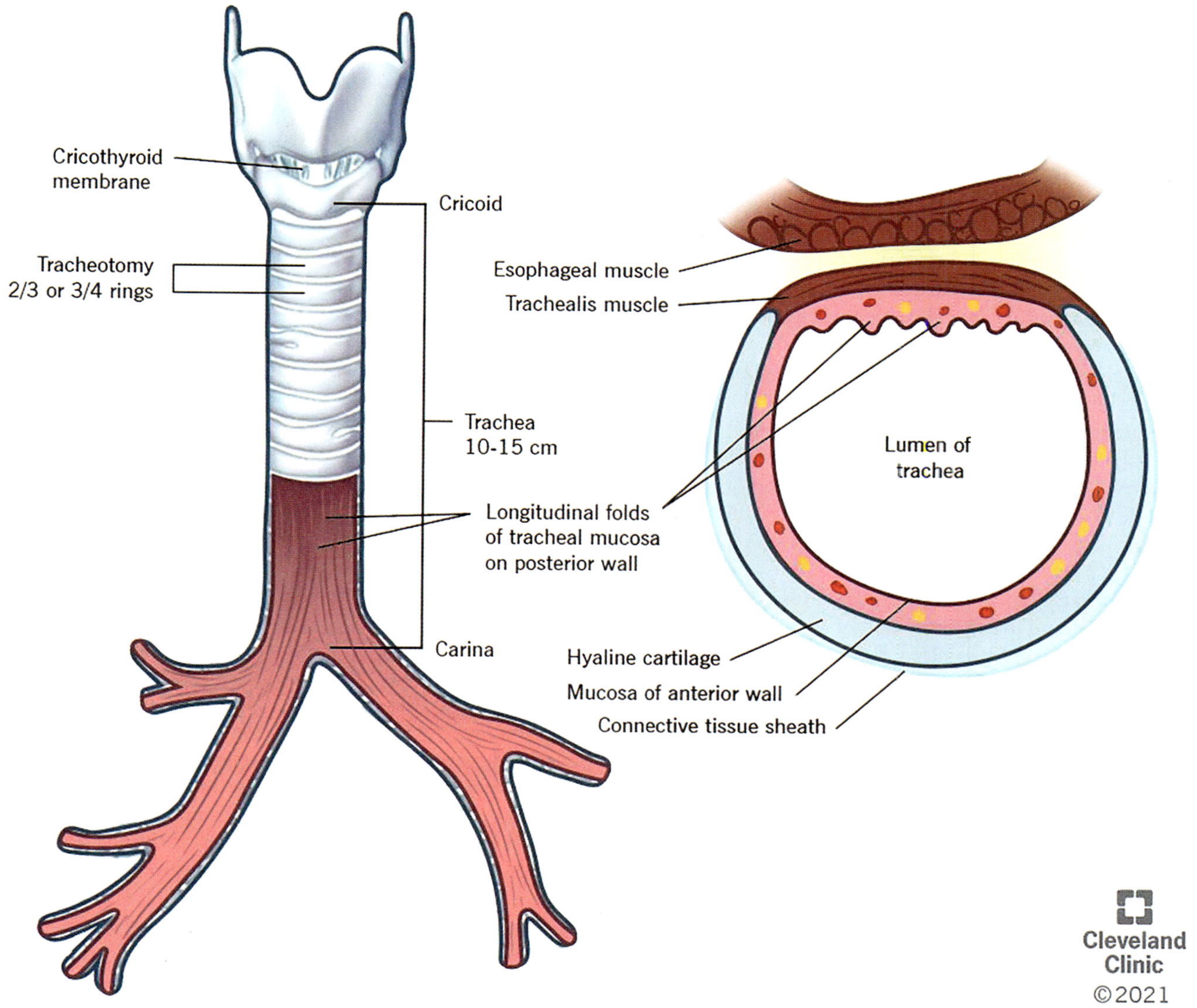

FIGURE 3.17. The trachea and extrapulmonary bronchi, and their relations. Trachea in cut away and in cross-section. Note longitudinal mucosal markings overlying the trachealis muscle posteriorly. (Reprinted with permission Cleveland Clinic Center for Medical Art & Photography ©2021. All Rights Reserved.)

measures 13 to 27 mm in diameter in males and 10 to 23 mm in women.[43] The trachea is comprised of 16 to 20 U-shaped hyaline cartilage rings[34] joined by fibroelastic tissue and closed posteriorly by the trachealis muscle.[6,42,43] The distance from the teeth to carina is 20 to 25 cm in the adult; 22 to 30 cm has also been reported.[41] The cervical part of the trachea rests in the midline but the intrathoracic portion deviates to the right to accommodate the aortic arch.[6,42,43] Classically, longitudinal mucosal markings can be seen posteriorly when the trachea is viewed through the bronchoscope, and these can be used to orient oneself during bronchoscopy (Figure 3.17).

How Is the Anatomy of the Pediatric Airway Different from that of the Adult?

Awake intubation is most often performed in the adult population, and this chapter is directed to this age group. Management of the pediatric airway does require additional consideration of the anatomic differences in children that will not be discussed here. The reader is directed to the pediatric sections of this book (Chapter 46) for further information.

WHAT DRUGS ARE USEFUL FOR AIRWAY ANESTHESIA? WHAT ARE THEIR TOXICITIES AND ASSOCIATED COMPLICATIONS?

Lidocaine, tetracaine, cocaine, benzocaine, and dyclonine have all been used to produce topical anesthesia of the airway, and lidocaine is commonly used to perform glossopharyngeal and SLN block. Dyclonine is a unique local anesthetic agent that was introduced in 1952 and is structurally distinct from the aminoesters and aminoamides. Although its successful use in awake bronchoscopic intubation in a patient with apparent allergy to local anesthetics has been described,[44] it has not been widely used for airway anesthesia and the product has since been discontinued in North America. Hence, our discussion will focus on the other aforementioned local anesthetic agents.

Lidocaine

Developed in 1944,[45] lidocaine is a member of the amide class of local anesthetics and is probably the most commonly used agent for regional anesthesia of the airway.[34,46] Oral lidocaine undergoes extensive first-pass metabolism in the liver[47] and approximately 35% of an oral dose reaches the systemic circulation.[48] It then undergoes significant first-pass hepatic metabolism by mixed function oxidases (CYP450)[47] into two active metabolites, monoethylglycinexylidide (MEGX) and glycylxylidide (GX), and several inactive metabolites.[49–52] MEGX is further metabolized into xylidide through hydrolysis.[51] Amide local anesthetics also bind plasma proteins to varying degrees and are generally weakly bound to abundant plasma proteins including albumin, and more extensively bound to α-1-acid glycoprotein.[52] In animal studies, MEGX has approximately 80% of the anti-arrhythmic activity of lidocaine while xylidide retains just 10% activity.[49,51] Hepatic dysfunction or reductions in hepatic blood flow, as well as congestive heart failure decrease the metabolism of amide local anesthetics and can lead to accumulation of both the parent compound and its active metabolites, promoting local anesthetic systemic toxicity (LAST).[46,48] Both the active and inactive metabolites are ultimately excreted by the kidneys; however renal insufficiency has little impact on the overall pharmacokinetics of local anesthetics.[45,50]

Airway topicalization with lidocaine rapidly produces anesthesia of the mucous membranes in approximately 2 minutes.[37,45] The duration of airway anesthesia ranges from 15 to 40 minutes.[53–55] Interestingly, Watanabe et al. found pre-treatment with intravenous glycopyrrolate 4 $\mu g \cdot kg^{-1}$ increased absorption and prolonged the duration of airway anesthesia with lidocaine (40 minutes vs. 20 minutes).[56] In most circumstances, excellent topical anesthesia of the airway in the adult can be produced by 4% (40 $mg \cdot mL^{-1}$) lidocaine. With 2% (20 $mg \cdot mL^{-1}$) lidocaine, topical anesthesia may be inadequate, and at 1% (10 $mg \cdot mL^{-1}$), lidocaine is insufficient for airway instrumentation.[57,58] Increasing the concentration beyond the optimum level of 4% does not affect the onset time or duration of effect.[57] Importantly, unlike local anesthetic infiltration, the addition of topical epinephrine penetrates mucous membranes poorly and does not slow the rate of anesthetic absorption.[59] The extent of systemic absorption depends on the site and technique of application, tissue vascularity, the total dose administered, the state of the mucosa, the concomitant use of drying agents,[56] the amount of mucous present, the rate and depth of respiration, the state of the circulation, the patient's disease state, dose per unit of body weight, and individual variation.[47,55,60–62] Absorption is quite rapid when local anesthetics are applied to the tracheobronchial tree[57,63] and alveolar absorption may approximate IV administration due to osmotic relationships in the pulmonary vascular bed designed to prevent the collection of fluid in the alveolar spaces.[57,64,65] Decreased rates of absorption occur in the upper airway secondary to decreased vascularity and surface area.[61]

The commonly accepted toxic plasma concentration of lidocaine is 5 $\mu g \cdot mL^{-1}$ or greater.[66,67] As plasma concentrations rise to this level and above, symptoms of systemic toxicity can occur including, but not limited to, light-headedness, tinnitus, perioral tingling, visual disturbances, and muscle twitching.[62,68] Seizures are most frequently seen at higher plasma concentrations, although they have occurred at plasma concentrations as low as 6 $\mu g \cdot mL^{-1}$.[61] Convulsions are classically followed by coma and respiratory arrest, arrhythmias, and cardiovascular collapse.[50,62,68] It should be noted, however, that excitatory manifestations of toxicity may be brief or not occur at all prior to loss of consciousness.[68,69] Clinical evidence of toxicity has been reported following lidocaine topicalization with doses between 6.0 and 9.3 $mg \cdot kg^{-1}$ lean body weight (LBW). Although a universally "safe" dose of lidocaine for topicalization has not, and likely cannot be definitively established, current guidelines suggest a maximum dose of topical lidocaine of about 9 $mg \cdot kg^{-1}$ LBW.[55] The terminal half-life of lidocaine is up to 2 hours; therefore, patients should remain nil per os for at least 2 hours following topicalization to guard against aspiration.[55] Hypersensitivity reactions to lidocaine, although exceedingly rare, may occur.[54] Methylparaben, used as a preservative, is structurally related to para-aminobenzoic acid (PABA, a known allergen), and can be responsible for some allergic reactions.[70] Methemoglobinemia has been reported in association with lidocaine administration, although these instances are also extremely rare.[71–73]

When the use of lidocaine is discussed in the context of topical anesthesia of the airway it is important to understand what the terms "aerosolization," "atomization," and "nebulization" mean. "Atomization" and "nebulization" are often used interchangeably and the terminology can be confusing. An aerosol can be defined as a suspension of particulate matter (such as droplets) in a gaseous medium (such as air or oxygen).[74] Aerosolization is the process of generating an aerosol. Atomizers use a driving gas and a Venturi to generate droplets from a solution that are typically 15 to 500 μm in diameter.[75] Jet and ultrasonic nebulizers incorporate baffles which selectively remove large droplets and deliver particles mostly 1 to 5 μm in diameter.[75] Deposition of the aerosol particles in the airway depends to a large extent on the particle or droplet size.[75] The peak deposition of aerosol droplets occurs in the peripheral airway for droplets of about 2 μm, in bronchioles for droplets of about 8 μm, in bronchi for droplets of about 15 μm, and in the upper airway for droplets larger than 40 μm.[76] Higher oxygen flow rates through nebulizers create smaller droplets (less than 30 μm) that travel further distally into the bronchial tree and increase the rate of absorption.[53] A droplet diameter between 1 and 5 μm is preferable for central and deep lung penetration[77] and a diameter <2 μm may be ideal for penetration to the most distal parts of the lung.[78] Particles <0.5 μm may avoid deposition altogether and be exhaled.[75] Droplets larger than 60 μm are preferred for airway anesthesia during awake intubation because they "rain out" in the proximal airway where topical anesthesia is required.[53] Therefore, when used for topical anesthesia of the airway, lidocaine is best delivered by atomizers rather than nebulizers.

In summary, it is important to consider the concentration and total dose of local anesthetic used, the topicalization method employed, the time course of administration, and the physiologic state and comorbidities of individual patients when evaluating the risk of toxicity for upper airway topicalization. The recommended maximum safe dose of topical lidocaine that can be applied to the airway has not been definitively established but is suggested to be approximately 9 mg·kg^{-1} LBW.[55] In practice, the smallest amount of anesthetic sufficient to achieve the desired effect should be used[79] and in general, the use of large doses for awake tracheal intubation is unnecessary. As always, clinical judgment is required and meticulous attention to detail should be employed when lidocaine is applied to the airway such that effective anesthesia is achieved without producing toxicity.

Tetracaine

Tetracaine, a long-acting amino-ester local anesthetic, was introduced in 1932 and is still used for spinal anesthesia and topical anesthesia.[45,60] It is hydrolyzed in the blood by plasma pseudocholinesterase to PABA[70] and diethylaminoethanol.[80] Allergic reaction, although rare, is more likely with the ester group of local anesthetics as compared to the amides, due in part to their metabolism into PABA.[70] The presence of atypical pseudocholinesterase is associated with decreased metabolism. Although once widely used for topical anesthesia of the airway, its use fell into disfavor after reports of toxic reactions and fatalities were published in the 1950s.[64,81]

Of the local anesthetics possessing topical action, tetracaine is among the most potent as well as the most toxic,[64] with tetracaine being about six times more toxic than cocaine.[59] When applied to the mucous membranes, it is rapidly absorbed into the circulation such that blood levels are almost comparable to those obtained after IV injection.[82] The maximal effective concentration of topical tetracaine is 1%.[57] The maximum safe dosage of tetracaine in the adult has never been clearly defined, however, aerosolized doses as low as 20 mg have been reported to cause toxicity and fatalities have occurred with doses of 100 mg.[64] A maximum dose of 20 mg of tetracaine hydrochloride has been recommended,[64,83,84] but some literature sources have cited maximum doses ranging between 50 and 100 mg.[85] Topical tetracaine produces excellent intubating conditions; however, because of its potential for severe toxicity and narrow therapeutic window, its use cannot be recommended,[86] especially when a much safer and equally effective alternative (lidocaine) is available.

Benzocaine: How Safe and Effective Is Benzocaine?

Benzocaine (ethyl aminobenzoate), is a water-insoluble ethyl ester of PABA and a local anesthetic that has been used to topicalize the airway.[84,87] It is most often available as a 20% spray that can produce topical anesthesia within 15 to 30 seconds of application, with a typical duration of 5 to 10[86] or 12 to 15 minutes.[87,88] It is also a component of Cetacaine®, a mixture containing 14% benzocaine, 2% tetracaine, and 2% butyl aminobenzoate (butamben).[89] Cetacaine also produces rapid onset topical anesthesia, but has extended duration of action (30-60 minutes) in comparison to benzocaine alone.[89]

Several reports of benzocaine-induced methemoglobinemia have been published since the 1950s and have limited the widespread clinical use of benzocaine.[73,90–92] Benzocaine has resulted in severe methemoglobinemia following the administration of as little as three or four 1-second sprays in adults.[87] The occurrence of benzocaine-induced methemoglobinemia appears to be unpredictable, idiosyncratic, and not directly related to dose.[93,94] Patients with active systemic infection,[95] G6PD or NADPH-dependent methemoglobin reductase deficiency[87] or who have primary relatives with a history of this reaction[96] may be at increased risk of this potentially fatal condition. A review of methemoglobinemia related to local anesthetics recommended that benzocaine should no longer be used.[73] Given its short duration of action and its potential for severe toxicity, the use of benzocaine as a topical anesthetic for airway management is difficult to justify when a much safer and equally effective alternative is available, namely lidocaine.

Cocaine: Does Cocaine Have a Role in Providing Topical Airway Anesthesia in Current Anesthesia Practice?

Cocaine (benzoylmethylecgonine) is an ester of benzoic acid and methylecgonine, extracted from the leaves of the coca plant.[97–99] It is the only local anesthetic that inhibits reuptake of norepinephrine and thereby produces vasoconstriction; hence its widespread use in the past for nasal procedures.[59,98,100] In addition, it is a sympathomimetic drug that causes the release of norepinephrine and epinephrine from the adrenal medulla and antagonizes voltage sodium channels in cardiac myocytes.[99] Cocaine is well absorbed through all mucous membranes[99,101] and metabolized by plasma butyrylcholinesterase and liver carboxylesterases into water-soluble metabolites which are excreted in the urine.[102] Peak plasma concentrations occur 20 to 60 minutes after nasal application[98,102] and the serum half-life after nasal application is approximately 90 minutes.[102] The maximum effective concentration of topical cocaine is 20%, and this solution produces an anesthetic effect within 0.3 minutes and has a duration of action of 54.5 minutes.[45] Typically, 1% to 10% cocaine is used clinically.[86]

The maximum recommended dose for topical nasal application is 3 mg·kg^{-1}.[53,102] However, toxic reactions have occurred after administration of as little as 10 to 30 mg.[98,100,103] Cocaine has been associated with hypertension, coronary artery spasm, angina, myocardial infarction, arrhythmias, sudden cardiac death, and myocardial contraction bands.[99,104,105] In addition, it has been stated that cocaine should be avoided or used cautiously in the presence of hypertension, hyperthyroidism, angina, or in patients taking monoamine oxidase inhibitors (MAOIs).[53] A survey of otolaryngoscopists published in 2004 reported 14 deaths associated with the administration of cocaine,[100] and this was compared to a similar survey published in 1977 which had reported 15 deaths. In contrast, topical cocaine was used without complications in a series of 92 bronchoscopies published in 2010.[106]

Oxymetazoline has been shown to be as effective as cocaine in the prevention of epistaxis caused by nasotracheal intubation,[107,108] as has normal saline,[108] phenylephrine/lidocaine,[103,109], and phenylephrine alone.[103] A study by Tarver et al. compared cocaine and lidocaine with oxymetazoline for nasal procedures and found no difference in local anesthetic efficacy.[110] Cocaine is listed as a schedule II controlled substance by the United States Drug Enforcement Agency and has a Black Box Warning due to is high potential for abuse and dependence.[102] Based on the available evidence, the disadvantages associated with the use of cocaine to produce nasal anesthesia for awake intubation far outweigh any potential advantage.

AIRWAY ANESTHESIA TECHNIQUES: TOPICAL ANESTHESIA AND NERVE BLOCKS

What Anesthetic Techniques Can Be Used to Anesthetize the Airway?

A description of the most commonly employed airway nerve blocks is described in the following section. Although a topicalization technique appears to be nearly universally preferred, airway nerve blocks can be an efficient and effective method of establishing airway anesthesia, particularly in patients with a soiled airway or "bloody" airway, provided the practitioner has the appropriate expertise and knowledge of local anatomy.

The recommended topicalization technique is described in the section ***What Technique Works Well for Awake Intubation?*** of this chapter.

Which Blocks Are Most Commonly Used?

Current literature on the amount of training and subsequent use of airway blocks among trainees and attending anesthesiologists is lacking. The most recent data available surveyed U.S. and Canadian anesthesiology residency programs about airway training in 2011.[111] Among the 88 of 147 schools who responded, topical anesthesia was employed almost universally (99%) to anesthetize the upper airway. Instruction in transtracheal injection was reported by 72%; SLN block, 53%; glossopharyngeal nerve block, 28%; and sphenopalatine/anterior ethmoid nerve blocks, 10%. Again, topical lidocaine provides excellent conditions for awake bronchoscopic intubation in most patients and current guidelines suggest that percutaneous airway nerve blocks be reserved for practitioners with adequate expertise in their use.[55]

Is there a role for ultrasound-guided regional techniques in nerve blocks of the airway?

Palpation of key landmarks for airway blocks may be difficult in the presence of obesity, variant anatomy, and anatomic distortion. The use of ultrasonography for nerve blocks of the airway was first published as a case report by Manikandan and colleagues in 2010, where it was applied to perform bilateral SLN blocks to supplement airway anesthesia prior to awake bronchoscopic intubation in a patient with a recent atlantoaxial fusion and obscured anatomical landmarks.[112] Using a high-frequency (5-10 MHz) linear probe placed transversely over the neck—initially at the submandibular triangle, then moved caudally and laterally—they systematically identified the external carotid artery, followed by the superior thyroid artery and SLA, which travels with the internal branch of the SLN to pierce the thyrohyoid membrane. The greater cornu of the hyoid was located medial to the SLA and a 22-gauge needle was introduced using an out-of-plane technique to deposit lidocaine in the plane between the greater cornu and the artery. A change in the patient's voice quality over a few minutes signaled onset of the block. Although achievable, the transverse approach and sonoanatomy is technically challenging due to the compact nature of the structures of the neck. Furthermore, significant variability in the origin of the superior thyroid and superior laryngeal arteries may make identification of these structures under ultrasound difficult, even for an experienced practitioner.[113–115] The close proximity of the air-filled trachea and larynx results in hyperechoic artifacts that may contribute to these difficulties.[116] Subsequent studies were unable to replicate images of the SLN using ultrasonography,[115,117,118] or noted an inability to visualize it due to limitations in spatial resolution.[119]

The introduction of small-footprint, high-frequency probes expanded the possible applications of ultrasound in the performance of airway nerve blocks. A technique developed by Kaur et al[120] used a high-frequency linear probe (8-15 MHz HST15 8/20) in the shape of a small hockey stick placed sagittally to initially identify the greater cornu of the hyoid bone in the submandibular area of 20 volunteers, positioned supine. The medial aspect of the probe is then rotated to rest obliquely across the neck, somewhat parallel to the mandible, and visualize the key structures including the superior horn of the thyroid cartilage inferolaterally and the SLN and SLA superiorly and medially, just prior to piercing the hyperechoic thyrohyoid membrane. Ultrasound-guided in-plane needling using cadavers confirmed the successful spread of dye along the SLN using this approach, highlighting its potential clinical utility. Successful use of this technique to facilitate awake bronchoscopic intubations in trauma patients with predicted difficult airways has been published in a case series.[121] Interestingly, a similar approach with a small footprint, 11-mm curvilinear transducer (8-5 MHz, C11 SonoSite, Bothell, WA) has been described, with visualization of both the SLN, artery, and vein between the strap muscles and thyrohyoid membrane when the probe is placed in a sagittal orientation on the lateral side of the neck, with the patient's head turned away.[122] An in-plane approach is taken with a 25 g needle and 2 mL of 2% lidocaine is injected around the nerve within the potential space between the thyroid membrane and thyrohyoid muscle after negative aspiration.

A more common approach that does not require visualization of the SLN is the ultrasound-guided deposition of local anesthetic within the "SLN space," first described by Barberet et al.[119] It is a potential space through which the internal branch of the SLN (ibSLN) travels bounded by the (i) thyrohyoid muscle anteriorly, (ii) thyrohyoid membrane posteriorly, (iii) thyroid cartilage inferiorly, and (iv) hyoid bone superiorly, as imaged in the parasagittal plane using a high-frequency linear probe. In his initial study, optimal images could be attained in 81% of subjects, and advanced age, obesity (BMI > 30 kg m^{-2}), and thick neck circumference (>40 cm) were factors associated with suboptimal views. The feasibility of targeting the SLN space using ultrasound rather than the nerve itself has since been tested in small cadaver studies using both in-plane and out-of-plane approaches, with some success.[118,123] To date, a single randomized controlled study has compared an ultrasound-guided ibSLN block of the SLN space to a traditional landmark technique for quality of airway anesthesia during awake nasal bronchoscopic intubation.[124] Twenty patients were included in each group and all patients received topicalization with 3 mL of nebulized 4% lidocaine, 3 mL 2% lidocaine transtracheal injection, and low-dose IV midazolam for sedation. Blinded observers of the flexible bronchoscopic intubation rated the quality of topical anesthesia significantly better in the ultrasound group, with the majority of patients in that group having no gag or cough response to intubation ($p < 0.001$), while 15 out of 20 in the landmark SLN block group experienced mild to moderate cough or gag with intubation.

While several studies have examined the utility of ultrasound for percutaneous cricothyrotomy and tracheotomy placement,[125–129] few studies have been published specifically on the use of ultrasound for performing translaryngeal airway blocks. Rare case reports have described successful identification of the midline and CTM using ultrasonography to facilitate translaryngeal block after failure of a traditional landmark technique in an obese patient[130] and in a patient with obscured landmarks due to an odontogenic abscess.[131] Krause et al. described an in-plane technique using a small curvilinear 8 to 5 MHz probe, wherein a 22 g needle could be advanced in a caudal direction through the CTM in the midline until the aspiration of free air, confirming placement in the trachea.[122] Of note, while a longitudinal approach allows simultaneous visualization of the CTM and tracheal rings, it may result in accidental nonmidline needle placement and complications including failure, tissue damage, and/or vascular injury.[132] In comparison, an transverse out-of-plane approach may allow for continuous imaging of the midline, but at the cost of visualizing the cricothyroid and thyroid cartilages themselves during needle advancement. Alternatively, preprocedural ultrasound scanning and skin marking may add to the safety of a landmark-guided approach.

Landmark-based extraoral (peristyloid) approaches to the glossopharyngeal nerve are associated with significant procedural risk due to its proximity to the vagus nerve, hypoglossal nerve, and internal carotid artery.[133] No ultrasound-guided glossopharyngeal nerve block techniques have been described for the purpose of awake intubation. However, ultrasound-guided glossopharyngeal nerve blockade has been safely applied in the treatment of chronic pain syndromes (Eagle's syndrome), intractable cancer pain, and could conceivably be applied for glossopharyngeal nerve blocks for airway managment.[134–137]

While further study of ultrasound-guided airway nerve blocks is certainly needed, these techniques have potential to provide high-quality airway anesthesia in clinical situations where external anatomical landmarks are obscured, or topicalization by other means is ineffective or not feasible.

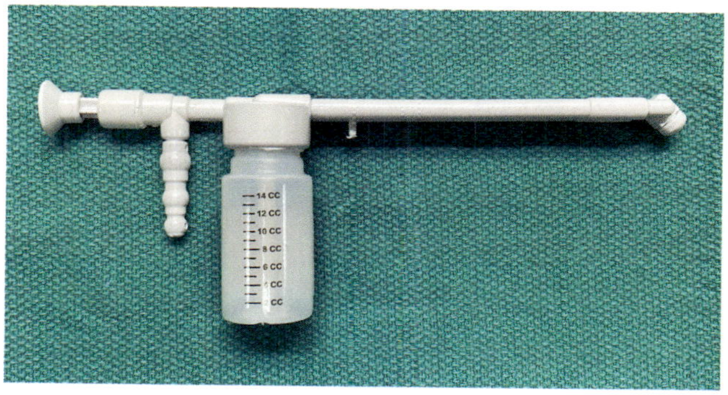

FIGURE 3.18. EZ-Spray (EZ-100m, Alcove Medical Corporation, Houston, Texas).

Topical Anesthesia (Video 28)

In 2011, Pott et al.[111] reported the results of a survey of airway training among U.S. and Canadian anesthesiology residency programs. Of those who responded to the survey (88 of 147 programs), topical anesthesia was employed almost universally (99%) to anesthetize the upper airway. In clinical practice, topical anesthesia is the main stay of anesthesia for awake intubation in most cases.

The posterior tongue, soft palate, tonsillar pillars, and oropharynx can typically be easily anesthetized topically using either Lidocaine 5% Ointment, Lidocaine 10% spray, or Lidocaine 4% solution via a mucosal atomizing device, an aerosol spraying device or by gargling.

Lidocaine 5% ointment can be used to provide anesthesia to the posterior third of the tongue. It can be applied to a tongue depressor and be placed on the posterior aspect of the patient's tongue. As the ointment rests on the tongue, it will begin to melt and spread the local anesthetic to a wider area. This can be a useful early first step in the topicalization process.

An aerosolized solution of lidocaine 4% can provide effective topicalization of the naso, oro, and hypopharynx. This can be administered via an aerosolization device, such as the disposable EZ-Spray (Figure 3.18; EZ-100m, Alcove Medical Corporation, Houston, TX). The device is connected to pressurize oxygen as the driving gas. The dose of local anesthetic in the reservoir should be monitored to avoid unintentional overdose and a risk of LAST.[138] Administration can also be accomplished using a MADgic © laryngotracheal mucosal atomization device (MAD) (Figure 3.19; Teleflex Medical, Morrisville, NC, USA). This device attaches to a standard luer-lock syringe attachment

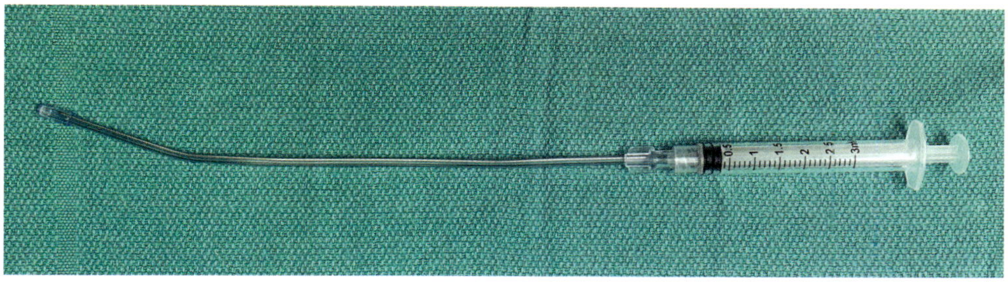

FIGURE 3.19. Laryngotracheal mucosal atomization device (MAD) (Teleflex Medical, Morrisville, NC, USA).

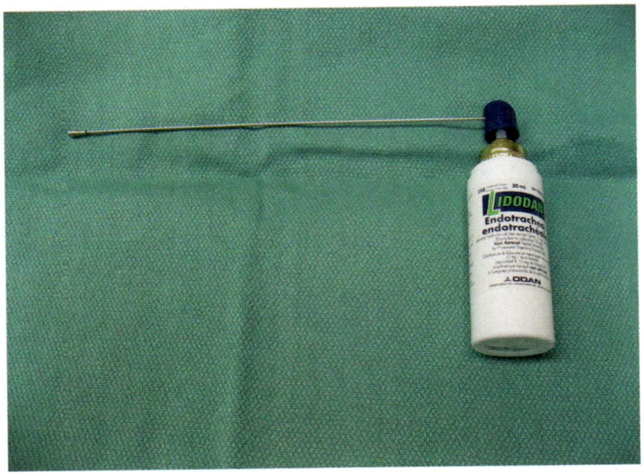

FIGURE 3.20. The 10% lidocaine aerosol fitted with a malleable stainless-steel nozzle (LidodanTM Endotracheal, Odan Laboratories Limited, Montreal, Quebec, Canada).

and consists of a plastic lumen with an integrated metallic malleable stylet that can allow targeting of the aerosol.

Lidocaine 10% spray is commercially available and marketed in Canada by Odan Laboratories Limited, Montreal, Quebec, Canada. This is a metered pump-action spray that delivers 10 mg of lidocaine per spray (Figure 3.20). It has a disposable metallic malleable spray nozzle. which can be used to direct the medication to the area of interest. This is particularly useful in emergency situations when the time needed for typical topicalization may be limited.

Glossopharyngeal Nerve Block

The glossopharyngeal nerve can be blocked in the oropharynx as it travels deep to the mucosa of the palatopharyngeal fold (posterior tonsillar pillar).[133,139–143] Alternatively, the lingual branches of the glossopharyngeal nerve, supplying primarily the posterior one-third of the tongue, can be blocked deep to the mucosa of the palatoglossal fold (anterior tonsillar pillar) with retrograde spread local anesthetic through the submucosa causing blockade of the pharyngeal and tonsillar branches in some cases.[143] An extraoral peristyloid approach to the glossopharyngeal nerve has also been described with and without ultrasound guidance.[134–136,144] While these blocks are safe and effective in experienced hands, they carry the potential for significant complications including intra-arterial injection, patient discomfort, hematoma formation, and anatomic distortion.[140] In addition, local anesthetic injected into the floor of the mouth anterior to the palatoglossal fold can result in an unintentional hypoglossal nerve block and impair the ability to swallow.[143,145] Ultimately, glossopharyngeal nerve blocks may be impractical in the setting of difficult intubation as an adequate mouth opening is required to expose the base of the tonsillar pillars, and patients with a strong gag reflex may require topicalization of the tongue and oropharynx in order to tolerate retraction of the tongue and placement of the needle tip.

Topicalization of the pharyngeal mucosa with atomized lidocaine and the application of 5% lidocaine ointment to the posterior one-third of the tongue is sufficient to abolish the gag reflex in the vast majority of individuals. With wide availability of these less invasive techniques, glossopharyngeal nerve blocks for the sole purpose of awake bronchoscopic intubation are rarely done in modern anesthetic practice and are reserved only for those with knowledge of local anatomy and adequate experience in their performance.[55,145]

Superior Laryngeal Nerve Block

The internal branch of the SLN travels just deep to the mucosa of the piriform fossae bilaterally. It can be blocked transmucosally at this location by using Krause or Jackson forceps to apply a cotton pledget soaked with 4% lidocaine against the mucosa in the piriform fossa for 1 to 2 minutes (Figure 3.21).[46,53] Anesthesia of the posterior third of the tongue is required prior to performing this block, and can be easily achieved with 5% lidocaine ointment applied to the base of the tongue using a simple wooden tongue depressor or similar instrument as discussed above.

Alternatively, ibSLN block can be performed using an external approach to the nerve as it penetrates the thyrohyoid membrane between the greater cornu of the hyoid bone and superior cornu of the thyroid cartilage, as has been historically taught

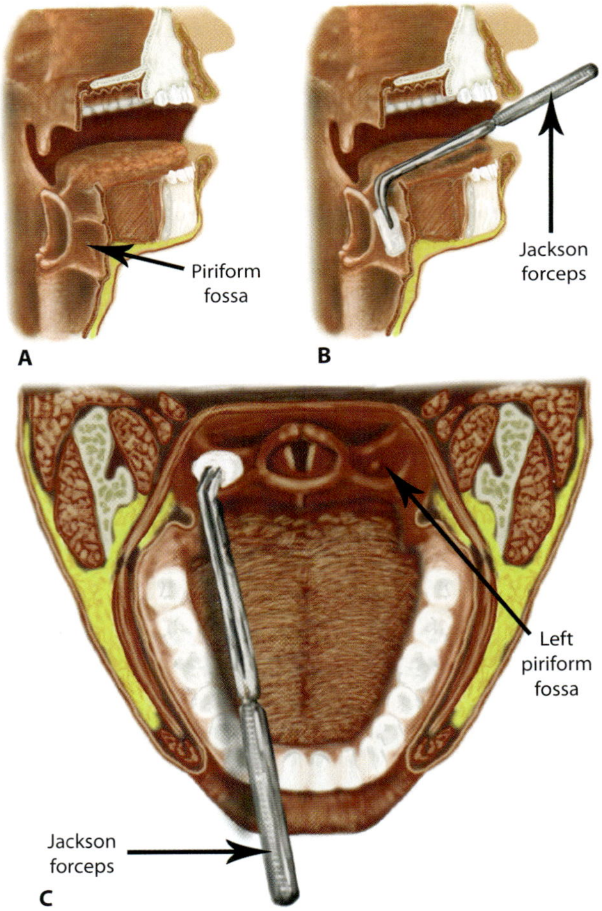

FIGURE 3.21. Schematic illustration of transmucosal superior laryngeal nerve block using Jackson forceps and a cotton pledget soaked in 4% lidocaine placed in **(A)** the piriform fossa and show the **(B)** lateral and **(C)** superior view of the block.

and recommended in the 1970s through 1990s.[46,53,139,144,146] This technique is rarely used in contemporary practice but may be useful in circumstances where the topical approach to the ibSLN is not possible due to restricted mouth opening, for example.[146] In the supine position with the neck extended, the patient's hyoid bone is palpated as a mobile bony structure superior to the thyroid cartilage. The hyoid is grasped between the thumb and index finger and displaced toward the side intended to be blocked (Figure 3.22).[144] Using the dominant hand, a 21- to 25-gauge needle is passed through the skin to contact the greater cornu of the hyoid and then walked caudally until it slips below the bone and into the thyrohyoid membrane. The needle is then advanced 2 to 3 mm to enter the paraglottic space, bounded laterally by the thyrohyoid membrane and medially by the mucosa of the piriform fossa. After negative aspiration, 2 to 3 mL of 2% lidocaine can then be injected as the needle is withdrawn.[34,133,146] If air is aspirated, the needle is likely within the laryngopharynx and the tip should be slowly withdrawn until the aspiration of air ceases. If blood is aspirated, the needle may have punctured the superior laryngeal vessels that travel with the SLN or the carotid artery. To remedy this, the needle should be withdrawn and redirected more anteriorly. An alternative approach using the superior cornu of the thyroid cartilage as the primary landmark can be performed if the hyoid bone cannot be adequately palpated.[46,144,146] Using a very similar technique, the needle is inserted to contact the greater cornu of the thyroid cartilage and then walked off the cartilage anteriorly and superiorly to pierce the thyrohyoid membrane (Figure 3.23).[146] A cadaver study by Canty and Poon demonstrated equivalent staining of the SLN with dye injected into the paraglottic space using either the hyoid bone or thyroid cartilage as a landmark.[147] Finally, the thyrohyoid

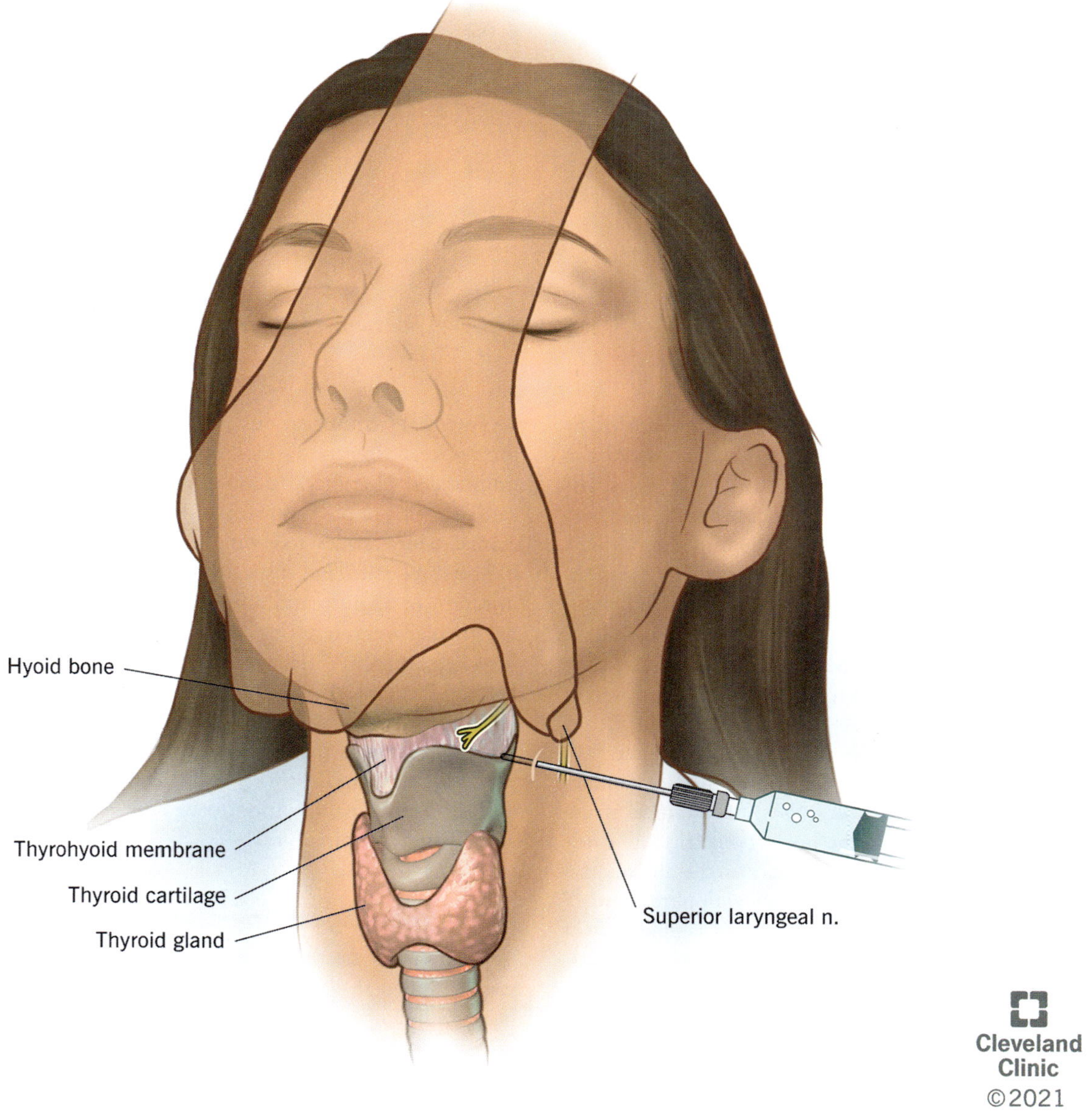

FIGURE 3.22. Schematic illustration of superior laryngeal nerve block. (Reprinted with permission Cleveland Clinic Center for Medical Art & Photography ©2021. All Rights Reserved.)

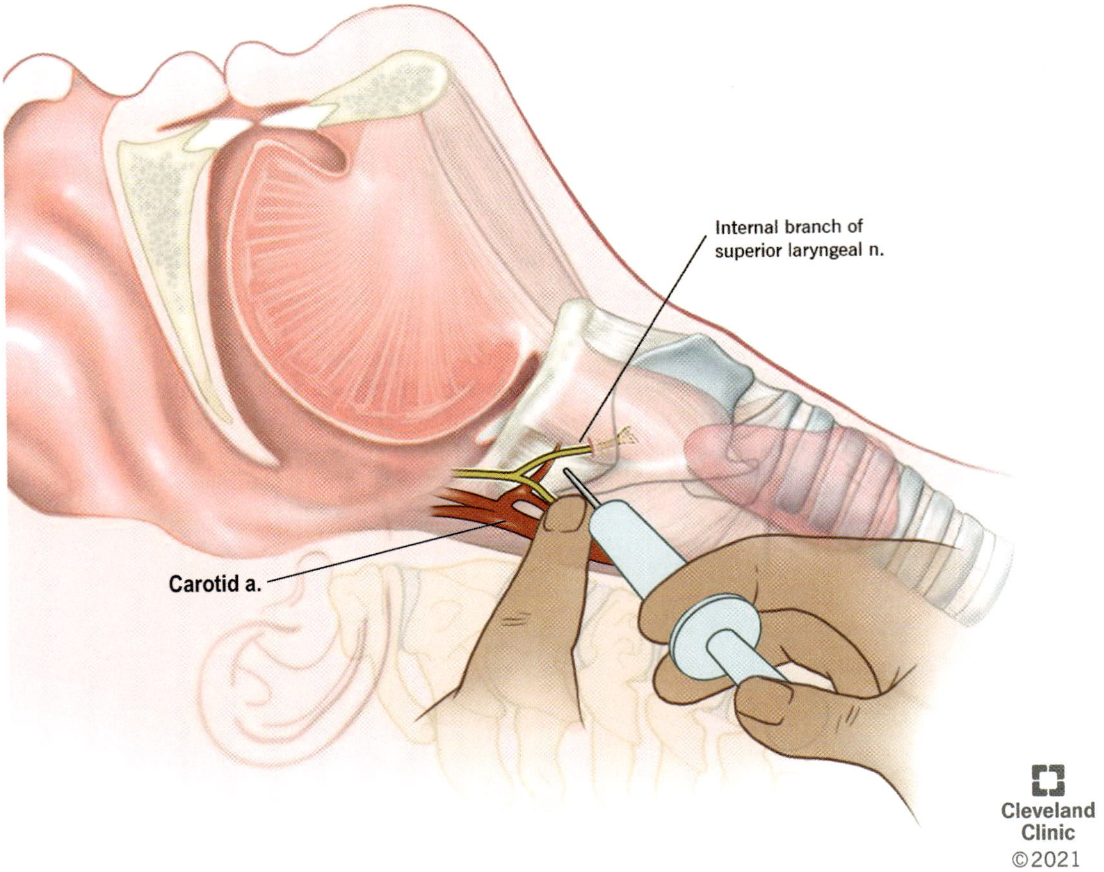

FIGURE 3.23. Alternative technique of superior laryngeal nerve block. (Reprinted with permission Cleveland Clinic Center for Medical Art & Photography ©2021. All Rights Reserved.)

membrane itself can be identified and directly punctured to perform the block. After palpating the thyroid notch in the midline, the superior edge of the thyroid cartilage is traced laterally for approximately 2 cm before puncturing the skin just above the cartilage and advancing the needle into a depth of 1 to 2 cm to pierce the thyrohyoid membrane at this location. The resistance felt as the needle pierces the membrane is helpful in both identifying it and indicating when the needle is at an appropriate depth to inject local anesthetic.[46,144] The onset time for SLN block is approximately 5 to 10 minutes.[86] Its duration of action has been reported to be at least 60 minutes,[140] but may be as long as 4 to 6 hours when 2% lidocaine is used.[86,146]

An ultrasound-guided approach can also be used to conduct an SLN Block (*see previous relevant section*). The critical structures in the ultrasound view are the hyoid bone, thyroid cartilage, thyrohyoid membrane, strap muscle, and the air-mucosal interface, which are generally easy to identify with ultrasound.[118] A linear high-frequency transducer is placed in a sagittal view of the upper border of the larynx and then is slowly translated lateral to a parasagittal view of the upper larynx, just anterior to the greater horn of the hyoid cartilage and the superior cornu of the thyroid cartilage (Figure 3.24). Local anesthetic, such as 2 mL of lidocaine 2% can be injected deep to the thyrohyoid muscle, but superficial to the thyrohyoid membrane (Figure 3.25). For the purpose of awake intubation, the nerve block would have to be completed bilaterally.

Potential complications of the SLN block include intra-arterial injection, local anesthetic toxicity, hematoma, unintended pharyngeal perforation, hypotension, and bradycardia.[53,133,140,144,146] A rare case of monocular blindness and cranial neuropathies following a landmark-based SLN block has been reported and suspected to be due to the unrecognized injection of air into and around the carotid artery and internal jugular vein resulting in pneumocephalus and ischemic optic neuropathy.[148] Hence, the carotid artery should always be palpated and displaced posteriorly[149] during the procedure to reduce the risk of intravascular injection (see Figure 3.23). Contraindications include local pathology, coagulopathy, and poor anatomic landmarks.[53,144] The block has also been thought (although not unanimously) to be contraindicated in patients at high risk of aspiration.[150]

Translaryngeal Anesthesia

Translaryngeal anesthesia for the purposes of awake intubation was described in an editorial by John Bonica in 1949, where he described its successful use in 1200 patients over the course of 3 years.[151] In a supine patient with the neck extended, the CTM is identified and a 20- to 23-gauge needle can be placed in the midline and directed posteriorly and somewhat caudally to enter the larynx (Figure 3.26).[6,46] Aiming the needle slightly caudally directs it away from the vocal cords which are located

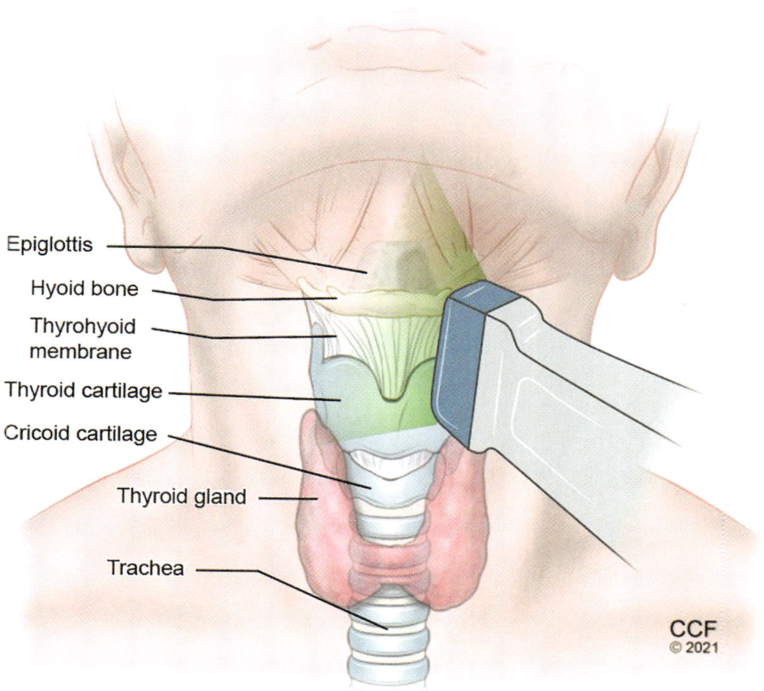

FIGURE 3.24. Transducer position for sagittal visualization of ultrasound guided superior laryngeal nerve block. (Reprinted with permission Cleveland Clinic Center for Medical Art & Photography ©2021. All Rights Reserved.)

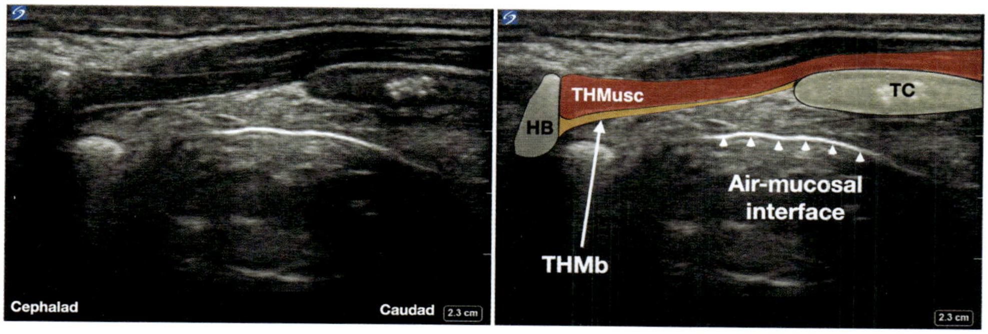

FIGURE 3.25. Ultrasound parasagittal view for ultrasound guided superior laryngeal nerve block. Injection should be into the plane between the thyrohyoid muscle and the thyrohyoid membrane. Air-mucosal interface (arrows), HB (hyoid bone), THMb (thyrohyoid membrane), TC (thyroid cartilage), THMusc (thyrohyoid muscle).

approximately 1 cm above the transverse plane at the midpoint of the CTM.[36] A loss of resistance is felt as the needle passes through the CTM, and correct position of the needle within the tracheal lumen is confirmed by the aspiration of air.[36,133] Alternatively, a 20-gauge angiocatheter can be used with the catheter advanced slightly over the needle tip after the aspiration of air. The needle is then withdrawn, leaving the catheter in place.[34] During inhalation (or at end exhalation), 2 to 5 mL of lidocaine 2% to 4% should then be rapidly injected with the expectation of vigorous coughing afterward.[34,36] Coughing aids the nebulization and spread of local anesthetic throughout the infraglottic area, as well as the inferior and superior surfaces of the vocal cords and the tracheobronchial tree. Spread of local anesthetic to supraglottic structures (epiglottis, vallecula, tongue, and pharynx) using this technique is possible, but unreliable. The extent of sensory blockade above the glottis is dependent on the magnitude of the cough response.[152] If the goal is to spread anesthetic into the supraglottic larynx and pharynx, then injection at end inhalation seems the most appropriate to achieve this.

Contraindications to needle puncture through the CTM include coagulopathy, presence of a large or other local pathology, and an inability to identify the membrane due to obscured landmarks as in the case of morbid obesity. Clearly, an inability to identify the CTM has implications for the efficacy of translaryngeal block as well as complications. Identification of

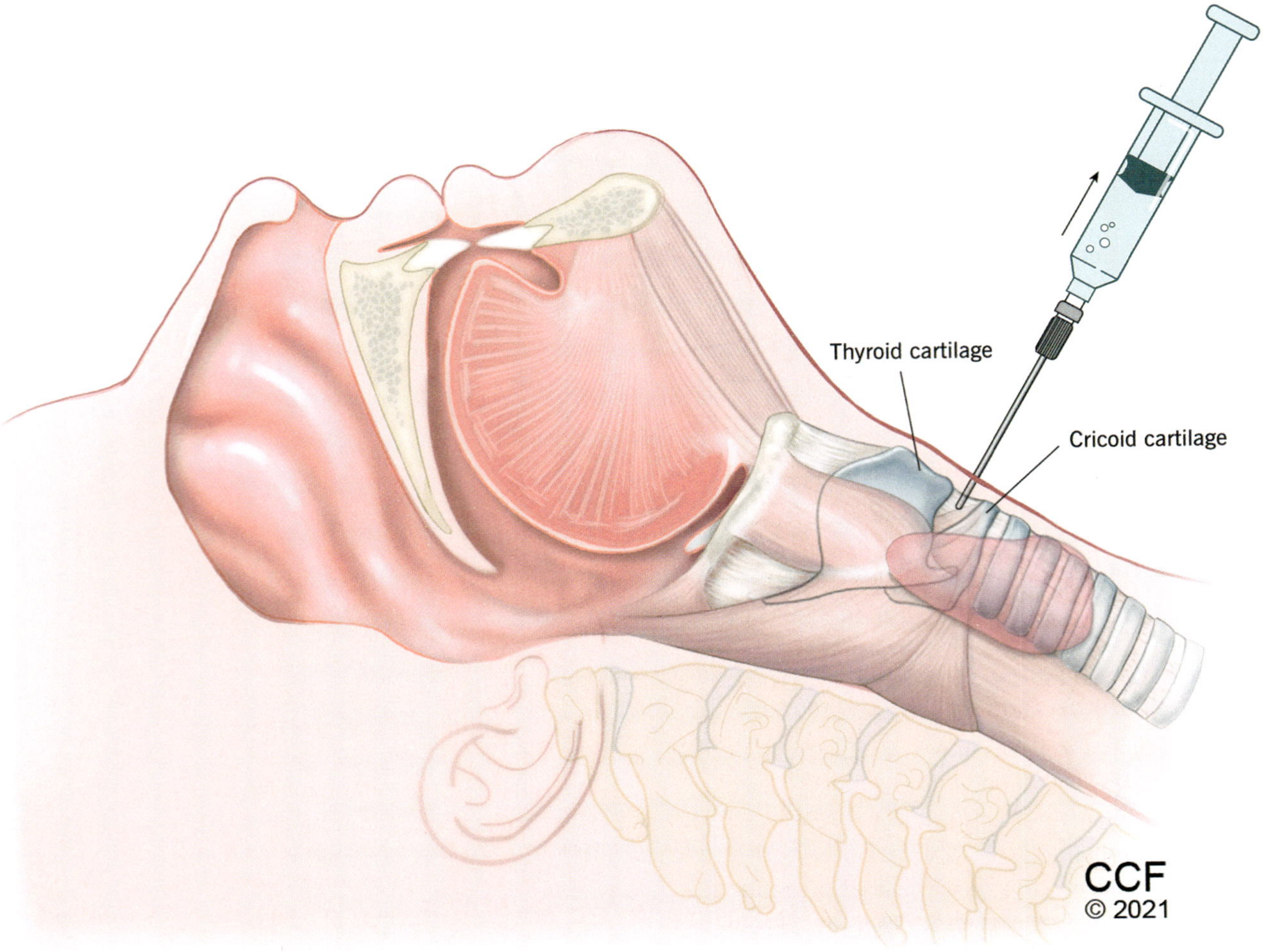

FIGURE 3.26. Needle position for a trans-cricothyroid injection. (Reprinted with permission Cleveland Clinic Center for Medical Art & Photography ©2021. All Rights Reserved.)

the CTM by anesthesia practitioners through palpation alone has been previously studied and associated with high failure rates.[153–155] The CTM was correctly identified in only 18% to 42% of study subjects overall, with success rates in subgroups ranging from 72% in nonobese males to 0% in obese females.[153,154] Patients with neck deformity or previous neck surgery were excluded from two of the studies.[153,155]

Ultrasound-guided landmarking of the CTM has gained prominence in recent years as a simple, yet effective technique to identify the CTM in a wide variety of patients. A meta-analysis comparing digital palpation and ultrasound-guided techniques for accuracy in identifying the CTM examined eight studies that included adult volunteers with normal anatomy,[155–158] cadavers or patients with poor surface landmarks (previous neck surgery, radiation or masses),[159–161] and pediatric subjects.[162] Ultrasound-guided approaches resulted in a significantly reduced failure rate compared to palpation, at the cost of a slightly longer procedural time that did not reach statistical significance.[163]

The cartilages of the larynx and trachea can be easily identified for preprocedural skin marking in most patients.[164] The patient is placed in a supine position with the neck extended. A linear high-frequency transducer is placed in the midline in a sagittal orientation in the suprasternal space. The tracheal rings can be seen as a series of similar-sized small hypoechoic circles ("string-of-black-pearls") lined posteriorly by a hyperechoic (bright) air-mucosal interface. Visualization cephalad reveals a more superficial and larger hypoechoic (dark) circle or oval shape represents the anterior aspect of the cricoid cartilage. As you proceed cephalad there will be a larger hypoechoic (dark) cartilage which represent the inferior aspect of the thyroid cartilage. The hyperechoic (white) air mucosal interface which lies between the thyroid and cricoid cartilages represents the CTM (Figure 3.27). An indelible surgical marker can be used to mark the skin at the mid-point of the CTM to verify the position before the landmark-based approach described above is used. A similar approach has been recommended for landmarking and preparation for FONA.[165]

Relative contraindications to translaryngeal anesthesia include those circumstances in which vigorous cough could be harmful, such as raised intracranial or intraocular pressure, open globe injuries of the eye, unstable cervical spine injuries, or advanced cardiac disease who may not tolerate reductions in preload (Valsalva) associated with prolonged coughing.[36] Potential complications include bleeding, subcutaneous emphysema, pneumomediastinum, pneumothorax, vocal cord damage, and

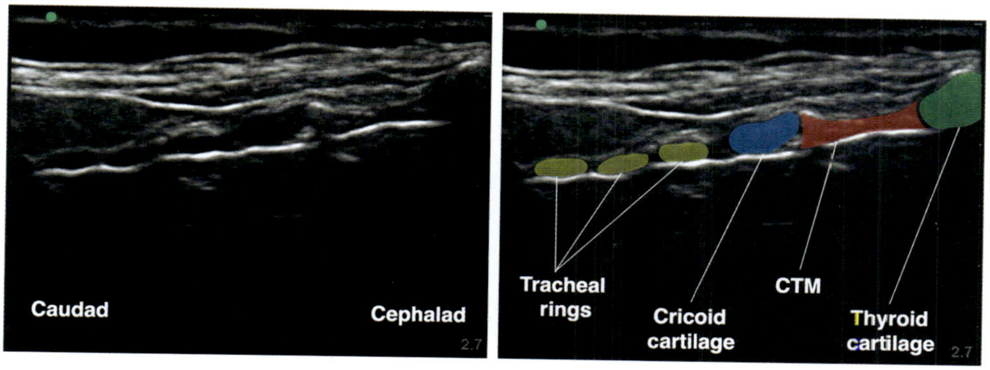

FIGURE 3.27. Ultrasound midline sagittal view of the suprasternal airway. CTM, cricothyroid membrane.

esophageal perforation.[166] Complications of laryngospasm and soft tissue infection, although rare, have also been reported.[36]

WHAT TECHNIQUE WORKS WELL FOR AWAKE INTUBATION?

A Suggested Step-by-Step Topicalization Procedure for an Awake Intubation

In general, the clinical scenarios in which an awake intubation may be necessary can be divided into two groups:

1. The emergency setting in which the risk of airway loss is high and time is limited ("no time").
2. The elective or urgent setting in which intubation is required and airway management is anticipated to be difficult. The risk is still high but there is time ("have time").

The *ideal* topicalization process has three basic components:

1. Lidocaine 5% ointment applied to the posterior third of the tongue
2. Atomized 3% to 4% lidocaine
3. Internal approach of SLN block

It may be necessary to modify this technique in the emergency setting.

In the elective or urgent setting of an anticipated difficult airway in which awake bronchoscopic intubation is planned ("have time"), profound regional anesthesia of the airway can be achieved using the following technique:

- A full explanation of the procedure is provided to the patient.
- Glycopyrrolate can be administered IM about 20 to 30 minutes (or IV at least 15 minutes) prior to planned airway manipulation. The tongue should appear dry prior to airway manipulation.
- If spinal movement is allowed and hemodynamics permit, the patient should be in the sitting or semi-sitting position. The airway practitioner should stand facing the patient.
- Oxygen is administered by nasal prongs with ETCO2 monitoring capability as well as pulse oximetry, non-invasive blood pressure and ECG monitoring.
- A remifentanil infusion can be initiated at 0.05 to 0.2 $\mu g \cdot kg^{-1} \cdot min^{-1}$. But, more than 0.1 $\mu g \cdot kg^{-1} \cdot min^{-1}$ is rarely required.
- Lidocaine 5% ointment is gently applied to the posterior third of the tongue using a tongue depressor. A layer of the ointment about 1 to 2 mm thick is placed on the distal centimeter of the tongue depressor.
- About 10 mL of aerosolized 3% or 4% lidocaine is then administered via the more patent nostril using an atomizer attached to a high-flow oxygen source. The spray delivered by the atomizer should be coordinated with respiration, with inhalation through the nose and exhalation through the mouth. The final few sprays are delivered through the mouth aiming the atomizer at the soft palate and tonsillar pillars.
- Alternatively, the aerosol can be administered via the mouth. When the atomized anesthetic is delivered entirely through the mouth it can be coordinated with deep inhalation or given continuously. The spray can be directed at the soft palate, the tonsillar pillars, and over the tongue into the pharynx and larynx. Gentle tongue traction performed by an assistant may be helpful.
- Cotton pledgets soaked in 4% aqueous lidocaine can then be gently advanced over the tongue into the piriform fossa on each side using Jackson forceps to confirm or supplement the block. As the pledget is removed, the mucosa of the oropharynx can be swabbed to confirm the absence of the gag reflex. This final step (SLN block) can be omitted at the discretion of the airway practitioner.
- Flexible bronchoscopy for intubation can then be performed.

Awake intubation under topical anesthesia, with and without sedation, can also be performed using video laryngoscopes and optical stylets. An airway regional anesthesia technique, similar to that described above, can be used for awake techniques using these devices.

In the emergency intubation setting, time is of the essence ("no time"). An explanation of the procedure should be provided to the patient as circumstances permit. In general, the use of sedation should be used sparingly or avoided as it may precipitate complete airway obstruction, and the time required for anti-sialagogues to provide mucosal drying is not available. Adequate regional anesthesia of the airway for awake intubation by DL can be readily achieved using 10% lidocaine spray. The spray is directed onto the posterior third of the tongue, the uvula, and the tonsillar pillars using the malleable, stainless-steel nozzle (Figure 3.20) and a tongue depressor to retract the tongue. Sprays can also be delivered into the piriform fossae; however, spraying into the larynx should be avoided as laryngospasm, cough, and a loss of patient cooperation may be precipitated. Where 10% lidocaine spray is not available, a device such as the MAD and 4% lidocaine can be substituted (Figure 3.19). If spinal movement is permissible and hemodynamics allow, then awake intubation by DL is most easily performed with the patient in the sitting position. Patients in respiratory distress are also reluctant or unable to lie flat. As time permits, it may be possible to achieve more profound anesthesia of the airway using some or all components of the three-step approach used for flexible bronchoscopic intubation as described above. Indirect intubation techniques in general require more profound airway anesthesia than does intubation by DL. Should a "can't intubate, can't oxygenate" crisis occur, then a cricothyrotomy will be necessary. Preparations for this eventuality include: (1) locating and marking the CTM (with or without ultrasound); (2) ensuring the necessary equipment is available; and (3) identifying who will perform the procedure.

SUMMARY

Awake intubation can be achieved rapidly with minimal patient discomfort. Effective topical anesthesia of the upper airway requires a sound knowledge of the airway anatomy, pharmacology, and regional anesthesia techniques. Manual dexterity, gentleness, and an appropriate bedside manner are also essential.

SELF-EVALUATION QUESTIONS

3.1. The internal branch of the superior laryngeal branch supplies sensory innervation to:

A. Base of the tongue

B. The laryngopharynx

C. The vocal cords

D. Posterior surface of the epiglottis

E. All of the above

3.2. The maximum effective concentration of topical lidocaine applied to the oropharynx is:

A. 1%

B. 2%

C. 4%

D. 10%

E. 15%

3.3. During translaryngeal anesthesia, correct needle placement is confirmed by:

A. Loss of resistance felt while puncturing the cricothyroid membrane

B. Aspiration of air through the syringe

C. Vigorous cough

D. Easy advancement of the angiocatheter over the needle

REFERENCES

1. Law JA, Broemling N, Cooper RM, et al. The difficult airway with recommendations for management–Part 2–the anticipated difficult airway. *Can J Anaesth*. 2013;60(11):1119-1138. doi:10.1007/s12630-013-0020-x.
2. Cook TM, Woodall N, Frerk C. Major complications of airway management in the UK: results of the Fourth National Audit Project of the Royal College of Anaesthetists and the Difficult Airway Society. Part 1: anaesthesia. *Br J Anaesth*. 2011;106(5):617-631. doi:10.1093/bja/aer058.
3. Morris IR. Functional anatomy of the upper airway. *Emerg Med Clin North Am*. 1988;6(4):639-669.
4. Standring S. Nose, nasal cavity and paranasal sinuses. In: Standring S, ed. *Gray's Anatomy*. 42nd ed. Amsterdam: Elsevier; 2021:686-701:chap 39.
5. Spiegel JH, Numa W. Nasal Trauma. In: Lalwani AK, ed. *Current Diagnosis & Treatment Otolaryngology—Head and Neck Surgery*. 4th ed. New York, NY: McGraw-Hill Education; 2020:chap 12.
6. Ellis H, Lawson A. *Anatomy for Anaesthetists*. 9th ed. Hoboken NJ: Wiley Press; 2014.
7. Yamamoto T, Flenner M, Schindler E. Complications associated with nasotracheal intubation and proposal of simple countermeasure. *Anaesthesiol Intensive Ther*. 2019;51(1):72-73. doi:10.5603/AIT.a2019.0002.
8. O'Reilly MJ, Reddick EJ, Black W, et al. Sepsis from sinusitis in nasotracheally intubated patients. A diagnostic dilemma. *Am J Surg*. 1984;147(5):601-604. doi:10.1016/0002-9610(84)90122-3.
9. Hall CE, Shutt LE. Nasotracheal intubation for head and neck surgery. *Anaesthesia*. 2003;58(3):249-256. doi:10.1046/j.1365-2044.2003.03034.x.
10. Tintinalli JE, Claffey J. Complications of nasotracheal intubation. *Ann Emerg Med*. 1981;10(3):142-144. doi:10.1016/s0196-0644(81)80379-4.
11. Watanabe S, Yaguchi Y, Suga A, Asakura N. A "bubble-tip" (Airguide) tracheal tube system: its effects on incidence of epistaxis and ease of tube advancement in the subglottic region during nasotracheal intubation. *Anesth Analg*. 1994;78(6):1140-1143. doi:10.1213/00000539-199406000-00019.
12. Earle R, Shanahan E, Vaghadia H, Sawka A, Tang R. Epistaxis during nasotracheal intubation: a randomized trial of the Parker Flex-Tip™ nasal endotracheal tube with a posterior facing bevel versus a standard nasal RAE endotracheal tube. *Can J Anaesth*. 2017;64(4):370-375.
13. Kim YC, Lee SH, Noh GJ, et al. Thermosoftening treatment of the nasotracheal tube before intubation can reduce epistaxis and nasal damage. *Anesth Analg*. 2000;91(3):698-701. doi:10.1097/00000539-200009000-00038.
14. Elwood T, Stillions DM, Woo DW, Bradford HM, Ramamoorthy C. Nasotracheal intubation: a randomized trial of two methods. *Anesthesiology*. 2002;96(1):51-53. doi:10.1097/00000542-200201000-00014.
15. Woodall NM, Harwood RJ, Barker GL. Complications of awake fibreoptic intubation without sedation in 200 healthy anaesthetists attending a training course. *Br J Anaesth*. 2008;100(6):850-855. doi:10.1093/bja/aen076.
16. Smith JE, Reid AP. Identifying the more patent nostril before nasotracheal intubation. *Anaesthesia*. 2001;56(3):258-262. doi:10.1046/j.1365-2044.2001.01717-3.x.
17. Özkan ASM, Akbas S, Toy E, Durmus M. North polar tube reduces the risk of epistaxis during nasotracheal intubation: a prospective, randomized clinical trial. *Curr Ther Res Clin Exp*. 2019;90:21-26. doi:10.1016/j.curtheres.2018.09.002.
18. Standring S. Pharynx. In: Standring S, ed. *Gray's Anatomy*. 42nd ed. Amsterdam: Elsevier; 2021:702-716:chap 40.
19. Isono S, Remmers JE, Tanaka A, Sho Y, Sato J, Nishino T. Anatomy of pharynx in patients with obstructive sleep apnea and in normal subjects. *J Appl Physiol (1985)*. 1997;82(4):1319-1326. doi:10.1152/jappl.1997.82.4.1319.
20. Ayuse T, Hoshino Y, Kurata S, et al. The effect of gender on compensatory neuromuscular response to upper airway obstruction in normal subjects under midazolam general anesthesia. *Anesth Analg*. 2009;109(4):1209-1218. doi:10.1213/ane.0b013e3181b0fc70.
21. Standring S. Mouth. In: Standring S, ed. *Gray's Anatomy*. 42nd ed. Amsterdam: Elsevier; 2021:636-663:chap 37.
22. Ovassapian A, Glassenberg R, Randel GI, Klock A, Mesnick PS, Klafta JM. The unexpected difficult airway and lingual tonsil hyperplasia: a case series and a review of the literature. *Anesthesiology*. 2002;97(1):124-132. doi:10.1097/00000542-200207000-00018.
23. Standring S. The anatomy of the peripheral nervous system. In: Standring S, ed. *Gray's Anatomy*. 42nd ed. Amsterdam: Elsevier; 2021:1464.e11-1464.e55:chap 80.
24. Standring S. Development of the head and neck. In: Standring S, ed. *Gray's Anatomy*. 42nd ed. Amsterdam: Elsevier; 2021:273-291:chap 17.
25. Standring S. Neck. In: Standring S, ed. *Gray's Anatomy*. 42nd ed. Amsterdam: Elsevier; 2021:573-606:chap 35.

26. Standring S. Infratemporal and pterygopalatine fossae and temporomandibular joint. In: Standring S, ed. *Gray's Anatomy*. 42nd ed. Amsterdam: Elsevier; 2021:664-685:chap 38.
27. Marcus BJ, Kaplan J, Collins KA. A case of Ludwig angina: a case report and review of the literature. *Am J Forensic Med Pathol*. 2008;29(3):255-259. doi:10.1097/PAF.0b013e31817efb24.
28. Kulkarni AH, Pai SD, Bhattarai B, Rao ST, Ambareesha M. Ludwig's angina and airway considerations: a case report. *Cases J*. 2008;1(1):19. doi:10.1186/1757-1626-1-19.
29. Standring S. Larynx. In: Standring S, ed. *Gray's Anatomy*. 42nd ed. Amsterdam: Elsevier; 2021:717-734:chap 41.
30. Nolan RT. Nasal intubation: an anatomical difficulty with Portex tubes. *Anaesthesia*. 1969;24(3):447-448. doi:10.1111/j.1365-2044.1969.tb02884.x.
31. Watton D, Hung OR. Unanticipated difficult nasal intubation due to a prominent anterior tubercle of the first cervical spine. *J Anesth Perioper Med*. 2016;3(6):276-279.
32. Reynolds JC, Ward PJ, Katzka DA, Parkman HP, Young MA. Mouth and Pharynx. In: Reynolds JC, ed. *Netter Collection of Medical Illustrations: Digestive System: Part I - Upper Digestive Tract*. 2nd ed. Amsterdam: Elsevier; 2017:69-141:chap 2.
33. Barash PG, Cahalan MK, Cullen BF, et al. *Clinical Anesthesia*. Philadelphia, PA: Wolters Kluwer Health; 2017.
34. Artime CA, Hagberg CA. Airway Management in the Adult. In: Gropper MA, Miller RD, Cohen NH, et al, eds. *Miller's Anesthesia*. 9th ed. Toronto, Canada: Elsevier; 2020:1373-1412:chap 44.
35. Dover K, Howdieshell TR, Colborn GL. The dimensions and vascular anatomy of the cricothyroid membrane: relevance to emergent surgical airway access. *Clin Anat*. 1996;9(5):291-295. doi:10.1002/(sici)1098-2353(1996)9:5<291::Aid-ca1>3.0.Co;2-g.
36. Gold MI, Buechel DR. Translaryngeal anesthesia: a review. *Anesthesiology*. 1959;20(2):181-185. doi:10.1097/00000542-195903000-00007.
37. Caparosa RJ, Zavatsky AR. Practical aspects of the cricothyroid space. *Laryngoscope*. 1957;67(6):577-591. doi:10.1288/00005537-195706000-00004.
38. Bennett JD, Guha SC, Sankar AB. Cricothyrotomy: the anatomical basis. *J R Coll Surg Edinb*. 1996;41(1):57-60.
39. Karle WE, Schindler JS. Surgical Management of the Difficult Adult Airway. In: Flint PW, Francis HW, Haughey BH, et al, eds. *Cummings Otolaryngology: Head and Neck Surgery*. 7th ed. Amsterdam: Elsevier; 2021:73-80:chap 6.
40. Ellis H. *Clinical Anatomy: A Revision and Applied Anatomy for Clinical Students*. 10th ed. Hoboken, NJ: Wiley-Blackwell; 2002:460.
41. Stone DJ, Bogdonoff DL. Airway considerations in the management of patients requiring long-term endotracheal intubation. *Anesth Analg*. 1992;74(2):276-287. doi:10.1213/00000539-199202000-00019.
42. Standring S. Pleura, lungs, trachea and bronchi. In: Standring S, ed. *Gray's Anatomy*. 42nd ed. Amsterdam: Elsevier; 2021:1020-1037:chap 54.
43. Kaminsky DA. Anatomy and Embryology. In: Kaminsky DA, ed. *Netter Collection of Medical Illustrations: Respiratory System*. 2nd ed. Amsterdam: Saunders, an imprint of Elsevier Inc; 2011:1-45:chap 1.
44. Bacon GS, Lyons TR, Wood SH. Dyclonine hydrochloride for airway anesthesia: awake endotracheal intubation in a patient with suspected local anesthetic allergy. *Anesthesiology*. 1997;86(5):1206-1207. doi:10.1097/00000542-199705000-00023.
45. Lin Y, Liu S. Local Anesthetics. In: Barash PG, Cullen BF, Stoelting RK, et al, eds. *Clinical Anesthesia*. 8th ed. Philadelphia, PA: Wolters Kluwer Health; 2017:572-574:chap 22.
46. Morris IR. Fibreoptic intubation. *Can J Anaesth*. 1994;41(10):996-1007; discussion 1007-8. doi:10.1007/bf03010944.
47. El-Boghdadly K, Pawa A, Chin KJ. Local anesthetic systemic toxicity: current perspectives. *Local Reg Anesth*. 2018;11:35-44. doi:10.2147/lra.S154512.
48. Boyes RN, Scott DB, Jebson PJ, Godman MJ, Julian DG. Pharmacokinetics of lidocaine in man. *Clin Pharmacol Ther*. 1971;12(1):105-116. doi:10.1002/cpt1971121105.
49. Narang PK, Crouthamel WG, Carliner NH, Fisher ML. Lidocaine and its active metabolites. *Clin Pharmacol Ther*. 1978;24(6):654-662. doi:10.1002/cpt1978246654.
50. Gitman M, Fettiplace MR, Weinberg GL, Neal JM, Barrington MJ. Local anesthetic systemic toxicity: a narrative literature review and clinical update on prevention, diagnosis, and management. *Plast Reconstr Surg*. 2019;144(3):783-795. doi:10.1097/prs.0000000000005989.
51. Kamal M, Naguib M. Local Anesthetics. In: Flood P, Rathmell JP, Shafer SL, eds. *Stoelting's Pharmacology and Physiology in Anesthetic Practice*. 5th ed. Philadelphia, PA: Wolters Kluwer; 2015:chap 10.
52. Lirk P, Picardi S, Hollmann MW. Local anaesthetics: 10 essentials. *Eur J Anaesthesiol*. 2014;31(11):575-585. doi:10.1097/eja.0000000000000137.
53. Walsh ME, Shorten GD. Preparing to perform an awake fiberoptic intubation. *Yale J Biol Med*. 1998;71(6):537-549.
54. Kirkpatrick MB. Lidocaine topical anesthesia for flexible bronchoscopy. *Chest*. 1989;96(5):965-967. doi:10.1378/chest.96.5.965.
55. Ahmad I, El-Boghdadly K, Bhagrath R, et al. Difficult Airway Society guidelines for awake tracheal intubation (ATI) in adults. *Anaesthesia*. 2020;75(4):509-528. doi:10.1111/anae.14904.
56. Watanabe H, Lindgren L, Rosenberg P, Randell T. Glycopyrronium prolongs topical anaesthesia of oral mucosa and enhances absorption of lignocaine. *Br J Anaesth*. 1993;70(1):94-95. doi:10.1093/bja/70.1.94.
57. Adriani J, Zepernick R, Arens J, Authement E. The comparative potency and effectiveness of topical anesthetics in man. *Clin Pharmacol Ther*. 1964;5:49-62. doi:10.1002/cpt19645149.
58. Ovassapian A. The flexible bronchoscope. A tool for anesthesiologists. *Clin Chest Med*. 2001;22(2):281-299. doi:10.1016/s0272-5231(05)70043-5.
59. Schenck NL. Local anesthesia in otolaryngology. A re-evaluation. *Ann Otol Rhinol Laryngol*. 1975;84(1 Pt 1):65-72. doi:10.1177/000348947508400110.
60. Efthimiou J, Higenbottam T, Holt D, Cochrane GM. Plasma concentrations of lignocaine during fibreoptic bronchoscopy. *Thorax*. 1982;37(1):68-71. doi:10.1136/thx.37.1.68.
61. Wu FL, Razzaghi A, Souney PF. Seizure after lidocaine for bronchoscopy: case report and review of the use of lidocaine in airway anesthesia. *Pharmacotherapy*. 1993;13(1):72-78.
62. Macfarlane AJR, Gitman M, Bornstein KJ, El-Boghdadly K, Weinberg G. Updates in our understanding of local anaesthetic systemic toxicity: a narrative review. *Anaesthesia*. 2021;76(Suppl 1):27-39. doi:10.1111/anae.15282.
63. Pelton DA, Daly M, Cooper PD, Conn AW. Plasma lidocaine concentrations following topical aerosol application to the trachea and bronchi. *Can Anaesth Soc J*. 1970;17(3):250-255. doi:10.1007/bf03004603.
64. Adriani J, Campbell D. Fatalities following topical application of local anesthetics to mucous membranes. *J Am Med Assoc*. 1956;162(17):1527-1530. doi:10.1001/jama.1956.02970340017006.
65. Scott DB, Littlewood DG, Covino BG, Drummond GB. Plasma lignocaine concentrations following endotracheal spraying with an aerosol. *Br J Anaesth*. 1976;48(9):899-902. doi:10.1093/bja/48.9.899.
66. Williams KA, Barker GL, Harwood RJ, Woodall NM. Combined nebulization and spray-as-you-go topical local anaesthesia of the airway. *Br J Anaesth*. 2005;95(4):549-553. doi:10.1093/bja/aei202.
67. Foo I, Macfarlane AJR, Srivastava D, et al. The use of intravenous lidocaine for postoperative pain and recovery: international consensus statement on efficacy and safety. *Anaesthesia*. 2021;76(2):238-250. doi:10.1111/anae.15270.
68. Sheppard H, Anandampillai R. Systemic toxic effects of local anaesthetics. *Anaesthesia & Intensive Care Medicine*. 2019;20(4):215-218. doi:10.1016/j.mpaic.2019.01.022.
69. Gitman M, Barrington MJ. Local anesthetic systemic toxicity: a review of recent case reports and registries. *Reg Anesth Pain Med*. 2018;43(2):124-130. doi:10.1097/aap.0000000000000721.
70. Bina B, Hersh EV, Hilario M, Alvarez K, McLaughlin B. True allergy to amide local anesthetics: a review and case presentation. *Anesth Prog*. Summer 2018;65(2):119-123. doi:10.2344/anpr-65-03-06.
71. Deas TC. Severe methemoglobinemia following dental extractions under lidocaine anesthesia. *Anesthesiology*. 1956;17(1):204. doi:10.1097/00000542-195601000-00028.
72. Karim A, Ahmed S, Siddiqui R, Mattana J. Methemoglobinemia complicating topical lidocaine used during endoscopic procedures. *Am J Med*. 2001;111(2):150-153. doi:10.1016/s0002-9343(01)00763-x.
73. Guay J. Methemoglobinemia related to local anesthetics: a summary of 242 episodes. *Anesth Analg*. 2009;108(3):837-845. doi:10.1213/ane.0b013e318187c4b1.
74. Fink J. Aerosol drug therapy. In: Kacmarek RM, Stoller JK, Heuer A, eds. *Egan's Fundamentals of Respiratory Care*. Amsterdam: Elsevier Mosby;2013:chap 36.
75. O'Callaghan C, Barry PW. The science of nebulised drug delivery. *Thorax*. 1997;52 (Suppl 2):S31-44. doi:10.1136/thx.52.2008.s31.
76. Chu SS, Rah KH, Brannan MD, Cohen JL. Plasma concentration of lidocaine after endotracheal spray. *Anesth Analg*. 1975;54(4):438-441. doi:10.1213/00000539-197507000-00007.
77. Le Brun PP, de Boer AH, Heijerman HG, Frijlink HW. A review of the technical aspects of drug nebulization. *Pharm World Sci*. 2000;22(3):75-81. doi:10.1023/a:1008786600530.
78. Newman SP, Pellow PG, Clarke SW. In vitro comparison of DeVilbiss jet and ultrasonic nebulizers. *Chest*. 1987;92(6):991-994. doi:10.1378/chest.92.6.991.

79. Berger R, McConnell JW, Phillips B, Overman TL. Safety and efficacy of using high-dose topical and nebulized anesthesia to obtain endobronchial cultures. *Chest.* 1989;95(2):299-303. doi:10.1378/chest.95.2.299.
80. IBM Corporation. Tetracaine. 2021. Micromedex Solutions. https://www.micromedexsolutions.com/micromedex2/librarian/PFDefaultActionId/evidencexpert.DoIntegratedSearch?navitem=topHome&isToolPage=true#. Accessed August 24, 2021.
81. Weisel W, Tella RA. Reaction to tetracaine (pontocaine) used as topical anesthetic in bronchoscopy; study of 1,000 cases. *J Am Med Assoc.* 1951;147(3):218-222. doi:10.1001/jama.1951.03670200010003.
82. Campbell D, Adriani J. Absorption of local anesthetics. *J Am Med Assoc.* 1958;168(7):873-877. doi:10.1001/jama.1958.03000070029006.
83. Patel D, Chopra S, Berman MD. Serious systemic toxicity resulting from use of tetracaine for pharyngeal anesthesia in upper endoscopic procedures. *Dig Dis Sci.* 1989;34(6):882-884. doi:10.1007/bf01540273.
84. Suzuki S, Gerner P, Lirk P. Local Anesthetics. In: Hemmings HC, Egan TD, eds. *Pharmacology and Physiology for Anesthesia: Foundations and Clinical Application.* 2nd ed. Amsterdam: Elsevier; 2019:390-411:chap 20.
85. Catterall W, Mackie K. Local anesthetics. In: Brunton LL, Chabner BA, Knollmann BC, eds. *Goodman and Gilman's The Pharmacological Basis of Therapeutics.* 10th ed. New York, NY: McGraw-Hill;2001.
86. Reed AP. Preparation for intubation of the awake patient. *Mt Sinai J Med.* 1995;62(1):10-20.
87. IBM Corporation. Benzocaine. 2021. Micromedex Solutions. https://www.micromedexsolutions.com/micromedex2/librarian/PFDefaultActionId/evidencexpert.DoIntegratedSearch?navitem=headerLogout#. Accessed September 3, 2021.
88. HURRICAINE® TOPICAL ANESTHETIC SPRAY. Beutlich Inc https://beutlich.com/stock/hurricaine-topical-anesthetic-spray/. Accessed September 1, 2021.
89. Cetylite Industries. Cetacaine® Topical Anesthetic Spray. Cetylite Industries. https://www.cetylite.com/medical/topical-anesthetics/cetacaine-topical-anesthetic-spray. Accessed September 1, 2021.
90. Nguyen ST, Cabrales RE, Bashour CA, et al. Benzocaine-induced methemoglobinemia. *Anesth Analg.* 2000;90(2):369-371. doi:10.1097/00000539-200002000-00024.
91. Rinehart RS, Norman D. Suspected methemoglobinemia following awake intubation: one possible effect of benzocaine topical anesthesia—a case report. *AANA J.* 2003;71(2):117-118.
92. Kwok S, Fischer JL, Rogers JD. Benzocaine and lidocaine induced methemoglobinemia after bronchoscopy: a case report. *J Med Case Rep.* 2008;2:16. doi:10.1186/1752-1947-2-16.
93. Chowdhary S, Bukoye B, Bhansali AM, et al. Risk of topical anesthetic-induced methemoglobinemia: a 10-year retrospective case-control study. *JAMA Intern Med.* 2013;173(9):771-776. doi:10.1001/jamainternmed.2013.75.
94. BheemReddy S, Messineo F, Roychoudhury D. Methemoglobinemia following transesophageal echocardiography: a case report and review. *Echocardiography.* 2006;23(4):319-321. doi:10.1111/j.1540-8175.2006.00159.x.
95. Vallurupalli S, Das S, Manchanda S. Infection and the risk of topical anesthetic induced clinically significant methemoglobinemia after transesophageal echocardiography. *Echocardiography.* 2010;27(3):318-323. doi:10.1111/j.1540-8175.2009.00994.x.
96. Spiller HA, Russell JL, Casavant MJ, Ho RY, Gerona RR. Identification of N-Hydroxy-para-aminobenzoic acid in a cyanotic child after benzocaine exposure. *Clin Toxicol (Phila).* 2014;52(9):976-979. doi:10.3109/15563650.2014.958615.
97. Harper SJ, Jones NS. Cocaine: what role does it have in current ENT practice? A review of the current literature. *J Laryngol Otol.* 2006;120(10):808-811. doi:10.1017/s0022215106001459.
98. Latorre F, Klimek L. Does cocaine still have a role in nasal surgery? *Drug Saf.* 1999;20(1):9-13. doi:10.2165/00002018-199920010-00002.
99. Maraj S, Figueredo VM, Lynn Morris D. Cocaine and the heart. *Clin Cardiol.* 2010;33(5):264-269. doi:10.1002/clc.20746.
100. Long H, Greller H, Mercurio-Zappala M, Nelson LS, Hoffman RS. Medicinal use of cocaine: a shifting paradigm over 25 years. *Laryngoscope.* 2004;114(9):1625-1629. doi:10.1097/00005537-200409000-00022.
101. Lange RA, Hillis LD. Cardiovascular complications of cocaine use. *N Engl J Med.* 2001;345(5):351-358. doi:10.1056/nejm200108023450507.
102. IBM Corporation. Cocaine. 2021. https://www.micromedexsolutions.com/micromedex2/librarian/CS/70CE8C/ND_PR/evidencexpert/ND_P/evidencexpert/DUPLICATIONSHIELDSYNC/31D91A/ND_PG/evidencexpert/ND_B/evidencexpert/ND_AppProduct/evidencexpert/ND_T/evidencexpert/PFActionId/evidencexpert.DoIntegratedSearch?SearchTerm=cocaine&UserSearchTerm=cocaine&SearchFilter=filterNone&navitem=searchGlobal#. Accessed September 5, 2021.
103. Gross JB, Hartigan ML, Schaffer DW. A suitable substitute for 4% cocaine before blind nasotracheal intubation: 3% lidocaine-0.25% phenylephrine nasal spray. *Anesth Analg.* 1984;63(10):915-918.
104. Osula S, Stockton P, Abdelaziz MM, Walshaw MJ. Intratracheal cocaine induced myocardial infarction: an unusual complication of fibreoptic bronchoscopy. *Thorax.* 2003;58(8):733-734. doi:10.1136/thorax.58.8.733.
105. Pergolizzi JV Jr, Magnusson P, LeQuang JAK, Breve F, Varrassi G. Cocaine and cardiotoxicity: a literature review. *Cureus.* 2021;13(4):e14594. doi:10.7759/cureus.14594.
106. Festic E, Johnson MM, Leventhal JP. The feasibility of topical cocaine use in fiberoptic bronchoscopy. *Acta Medica Academica.* 2010;39(1):1-6.
107. Katz RI, Hovagim AR, Finkelstein HS, Grinberg Y, Boccio RV, Poppers PJ. A comparison of cocaine, lidocaine with epinephrine, and oxymetazoline for prevention of epistaxis on nasotracheal intubation. *J Clin Anesth.* 1990;2(1):16-20. doi:10.1016/0952-8180(90)90043-3.
108. Rector FT, DeNuccio DJ, Alden MA. A comparison of cocaine, oxymetazoline, and saline for nasotracheal intubation. *AANA J.* 1987;55(1):49-54.
109. Latorre F, Otter W, Kleemann PP, Dick W, Jage J. Cocaine or phenylephrine/lignocaine for nasal fibreoptic intubation? *Eur J Anaesthesiol.* 1996;13(6):577-581. doi:10.1046/j.1365-2346.1996.00015.x.
110. Tarver CP, Noorily AD, Sakai CS. A comparison of cocaine vs. lidocaine with oxymetazoline for use in nasal procedures. *Otolaryngol Head Neck Surg.* 1993;109(4):653-659. doi:10.1177/019459989310900404.
111. Pott LM, Randel GI, Straker T, Becker KD, Cooper RM. A survey of airway training among U.S. and Canadian anesthesiology residency programs. *J Clin Anesth.* 2011;23(1):15-26. doi:10.1016/j.jclinane.2010.06.009.
112. Manikandan S, Neema PK, Rathod RC. Ultrasound-guided bilateral superior laryngeal nerve block to aid awake endotracheal intubation in a patient with cervical spine disease for emergency surgery. *Anaesth Intensive Care.* 2010;38(5):946-948. doi:10.1177/0310057x1003800523.
113. Vázquez T, Cobiella R, Maranillo E, et al. Anatomical variations of the superior thyroid and superior laryngeal arteries. *Head Neck.* 2009;31(8):1078-1085. doi:10.1002/hed.21077.
114. Herrera-Núñez M, Menchaca-Gutiérrez JL, Pinales-Razo R, et al. Origin variations of the superior thyroid, lingual, and facial arteries: a computed tomography angiography study. *Surg Radiol Anat.* 2020;42(9):1085-1093. doi:10.1007/s00276-020-02507-6.
115. Vaghadia H, Lawson R, Tang R, Sawka A. Failure to visualise the superior laryngeal nerve using ultrasound imaging. *Anaesth Intensive Care.* 2011;39(3):503; author reply 503.
116. Tsui B, Ip V, Walji A. Airway sonography in live models and cadavers. *J Ultrasound Med.* 2013;32(6):1049-1058. doi:10.7863/ultra.32.6.1049.
117. Singh M, Chin KJ, Chan VW, Wong DT, Prasad GA, Yu E. Use of sonography for airway assessment: an observational study. *J Ultrasound Med.* 2010;29(1):79-85. doi:10.7863/jum.2010.29.1.79.
118. Stopar-Pintaric T, Vlassakov K, Azman J, Cvetko E. The thyrohyoid membrane as a target for ultrasonography-guided block of the internal branch of the superior laryngeal nerve. *J Clin Anesth.* 2015;27(7):548-552. doi:10.1016/j.jclinane.2015.07.016.
119. Barberet G, Henry Y, Tatu L, et al. Ultrasound description of a superior laryngeal nerve space as an anatomical basis for echoguided regional anaesthesia. *Br J Anaesth.* 2012;109(1):126-128. doi:10.1093/bja/aes203.
120. Kaur B, Tang R, Sawka A, Krebs C, Vaghadia H. A method for ultrasonographic visualization and injection of the superior laryngeal nerve: volunteer study and cadaver simulation. *Anesth Analg.* 2012;115(5):1242-1245. doi:10.1213/ANE.0b013e318265f75d.
121. Sawka A, Tang R, Vaghadia H. Sonographically guided superior laryngeal nerve block during awake fiberoptic intubation. *A A Case Rep.* 2015;4(8):107-110. doi:10.1213/xaa.0000000000000136.
122. Krause M, Khatibi B, Sztain JF, Rahman P, Shapiro AB, Sandhu NS. Ultrasound-guided airway blocks using a curvilinear probe. *J Clin Anesth.* 2016;33:408-412. doi:10.1016/j.jclinane.2016.04.058.
123. Lan C, Cheng W, Yang Y. A new method for ultrasound-guided superior laryngeal nerve block. *Tzu Chi Medical Journal.* 2013;25(3):161-163. doi:10.1016/j.tcmj.2013.05.001.
124. Ambi US, Arjun BK, Masur S, Endigeri A, Hosalli V, Hulakund SY. Comparison of ultrasound and anatomical landmark-guided technique for superior laryngeal nerve block to aid awake fibre-optic intubation: A prospective randomised clinical study. *Indian J Anaesth.* 2017;61(6):463-468. doi:10.4103/ija.IJA_74_17.
125. Guinot PG, Zogheib E, Petiot S, et al. Ultrasound-guided percutaneous tracheostomy in critically ill obese patients. *Crit Care.* 2012;16(2):R40. doi:10.1186/cc11233.

126. Kupeli I, Nalbant RA. Comparison of 3 techniques in percutaneous tracheostomy: Traditional landmark technique; ultrasonography-guided long-axis approach; and short-axis approach - Randomised controlled study. *Anaesth Crit Care Pain Med.* 2018;37(6):533-538. doi:10.1016/j.accpm.2017.11.011.
127. Gobatto ALN, Besen B, Tierno P, et al. Ultrasound-guided percutaneous dilational tracheostomy versus bronchoscopy-guided percutaneous dilational tracheostomy in critically ill patients (TRACHUS): a randomized noninferiority controlled trial. *Intensive Care Med.* 2016;42(3):342-351. doi:10.1007/s00134-016-4218-6.
128. Alansari M, Alotair H, Al Aseri Z, Elhoseny MA. Use of ultrasound guidance to improve the safety of percutaneous dilatational tracheostomy: a literature review. *Crit Care.* 2015;19(1):229. doi:10.1186/s13054-015-0942-5.
129. Green JS, Tsui BC. Applications of ultrasonography in ENT: airway assessment and nerve blockade. *Anesthesiol Clin.* 2010;28(3):541-553. doi:10.1016/j.anclin.2010.07.012.
130. De Oliveira GS Jr, Fitzgerald P, Kendall M. Ultrasound-assisted translaryngeal block for awake fibreoptic intubation. *Can J Anaesth.* 2011;58(7):664-665. doi:10.1007/s12630-011-9501-y.
131. Iida T, Suzuki A, Kunisawa T, Iwasaki H. Ultrasound-guided superior laryngeal nerve block and translaryngeal block for awake tracheal intubation in a patient with laryngeal abscess. *J Anesth.* 2013;27(2):309-310. doi:10.1007/s00540-012-1492-1495.
132. Kleine-Brueggeney M, Greif R, Ross S, et al. Ultrasound-guided percutaneous tracheal puncture: a computer-tomographic controlled study in cadavers. *Br J Anaesth.* 2011;106(5):738-742. doi:10.1093/bja/aer026.
133. Pintaric TS. Upper airway blocks for awake difficult airway management. *Acta Clin Croat.* 2016;55(Suppl 1):85-89.
134. Maher T, Shankar H. Ultrasound-guided peristyloid steroid injection for eagle syndrome. *Pain Pract.* 2017;17(4):554-557. doi:10.1111/papr.12497.
135. Ažman J, Stopar Pintaric T, Cvetko E, Vlassakov K. Ultrasound-guided glossopharyngeal nerve block: a cadaver and a volunteer sonoanatomy study. *Reg Anesth Pain Med.* 2017;42(2):252-258. doi:10.1097/aap.0000000000000561.
136. Bedder MD, Lindsay D. Glossopharyngeal nerve block using ultrasound guidance: a case report of a new technique. *Reg Anesth.* 1989;14(6):304-307.
137. Sundaram S, Punj J. Randomized controlled trial comparing landmark and ultrasound-guided glossopharyngeal nerve in eagle syndrome. *Pain Med.* 2020;21(6):1208-1215. doi:10.1093/pm/pnz370.
138. Wang H, Ford RZ, Milne AD. Differences in aerosol flow rates between disposable and reusable atomizers used for airway topicalization: implications for local anesthetic toxicity. *Can J Anaesth.* 2021;68(2):270-271. doi:10.1007/s12630-020-01856-5.
139. Morris IR. Pharmacologic aids to intubation and the rapid sequence induction. *Emerg Med Clin North Am.* 1988;6(4):753-768.
140. DeMeester TR, Skinner DB, Evans RH, Benson DW. Local nerve block anesthesia for peroral endoscopy. *Ann Thorac Surg.* 1977;24(3):278-283. doi:10.1016/s0003-4975(10)63757-5.
141. Amri P, Nikbakhsh N, Modaress SR, Nosrati R. Upper airway nerve block for rigid bronchoscopy in the patients with tracheal stenosis: a case series. *Anesth Pain Med.* 2020;10(4):e99796. doi:10.5812/aapm.99796.
142. Barton S, Williams JD. Glossopharyngeal nerve block. *Arch Otolaryngol.* 1971;93(2):186-188. doi:10.1001/archotol.1971.00770060272014.
143. Woods Andrew M, Lander Christopher J. Abolition of gagging and the hemodynamic response to awake laryngoscopy. *Anesthesiology.* 1987;67(3S):A220-A220. doi:10.1097/00000542-198709001-00220.
144. Simmons ST, Schleich AR. Airway regional anesthesia for awake fiberoptic intubation. *Reg Anesth Pain Med.* 2002;27(2):180-192. doi:10.1053/rapm.2002.30659.
145. Sitzman BT, Rich GF, Rockwell JJ, Leisure GS, Durieux ME, DiFazio CA. Local anesthetic administration for awake direct laryngoscopy. Are glossopharyngeal nerve blocks superior? *Anesthesiology.* 1997;86(1):34-40. doi:10.1097/00000542-199701000-00006.
146. Gotta AW, Sullivan CA. Anaesthesia of the upper airway using topical anaesthetic and superior laryngeal nerve block. *Br J Anaesth.* 1981;53(10):1055-1058. doi:10.1093/bja/53.10.1055.
147. Canty DJ, Poon L. Superior laryngeal nerve block: an anatomical study comparing two techniques. *J Clin Anesth.* 2014;26(7):517-522. doi:10.1016/j.jclinane.2014.03.005.
148. Akhaddar A, Baallal H, Hammoune N, Bouabbadi S, Adraoui A, Belfquih H. Unilateral blindness following superior laryngeal nerve block for awake tracheal intubation in a case of posterior cervical spine surgery. *Surg Neurol Int.* 2020;11:277. doi:10.25259/sni_505_2020.
149. Artime CA, Roy S, Hagberg CA. The difficult airway. *Otolaryngol Clin North Am.* 2019;52(6):1115-1125. doi:10.1016/j.otc.2019.08.009.
150. Walts LF, Kassity KJ. Spread of local anesthesia after upper airway block. *Arch Otolaryngol.* 1965;81:77-79. doi:10.1001/archotol.1965.00750050082017.
151. Bonica JJ. Transtracheal anesthesia for endotracheal intubation. *Anesthesiology.* 1949;10(6):736-738. doi:10.1097/00000542-194911000-00010.
152. Kundra P, Kutralam S, Ravishankar M. Local anaesthesia for awake fibreoptic nasotracheal intubation. *Acta Anaesthesiol Scand.* 2000;44(5):511-516. doi:10.1034/j.1399-6576.2000.00503.x.
153. Lamb A, Zhang J, Hung O, et al. Accuracy of identifying the cricothyroid membrane by anesthesia trainees and staff in a Canadian institution. *Can J Anaesth.* 2015;62(5):495-503. doi:10.1007/s12630-015-0326-y.
154. Aslani A, Ng SC, Hurley M, McCarthy KF, McNicholas M, McCaul CL. Accuracy of identification of the cricothyroid membrane in female subjects using palpation: an observational study. *Anesth Analg.* 2012;114(5):987-992. doi:10.1213/ANE.0b013e31824970ba.
155. Altun D, Ali A, Koltka K, et al. Role of ultrasonography in determining the cricothyroid membrane localization in the predicted difficult airway. *Ulus Travma Acil Cerrahi Derg.* 2019;25(4):355-360. Öngörülen zor havayolunda krikotiroit membran lokalizasyonunun belirlenmesinde ultrasonografinin rolü. doi:10.14744/tjtes.2019.65250.
156. Bowness J, Taylor A, Saint-Grant AL, et al. Identifying the cricothyroid membrane: a comparison of palpation, laryngeal handshake and ultrasound. *Trends in Anaesthesia and Critical Care.* 2020;30:E56. doi:10.1016/j.tacc.2019.12.139.
157. You-Ten KE, Wong DT, Ye XY, Arzola C, Zand A, Siddiqui N. Practice of ultrasound-guided palpation of neck landmarks improves accuracy of external palpation of the cricothyroid membrane. *Anesth Analg.* 2018;127(6):1377-1382. doi:10.1213/ane.0000000000003604.
158. Yıldız G, Göksu E, Şenfer A, Kaplan A. Comparison of ultrasonography and surface landmarks in detecting the localization for cricothyroidotomy. *Am J Emerg Med.* 2016;34(2):254-256. doi:10.1016/j.ajem.2015.10.054.
159. Siddiqui N, Arzola C, Friedman Z, Guerina L, You-Ten KE. Ultrasound improves cricothyrotomy success in cadavers with poorly defined neck anatomy: a randomized control trial. *Anesthesiology.* 2015;123(5):1033-1041. doi:10.1097/aln.0000000000000848.
160. Siddiqui N, Yu E, Boulis S, You-Ten KE. Ultrasound is superior to palpation in identifying the cricothyroid membrane in subjects with poorly defined neck landmarks: a randomized clinical trial. *Anesthesiology.* 2018;129(6):1132-1139. doi:10.1097/aln.0000000000002454.
161. Kristensen MS, Teoh WH, Rudolph SS, et al. Structured approach to ultrasound-guided identification of the cricothyroid membrane: a randomized comparison with the palpation method in the morbidly obese. *Br J Anaesth.* 2015;114(6):1003-1004. doi:10.1093/bja/aev123.
162. Forshaw N, Navaratnarajah J, Dobby N. Identifying the cricothyroid membrane in children: palpation versus ultrasound. *British Journal of Anaesthesia.* 2018;121(1):E13. doi:10.1016/j.bja.2018.02.057.
163. Hung KC, Chen IW, Lin CM, Sun CK. Comparison between ultrasound-guided and digital palpation techniques for identification of the cricothyroid membrane: a meta-analysis. *Br J Anaesth.* 2021;126(1):e9-e11. doi:10.1016/j.bja.2020.08.012.
164. You-Ten KE, Siddiqui N, Teoh WH, Kristensen MS. Point-of-care ultrasound (POCUS) of the upper airway. *Can J Anaesth.* 2018;65(4):473-484.
165. Rai Y, You-Ten E, Zasso F, De Castro C, Ye XY, Siddiqui N. The role of ultrasound in front-of-neck access for cricothyroid membrane identification: A systematic review. *J Crit Care.* 2020;60:161-168. doi:10.1016/j.jcrc.2020.07.030.
166. Danzl DF, Thomas DM. Nasotracheal intubations in the emergency department. *Crit Care Med.* 1980;8(11):677-682. doi:10.1097/00003246-198011000-00019.

CHAPTER 4

Pharmacology of Intubation

Karim Wafa, Jonathan G. Bailey, and Orlando R. Hung

CASE PRESENTATION

A 41-year-old female with acute cholecystitis presents to the operating room (OR) for laparoscopic cholecystectomy. The patient's medical history is significant for type II diabetes, gastroesophageal reflux disease, obesity (BMI 52 kg·m^{-2}) and obstructive sleep apnea (OSA) with no surgical history. She has been using a continuous positive airway pressure machine regularly for the past 3 years and her serum glucose levels have been well controlled (A1C 6.5%). When asked, she endorsed symptoms of free reflux, waking her up in the night 3 to 4 times a week. She is on pantoprazole 40 mg PO once daily and has no allergies. She is alert and in no distress but has had multiple episodes of vomiting in the past 24 hours. Her last meal was over 24 hours ago. A focused cardiovascular and respiratory exam were unremarkable, and her vitals were all within normal limits. An airway exam was completed and showed a Mallampati class III, good mouth opening (>5 cm), good thyromental distance (6 cm), good mandibular protrusion, and normal neck extension. There were no missing, loose, or protruding teeth.

Given her history of free reflux and vomiting, you decide to proceed with a rapid sequence intubation (RSI) and intubation. After appropriate patient positioning and denitrogenation, you induce the patient. On direct laryngoscopy, a grade 3b view is obtained where you are unable to secure the airway. After another two unsuccessful attempts with a styletted smaller ETT followed by video-laryngoscopy, you declare a failed airway and decide to wake the patient up.

How Will Your Choice of Neuromuscular Blocking Agent for the RSI Impact This Decision?

The ideal muscle relaxant to facilitate intubation in a situation requiring an RSI should have a rapid onset, a short duration of action, and be immediately reversible. The two most commonly used neuromuscular blocking agents for rapid sequence inductions are the nondepolarizing neuromuscular blocking agent rocuronium and the depolarizing neuromuscular blocking agent succinylcholine. Succinylcholine was the agent of choice when no contraindications exist, given its short duration of action of 5 to 8 minutes and its rapid onset of drug effect (<60 seconds). The side effects of succinylcholine include fasciculations, hyperkalemia, bradycardia, increased intraocular pressure, and malignant hyperthermia (MH). Rocuronium has been commonly used given that at larger doses (1-1.2 mg·kg^{-1}) a similar onset time to succinylcholine can be achieved (1 minute), but the major drawback to the use of rocuronium for RSI in the context of a potentially difficult airway is its long duration of action compared with succinylcholine. This has changed with the advent of sugammadex which at adequate doses can reverse rocuronium-induced profound neuromuscular blockade in 2.7 minutes. Normal healthy individuals theoretically have 8 minutes of apneic reserve; however, in critically ill, morbidly obese, pediatric, or pregnant patients that reserve is significantly reduced increasing their risk of hypoxemia prior to the return of spontaneous breathing.

Despite the rapid reversal of neuromuscular blockade by sugammadex, we would not recommend the sole reliance on sugammadex to rescue the failed airway post administration of rocuronium (see section "Reversal of NDMR by Sugammadex" for more detail).

PHYSIOLOGY OF TRACHEAL INTUBATION

What Are the Physiological Responses to Tracheal Intubation?

The goal of tracheal intubation is to provide a successful and definitive airway. Unfortunately, laryngoscopy and intubation can result in a cascade of physiological and pathophysiological reflex responses. These responses are initiated by stimulation of afferent receptors in the posterior pharynx supplied by the glossopharyngeal and vagus nerves. The central nervous system (CNS), cardiovascular system, and respiratory system all respond predictably to these afferent stimuli, and in selected patients, the resultant physiologic manifestations may adversely affect the patients' outcome. Though little data exists to suggest that patient outcomes are altered by attenuating the increases in intracranial pressure (ICP), stimulation of the autonomic nervous system with increases in the heart rate and blood pressure, and stimulation of the upper and lower respiratory tract resulting in increases in airway resistance, in light of the possible adverse effects in a compromised patient, it seems prudent and logical to attempt to attenuate these responses.

The CNS responds to airway manipulation by increasing cerebral metabolic oxygen demand ($CMRO_2$) and cerebral blood flow (CBF). If the intracranial compliance is decreased ("tight brain"), the increase in CBF may increase the ICP further. This response is important in situations in which there is a loss of autoregulation such that blood flow to the brain, or regions of the brain, becomes pressure-passive (i.e., increases in blood pressure result in increases in ICP).

Laryngoscopy stimulates protective reflexes and predictably leads to cardiovascular and respiratory system responses mediated by the sympathetic nervous system. In children, this process is believed to be primarily a monosynaptic reflex promoting vagal stimulation of the sinoatrial node resulting in bradycardia. For further details see Chapter 3. These responses may be detrimental in patients with myocardial ischemia ("tight coronaries"), known as intracerebral or aortic aneurysms, major vessel dissection, or those with major vascular injuries. Hypertension may also lead to significant increases in ICP if autoregulation has been lost (e.g., acute severe head injury or intracranial hemorrhage).

The respiratory system may respond in three important ways to laryngoscopy and intubation: activation of the upper-airway reflexes leading to laryngospasm, coughing, and bronchospasm ("tight lungs"). Laryngospasm, a forceful involuntary spasm of the laryngeal musculature, may produce difficulty with intubation as well as ventilation. Persistent and life-threatening laryngospasm is treated with a gentle continuous positive airway pressure with 100% oxygen, intravenous (IV) lidocaine (1.5 mg·kg^{-1}), or if persistent, neuromuscular blockade (e.g., succinylcholine at 10% of the intubating dose). Negative intrathoracic pressure created by inspiration attempts against a closed glottis (laryngospasm) may result in negative pressure pulmonary edema (see Chapter 62). Coughing may produce significant adverse effects in patients with increased ICP, an unstable cervical spine injury, or penetrating eye injuries.

Activation of the lower airway reflexes leads to an increase in airway resistance. This reaction is most often manifested by bronchospasm brought about by reflexes, irritants, or antigens. Whether mitigation of these reflexes improves patient outcomes is not known. Prelaryngoscopy administration of drugs is capable of mitigating these potentially harmful physiologic effects.

Current evidence that this symphony of adverse advents can be mitigated is most compelling for the IV administration of anesthetics, including lidocaine, opioids, and muscle relaxants, and much less so for atropine, except in the case of selected pediatric patients. This chapter provides a general discussion of the appropriate pharmacological agents used in airway management and their relevant properties. It should be emphasized that the goal of this chapter is not to discuss the rationale of using a specific sedative or muscle relaxant in an anticipated difficult airway. Rather, this discussion will center on the use of drugs to facilitate tracheal intubation and mitigate adverse physiological consequences.

PHARMACOLOGICAL AGENTS USED PRIOR TO INDUCTION OF ANESTHESIA

What Are the Common Agents Used Prior to Induction of Anesthesia for Intubation?

Prelaryngoscopy agents (also known as "pretreatment agents") are used to attenuate the adverse physiologic responses to laryngoscopy and intubation. Pretreatment agents fall into the following categories: beta blockers, local anesthetics, opioids, alpha 2 agonists, and defasciculating agents. Ideally, all pretreatment agents should be administered shortly before (typically about 3 minutes and up to 10 minutes for alpha 2 agonists) induction to synchronize the onset of peak drug effects of all drugs administered in the airway management sequence.

While short-acting beta-blockers, such as esmolol, have been shown to be beneficial in attenuating the sympathetic response to laryngoscopy,[1] they are not effective in attenuating to any associated rise in ICP. They may potentially increase airway resistance, especially in patients with reactive airways disease. Furthermore, beta-blockers are also negative inotropes and in some clinical situations, particularly in emergencies in which maximum cardiac reserve should be preserved, the combination of beta-blockers and the negative cardiovascular effects of most induction agents could be catastrophic.

What Is the Role of Dexmedetomidine as a Premedication for Laryngoscopy?

Dexmedetomidine is an alpha 2 adrenoreceptor agonist, which regulates heart rate and blood pressure, with anesthetic, analgesic, and sedative properties. These effects are achieved by inhibiting the release of norepinephrine, both peripherally and centrally, decreasing sympathetic nervous system activity. Dexmedetomidine is shorter-acting than clonidine and is more selective for alpha 2 adrenoreceptor versus alpha 1 adrenoreceptors.[2]

A meta-analysis published by De Cassai et al. analyzed the impact of dexmedetomidine on the hemodynamic response during tracheal intubation.[3] The meta-analysis included 99 studies with a total of 6833 randomized patients. Dexmedetomidine doses ranged from a high dose (greater than or equal to 0.7 $\mu g \cdot kg^{-1}$), medium dose (0.40-0.69 $\mu g \cdot kg^{-1}$), to a low dose (less than 0.4 $\mu g \cdot kg^{-1}$). The majority of the studies used 0.5 $\mu g \cdot kg^{-1}$ or 1 $\mu g \cdot kg^{-1}$ bolus dosing of dexmedetomidine.[3]

For the primary outcome, patients who received dexmedetomidine as a premedication prior to laryngoscopy had a lower heart rate and blood pressure. Of note, premedication with an anticholinergic agent prior to intubation did not reduce the risk of intraoperative bradycardia and/or hypotension. The secondary outcomes of the meta-analysis assessed intraoperative complications which included intraoperative hypotension and bradycardia as well as postoperative shivering, nausea and vomiting, pain, bradycardia, and hypotension. The study found that while premedication with dexmedetomidine increased the risk of intraoperative hypotension and bradycardia, there were no differences in postoperative hypotension and bradycardia. Additionally, dexmedetomidine use was associated with reduced risk of postoperative shivering, nausea and vomiting, and pain and required less analgesics on the first postoperative day. In the meta-analysis 1 out of 12 patients developed significant bradycardia and as such, the authors caution against the use of dexmedetomidine in select patients, especially in those with the high vagal tone, given the high risk of bradycardia and hypotension.[3]

What Is the Rationale of Using Intravenous Lidocaine for Tracheal Intubation?

Local anesthetics bind to closed, inactivated sodium channels and prevent subsequent channel activation. Sodium channels in the closed inactivated state are not permeable to sodium and therefore action potentials cannot be generated. Local anesthetic agents are a combination of a lipophilic benzene ring and a hydrophilic amine either linked by an amide or an ester bridge. Lidocaine is a low-potency, rapid-onset, and intermediate-acting amide local anesthetic. The literature is replete with articles that offer varying conclusions as to the efficacy of lidocaine when used in the pretreatment phase of tracheal intubation to attenuate various adverse effects of laryngoscopy and intubation.

Attenuation of the elevation of ICP related to airway manipulation is ascribed to lidocaine's ability to increase the depth of anesthesia, decrease $CMRO_2$ demand globally, decrease CBF, and increase cerebrovascular resistance. Patients with intracranial pathology may have an abnormal intracranial pressure–volume relationship, which can predispose them to abrupt, extreme, and prolonged elevations of ICP. Such increases can contribute to secondary injury of the brain, such as herniation of the brain and impaired perfusion leading to ischemia. Indirect evidence exists that lidocaine can attenuate the intracranial hypertensive response to laryngoscopy and intubation. For instance, intracranial hypertension associated with tracheal suctioning is suppressed by IV lidocaine.[4–7] Intratracheal lidocaine is equally effective.[6] Lidocaine (1.5 $mg \cdot kg^{-1}$) administered 3 minutes before intubation suppresses the cough reflex and attenuates the increase in airway resistance resulting from laryngoscopy and endotracheal intubation.

There is evidence that local anesthetic attenuates the hemodynamic response to laryngoscopy. Pretreatment with local anesthetics decreases the chance of arrhythmias and ischemic ECG changes following laryngoscopy.[8] A systematic review of 37 trials found that IV lidocaine attenuates the hemodynamic response to laryngoscopy in all age groups.[9]

Lidocaine's effect on antigenic-mediated bronchospasm is more controversial. Lidocaine and other local anesthetics may lead to bronchoconstriction in patients with reactive airway disease when given via the inhalational route[10] (see Chapter 3 for a full discussion of this evidence). In normal individuals, lidocaine does not alter airway resistance and has been shown to produce mild bronchodilation.[11] In three similar trials, Groeben and colleagues[12–14] showed that IV lidocaine attenuated the response to an inhalational histamine challenge in patients with mild asthma. The inhalational administration of lidocaine to such patients, however, was met with short-lived initial increases in airway resistance.[13] In a randomized controlled trial of 60 asthmatic patients, administration of IV lidocaine did not significantly reduce airway resistance after intubation.[15] If pretreating is deemed necessary, IV lidocaine (1.5 $mg \cdot kg^{-1}$) 3 minutes before induction is advocated for adult patients with reactive airway disease (i.e., "tight lungs") or those with elevated ICP (i.e., "tight brains"). The onset of action is 45 to 90 seconds after an IV bolus administration of lidocaine and the duration of effect is 10 to 20 minutes.[16]

Lidocaine has a wide safety margin, particularly at a dose of 1.5 $mg \cdot kg^{-1}$; however, particular attention should be directed toward cumulative local anesthetic dose when regional techniques or local infiltration by the surgical team occurs.[17] The primary toxic effect is the development of seizures, which usually occur at much higher doses. IV lidocaine at rates of 1.5 to 3.0 $mg \cdot kg^{-1} \cdot min^{-1}$ resulted in seizures in healthy volunteers once the total dose reached 6 to 8 $mg \cdot kg^{-1}$.[18,19] The maximum dose for subcutaneous lidocaine is generally considered to be 4.5 $mg \cdot kg^{-1}$ [20] plain or 7 $mg \cdot kg^{-1}$ with epinephrine.[16,20] However, even healthy volunteers often experience some neurologic

TABLE 4.1. Pharmacokinetics of Opioids in Clinical Use[16,22,25–27]

	Morphine	Hydromorphone	Fentanyl	Sufentanil	Remifentanil
pK_a	7.9	8.59	8.4	8.0	7.3
% Ionization	23	–	8.5	20	58
% Protein bound	35	8-19	84	93	66-93
Rapid redistribution, $t_{½\pi}$ (min)	–	–	1.2-1.9	1.4	0.4-0.5
Distribution, $t_{½\alpha}$ (min)	1.5-4.4	–	9.2-19	17	2-3.7
Elimination, $t_{½\beta}$ (h)	1.7-3.3	2.5-3.0	3.1-6.6	2.2-4.6	0.17-0.33
Onset effect (min)	5-10	5	Immediate	1-3	1 to 3
Peak effect (min)	20	10-20	3-5	5.6	1.8
Duration (min)	4-5 hours	4-5 hours	30-60	~40	3-10
Induction dose ($\mu g \cdot kg^{-1}$)	–	–	1-4	0.2-0.4	1-3

symptoms, such as perioral numbness/tingling, auditory disturbances, and dizziness, with IV bolus doses as low as 1 $mg \cdot kg^{-1}$.[21]

Why Do We Use Opioids Prior to Tracheal Intubation?

Opium, derived from the seeds of the poppy *Papaver somniferum*, is composed of more than 20 alkaloids, some of which serve as the foundation molecules for modern opioids. A German pharmacist isolated the first alkaloid from opium in 1806 and named it morphine after the Greek god of dreams, Morpheus.[22] A broad definition of the term *opioid* includes all drugs, synthetic and natural, which interact with opioid receptors, whether endogenous, exogenous, agonist, or antagonists. The use of natural opiates has been around for thousands of years; however, it wasn't until 1962, with the recent development of synthetic opioids that opioids were used in anesthesia.[23] Opioids were used for their ability to reduce the hypnotic agent dose thereby providing a more hemodynamically stable induction of anesthesia. As a result, they were soon incorporated into what came to be known as balanced anesthesia technique.[23] With the advent of newer, more rapid-acting agents (such as remifentanil), they continue to play an important role in airway management.

Opioids act throughout the nervous system, including the dorsal horn of the spinal cord (substantia gelatinosa), periaqueductal gray matter, and the periphery. They inhibit presynaptic release and postsynaptic response to excitatory neurotransmitters, such as acetylcholine (ACh) and substance P, by altering the potassium and calcium conductance.[22] As such, they are useful in attenuating adverse responses to airway manipulation in patients with "tight brains" and "tight coronaries."

Although highly selective, opioid effects typically involve complex interactions among various receptor sites. Mu (μ), kappa (κ), and delta (δ) receptor classes and their subtypes have been firmly established.[24] Most clinically useful opioids are highly selective μ agonists, which are responsible for the bulk of supraspinal and spinal analgesia.

Opioids are typically of low molecular weight but vary widely in their lipid solubility, percent of ionization, and degree of binding to proteins (Table 4.1). Commonly used opioids for induction (fentanyl, sufentanil, and remifentanil) are more lipid soluble, which accounts for their speed of onset of action. Redistribution is responsible for the termination of their CNS drug action. Metabolism of most opioids occurs through a two-stage hepatic process that generally results in an inactive metabolite. The exception is remifentanil, which contains an ester linkage and is rapidly hydrolyzed by nonspecific esterases in the blood and tissue.

Physiologically, opioids exert their effect on all organ systems. Venodilation and depressed sympathetic reflexes typically result in a decrease in heart rate and blood pressure. Unlike some opioids (most notably morphine) fentanyl, sufentanil, and remifentanil do not release histamine. This is partly why they cause less hypotension than morphine. All opioids depress ventilation by blunting the carbon dioxide response at the respiratory center, raising the apneic threshold, and depressing the slope of the CO_2 response curve (Figure 4.1).

The primary reason to include an opioid in the intubation sequence is their ability to significantly attenuate the sympathetic response that occurs with manipulation of the airway. Unfortunately, the rapid administration of fentanyl and its

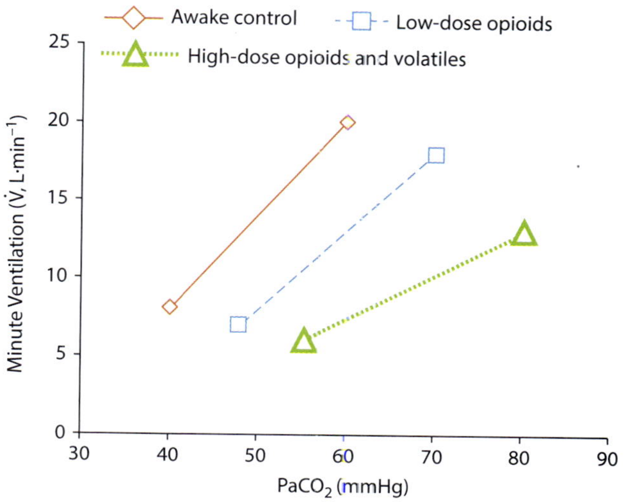

FIGURE 4.1. Carbon dioxide (CO_2) ventilatory response curve. In health, awake controls increasing partial pressure of carbon dioxide in arterial blood ($PaCO_2$) results in an increase in minute ventilation ($\dot{V}$). Increasing plasma concentration of opioids shifts the CO_2 response curve to the right. High concentrations eventually result in depression of the slope of the curve.[22]

derivatives has been associated with brief episodes of coughing and chest wall rigidity.[28–30]. Large induction doses of an opioid (e.g., sufentanil 3 μg·kg^{-1}) can decrease pulmonary compliance in 50% to 86% of patients and potentially induce glottic closure interfering with ventilation of the patient.[28–31] Doses of this magnitude are seldom if ever employed in emergency airway management, in or out of the OR.

What Types of Opioids Are Commonly Used for Tracheal Intubation?

The hemodynamic and intracranial responses to tracheal intubation are usually short-lived. Therefore, the "ideal" choice of an opioid for tracheal intubation should be based on its pharmacokinetic and pharmacodynamic characteristics, namely, a rapid onset and a brief duration of drug effect. While there are currently many opioids available, the following discussion will be restricted to only those opioids with a rapid onset and short duration of drug effect.

Fentanyl

Like meperidine, fentanyl is a phenylpiperidine-derived synthetic opioid agonist. It is roughly 100 times more potent than morphine. Fentanyl in large doses (10-30 μg·kg^{-1}) causes chest wall rigidity in 35% to 85% of patients.[28,30,32] This side effect is present in all age groups.[33] Rigidity is a unique and idiosyncratic response to opioids and is probably related to the dose and speed of administration. Although the exact mechanism is unknown, an animal study demonstrated opioid-induced muscle rigidity coincident with activation of central μ-receptors.[34] Others have suggested mechanisms involving the cerulospinal noradrenergic system[35,36] and the neurochemical system affected in Parkinson's disease.[37]

Tagaito et al.[38] found that increasing doses of fentanyl reduced the incidence of respiratory and laryngeal responses to laryngeal irritation under propofol anesthesia. Fentanyl is a short-acting opioid owing to redistribution of the drug, although accumulation with repeated dosing or after a long duration of infusion can limit its use.[27] Peak drug effect occurs 3 to 5 minutes following IV administration with an equilibration half-time between the plasma and brain of 5 minutes.[27] Doses recommended for attenuating the adverse effects of airway manipulation range from 1 to 4 μg·kg^{-1}. One must be prepared to treat dose-related hypotension and respiratory depression that may occur with fentanyl administration; especially in the absence of surgical stimulation post-induction and intubation.

Fentanyl may decrease airway reflexes associated with the placement of an extraglottic device (EGD); however, the doses required may interfere with spontaneous ventilation once the EGD is placed. Fentanyl 1 μg·kg^{-1}, when given 5 minutes prior to placement of an EGD, has been shown to increase the rate of apneas and the need for positive pressure ventilation, while the frequency of laryngospasm and breath holding were similar to placebo.[39] One study estimated that the ED_{50} of fentanyl is 0.5 μg·kg^{-1} and the ED_{95} is 7.5 μg·kg^{-1} for insertion of an EGD following propofol induction.[40] Thus, the need for optimal conditions and the absence of airway reflexes must be weighed against the effects of large doses of opioids.

Sufentanil

A thienyl derivative of fentanyl, sufentanil is 10 to 15 times more potent than fentanyl. Sufentanil is a highly specific μ agonist with similar pharmacokinetic properties as fentanyl. It is extremely lipophilic permitting rapid penetration of the blood–brain barrier and onset of CNS effects. Sufentanil 0.3 to 1 μg·kg^{-1}, administered 1 to 3 minutes prior to intubation, will blunt the response to laryngoscopy. Rigidity has been reported with larger doses.[32] The difficult ventilation associated with opioid rigidity may be due in part to vocal cord closure when administered in doses of 3 μg·kg^{-1}.[29,31]

Remifentanil

Remifentanil is a structurally unique opioid. It is a piperidine analog with a methyl ester side chain. The ester linkage renders it susceptible to cleavage by nonspecific plasma and tissue esterases.[41] The rapid metabolism of remifentanil, rather than redistribution, is responsible for its ultrashort duration of action; and with limited redistribution, there is no accumulation. It is rapidly cleared from the plasma (3 L·min^{-1}).[32] Remifentanil is not, however, a substrate for pseudocholinesterase and therefore it is unaffected by pseudocholinesterase deficiency.

Remifentanil is a potent μ receptor agonist with a similar potency to fentanyl. Doses of 0.25 to 3 μg·kg^{-1} have successfully attenuated the response to laryngoscopy.[42–47] At higher doses, centrally mediated depression of sympathetic tone and vagally induced bradycardia may occur. This bradycardia can be attenuated by the prior administration of glycopyrrolate or other antimuscarinics.[22] Peak respiratory depression occurs 5 minutes after bolus dosing, and lasts 10 minutes after 1.5 μg·kg^{-1} and 20 minutes after 2 μg·kg^{-1} .[48] Remifentanil, like other opioids, may cause chest wall rigidity depending on the dose and speed of administration.[49]

The clinical utility of remifentanil is reflected in its distinctive pharmacokinetic characteristics. Its rapid onset, brief duration, and easily titratable nature have enhanced its profile for airway management, particularly in emergency settings, and for short surgical procedures. A small dose of remifentanil (0.25 μg·kg^{-1}) can provide excellent conditions for laryngeal mask airway insertion with minimal hemodynamic disturbance.[50] The trachea may be successfully intubated without muscle relaxants with the combination of remifentanil and an induction agent. Remifentanil, 2 to 4 μg·kg^{-1}, in this setting, provides good to excellent intubating conditions .[44,51–53] Remifentanil has been found to be superior to lidocaine and esmolol at attenuating the hemodynamic responses to intubation.[54]

What Is Opioid-Free Anesthesia?

While opioids have been used regularly in the perioperative period, they have multiple side effects which may limit their use. Some of the acute side effects of opioids include nausea, pruritis, respiratory depression, and constipation.[55] As a result, patients with opioid-related side effects have longer hospital stays, higher readmission rates, and unplanned hospital admissions.[55] Additionally, opioids are associated with addiction and overprescription of opioids has contributed to the opioid crisis.[55]

Given the known side effects of opioids, there has been a movement to eliminate the use of opioids in the perioperative period in an attempt to improve postoperative patient outcomes. The founding idea is based on that pain and nociception are two different entities. Pain is defined as a conscious unpleasant perception of a noxious stimulus whereas nociception is identified as the activation of noxious receptors.[56] The surgical response under anesthesia is therefore not defined as pain but as a sympathetic response to nociception. As such, advocates of opioid-free anesthesia promote using pharmacologic agents in the intraoperative period which control the autonomic nervous system's response to stimulation of noxious receptors also termed antinociception.[56,57]

There is a continuum with regards to opioid-free anesthesia from opioid-minimizing to opioid-elimination; where some advocate for reduced opioid use while others promote eliminating opioids from anesthetic practice. Regardless of the philosophy, the strategy includes the use of opioid-sparing adjuncts in a multimodal approach to target different nociceptive pathways and include NMDA antagonists (ketamine, lidocaine, and magnesium), sodium channel blockers (local anesthetics–regional techniques vs. Intravenous administration), anti-inflammatory drugs (NSAIDs, dexamethasone) and alpha 2 agonists (dexmedetomidine and clonidine).[56] Beta-blockers have also been used in opioid-free anesthesia to blunt the sympathetic response to surgery maintaining hemodynamic stability.[56,58,59] However, there is limited evidence to support the use of beta blockers in opioid-free anesthesia.

What Are the Purported Benefits of Opioid-Free Anesthesia?

Despite the goal of reducing prolonged opioid use following discharge, evidence is lacking to support an association with intraoperative opioid use to manage moderate to severe pain in the immediate postoperative period and prolonged postoperative opioid use.[60] An opioid-free or opioid-sparing approach has been shown to decrease postoperative nausea and vomiting (PONV) rates. A recent meta-analysis of 23 trials, found reduced PONV rates in the opioid-reduced groups. The same review found no difference in postoperative pain or length of stay between groups; however, the vast majority of included studies used opioid analgesia in the postoperative phase.[61] It has also been suggested that opioid-free anesthesia reduces opioid-induced hyperalgesia. The meta-analysis found a reduction in mechanical wound hyperalgesia in the opioid-free group, based on very low-quality data.[61]

What Are the Potential Adverse Events Associated with Opioid-Free Anesthesia?

While opioids do have known side effects which have to be weighed against the benefits when used, opioid-free anesthesia also has limitations. Adding multiple adjunct agents in higher doses to compensate for an opioid-free anesthetic, predisposes patients to an increased risk of adverse medication interaction.[60,62] The titrated use of short-acting beta-blockers in the intraoperative period, while may help control the sympathetic response to nociception, but they do have hemodynamic consequences that may have deleterious effects in the intraoperative phase that limit their use.

The addition of dexmedetomidine to a general anesthetic compared to remifentanil was associated with less pain, shivering, and PONV; however, the time to extubation and recovery-room length of stay were significantly longer.[63] In a randomized trial completed by Beloeil et al.[64] they investigated the effects of nonopioid anesthesia with dexmedetomidine versus a balanced anesthetic with intraoperative remifentanil plus morphine on postoperative related adverse events. The study was stopped prematurely due to five cases of severe bradycardia in the dexmedetomidine group. The dexmedetomidine group also had more adverse postoperative events and hypoxemia.

Finally, due to the ceiling effects of most nonopioid analgesic adjuncts, pain control may be compromised by eliminating opioids when analgesic needs exceed the analgesia offered by available adjuncts.[62] Additionally, some adjuncts have narrow therapeutic windows, mandating closer monitoring if they are continued in the postoperative period (e.g., IV lidocaine).[17]

What Is a Strategy for Opioid-Sparing Multimodal Anesthesia?

Whether you support the use of opioid-free anesthesia or not, it's important to keep the primary goal in mind which is the provision of safe and effective anesthesia. Given the currently available evidence, we are more in favor of a multimodal analgesic approach which includes opioids when appropriate. This is more in keeping with an opioid-sparing technique whereby, excessive opioid use is avoided. The combination of drugs with different mechanisms of action promotes an additive beneficial effect and reduces unwanted side effects. This strategy is supported by the most recent Enhanced Recovery after Surgery Guidelines whereby analgesia is best provided by opioid-sparing versus opioid-free.[60,65]

In favor of minimizing intraoperative opioid use as part of an opioid-sparing strategy, practitioners can choose to omit opioids during induction. There are many published protocols for the use of adjunct agents for an opioid-free induction of anesthesia in a variety of surgeries.[66–68] We suggest using a combination of the adjuncts found in Table 4.2 based on the patient's comorbidities, hemodynamic goals, and the predicted analgesic requirements based on both patient and procedural factors.

INDUCTION AGENTS

The ideal induction agent would quickly render the patient unconscious, unresponsive, and amnestic in one arm/heart/brain circulation time. Such an agent would also provide analgesia, maintain stable cerebral perfusion pressure (CPP) and cardiovascular hemodynamics, be immediately reversible, and have few if any, adverse side effects. Unfortunately, such an induction agent does not exist.

Most induction agents are highly lipophilic, and therefore have a rapid onset of effect within 30 to 45 seconds of IV administration. Their clinical effect is likewise terminated quickly

TABLE 4.2. Drug Adjuncts for an Opioid-Free Induction[68,69]

Category	Medication	Dose	Select Side effects
NMDA antagonists			
	Ketamine	0.1 mg·kg^{-1}	Tachycardia, hypertension, emergence delirium
	Magnesium	40 mg·kg^{-1}	Hypotension
Sodium channel blockers			
	Lidocaine	1 to 1.5 mg·kg^{-1}	Bradycardia, atrioventricular block, hypotension, agitation, confusion, seizure
Anti-inflammatory			
	Dexamethasone	10 mg	Agitation, peptic ulcer, hyperglycemia
Alpha 2 agonists			
	Dexmedetomidine	0.25 μg·kg^{-1} 10 minutes prior to induction (Max dose 20 μg)	Bradycardia, hypotension, hypertension, agitation, respiratory depression

as the drug rapidly redistributes from the CNS to less well-perfused tissues. All induction agents have the potential to cause myocardial depression and hypotension. These effects depend on the particular drug and the patient's underlying physiologic condition. The faster the drug is administered, the larger the amount of the drug that will be delivered to those organs with the greatest blood flow (such as the brain and heart) and the more pronounced the effect is. The choice of drug and the dose must be individualized to each patient to capitalize on desired effects while minimizing adverse effects.

The induction agents include short-acting barbiturates: thiopental and methohexital; benzodiazepines: principally midazolam; and miscellaneous agents: etomidate, ketamine, and propofol (Table 4.3). Opioids can function as anesthetic induction agents when used in very large doses (e.g., fentanyl 30 μg·kg^{-1}), but are rarely, if ever, used for that purpose during routine or emergency intubation, so will not be discussed in this chapter.

All of the induction agents discussed in this chapter share similar pharmacokinetic characteristics. The duration of observed clinical effect of each drug is measured in minutes and is due to the redistribution of the drug from the central circulation (brain) to larger, but less well-perfused tissues, for example, fat and muscle. The elimination half-life ($t_{1/2\beta}$, usually measured in hours) is characterized by each drug's re-entry from fat and lean muscle into plasma down a concentration gradient followed by hepatic metabolism, which precedes renal excretion. It generally requires four to five elimination half-lives to clear the drug completely from the body.

Because the target organ is the brain, and the desired effect is produced rapidly following IV bolus administration of the drug, dosing of induction agents in normal-sized and obese adults should be based on lean body weight in kilograms. Hypovolemia results in the patient having a contracted central compartment; therefore, lower doses of induction agents are necessary to achieve adequate levels at the target organ (brain). Aging affects the pharmacokinetics of induction agents. In older adults, lean body mass and total body water decrease while total body fat increases, resulting in an increased volume of distribution, an increase in $t_{1/2\beta}$, and an increased duration of drug effect. Older adults are also much more sensitive to the hemodynamic and respiratory depressant effects of these agents, and consequently, most induction doses should be reduced.

BARBITURATES

Barbiturates are derived from barbituric acid, a cyclic compound obtained by the combination of urea and malonic acid. These agents act at the barbiturate receptor, which forms part of the GABA-receptor complex to enhance and mimic the action of GABA. In North America, the use of barbiturates for airway management is very uncommon; however, they remain in common use in many countries around the world. The most commonly used barbiturates are thiopental and methohexital. Thiopental is no longer available in North America and as such will not be discussed further.[70]

Methohexital is still available in some parts of North America for use in patients undergoing electroconvulsive therapy (ECT) because of its desirable rapid onset of anesthesia, short duration of action, and minimal anticonvulsant properties.[71] Methohexital shares similar clinical pharmacologic properties with thiopental although it is significantly less lipid soluble and is 2 to 3 times more potent than thiopental. The elimination of methohexital is 3 to 4 times faster than thiopental.[72]

There is a 10% to 20% incidence of nausea and vomiting that occurs during recovery from a barbiturate induction. Methohexital has a greater incidence than thiopental of twitching and hiccups (excitatory phenomena) that may be misdiagnosed as seizures.[73]

BENZODIAZEPINES

Discuss the Clinical Pharmacology of Benzodiazepines

Although chemically distinct from barbiturates, benzodiazepines also exert their effects via the GABA-receptor complex. Benzodiazepines are allosteric modulators of the $GABA_A$ receptor; specifically, benzodiazepines bind to an allosteric site on the $GABA_A$ receptor complex thereby increasing the receptor

TABLE 4.3. Commonly Used Induction Drugs[22,70]

Drugs	Dose	Effect Onset	Peak	Duration	Half-Life	Metabolism	Elimination
Propofol	IV: 1.5-2.5 mg·kg^{-1}	30 seconds	-	3-10 minutes	Biphasic – initial 40 minutes; Terminal 4-7 hours	Hepatic	Renal
Methohexital	IV: 1.5 mg·kg^{-1}	Immediate	-	5-15 minutes	1.6-3.9 hours	Hepatic	Renal
Ketamine	IV: 1-2 mg·kg^{-1}	IV: 30 seconds	IV: 1 min	IV: 10-20 minutes	Biphasic – initial 11 minutes and terminal is 2.5 hours	Hepatic	Renal
	IM: 4-8 mg·kg^{-1}	IM 3-4 minutes	IM: 5-30 minutes	IM: 12-25 minutes (Recovery to orientation is longer)			
Etomidate	IV: 0.2-0.4 mg·kg^{-1}	30-60 seconds	1minute	3-5 minutes	2.9-5.3 hours	Hepatic and plasma esterases	Renal
Midazolam	IV: 0.1-0.3 mg·kg^{-1}	3-5 minutes	3-5 minutes	15-80 minutes	1-4 hours	Hepatic	Renal
Dexmedetomidine (adjunct)	IV: 0.5-1 µg·kg^{-1}	5-10 minutes	15-30 minutes	60-120 minutes	2-3 hours	Hepatic	Renal
Lidocaine (adjunct)	IV: 0.5-2 mg·kg^{-1}	45-90 seconds		10-20 minutes	Biphasic – initial 7-30 minutes; Terminal: 1.5-2 hours	Hepatic	Renal

complex affinity for GABA.[74] The benzodiazepines provide amnesia, anxiolysis, sedation, anticonvulsant effects, and hypnosis (sleep). This potent, dose-related amnestic property is perhaps their greatest asset.

The lipophilicity of benzodiazepines varies widely. Greater lipid solubility confers a more rapid onset of action because of the brain's high lipid content. The two benzodiazepines most clinically used during airway manipulation are midazolam and diazepam. Of the two, midazolam is the more lipid soluble. However, many studies have shown that the onset of effect is 2.5 times slower for midazolam than diazepam.[75] Induction of anesthesia with midazolam alone has been described. With doses of 0.15 to 0.2 mg·kg^{-1} induction of anesthesia occurs after 1.5 minutes (0.3-8 minutes) with opioid premedication or 2 to 2.5 minutes without. Therefore, the time to clinical effectiveness of benzodiazepines is longer than any of the other induction agents, which hinders their role in emergency airway management. The termination of action of midazolam and diazepam is due to redistribution and subsequent hepatic metabolism via cytochrome P450–3A4 microsomal oxidation. Midazolam has one insignificant active metabolite and a $t_{1/2elim}$ of 2 to 4 hours. Diazepam has two active metabolites, both of which can prolong its sedative effect but more importantly are metabolized and excreted more slowly than diazepam and account for its prolonged $t_{1/2\beta}$ of 20 to 40 hours. The benzodiazepines do not release histamine, and allergic reactions are very rare. Clearance will be prolonged in older adults, critically ill patients, obese patients, or patients with renal disease or low cardiac output.[76]

What Are the Clinical Uses and Adverse Effects of Benzodiazepines?

The primary indications for benzodiazepines are anxiolysis, amnesia, sedation, and seizure management. Because of their dose-related reduction in systemic vascular resistance and direct myocardial depression, dosage must be adjusted in volume-depleted or hemodynamically compromised patients. Unlike the other induction agents, including those that cause hypotension, midazolam is generally under-dosed during emergency induction. The dose of midazolam for induction of anesthesia is 0.1 to 0.3 mg·kg^{-1}.[77–80] Doses of 0.15 to 0.2 mg·kg^{-1} are purported not to cause hypotension in normal individuals.[76]

Most often midazolam is used as an adjunct to other induction agents. Its amnestic effects may be advantageous during RSI, particularly is the case of hemodynamic instability where lower doses of induction agents will be used. Midazolam causes anterograde amnesia in a dose-dependent manner (2-10 mg IV); however, there is no evidence that it causes retrograde amnesia.[81,82]

Many practitioners avoid the use of midazolam in older patients during the perioperative period for the fear of causing harm by increasing the risk of delirium. In an analysis of a database created from prospective data by Wang et al. involving 1266 patients 65 years or older who underwent elective major noncardiac surgery, premedication with midazolam was not associated with a higher incidence of delirium on the first postoperative day.[83] Midazolam was administered IV approximately 15 minutes before surgery and the dose used was 1.99 +/−1.03 mg (mean +/− standard deviation). Additionally, a retrospective population-based cohort study by Memtsoudis et al. showed that while the use of long-acting benzodiazepines was associated with increased odds of postoperative delirium in patients 65 years or older undergoing elective total hip/knee arthroplasty surgery, that was not the case for short-acting benzodiazepines. Interestingly, the use of short-acting benzodiazepines in both elective total hip/knee arthroplasty surgery reduced the odds of postoperative delirium. This effect was abolished if long-acting benzodiazepines were also used. Rather than being protective against delirium, the reduced odds ratio associated with short-acting benzodiazepines likely represents a selection bias whereas benzodiazepines were given in patients at lower risk of delirium but avoided in patients deemed high risk of delirium.[84] While these data support the avoidance of long-acting benzodiazepines, these studies suggest that premedication with midazolam was not associated with a higher incidence of delirium in the early postoperative period.

More studies are being conducted on the impact of perioperative administration of midazolam on outcomes of older patients one of which is a multicenter, randomized, placebo-controlled, double-blinded, interventional trial which is being conducted in Germany on patient satisfaction after premedication with midazolam in elderly patients.[85]

ETOMIDATE

Discuss the Clinical Pharmacology of Etomidate

Etomidate is a carboxylated imidazole derivative that is primarily an IV hypnotic agent used for the rapid induction of anesthesia. It is available in a 0.2% solution dissolved in 35% propylene glycol. It inhibits the reticular activating system, mimicking GABA at the GABA-receptor complex. Etomidate owes its rapid onset to its high lipid solubility and large nonionized portion at physiological pH.[32] Its rapid redistribution leads to prompt awaking following administration. The elimination half-life of etomidate is 2 to 5 hours. It is rapidly hydrolyzed by hepatic metabolism and plasma esterases to water-soluble inactive metabolites excreted primarily by the kidneys.

Etomidate is a potent direct cerebral vasoconstrictor.[86] It attenuates underlying elevated ICP by decreasing CBF and $CMRO_2$. Its hemodynamic stability preserves CPP. The use of etomidate in patients with seizure disorders should be limited to the induction of anesthesia and not its maintenance. Etomidate has been shown to increase electroencephalographic activity in certain leads[87] and is less effective than other agents in attenuating the motor activity associated with seizures.[88] Etomidate has no analgesic properties.

The respiratory system may be centrally stimulated by etomidate, so the administration is not usually associated with apnea unless opioids are co-administered.[32,89] Etomidate lacks any direct bronchodilatory properties. Eames and colleagues[90] prospectively demonstrated that 2.5 mg·kg^{-1} of propofol was superior to either 0.4 mg·kg^{-1} etomidate or 5 mg·kg^{-1} thiopental in decreasing mean airway pressure during bronchoscopy in 75 patients.

Etomidate is touted as *the* most hemodynamically stable induction agent.[91–93] It mildly decreases systemic vascular resistance but appears to have no direct effect on cardiac output or contractility. Gauss and colleagues[94] conducted an echocardiographic assessment of the hemodynamics of various induction agents and showed that etomidate produced no changes in the hemodynamic variables measured.

What Are the Adverse Effects of Etomidate?

Etomidate is associated with nausea and vomiting during recovery in 30% to 40% of patients undergoing general anesthesia. Pain on injection is common because of the propylene glycol solvent. The incidence can be as high as 80%.[95] Myoclonic movements due to an imbalance of inhibition and excitation in the thalamocortical tract are common and have been confused with seizure activity.[87] It is of no clinical consequence and generally terminates promptly. The occurrence of hiccups, usually during awakening, is highly variable, ranging between 0% and 70%.[96]

The most significant and controversial side effect of etomidate is its reversible blockade of 11-beta-hydroxylase. Etomidate causes reversible adrenocortical suppression by interfering with 11-beta-hydroxylation of 11-deoxycortisol, which prevents its conversion to cortisol. It decreases both serum cortisol and aldosterone levels. Single bolus induction doses of etomidate have transiently inhibited cortisol and aldosterone synthesis.[97–99] Studies of elective surgical patients receiving etomidate showed a reduction in serum cortisol levels but no change in mortality.[100] A retrospective study and an randomized controlled trial (RCT) of critically ill trauma patients also found evidence of adrenal suppression without a significant change in mortality.[101,102] Adrenal suppression is of the greatest concern in septic patients. One systematic review including mainly RCT studies found an increase in mortality when a single dose of etomidate was used for septic patients.[103] This is especially true for patients requiring multiple vasopressors and those with an intra-abdominal source of infection.[104] However, several large cohort studies did not find a difference in mortality in septic patients who received a single dose of etomidate.[105–107]

What Is the Role of Etomidate as an Induction Agent for Tracheal Intubation?

Etomidate has been largely abandoned for most indications due to its reversible adrenal suppression. As per the discussion above, use of etomidate is not advised in septic patients and use in trauma patients is controversial at best. Furthermore, ketamine offers similar hemodynamic stability in these patient groups.[102] There is some evidence that etomidate provides better quality seizures during electroconvulsive therapy.[108]

As with any induction agent, dosage must be adjusted in hemodynamically compromised patients. In euvolemic and hemodynamically stable patients, the normal induction dose of etomidate is 0.2 to 0.4 mg·kg^{-1}. In compromised patients, the induction dose should be reduced commensurate with the patient's clinical status.

The use of etomidate to facilitate airway management in the patient with status epilepticus is not contraindicated, as it does depress the level of consciousness, and long-term medication with benzodiazepines or propofol ordinarily follows the intubation.

KETAMINE

Discuss the Clinical Pharmacology of Ketamine

Ketamine, an arylcyclohexylamine, is a structural analog of phencyclidine, which may account for psychomimetic side effects, such as hallucinations and nightmares. The compound has a chiral center producing stereoisomers and is commercially available as a racemic mixture. It is fairly lipid soluble and minimally protein bound accounting for its rapid onset (45-60 seconds). Ketamine is extensively absorbed by the liver and metabolized by the cytochrome P-450 biotransformation system. The primary metabolite, norketamine, has roughly 1/5 the potency of the parent molecule. Its high lipid solubility produces rapid redistribution and short duration of effect. Rapid hepatic metabolism is responsible for the short elimination half-life of 2 to 3 hours. Ketamine has been touted as a "complete" anesthetic by many, as it provides analgesia, amnesia, and hypnosis (unconsciousness). Besides blocking polysynaptic spinal cord reflexes, ketamine is a noncompetitive antagonist of *N*-methyl-D-aspartate (NMDA) receptors at the GABA-receptor complex, promoting the inhibition of excitatory neurotransmitters in selected areas of the brain. An interaction between ketamine and a number of opioid receptors may be partially responsible for its analgesic properties. Ketamine produces dissociative anesthesia by electrophysiologically separating the thalamus from the limbic system. Patients may appear conscious but are unable to respond to, and are unaware of stimuli. Ketamine centrally stimulates the sympathetic nervous system, which in turn releases catecholamines, augmenting the heart rate and blood pressure in those patients who are not catecholamine-depleted secondary to the demands of their underlying disease. Similar to most other anesthetics, however, ketamine in the face of catecholamine depletion causes dose-dependent myocardial depression.

Traditionally, ketamine's direct stimulation of the CNS is thought to increase cerebral metabolism, $CMRO_2$, and CBF, thus potentially increasing ICP in patients with CNS injury. These generalizations may not be valid. Albanese and colleagues[109] studied the effects of ketamine (5 mg·kg^{-1}) in eight patients with traumatic brain injury who were ventilated and sedated with propofol. There was a significant decrease in the ICP, while the CPP and middle cerebral artery blood flow velocities were unchanged. One systematic review comparing propofol, ketamine, etomidate, and midazolam for sedation of patients in the ICU with traumatic brain injuries found no difference in ICP or CPP.[110] There is some evidence that the antagonist behavior of ketamine at NMDA receptors may have a neuroprotective benefit.[111] Ketamine has been used to decrease the hemodynamic response to endotracheal suctioning in the ICU for traumatic brain injury patients.[112] Ketamine is unlikely to cause a significant rise in ICP with induction and intubation, given that suctioning did not result in significant variation in mean arterial pressure, CPP, or CBF velocity.[112] Unfortunately, the evidence with respect to the use of ketamine for induction of anesthesia specifically in the patient with intracranial hypertension is lacking. However, it can be said that ketamine may be used in the sedated, mechanically ventilated patient with little concern for worsening intracranial hypertension.[113–115] Ketamine's long-term exclusion from the induction of patients with decreased intracranial compliance may be an overgeneralization.

A key feature of ketamine is its effects on the respiratory system. Despite inducing profound anesthesia, upper airway reflexes and central respiratory drive are preserved to a degree following ketamine administration; although with high doses, hypoventilation and apnea will occur. In addition, ketamine directly relaxes bronchial smooth muscle, producing bronchodilation. Ketamine has been successfully used to treat status asthmaticus and less severe bronchospasm.[116–119] Hemmingsen and colleagues[117] in a placebo-controlled trial showed that ketamine (1 $mg{\cdot}kg^{-1}$) successfully relieved bronchospasm in ventilated subjects.

With Its Unique Characteristics, What Is the Role of Ketamine as an Induction Agent for Airway Management?

Ketamine is the traditional induction agent for patients with reactive airways disease who require tracheal intubation. Because of its unique pharmacologic profile, ketamine may also be considered for induction in hypovolemic patients and for patients with hemodynamic instability due to cardiac tamponade or distributive shock. In normotensive or hypertensive patients with ischemic heart disease, catecholamine release may adversely increase myocardial oxygen demand. For patients with known ischemic heart disease being induced for coronary artery bypass grafting, ketamine was found to increase heart rate by an average 20 bpm and mean arterial blood pressure by an average 40 mmHg. Systolic function, diastolic function, and stroke volume index were all reduced based on pre and postinduction echocardiography.[120] Therefore, ischemic heart disease and hypertension are relative contraindications to the use of ketamine for induction.

Based on the previous discussion, the use of ketamine in patients with elevated ICP remains controversial. Traditional teaching would have us avoid ketamine despite there being little to no evidence to support such a practice.

The induction dose of ketamine is 1 to 2 $mg{\cdot}kg^{-1}$. This dose needs to be adjusted for hypovolemic and/or hypotensive patients. Ketamine may be mixed with propofol as a 50:50 mixture (5 $mg{\cdot}mL^{-1}$ of each), "ketofol," a combination that produces less hypotension, but more respiratory depression than propofol alone.[121]

Ketamine is commonly used in low- and middle-income countries for induction and maintenance of anesthesia. The scarcities of vasopressors, advanced airway equipment, and anesthesia providers with advanced airway training make the stable hemodynamic profile and ability to maintain airway reflexes very desirable. Despite the paucity of other medications and equipment, ketamine is relatively available.[122]

What Are the Adverse Effects of Ketamine?

Because of its stimulating effects, ketamine enhances laryngeal reflexes and increases pharyngeal and bronchial secretions. These secretions may precipitate laryngospasm and be bothersome during upper airway examination in the difficult airway patient or procedural sedation. An antimuscarinic agent such as glycopyrrolate may be administered in conjunction with ketamine to promote a drying effect. The maintenance of airway reflexes does not negate the need for intubation and airway protection when faced with patients at risk for aspiration.

It is found that 5% to 30% of patients will experience hallucinations or dreams on emergence from ketamine. They are more common in adults than children and can be eliminated by the concomitant or subsequent administration of a benzodiazepine.[113]

PROPOFOL

Discuss the Clinical Pharmacology of Propofol

Propofol (2,6-disopropylphenol) is an alkylphenol derivative with hypnotic properties. Propofol is supplied in an emulsion of 10% soybean oil, 2.25% glycerol, and 1.2% egg lecithin.[123] It is highly lipid soluble and hence rapidly acting. The initial redistribution half-life is 2 to 8 minutes. It is rapidly metabolized to inactive, water-soluble metabolites.

Propofol enhances GABA activity at the GABA-receptor complex. It decreases $CMRO_2$ and ICP .[124–126] Propofol causes a direct reduction in blood pressure through vasodilation and direct myocardial depression, resulting in a decrease in CPP, which may be detrimental in a compromised patient.[127] Propofol has profound anticonvulsant properties.[128] It is a potent depressor of ventilation, inhibiting hypoxic and hypercarbic ventilatory drive.

What Is the Role of Propofol as an Induction Agent for Tracheal Intubation?

Propofol is an excellent induction agent in hemodynamically stable patients. Its potential for hypotension and reduction in CPP may reduce its role as an induction agent for rapid sequence intubation/induction (RSI). However, it remains a commonly used agent in this setting as the adverse hemodynamic changes and other pharmacological effects of propofol are very predictable. Altered dosing for unstable patients or using it in conjunction with ketamine, "ketofol," helps to attenuate the undesirable hemodynamic effects.

There are no absolute contraindications to the use of propofol. The company product monograph lists egg and soy allergies as contraindications due to the presence of 1.2% egg lecithin and 10% soybean oil.[129] Similarly, there are concerns for patients with peanut allergies because of the cross-reactivity between soy and peanut antigens. Nevertheless, propofol administration is likely safe in these patients since several studies have found that patients do not react to propofol, even if they are sensitized to egg, soy, or peanuts.[130,131]

The induction dose of propofol is 1 to 2 $mg \cdot kg^{-1}$ in a euvolemic, normotensive patient. Because of its predictable tendency to reduce mean arterial blood pressure, smaller doses are generally used when propofol is given as an induction agent for emergency induction. Propofol can cause mild clonus but to a lesser degree than thiopental, etomidate, or methohexital.[87]

The pain associated with the injection of propofol is comparable to that of methohexital, less than etomidate, and more than thiopental.[22] This effect can be attenuated by injecting the medication through a rapidly running IV infusion in a large vein. Alternatively, pretreatment with a small dose of 1% lidocaine (4 mL)[132] or mixing the propofol with a small amount of 1% lidocaine (2-4 mL) prior to injection[133] has both been shown to minimize the discomfort. In a systematic review, combination therapy using two different agents was most effective for control of pain on injection of propofol. Both opioids and 5-HT3 antagonists were effective single-agent therapies.[134]

What Are the Newest Induction Agents that Are Currently Under Investigation?

Given the limitations of the currently available induction agents, there are ongoing efforts to develop the "ideal" induction agent. Many of these agents will likely not become widely used, however, being up-to-date with the development of new agents will help you understand the limitations of our current agents and predict changes in future practice.

$GABA_A$ Receptor Agonists

Benzodiazepine

Remimazolam (CNS 7056) is a new ester-hydrolyzed benzodiazepine that has completed a Phase IIa trial.[135] It is an ultra-short-acting IV benzodiazepine with rapid onset.[136] Its onset of action is 1.5 to 2.5 minutes compared to 5 minutes for midazolam.[135] Its sedative effect lasts for 10 minutes in comparison to 40 minutes after the administration of midazolam.[137] Remimazolam has been approved in Japan on January 23, 2020, for use in general anesthesia.[136] It has been approved in the United States on July 2, 2020, and in the European Union on April 20, 2021, for procedural sedation in adult patients.[138,139] It is currently being reviewed by regulatory agencies for general anesthesia in South Korea and procedural sedation in China.

JM-1232 (-) (also known as MR04A3 when administered as a 1% aqueous preparation) is an isoindoline derivative benzodiazepine.[137] It is chemically different from other benzodiazepines but is a full agonist of the $GABA_A$ receptor. It has shown a favorable safety profile in humans and may have analgesic effects.[140,141]

Etomidate derivatives

As discussed above, etomidate has fallen out of favor due to its propensity to cause adrenocortical suppression. Methoxycarbonyl-etomidate (MOC-etomidate) is a rapidly metabolized analog of etomidate, which causes only very brief adrenocortical suppression.[137] In a lipopolysaccharide sepsis model in rats, MOC-etomidate caused less adrenal suppression and lower mortality than etomidate.[142] It shows similar hemodynamic stability as etomidate.[137]

Carboetomidate is an analog of etomidate where the nitrogen atom on the imidazole ring has been removed, decreasing its ability to interact with 11-beta-hydroxylase (the enzyme responsible for adrenal suppression) by three orders of magnitude.[137] In rat models of sepsis, carboetomidate causes less adrenal suppression and less proinflammatory cytokine production than etomidate.[143] While having significantly lower adrenocortical suppression, both MOC-etomidate and carboetomidate demonstrate reduced anesthetic potency.[144]

Cyclopropyl methoxycarbonyl metomidate, initially known as CPMM now known as ABP-700, is a second-generation etomidate analog. In animal studies, ABP-700 has been shown to be more potent with a longer half-life when compared with MOC-etomidate.[145] Additionally, ABP-700 does not accumulate after a prolonged infusion and has been shown to be safe in Phase I clinical trial.[146,147]

AZD3043

AZD3043 is an allosteric modulator of the γ-aminobutyric acid type A ($GABA_A$) receptor. This is a member of the new class of agents referred to as a "soft" drug characterized by their rapid degradation to inactive metabolites. AZD3043 is rapidly hydrolyzed by esterases, including butyrylcholinesterases, present in blood and liver.[148] AZD3043 induces anesthesia with good hemodynamic stability and minimal respiratory depression. In Phase I trials, boluses of AZD3043 were associated with a dose-dependent increase in heart rate and blood pressure. Apnea occurred at higher bolus doses but lasted a maximum of 97 seconds, not requiring assisted ventilation.[149] Onset and recovery were both rapid, although dose-dependent.[149] Similar hemodynamic and respiratory stability was observed during infusions of AZD3043, along with a relatively short recovery period in doses high enough to achieve a bispectral index (BIS) $<60\%$.[148,149]

Alfaxalone

Alfaxalone is a short-acting $GABA_A$ receptor agonist with a fast-onset anesthetic and sedative effect. It has anticonvulsant and neuroprotective properties. It was initially used as a short-acting IV anesthetic between 1972 and 1984 but was withdrawn from the market due to hypersensitivity reactions. This adverse side effect was attributed to its solvent, Cremophor EL.[150] Alfaxalone has since returned as a potential new anesthetic agent with a new betadex formulation (7-sulfobutyl ether beta-cyclodextrin). In a Phase I study assessing the pharmacokinetic and pharmacodynamic of the new formulation, plasma levels associated with anesthesia after a single bolus injection were similar to those of the previous formulation of Alfaxalone. Additionally, there were no adverse effects noted during the study with minimal cardiovascular effects.[151]

NEUROMUSCULAR BLOCKING AGENTS

Neuromuscular blocking agents are the cornerstone of emergency airway management and are used to obtain total muscle relaxation to facilitate rapid endotracheal intubation while minimizing the risks of aspiration or other adverse physiologic events. Neuromuscular blocking agents do not provide analgesia, sedation, or amnesia, and an induction or sedative agent must be used in combination during RSI in patients who are not completely unresponsive. Similarly, appropriate sedation is essential when neuromuscular blockade is maintained for controlled mechanical ventilation following intubation.

How Are Neuromuscular Blocking Agents Classified According to Their Pharmacology?

In order to understand the pharmacology of neuromuscular blocking agents, it is important to understand their effects on the postjunctional, cholinergic, nicotinic receptors at the neuromuscular junction. Under normal circumstances, the neuron synthesizes acetylcholine (ACh) from choline and acetate and packages it in vesicles. Each vesicle contains 5000 to 10,000 ACh molecules. Calcium enters the nerve through channels that open in response to the action potential propagating the length of the nerve. Calcium permits the binding of specific proteins to the vesicles necessary for them to bind to the nerve end membrane. Binding produces fusion and the release of ACh. The ACh migrates across the synaptic cleft and attaches to nicotinic ACh receptors, promoting muscle fiber depolarization and producing muscle contraction. ACh then detaches from the receptor to be eligible for reuptake into the nerve terminal or hydrolysis by acetylcholinesterase, which also resides in the cleft.

Neuromuscular blocking agents are either ACh agonists (depolarizers of the motor end plate) or antagonists (nondepolarizers of the motor end plate). The antagonists attach to the receptors and competitively block ACh from accessing ACh receptors. Because they are in competition with ACh for the motor end plate, they can be displaced from the end plate by increasing concentrations of ACh, the end result of reversal agents (the cholinesterase inhibitors), such as neostigmine and edrophonium, which inhibit acetylcholinesterase and allow ACh accumulation and the return of neuromuscular function.

In clinical practice, there are two classes of neuromuscular blocking agents: the competitive and noncompetitive (or depolarizing) neuromuscular blocking agents, of which succinylcholine is the prototype and the only one in common clinical use. The competitive or nondepolarizing agents are divided into two main classes: the benzylisoquinolinium compounds and the aminosteroid compounds. The benzylisoquinolines, *d*-tubocurarine, metocurine, atracurium, cisatracurium, and mivacurium share common properties. The aminosteroids, vecuronium, pancuronium, rapacuronium, and rocuronium also share common attributes that are distinct from those of the benzylisoquinolines.

The ideal muscle relaxant to facilitate tracheal intubation would have a rapid onset, a short duration of action, no significant adverse side effects, metabolism and excretion independent of liver and kidney function, immediate reversibility, and a low cost. Unfortunately, such an agent does not exist. Succinylcholine comes closest to meeting all these desirable goals. Despite the historic and well-known adverse effects of succinylcholine and the continuous advent of new competitive neuromuscular blocking agents, succinylcholine remains an essential drug in facilitating tracheal intubation.

DEPOLARIZING NEUROMUSCULAR BLOCKING AGENT

What Are the Clinical Pharmacological Characteristics of Succinylcholine That Make It a Unique Neuromuscular Blocking Agent?

Succinylcholine is chemically similar to ACh. It consists of two molecules of ACh linked by an ester bridge and, as does ACh, succinylcholine stimulates the nicotinic and muscarinic cholinergic receptors of the sympathetic and parasympathetic nervous systems. Once succinylcholine reaches the neuromuscular junction, it binds tightly to the ACh receptors. ACh receptors related to neuromuscular transmission are located in three areas:

- The presynaptic receptors, responsible for regulation of ACh vesicles release, generate an action potential along the neuron.
- The postsynaptic receptors: the principle paralyzing component of succinylcholine occurs at the postsynaptic receptor. The resultant depolarization and subsequent desensitization to further stimulation produced by succinylcholine occurs because, unlike ACh, succinylcholine is not rapidly hydrolyzed by acetylcholinesterase. Succinylcholine is resistant to degradation by cleft acetylcholinesterase and is susceptible to rapid hydrolysis by pseudocholinesterase, an enzyme of the liver and plasma not present at the neuromuscular junction. Therefore, diffusion away from the neuromuscular junction motor end plate and back into the vascular compartment is ultimately responsible for succinylcholine metabolism. This also explains why only a fraction of the initial IV dose of succinylcholine ever reaches the motor end plate to promote paralysis.
- Extrajunctional receptors, although numerous, are generally not of clinical significance. In pathological states such as denervation injuries or severe muscle crush injury, these receptors become unregulated and proliferate. The depolarization of the extrajunctional receptors in large numbers can result in clinically significant hyperkalemia.

Succinylmonocholine, the initial metabolite of succinylcholine, sensitizes the cardiac muscarinic receptors in the sinus node to repeat doses of succinylcholine, which may then lead to atropine-responsive bradycardia.

What Are the Indications and Contraindications for Succinylcholine?

Succinylcholine remains the neuromuscular blocking agent of choice for emergency RSI because of its rapid onset and relatively brief duration of action. A personal or family history of MH is an absolute contraindication to the use of succinylcholine. Patients judged to be at risk for succinylcholine-related hyperkalemia also represent absolute contraindications to its use. Under these circumstances, to facilitate tracheal intubation rapidly, a large dose of a competitive, nondepolarizing neuromuscular blocking agent should be used.[152]

How Can Succinylcholine Be Used Safely?

In the normal-sized adult patient, the recommended dose of succinylcholine for intubation is 1 to 2 $mg \cdot kg^{-1}$. In a rare, life-threatening circumstance when succinylcholine must be given IM because of inability to secure venous access, a dose of 3 to 4 $mg \cdot kg^{-1}$ IM may be used.

The intubating dose is typically felt to be 2 to 3 times the dose that produces on average 95% decrease in twitch height of the adductor pollicis muscle (effective dose or ED_{95}). The ED_{95} of succinylcholine is 0.3 to 0.6 $mg \cdot kg^{-1}$ in adults,[153,154] 0.5 $mg \cdot kg^{-1}$ in children, and 0.7 $mg \cdot kg^{-1}$ in infants and neonates.[155] Therefore, an appropriate intubating dose of succinylcholine for a normal-sized adult is 1 $mg \cdot kg^{-1}$. For obese patients dosing appears to be more successful if the total body weight is used rather than the ideal body weight.[156] The average onset time is 1 minute. Defasciculation with a nondepolarizing muscle relaxant (NDMR) will decrease the potency of succinylcholine by 50%. Therefore, if one intends to prevent fasciculations by pretreating with a nondepolarizing agent, a succinylcholine dose of 1.5 to 2 $mg \cdot kg^{-1}$ is required for intubation.[154]

The mean elimination half-life of succinylcholine is 43 seconds.[157] The rate of metabolism determines the duration of action. A normal adult has a theoretical 8-minute apneic reserve of oxygen. The mean time to return to spontaneous ventilation after an intubating dose of succinylcholine (1 $mg \cdot kg^{-1}$) is approximately 5 to 8 minutes.[158] Hayes and colleagues did, however, have 10% of their patients desaturate before the return of spontaneous ventilation.[158] The airway practitioner still has to provide mechanical ventilation until respiratory muscle function returns.

What Are the Adverse Effects of Succinylcholine and How Can We Minimize These Side Effects?

The recognized side effects of succinylcholine include fasciculations, hyperkalemia, bradycardia, asystole, prolonged neuromuscular blockade, MH, and masseter muscle spasm. Each of these will be discussed separately.

Fasciculations

Fasciculations are involuntary, unsynchronized muscle contractions caused by depolarization of ACh receptors. Fasciculations cause muscle damage that manifests itself as myalgia, increased creatinine kinase, myoglobinemia, and an increase in catecholamines leading to increases in heart rate and blood pressure. These uncontrolled muscle contractions increase oxygen consumption and carbon dioxide production, and can lead to increased cardiac output, and potentially CBF and ICP. The increase in oxygen consumption has been theorized to produce more rapid desaturation in patients where succinylcholine is employed compared to those where a nondepolarizer is used.[159,160]

Virtually all patients receiving succinylcholine will experience fasciculations. Data from 52 randomized trials show that fasciculations occur in 94% (range, 73-100%) of patients receiving succinylcholine and myalgias in 51% (range, 10-83%) at 24 hours.[161] However, 15% to 20% subjects undergoing surgery without being exposed to succinylcholine will suffer from postoperative myalgias.[162] Not only is the link between fasciculations and myalgias controversial,[161] there is no evidence that the severity of fasciculations corresponds with more severe myalgias,[163] nor does it appear to be a dose-related side effect.

Small doses of NDMRs given prior to succinylcholine have clearly been shown to decrease the incidence and intensity of fasciculations.[164-169] Traditionally, 10% of the intubating dose of an NDMR has been given to pretreat for fasciculations. However, at this dose, a significant number of patients experience weakness. The limited evidence that exists does not suggest a dose response effect, meaning that there is no advantage to increasing the pretreatment dose from 10% to 30% of the intubating dose.[161]

Lidocaine is an alternative to NDMRs for defasciculation. At doses of 1.5 $mg \cdot kg^{-1}$, lidocaine effectively decreases the incidence of fasciculation and myalgia following the administration of succinylcholine.[163,169] Lidocaine appears to work by preventing ionic exchange across the sodium channels. Sodium channel blockers (lidocaine, phenytoin), rocuronium, and gallamine have all been shown to reduce succinylcholine-related myalgia with a number needed to treat (NNT) of 3 in randomized trials. NSAIDs have a NNT of 2.5 to reduce myalgia.[161]

Hyperkalemia

Under normal circumstances, serum potassium increases minimally when succinylcholine is administered (0-0.5 $mEq \cdot L^{-1}$) due to depolarization of the myocytes. A pathological response to succinylcholine can occur, however, resulting in rapid and dramatic increases in serum potassium. These pathologic hyperkalemic responses occur by two distinct mechanisms: receptor upregulation and rhabdomyolysis. In either situation, potassium increase may approach 4 times the normal efflux of potassium, resulting in hyperkalemic dysrhythmias, or cardiac arrest.[170] Gronert[170] reviewed 129 cases of cardiac arrest from hyperkalemia; 57 were due to rhabdomyolysis and 78 were due to upregulation. The mortality was higher in those cases of rhabdomyolysis (30%) compared to cases of upregulation (11%).

Receptor upregulation occurs in burn victims, patients that suffer denervation injury, and patients with sepsis or widespread inflammation. In burn victims, extrajunctional receptor sensitization becomes clinically significant at 4 to 5 days post-burn. It lasts for an indefinite period of time, although the 'at risk' period is deemed to have passed at the point healing of the burned area is complete. It is prudent not to administer succinylcholine to postburned patients if any question exists regarding the status of their burn. The percent of body surface area burned does not determine the magnitude of hyperkalemia; significant hyperkalemia has been reported in patients with as little as 8% total body surface area burn.[171] Most emergency intubations for burns are performed well within the safe 4-day window after the burn occurs. There have been no reports of hyperkalemia in the first 24 hours post-burn. It seems rational to avoid the administration of succinylcholine until the burn has completely healed.

The patient who suffers a denervation event secondary to a lower motor neuron or upper motor neuron injury is at risk for hyperkalemia. Following lower motor neuron denervation injuries, patients exhibit a sensitivity to succinylcholine, which begins 3 to 4 days postinjury[172] and patients suffering from severe polyneuropathies display increased potassium release following the administration of succinylcholine.[173,174] Upper motor neuron lesions, such as stroke and traumatic closed head injuries, display a similar sensitivity to succinylcholine, usually 3 to 5 days after the event.[172] As long as any neuromuscular disease is active, one ought to expect that there will be augmentation of the extrajunctional receptors and risk for hyperkalemia with the use of succinylcholine. Congenital upper motor neuron and lower motor neuron lesions, such as cerebral palsy and myelomeningocele, do not exhibit an altered response to succinylcholine.[175,176] The duration of the upregulation and altered response to succinylcholine in neuromuscular disorders is not clear. Upregulation has been observed 3 years following an injury and may last even longer in progressive disease types.[172] Unlike fasciculations, the hyperkalemic response cannot be attenuated by administering defasciculating doses of NDMRs, and therefore, these specific clinical situations should be considered absolute contraindications to succinylcholine during the specified time periods.

Infection or inflammation can alter the neuromuscular junction response to muscle relaxants.[172] This situation is complicated by the intensive care unit environment where total body disuse atrophy, and chemical denervation of the ACh receptors can occur if muscle relaxants are chronically infused. Exaggerated hyperkalemic responses to succinylcholine have been observed in patients with life-threatening infections.[177,178] The at-risk time period appears to be 5 days after the illness has begun and continues indefinitely as long as the disease process is active.

Succinylcholine is absolutely contraindicated in patients with inherited myopathies such as Duchenne and Becker muscular dystrophies. The combination of the succinylcholine-induced contractures and the fragile muscle membrane of the myopathic patients predisposes them to rhabdomyolysis.[179] In children up to 10 years of age, an elevated creatine kinase is a highly sensitive indicator of muscular dystrophy.[180] Myopathic rhabdomyolysis and hyperkalemia-induced cardiac arrest are associated with a significant degree of mortality. The hyperkalemic efflux can be 4 times the expected normal response. Any inappropriate response by young males following the use of succinylcholine should alert the practitioner to the possibility of undiagnosed Duchenne muscular dystrophy.[181]

Bradycardia

Bradycardia following the administration of succinylcholine is seen most commonly in children because of their heightened vagotonic state. This is especially so as the sympathetic nervous system does not mature until 4 to 6 months of age. Bradycardia is attenuated or abolished by administering 0.02 $mg{\cdot}kg^{-1}$ of atropine or 0.01 $mg{\cdot}kg^{-1}$ of glycopyrrolate[47] as pretreatment before administering succinylcholine. The age above which prophylactic atropine is no longer needed is unknown. McAuliffe and colleagues[182] have shown that the incidence of bradycardia following succinylcholine in children 1 to 12 years of age is lower than previously thought; stating that atropine pretreatment may not be necessary. Expert opinion has gravitated to this same recommendation: treat bradycardia if it preexists or occurs following succinylcholine administration rather than employing routine pretreatment. Regardless of the age, repeated doses of succinylcholine may produce the profound vagally mediated bradycardia requiring the administration of antimuscarinics.

Prolonged Neuromuscular Blockade

Prolonged neuromuscular blockade may result from an acquired reduction in pseudocholinesterase concentration, a congenital absence of pseudocholinesterase, or the presence of an atypical form of pseudocholinesterase, all of which will delay the degradation of succinylcholine and prolong paralysis. Reduced concentrations of pseudocholinesterase may be a result of liver disease, pregnancy, burns, oral contraceptives, uremia, drug abuse, or plasmapheresis. This quantitative loss of pseudocholinesterase is rarely clinically significant. Atypical or abnormal genetic variants of pseudocholinesterase can be uncovered by testing. The patient who is a homozygous for atypical pseudocholinesterase (1:1500) may have paralysis for 3 to 6 hours after a single dose of succinylcholine.

Increase in Intraocular Pressure

Elevated intraocular pressure results from muscle contractures of the orbital muscles that occur following stimulation of the postsynaptic ACh receptors. Succinylcholine can increase the intraocular pressure by 6 to 8 mmHg,[183] which leads to the recommendation that succinylcholine not be used in patients with an open eye injury. While there have been anecdotal personal communications of vitreous extrusion in the presence of an opened globe injury related to the administration of succinylcholine or during intubation, there are no available case reports.[184] The use of succinylcholine has been advocated in patients for whom the prompt securing of the airway is indicated in the face of open-globe injuries.[184] The more pressing concern should be protection and the prevention of the deleterious side effects of intubation, such as hypoxia and coughing. If induction with succinylcholine is planned, several agents can attenuate the increase in intraocular pressure. These include thiopental,[185] propofol,[186] opioids,[187] nifedipine,[188] lidocaine,[189] and dexmedetomidine.[190]

Malignant Hyperthermia (MH)

A personal or family history of MH is an absolute contraindication to the use of succinylcholine. MH is an acute hypermetabolic disorder of skeletal muscle. The incidence of MH ranges from 1:50000 to 1:4000.[191] It is an inherited syndrome typified by alteration of the Ry1 ryanodine receptor, which modulates calcium release from the sarcoplasmic reticulum. It can be triggered by halogenated anesthetics and succinylcholine. Following the initiating event, its onset can be acute and progressive or delayed for hours. Generalized awareness of MH, earlier diagnosis, and the availability of dantrolene have decreased mortality to approximately 10%.[192]

MH is characterized by an acute loss of intracellular calcium control. This results in a cascade of rapidly progressive events manifested primarily by increased metabolism (increased oxygen consumption and carbon dioxide production) as well as muscular rigidity, autonomic instability, hypoxia, hypotension, severe lactic acidosis, hyperkalemia, and myoglobinemia. An elevation in temperature is a highly variable manifestation. The treatment for MH consists of discontinuing known or suspected precipitant and the immediate administration of dantrolene. Dantrolene is essential for successful resuscitation and should be given as soon as the diagnosis is entertained. The initial dose is 2.5 $mg{\cdot}kg^{-1}$ and is repeated every 5 minutes until muscle relaxation occurs or a maximum dose of 10 $mg{\cdot}kg^{-1}$ is administered. Dantrolene is free of any serious side effects. Additionally, measures to control body temperature, manage hyperkalemia, maintain acid–base balance, and enhance urinary output to preserve renal function must be instituted as soon as possible.

All cases of MH require constant monitoring of pH, arterial blood gases, and serum potassium. Immediate and aggressive management of hyperkalemia with the administration of calcium gluconate, glucose, insulin, and sodium bicarbonate may be necessary. Following an acute MH crisis, intensive care monitoring is recommended for 24 to 36 hours. Arterial blood pH, myoglobinemia, and creatine kinase should be serially monitored. Recrudescence occurs in 25% of MH cases.[191] Patients should be maintained on dantrolene (1 $mg{\cdot}kg^{-1}$ every 6-8 hours) for the first 24 hours after a crisis.

Masseter Muscle Rigidity

Masseter muscle rigidity (MMR) is defined as the transient inability to distract the mandible from the maxilla such that the mouth cannot be opened or opened only with force.[193] The incidence of MMR following succinylcholine is 0.3% to 1%.[194] Pretreatment with defasciculating doses of NDMRs will not prevent MMR. MMR typically subsides in 2 to 3 minutes. More than 50% of patients with MMR are susceptible to MH based on caffeine–halothane contracture studies.[195] In the setting of the OR where an operation is contemplated, a continuance of a nontriggering anesthetic following tracheal intubation is reasonable if proper monitoring is available (end-tidal carbon dioxide, temperature, creatine kinase, and myoglobin) and the anesthesia practitioner is comfortable treating MH,[194] otherwise, the anesthetic should be discontinued and patient monitored for signs of MH.

NONDEPOLARIZING (COMPETITIVE) NEUROMUSCULAR BLOCKING AGENTS

Discuss the Clinical Pharmacology of Nondepolarizing Neuromuscular Blocking Agents

NDMRs competitively antagonize the action of ACh transmission at the postjunctional, cholinergic, nicotinic receptors at the neuromuscular junction. They are incapable of inducing the conformational change necessary to initiate depolarization of the neuromuscular junction. NDMRs prevent ACh access to both alpha subunits of the nicotinic receptor required for depolarization and muscle contraction. This competitive blockade is characterized by the absence of fasciculations and the ability to reverse the block.

Reversal is accomplished by the administration of acetylcholinesterase inhibitors that prevent the metabolism of ACh allowing its reaccumulation at the neuromuscular junction competing with the NDMR and gaining access to the receptor promoting depolarization at the motor end plate, promoting a muscle contraction. Unfortunately, all acetylcholinesterase inhibitors (AChEIs) have an inherent ceiling effect that limits their ability to reverse the neuromuscular blockade. AChEIs reach their maximum possible effect when all acetylcholinesterases are blocked, which occurs near to clinically used dosages.[22] Because of this ceiling effect, AChEIs must be administered once a spontaneous recovery from the neuromuscular blockade is well underway. In order to achieve recovery of a train of four ratio >0.9, AChEIs should be administered once four twitches are present.[22,196]

Metabolism and elimination of NDMRs occur through a variety of biochemical pathways involving the liver, kidney, and Hofmann degradation. Hofmann degradation, a nonenzymatic degradation, is largely responsible for the metabolism of cisatracurium and atracurium.

Mivacurium is a benzylisoquinoline derivative that unlike the rest of the NDMRs is metabolized by pseudocholinesterase. Intubating doses range from 0.15 to 0.2 $mg{\cdot}kg^{-1}$ with a short onset time and brief duration. Mivacurium duration will be prolonged in patients with atypical pseudocholinesterase. In addition, mivacurium releases histamine that can induce hypotension.

Cisatracurium, as previously mentioned, undergoes Hofmann degradation and elimination, rendering it virtually independent of liver and renal function. It is devoid of autonomic side effects. Cisatracurium has a relatively long onset time and intermediate duration (Table 4.4).

Rocuronium, an aminosteroid, is eliminated primarily by the liver. It has an ED_{95} of 0.3 $mg{\cdot}kg^{-1}$. A dose of 0.6 $mg{\cdot}kg^{-1}$ can provide good intubating conditions in 90 seconds. In order to provide good intubating conditions in 60 seconds, similar to that of succinylcholine, a larger dose (1-1.2 $mg{\cdot}kg^{-1}$) is commonly required for an RSI.[152] However, it has an intermediate duration of action.

Vecuronium is an analog of pancuronium, only differing by the loss of an acetylcholine moiety. This subtle change in chemical structure provides improved hemodynamic stability. All steroidal NDMRs have the potential to cause tachycardia after administration.[197] This is likely the result of blocking the cardiac vagus via muscarinic M2 receptors and by blocking neuronal reuptake of norepinephrine causing tachycardia and hypertension.[197–199] The strength of this interaction varies among NDMRs of the vecuronium group (rocuronium, pipecuronium, vecuronium), with rocuronium having the least affinity for cardiac M2 receptors.[197] All of the agents in the vecuronium group have less affinity than pancuronium.[197] Tachycardia secondary to rocuronium administration will likely respond to sugammadex reversal.[200]

Based on the most recently revised Guidelines to the Practice of Anesthesia published in 2020 the use of neuromuscular monitoring when neuromuscular blocking agents are administered is now a "must." As such, neuromuscular blockade monitors are now "required" equipment to be in continuous use when neuromuscular blocking agents are in use.[201]

TABLE 4.4. Commonly Used NDMRs, Their Therapeutic Intubating Doses, Pretreatment Doses for Preventing Fasciculation and Myalgias, and Their Basic Pharmacokinetics[22]

	Intubating Dose ($mg{\cdot}kg^{-1}$)	Pretreatment ($mg{\cdot}kg^{-1}$)	Onset (minutes)	Duration (minutes)	Elimination Pathway
Rocuronium	0.6-1.2	0.03-0.06	1-3	30-70	Renal 30%; Hepatic 70%
Vecuronium	0.1	0.005-0.01	3-4	25-50	Renal 10-50%; Hepatic 30-50%
Cisatracurium	0.15–0.20	0.005	4-7	35-50	Hofmann elimination 30%; Ester hydrolysis 60%
Mivacurium	0.2	0.008	3-4	15-20	Plasma cholinesterase

Reversal of NDMR by Sugammadex

Sugammadex is a modified gamma-cyclodextrin approved for the reversal of steroidal NDMRs in Canada in February 2016 and in the United States in December 2015. Cyclodextrins are cyclic oligosaccharides, whose 3D structures resemble a doughnut.[202] They have a hydrophobic interior and hydrophilic exterior, the hydrophobic portion traps drugs within the cyclodextrin cavity. Sugammadex is a muscle relaxant-binding agent; it does not interact with nicotinic receptors or with acetylcholinesterases and acts independently of the degree of neuromuscular blockade. Sugammadex encapsulates and inactivates steroidal NDMRs (rocuronium and vecuronium) the resultant complex being excreted in the urine.[203] Sugammadex does not appear to have any significant respiratory effects; however, it is known to induce hypersensitivity and anaphylactic reactions.[204] Approval of sugammadex in the United States was delayed due to concerns about hypersensitivity reactions. There have been 15 reported cases of hypersensitivity to sugammadex (11 anaphylactic), usually occurring within 5 minutes of administration.[205] However, after a further randomized, double-blind, parallel-group, repeat-dose trial the US Food and Drug Administration (FDA) approved sugammadex in December 2015.[206]

Of note, sugammadex may cause cardiac arrhythmias which may include bradycardia, asystole ventricular fibrillation, and ventricular tachycardia.[207–209] Additionally, sugammadex binds and inhibits oral contraceptives. The use of sugammadex is equivalent to one missed daily dose of an oral contraceptive. As such, a woman of childbearing age should be counseled to use alternative contraceptive methods for 7 days postexposure.[210]

The recommended doses of sugammadex required to reverse rocuronium-induced neuromuscular blockade depend on the depth of neuromuscular block at the time of reversal. The suggested doses are as follows: 16 $mg{\cdot}kg^{-1}$ for immediate reversal after 1.2 $mg{\cdot}kg^{-1}$ of rocuronium also known as a profound block, 4 $mg{\cdot}kg^{-1}$ for reversal of deep neuromuscular block (posttetanic count of 1-2), and 2 $mg{\cdot}kg^{-1}$ for reversal of moderate neuromuscular blockade if train-of-four (TOF) count is 2.[22] Reversal of profound rocuronium blockade (1.2 $mg{\cdot}kg^{-1}$) with sugammadex (16 $mg{\cdot}kg^{-1}$) was significantly faster than spontaneous recovery from succinylcholine (1 $mg{\cdot}kg^{-1}$).[211] Rocuronium binds tightly to sugammadex rendering recurarization as unlikely. However, if an inadequate dose of sugammadex is administered, unbound rocuronium redistributed from peripheral compartments may hinder the efficacy of sugammadex.[212] The time from profound neuromuscular blockade to recovery was 2.7 minutes after administration of sugammadex.[213]

In the event of a "can't intubate, can't oxygenate" (CICO) situation the rescue reversal of rocuronium at an RSI dose of 1.2 $mg{\cdot}kg^{-1}$ may not result in the return of spontaneous ventilation prior to significant oxygen desaturation. This was demonstrated in a simulation study by Naguib et al.[214] which showed that post rocuronium reversal by sugammadex the duration of hemoglobin oxygen saturation, loss of responsiveness, and intolerable ventilatory depression (a respiratory rate of less than or equal to 4 breaths per minute) were dependent on body habitus. In obese and morbidly obese patients, there was a high probability of intolerable ventilatory depression past the time when oxygen desaturation below 90% occurred. This duration of intolerable ventilatory depression lasted as long as 15 minutes in 5% of individuals. As such, the focus during a CICO situation should be centered around oxygenation and ventilation. Although sugammadex is a useful addition to the armamentarium of airway practitioners, the intelligent use of muscle relaxants ought to limit the need for such an agent in the setting of anticipated difficult and failed airway management.

Sugammadex is entirely cleared by the kidneys with a clearance rate of 75 to 120 $mL{\cdot}min^{-1}$. In a phase 1 study, exposure of sugammadex in patients with moderate (CrCL 30-50 $mL{\cdot}min^{-1}$) to severe renal impairment (less than 30 $mL{\cdot}min^{-1}$) is increased.[210,215] In the same study, sugammadex at a dose of 4 $mg{\cdot}kg^{-1}$ was well tolerated in patients with renal impairment with a safety profile similar to healthy individuals. The mean sugammadex exposure due to reduced clearance was increased by 2.42 and 5.42 times in moderate and severe renal impairment, respectively, when compared with healthy individuals.[215] In patients with renal failure, time for recovery of the TOF ratio to 0.9 was prolonged (5.6 +/− 3.6 vs. 2.7 +/−1.3 minutes).[216] While these results may suggest that sugammadex is safe in patients with moderate renal impairment there is insufficient evidence to support the use of sugammadex in patients with severe renal impairment. Sugammadex-rocuronium complex is mainly eliminated via urine excretion[70] and the effectiveness of dialysis in removing sugammadex and rocuronium from plasma has not been demonstrated consistently. As such, it is prudent to avoid sugammadex in patients with a creatinine clearance of <30 mL per minute. Currently, there is a phase 1 study assessing the concentration of sugammadex and sugammadex-rocuronium complex in surgical patients with routine outpatient hemodialysis[217]; however, no results have been reported yet.

NDMR can also be antagonized by cholinesterase inhibitors (anticholinesterases), such as carbamoyl esters (neostigmine, physostigmine, and pyridostigmine) or quaternary ammonium alcohols (edrophonium).[22] By inhibiting cholinesterases at the motor end-plate of skeletal muscle ACh levels are amplified competing with the NMDR for nicotinic receptor binding. Cholinesterase inhibitors also increase ACh levels at postganglionic muscarinic receptors resulting in unwanted side effects like bradycardia, hypotension, bronchospasm, and sialorrhea.[218] As such, a muscarinic antagonist (atropine or glycopyrrolate) must be co-administered with cholinesterase inhibitors to avoid these side effects during NDMR reversal. Furthermore, cholinesterase inhibitors are not recommended to reverse NDMR at a deep level of neuromuscular blockade (posttetanic count of 1 to 2) and as such, have no role in managing emergent NMDR reversal in CICO situations.[22]

What Are the Indications and Contraindications of NDMRs?

The NDMRs serve a multipurpose role in emergency airway management. They can be used as pretreatment agents to attenuate the many undesirable side effects associated with muscle fasciculations (e.g., the increase in ICP, IOP, etc.) following the use of succinylcholine. They serve as the muscle relaxant of choice if succinylcholine is contraindicated or unavailable, or to maintain postintubation paralysis when the succinylcholine block wears off. NDMRs should be used with caution in the face of difficult ventilation/intubation; however, they are not contraindicated in this scenario. As stated in the previous section, reversal of NDMRs with sugammadex may not occur before significant desaturation. Therefore, awake intubation is the safest option (see Chapter 3). Nevertheless, NDMRs improve face-mask ventilation and intubation conditions and allow for additional attempts at intubation under optimized conditions.[219] When the use of NDMRs is planned in a patient with predictors of difficult ventilation, multiple backup options should be planned, a skilled assistant should be nearby, and sugammadex should be immediately available.[219]

How Can We Use NDMRs Effectively for Rapid Sequence Induction and Intubation?

NDMRs are the only option for RSI when succinylcholine is contraindicated or not available. In these situations, NDMRs can be used for emergency RSI. The drug of choice is rocuronium 1 to 1.2 $mg{\cdot}kg^{-1}$ based on its time to onset. If rocuronium is not available, vecuronium 0.15 $mg{\cdot}kg^{-1}$ is a reasonable alternative (Table 4.4).

How Do We Decide When to Use a Nondepolarizing Muscle Relaxant Versus Succinylcholine for Tracheal Intubation?

The use of neuromuscular blocking agents to facilitate tracheal intubation results in an increased success rate and fewer complications.[152,220–222] The ideal neuromuscular blocking agent has rapid-onset, quick-offset, is reversible and absent of clinically relevant side effects.[223,224] Succinylcholine is superior to the slower onset NDMRs such as pancuronium, atracurium, and vecuronium.[225] The most commonly used muscle relaxants in a rapid sequence induction/intubation are succinylcholine and rocuronium based on their pharmacokinetic and pharmacodynamic profiles. While rocuronium provides a comparable onset time when compared with succinylcholine, it has a prolonged duration of action.[22] Previously, the decision to use rocuronium versus succinylcholine was debated; however, with the introduction of sugammadex there is no evidence of outcome benefit to recommend succinylcholine over rocuronium.[219]

Are There any New Muscle Relaxants or Adjuncts with a Better Pharmacodynamic Profile?

The next generation of neuromuscular blocking drugs aims for a rapid onset with a short duration of action, mimicking succinylcholine, but with minimal side effects.

Gantacurium

Among the new generation of muscle relaxants are fumarate compounds, olefinic (double-bonded) isoquinolinium diesters. The first candidate is the asymmetrical mixed tetrahydroisoquinolinium chlorofumarate, Gantacurium (GW280430A). It is an NDMR with an ultrashort duration of action, developed to replace succinylcholine. Belmont[226] has estimated the ED_{95} to be 0.19 $mg{\cdot}kg^{-1}$. The onset of action at doses 2.5 to 3 times the ED_{95} was within 90 seconds with transient cardiovascular adverse effects suggestive of histamine release.[226] Spontaneous recovery to a train-of-four of 0.9 was evident 12 to 15 minutes after large doses ($3 \times ED_{95}$).[227] Gantacurium's metabolism is nonenzymatic, partially due to rapid formation of an inactive cysteine product, while the ester moiety undergoes a slower ester hydrolysis to inactive metabolites.[227] The metabolism of Gantacurium via spontaneous cysteine adduction is pH, temperature, and organ independent.[228] Fumarates unique nondepolarizing neuromuscular blocking agents that are antagonized by cysteine.[228] Histamine release, occurring at doses of $4 \times ED_{95}$, when administered in combination with volatile anesthetics, resulted in a 17% reduction in blood pressure.[229] Gantacurium has very little vagolytic effect and ganglion blockade.[229] Perhaps the most interesting aspect of Gantacurium is that its effect can be reversed by exogenous L-cysteine rapidly (12-15 seconds) and the reaction is irreversible. This reversal was possible even at the onset of complete muscle paralysis in both dogs and monkeys.[229] A Phase-2 trial in adults has been completed,[230] but no results have yet been published.

CW002

The discovery that fumarate muscle relaxants could be reversed by L-cysteine led to the development of an intermediate-acting fumarate NDMR, CW002. It is a nonhalogenated, symmetrical, benzylisoquinolinium fumarate diester developed from 2007 to 2008. CW002 is an analog of Gantacurium, with a slight alteration in its chemical structure that results in a slower interaction with endogenous L-cysteine and therefore possesses a longer duration of action. Phase I clinical trials began in 2012[231] and subsequent clinical trials are ongoing.[232–234]

Preliminary results indicate an ED_{95} of 0.07 mg·kg^{-1}. Doses of 1.5 to 2.0 times the ED_{95} resulted in an onset time of 2.9 minutes, and a duration of action of 55 minutes. Animal studies have shown a good safety profile. While no human studies have assessed L-cysteine reversal of CW002, in Rhesus monkeys a dose 50 mg·kg^{-1} of L-cysteine was able to successfully reverse the neuromuscular blockade of CW002 administered at 4-5 × the ED50 in 2 to 3 minutes.[235]

CW011

CW011 is a nonhalogenated, olefinic diester analog of gantacurium with a similar onset, but the intermediate duration of action.[232,233] CW011 has a higher potency as demonstrated in animal studies with an ED95 of 0.025 mg·kg^{-1}. It has a duration of action of 20.8 minutes with a 4-5 × the ED95.[232] No human studies have been conducted for CW011 to date.[236]

Calabadions

Calabadions are part of the Cucurbit[n]uril class of complex molecules, which were traditionally used as drug delivery vehicles. These molecules have been found to bind to the tertiary amine groups of both benzylisoquinolinium and steroidal NDMRs, preventing binding to the neuromuscular nicotinic receptors.[229] Where sugammadex works only on steroidal NDMRs, calabadions work on both classes. In a rat model, calabadion 1 has shown a favorable safety profile, having little to no cardiovascular or respiratory effects.[237] Calabadion 2 is the second-generation acyclic member of the calabadion family. In rats, calabadion 2 was found to be superior to sugammadex in terms of time to breathing onset and train-of-four recovery even after profound paralysis with rocuronium, vecuronium, and cisatracurium.[238] This effect is attributed to its larger hydrophobic cavity which contains two naphthalene walls as compared with the two benzene walls of calabadion 1.[239]

■ What Is the Incidence of Awareness When Using Neuromuscular Blockers and What Are the Risk Factors for Awareness?

Traditionally, we have believed that awareness under anesthesia was especially associated with: emergency cesarian sections under general anesthesia, largely opioid-dependent cardiac anesthesia, and trauma victims in shock. NAP5 has amplified our understanding of awareness under anesthesia. According to the 5th National Audit Project (NAP5), the overall incidence of accidental awareness during anesthesia is 1:19,600 (0.005%); however, when neuromuscular blocking agents were used the incidence was more than twice that, increasing to 1:8200 (0.012%).[240] Risk factors for awareness included female sex (remains higher than males when obstetric cases are excluded), age (younger adults, but not children), obesity, anesthesiologist experience (junior trainees), previous awareness, after-hours procedures, emergencies, type of surgery (obstetric, cardiac, thoracic), and use of neuromuscular blocking agents.[240,241]

The BIS monitor is the most widely used brain function monitor to assess anesthetic depth. Its use has been demonstrated to lower the incidence of intraoperative awareness when total intravenous anesthesia (TIVA)[242,243] was in use; however, there are no studies that assess its use during awake or difficult intubations. While the BIS can be a useful tool, the focus during the management of emergency or difficult airway should be centered on oxygenation and proper positioning. Clearly, the risk of awareness of an intubation ought to be balanced against the hemodynamic status of the patient in that emergency rapid sequence intubation of a patient with actual or potential hemodynamic instability where the dose of induction agent is intentionally reduced or eliminated carries a significant risk for awareness.

AWAKE INTUBATION

For patients with predictors of difficult face-mask ventilation and difficult intubation, or those with extreme hemodynamic instability, intubating the conscious patient may be the safest option. The goal during this process is to establish a protected airway while maintaining spontaneous ventilation and hemodynamic stability and preventing aspiration and minimizing patient discomfort. Many agents have been used to achieve these goals some of which are ketamine, propofol, dexmedetomidine, opioids and benzodiazepines.

In this section we will briefly discuss the pharmacology of the agents used during awake intubation other than local anesthetics. For a full discussion of preparation, techniques, and agents for awake intubation, please refer to Chapter 3.

■ Which Agents Can Be Administered to Facilitate an Awake Intubation?

It is imperative to recognize that patients presenting emergently with severe, obstructing upper airway conditions (e.g., epiglottitis, Ludwig's Angina, angioedema, etc) may suddenly and totally obstruct with ANY IV agent including benzodiazepines, opioids, or ketamine. All are absolutely contraindicated in this setting unless the intention is the immediate performance of an awake front-of-neck airway (FONA).

Remifentanil

All opioids are capable of attenuating adverse airway reflexes during an awake intubation. However, it should be recognized that topical anesthesia alone is sufficient to perform the task with total patient comfort, provided time is taken and all glossopharyngeal and vagal sensations of the upper airway being blocked. Recognize that the opioid is only employed to accommodate for a "patchy" block.

Remifentanil's pharmacokinetic properties make it an easily titratable option for the attenuation of reflex gag and reflex glottis closure during awake intubation. Suppression of these reflexes while maintaining patient comfort without compromising spontaneous ventilation for awake tracheal intubation is the goal. Remifentanil via continuous infusion (0.07-0.25 μg·kg^{-1}·min^{-1}) has been reported.[244–246] Even though some other authors recommend infusion doses above 0.1 μg·kg^{-1}·min^{-1}, the authors feel strongly based on clinical experience that this ceiling should not be exceeded. The equilibration half-time of remifentanil from the plasma to effect sites is rapid at 1.0 to 1.5 minutes.[247] Similarly, its context-sensitive half-time remains short even after long infusions (3 minutes after a 3-hour infusion).[247] Aside from bradycardia, remifentanil offers a stable hemodynamic profile. However, compared to propofol infusions, remifentanil infusions produce greater respiratory depression at lower levels of sedation.[247] Boluses of remifentanil result in a high incidence of apnea and chest wall rigidity.[247]

Dexmedetomidine

Dexmedetomidine is increasingly used for sedation during awake intubation because of its ability to produce sedation without respiratory depression. Hypercarbic respiratory drive is maintained and the carbon dioxide threshold for apnea is decreased rather than increased.[248] In addition, dexmedetomidine is an antisialagogue, which improves conditions for awake intubation.[248] For awake intubation, patients typically receive a bolus of 1 $\mu g \cdot kg^{-1}$ over 10 minutes followed by a continuous infusion of 0.3 to 0.7 $\mu g \cdot kg^{-1} \cdot hr^{-1}$.[249,250] Doses as high as 5 to 15 $\mu g \cdot kg^{-1} \cdot hr^{-1}$ have been used to facilitate tracheal procedures while maintaining spontaneous respiration, using dexmedetomidine as a single agent total IV anesthesia.[251] High doses of dexmedetomidine seem to be restricted by bradycardia.[252]

Compared to propofol, midazolam, and sufentanil, patients receiving dexmedetomidine reacted less during awake intubation.[249,250] Compared to sufentanil, patients had less hypertension, pain, memory of events, and respiratory depression.[250] Compared to propofol, patients had fewer airway events and had less heart rate response when receiving dexmedetomidine.[249] Additionally, patients receiving dexmedetomidine, with or without midazolam, had fewer oxygen desaturation events when compared with propofol and opioids.[253] In patients receiving fentanyl and ketamine versus. dexmedetomidine, there was no significant difference found in patient discomfort score, intubation time, SpO2, and recall of intubation event.[254] Compared to remifentanil, dexmedetomidine significantly reduced the incidence of hypoxemia and patient recall of intubation.[255] There was no difference between remifentanil and dexmedetomidine for the first intubation success rate or changes in hemodynamic parameters during the intubation.[255] However, dexmedetomidine is less titratable than remifentanil since its onset of action is slow (about 15 minutes) and the peak effect is only reached after 60 minutes of infusion (redistribution half-life 6 minutes).[248]

Benzodiazepines

Benzodiazepines are often used for awake intubation because of their amnesic and anxiolytic properties. Early case series used diazepam for awake intubation, whereas newer studies generally use midazolam, generally in combination with opioids.[256] Three case series describe the use of midazolam for awake intubation. These series found that many patients coughed during the procedure, despite the administration of topical anesthesia and between 10% and 14% patients experienced oxygen desaturation below 90%.[256–259] In one series that used midazolam 1 to 3 mg before airway topicalization and up to 5 mg IV while advancing the ETT over the bronchoscope, oxygen saturation dropped below 90% in 14.3% of the 57 patients, and 21% experienced moderate or severe coughing.[257]

Ketamine

Ketamine's preservation of central respiratory drive makes it appealing for awake upper airway evaluation in the difficult airway patient. However, because ketamine increases oral secretions, and airway reflexes are maintained its use in awake intubation has been limited.[252] One RCT compared remifentanil alone, ketamine alone and remifentanil/ketamine in combination. A dose of 0.3 $mg \cdot kg^{-1}$ of ketamine was used in both groups. The remifentanil/ketamine group had a higher rate of intense cough than the remifentanil only group, but no other differences. The ketamine alone group had unacceptably high rates of intense cough (60%), agitation (15%), inadequate level of sedation (10%), and recall of discomfort (60%).[260]

Propofol

Propofol infusions have also been described for awake intubation. Propofol is easily titratable with short-term infusions, having a time to peak effect of 1.5 to 1.9 minutes.[261] Propofol does depress the slope of the CO2 response curve and shift it to the right.[262] Propofol infusions when combined with opioids decrease minute ventilation more than opioids alone.[262] Propofol infusions at 1 to 2 $mg \cdot kg^{-1} \cdot hr^{-1}$ have been used successfully.[256] When compared to midazolam and fentanyl, there were no differences in intubating conditions, time to intubate or coughing, but the propofol group was more sedated.[256] Several studies have assessed propofol target-controlled infusion (TCI) systems, alone and in combination with remifentanil. Plasma concentrations of 1 to 3.9 $\mu g \cdot mL^{-1}$ have been used successfully though the rate of respiratory depression begins to increase above concentrations of 3.5 $\mu g \cdot mL^{-1}$ and unacceptably high rates of respiratory depression occur at >5.0 $\mu g \cdot mL^{-1}$ plasma concentration.[256] When propofol TCI is used in combination with remifentanil TCI plasma concentrations of 0.8 to 2.0 $\mu g \cdot mL^{-1}$ and 1.5 to 3.2 $\mu g \cdot mL^{-1}$ respectively have been used.[256] When propofol TCI was compared to remifentanil TCI, endoscopy/intubation scores were better, endoscopy/intubation time was shorter, and patient comfort scores were better in the remifentanil groups. The patients receiving remifentanil remembered more but satisfaction scores were similar.[263] One RCT comparing propofol TCI to dexmedetomidine infusion (1.0 $\mu g \cdot kg^{-1}$) reported that the patients receiving dexmedetomidine had better intubating conditions, less airway obstruction, and better comfort scores. However, the success rate, time to intubation, and patient satisfaction were the same between groups.[264] TCI technology was first described three decades ago and is approved in over 90 countries around the world.[265] TCI technology has not been approved by the FDA.[265] This was initially due to the FDA expressing concerns about computer-based drug delivery which discouraged manufacturers from pursuing approval of TCI in the United States.[267] Additionally, the patent protecting TCI technology has expired which reduces the incentive for companies to shoulder the potential financial cost of seeking approval for the technology in the United States.[266] TCI has received a partial approval in Canada with no active marketing.[265] Prior to incorporating TCI into their clinical practice, practitioners should seek specific education in TCI equipment, models, limitations, and pharmacokinetics. A complete discussion of TCI pharmacokinetics and models is outside the scope of this chapter.

SUMMARY

Tracheal intubation and manipulation of the airway are associated with significant physiological changes. Although it is unknown if pharmacological attenuation of these responses improves outcomes, it seems both reasonable and logical to minimize these responses, particularly in compromised patients: "tight coronaries," "tight brain," and "tight lungs." This chapter provides a general discussion of the appropriate pharmacological agents and their relevant properties. Successful and safe use of these drugs requires a clear understanding of the patient's physiology, the pharmacokinetic and pharmacodynamic properties of the drugs, as well as the associated side effects.

SELF-EVALUATION QUESTIONS

4.1. Which of the following is a **TRUE** statement about the elimination of remifentanil?

A. It is metabolized by hepatic enzymes.

B. It is primarily removed from the body unchanged by the kidneys.

C. It is metabolized primarily by plasma and tissue esterases.

D. It is primarily removed from the body by Hofmann degradation.

E. It is metabolized primarily by plasma pseudocholinesterases.

4.2. The suggested doses for the reversal of rocuronium-induced deep neuromuscular blockade by sugammadex is:

A. 16 $mg{\cdot}kg^{-1}$

B. 12 $mg{\cdot}kg^{-1}$

C. 4 $mg{\cdot}kg^{-1}$

D. 2 $mg{\cdot}kg^{-1}$

E. 1 $mg{\cdot}kg^{-1}$

4.3. All the following statements about the reversal of rocuronium by sugammadex are true **EXCEPT**:

A. In a CICO situation, reversal of rocuronium by sugammadex is reliable in restoring adequate spontaneous ventilation prior to significant desaturation.

B. Both sugammadex and rocuronium carry a risk of a hypersensitivity and anaphylactic reaction.

C. It is prudent to avoid sugammadex in patients with a creatinine clearance of <30 $mL{\cdot}min^{-1}$.

D. Sugammadex binds and inhibit oral contraceptives.

E. Sugammadex encapsulates and inactivates rocuronium and vecuronium; the resultant complex is excreted in the urine.

4.4. All of the following are true about dexmedetomidine **EXCEPT**:

A. Dexmedetomidine is an alpha 2 adrenoreceptor agonist.

B. Dexmedetomidine is longer acting than clonidine and is more selective for alpha 2 adrenoreceptor versus alpha 1 adrenoreceptors

C. Dexmedetomidine use is associated with reduced risk of postoperative shivering, nausea and vomiting, and pain.

D. Dexmedetomidine maintains hypercarbic respiratory drive.

E. Dexmedetomidine is an antisialagogue.

REFERENCES

1. Figueredo E, Garcia-Fuentes EM. Assessment of the efficacy of esmolol on the haemodynamic changes induced by laryngoscopy and tracheal intubation: a meta-analysis. *Acta Anaesthesiol Scand.* 2001;45:1011-1022.
2. Demiri M, Antunes T, Fletcher D, Martinez V. Perioperative adverse events attributed to α2-adrenoceptor agonists in patients not at risk of cardiovascular events: systematic review and meta-analysis. *Br J Anaesth.* 2019;123:795-807.
3. De Cassai A, Boscolo A, Geraldini F, et al. Effect of dexmedetomidine on hemodynamic responses to tracheal intubation: a meta-analysis with meta-regression and trial sequential analysis. *J Clin Anesth.* 2021;72:110287.
4. Donegan MF, Bedford RF. Intravenously administered lidocaine prevents intracranial hypertension during endotracheal suctioning. *Anesthesiology.* 1980;52:516-518.
5. Robinson N, Clancy M. In patients with head injury undergoing rapid sequence intubation, does pretreatment with intravenous lignocaine/lidocaine lead to an improved neurological outcome? A review of the literature. *Emerg Med J.* 2001;18:453-457.
6. White PF, Schlobohm RM, Pitts LH, Lindauer JM. A randomized study of drugs for preventing increases in intracranial pressure during endotracheal suctioning. *Anesthesiology.* 1982;57:242-244.
7. Yano M, Nishiyama H, Yokota H, Kato K, Yamamoto Y, Otsuka T. Effect of lidocaine on ICP response to endotracheal suctioning. *Anesthesiology.* 1986;64:651-653.
8. Khan FA, Ullah H. Pharmacological agents for preventing morbidity associated with the haemodynamic response to tracheal intubation. *Cochrane Database Syst Rev.* 2013;7:CD004087-CD.
9. Qi DY, Wang K, Zhang H, et al. Efficacy of intravenous lidocaine versus placebo on attenuating cardiovascular response to laryngoscopy and tracheal intubation: a systematic review of randomized controlled trials. *Minerva Anestesiol.* 2013;79:1423-1435.
10. McAlpine LG, Thomson NC. Lidocaine-induced bronchoconstriction in asthmatic patients. Relation to histamine airway responsiveness and effect of preservative. *Chest.* 1989;96:1012-1015.
11. Kirkpatrick MB, Sanders RV, Bass JB Jr. Physiologic effects and serum lidocaine concentrations after inhalation of lidocaine from a compressed gas-powered jet nebulizer. *Am Rev Respir Dis.* 1987;136:447-449.
12. Groeben H, Foster WM, Brown RH. Intravenous lidocaine and oral mexiletine block reflex bronchoconstriction in asthmatic subjects. *Am J Respir Crit Care Med.* 1996;154:885-888.
13. Groeben H, Silvanus MT, Beste M, Peters J. Both intravenous and inhaled lidocaine attenuate reflex bronchoconstriction but at different plasma concentrations. *Am J Respir Crit Care Med.* 1999;159:530-535.
14. Groeben H, Silvanus MT, Beste M, Peters J. Combined intravenous lidocaine and inhaled salbutamol protect against bronchial hyperreactivity more effectively than lidocaine or salbutamol alone. *Anesthesiology.* 1998;89:862-868.
15. Maslow AD, Regan MM, Israel E, et al. Inhaled albuterol, but not intravenous lidocaine, protects against intubation-induced bronchoconstriction in asthma. *Anesthesiology.* 2000;93:1198-1204.
16. McEvoy G. AHFS drug information 2006. Bethesda, MD: American Society of Health-System Pharmacists; 2006.
17. Foo I, Macfarlane AJR, Srivastava D, et al. The use of intravenous lidocaine for postoperative pain and recovery: international consensus statement on efficacy and safety. *Anaesthesia.* 2021;76:238-250.

18. Usubiaga JE, Wikinski J, Ferrero R, Usubiaga LE, Wikinski R. Local anesthetic-induced convulsions in man an electroencephalographic study. *Anesthesia and Analgesia Current Researches*. 1966;45:611-620.
19. DeToledo JC. Lidocaine and seizures. *Therapeutic Drug Monitoring*. 2000;22:320-322.
20. Butterworth IV JF, Mackey DC, Wasnick JD. Morgan & Mikhail's Clinical Anesthesiology. 5th ed. United States: McGraw-Hill; 2013.
21. Heinonen JA, Litonius E, Salmi T, et al. Intravenous Lipid Emulsion given to volunteers does not affect symptoms of lidocaine brain toxicity. *Basic & Clinical Pharmacology & Toxicology*. 2015;116:378-383.
22. Barash P, Cullen B, Stoelting R, et al. *Clinical Anesthesia*, 8th ed. Philadelphia, PA: Lippincott Williams & Wilkins; 2017.
23. Forget P. Opioid-free anaesthesia. Why and how? A contextual analysis. *Anaesth Crit Care Pain Med*. 2019;38:169-172.
24. Atcheson R, Lambert DG. Update on opioid receptors. *Br J Anaesth*. 1994;73:132-134.
25. *Product Monograph: Fentanyl Citrate Injection*. Sandoz Canada; 2014.
26. ULTIVA® (remifentanil hydrochloride) for Injection. Prescribing Information Glaxo Group Limited; 2015.
27. Shafer SL, Varvel JR. Pharmacokinetics, pharmacodynamics, and rational opioid selection. *Anesthesiology*. 1991;74:53-63.
28. Bailey PL, Wilbrink J, Zwanikken P, Pace NL, Stanley TH. Anesthetic induction with fentanyl. *Anesth Analg*. 1985;64:48-53.
29. Bennett JA, Abrams JT, Van Riper DF, Horrow JC. Difficult or impossible ventilation after sufentanil-induced anesthesia is caused primarily by vocal cord closure. *Anesthesiology*. 1997;87:1070-1074.
30. Streisand JB, Bailey PL, LeMaire L, et al. Fentanyl-induced rigidity and unconsciousness in human volunteers. Incidence, duration, and plasma concentrations. *Anesthesiology*. 1993;78:629-634.
31. Abrams JT, Horrow JC, Bennett JA, Van Riper DF, Storella RJ. Upper airway closure: a primary source of difficult ventilation with sufentanil induction of anesthesia. *Anesth Analg*. 1996;83:629-632.
32. Stoelting RK. Pharmacology and physiology in anesthetic practice, 3rd ed. Philadelphia, PA: Lippincott-Raven; 1999.
33. Muller P, Vogtmann C. Three cases with different presentation of fentanyl-induced muscle rigidity—a rare problem in intensive care of neonates. *Am J Perinatol*. 2000;17:23-26.
34. Vankova ME, Weinger MB, Chen DY, Bronson JB, Motis V, Koob GF. Role of central mu, delta-1, and kappa-1 opioid receptors in opioid-induced muscle rigidity in the rat. *Anesthesiology*. 1996;85:574-583.
35. Liu RH, Fung SJ, Reddy VK, Barnes CD. Localization of glutamatergic neurons in the dorsolateral pontine tegmentum projecting to the spinal cord of the cat with a proposed role of glutamate on lumbar motoneuron activity. *Neuroscience*. 1995;64:193-208.
36. Lui PW, Lee TY, Chan SH. Involvement of locus coeruleus and noradrenergic neurotransmission in fentanyl-induced muscular rigidity in the rat. *Neurosci Lett*. 1989;96:114-119.
37. Mets B. Acute dystonia after alfentanil in untreated Parkinson's disease. *Anesth Analg*. 1991;72:557-558.
38. Tagaito Y, Isono S, Nishino T. Upper airway reflexes during a combination of propofol and fentanyl anesthesia. *Anesthesiology*. 1998;88:1459-1466.
39. Joshi GP, Kamali A, Meng J, Rosero E, Gasanova I. Effects of fentanyl administration before induction of anesthesia and placement of the Laryngeal Mask Airway: a randomized, placebo-controlled trial. *J Clin Anesth*. 2014;26:136-142.
40. Wong THK, Critchley LAH, Lee A, Khaw KS, Kee WDN, Gin T. Fentanyl dosage and timing when inserting the Laryngeal Mask Airway. *Anaesth Intensive Care*. 2010;38:55-64.
41. Egan TD, Lemmens HJ, Fiset P, et al. The pharmacokinetics of the new short-acting opioid remifentanil (GI87084B) in healthy adult male volunteers. *Anesthesiology*. 1993;79:881-892.
42. Batra YK, Al Qattan AR, Ali SS, Qureshi MI, Kuriakose D, Migahed A. Assessment of tracheal intubating conditions in children using remifentanil and propofol without muscle relaxant. *Paediatr Anaesth*. 2004;14:452-456.
43. Blair JM, Hill DA, Wilson CM, Fee JP. Assessment of tracheal intubation in children after induction with propofol and different doses of remifentanil. *Anaesthesia*. 2004;59:27-33.
44. Grant S, Noble S, Woods A, Murdoch J, Davidson A. Assessment of intubating conditions in adults after induction with propofol and varying doses of remifentanil. *Br J Anaesth*. 1998;81:540-543.
45. Habib AS, Parker JL, Maguire AM, Rowbotham DJ, Thompson JP. Effects of remifentanil and alfentanil on the cardiovascular responses to induction of anaesthesia and tracheal intubation in the elderly. *Br J Anaesth*. 2002;88:430-433.
46. Maguire AM, Kumar N, Parker JL, Rowbotham DJ, Thompson JP. Comparison of effects of remifentanil and alfentanil on cardiovascular response to tracheal intubation in hypertensive patients. *Br J Anaesth*. 2001;86:90-93.
47. McAtamney D, O'Hare R, Hughes D, Carabine U, Mirakhur R. Evaluation of remifentanil for control of haemodynamic response to tracheal intubation. *Anaesthesia*. 1998;53:1223-1227.
48. Glass PS, Hardman D, Kamiyama Y, et al. Preliminary pharmacokinetics and pharmacodynamics of an ultra-short-acting opioid: remifentanil (GI87084B). *Anesth Analg*. 1993;77:1031-1040.
49. Joshi GP, Warner DS, Twersky RS, Fleisher LA. A comparison of the remifentanil and fentanyl adverse effect profile in a multicenter phase IV study. *J Clin Anesth*. 2002;14:494-499.
50. Lee MP, Kua JS, Chiu WK. The use of remifentanil to facilitate the insertion of the laryngeal mask airway. *Anesth Analg*. 2001;93:359-362.
51. Alexander R, Olufolabi AJ, Booth J, El-Moalem HE, Glass PS. Dosing study of remifentanil and propofol for tracheal intubation without the use of muscle relaxants. *Anaesthesia*. 1999;54:1037-1040.
52. Erhan E, Ugur G, Alper I, Gunusen I, Ozyar B. Tracheal intubation without muscle relaxants: remifentanil or alfentanil in combination with propofol. *Eur J Anaesthesiol*. 2003;20:37-43.
53. Klemola UM, Mennander S, Saarnivaara L. Tracheal intubation without the use of muscle relaxants: remifentanil or alfentanil in combination with propofol. *Acta Anaesthesiol Scand*. 2000;44:465-469.
54. Min JH, Chai HS, Kim YH, et al. Attenuation of hemodynamic responses to laryngoscopy and tracheal intubation during rapid sequence induction: remifentanil vs. lidocaine with esmolol. *Minerva Anestesiologica*. 2010;76:188-192.
55. Chia PA, Cannesson M, Bui CCM. Opioid free anesthesia: feasible? *Curr Opin Anaesthesiol*. 2020;33:512-517.
56. Beloeil H. Opioid-free anesthesia. *Best Pract Res Clin Anaesthesiol*. 2019;33:353-360.
57. Bugada D, Lorini LF, Lavand'homme P. Opioid free anesthesia: evidence for short and long-term outcome. *Minerva Anestesiol*. 2021;87:230-237.
58. Collard V, Mistraletti G, Taqi A, et al. Intraoperative esmolol infusion in the absence of opioids spares postoperative fentanyl in patients undergoing ambulatory laparoscopic cholecystectomy. *Anesth Analg*. 2007;105:1255-1262.
59. Gelineau AM, King MR, Ladha KS, Burns SM, Houle T, Anderson TA. Intraoperative esmolol as an adjunct for perioperative opioid and postoperative pain reduction: a systematic review, meta-analysis, and meta-regression. *Anesth Analg*. 2018;126:1035-49.
60. Kharasch ED, Clark JD. Opioid-free anesthesia: time to regain our balance. *Anesthesiology*. 2021;134:509-514.
61. Frauenknecht J, Kirkham KR, Jacot-Guillarmod A, Albrecht E. Analgesic impact of intra-operative opioids vs. opioid-free anaesthesia: a systematic review and meta-analysis. *Anaesthesia*. 2019;74:651-662.
62. Shanthanna H, Ladha KS, Kehlet H, Joshi GP. Perioperative opioid administration. *Anesthesiology*. 2021;134:645-659.
63. Grape S, Kirkham KR, Frauenknecht J, Albrecht E. Intra-operative analgesia with remifentanil vs. dexmedetomidine: a systematic review and meta-analysis with trial sequential analysis. *Anaesthesia*. 2019;74:793-800.
64. Beloeil H, Garot M, Lebuffe G, et al. Balanced opioid-free anesthesia with dexmedetomidine versus balanced anesthesia with remifentanil for major or intermediate noncardiac surgery. *Anesthesiology*. 2021;134:541-551.
65. Gustafsson UO, Scott MJ, Hubner M, et al. Guidelines for perioperative care in elective colorectal surgery: Enhanced Recovery After Surgery (ERAS(®)) society recommendations: 2018. *World J Surg*. 2019;43:659-695.
66. Boysen PG 2nd, Pappas MM, Evans B. An Evidence-based opioid-free anesthetic technique to manage perioperative and periprocedural pain. *Ochsner J*. 2018;18:121-125.
67. Léger M, Pessiot-Royer S, Perrault T, et al. The effect of opioid-free anesthesia protocol on the early quality of recovery after major surgery (SOFA trial): study protocol for a prospective, monocentric, randomized, single-blinded trial. *Trials*. 2021;22:855.
68. Mulier JP, Dillemans B. Anaesthetic factors affecting outcome after bariatric surgery, a retrospective levelled regression analysis. *Obes Surg*. 2019;29:1841-1850.
69. Mulier JP, Zadonsky I. 2017 "OFAM (opioid free anesthesia mixture)-keep it simple 2017 [cited January 2022]. Available from: https://www.researchgate.net/publication/320271760_2017_OFAM_opioid_free_anesthesia_mixture-keep_it_simple.
70. Flood P, Rathmell J, Urman R. Stoelting's Pharmacology & Physiology in Anesthetic Practice, 6th ed. Philadelphia, PA: Wolters Kluwer; 2022.
71. Uppal V, Dourish J, Macfarlane A. Anaesthesia for electroconvulsive therapy. CEACCP 2010.
72. Beskow A, Werner O, Westrin P. Faster recovery after anesthesia in infants after intravenous induction with methohexital instead of thiopental. *Anesthesiology*. 1995;83:976-979.

73. Todd MM, Drummond JC, U HS. The hemodynamic consequences of high-dose methohexital anesthesia in humans. *Anesthesiology.* 1984;61:495-501.
74. Nielsen S. Benzodiazepines. *Curr Top Behav Neurosci.* 2017;34:141-159.
75. Mould DR, DeFeo TM, Reele S, et al. Simultaneous modeling of the pharmacokinetics and pharmacodynamics of midazolam and diazepam. *Clin Pharmacol Ther.* 1995;58:35-43.
76. Hypnovel (midazolam). Sydney, AU: Roche Products Pty Limited; 2015.
77. Berggren L, Eriksson I. Midazolam for induction of anaesthesia in outpatients: a comparison with thiopentone. *Acta Anaesthesiol Scand.* 1981;25:492-496.
78. Driessen JJ, Booij LH, Crul JF, Vree TB. [Comparative study of thiopental and midazolam for induction of anesthesia]. *Anaesthesist.* 1983;32(10):478-482.
79. Jensen S, Schou-Olesen A, Huttel MS. Use of midazolam as an induction agent: comparison with thiopentone. *Br J Anaesth.* 1982;54:605-607.
80. Izuora KL, Ffoulkes-Crabbe DJ, Kushimo OT, Orumwense TO, Lawani-Osunde AS, Chukwuani CM. Open comparative study of the efficacy, safety and tolerability of midazolam versus thiopental in induction and maintenance of anaesthesia. *West Afr J Med.* 1994;13:73-80.
81. Bulach R, Myles PS, Russnak M. Double-blind randomized controlled trial to determine extent of amnesia with midazolam given immediately before general anaesthesia. *Br J Anaesth.* 2005;94:300-305.
82. Twersky RS, Hartung J, Berger BJ, McClain J, Beaton C. Midazolam enhances anterograde but not retrograde-amnesia in pediatric-patients. *Anesthesiology.* 1993;78:51-55.
83. Wang ML, Min J, Sands LP, Leung JM. Midazolam premedication immediately before surgery is not associated with early postoperative delirium. *Anesth Analg.* 2021;133:765-771.
84. Memtsoudis S, Cozowicz C, Zubizarreta N, et al. Risk factors for postoperative delirium in patients undergoing lower extremity joint arthroplasty: a retrospective population-based cohort study. *Regional Anesthesia & Pain Medicine.* 2019;44:934-943.
85. Kowark A, Rossaint R, Keszei AP, et al. Impact of PReOperative Midazolam on OuTcome of Elderly patients (I-PROMOTE): study protocol for a multicentre randomised controlled trial. *Trials.* 2019;20:430.
86. Milde LN, Milde JH, Michenfelder JD. Cerebral functional, metabolic, and hemodynamic effects of etomidate in dogs. *Anesthesiology.* 1985;63:371-377.
87. Reddy RV, Moorthy SS, Dierdorf SF, Deitch RD Jr, Link L. Excitatory effects and electroencephalographic correlation of etomidate, thiopental, methohexital, and propofol. *Anesth Analg.* 1993;77:1008-1011.
88. Avramov MN, Husain MM, White PF. The comparative effects of methohexital, propofol, and etomidate for electroconvulsive therapy. *Anesth Analg.* 1995;81:596-602.
89. Choi SD, Spaulding BC, Gross JB, Apfelbaum JL. Comparison of the ventilatory effects of etomidate and methohexital. *Anesthesiology.* 1985;62:442-447.
90. Eames WO, Rooke GA, Wu RS, Bishop MJ. Comparison of the effects of etomidate, propofol, and thiopental on respiratory resistance after tracheal intubation. *Anesthesiology.* 1996;84:1307-1311.
91. Choi YF, Wong TW, Lau CC. Midazolam is more likely to cause hypotension than etomidate in emergency department rapid sequence intubation. *Emerg Med J.* 2004;21:700-702.
92. Jellish WS, Riche H, Salord F, Ravussin P, Tempelhoff R. Etomidate and thiopental-based anesthetic induction: comparisons between different titrated levels of electrophysiologic cortical depression and response to laryngoscopy. *J Clin Anesth.* 1997;9:36-41.
93. Guldner G, Schultz J, Sexton P, Fortner C, Richmond M. Etomidate for rapid-sequence intubation in young children: hemodynamic effects and adverse events. *Acad Emerg Med.* 2003;10:134-139.
94. Gauss A, Heinrich H, Wilder-Smith OH. Echocardiographic assessment of the haemodynamic effects of propofol: a comparison with etomidate and thiopentone. *Anaesthesia.* 1991;46:99-105.
95. Holdcroft A, Morgan M, Whitwam JG, Lumley J. Effect of dose and premedication on induction complications with etomidate. *Br J Anaesth.* 1976;48:199-205.
96. Ghoneim MM, Yamada T. Etomidate: a clinical and electroencephalographic comparison with thiopental. *Anesth Analg.* 1977;56:479-485.
97. Duthie DJ, Fraser R, Nimmo WS. Effect of induction of anaesthesia with etomidate on corticosteroid synthesis in man. *Br J Anaesth.* 1985;57:156-159.
98. Wagner RL, White PF. Etomidate inhibits adrenocortical function in surgical patients. *Anesthesiology.* 1984;61:647-651.
99. Wagner RL, White PF, Kan PB, Rosenthal MH, Feldman D. Inhibition of adrenal steroidogenesis by the anesthetic etomidate. *N Engl J Med.* 1984;310:1415-1421.
100. Hohl CM, Kelly-Smith CH, Yeung TC, Sweet DD, Doyle-Waters MM, Schulzer M. The effect of a bolus dose of etomidate on cortisol levels, mortality, and health services utilization: a systematic review. *Ann Emerg Med.* 2010;56:105-113.
101. Hinkewich C, Green R. The impact of etomidate on mortality in trauma patients. *Journal Canadien D Anesthesie.* 2014;61:650-655.
102. Jabre P, Combes X, Lapostolle F, et al. Etomidate versus ketamine for rapid sequence intubation in acutely ill patients: a multicentre randomised controlled trial. *Lancet.* 2009;374:293-300.
103. Chan CM, Mitchell AL, Shorr AF. Etomidate is associated with mortality and adrenal insufficiency in sepsis: a meta-analysis. *Critical Care Medicine.* 2012;40:2945-2953.
104. Rech M, Bennett S, Chaney W, Sterk E. Risk factors for mortality in septic patients who received etomidate. *Am J Emerg Med.* 2015;33:1340-1343.
105. Gu W-J, Wang F, Tang L, Liu J-C. Single-dose etomidate does not increase mortality in patients with sepsis a systematic review and meta-analysis of randomized controlled trials and observational studies. *Chest.* 2015;147:335-346.
106. Alday NJ, Jones GM, Kimmons LA, Phillips GS, McCallister JW, Doepker BA. Effects of etomidate on vasopressor use in patients with sepsis or severe sepsis: a propensity-matched analysis. *J Crit Care.* 2014;29:517-522.
107. McPhee LC, Badawi O, Fraser GL, et al. Single-dose etomidate is not associated with increased mortality in ICU patients with sepsis: analysis of a large electronic ICU database. *Critical Care Medicine.* 2013;41:774-783.
108. Singh PM, Arora S, Anuradha Borle A, Varma P, Trikha A, Goudra BG. Evaluation of etomidate for seizure duration in electroconvulsive therapy: a systematic review and meta-analysis. *J ECT.* 2015;31:213-225.
109. Albanese J, Arnaud S, Rey M, Thomachot L, Alliez B, Martin C. Ketamine decreases intracranial pressure and electroencephalographic activity in traumatic brain injury patients during propofol sedation. *Anesthesiology.* 1997;87:1328-1334.
110. Roberts DJ, Hall RI, Kramer AH, Robertson HL, Gallagher CN, Zygun DA. Sedation for critically ill adults with severe traumatic brain injury: a systematic review of randomized controlled trials. *Critical Care Medicine.* 2011;39:2743-2751.
111. Hirota K, Lambert DG. Ketamine: its mechanism(s) of action and unusual clinical uses. *Br J Anaesth.* 1996;77:441-444.
112. Caricato A, Tersali A, Pitoni S, et al. Racemic ketamine in adult head injury patients: use in endotracheal suctioning. *Critical Care.* 2013;17.R267
113. Zeiler FA, Teitelbaum J, West M, Gillman LM. The Ketamine Effect on ICP in Traumatic Brain Injury. *Neurocrit Care.* 2014;21:163-173.
114. Zeiler FA, Teitelbaum J, West M, Gillman LM. The ketamine effect on intracranial pressure in nontraumatic neurological illness. *J Crit Care.* 2014;29:1096-1106.
115. Wang X, Ding X, Tong Y, et al. Ketamine does not increase intracranial pressure compared with opioids: meta-analysis of randomized controlled trials. *J Anesth.* 2014;28:821-827.
116. Hemming A, MacKenzie I, Finfer S. Response to ketamine in status asthmaticus resistant to maximal medical treatment. *Thorax.* 1994;49:90-91.
117. Hemmingsen C, Nielsen PK, Odorico J. Ketamine in the treatment of bronchospasm during mechanical ventilation. *Am J Emerg Med.* 1994;12:417-420.
118. Hirshman CA, Downes H, Farbood A, Bergman NA. Ketamine block of bronchospasm in experimental canine asthma. *Br J Anaesth.* 1979;51:713-738.
119. L'Hommedieu CS, Arens JJ. The use of ketamine for the emergency intubation of patients with status asthmaticus. *Ann Emerg Med.* 1987;16:568-571.
120. Jakobsen CJ, Torp P, Vester AE, Folkersen L, Thougaard A, Sloth E. Ketamine reduce left ventricular systolic and diastolic function in patients with ischaemic heart disease. *Acta Anaesthesiologica Scandinavica.* 2010;54:1137-1144.
121. Kennedy MJ, Smith LJ. A comparison of cardiopulmonary function, recovery quality, and total dosages required for induction and total intravenous anesthesia with propofol versus a propofol-ketamine combination in healthy Beagle dogs. *Vet Anaesth Analg.* 2015;42:350-359.
122. Dong TT, Mellin-Olsen J, Gelb AW. Ketamine: a growing global health-care need. *Br J Anaesth.* 2015;115:491-493.
123. Bryson HM, Fulton BR, Faulds D. Propofol. An update of its use in anaesthesia and conscious sedation. *Drugs.* 1995;50:513-559.
124. Cavazzuti M, Porro CA, Barbieri A, Galetti A. Brain and spinal cord metabolic activity during propofol anaesthesia. *Br J Anaesth.* 1991;66:490-495.
125. Lagerkranser M, Stange K, Sollevi A. Effects of propofol on cerebral blood flow, metabolism, and cerebral autoregulation in the anesthetized pig. *J Neurosurg Anesthesiol.* 1997;9:188-193.

126. Pinaud M, Lelausque JN, Chetanneau A, Fauchoux N, Menegalli D, Souron R. Effects of propofol on cerebral hemodynamics and metabolism in patients with brain trauma. *Anesthesiology*. 1990;73:404-409.
127. Searle NR, Sahab P. Propofol in patients with cardiac disease. *Can J Anaesth*. 1993;40:730-747.
128. Ebrahim ZY, Schubert A, Van Ness P, Wolgamuth B, Awad I. The effect of propofol on the electroencephalogram of patients with epilepsy. *Anesth Analg*. 1994;78:275-279.
129. Diprivan Product Information 2012 [cited Nov 2015]. Available from: https://gp2u.com.au/static/pdf/D/DIPRIVAN-PI.pdf.
130. Molina-Infante J, Arias A, Vara-Brenes D, et al. Propofol administration is safe in adult eosinophilic esophagitis patients sensitized to egg, soy, or peanut. *Allergy*. 2014;69:388-394.
131. Wiskin AE, Smith J, Wan SKY, Nally MWJ, Shah N. Propofol anaesthesia is safe in children with food allergy undergoing endoscopy. *Br J Anaesth*. 2015;115:145-146.
132. King SY, Davis FM, Wells JE, Murchison DJ, Pryor PJ. Lidocaine for the prevention of pain due to injection of propofol. *Anesth Analg*. 1992;74:246-249.
133. Johnson RA, Harper NJ, Chadwick S, Vohra A. Pain on injection of propofol. Methods of alleviation. *Anaesthesia*. 1990;45:439-442.
134. Bakhtiari E, Mousavi SH, Gharavi Fard M. Pharmacological control of pain during propofol injection: a systematic review and meta-analysis. *Expert Rev Clin Pharmacol*. 2021;14:889-899.
135. Borkett KM, Riff DS, Schwartz HI, et al. A phase IIa, randomized, double-blind study of remimazolam (CNS 7056) versus midazolam for sedation in upper gastrointestinal endoscopy. *Anesthesia and Analgesia*. 2015;120:771-780.
136. Keam SJ. Remimazolam: first approval. *Drugs*. 2020;80:625-633.
137. Sneyd JR, Rigby-Jones AE. New drugs and technologies, intravenous anaesthesia is on the move (again). *Br J Anaesth*. 2010;105:246-254.
138. Drug Approval Package: BYFAVO 2020 [cited January 2022]. Available from: https://www.accessdata.fda.gov/drugsatfda_docs/nda/2020/212295Orig1s000TOC.cfm.
139. Byfavo 2021. Accessed January 2022. https://www.ema.europa.eu/en/medicines/human/EPAR/byfavo#assessment-history-section.
140. Sneyd JR, Rigby-Jones AE, Cross M, et al. First human administration of MR04A3: a novel water-soluble nonbenzodiazepine sedative. *Anesthesiology*. 2012;116:385-395.
141. Chiba S, Nishiyama T, Yamada Y. The antinociceptive effects and pharmacological properties of JM-1232(-): a novel isoindoline derivative. *Anesthesia and Analgesia*. 2009;108:1008-1014.
142. Santer P, Pejo E, Feng Y, Chao W, Raines DE. Cyclopropyl-methoxycarbonyl metomidate: studies in a lipopolysaccharide inflammatory model of sepsis. *Anesthesiology*. 2015;123:368-376.
143. Pejo E, Feng Y, Chao W, Cotten JF, Ge RL, Raines DE. Differential effects of etomidate and its pyrrole analogue carboetomidate on the adrenocortical and cytokine responses to endotoxemia. *Critical Care Medicine*. 2012;40:187-192.
144. Jiang JH, Xu XQ, Jiang WG, et al. Discovery of the EL-0052 as a potential anesthetic drug. *Comput Struct Biotechnol J*. 2021;19:710-718.
145. Husain SS, Pejo E, Ge R, Raines DE. Modifying methoxycarbonyl etomidate inter-ester spacer optimizes in vitro metabolic stability and in vivo hypnotic potency and duration of action. *Anesthesiology*. 2012;117:1027-1036.
146. Pejo E, Liu J, Lin X, Raines DE. Distinct hypnotic recoveries after infusions of methoxycarbonyl etomidate and cyclopropyl methoxycarbonyl metomidate: the role of the metabolite. *Anesth Analg*. 2016;122:1008-1014.
147. Struys M, Valk BI, Eleveld DJ, et al. A phase 1, single-center, double-blind, placebo-controlled study in healthy subjects to assess the safety, tolerability, clinical effects, and pharmacokinetics-pharmacodynamics of intravenous cyclopropyl-methoxycarbonylmetomidate (ABP-700) after a single ascending bolus dose. *Anesthesiology*. 2017;127:20-35.
148. Kalman S, Koch P, Ahlen K, et al. First human study of the investigational sedative and anesthetic drug AZD3043: a dose-escalation trial to assess the safety, pharmacokinetics, and efficacy of a 30-minute infusion in healthy male volunteers. *Anesthesia and Analgesia*. 2015;121:885-893.
149. Norberg A, Koch P, Kanes SJ, et al. A bolus and bolus followed by infusion study of AZD3043, an investigational intravenous drug for sedation and anesthesia: safety and pharmacodynamics in healthy male and female volunteers. *Anesthesia and Analgesia*. 2015;121:894-903.
150. Feng AY, Kaye AD, Kaye RJ, Belani K, Urman RD. Novel propofol derivatives and implications for anesthesia practice. *J Anaesthesiol Clin Pharmacol*. 2017;33:9-15.
151. Goodchild CS, Serrao JM, Sear JW, Anderson BJ. Pharmacokinetic and pharmacodynamic analysis of alfaxalone administered as a bolus intravenous injection of phaxan in a phase 1 randomized trial. *Anesth Analg*. 2020;130:704-714.
152. Andrews JI, Kumar N, van den Brom RH, Olkkola KT, Roest GJ, Wright PM. A large simple randomized trial of rocuronium versus succinylcholine in rapid-sequence induction of anaesthesia along with propofol. *Acta Anaesthesiol Scand*. 1999;43:4-8.
153. Kopman AF, Klewicka MM, Neuman GG. An alternate method for estimating the dose-response relationships of neuromuscular blocking drugs. *Anesth Analg*. 2000;90:1191-1197.
154. Szalados JE, Donati F, Bevan DR. Effect of d-tubocurarine pretreatment on succinylcholine twitch augmentation and neuromuscular blockade. *Anesth Analg*. 1990;71:55-59.
155. Meakin G, McKiernan EP, Morris P, Baker RD. Dose-response curves for suxamethonium in neonates, infants and children. *Br J Anaesth*. 1989;62:655-658.
156. Lemmens HJ, Brodsky JB. The dose of succinylcholine in morbid obesity. *Anesth Analg*. 2006;102:438-442.
157. Roy JJ, Donati F, Boismenu D, Varin F. Concentration-effect relation of succinylcholine chloride during propofol anesthesia. *Anesthesiology*. 2002;97:1082-1092.
158. Hayes AH, Breslin DS, Mirakhur RK, Reid JE, O'Hare RA. Frequency of haemoglobin desaturation with the use of succinylcholine during rapid sequence induction of anaesthesia. *Acta Anaesthesiol Scand*. 2001;45:746-749.
159. Weingart SD, Levitan RM. Preoxygenation and prevention of desaturation during emergency airway management. *Ann Emerg Med*. 2012;59:165-175.
160. Taha SK, El-Khatib MF, Baraka AS, et al. Effect of suxamethonium vs rocuronium on onset of oxygen desaturation during apnoea following rapid sequence induction. *Anaesthesia*. 2010;65:358-361.
161. Schreiber JU, Lysakowski C, Fuchs-Buder T, Tramer MR. Prevention of succinylcholine-induced fasciculation and myalgia: a meta-analysis of randomized trials. *Anesthesiology*. 2005;103:877-884.
162. Mikat-Stevens M, Sukhani R, Pappas AL, Fluder E, Kleinman B, Stevens RA. Is succinylcholine after pretreatment with d-tubocurarine and lidocaine contraindicated for outpatient anesthesia? *Anesth Analg*. 2000;91:312-316.
163. Wong SF, Chung F. Succinylcholine-associated postoperative myalgia. *Anaesthesia*. 2000;55:144-152.
164. D'Honneur G, Gall O, Gerard A, Rimaniol JM, Lambert Y, Duvaldestin P. Priming doses of atracurium and vecuronium depress swallowing in humans. *Anesthesiology*. 1992;77:1070-1073.
165. Harvey SC, Roland P, Bailey MK, Tomlin MK, Williams A. A randomized, double-blind comparison of rocuronium, d-tubocurarine, and "mini-dose" succinylcholine for preventing succinylcholine-induced muscle fasciculations. *Anesth Analg*. 1998;87:719-22.
166. Martin R, Carrier J, Pirlet M, Claprood Y, Tetrault JP. Rocuronium is the best non-depolarizing relaxant to prevent succinylcholine fasciculations and myalgia. *Can J Anaesth*. 1998;45:521-525.
167. Mencke T, Schreiber JU, Becker C, Bolte M, Fuchs-Buder T. Pretreatment before succinylcholine for outpatient anesthesia? *Anesth Analg*. 2002;94:573-576.
168. Motamed C, Choquette R, Donati F. Rocuronium prevents succinylcholine-induced fasciculations. *Can J Anaesth*. 1997;44:1262-1268.
169. Pace NL. Prevention of succinylcholine myalgias: a meta-analysis. *Anesth Analg*. 1990;70:477-483.
170. Gronert GA. Cardiac arrest after succinylcholine: mortality greater with rhabdomyolysis than receptor upregulation. *Anesthesiology*. 2001;94:523-529.
171. Viby-Mogensen J, Hanel HK, Hansen E, Graae J. Serum cholinesterase activity in burned patients. II: anaesthesia, suxamethonium and hyperkalaemia. *Acta Anaesthesiol Scand*. 1975;19:169-179.
172. Martyn JA, White DA, Gronert GA, Jaffe RS, Ward JM. Up-and-down regulation of skeletal muscle acetylcholine receptors. Effects on neuromuscular blockers. *Anesthesiology*. 1992;76:822-843.
173. Feldman JM. Cardiac arrest after succinylcholine administration in a pregnant patient recovered from Guillain-Barre syndrome. *Anesthesiology*. 1990;72:942-944.
174. Fergusson RJ, Wright DJ, Willey RF, Crompton GK, Grant IW. Suxamethonium is dangerous in polyneuropathy. *Br Med J (Clin Res Ed)*. 1981;282:298-299.
175. Dierdorf SF, McNiece WL, Rao CC, et al. Effect of succinylcholine on plasma potassium in children with cerebral palsy. *Anesthesiology*. 1985;62:88-90.
176. Dierdorf SF, McNiece WL, Rao CC, Wolfe TM, Means LJ. Failure of succinylcholine to alter plasma potassium in children with myelomeningocoele. *Anesthesiology*. 1986;64:272-273.
177. Khan TZ, Khan RM. Changes in serum potassium following succinylcholine in patients with infections. *Anesth Analg*. 1983;62:327-331.

178. Kohlschutter B, Baur H, Roth F. Suxamethonium-induced hyperkalaemia in patients with severe intra-abdominal infections. *Br J Anaesth.* 1976;48:557-562.
179. Donati F. Succinylcholine in modern anesthesia. *Anesthesiology Rounds.* 2002;1.
180. Larach MG, Rosenberg H, Gronert GA, Allen GC. Hyperkalemic cardiac arrest during anesthesia in infants and children with occult myopathies. *Clin Pediatr.* 1997;36:9-16.
181. Smith CL, Bush GH. Anaesthesia and progressive muscular dystrophy. *Br J Anaesth.* 1985;57:1113-1118.
182. McAuliffe G, Bissonnette B, Boutin C. Should the routine use of atropine before succinylcholine in children be reconsidered? *Can J Anaesth.* 1995;42:724-729.
183. Cunningham AJ, Barry P. Intraocular pressure—physiology and implications for anaesthetic management. *Can Anaesth Soc J.* 1986;33:195-208.
184. Vachon CA, Warner DO, Bacon DR. Succinylcholine and the open globe. Tracing the teaching. *Anesthesiology.* 2003;99:220-223.
185. Mirakhur RK, Shepherd WFI, Darrah WC. Propofol or thiopentone: effects on intraocular-pressure associated with induction of anesthesia and tracheal intubation (facilitated with suxamethonium). *Br J Anaesth.* 1987;59:431-436.
186. Eti Z, Yayci A, Umuroglu T, Gögüş FY, Bozkurt N. The effect of propofol and alfentanil on the increase in intraocular pressure due to succinylcholine and intubation. *Eur J Ophthalmol.* 2000;10:105-109.
187. Alexander R, Hill R, Lipham WJ, Weatherwax KJ, El-Moalem HE. Remifentanil prevents an increase in intraocular pressure after succinylcholine and tracheal intubation. *Br J Anaesth.* 1998;81:606-607.
188. Indu B, Batra YK, Puri GD, Singh H. Nifedipine attenuates the intraocular-pressure response to intubation following succinylcholine. *Can J Anaesth.* 1989;36:269-272.
189. Lerman J, Kiskis AA. Lidocaine attenuates the intraocular-pressure response to rapid intubation in children. *Can Anaesth Soc J.* 1985;32:339-345.
190. Mowafi HA, Aldossary N, Ismail SA, Alqahtani J. Effect of dexmedetomidine premedication on the intraocular pressure changes after succinylcholine and intubation. *Br J Anaesth.* 2008;100:485-489.
191. Rosenbaum HK, Miller JD. Malignant hyperthermia and myotonic disorders. *Anesthesiol Clin North Am.* 2002;20:623-664.
192. Rosenberg H FJ, Brandom BW. Malignant hyperthermia and other pharmaco-genetic disorders. In: Barash PG CB, Stoelting RK, eds. *Clinical Anesthesia,* 4th ed. Philadelphia: Lippincott Williams & Wilkins; 2001:521–549.
193. Rosenberg H. Trismus is not trivial. *Anesthesiology.* 1987;67:453-455.
194. Littleford JA, Patel LR, Bose D, Cameron CB, McKillop C. Masseter muscle spasm in children: implications of continuing the triggering anesthetic. *Anesth Analg.* 1991;72:151-60.
195. O'Flynn RP, Shutack JG, Rosenberg H, Fletcher JE. Masseter muscle rigidity and malignant hyperthermia susceptibility in pediatric patients. An update on management and diagnosis. *Anesthesiology.* 1994;80:1228-1233.
196. Donati F. Residual paralysis: a real problem or did we invent a new disease? *Can J Anaesth.* 2013;60:714-729.
197. Appadu BL, Lambert DG. Studies on the interaction of steroidal neuromuscular blocking-drugs with cardiac muscarinic receptors. *Br J Pharmacol.* 1994;2:86-88.
198. Stevens JB, Hecker RB, Talbot JC, Walker SC. The haemodynamic effects of rocuronium and vecuronium are different under balanced anaesthesia. *Acta Anaesthesiologica Scandinavica.* 1997;41:502-505.
199. Bowman WC. Neuromuscular block. *Br J Pharmacol.* 2006;147:S277-S86.
200. Orioli Guimarães E, Saldanha M, Fortes T, Grisolia M, Miranda M, Alves Bersot C. Sugammadex in the management of sinus tachycardia after rocuronium administration: a case report. *Open Journal of Anesthesiology.* 2014;4:203-206.
201. Dobson G, Chow L, Filteau L, et al. Guidelines to the practice of anesthesia - revised edition 2020. *Can J Anaesth.* 2020;67:64-99.
202. Brull SJ, Naguib M. Selective reversal of muscle relaxation in general anesthesia: focus on sugammadex. *Drug Des Devel Ther.* 2009;3:119-129.
203. Yang LP, Keam SJ. Sugammadex: a review of its use in anaesthetic practice. *Drugs.* 2009;69:919-942.
204. Baldo BA, McDonnell NJ. Sugammadex and anaphylaxis in the operating theater. *Rev Esp Anestesiol Reanim.* 2014;61:239-245.
205. Tsur A, Kalansky A. Hypersensitivity associated with sugammadex administration: a systematic review. *Anaesthesia.* 2014;69:1251-1257.
206. FDA Approves BRIDION® to Reverse Effects of Neuromuscular Blockers (US) 2015 [cited March 2023]. Available from: https://uk.practicallaw.thomsonreuters.com/2-621-3424?transitionType=Default&contextData=(sc.Default).
207. Hunter JM, Naguib M. Sugammadex-induced bradycardia and asystole: how great is the risk? *Br J Anaesth.* 2018;121:8-12.
208. Bhavani SS. Severe bradycardia and asystole after sugammadex. *Br J Anaesth.* 2018;121:95-96.
209. FDA Adverse Event Reporting System (FAERS) 2017. Acessed January 2022. https://www.fda.gov/Drugs/InformationOnDrugs/ucm135151.htm.
210. Zwiers A, van den Heuvel M, Smeets J, Rutherford S. Assessment of the potential for displacement interactions with sugammadex: a pharmacokinetic-pharmacodynamic modelling approach. *Clin Drug Investig.* 2011;31:101-111.
211. Lee C, Jahr JS, Candiotti KA, Warriner B, Zornow MH, Naguib M. Reversal of profound neuromuscular block by sugammadex administered three minutes after rocuronium: a comparison with spontaneous recovery from succinylcholine. *Anesthesiology.* 2009;110:1020-1025.
212. Craig RG, Hunter JM. Neuromuscular blocking drugs and their antagonists in patients with organ disease. *Anaesthesia.* 2009;64 (Suppl 1):55-65.
213. Chambers D, Paulden M, Paton F, et al. Sugammadex for the reversal of muscle relaxation in general anaesthesia: a systematic review and economic assessment. *Health Technol Assess.* 2010;14(39):1-211.
214. Naguib M, Brewer L, LaPierre C, Kopman AF, Johnson KB. The myth of rescue reversal in "Can't Intubate, Can't Ventilate" scenarios. *Anesth Analg.* 2016;123:82-92.
215. Min KC, Lasseter KC, Marbury TC, et al. Pharmacokinetics of sugammadex in subjects with moderate and severe renal impairment. *Int J Clin Pharmacol Ther.* 2017;55:746-752.
216. de Souza CM, Tardelli MA, Tedesco H, et al. Efficacy and safety of sugammadex in the reversal of deep neuromuscular blockade induced by rocuronium in patients with end-stage renal disease: a comparative prospective clinical trial. *Eur J Anaesthesiol.* 2015;32:681-686.
217. Identifier NCT04556721, A Pharmacokinetic Study of Sugammadex in Dialysis Patients 2000. Cited January 2022. https://clinicaltrials.gov/ct2/show/NCT04556721.
218. Hristovska AM, Duch P, Allingstrup M, Afshari A. Efficacy and safety of sugammadex versus neostigmine in reversing neuromuscular blockade in adults. *Cochrane Database Syst Rev.* 2017;8:Cd012763.
219. Law JA, Duggan LV, Asselin M, et al. Canadian Airway Focus Group updated consensus-based recommendations for management of the difficult airway: Part 2. Planning and implementing safe management of the patient with an anticipated difficult airway. *Can J Anaesth.* 2021;68:1405-1436.
220. Kovacs G, Law JA, Ross J, et al. Acute airway management in the emergency department by non-anesthesiologists. *Can J Anaesth.* 2004;51:174-180.
221. Laurin EG, Sakles JC, Panacek EA, Rantapaa AA, Redd J. A comparison of succinylcholine and rocuronium for rapid-sequence intubation of emergency department patients. *Acad Emerg Med.* 2000;7:1362-1369.
222. Mazurek AJ, Rae B, Hann S, Kim JI, Castro B, Cote CJ. Rocuronium versus succinylcholine: are they equally effective during rapid-sequence induction of anesthesia? *Anesth Analg.* 1998;87:1259-1262.
223. Savarese JJ, Kitz RJ. Does clinical anesthesia need new neuromuscular blocking agents? *Anesthesiology.* 1975;42:236-239.
224. Raghavendra T. Neuromuscular blocking drugs: discovery and development. *J R Soc Med.* 2002;95:363-367.
225. Mehta MP, Sokoll MD, Gergis SD. Accelerated onset of non-depolarizing neuromuscular blocking drugs: pancuronium, atracurium and vecuronium. A comparison with succinylcholine. *Eur J Anaesthesiol.* 1988;5:15-21.
226. Belmont MR, Lien CA, Tjan J, et al. Clinical pharmacology of GW280430A in humans. *Anesthesiology.* 2004;100:768-773.
227. Naguib M, Brull SJ. Update on neuromuscular pharmacology. *Curr Opin Anaesthesiol.* 2009;22:483-490.
228. Lien CA, Savard P, Belmont M, Sunaga H, Savarese JJ. Fumarates: unique nondepolarizing neuromuscular blocking agents that are antagonized by cysteine. *J Crit Care.* 2009;24:50-57.
229. Heerdt PM, Sunaga H, Savarese JJ. Novel neuromuscular blocking drugs and antagonists. *Curr Opin Anaesthesiol.* 2015;28:403-410.
230. Identifier NCT00235976, The Efficacy and Safety of Gantacurium Chloride for Injection in Tracheal Intubation in Healthy Adult Patients Undergoing Surgery Under General Anesthesia. Accessed January 2022. https://clinicaltrials.gov/ct2/show/record/NCT00235976.
231. Identifier NCT01338935, Phase I Clinical Trial to Evaluate the Safety, Pharmacokinetics and Efficacy of CW002 (CW002). Accessed January 2022. https://clinicaltrials.gov/ct2/show/NCT01338935.
232. Savarese JJ, McGilvra JD, Sunaga H, et al. Rapid chemical antagonism of neuromuscular blockade by L-cysteine adduction to and inactivation of the olefinic (double-bonded) isoquinolinium diester compounds gantacurium (AV430A), CW 002, and CW 011. *Anesthesiology.* 2010;113:58-73.

233. de Boer HD, Carlos RV. New drug developments for neuromuscular blockade and reversal: gantacurium, CW002, CW011, and calabadion. *Curr Anesthesiol Rep*. 2018;8:119-124.
234. Heerdt PM, Sunaga H, Owen JS, et al. Dose-response and cardiopulmonary side effects of the novel neuromuscular-blocking drug CW002 in man. *Anesthesiology*. 2016;125:1136-1143.
235. Sunaga H, Savarese JJ, McGilvra JD, et al. Preclinical pharmacology of CW002: a nondepolarizing neuromuscular blocking drug of intermediate duration, degraded and antagonized by l-cysteine-additional studies of safety and efficacy in the anesthetized rhesus monkey and cat. *Anesthesiology*. 2016;125:732-743.
236. Stäuble CG, Blobner M. The future of neuromuscular blocking agents. *Curr Opin Anaesthesiol*. 2020;33:490-498.
237. Hoffmann U, Grosse-Sundrup M, Eikermann-Haerter K, et al. A new agent to reverse the effects of benzylisoquinoline and steroidal neuromuscular-blocking agents. *Anesthesiology*. 2013;119:317-325.
238. Haerter F, Simons J, Foerster U, et al. Comparative effectiveness of calabadion and sugammadex to reverse non-depolarizing neuromuscular-blocking agents. *Anesthesiology*. 2015;123(6):1337-1349.
239. Zhang B, Zavalij PY, Isaacs L. Acyclic CB[n]-type molecular containers: effect of solubilizing group on their function as solubilizing excipients. *Org Biomol Chem*. 2014;12:2413-2422.
240. Pandit JJ, Andrade J, Bogod DG, et al. 5th National Audit Project (NAP5) on accidental awareness during general anaesthesia: summary of main findings and risk factors. *Br J Anaesth*. 2014;113:549-559.
241. Pandit JJC, Tim M. Accidental awareness during general anaesthesia in the United Kingdom and Ireland. 5th National Audit Project of The Royal College of Anaesthetists and the Association of Anaesthetists of Great Britain and Ireland London, UK: The Royal College of Anaesthetists; 2014.
242. Gao W-W, He Y-H, Liu L, Yuan Q, Wang Y-F, Zhao B. BIS Monitoring on intraoperative awareness: a meta-analysis. *Curr Med Sci*. 2018;38:349-353.
243. Lewis SR, Pritchard MW, Fawcett LJ, Punjasawadwong Y. Bispectral index for improving intraoperative awareness and early postoperative recovery in adults. *Cochrane Database Syst Rev*. 2019;9:Cd003843.
244. Donaldson AB, Meyer-Witting M, Roux A. Awake fibreoptic intubation under remifentanil and propofol target-controlled infusion. *Anaesth Intensive Care*. 2002;30:93-95.
245. Machata AM, Gonano C, Holzer A, et al. Awake nasotracheal fiberoptic intubation: patient comfort, intubating conditions, and hemodynamic stability during conscious sedation with remifentanil. *Anesth Analg*. 2003;97:904-908.
246. Puchner W, Egger P, Puhringer F, Lockinger A, Obwegeser J, Gombotz H. Evaluation of remifentanil as single drug for awake fiberoptic intubation. *Acta Anaesthesiol Scand*. 2002;46:350-354.
247. Beers R, Camporesi E. Remifentanil update - Clinical science and utility. *CNS Drugs*. 2004;18:1085-1104.
248. Afonso J, Reis F. Dexmedetomidine: current role in anesthesia and intensive care Dexmedetomidina: papel atual em anestesia e cuidados intensivos. *Revista Brasileira de Anestesiologia*. 2012;62:125-133.
249. He X-Y, Cao J-P, He Q, Shi X-Y. Dexmedetomidine for the management of awake fibreoptic intubation. *Cochrane Database Syst Rev*. 2014;1:CD009798-CD.
250. Shen S-L, Xie Y-h, Wang W-Y, Hu S-F, Zhang Y-L. Comparison of dexmedetomidine and sufentanil for conscious sedation in patients undergoing awake fibreoptic nasotracheal intubation: a prospective, randomised and controlled clinical trial. *Clin Respir J*. 2014;8:100-107.
251. Ramsay MAE, Luterman DL. Dexmedetomidine as a total intravenous anesthetic agent. *Anesthesiology*. 2004;101:787-790.
252. Panzer O, Moitra V, Sladen RN. Pharmacology of sedative-analgesic agents: dexmedetomidine, remifentanil, ketamine, volatile anesthetics, and the role of peripheral Mu antagonists. *Anesthesiol Clin*. 2011;29:587-605.
253. Cabrini L, Baiardo Redaelli M, Ball L, et al. Awake fiberoptic intubation protocols in the operating room for anticipated difficult airway: a systematic review and meta-analysis of randomized controlled trials. *Anesth Analg*. 2019;128:971-980.
254. Verma AK, Verma S, Barik AK, Kanaujia V, Arya S. Intubating conditions and hemodynamic changes during awake fiberoptic intubation using fentanyl with ketamine versus dexmedetomidine for anticipated difficult airway: a randomized clinical trial. *Braz J Anesthesiol*. 2021;71:259-264.
255. Tang ZH, Chen Q, Wang X, et al. A systematic review and meta-analysis of the safety and efficacy of remifentanil and dexmedetomidine for awake fiberoptic endoscope intubation. *Medicine*. 2021;100:e25324.
256. Johnston KD, Rai MR. Conscious sedation for awake fibreoptic intubation: a review of the literature. *Can J Anaesth*. 2013;60:584-599.
257. Sidhu VS, Whitehead EM, Ainsworth QP, Smith M, Calder I. A technique of awake fiberoptic intubation - experience in patients with cervical-spine disease. *Anaesthesia*. 1993;48:910-913.
258. Reasoner DK, Warner DS, Todd MM, Hunt SW, Kirchner J. A comparison of anesthetic techniques for awake intubation in neurosurgical patients. *J Neurosurg Anesthesiol*. 1995;7:94-99.
259. Joo HS, Kapoor S, Rose DK, Naik VN. The intubating laryngeal mask airway after induction of general anesthesia versus awake fiberoptic intubation in patients with difficult airways. *Anesthesia and Analgesia*. 2001;92:1342-1346.
260. Belda I, Cubas MG, Rivas E, Valero R, Martínez-Pallí G, Balust J. Remifentanil target controlled infusion (TCI) vs ketamine or ketamine in combination with remifentanil TCI for conscious sedation in awake fiberoptic intubation: a randomized controlled trial. *Eur J Anaesthesiol*. 2011;28.
261. Kim J-Y, Park S-Y, Park S-K, Kim J-S, Min S-K. Titration of the plasma effect site equilibrium rate constant of propofol; a link method of 'Concentration-Probability-Time'. *Korean J Anesthesiol*. 2010;58:31-38.
262. Pavlin DJ, Coda B, Shen DD, et al. Effects of combining propofol and alfentanil on ventilation, analgesia sedation and emesis in human volunteers. *Anesthesiology*. 1996;84:23-37.
263. Rai MR, Parry TM, Dombrovskis A, Warner OJ. Remifentanil target-controlled infusion vs propofol target-controlled infusion for conscious sedation for awake fibreoptic intubation: a double-blinded randomized controlled trial. *Br J Anaesth*. 2008;100:125-130.
264. Tsai CJ, Chu KS, Chen TI, Lu DV, Wang HM, Lu IC. A comparison of the effectiveness of dexmedetomidine versus propofol target-controlled infusion for sedation during fibreoptic nasotracheal intubation. *Anaesthesia*. 2010;65:254-259.
265. Absalom AR, Glen JI, Zwart GJ, Schnider TW, Struys MM. Target-controlled infusion: a mature technology. *Anesth Analg*. 2016;122:70-78.
266. Egan TD, Westphal M, Minto CF, Schnider TW. Moving from dose to concentration: as easy as TCI! *Br J Anaesth*. 2020;125:847-849.
267. Egan TD, Shafer SL. Target-controlled infusions for intravenous anesthetics: surfing USA not! *Anesthesiology*. 2003;99:1039-1041.

CHAPTER 5

Aspiration: Risks and Prevention

Saul Pytka

INTRODUCTION

Pulmonary aspiration, an uncommon occurrence in nonemergency airway management, may lead to a spectrum of sequelae, from no discernable effects to significant morbidity and mortality. In this chapter, we will outline the known factors that increase the risks of aspiration and how airway management may be optimized to reduce the risks to the patient.

Although reported in the literature as a relatively uncommon complication of nonemergency airway management, a majority of airway practitioners will acknowledge that the risk of aspiration is a major concern to them in daily practice. Most would acknowledge that if they have not had an episode of aspiration in one of their patients, they know a colleague who has had to deal with the complication.[1] Kluger reported in 1998 that over 71% of all anesthesiologists responding to a national mail-in survey in New Zealand had had at least one case of aspiration in their careers.

HISTORICAL PERSPECTIVE

When Was Gastric Aspiration First Described in Anesthesia Practice?

Although aspiration has been referenced in the anesthesia literature since the mid-1800s, Mendelson was the first to describe in a detailed manner the occurrence of aspiration in conjunction with the delivery of anesthesia.[2] Since that time, a plethora of publications have followed, outlining the risks and ways of preventing the problem. Unfortunately, much of the information is conflicting, and conclusions have been derived from studies with surrogate endpoints that may have very little to do with actual clinical risks. For example, the often-quoted study by Roberts and Shirley[3] suggested a gastric volume of greater than 25 mL and pH of less than 2.5, as a specific risk factor for aspiration. This postulation was accepted by subsequent investigators who directed their efforts for prevention of aspiration to the assumption that these specific values were critical factors in predicting the outcome of aspiration. What Was Sellick's Approach to Minimize the Risk of Gastric Aspiration?

In the discussion section of his 1961 paper advocating the use of cricoid pressure during the induction of anesthesia to prevent the aspiration of gastric contents, Sellick examined alternatives available at the time.[4] He identified inhalational induction in the supine or lateral position (with head-down tilt) and rapid IV induction of anesthesia in the sitting position. He commented that, with inhalational induction, vomiting usually occurred in lighter stages of anesthesia when protective reflexes were hopefully still present and noted that any difficulty during induction predisposed to regurgitation and anoxia. Rapid IV induction in the sitting position often led to cardiovascular collapse in critically ill patients, and pulmonary aspiration was made more likely by the sitting position, if gastric reflux occurred. Sellick advocated the use of cricoid pressure during induction of anesthesia as a third option.

Sellick suggested that the stomach should be emptied before induction and the nasogastric tube then be removed. He was of the opinion that the nasogastric tube would prevent esophageal occlusion with cricoid pressure. The patient was positioned with the head and neck fully extended and, following denitrogenation, induction ideally occurred with an IV barbiturate-muscle relaxant combination. Cricoid pressure was instituted before induction, moderate pressure was applied during induction, and this was increased to firm pressure once consciousness was lost. Sellick suggested that the lungs may be ventilated without risk of gastric regurgitation. Once intubation was completed and the cuff inflated, cricoid pressure could be safely released.

In his description of cricoid pressure, Sellick reported its application in 23 high-risk cases.[4] He noted no instance of pulmonary aspiration in any patient but did report that, in three cases, release of cricoid pressure after intubation was followed immediately by reflux into the pharynx of gastric or esophageal contents, suggesting that cricoid pressure had indeed been effective.

INCIDENCE AND RISK

What Is the Incidence of Aspiration in Anesthesia Practice?

The difficulty in determining the actual incidence of aspiration relates to a number of factors. First, because it occurs rarely, studies addressing the topic need to be very large. Most, if not all, of the better studies to date have been derived from large computerized databases. Second, aspiration is not always easy to recognize and, as will be illustrated below, rarely leads to clinical findings, let alone serious sequelae. Hence, it is an event likely to be missed and therefore underreported.

The recognition of gastric material in the pharynx does not alone support a diagnosis of aspiration. Despite the evident regurgitation, pulmonary aspiration may not have occurred. Even if foreign material is seen below the level of the true vocal cords, there may be a wide spectrum of clinical consequences. Silent aspiration may occur, wherein the patient exhibits no signs or symptoms of aspiration and there are no disruptions of physiological parameters. Indeed, it has been reported that asymptomatic aspiration may occur in up to 45% of normal subjects during sleep, and as many as 70% of people who have a blunted level of consciousness and responsiveness.[5]

Aspiration may become symptomatic, with cough and audible wheeze. Acute lung injury may be associated with tachypnea, increase in alveolar-arterial (A-a) gradient, hypoxemia, and radiological evidence of lung injury—with infiltrates and/or atelectasis. Frank respiratory failure may ensue, with the development of acute respiratory distress syndrome (ARDS), the need for ventilatory support, and (rarely) death.

Although many papers have reviewed the topic of aspiration, there has been a notable absence of consistent end points. In 1993, Warner et al.[6] published a retrospective review of 215,488 general anesthetics over a period of 6 years. Aspiration was defined as:

> *...either the presence of bilious secretions, or particulate matter, in the tracheobronchial tree; or, in patients who did not have their tracheobronchial airways directly examined after regurgitation, the presence of an infiltrate on postoperative chest roentgenogram that was not identified by preoperative roentgenogram, or physical examination.*

Of the anesthetics included, 202,061 were elective and the remaining 13,427 were emergency cases. There were 52 and 15 aspirations in these two groups, respectively. The overall incidence of aspiration was 1:3216. Aspiration occurred in 1:3886 of elective surgeries and 1:895 of emergency procedures. Sixty-seven cases of significant aspiration were recognized; one patient died from surgical causes intraoperatively. Of the remaining 66 patients, 42 (64%) experienced no obvious sequelae from the aspiration and 13 (20%) required mechanical ventilation with 6 (9%) needing prolonged (>24 h) mechanical support. Of the latter group, three died of complications from their aspiration, giving a death rate of 1:71,829.

In 1996, Mellin-Olsen et al.[7] reported a prospective review of 85,594 cases over a 5-year period. They defined aspiration as "what the anesthetist has interpreted as such during, or immediately after the anesthetic procedures, based on clinical signs like gastric content, in the pharynx/larynx/trachea and a drop in O_2 saturation." In their study, a total of 25 cases of aspiration were recorded; 52,650 patients had received a general anesthetic, with the remainder undergoing either regional or IV sedation. All cases of aspiration occurred in the general anesthetic population, giving an incidence of 1:2106. The incidence of aspiration was 1:3303 in elective procedures under general anesthetic and 1:809 for emergency procedures, both rates similar in magnitude to those reported by Warner et al.[6] In the patients who had aspirated, there were similar complications to those described by Warner and colleagues.[6] No deaths occurred and 22/25 patients had either no or minimal sequelae; three experienced more serious consequences. One patient required ventilation for 7 days, but made a complete recovery from his lung injury.

Olsson et al.[8] reported a similar retrospective review, with an incidence of aspiration of 1:2131 and a mortality rate of 1:46,000. Finally, Sakai et al.[9] conducted a 4-year retrospective review of 99,441 anesthetics at a single American university hospital. There were 14 cases of confirmed pulmonary aspiration for an incidence of 0.014% or 1:7103 overall. Seven cases of aspiration occurred in gastroesophageal procedures, and patients in whom aspiration occurred had one or more identifiable risk factors. Six patients developed pulmonary complications related to the aspiration and one died. All these studies reaffirm that aspiration is a relatively uncommon occurrence and the mortality due to aspiration in the perioperative period is rare.

Kluger and Short[10] reported, in 1999, the analysis of data from the Australian Anaesthetic Incident Monitoring Study (AIMS). AIMS is a voluntary, anonymous reporting system of anesthesia-related incidents, collected in a central database. Unfortunately, the nature of this type of study does not allow for a denominator (i.e., the total number of anesthetics performed by all reporting practitioners) and the incidence is unavailable. Of the 5000 reported events, 133 dealt with aspiration. Aspiration was deemed to have occurred if *"any obvious non-respiratory secretions were suctioned via a tracheal tube, there was chest X-ray evidence of new pathology after an incident, and/or there were signs of new wheeze or crackles after an episode of regurgitation or vomiting."* In this group of 133 aspirations, five deaths were recorded. Of interest, aspiration did occur in a number of patients undergoing regional anesthesia in the AIMS study (7 out of the 133), whereas none were reported to have occurred in almost 31,000 regional and sedation cases in the paper by Mellin-Olsen et al.[7]

The American Society of Anesthesiologists (ASA) Closed Claims Database reviewed the incidence of aspiration as a cause of liability to anesthesiologists and in 2000, Cheney[11] reported that aspiration represented 3.5% of all claims as a primary or secondary event, and in half of those it was the offending event leading to a claim. Seven percent of the aspiration claims were during regional anesthesia. In an updated report published in 2011, reviewing 8954 claims registered from 1970 to 2007, aspiration had become the third most common adverse respiratory event leading to anesthesia claims, now representing nearly one in five events leading to a claim.[12]

In 2011, the 4th National Audit Project (NAP4) of the Royal College of Anaesthetists and the Difficult Airway Society reported the first prospective study of reporting all cases of major complications associated with airway management in the United Kingdom in Anesthesia, ICU, and the ER between 2008 and 2009.[13] It was estimated that approximately 3 million patients undergo anesthesia alone per year. Detailed assessments of the cases led to identification of common issues and suggestions on preventative strategies. Of note, aspiration of gastric contents represented 50% of all anesthesia-related airway-associated deaths. Aspiration is the commonest primary cause of death and brain injury among the anesthesia patient population, and a significant secondary cause associated with other airway events. Of the aspiration cases, 90% had predictable risk factors that did play a role in management strategy. Sixty-one percent occurred during induction or airway instrumentation. Of note, aspiration of blood clot after was also reported as a cause of death.

In conclusion, the incidence of aspiration in a surgical population is consistently estimated at between 1:2000 and 1:4000, depending on the population studied, and when the data had been reported. Emergency surgery increases the risk of aspiration fourfold, or more, compared to elective operation yet overall mortality remains low.

What Are the Risk Factors That Contribute to Aspiration?

In published studies measuring the incidence of aspiration, the most common association was with emergency surgery.[6–8,10,11] Olsson et al.[8] reported that the timing of surgery also correlated with an increased incidence of aspiration, with a sixfold increase in the rate of aspiration between 18:00 and 06:00 hours. The causative factors that relate to the increased risk of aspiration with emergency surgery are not outlined in the studies, but numerous issues, such as lack of fasting, stress, depression of GI motility, less staff availability, higher dependence upon less-experienced anesthesia staff, and fatigue may all play contributing roles. A preponderance of the cases of aspiration reported by Olsson et al.[8] occurred in patients who had abdominal surgery performed, with esophageal and upper abdominal procedures predominating. The incidence of aspiration in cesarean section was 1:661. Interestingly roughly 10 years later, Warner et al.[6] reported no cases of aspiration during cesarean section. In another paper reviewing the incidence of aspiration in children, Warner et al.[14] reviewed 63,180 anesthetics in children under the age of 18 and also found the incidence of aspiration in the emergency patient (1:373) to be significantly higher than that in the elective situation (1:4544).

There are reports that examine the incidence of aspiration in the prehospital and emergency department (ED) settings. In the prehospital setting, the rates of occurrence of aspiration vary from 6% to 90%, depending on the study populations and facilities, and whether the study considered survivors, nonsurvivors, or postmortem examinations.[15,16] Often, aspiration had already occurred prior to attempted intervention and provision of care. In some papers, the incidence of failure to intubate the trachea is as high as 47%.[17,18] In the study by Gausche et al.,[17] patients were randomized into intubation group versus transport by bag mask. There was an intubation success rate by the paramedics of only 57% and the only aspirations occurred in the intubation group. The outcomes between the two groups, in terms of survival, were similar. In the prehospital literature, the source of aspirate in trauma patients differs from that of the emergency surgical population. In the study by Lockey et al.,[15] 34%, or a total of 18 of the trauma patients, had evidence suggestive of aspiration. Of these, 15 had blood contaminating their airway, while only three had evidence of gastric contents. All had significant head injuries, with a Glasgow Coma Scale of 8 or less.[15]

Taryle et al.[19] reviewed 43 consecutive intubations in the ED in a major teaching institution and reported a total of 38 complications in half of the patients (22/43). Aspiration occurring prior to airway manipulation was not included. There was a total of eight aspirations, the second most common complication after prolonged intubating time. Sakles et al.[20] reported a 1-year review of all intubations in an ED that had a census of 60,000 patients per year. In 610 consecutive intubations, 49 patients had a total of 57 immediate complications. Although there were ten cases of vomiting, they did not report any occurrences of aspiration. Reporting on airway complications during emergency intubation occurring outside of the operating room, Mort[21] noted that fewer aspirations occurred in the ED than on the wards or the medical ICU. The obstetrical population will be discussed later in this chapter.

A review of aspiration in the pediatric population, published by the Pediatric Sedation Research Consortium, looked at the incidence of aspiration and major adverse events occurring during procedural sedation in patients known to have been NPO versus those not fulfilling NPO guidelines.[22] This prospective review of over 139,000 encounters showed a very low incidence of aspiration in either group, with no difference between fasted and nonfasted patients (0.97 vs. 0.79 per 10,000). Major adverse events did not appear to correlate to the NPO status either, with an occurrence of 5.57 versus 5.91 per 10,000, respectively, echoing the findings of Brady et al.[23] in their 2009 Cochrane review on the same topic. As the literature has indicated in the past, the incidence of aspiration and adverse events were associated with age (neonates and infants), ASA status, emergency versus nonemergency, and procedure type.[22]

■ What Happens During an Aspiration That Determines Its Severity?

The consequences of aspiration can occur as a result of a chemical injury to the airway mucosa from either acid or bile. Injury may occur from particulate material in the aspirate causing either airway obstruction, or an inflammatory response. Finally, there may be pneumonia secondary to contamination from bacteria in the stomach or upper airway. (See also Chapter 41.)

Injury resulting from aspiration is often that of an acute chemical burn and is a function of both volume and pH of the aspirate. Subsequent release of inflammatory substances, such as cytokines and interleukins from injured tissue, provokes neutrophil migration to the affected areas and further airway reaction. Airway edema and capillary leak in the alveoli can increase airway resistance and worsen lung compliance. The end result is ventilation–perfusion mismatching, hypoxemia, and inflammatory infiltration and/or atelectasis.

The initial chemical burn effect occurs within seconds, followed by neutralization of the acid within 15 seconds. The sudden onset of bronchospasm and laryngospasm may occur.

Histologically, rapid inflammation occurs, with alveolar wall thickening and cellular infiltration into the alveoli and interstitium. Hemorrhage can occur in the interstitium and alveoli. Alveolar wall disruption and rupture and significant intra-alveolar edema and fluid can follow.

Full evolution of injury can take several days. Repair of the injury is of the order of 3 to 7 days. Particulate materials can induce a local reaction themselves and lead to pneumonia. Indeed, attempts to neutralize the gastric pH with particulate antacids may aggravate reaction in the lung due to the particles rather than from the acid itself. Particulate materials of sufficient size or number can produce substantive airway obstruction in their own right.

Pneumonia may follow, related to organisms from the upper airway, esophagus, and stomach. This is usually of a mixed flora, with anaerobes and aerobes present. Depending on the organism and the premorbid condition of the patient, this may progress to lung abscess. This is unlikely in the healthy patient. Differentiating between inflammatory pneumonitis and pneumonia may be difficult. The clinical and radiological picture may be similar. Pneumonitis is usually acute, resolving within hours to a day. If the presentation is one of progression without resolution, lasting days, with fever and purulent sputum, a diagnosis of pneumonia is more likely.[24–28]

PATIENT POPULATIONS AT RISK

■ What Is the Relevance of the Issues of Gastric Volume, pH, and Constituency of the Gastric Contents?

Roberts and Shirley[3] concluded that a pH of <2.5 and a gastric volume of 25 mL (or 0.4 $mL{\cdot}kg^{-1}$) correlated with aspiration and resultant pneumonitis. In their study, an acid solution was injected directly into the bronchus of a monkey and extrapolations were made regarding the volume and pH that would place humans at risk. These conclusions have been challenged by numerous investigators.[29,30] Schreiner[30] in 1998 pointed out that over 30% to 60% of patients have a gastric fluid volume greater than 0.4 $mL{\cdot}kg^{-1}$ (median 0.3, but as high as 4.5 $mL{\cdot}kg^{-1}$), yet the incidence of aspiration is quite rare. Indeed, it has been demonstrated that the incidence of gastroesophageal reflux (GER) is not associated with residual gastric volume (RGV).[31] Rather, it has been shown that GER during anesthesia is related to episodes of straining on an endotracheal tube when inadequate anesthesia has been provided.[32]

Maltby et al.[29] argue that the risk of aspiration is due to loss of the barrier pressure at the gastroesophageal sphincter (GES), also referred to as the lower esophageal sphincter (LES). Normally, stomach contents are prevented from refluxing into the esophagus by the pressure exerted by the LES. The difference between LES pressure and intragastric pressure is the barrier pressure. The stomach is a very compliant structure and intragastric pressure can remain stable until volumes greater than 1000 mL are present.[33] Indeed, as intragastric pressure rises, because of its anatomical design, so does LES pressure, maintaining the barrier pressure. In one study, measurements of the intragastric pressure and LES pressure during laparoscopy demonstrated that a rise in mean gastric pressure from 5.2 to 15.7 was matched by a rise in LES tone from 31.2 to 47.0 cm H_2O.[34]

There is a clear association between aspiration and vomiting or gagging.[1,6–8,10] With active vomiting, or gagging, the sudden onset of high intragastric pressure is associated with relaxation of both the lower and upper esophageal sphincter mechanisms. This combination enhances the risk of pulmonary aspiration.

The higher the baseline intragastric pressure, the greater the tendency for GER and pulmonary aspiration. With an intestinal obstruction, for example, the intragastric pressure is high in association with the large RGV. This accounts for the high incidence of aspiration in this patient population and the finding that it is one of the most common factors associated with aspiration in most publications. By the same reasoning, patients with a documented hiatal hernia, or a history of GER disease (GERD), are also exposed to a higher risk of regurgitation and aspiration.[10]

Active vomiting, in association with an unprotected airway, is most likely to occur during induction of anesthesia (see Chapter 41), with airway manipulation prior to placement of the endotracheal tube, and at the end of a procedure as the patient is awakening and the airway is no longer protected. Inadequate levels of anesthesia at these times and difficulty securing an airway are the essential elements favoring the occurrence of aspiration. Two-thirds of aspiration events are reported during induction and extubation, equally divided between the two periods.[6]

■ How Important Is a History of Heartburn? Acid Taste or Burping? A History of GERD? How Much Reflux Is Significant?

Reflux occurs when the barrier pressure fails to prevent gastric contents moving from the stomach into the esophagus. Intuitively, those with a clear history of reflux should be at greater risk of aspiration. Kluger and Short[10] found that a history of reflux and hiatal hernia were the ninth and tenth most common predisposing factors for aspiration, representing seven and six cases, respectively, in the database of 133 total cases of aspiration. The patient with a history of acid reflux, with complaints of acid taste or choking at night, is deemed by many practitioners to be at greater risk of aspiration than one with only complaints of heartburn. The latter may simply suggest gastric mucosal pathology. However, no specific data are available to indicate that one symptom is more helpful than another in identifying who is at greater risk. Again, the larger the volume of reflux, the more significant is likely to be the risk of aspiration.

What Clinical Situations and Characteristics Predispose to Aspiration?

Emergency Surgery

Emergency surgery is the most significant risk factor associated with aspiration in the studies outlined earlier, increasing the incidence of aspiration by four- to sixfold.[6]

ASA Physical Status

When Warner et al.[6] compared the ASA status to the risk of aspiration in elective situations, the risk or aspiration increased by almost sevenfold as ASA status rose from I to IV or V. In emergency situations, the occurrence of aspiration increased from 1:2949 for ASA I patients to 1:343 for ASA IV and V patients, or almost a ninefold increment (Table 5.1). Olsson et al.[8] also reported an increased risk of aspiration and increased morbidity with increasing ASA status. Most, if not all, of the reported aspiration-associated deaths occur in ASA IV and V patients.

Airway and Intubation Difficulties

Difficult intubation is associated with an increased risk of aspiration. Vomiting during airway interventions is frequently associated with aspiration, far more so than passive regurgitation. In Olsson's paper,[8] out of 15 cases of aspiration in elective patients with no risk factors predisposing to aspiration could be identified from the chart review, 10 (67%) had difficulty with intubation preceding the vomiting and aspiration. In total, 58 out of the 87 patients who aspirated did so due to difficulty with intubation or, with airway manipulation. Warner et al.[6] described aspiration in 69% of his patients in whom active vomiting or gagging occurred during intubation or extubation. Mort[21] demonstrated that when the number of intubation attempts went from ≤2 to >2, a significant increase in complications occurred. The incidence of regurgitation rose from 1.9% to 22% and aspiration from 0.8% to 13%, directly correlated with an increase in the number of intubation attempts.[21] Sakai et al.[9] reported that 5 of 16 reported aspirations occurred during laryngoscopy or airway interventions including the exchange of airway devices in at-risk patients.

In summary, there are multiple studies describing morbidity and mortality associated with airway interventions and difficulties.[21,35–37]

TABLE 5.1. Risk of Pulmonary Aspiration in Elective and Emergency General Anesthetics by ASA Physical Status Classification[6]

ASA Physical Status	Elective	Emergency	*p*
I	4/36,916 (1:9229)	1/2949 (1:2,949)	.319
II	11/82,436 (1:7494)	3/5036 (1:1,679)	.043
III	31/74,301 (1:2397)	8/4413 (1:552)	<.001
IV and V	6/8409 (1:1401)	3/1029 (1:343)	.066
Total	52/202,061 (1:3886)	15/13,427 (1:895)	<.001

Obesity

There was no correlation between obesity and aspiration in the studies by Warner et al.[6] or Mellin-Olson et al.[7] However, Olsson et al.[8] did find obesity to be a contributing factor for aspiration risk and obesity is frequently listed as an aspiration-associated factor in many other references. The association of obesity with an elevated risk of aspiration may relate to a high incidence of pertinent comorbidities. For example, delayed gastric emptying is known to be associated with diabetes, which is a more frequent finding in the obese. Other factors related to the obese include GER, difficult intubation, and inadequate anesthesia at the time of induction. This may account for the larger number of obese patients reported in aspiration populations.[10]

Obese patients have the same gastric emptying rate for liquids as nonobese patients. Depending on the meal content, the gastric emptying in obese patients for solids may be faster, slower, or the same as in the nonobese.[29,38–41] Maltby et al.[29] reported that obesity did not slow gastric emptying in the absence of other predisposing comorbid conditions and suggested that fasting guidelines should be applied to obese patients using the same criterion as for the nonobese. In their paper, obese patients, with no comorbid conditions, were randomized into fasting and nonfasting groups. The latter received a 300-mL clear fluid challenge preoperatively, with no difference in RGV demonstrated postintubation between the two groups. A study reviewing anesthesia for electroconvulsive therapy in 50 obese patients reported no cases of aspiration in 660 procedures.[42]

By contrast to the above, in the NAP4, obesity represented a disproportionate number of case reports of airway-related morbidity and mortality, with a proportion that is twice that of the nonobese population. Among reported misadventures, aspiration was increased in frequency compared to the nonobese, along with difficulty in securing the airway with intubation, and airway obstruction on emergence or recovery. The risks increased with increasing BMI. Indeed, BMI >30 and BMI >40 were twice and four times as likely than the overall populations to suffer airway complications, including aspiration. Review of these cases led to the conclusion that lack of anticipation of difficulties, use of inappropriate airway choices, failure to be prepared for use of alternative modes of airway intervention were among other failures in the management of the obese airway.[13]

Pregnancy

It has been well accepted that the obstetrical population is at increased risk of aspiration. This has been felt to be secondary to a number of factors. Hormones, particularly progesterone, cause relaxation of the LES and impair gastric emptying.

Mechanical effects of the gravid uterus alter the position of the stomach and, as term approaches, create a gastric "pinchcock," partially obstructing the gastroduodenal junction. The gravid uterus also increases intra-abdominal pressure, which then increases intragastric pressure. It has been demonstrated that the intragastric pressure in pregnancy is increased to 17.2 cm H_2O from the nonpregnant level of 7.3 cm H_2O. Women experiencing heartburn in pregnancy have a drop in the LES tone from the normal in pregnancy of 44 cm H_2O to 24 cm H_2O. Heartburn in pregnancy is reported in some series to be between 45% and 70%, with 27% of these patients having hiatal hernias. The onset of labor with pain and stress, coupled with the presence of opioid analgesics, are independent factors associated with a reduction in gastric emptying. Increased difficulty with intubation occurs in the parturient related to hormonally induced mucosal edema and increased breast mass. For many reasons, the parturient is at an increased risk for aspiration.[3,43–45]

Interestingly, however, this risk has significantly decreased since Mendelson reported a maternal death rate from aspiration during C-section of 1:667.[2,5] This may well be due to the increased use of regional anesthesia and the application of rapid sequence induction (RSI) techniques, with cricoid pressure and cuffed endotracheal tubes.[46] The use of pharmacologic interventions, although not proven to alter the incidence, may also be a contributing factor. The adoption of difficult airway practices that discourage persistent failing attempts at intubation may be an important factor.

A number of recent publications support the contention that the risk of aspiration has become a much smaller contributor to maternal morbidity and mortality. Mhyre et al.[47] reviewed all reported maternal deaths in the state of Michigan, USA, between 1985 and 2003. Of the 855 recorded deaths over that time, 15 were felt to be associated with anesthesia in either a related or contributing form. Of the 15 cases, only one was felt to be due to aspiration. This occurred in the recovery area following cesarean delivery of a stillbirth. The rest of the deaths had no association with aspiration. Interestingly, all anesthesia-related deaths from airway issues occurred during emergence from general anesthesia or in the recovery room. None occurred during induction.

In a recent prospective observational study, McDonnell et al.[48] reported on the incidence of problems associated with airway management in the parturient, during the period 2005 to 2006, in 13 hospitals with just under 50,000 deliveries per year. During that period, 1095 general anesthetics were performed. In that series, eight cases reported regurgitation (0.7%), with one case of aspiration confirmed (0.1%). Two of the regurgitation cases occurred in elective Caesarian sections. Of the eight regurgitation cases, four occurred during induction and five at emergence (one patient regurgitated at both times). Interestingly, the incidence of difficult intubation was 3.3%, with failed intubation of 0.36%. The latter was managed with a laryngeal mask airway (LMA).

The low incidence of aspiration is supported by the Closed Claims Analysis of the ASA.[49] From 1990 onward, only two cases of aspiration were implicated in a maternal death or permanent brain damage, with one of these being in association with general anesthesia, the other with regional anesthesia.

In conclusion, the incidence of aspiration in obstetrics continues to decline as a source of morbidity and mortality. Increased use of regional anesthesia, a larger number of skilled practitioners comfortable with airway management options, better monitoring, and the use of prophylaxis may all be contributing factors.

Age

Although Warner et al.[6] did not find age to be an independent risk factor for aspiration, Olsson et al.[8] reported that extremes of age increased the risk of aspiration. Warner et al.[14] reviewed 63,180 anesthetics in children under the age of 18. The incidence of aspiration in that population was not dissimilar to adults, except that there was an increased incidence of aspiration in patients less than 3 years of age. Over 91% of the patients who experienced aspirations in this population had either a bowel obstruction or ileus perhaps skewing the incidence in young children, although there is also some uncertainty as to the effectiveness of the LES in this population. Distended stomachs from both fluids and air entrained during crying or using a pacifier predisposes to gastric reflux when these infants cry or gag. The efficacy and method of application of cricoid pressure during RSI in small children has not been defined.

Borland found that the incidence of aspiration in the pediatric population was 10.2:10,000, higher than Warner's reported 3.8:10,000.[14,50]

Decreased Levels of Consciousness and Neurological Disease

It is recognized that the incidence of aspiration of extraglottic (e.g., blood) and lower GI tract (e.g., stomach contents) contaminants is increased in patients with a reduced level of consciousness.[8,15] In these patient populations, loss of function of the LES and upper esophageal sphincter and delayed gastric emptying combine with a reduction of upper airway protective reflexes to promote both regurgitation and aspiration.[51,52] This has relevance for the postanesthetic period as well, as it has been shown that patients left in the supine position with a reduced level of consciousness have an increased incidence of aspiration.

Patients with other underlying neurological diseases, such as Parkinson's disease and multiple sclerosis, are also at increased risk of aspiration due to impairment of their protective airway reflexes.[53] The diabetic with autonomic neuropathy has been demonstrated to have delayed gastric emptying, sometimes manifested by early postprandial satiety, but it is usually asymptomatic. Diabetics have a theoretically increased incidence of difficult laryngoscopy and intubation due to glycosylation of collagen in the joints of the cervical spine, resulting in diabetic stiff joint syndrome.[54] In spite of speculation that diabetics ought to be at increased risk of regurgitation and aspiration,[55,56] no studies have found diabetes to be an independent risk factor for aspiration.[1,6–8,10,11,14,50]

Bowel Obstruction or Other Gastrointestinal Pathology

As discussed above, increased gastric volume predisposes patients to an increased risk of aspiration. Gastric obstruction, and or ileus, is one of the commonest clinical findings associated with aspiration.[8,10,14] The incidence of aspiration in esophageal endoscopy is 1:188, and appendectomy 1:751.

Full Stomach

Even in the absence of bowel pathology, recent ingestion of a meal has been documented to be a risk factor for aspiration.[6,8,10,14] Guidelines for fasting have been developed for the elective population. However, fasting does not guarantee an empty stomach and RGVs can be quite variable.

Is There a Difference in Gastric Emptying in Emergency Patients or Those Who Have Received Opioids?

Trauma patients have been shown to have delayed gastric emptying up to a week after injury. Patients who are critically ill, in ICU, also have significantly delayed gastric emptying.[57] Neurological injury, either head or spinal cord, is associated with significant delays in gastric emptying related, in part, to catecholamine surge.[58]

Opioids, irrespective of the manner of administration, have been shown to decrease gastric emptying significantly.[59–61]

Finally, alcohol ingestion, which is not uncommon in the population presenting urgently after trauma, significantly delays gastric emptying; this is true even when the ingested alcohol is of relatively small volume (300 mL) and of low alcohol content (4%-10%).[62]

STRATEGIES AIMED AT MINIMIZING ASPIRATION RISK

What Are the Current Fasting Guidelines? What Evidence Supports Their Use?

The American Society of Anesthesiologists has published an updated set of fasting guidelines,[63] generated from a review of the available literature and expert opinion. These guidelines are consistent with those advanced in 1999,[64] and were developed with the healthy patient in mind, booked for elective surgery. They are not intended to be applied to patients with comorbidities that would increase the risk of aspiration. There is a striking paucity of evidence around the relationships between fasting times, gastric volume, gastric fluid pH, and the risk of pulmonary aspiration. The consensus guidelines recommended the following:

> For clear fluids, the Task Force recommended a minimum 2-hour period of preoperative abstinence for healthy infants, children, and adults. Clear fluids consist of water, black tea or coffee, pulp-free juices, fat- and protein-free drinks, and carbonated drinks but should not contain alcohol. There is controversy as to the benefits of ingestion of carbohydrate-containing beverages. Some investigators feel that they may reduce gastric volume and raise pH, although this difference is not of clinical significance. There is also some evidence to suggest that fasting itself may have detrimental effects, particularly in the pediatric population, resulting in greater anxiety and hunger.
>
> For breast milk, the Task Force recommended a fasting period, for both infants and neonates, of 4 hours. Commercial milk and infant formula have a recommended fasting period of 6 hours.
>
> A minimum period of 6 hours is recommended from the last ingestion of solids until the provision of anesthesia for elective surgery following a light meal (citing toast and a clear liquid as an example of a light meal). Indeed, some studies have noted that solids, particularly fats, can be found in the stomach for periods of over 8 hours after a meal. The Task Force recommended that consideration should be taken into account of the amount and type of food prior to the provision of anesthetic care after consumption of meals other than what is considered "light" (i.e., clear liquids and toast).[65,66] These guidelines recommend that the fasting period following the intake of a meal containing fried or fatty foods should be 8 hours or more.

There is controversy as to the application of these guidelines in the parturient,[67] a complex group, as there is always a potential need for emergency surgery. It would seem reasonable to allow the moderate intake of clear fluids or ice chips for the low-risk parturient. However, the high-risk parturient, either due to comorbidities or at increased risk of requiring an operative delivery, should be fasted.[68] For elective cesarean sections, a fast of 8 hours following solids is recommended.

What Role Do Pharmacological Agents Play at Minimizing Aspiration Risk?

Although evidence exists to support the contention that pharmacological agents reduce gastric acid production, gastric volume, or both, no evidence exists to support their use in preventing or reducing the incidence of aspiration or improving outcome if aspiration was to occur. Furthermore, the administration of many of the pharmacological agents could not be justified on the basis of cost-benefit analysis. Subsequently, the ASA Task Force has not recommended the routine use of any pharmacological interventions for the prevention of aspiration in patients with no apparent increased risk for aspiration, including gastrointestinal stimulants, histamine-2 (H-2) receptor antagonists, or proton pump inhibitors.

Similarly, there are no recommendations regarding the "at-risk" patient, other than the use of nonparticulate antacids in the obstetrical population. The majority of studies looking at the efficacy of these drugs have been carried out in the healthy, low-risk populations.

H-2 antagonists, such as ranitidine, famotidine, and nizatidine, act by binding competitively to the histamine receptors on the gastric parietal cell. They are effective in increasing gastric pH and reducing gastric volume within 2 to 3 hours of administration. Unfortunately, the effect of the drug diminishes after a few days as tolerance develops.[69]

Proton pump inhibitors interfere with the H^+/K^+ ATPase pump on the parietal cells. They are less effective than H-2 antagonists if the intent is to use them for a single dose as they require at least two doses to be effective, both the night before and the morning of surgery. Tachyphylaxis does not appear to develop with these agents.

Although reductions in gastric acid and volume have been shown with these agents, they do not reduce the harm from biliary fluid or particulate matter aspiration. Evidence from the animal literature suggests that pulmonary injury from bile is as significant, if not more so, than acid alone.[70] Bile, with a pH of 7.19, caused severe chemical pneumonitis and edema in one animal study.[70]

Prokinetic agents are used to accelerate emptying of the stomach, thereby reducing RGV. The most commonly used of these is metoclopramide. It has multiple effects, including prokinetic properties, antiemetic properties, and finally, an effect on increasing the tone of the LES. It acts by antagonizing dopamine and serotonin receptors. Depending on the receptor subtype, it may also act as an agonist. Its antiemetic effects are largely due to the 5HT3 antagonism and the prokinetic effects from the 5HT4 agonism. Its prokinetic properties, however, are quickly inhibited by the presence of opioids and anticholinergic agents.

Of interest, the antibiotic erythromycin has been shown to be an effective agent in stimulating gastric motility, thereby increasing the rate of gastric emptying. It exerts its effect via the motilin receptor. Unlike metoclopramide, it has no extrapyramidal side effects and its prokinetic properties are not inhibited by opioids or anticholinergics. Doses of 1 to 2 $mg{\cdot}kg^{-1}$ have been reported to be effective in reducing gastric fluid volume.[71,72]

The use of antacids has been demonstrated to reduce the pH of gastric contents for variable lengths of time. As discussed earlier in this chapter, the administration of particulate antacids can be problematic. The use of clear nonparticulate antacids has been in wide use for more than two decades, primarily in the obstetrical population. Sodium citrate is in routine use, prior to elective or emergency obstetrical procedures. Bicitra is a commercially available form of sodium citrate. The mechanism of action is by conversion to sodium bicarbonate. Rebound acidity will occur with prolonged use, increasing the volume of acid production.[73]

What Is the Role of Ultrasound in Assessing Gastric Volume and Aspiration Risk?

Carp et al.[74] tested the ability of high-resolution ultrasound imaging to identify the stomach contents of nonpregnant volunteers and parturients and demonstrated that it was capable of identifying both the gastric volumes and content. Perlas et al. evaluated the feasibility of using bedside ultrasonography for assessing gastric content and volume.[75] They reported that the gastric antrum could be consistently identified and assessment of the antrum provided the most reliable quantitative information for gastric volume; the antral cross-sectional area (CSA) correlated with volume in a close-to-linear fashion, particularly when subjects were in the right lateral decubitus position. They concluded that bedside two-dimensional ultrasonography could be a useful noninvasive tool to determine gastric content and volume. In a review of a number of studies on the topic, Van de Putte and Perlas[76] also reported that the antrum is the gastric region that is most amenable to sonographic examination and that its evaluation accurately reflects the content of the entire organ.

Ultrasonographic measurement of antral CSA is feasible and reliable in the majority of critically ill patients. Hamada et al.[77] assessed the feasibility and validity of ultrasonographic measurement of antral CSA (us-CSA) in 55 critically ill patients who had an abdominal CT scan within an hour of the ultrasound assessment. Antral us-CSA measurements were feasible in 95% of cases and were positively correlated with gastric volume measured by the CT scan when performed in "good" conditions (65%) ($r = 0.43$). There was good reproducibility of measurements and there was clinically acceptable agreement between measurements performed by radiologists and intensivists.

Mathematical models are available to predict gastric volume based on antral CSA in adults and they are thought to be both accurate and clinically applicable. A semiquantitative three-point (grade 0-2) grading system has also been reported as a simple screening tool to differentiate low- from high-volume states.[78] This three-point grading system is based solely on qualitative evaluation of the gastric antrum that is scanned in both the supine and right lateral decubitus positions. A grade 0 antrum appears empty in both positions, and suggests no gastric content is present. A grade 1 antrum appears empty in the supine position, but fluid is visible in the RLD, consistent with a small volume (<100 mL) of gastric fluid. A grade 2 antrum is that in which clear fluid is evident in both patient positions consistent with a higher volume (>100 mL). Ultrasound assessment of gastric volume by anesthesia practitioners is highly reproducible with high intrarater and interrater reliability. Kruisselbrink et al.[79] assessed the intrarater and interrater reliability of a method of gastric volume assessment based on gastric antral area and determined that reliability was nearly perfect and the two methods were essentially equivalent.

As a new diagnostic tool, gastric sonography needs to be characterized in terms of its validity (does it assess what it intends to assess, and how accurately), reliability (how reproducible are the results), and interpretability (i.e., what are the clinical implications of specific findings). Most studies to date deal with validity considerations and suggest that bedside ultrasound accurately determines RGV. Even though several descriptions of the type of content have been published, the sensitivity and specificity of a qualitative exam remain to be studied in a systematic manner. As data on the validity and reliability of gastric sonography become increasingly available, the next important question is to correlate ultrasound assessment with aspiration risk to tailor anesthetic management in appropriate cases. Gastric ultrasound may ultimately prove to be very useful in aiding anesthesia practitioners in the determination of aspiration risk at the bedside and more appropriately guiding anesthetic management (also see Chapters 41 and 64).

What Is the Role of Rapid Sequence Induction in Airway Management?

Rapid sequence induction (RSI) with cricoid pressure has been deployed widely in anesthesia and emergency care for close to five decades and has been described as the standard of care in anesthesia for patients at risk for gastric regurgitation.[80] As well, it has been cited to be the most common method of airway management by emergency physicians for critically ill and injured emergency patients and is also the principal salvage technique when other oral or nasal intubation methods fail in the emergency department.[8] Although it is characterized by a high success rate and a low rate of serious complications, its use has been challenged recently by authors in both anesthesia and emergency medicine who point out that the evidence base supporting its use is largely comprised of nonrandomized historical controls, case series, uncontrolled studies, and expert opinion, and that the use of cricoid pressure may complicate airway management.[20,81–84]

The use of a rapid sequence technique results in fewer attempts, more rapid intubations, and higher success rates when compared to intubation with no sedation or sedation alone, both in hospital and in the prehospital setting.[85–87] Concerns about the role of rapid sequence techniques in the prehospital setting for the care of severely head-injured patients relate to the potential for hypoxemia under some circumstances. The major issues seem to be the occurrence of severe hypoxemia during induction in patients who were not hypoxemic before induction and the excess morbidity and mortality in those patients. An effective strategy for maintenance of oxygenation is needed before it can be concluded that rapid sequence intubation is of value in the out-of-hospital care of patients with serious closed head injury.[85–89]

Describe the Technique of RSI

The patient should be placed supine at a height that is most convenient for the airway practitioner performing laryngoscopy. The head should be placed in the "sniffing" position with a firm pillow under the occiput. Although the benefit of the "sniffing" position compared to simple extension was recently challenged by Adnet et al.,[90] it did provide an advantage in patients who were obese or in whom there was at least one factor predictive of difficult intubation.

Denitrogenation

The usual method for denitrogenating (often referred to as preoxygenation) patients involves having the patient breathe 100% oxygen at tidal volumes through a tight-fitting face mask for 3 to 5 minutes. An alternative strategy is to have patients take four vital capacity breaths, but there is evidence that the former methodology is preferable.[91] Having said that, two reviews have concluded that having the patient take eight deep breaths (8 DB) in 60 seconds provides a similar duration of safe apnea as does 3 to 5 minutes of tidal volume ventilation.[92,93] For this reason, whenever possible, it is recommended that either the tidal-volume breathing or the 8 DB technique be employed. The same reviews concluded that denitrogenation of obese patients in the head-up compared to supine position also provided a longer period of safe apnea after the induction of anesthesia.

Cricoid Pressure

The cricoid cartilage should be identified by the assistant during denitrogenation, before induction of anesthesia, and the accuracy of the landmark should be confirmed by the airway practitioner. Cricoid pressure may be gently applied at the start of the induction sequence and the pressure increased to the amount recommended concurrent with the induction of anesthesia. The pressure should not be released until the cuff is inflated and the intratracheal position of the tube has been confirmed.

Nasogastric Tubes and Gastric Evacuation

Sellick[4] recommended evacuating the stomach content with a gastric tube and then removing the tube before induction of anesthesia. Stept and Safar[94] argued that there was little evidence to support an effect of the tube on esophageal sphincter competence and suggested that the risk would be outweighed by the advantage of continuous gastric decompression when the tube was left in situ. Satiani et al.[95] demonstrated no difference in the incidence of regurgitation with or without a nasogastric tube. Salem and colleagues[96] demonstrated the effectiveness of cricoid pressure in preventing reflux in both infant and adult cadavers with nasogastric tubes in place. It is recommended that if a nasogastric tube has been placed to empty the stomach, it should be left in place and open to atmosphere to limit increases in intragastric pressure during induction of anesthesia.

The Choice of Sedatives/Hypnosis During RSI

Despite wide acceptance and use of RSI, no single agent has emerged as the drug of choice for sedation and hypnosis during RSI. A deeper plane of anesthesia may improve intubating conditions in emergency patients undergoing RSI by complementing incomplete muscle paralysis.[97]

The use of etomidate, ketamine, a benzodiazepine, or no sedative agent prior to neuromuscular blockade is associated with a lower likelihood of successful intubation on the first attempt, as compared with thiopental, methohexital, or propofol.[97] The use of the benzodiazepine midazolam alone is associated with a prolonged delay to time of laryngoscopy and doses >0.1 mg·kg^{-1} are associated with a dose-related incidence of hypotension.[97–100]

Etomidate, thiopental, and propofol have a favorable effect on intraocular pressure (IOP) and intracranial pressure (ICP).[101–103] Barbiturates provide cerebral protective qualities against ischemia caused by elevated ICP. However, barbiturates may significantly lower mean arterial blood pressure and thereby lower cerebral perfusion pressure, potentially compromising collateral blood flow to ischemic regions of the brain.[101] Although propofol also reduces ICP, it reduces mean arterial pressure (MAP) more than barbiturates and can thus cause a significant reduction of cerebral perfusion pressure.[104] Etomidate, in contrast to barbiturates and propofol, reduces ICP to a similar degree while maintaining or increasing MAP and cerebral perfusion pressure, but there is evidence of neurotoxicity in experimental models.[105,106]

Ketamine, when used in the presence of hypovolemic shock, can be unpredictable in its effect on the hemodynamic profile. It possesses both indirect sympathomimetic stimulation and direct myocardial depressant properties, which support or raise systemic blood pressure in the acutely injured and hypovolemic patient. However, a patient who has been physiologically stressed for an extended period may be depleted of endogenous catecholamines, thereby rendering indirect autonomic stimulation ineffective and allowing the direct myocardial depressant effects to dominate.

Although it clearly has some advantages in a compromised patient, a significant disadvantage of etomidate is that it does not blunt the sympathetic response to endotracheal intubation.[107] This may result in hypertension and tachycardia during endotracheal intubation secondary to sympathetic stimulation. This response may raise ICP and increase myocardial work. Mitigation of this effect is achieved with the use of 1.5 to 5 μg·kg^{-1} of fentanyl in conjunction with etomidate.[108]

Lidocaine is widely used as a pretreatment agent to decrease the magnitude of increase of ICP in patients with closed head injury (with or without increased ICP). In fact, the evidence that IV lidocaine reduces the magnitude of the increase in ICP with elective tracheal intubation or suctioning in patients with increased ICP is indirect, and there is no evidence that it renders this effect in head-injured patients undergoing RSI.[109] As well, when it was administered intravenously in a dose of 1 mg·kg^{-1} in healthy patients receiving thiopental and succinylcholine for induction of anesthesia, lidocaine use was associated with a decrease in mean arterial pressure of 30 mmHg.[110]

The Choice of Muscle Relaxant During Rapid Sequence Techniques

Succinylcholine is widely used in anesthesia and emergency medicine during rapid sequence techniques. Doses approximating 1 mg·kg^{-1} have been conventionally used for intubation; the average time to return to 50% of twitch height following this dose is 8 to 9 minutes, and 10 to 11 minutes for a return to 90% of twitch height. A number of authors have explored the use of smaller doses to decrease the time to recovery and to limit the dose-dependent sequelae. El-Orbany et al.[82] assessed onset times and time to twitch recovery for succinylcholine in doses of 0.3, 0.4, 0.5, 0.6, and 1 mg·kg^{-1} after anesthesia was induced with fentanyl and propofol. Onset times ranged between 82 and 52 seconds, decreasing with increasing doses of succinylcholine but not differing between 0.6 and 1 mg·kg^{-1}. Intubation conditions were often unacceptable after 0.3 and 0.4 mg·kg^{-1} doses, but acceptable conditions were achieved in all patients receiving more than 0.5 mg·kg^{-1}; intubation conditions in patients receiving 0.6 mg·kg^{-1} and 1.0 mg·kg^{-1} were identical. The times to twitch recovery and to regular spontaneous reservoir bag movements were significantly shorter in the 0.6 mg·kg^{-1} dose group compared with patients receiving 1 mg·kg^{-1}. Naguib et al.[111] carried out a similar study administering succinylcholine 0.3 to 1.0 mg·kg^{-1} after anesthesia was induced with fentanyl and propofol. Intubating conditions were acceptable (excellent plus good grade combined) in 30%, 92%, 94%, and 98% of patients after 0.0, 0.3, 0.5, and 1.0 mg·kg^{-1} succinylcholine, respectively. The calculated doses of succinylcholine that were required to achieve acceptable intubating conditions in 90% and 95% of patients at 60 seconds were 0.24 mg·kg^{-1} and 0.56 mg·kg^{-1}, respectively.

While these results may have significant clinical implications, more studies are needed to examine the effectiveness of these smaller doses of succinylcholine in different patient populations, including obese, pregnant, pediatric, trauma, and critically ill patients. It must also be emphasized that the goal is "100% acceptable intubating conditions," particularly in an emergency.

Since there are significant side effects associated with the use of succinylcholine, there is considerable enthusiasm in anesthesia practice to replace succinylcholine with a nondepolarizing muscle relaxant. At this time, rocuronium has emerged as the most likely nondepolarizer to fill this role. Rocuronium 1 mg·kg^{-1} given after induction in a rapid sequence technique is clinically equivalent to succinylcholine 1 mg·kg^{-1}.[112] The incidences of clinically acceptable intubating conditions with rocuronium and succinylcholine were 93.2% and 97.1%, respectively. Clinically acceptable conditions occurred less frequently when rocuronium 0.6 mg·kg^{-1} was used. The use of propofol 2.5 mg·kg^{-1} combined with rocuronium 0.6 mg·kg^{-1} results in satisfactory intubating conditions in 90% of patients within 61 seconds (range 50-81 seconds).[113] The use of either thiopental (5.0 mg·kg^{-1}) or etomidate (0.3 mg·kg^{-1}) combined with rocuronium 0.6 mg·kg^{-1} results in a longer time to achieve, and a lower incidence of satisfactory intubating conditions than that achieved with propofol/rocuronium combinations.[114] The addition of alfentanil 10 μg·kg^{-1} to these doses of etomidate and thiopental results in an increased likelihood of acceptable intubation conditions at 60 seconds following rocuronium administration.[115]

Three separate Cochrane reviews were conducted by Perry et al.[116–118] to determine if rocuronium (1.2 mg·kg^{-1}) could provide comparable intubating conditions to succinylcholine during RSI intubation. The investigators found no statistical difference in intubation conditions when succinylcholine was compared to 1.2 mg·kg^{-1} rocuronium; however, succinylcholine was clinically superior as it has a shorter duration of action. The time to full twitch recovery following paralyzing doses of rocuronium may be in excess of 1 hour, a factor that may exceed the comfort level of some practitioners. The availability and use of *Sugammadex* (see the section below and Chapter 4) would be a potential solution in the situation where rocuronium is required for RSI, rather than succinylcholine but concern exists due to the prolonged neuromuscular block from the dose of rocuronium required.[119]

Positive Pressure Ventilation During RSI

In the eighteenth century, application of pressure in the cricoid area was advocated to allow for ventilation of the lungs without causing gastric distention.[120] Sellick,[4] in his description of cricoid pressure, also recommended ventilating the lungs while awaiting onset of muscle paralysis. On the other hand, Stept and Safar[94] recommended against the use of ventilation after application of cricoid pressure and conventional practice had until recently favored this recommendation. However, there is now evidence that not only is there a benefit to ventilating the patient's lungs during the period of apnea but also that it can be done safely.

The average time to return to 90% of twitch height following an intubating dose of succinylcholine is considerably longer than it will take most patients to have oxygen desaturation, even under ideal circumstances.[121] Using a simulator model, Hardman et al.[122] have identified the factors that shorten the time to desaturate with apnea. The factors that have a moderate effect are a reduced ventilatory minute volume preceding apnea and a reduced duration of denitrogenation. Those that have a large effect are increased oxygen consumption and reduced functional residual capacity. All of those factors are likely to be relevant in many instances of RSI.

There is a relationship between airway pressure and gastric inflation.[123,124] In subjects face-mask ventilation (FMV) without cricoid pressure, airway pressures below 15 cm H_2O rarely cause stomach inflation. Similarly, pressures ≤10 cm H_2O will not cause gastric distention but may provide insufficient ventilation; pressures ≥15 cm H_2O are generally adequate.[125] Pressures between 15 and 20 cm H_2O will result in gastric insufflation in some patients, and pressures ≥20 cm H_2O do so in most patients.[123,125] Application of cricoid pressure during FMV increases the maximum pressure that may be generated during FMV, without air entering the stomach, to about 45 cm H_2O.[124]

Petito and Russell[126] measured the ability of cricoid pressure to prevent gastric inflation during FMV of the lungs. Fifty patients were randomized to either have or not have cricoid pressure applied during a 3-minute period of standardized FMV. Patients who had cricoid pressure applied had less gas in the stomach after mask ventilation. However, more patients who had cricoid pressure applied (36% vs. 12%) were considered more difficult to ventilate and these patients tended to have more air in the stomach when compared to those considered easy to ventilate with applied cricoid pressure.

In summary, adequate ventilation of the lungs may be achieved with ventilation pressures of about 15 cm H_2O. As applied pressures increase to ≥20 cm H_2O, gastric insufflation will occur. The application of cricoid pressure significantly reduces the volume of air entering the stomach at low-to-moderate ventilation pressures. It allows for continued ventilation of the lungs even in situations where past convention would have discouraged it, such as in RSI. Ventilating the lungs while awaiting the onset of muscle block is a prudent and useful maneuver to prevent oxygen desaturation, and there is an evidence base that supports this intervention. In order to prevent gastric insufflation, every effort should be made to ventilate the lungs at the lowest pressure possible.

Another method to reduce the onset of oxygen desaturation, or increase the safe apneic time, is the use of apneic oxygenation. This occurs when a patent airway exists, between the lung and the upper airway. With a nasopharyngeal catheter insufflating O_2 at 5 L·min^{-1} after onset of apnea following denitrogenation, Taha demonstrated that SpO_2 would remain at 100% for 6 minutes.[127] In the control, with no O_2 flow via cannula, the mean time for SpO_2 to drop to 95% was 3.6 minutes. A similar result occurred in a study conducted by Ramachandran et al.[128] in which they randomized obese males into two groups (n = 15 per group). The study group had nasal cannula with free flow of O_2 at 5 L·min^{-1} and the second was a control group. Both were denitrogenated in a standard fashion, induced with propofol/remifentanil/succinylcholine then underwent a simulated difficult laryngoscopy. Oxygen saturations were measured against time. The mean time to oxygen desaturation for the control group (SpO_2 <95%) was 3.49 minutes, whereas the study group had a mean time to 95% saturation of 5.29 minutes. In the study group, eight still had a SpO_2 >95% at 6 minutes versus only 1 in the control population. Finally, the lowest oxygen saturation in the study oxygenated group was 94.3% versus 87.7% in the control population.

More recently, the use of high-flow nasal cannula (HFNC), of flows of 40 to 70 L·min^{-1}, has reported that apneic oxygenation has increased time up to 30 minutes.

CRICOID PRESSURE

Discuss the Applied Anatomy of Cricoid Pressure

The cricoid cartilage is shaped like a signet ring with the narrow part of the ring being oriented anteriorly. The anterior arch of the cricoid cartilage is attached to the thyroid cartilage by the cricothyroid membrane. Laterally, the cricothyroid muscles are situated in the cricothyroid gap (see Figure 3.13). The inferior horns of the thyroid cartilage articulate with the lateral surfaces of the cricoid cartilage. The cricoid cartilage is attached to the first tracheal ring by the cricotracheal ligament. The esophagus begins at the lower border of the posterior aspect of the cricoid cartilage. Sellick proposed the application of cricoid pressure during induction of anesthesia to prevent regurgitation of gastric or esophageal contents by compressing the esophagus between the cricoid and the cervical spine, obliterating the esophageal lumen.[4] To perform the maneuver, the neck was extended, increasing the anterior convexity of the cervical spine and stretching the esophagus. Sellick hypothesized that this prevented lateral displacement of the esophagus when cricoid pressure was applied. However, Vanner and Pryle[129] reported that contrast CT scanning in one patient revealed that when cricoid pressure was applied, although the cricoid cartilage and cervical vertebrae were approximated, only part of the esophageal lumen was obliterated. Smith and Boyer[130] reviewed 51 cervical CT scans of normal patients to assess the anatomic relationships between the cricoid cartilage and the esophagus. Lateral esophageal displacement relative to the cricoid cartilage was evident in half (25 of 51) of the patients; 64% of those with lateral displacement had esophageal displacement beyond the lateral border of the cricoid cartilage. Smith et al.[131] subsequently reported on MRI taken of 22 volunteers with and without cricoid pressure applied. The esophagus was again seen to be displaced laterally relative to the cricoid cartilage in 52.6% of the subjects; this increased to 90.5% with the application of cricoid pressure. Lateral laryngeal displacement and airway compression were observed in 66.7% and 81% of the necks, respectively, with the application of cricoid pressure. Boet et al.[132] studied esophageal patency with and without cricoid pressure in 20 conscious volunteers using MRI. Target cricoid pressure was achieved in 16 of 20 individuals, corresponding to a mean percentage reduction in cricovertebral distance of 43% (range 25%-80%). Incomplete esophageal occlusion was seen in 10 of 16, or 62.5% of individuals when what was deemed to be appropriate cricoid pressure was applied. Incomplete esophageal occlusion was always associated with a lateral deviation of the esophagus. Rice et al.[133] investigated the anatomic impact of cricoid pressure in 24 awake adult volunteers using MRI with and without applied pressure. With cricoid pressure applied, the mean anteroposterior diameter of the hypopharynx was reduced by 35% and the lumen likely obliterated, and this compression was maintained even when the cricoid ring was lateral to the vertebral body. The location of the esophagus was irrelevant to the efficiency of the cricoid pressure with regard to the prevention of gastric regurgitation into the pharynx. The magnetic resonance images showed that compression of the alimentary tract occurs with midline and lateral displacement of the cricoid cartilage relative to the underlying vertebral body. Finally, Zeidan et al.[134] used real-time visual and mechanical means to assess the patency of the esophageal entrance with and without cricoid pressure in 107 patients who were anesthetized and paralyzed. Attempts to insert two gastric tubes (GT) into the esophagus were made by a "blinded" operator with and without cricoid pressure, the timing of which was randomized while images were recorded with a GlideScope. A successful insertion of a GT in the presence of cricoid pressure was considered evidence of a patent esophageal entrance and ineffective cricoid pressure, whereas an unsuccessful insertion of a GT was considered evidence of an occluded esophageal entrance and effective cricoid pressure. Advancement of either size GT into the esophagus could not be accomplished during cricoid pressure in any patient but was easily done in all subjects when cricoid pressure was not applied. This occurred whether the esophageal entrance was in a midline position or in a left or right lateral position relative to the glottis. Esophageal patency was visually observed in the absence of cricoid pressure, whereas occlusion of the esophageal entrance was observed during cricoid pressure in all patients. The efficacy of the maneuver was independent of the position of the esophageal entrance relative to the glottis, whether midline or lateral.

There is a potential for lateral positioning and displacement of the esophagus relative to the cricoid cartilage and this may possibly explain case reports in which, despite the application of cricoid pressure during RSI, regurgitation and aspiration occurred.[83] It is also possible that the failure to prevent aspiration was attributable in some of these instances to the improper application of the technique rather than the failure of the technique. The esophageal lumen may be occluded with the application of cricoid pressure even when the esophagus rests partially lateral to the midline or is displaced laterally with the pressure application, and some of the effects of the applied pressure in occluding the lumen of the upper gastrointestinal tract may occur at the hypopharynx.

What Is the Sellick Technique?

Sellick[135] outlined a number of steps in his original description of cricoid pressure applied concurrently with anesthetic induction. The patient was placed in the tonsillectomy position with the cervical spine in extension. Before induction of anesthesia, the cricoid was palpated and lightly held between the thumb and index finger; as induction commenced, pressure was exerted on the cricoid cartilage mainly by the index finger. As the patient lost consciousness, Sellick recommended firm pressure sufficient to seal the esophagus. Cricoid pressure was initially felt to be contraindicated by Sellick in the setting of active vomiting, in the belief that the esophagus may be damaged by vomit under high pressure. He later modified this stand, stating that he felt the risk of rupture to be almost nonexistent.[135] Since his original description, the technique has been exposed to much study and critique. Data have now accumulated to provide evidence to support many of Sellick's recommendations.

Does Cricoid Pressure Reliably Protect Against Regurgitation and Aspiration?

There are no outcome studies confirming the clinical benefit of cricoid pressure when used either in anesthesia or resuscitation. Brimacombe and Berry[80] cited numerous case reports documenting the occurrence of aspiration despite the application of cricoid pressure. There are also multiple studies documenting a negative impact of cricoid pressure on patient interventions, usually relating to airway management. There is also a single case report in the literature attributing rupture of the esophagus to cricoid pressure.[136] It involved an elderly female subjected to laparotomy after repeated episodes of hematemesis. The patient, who vomited on induction, was positioned laterally, cricoid pressure was released, and the trachea was intubated after pharyngeal suctioning. At surgery, a longitudinal split was found in the lower esophagus. It was concluded, by the reporting authors, that the esophageal rupture represented an esophageal injury attributable to the cricoid pressure. However, the diagnosis of rupture of the esophagus as a result of the repeated episodes of hematemesis represents as likely a cause, as the stomach adjacent to the area of esophageal injury was noted to be bruised and swollen during the surgery, suggesting a temporally more remote injury.

There are a number of factors that would explain why cricoid pressure cannot provide absolute protection against aspiration, in addition to the anatomic factors already outlined. The landmarks on the patient's neck may not be identified properly and, as a result, pressure not exerted on the cricoid cartilage itself. Cricoid pressure may not have been commenced prior to induction, allowing for an interval between loss of consciousness and application of pressure, during which the patient is at risk for aspiration. Personnel may be inadequately trained. Cricoid pressure may be released inadvertently before the trachea is intubated and the cuff inflated. Finally, it may be difficult to maintain occlusive pressures for prolonged periods and the maneuver may become less effective in preventing aspiration during instances of difficult intubation.

There is evidence that cricoid pressure may decrease the barrier pressure of the lower esophageal sphincter (LES) as well, increasing the risk of passive regurgitation. Tournadre et al.[137] showed that LES pressure decreased from 24 mmHg to 15 mmHg at 20 N of cricoid pressure and to 12 mmHg when 40 N of cricoid pressure was applied.

There is a paucity of data to evaluate the role of cricoid pressure in preventing patient complications and evidence that it may make securing the airway more difficult in some circumstances. At present, it is still recommended as part of the airway algorithm,[138,139] and in the opinion of the authors, it still plays an important role.

How Much Cricoid Pressure Is Needed to Prevent Gastric Regurgitation?

Twenty newtons (N) of applied cricoid pressure are probably adequate in many instances, and 30 N is more than enough to prevent regurgitation into the pharynx in most patients. Pressures greater than 30 N (approximately 3 kg, or 7 lb) are unlikely to be necessary.[41,140–142] The originally described forces (40 N) would rarely be necessary to prevent gastric regurgitation.

How Do You Measure the Performance of Cricoid Pressure?

Meek et al.[143] investigated the cricoid pressure technique of anesthetic assistants. A large variation in the force applied (from <10 N to >90 N) was observed. Performance was improved markedly by providing simple instruction and further improved by practical training in the application of target force on a simulator. Meek et al.[144] also studied six operating room assistants performing simulated cricoid pressure (on a model of the larynx) to determine how long and under what conditions cricoid pressure could be sustained. Subjects were asked to maintain forces of 20, 30, and 40 N for a target time of 20 minutes with the arm either extended or flexed; most could not do so. Mean times to release of cricoid pressure varied from 3.7 minutes (flexed) to 7.6 minutes (extended) at 40 N, to 6.4 to 10.2 minutes at 30 N, and 13.2 to 14.6 minutes at 20 N, respectively. These findings suggest that the ability to generate forces sufficient to provide esophageal occlusion and airway protection is limited.

Is Bimanual Cricoid Pressure Better than a One-Handed Technique?

Flexion of the head on the neck may occur as a result of cricoid pressure and this may impede laryngoscopy. Bimanual (two-handed) cricoid pressure with the free hand of the assistant placed behind and supporting the neck or alternatively, with the use of a small support placed behind the patient's neck, has been recommended to overcome the tendency to neck flexion.[145] However, Vanner et al.[146] found no benefit for laryngoscopy when a cushion was placed behind the neck to prevent neck flexion during the application of cricoid pressure. Cook[147] compared the view of the larynx at laryngoscopy in 121 patients with one- or two-handed cricoid pressure applied. In 28 cases, the laryngeal view was better with one-handed cricoid pressure, and in 11 cases, the laryngeal view was better with two-handed cricoid pressure. In 81 cases, the view was unaffected by the type of cricoid pressure applied. Two-handed cricoid pressure was not demonstrated to routinely provide an advantage over the one-handed technique.

Yentis[148] also studied the effect of the two different methods of cricoid pressure on laryngoscopic view in 94 patients and reached contrary conclusions to those of Cook.[147] In 21 cases, a better laryngoscopic view was obtained with the bimanual technique; in 8 cases, it was better with the single-handed technique; and in 65 cases, the method of cricoid pressure made no difference. The force applied may have some impact on both the amount of neck flexion and the balancing potential of a bimanual technique. In the study by Yentis,[148] considerably larger forces were applied (50-55 N) than in either Vanner's (30 N) or Cook's (40 N) studies. It is possible that more neck flexion occurred with the larger applied force and more benefit was thus realized when a bimanual technique was employed.

In summary, the technique of cricoid pressure that produces the best laryngoscopic view in an individual patient cannot be predicted. However, an alternative technique should be considered if it is suspected that the technique of cricoid pressure application is having a deleterious effect on direct laryngoscopy.

Does It Matter Which Hand Is Used to Apply Cricoid Pressure?

Cook et al.[149] assessed the cricoid force applied by trained anesthesia assistants and the ability to maintain the applied force, and compared the two hands. Overall, the assistants applied a lower force than is classically taught but were able to maintain the force with either hand for a sustained period. The use of the left hand resulted in slightly lower applied forces but the differences were not felt to be clinically relevant. Thus, no recommendation can be made regarding position of the assistants as it relates to the handedness of the cricoid pressure.

How Does Cricoid Pressure Affect Ventilation and Airway Interventions?

A concern about cricoid pressure in general, and at higher applied pressures, in particular, has been the potential for compromise of either the quality of the airway or the effectiveness of airway interventions.[150–152] In a recent report of 23 failed intubations over a 17-year period in one maternity unit, cricoid pressure was maintained during the failed intubation drill.[153] In 14 patients (60%), ventilation via a face mask was not difficult, indicating that cricoid pressure was at least not harmful in these patients. In the remaining nine patients, ventilation was difficult in seven (30%) and impossible in two (9%). Although some patients had laryngeal edema, it is possible that cricoid pressure contributed to the difficult ventilation in these patients.[150]

Vanner[152] reported that difficulty breathing occurred in about half of awake patients with 40 N forces applied, and Lawes et al.[154] reported that airway obstruction occurred in about 10% of patients. Hartsilver and Vanner[155] investigated whether airway obstruction is related strictly to the force applied or whether the technique of application was also relevant. They recorded expired tidal volumes and inflation pressures during mask ventilation in anesthetized patients. Airway obstruction occurred in 2% of patients with pressure applied at 30 N and in 35% with 44 N. If the force is applied in an upward and backward direction, obstruction at 30 N occurs in 56%.

Aoyama et al.[156] assessed the effect of cricoid pressure (prior to insertion) on the positioning of and ventilation through the laryngeal mask airway (LMA). Ventilation was considered adequate in all patients in the group with no cricoid pressure applied but in only 25% of those with pressure applied. Using a flexible bronchoscope, the glottis was visible below the aperture bars of the LMA in all patients when no pressure was applied, suggesting correct placement. Correct placement was evident in only 15% of patients who had the LMA placed with cricoid pressure applied. Evaluation using a flexible bronchoscope showed that the mask was not inserted far enough in the remaining 85% of patients. Radiographs taken showed that the tip of the mask in the no-cricoid-pressure group was located below the level of the cricoid cartilage (C6 or C7 vertebra), whereas the mask tip in the cricoid pressure group was above this level (C4 or C5).

Asai et al.[157] studied 50 patients to assess if the cricoid pressure applied after placement of the laryngeal mask prevented gastric insufflation, without affecting ventilation.

Cricoid pressure significantly decreased mean expiratory volume delivered through an LMA. This inhibitory effect was greater when the pressure was applied without support of the neck. Cricoid pressure also reduced the incidence of gastric insufflation. In no patient was the mask dislodged. The inhibitory effect of cricoid pressure on ventilation without support of the neck was greater than cricoid pressure with support of the neck.

MacG Palmer and Ball[158] studied the effect of cricoid pressure on airway anatomy in 30 anesthetized patients examined using a flexible bronchoscope through an LMA. They assessed the effect of 20, 30, and 44 N on the internal appearance of the cricoid and vocal cords. At 44 N, cricoid deformation occurred in 90% of patients and 50% had cricoid occlusion; 43% had cricoid occlusion at 30 N and 23% at 20 N. Associated difficulty in ventilation was present in 50% of patients and 60% had vocal cord closure with associated difficult ventilation, at forces up to 44 N.[159–161]

Smith and Boyer[130] evaluated the ease of rigid fiber-optic (WuScope System) intubation in anesthetized adults receiving cricoid pressure. Each patient had their trachea intubated under two conditions: with and without cricoid pressure. An easy intubation occurred in 91% of patients without cricoid pressure and in 66% of patients with cricoid pressure applied. Cricoid pressure compressed the vocal cords in 27% of patients and impeded tracheal tube placement in 15%. In three patients (9%), pressure had to be released in order to successfully intubate their tracheas.

Hodgson et al.[130,162] assessed the effect of application of cricoid pressure on the success of lightwand (SurchLite) intubation in 60 adult female patients presenting for abdominal hysterectomy. All 30 patients allocated to intubation without cricoid pressure were intubated successfully, at the first attempt, within a median time of 28 seconds. Lightwand intubation with cricoid pressure was successful in 26 of 30 patients at the first attempt, but the median time to successful intubation was significantly longer at 48.5 seconds. Three patients required two attempts for successful intubation, and one could not be intubated with the lightwand while the cricoid pressure was applied.

Turgeon et al.[161] assessed the impact of cricoid pressure on laryngoscopy and intubation, comparing the experience with and without applied pressure in 700 patients, and found no appreciable effect on tracheal intubation success, laryngeal view, or time to tracheal intubation. However, Noguchi et al.,[163] in a study designed to examine the effect of cricoid pressure on passing a bougie, reported that cricoid pressure significantly worsened the laryngeal view. Finally, Harris et al.[164] evaluated the effects of cricoid pressure and laryngeal manipulation on laryngeal view using a Macintosh laryngoscope during prehospital airway management in 402 patients cared for by a physician-led prehospital trauma service. The majority (98.8%) of the tracheal intubations were successful on the first or second attempt and cricoid pressure was maintained in most. In 22 intubations, cricoid pressure was removed when difficulty was experienced and the laryngeal view improved in 50% of these. Bimanual laryngeal manipulation was used after cricoid pressure release in 25 intubations and the view improved in 60% of these. Backwards upward, rightward pressure (BURP) was applied in 14 intubations after release of the cricoid pressure, and the laryngeal view improved in 64%. Two patients regurgitated when cricoid pressure was released. Both had prolonged periods of bag valve mask ventilation and difficult intubations. The results suggest that cricoid pressure should be removed if the laryngeal view obtained is not sufficient to allow immediate intubation but that, in a significant proportion of patients, the view will remain sub-optimal, implying that the cricoid pressure did not degrade the view in many. Further manipulation of the larynx is likely to improve the chances of successful tracheal tube placement in many of these patients after the release of cricoid pressure.

Corda et al.[165] assessed the impact of cricoid pressure on glottic visualization during GlideScope video-laryngoscopy (GVL) in 100 patients undergoing general anesthesia. There was no difference overall in glottic grade when cricoid pressure was applied with views improving in 39% of patients and worsening in 20%. However, glottic opening area was reduced when cricoid pressure was applied compared to during video-laryngoscopy alone. There were no glottis views worse than a grade 2b registered in any patient during the study. Cricoid pressure does not appear to compromise the effectiveness of the GVL.

In summary, properly applied cricoid pressure has a limited impact on the ability to ventilate the lungs, the quality of the airway realized, and may decrease the effectiveness of airway interventions. As applied pressures are increased, the potential for compromise of both the airway and airway interventions is also increased. At the time of publication, cricoid pressure remains in the difficult airway algorithm of the ASA, the Difficult Airway Society guidelines of the United Kingdom, and the guidelines from the Canadian Airway Focus Group.[139,166] However, emphasis is now on the release of cricoid pressure if airway intervention becomes difficult.[139,166,167]

What Is the Impact of Cricoid Pressure on Cervical Spine Movement?

In the setting of potential or actual cervical injury, concerns have been expressed that the application of cricoid pressure may result in cervical spine displacement, causing or worsening cord injury. Although cricoid pressure is widely used during airway management in trauma settings, there are no data either affirming its safety or implying that it actually poses a risk. Gabbott[168] assessed the impact of single-handed cricoid pressure applied concurrent with manual in-line stabilization of the neck in a neutral position in 30 healthy patients undergoing general anesthesia with neuromuscular paralysis. Vertical displacement was measured from the midpoint of the neck (directly below the cricoid cartilage), and mean neck displacement (vertebral) was 4.6 mm with a range of 0 to 8 mm.

Helliwell and Gabbott[169] then measured the effect of single-handed cricoid pressure on cervical spine movement after applying manual in-line stabilization in cadavers. The median vertical displacement measured from the body of C5 was 0.5 mm (range 0-1.5 mm). There was no disruption of the lines formed by the anterior or posterior borders of the cervical bodies. In this second study, Gabbott was unable to demonstrate that single-handed cricoid pressure caused clinically significant displacement of the cervical spine in a cadaver model.[168]

Wood[170] studied the effect of cricoid pressure on the view obtained at direct laryngoscopy with concurrent cervical stabilization maneuvers. Laryngoscopic view was best in the unrestrained position, with 77.4% of these views being grade 1. More frequently, grade 3 views were obtained in the presence of cervical stabilization with or without cricoid pressure. When in the stabilized position, application of cricoid pressure improved the view in 26% of patients. Wood concluded that cricoid pressure may actually improve the view of the larynx when the neck is stabilized, even though it is often detrimental to the view in the absence of stabilization.

In summary, there is no evidence that would either encourage or discourage the use of cricoid pressure in the setting of real or potential cervical injury. However, its use in this setting is common and there is no evidence of harm caused. Cricoid pressure may actually facilitate laryngoscopy when cervical immobilization is employed, in much the same fashion that anterior laryngeal pressure does.

OTHER CONSIDERATIONS

What Is the Aspiration Risk Associated with the Use of Extraglottic Devices?

Most of the following discussion on extraglottic devices (EGD) (also known as supraglottic devices [SGD], refer to Chapter 13 for details) will involve the LMA, which has the largest body of literature. It should be noted that the recent literature supports the use of second-generation EGD, which includes the LMA®-ProSeal™, LMA®-Supreme™, Laryngeal Tube®, and i-gel®, to name a few. An EGD ideally should produce reliable first-time placement, high seal quality, separation of GI and respiratory tracts and, importantly, ability to intubate through the device with an optically guided technique.[171]

The LMA® has enjoyed decades of widespread use in anesthesia worldwide and has been hailed for its ease of use, efficacy, and low incidence of complications. As its use expanded, so did the nature of its application and it began to be employed for positive pressure ventilation, prolonged anesthesia (more than 2 hours duration), laparoscopic and nonlaparoscopic abdominopelvic surgery, and for surgery in the prone position. These applications have been labeled nonconventional applications and as these patterns of practice have become more common, increasing concerns about aspiration are being expressed. In the NAP4 report, of the approximately 3 million administered in the United Kingdom, EGD represented 56% of all airway management techniques, with an endotracheal tube used in 38%.[13]

Investigators have addressed these concerns in three ways:

1. Esophageal pH probes have been employed to determine the incidence and extent of GER during anesthesia with LMAs in place;
2. Deliberate pharyngeal soiling has been used to measure the protection afforded to the respiratory tract by the LMA. Clinical studies have compared the incidence of reflux with LMAs, endotracheal tubes, and alternative airways;
3. Finally, retrospective series and case reports have addressed the incidence of aspiration associated with LMA use and describe the clinical events and sequelae when aspiration occurred. The bulk of the published literature refers to the LMA®-Classic™ and more recently, the newer iterations of the LMA, including the LMA-ProSeal (PLMA) and the intubating LMA (LMA®-Fastrach™).

Roux et al.[172] studied esophageal reflux using esophageal pH probes in 60 patients administered anesthesia with either a face mask or an LMA. They concluded that the use of the LMA was associated with an increased incidence of gastric reflux in the lower esophagus, but not mid-esophagus, and that reflux was not influenced by either volume of air or pressure inside the LMA cuff. Joshi et al.[173] found no evidence of gastric content in the hypopharynx using pH probes in a study that compared the LMA with the endotracheal tube in spontaneously breathing patients. Ho et al.[174] reported that the use of positive pressure ventilation in a similar model did not increase the risk of reflux. Hagberg et al.[175] studied both reflux and tracheal aspiration using pH electrodes measuring in the proximal and distal esophagus and the trachea. The patients were managed with either an LMA or a Combitube®. No changes in esophageal or pharyngeal pH were observed, but 12% of the LMA group and 4% of the Combitube' group had pH changes in the trachea. No patient demonstrated clinical signs or symptoms of aspiration.

Using pH probes, McCrory and McShane[176] determined the incidence and level of reflux during spontaneous respiration with the LMA and compared the supine and lithotomy positions. The pH was measured in both the esophagus and the bowl of the LMA. Reflux into the esophagus occurred in 38% of the patients in the supine position and 100% of the patients in the lithotomy position. A change in pH was also measured in the bowl of the LMA in 57% of patients in the lithotomy position, but was not seen in the supine patients.

Cheong et al.[177] compared the incidence of reflux and regurgitation in adults at the time of LMA removal and compared the incidence when two strategies were employed for removal. In one group, the LMA was removed when signs of rejection were observed (swallowing, struggling, restlessness) and in the second, when the patients could open their mouth to command. A pH probe was used to assess reflux, and a gelatin capsule containing methylene blue swallowed before anesthesia induction was used to identify regurgitation. Instances of reflux measured with the pH probe were more common in the late-removal group. There were no regurgitation events observed in either group.

Evans et al.[178] assessed the ability of the LMA-ProSeal to isolate the respiratory tract from the digestive tract. Methylene blue-dyed saline was instilled into the hypopharynx via the drainage tube once the mask was in place in 102 patients. A flexible bronchoscope was used to view the bowl of the mask to assess for evidence of methylene blue. Although an effective barrier was observed in all patients initially, mask displacement occurred in two patients (2%) and dye leaked into the bowl of the mask.

Verghese and Brimacombe[179] surveyed the use of the LMA in 11,910 patients, with special emphasis on nonconventional use of the LMA, and the occurrence of airway-related complications. Of the 11,910 uses recorded, 2222 were considered to be nonconventional. Eighteen of the 44 documented critical incidents related to the airway included laryngospasm (8), regurgitation (4), bronchospasm (3), vomiting (2), and aspiration (1). There was no difference between the rates of occurrence of critical incidents in conventional (0.16%) versus nonconventional (0.14%) use of the LMA. Brimacombe and Berry[180] performed a meta-analysis of the published literature relevant to the association of LMA use and aspiration. In the reviewed papers, there were three cases of aspiration in 12,901 patients with no death or permanent disabilities recorded.

Keller et al.[181] described three cases of aspiration: the first death and the first case of severe permanent neurological injury associated with aspiration and the use of the LMA. All three patients were considered by the authors to be at increased risk of aspiration; two had previous gastric surgery and the third had a hiatus hernia. Keller also reported a literature review designed to assess risk factors for LMA-associated aspiration. Twenty case reports were identified in the literature. In 14 cases, there were factors that could increase the risk of aspiration, including inadequate depth of anesthesia (7), intra-abdominal surgery (3), upper GI tract disease (2), lithotomy position (2), exchanging the LMA (2), a full stomach (1), multiple trauma (1), multiple insertion attempts (1), obesity (1), opioid use (1), and cuff deflation (1).

NAP4 reported numerous cases of severe outcomes related to airway complications where EGD was used inappropriately, particularly in morbidly obese patients and those with high risk of aspiration.[13] The greatest complications occurred with the first-generation LMA, such as the LMA-Classic, and fewer with the second-generation devices, such as the LMA-ProSeal and i-gel.

In summary, there is evidence that gastric reflux into the lower esophagus occurs with some frequency during anesthesia provided with an EGD even in healthy patients without obvious risk factors. Reflux to higher levels of the esophagus or into the pharynx appears to be less common but does occur. It may be increased by patient positioning, such as the lithotomy and lateral decubitus positions. Although the EGD cuff may provide a protective barrier to refluxing materials, the barrier is not absolute and aspiration may occur even with second-generation devices in place. The incidence of aspiration associated with EGD use seems low and not significantly altered when the EGD is used in an unconventional manner. However, it is likely that many cases of EGD-associated aspirations have occurred and gone unreported. When aspirations are reported, it is common that factors traditionally associated with a higher risk of aspiration are present.

In the opinion of the authors, and supported by the recommendations of the NAP4 report, in situations where the patient is at an increased or high risk of aspiration, it would seem prudent to employ alternate methods to EGD when managing the airway, specifically, endotracheal intubation with RSI.

Is It Safe to Use a Lightwand Intubation Technique in Patients at Risk of Aspiration?

Light-guided intubation has proven its efficacy in many clinical situations. Studies have shown that the technique is both safe and effective, with minimal trauma and its ability to secure the airway in clinical situations where anatomical features make the use of the laryngoscope less likely to be successful. Indeed, features that predict difficult laryngoscopy have little or no correlation with the ease or difficulty of light-guided intubation.[182]

The question of the safety of this technique in the patient at risk of aspiration is one not well addressed in the literature. Only one paper exists, which reviews the use of this technique in the presence of cricoid pressure and RSI in a randomized trial, and it suggests that the use of the device is hampered by the presence of cricoid pressure.[162] Sixty healthy patients were randomized into a cricoid pressure group and a noncricoid pressure group. Of the noncricoid pressure group, there was a 100% success rate on the first attempt. In the cricoid pressure group of 30 patients, only 26 were intubated on the first attempt, three on the second, and one failed. The conclusion was that the light-guided technique should not be used as a first-line choice for RSI.

As discussed earlier, a failed or difficult intubation increases the risk of aspiration. Under circumstances where a difficult laryngoscopic intubation is predicted, one could argue that the use of a light-guided technique might represent a safer choice. Hung et al.[183] reported that the success of a lightwand device, Trachlight™ (see Chapter 12) was at least as good, if not better than, as the laryngoscope in a series of 950 patients randomized into Trachlight™ and direct laryngoscope intubation. In another study, Hung et al.[182] studied 265 patients deemed to be difficult laryngoscopic intubations. Of these, 206 were felt to be difficult either because of previously documented problems or anatomical factors predicting difficulty, such as cervical fusion, small mandibles, and limited mouth opening. The remaining 59 were unanticipated failed direct laryngoscopic intubations whose airways were secured with the light-guided technique. A total of two failures occurred, both of which could have been predicted due to anatomical abnormalities that made the transillumination difficult (obese patients).

Clearly, clinical judgment is required. In addition, coughing and gagging in relation to prolonged attempts at laryngoscopy are as likely, if not more so, to expose the patient to the potential of aspirating than if the assistant releases cricoid pressure momentarily to facilitate insertion of a lightwand device.

Unfortunately, apart from the solitary paper cited above, there is not enough evidence to draw a firm conclusion.

Is Awake Intubation with an Anesthetized Airway Associated with a Lower Risk of Aspiration than Under General Anesthesia?

Airway anesthesia is a routine part of awake intubation. Many sources caution against these airway anesthesia techniques in the patient with a "full stomach," fearing that anesthetizing the upper airway impairs protective reflexes leaving the patient at risk should regurgitation occur.[184–187] The question then arises how should one proceed with a patient who has an anticipated difficult airway in the presence of the elevated risk of regurgitation? Only one relevant study[185] has been published in 1989. The tracheas of 123 patients at high risk for aspiration were intubated awake, but sedated, with a flexible bronchoscope. In 114 cases, the vocal cords were anesthetized by either injection of 4% lidocaine through the working channel of the bronchoscope or by transtracheal injection of lidocaine. No local anesthetics were used on 15 occasions. Topical anesthesia was applied to the oropharynx by benzocaine–amethocaine (Cetacaine) spray and benzocaine ointment for oral intubations. Patients having nasal intubations received topical 4% cocaine to the nasal mucosa. No incidences of aspiration were identified in this study.

While many use propofol boluses for "awake" intubation, this technique must be used with great caution. Propofol and other sedatives, including dexmedetomidine, decrease LES tone, predisposing to aspiration. In addition, the patient with airway compromise may depend on voluntary muscle tone for airway patency.[187]

Clearly, each situation is unique. An anesthetized airway in an awake patient can prevent gagging, retching, and coughing during intubation. In addition, the awake, cooperative patient maintains the LES tone, can anticipate vomiting, and assist in maneuvers to prevent aspiration, such as turning the head to the side, opening the mouth for suctioning, etc.[185] On the other hand, sedation can produce an uncooperative patient that in addition has depressed airway reflexes.

In the patient at high risk for aspiration, one must weigh each technique carefully in securing an airway while minimizing the risk of aspiration.

How Should Aspiration Be Managed?

When aspiration is suspected, prompt measures should be taken to prevent further aspiration. The head of the bed should immediately be adjusted to a 30-degree head-down position and the patient's head turned to the left side to facilitate drainage of secretions. The upper airway should be suctioned thoroughly. If the patient aspirates on induction, intubation should follow immediately with aggressive tracheal suctioning before ventilation, if possible. If intubation was not intended (as in procedural sedation) and the patient is spontaneously breathing, then supplemental oxygen by face mask should be applied after suctioning as one prepares for further assessment.[5,188,189]

As was mentioned earlier, damage to the lungs after the aspiration of gastric contents occurs within seconds, with subsequent neutralization of acid within 15 seconds. Consequently, bronchoscopy is not indicated except to remove large particulate matter.

The decision to proceed with or cancel the surgery should depend on the severity of the aspiration, the patient's clinical status, and the urgency of the procedure. Once able to communicate, the patient should be notified that aspiration has occurred and observed for signs of pneumonitis and pneumonia over the ensuing days.

Since gastric acid normally prevents the growth of bacteria, antibiotics are not indicated simply because aspiration has occurred. The incidence of progression to bacterial pneumonia following chemical lung injury is unknown. Symptoms of pneumonitis include wheezing, coughing, dyspnea, and cyanosis. Further complications may include pulmonary edema, hypotension, hypoxemia, and severe ARDS.[27] Treatment of pneumonitis largely consists of supportive therapy, varying from simple oxygen supplementation to full ventilatory support.

The ventilation techniques used are beyond the scope of this chapter; however, the primary goals should be to promote oxygenation and prevent further lung parenchymal damage. As with most types of acute lung injury, avoidance of barotrauma by delivering low lung volume ventilation with less than 6 $mL \cdot kg^{-1}$ coupled with cautious use of PEEP are important. In a porcine animal model where acid aspiration was induced, high levels of PEEP led to histologic evidence of more severe lung injury than did recruitment maneuvers.[190]

Should Corticosteroids Be Administered Following the Aspiration of Gastric Contents?

The use of steroids following aspiration has been historically based on theoretical considerations, which remain unproven. These relate to anti-inflammatory properties, stabilizing effects on lysosomal membranes, ability to reduce platelet aggregation, and an improvement of peripheral release of oxygen from erythrocytes.[191] Studies conducted in the 1960s, 1970s, and 1980s consistently failed to prove a benefit of high-dose steroids after aspiration.[192–194] Nevertheless, the practice continues[27] despite a significantly higher death rate from secondary infections in the group receiving steroids.[195]

The use of high-dose steroids has not been proven effective and can adversely affect mortality in the critically ill population.[5,195] Therefore, its use in episodes of aspiration is not recommended.

Should Antibiotics Be Administered Empirically to Prevent Pneumonia Following the Aspiration of Gastric Contents?

The majority of literature on the treatment of aspiration pneumonia is related to the aspiration of colonized oropharyngeal secretions,[27] not gastric contents. Treatment should focus on supportive care to maintain oxygenation followed by organism-specific antibiotic therapy should bacterial pneumonia develop. The incidence of postaspiration pneumonia is more common in debilitated patients with comorbid conditions, and patients who have been on ventilatory support, due to leakage around the tracheal tube cuff that occurs in these patients.

The prophylactic use of antibiotics following aspiration has not been demonstrated to prevent pneumonia and is not recommended.[196] Some exceptions may include patients with bowel obstruction[27] and elderly or debilitated patients.[196] The choice of antibiotics varies according to the syndrome and the clinical situation. For example, institutionalized elderly patients with aspiration pneumonia more commonly have anaerobic microorganisms[197] than other population.

The recommendations for antibiotic selection change frequently and current guidelines for antibiotic therapy should be consulted. Such guidelines have been published by the following medical societies: American Thoracic Society,[198] Infectious Diseases Society of America,[199] Canadian Infectious Disease Society,[200] and the Canadian Thoracic Society.[200] Most commonly, it is recommended that antibiotic selection be guided by culture and sensitivity determinations.[27]

How Long Should the Patient Be Observed Following the Aspiration of Gastric Contents Episode?

In a retrospective study of the perioperative course of 172,334 patients receiving general anesthesia, Warner et al.[6] reviewed 67 cases of aspiration. Forty-two of these patients who were asymptomatic at 2 hours postaspiration or procedure never manifested any sequelae, acute or delayed. Eighteen of these were day surgeries, and 12 were discharged home on the day of surgery. Twenty-four patients developed symptoms within 2 hours including cough or wheeze (17), decrease in arterial oxygen saturation of >10% on room air (10), an increase in the A-a gradient >300 (1), or radiographic changes (12). Of the 24 with symptoms, 18 required respiratory support or ICU admission, with 6 being ventilated for more than 24 hours because of the development of ARDS. Only one patient developed pneumonia and required antibiotics.

Patients who have been discharged home after suspected episodes of aspiration should be informed of the symptoms of pulmonary complications and instructed to report them promptly should they occur.

SUMMARY

The prevention of aspiration is a significant focus of the airway practitioner. Certain factors markedly increase the risk of this event occurring. Some are inherent to the patients themselves, primarily premorbid conditions known to predispose to aspiration, some related to the patients' pathology and planned intervention, such as emergency surgery, bowel pathology, high ASA risk scores, pregnancy, difficult airway, and decreased level of consciousness. Airway management in the semiconscious patient may lead to coughing and gagging during attempts to secure the airway, accounting for over two-thirds of the perioperative aspirations.

Recognition of high-risk patients is important. Maneuvers to reduce gastric acidity and volume, both pharmacologically and with drainage, may have their role but need to be targeted to specific situations. Bile and particulate materials are potentially as harmful to the lung as is the acid that tends to be the primary focus. Thus, use of particulate antacids has been abandoned in the perioperative setting.

Although the efficacy of the Sellick maneuver has come under recent criticism, it is still a standard of care in the protection of the airway at risk in airway algorithms. A well-trained assistant is crucial. Under conditions when it hampers intubation or ventilation, it should be emphasized that cricoid pressure should be released. The wisdom of the use of extraglottic devices in the high aspiration-risk patient, when other options are available, should be critically analyzed.

Although obesity has not been felt to be a risk factor for aspiration in the past, the high representation of obesity in the NAP4 study with airway-related complications and death, and aspiration compared to the nonobese, requires careful thought into management strategies in the population.

Finally, in the unlikely event that aspiration does occur, guidelines that are evidence based should be used in the assessment and management of these patients.

SELF-EVALUATION QUESTIONS

5.1. How much cricoid pressure has been shown to prevent gastric regurgitation?

A. 10 N
B. 20 N
C. 30 N
D. 40 N
E. 50 N

5.2. Which of the following is **NOT** true about cricoid pressure and airway techniques?

A. The difficulty in ventilation using the LMA is dependent on the amount of pressure applied.
B. Cricoid pressure reduces the incidence of gastric insufflation when using an LMA.
C. Improper LMA placement can occur when cricoid pressure is applied.
D. Ventilation via a face mask has not been shown to be affected by cricoid pressure.
E. In the event of difficulty with laryngoscopy, cricoid pressure should be released.

5.3. Which of the following is NOT a known factor that increases the risk of aspiration?

A. Emergency surgery
B. Timing of surgery
C. Lack of fasting
D. Pregnant patients
E. Children

REFERENCES

1. Kluger MT, Willemsen G. Anti-aspiration prophylaxis in New Zealand: a national survey. *Anaesth Intensive Care.* 1998;26:70-77.
2. Mendelson C. The aspiration of stomach contents into the lungs during obstetric anesthesia. *Am J Obstet Gynecol.* 1946;52:191-205.
3. Roberts RB, Shirley MA. Reducing the risk of acid aspiration during cesarean section. *Anesth Analg.* 1974;53:859-868.
4. Sellick BA. Cricoid pressure to control regurgitation of stomach contents during induction of anaesthesia. *Lancet.* 1961;2:404-406.
5. Engelhardt T, Webster NR. Pulmonary aspiration of gastric contents in anaesthesia. *Br J Anaesth.* 1999;83:453-460.
6. Warner MA, Warner ME, Weber JG. Clinical significance of pulmonary aspiration during the perioperative period. *Anesthesiology.* 1993;78:56-62.
7. Mellin-Olsen J, Fasting S, Gisvold SE. Routine preoperative gastric emptying is seldom indicated. A study of 85,594 anaesthetics with special focus on aspiration pneumonia. *Acta Anaesthesiol Scand.* 1996;40:1184-1188.
8. Olsson GL, Hallen B, Hambraeus-Jonzon K. Aspiration during anaesthesia: a computer-aided study of 185,358 anaesthetics. *Acta Anaesthesiol Scand.* 1986;30:84-92.
9. Sakai T, Planinsic RM, Quinlan JJ, Handley LJ, Kim TY, Hilmi IA. The incidence and outcome of perioperative pulmonary aspiration in a university hospital: a 4-year retrospective analysis. *Anesth Analg.* 2006;103:941-947.
10. Kluger MT, Short TG. Aspiration during anaesthesia: a review of 133 cases from the Australian Anaesthetic Incident Monitoring Study (AIMS). *Anaesthesia.* 1999;54:19-26.
11. Cheney FW. Aspiration: a liability hazard for the anesthesiologist? *ASA Newslett.* 2000;64(6):5-6.
12. Baillie R, Posner KL. New trends in adverse respiratory events from ASA Closed Claims Project. *Newsl Am Soc Anesthesiol.* 2011;75:28-29.

13. Cook TM, Woodall N, Frerk C, Fourth National Audit P. Major complications of airway management in the UK: results of the Fourth National Audit Project of the Royal College of Anaesthetists and the Difficult Airway Society. Part 1: anaesthesia. *Br J Anaesth.* 2011;106:617-631.
14. Warner MA, Warner ME, Warner DO, Warner LO, Warner EJ. Perioperative pulmonary aspiration in infants and children. *Anesthesiology.* 1999;90:66-71.
15. Lockey DJ, Coats T, Parr MJ. Aspiration in severe trauma: a prospective study. *Anaesthesia.* 1999;54:1097-1098.
16. McNicholl BP. The golden hour and prehospital trauma care. *Injury.* 1994;25:251-254.
17. Gausche M, Lewis RJ, Stratton SJ, et al. Effect of out-of-hospital pediatric endotracheal intubation on survival and neurological outcome: a controlled clinical trial. *JAMA.* 2000;283:783-790.
18. Nolan JD. Prehospital and resuscitative airway care: should the gold standard be reassessed? *Curr Opin Crit Care.* 2001;7:413-421.
19. Taryle DA, Chandler JE, Good JT Jr, Potts DE, Sahn SA. Emergency room intubations—complications and survival. *Chest.* 1979;75:541-543.
20. Sakles JC, Laurin EG, Rantapaa AA, Panacek EA. Airway management in the emergency department: a one-year study of 610 tracheal intubations. *Ann Emerg Med.* 1998;31:325-332.
21. Mort TC. Emergency tracheal intubation: complications associated with repeated laryngoscopic attempts. *Anesth Analg.* 2004;99:607-613, table of contents.
22. Beach ML, Cohen DM, Gallagher SM, Cravero JP. Major adverse events and relationship to nil per os status in pediatric sedation/anesthesia outside the operating room: a report of the pediatric sedation research consortium. *Anesthesiology.* 2016;124:80-88.
23. Brady M, Kinn S, Ness V, O'Rourke K, Randhawa N, Stuart P. Preoperative fasting for preventing perioperative complications in children. *Cochrane Database Syst Rev.* 2009:CD005285.
24. Coriat P, Labrousse J, Vilde F, Tenaillon A, Lissac J. Diffuse interstitial pneumonitis due to aspiration of gastric contents. *Anaesthesia.* 1984;39:703-705.
25. Knight PR, Druskovich G, Tait AR, Johnson KJ. The role of neutrophils, oxidants, and proteases in the pathogenesis of acid pulmonary injury. *Anesthesiology.* 1992;77:772-778.
26. Knight PR, Rutter T, Tait AR, Coleman E, Johnson K. Pathogenesis of gastric particulate lung injury: a comparison and interaction with acidic pneumonitis. *Anesth Analg.* 1993;77:754-760.
27. Marik PE. Aspiration pneumonitis and aspiration pneumonia. *N Engl J Med.* 2001;344:665-671.
28. Smith G, Ng A. Gastric reflux and pulmonary aspiration in anaesthesia. *Minerva Anestesiol.* 2003;69:402-406.
29. Maltby JR, Pytka S, Watson NC, Cowan RA, Fick GH. Drinking 300 mL of clear fluid two hours before surgery has no effect on gastric fluid volume and pH in fasting and non-fasting obese patients. *Can J Anaesth.* 2004;51:111-115.
30. Schreiner MS. Gastric fluid volume: is it really a risk factor for pulmonary aspiration? *Anesth Analg.* 1998;87:754-756.
31. Hardy JF, Lepage Y, Bonneville-Chouinard N. Occurrence of gastroesophageal reflux on induction of anaesthesia does not correlate with the volume of gastric contents. *Can J Anaesth.* 1990;37:502-508.
32. Illing L, Duncan PG, Yip R. Gastroesophageal reflux during anaesthesia. *Can J Anaesth.* 1992;39:466-470.
33. Guyton AD, Hall JE. *Textbook of Medical Physiology.* 10th ed. Philadelphia, PA: WB Saunders Company; 2000:728-733.
34. Jones MJ, Mitchell RW, Hindocha N. Effect of increased intra-abdominal pressure during laparoscopy on the lower esophageal sphincter. *Anesth Analg.* 1989;68:63-65.
35. Mort TC. The incidence and risk factors for cardiac arrest during emergency tracheal intubation: a justification for incorporating the ASA Guidelines in the remote location. *J Clin Anesth.* 2004;16:508-516.
36. Rose DK, Cohen MM. The airway: problems and predictions in 18,500 patients. *Can J Anaesth.* 1994;41:372-383.
37. Schwartz DE, Matthay MA, Cohen NH. Death and other complications of emergency airway management in critically ill adults. A prospective investigation of 297 tracheal intubations. *Anesthesiology.* 1995;82:367-376.
38. Dubois A. Obesity and gastric emptying. *Gastroenterology.* 1983;84:875-876.
39. Horowitz M, Collins PJ, Cook DJ, Harding PE, Shearman DJ. Abnormalities of gastric emptying in obese patients. *Int J Obes.* 1983;7:415-421.
40. Maddox A, Horowitz M, Wishart J, Collins P. Gastric and oesophageal emptying in obesity. *Scand J Gastroenterol.* 1989;24:593-598.
41. Wright RA, Krinsky S, Fleeman C, Trujillo J, Teague E. Gastric emptying and obesity. *Gastroenterology.* 1983;84:747-751.
42. Kadar AG, Ing CH, White PF, Wakefield CA, Kramer BA, Clark K. Anesthesia for electroconvulsive therapy in obese patients. *Anesth Analg.* 2002;94:360-361, table of contents.
43. Ewah B, Yau K, King M, Reynolds F, Carson RJ, Morgan B. Effect of epidural opioids on gastric emptying in labour. *Int J Obstet Anesth.* 1993;2:125-128.
44. Macfie AG, Magides AD, Richmond MN, Reilly CS. Gastric emptying in pregnancy. *Br J Anaesth.* 1991;67:54-57.
45. Shinder SM, Levinson G. *Anesthesia for Obstetrics.* 2nd ed. Philadelphia, PA: Lippincott Williams & Wilkins; 1987:300-315.
46. Vanner R. Cricoid pressure. *Int J Obstet Anesth.* 2009;18:103-105.
47. Mhyre JM, Riesner MN, Polley LS, Naughton NN. A series of anesthesia-related maternal deaths in Michigan, 1985-2003. *Anesthesiology.* 2007;106:1096-1104.
48. McDonnell NJ, Paech MJ, Clavisi OM, Scott KL. Difficult and failed intubation in obstetric anaesthesia: an observational study of airway management and complications associated with general anaesthesia for caesarean section. *Int J Obstet Anesth.* 2008;17:292-297.
49. Davies JM, Posner KL, Lee LA, Cheney FW, Domino KB. Liability associated with obstetric anesthesia: a closed claims analysis. *Anesthesiology.* 2009;110:131-139.
50. Borland LM, Sereika SM, Woelfel SK, et al. Pulmonary aspiration in pediatric patients during general anesthesia: incidence and outcome. *J Clin Anesth.* 1998;10:95-102.
51. Kao CH, ChangLai SP, Chieng PU, Yen TC. Gastric emptying in head-injured patients. *Am J Gastroenterol.* 1998;93:1108-1112.
52. Saxe JM, Ledgerwood AM, Lucas CE, Lucas WF. Lower esophageal sphincter dysfunction precludes safe gastric feeding after head injury. *J Trauma.* 1994;37:581-584; discussion 4-6.
53. Hardoff R, Sula M, Tamir A, et al. Gastric emptying time and gastric motility in patients with Parkinson's disease. *Mov Disord.* 2001;16:1041-1047.
54. Erden V, Basaranoglu G, Delatioglu H, Hamzaoglu NS. Relationship of difficult laryngoscopy to long-term non-insulin-dependent diabetes and hand abnormality detected using the 'prayer sign'. *Br J Anaesth.* 2003;91:159-160.
55. Kalinowski CP, Kirsch JR. Strategies for prophylaxis and treatment for aspiration. *Best Pract Res Clin Anaesthesiol.* 2004;18:719-737.
56. McAnulty GR, Robertshaw HJ, Hall GM. Anaesthetic management of patients with diabetes mellitus. *Br J Anaesth.* 2000;85:80-90.
57. Heyland DK, Tougas G, King D, Cook DJ. Impaired gastric emptying in mechanically ventilated, critically ill patients. *Intensive Care Med.* 1996;22:1339-1344.
58. Kao CH, Ho YJ, Changlai SP, Ding HJ. Gastric emptying in spinal cord injury patients. *Dig Dis Sci.* 1999;44:1512-1515.
59. Kelly MC, Carabine UA, Hill DA, Mirakhur RK. A comparison of the effect of intrathecal and extradural fentanyl on gastric emptying in laboring women. *Anesth Analg.* 1997;85:834-838.
60. Murphy DB, Sutton JA, Prescott LF, Murphy MB. Opioid-induced delay in gastric emptying: a peripheral mechanism in humans. *Anesthesiology.* 1997;87:765-770.
61. Porter JS, Bonello E, Reynolds F. The influence of epidural administration of fentanyl infusion on gastric emptying in labour. *Anaesthesia.* 1997;52:1151-1156.
62. Franke A, Nakchbandi IA, Schneider A, Harder H, Singer MV. The effect of ethanol and alcoholic beverages on gastric emptying of solid meals in humans. *Alcohol Alcohol.* 2005;40:187-193.
63. American Society of Anesthesiologists C. Practice guidelines for preoperative fasting and the use of pharmacologic agents to reduce the risk of pulmonary aspiration: application to healthy patients undergoing elective procedures: an updated report by the American Society of Anesthesiologists Committee on Standards and Practice Parameters. *Anesthesiology.* 2011;114:495-511.
64. Practice guidelines for preoperative fasting and the use of pharmacologic agents to reduce the risk of pulmonary aspiration: application to healthy patients undergoing elective procedures: a report by the American Society of Anesthesiologist Task Force on Preoperative Fasting. *Anesthesiology.* 1999;90:896-905.
65. Brady M, Kinn S, Stuart P. Preoperative fasting for adults to prevent perioperative complications. *Cochrane Database Syst Rev.* 2003:CD004423.
66. Soreide E, Eriksson LI, Hirlekar G, et al. Pre-operative fasting guidelines: an update. *Acta Anaesthesiol Scand.* 2005;49:1041-1047.
67. O'Sullivan G, Scrutton M. NPO during labor. Is there any scientific validation? *Anesthesiol Clin North Am.* 2003;21:87-98.
68. Practice guidelines for obstetric anesthesia: an updated report by the American Society of Anesthesiologists Task Force on Obstetric Anesthesia. *Anesthesiology.* 2007;106:843-863.

69. Hatlebakk JG, Berstad A. Pharmacokinetic optimisation in the treatment of gastro-oesophageal reflux disease. *Clin Pharmacokinet*. 1996;31:386-406.
70. Porembka DT, Kier A, Sehlhorst S, Boyce S, Orlowski JP, Davis K Jr. The pathophysiologic changes following bile aspiration in a porcine lung model. *Chest*. 1993;104:919-924.
71. Sturm A, Holtmann G, Goebell H, Gerken G. Prokinetics in patients with gastroparesis: a systematic analysis. *Digestion*. 1999;60:422-427.
72. Zatman TF, Hall JE, Harmer M. Gastric residual volume in children: a study comparing efficiency of erythromycin and metoclopramide as prokinetic agents. *Br J Anaesth*. 2001;86:869-871.
73. Gibbs CP, Schwartz DJ, Wynne JW, Hodd CI, Kuck EJ. Antacid pulmonary aspiration in the dog. *Anesthesiology*. 1979;51:380-385.
74. Carp H, Jayaram A, Stoll M. Ultrasound examination of the stomach contents of parturients. *Anesth Analg*. 1992;74:683-687.
75. Perlas A, Chan VW, Lupu CM, Mitsakakis N, Hanbidge A. Ultrasound assessment of gastric content and volume. *Anesthesiology*. 2009;111:82-89.
76. Van de Putte P, Perlas A. Ultrasound assessment of gastric content and volume. *Br J Anaesth*. 2014;113:12-22.
77. Hamada SR, Garcon P, Ronot M, Kerever S, Paugam-Burtz C, Mantz J. Ultrasound assessment of gastric volume in critically ill patients. *Intensive Care Med*. 2014;40:965-972.
78. Perlas A, Davis L, Khan M, Mitsakakis N, Chan VW. Gastric sonography in the fasted surgical patient: a prospective descriptive study. *Anesth Analg*. 2011;113:93-97.
79. Kruisselbrink R, Arzola C, Endersby R, Tse C, Chan V, Perlas A. Intra- and interrater reliability of ultrasound assessment of gastric volume. *Anesthesiology*. 2014;121:46-51.
80. Brimacombe JR, Berry AM. Cricoid pressure. *Can J Anaesth*. 1997;44:414-425.
81. Bair AE, Filbin MR, Kulkarni RG, Walls RM. The failed intubation attempt in the emergency department: analysis of prevalence, rescue techniques, and personnel. *J Emerg Med*. 2002;23:131-140.
82. El-Orbany MI, Joseph NJ, Salem MR, Klowden AJ. The neuromuscular effects and tracheal intubation conditions after small doses of succinylcholine. *Anesth Analg*. 2004;98:1680-1685, table of contents.
83. Ellis DY, Harris T, Zideman D. Cricoid pressure in emergency department rapid sequence tracheal intubations: a risk-benefit analysis. *Ann Emerg Med*. 2007;50:653-665.
84. Sloane C, Vilke GM, Chan TC, Hayden SR, Hoyt DB, Rosen P. Rapid sequence intubation in the field versus hospital in trauma patients. *J Emerg Med*. 2000;19:259-264.
85. Pearson S. Comparison of intubation attempts and completion times before and after the initiation of a rapid sequence intubation protocol in an air medical transport program. *Air Med J*. 2003;22:28-33.
86. Ricard-Hibon A, Chollet C, Leroy C, Marty J. Succinylcholine improves the time of performance of a tracheal intubation in prehospital critical care medicine. *Eur J Anaesthesiol*. 2002;19:361-367.
87. Rocca B, Crosby E, Maloney J, Bryson G. An assessment of paramedic performance during invasive airway management. *Prehosp Emerg Care*. 2000;4:164-167.
88. Davis DP, Dunford JV, Poste JC, et al. The impact of hypoxia and hyperventilation on outcome after paramedic rapid sequence intubation of severely head-injured patients. *J Trauma*. 2004;57:1-8; discussion 10.
89. Dunford JV, Davis DP, Ochs M, Doney M, Hoyt DB. Incidence of transient hypoxia and pulse rate reactivity during paramedic rapid sequence intubation. *Ann Emerg Med*. 2003;42:721-728.
90. Adnet F, Baillard C, Borron SW, et al. Randomized study comparing the "sniffing position" with simple head extension for laryngoscopic view in elective surgery patients. *Anesthesiology*. 2001;95:836-841.
91. Gambee AM, Hertzka RE, Fisher DM. Preoxygenation techniques: comparison of three minutes and four breaths. *Anesth Analg*. 1987;66:468-470.
92. Neilipovitz DT, Crosby ET. No evidence for decreased incidence of aspiration after rapid sequence induction. *Can J Anaesth*. 2007;54:748-764.
93. Tanoubi I, Drolet P, Donati F. Optimizing preoxygenation in adults. *Can J Anaesth*. 2009;56:449-466.
94. Stept WJ, Safar P. Rapid induction-intubation for prevention of gastric-content aspiration. *Anesth Analg*. 1970;49:633-636.
95. Satiani B, Bonner JT, Stone HH. Factors influencing intraoperative gastric regurgitation: a prospective random study of nasogastric tube drainage. *Arch Surg*. 1978;113:721-723.
96. Salem MR, Wong AY, Fizzotti GF. Efficacy of CP in preventing aspiration of gastric contents in paediatric patients. *Br J Anaesth*. 1972;44:401-404.
97. Sivilotti ML, Filbin MR, Murray HE, Slasor P, Walls RM. Does the sedative agent facilitate emergency rapid sequence intubation? *Acad Emerg Med*. 2003;10:612-620.
98. Adams P, Gelman S, Reves JG, Greenblatt DJ, Alvis JM, Bradley E. Midazolam pharmacodynamics and pharmacokinetics during acute hypovolemia. *Anesthesiology*. 1985;63:140-146.
99. Davis DP, Kimbro TA, Vilke GM. The use of midazolam for prehospital rapid-sequence intubation may be associated with a dose-related increase in hypotension. *Prehosp Emerg Care*. 2001;5:163-168.
100. Sivilotti ML, Ducharme J. Randomized, double-blind study on sedatives and hemodynamics during rapid-sequence intubation in the emergency department: the SHRED Study. *Ann Emerg Med*. 1998;31:313-324.
101. Michenfelder JD, Milde JH, Sundt TM Jr. Cerebral protection by barbiturate anesthesia. Use after middle cerebral artery occlusion in Java monkeys. *Arch Neurol*. 1976;33:345-350.
102. Mirakhur RK, Elliott P, Shepherd WF, Archer DB. Intra-ocular pressure changes during induction of anaesthesia and tracheal intubation. A comparison of thiopentone and propofol followed by vecuronium. *Anaesthesia*. 1988;43(Suppl):54-57.
103. Thomson MF, Brock-Utne JG, Bean P, Welsh N, Downing JW. Anaesthesia and intra-ocular pressure: a comparative of total intravenous anaesthesia using etomidate with conventional inhalation anaesthesia. *Anaesthesia*. 1982;37:758-761.
104. Hartung HJ. Intracranial pressure in patients with craniocerebral trauma after administration of propofol and thiopental. *Anaesthesist*. 1987;36:285-287.
105. McCollum JS, Dundee JW. Comparison of induction characteristics of four intravenous anaesthetic agents. *Anaesthesia*. 1986;41:995-1000.
106. Moss E, Powell D, Gibson RM, McDowall DG. Effect of etomidate on intracranial pressure and cerebral perfusion pressure. *Br J Anaesth*. 1979;51:347-352.
107. Giese JL, Stockham RJ, Stanley TH, Pace NL, Nelissen RH. Etomidate versus thiopental for induction of anesthesia. *Anesth Analg*. 1985;64:871-876.
108. Weiss-Bloom LJ, Reich DL. Haemodynamic responses to tracheal intubation following etomidate and fentanyl for anaesthetic induction. *Can J Anaesth*. 1992;39:780-785.
109. Robinson N, Clancy M. In patients with head injury undergoing rapid sequence intubation, does pretreatment with intravenous lignocaine/lidocaine lead to an improved neurological outcome? A review of the literature. *Emerg Med J*. 2001;18:453-457.
110. Asfar SN, Abdulla WY. The effect of various administration routes of lidocaine on hemodynamics and ECG rhythm during endotracheal intubation. *Acta Anaesthesiol Belg*. 1990;41:17-24.
111. Naguib M, Samarkandi A, Riad W, Alharby SW. Optimal dose of succinylcholine revisited. *Anesthesiology*. 2003;99:1045-1049.
112. Andrews JI, Kumar N, van den Brom RH, Olkkola KT, Roest GJ, Wright PM. A large simple randomized trial of rocuronium versus succinylcholine in rapid-sequence induction of anaesthesia along with propofol. *Acta Anaesthesiol Scand*. 1999;43:4-8.
113. Dobson AP, McCluskey A, Meakin G, Baker RD. Effective time to satisfactory intubation conditions after administration of rocuronium in adults. Comparison of propofol and thiopentone for rapid sequence induction of anaesthesia. *Anaesthesia*. 1999;54:172-176.
114. Skinner HJ, Biswas A, Mahajan RP. Evaluation of intubating conditions with rocuronium and either propofol or etomidate for rapid sequence induction. *Anaesthesia*. 1998;53:702-706.
115. Fuchs-Buder T, Sparr HJ, Ziegenfuss T. Thiopental or etomidate for rapid sequence induction with rocuronium. *Br J Anaesth*. 1998;80:504-506.
116. Perry J, Lee J, Wells G. Rocuronium versus succinylcholine for rapid sequence induction intubation. *Cochrane Database Syst Rev*. 2003:CD002788.
117. Perry JJ, Lee JS, Sillberg VA, Wells GA. Rocuronium versus succinylcholine for rapid sequence induction intubation. *Cochrane Database Syst Rev*. 2008:CD002788.
118. Tran DT, Newton EK, Mount VA, Lee JS, Wells GA, Perry JJ. Rocuronium versus succinylcholine for rapid sequence induction intubation. *Cochrane Database Syst Rev*. 2015:CD002788.
119. Naguib M. Sugammadex: another milestone in clinical neuromuscular pharmacology. *Anesth Analg*. 2007;104:575-581.
120. Salem MR, Sellick BA, Elam JO. The historical background of cricoid pressure in anesthesia and resuscitation. *Anesth Analg*. 1974;53:230-232.
121. Farmery AD, Roe PG. A model to describe the rate of oxyhaemoglobin desaturation during apnoea. *Br J Anaesth*. 1996;76:284-291.
122. Hardman JG, Wills JS, Aitkenhead AR. Factors determining the onset and course of hypoxemia during apnea: an investigation using physiological modelling. *Anesth Analg*. 2000;90:619-624.
123. Lawes EG, Campbell I, Mercer D. Inflation pressure, gastric insufflation and rapid sequence induction. *Br J Anaesth*. 1987;59:315-318.

124. Ruben H, Knudsen EJ, Carugati G. Gastric inflation in relation to airway pressure. *Acta Anaesthesiol Scand.* 1961;5:107-114.
125. Bouvet L, Albert ML, Augris C, et al. Real-time detection of gastric insufflation related to facemask pressure-controlled ventilation using ultrasonography of the antrum and epigastric auscultation in nonparalyzed patients: a prospective, randomized, double-blind study. *Anesthesiology.* 2014;120:326-334.
126. Fetito SP, Russell WJ. The prevention of gastric inflation--a neglected benefit of cricoid pressure. *Anaesth Intensive Care.* 1988;16:139-143.
127. Taha SK, Siddik-Sayyid SM, El-Khatib MF, Dagher CM, Hakki MA, Baraka AS. Nasopharyngeal oxygen insufflation following pre-oxygenation using the four deep breath technique. *Anaesthesia.* 2006;61:427-430.
128. Ramachandran SK, Cosnowski A, Shanks A, Turner CR. Apneic oxygenation during prolonged laryngoscopy in obese patients: a randomized, controlled trial of nasal oxygen administration. *J Clin Anesth.* 2010;22:164-168.
129. Vanner RG, Pryle BJ. Nasogastric tubes and cricoid pressure. *Anaesthesia.* 1993;48:1112-1113.
130. Smith CE, Boyer D. Cricoid pressure decreases ease of tracheal intubation using fibreoptic laryngoscopy (WuScope System. *Can J Anaesth.* 2002;49:614-619.
131. Smith KJ, Dobranowski J, Yip G, Dauphin A, Choi PT. Cricoid pressure displaces the esophagus: an observational study using magnetic resonance imaging. *Anesthesiology.* 2003;99:60-64.
132. Boet S, Duttchen K, Chan J, et al. Cricoid pressure provides incomplete esophageal occlusion associated with lateral deviation: a magnetic resonance imaging study. *J Emerg Med.* 2012;42:606-611.
133. Rice MJ, Mancuso AA, Gibbs C, Morey TE, Gravenstein N, Deitte LA. Cricoid pressure results in compression of the postcricoid hypopharynx: the esophageal position is irrelevant. *Anesth Analg.* 2009;109:1546-1552.
134. Zeidan AM, Salem MR, Mazoit JX, Abdullah MA, Ghattas T, Crystal GJ. The effectiveness of cricoid pressure for occluding the esophageal entrance in anesthetized and paralyzed patients: an experimental and observational glidescope study. *Anesth Analg.* 2014;118:580-586.
135. Sellick BA. Rupture of the oesophagus following cricoid pressure? *Anaesthesia.* 1982;37:213-214.
136. Ralph SJ, Wareham CA. Rupture of the oesophagus during cricoid pressure. *Anaesthesia.* 1991;46:40-41.
137. Tournadre JP, Chassard D, Berrada KR, Bouletreau P. Cricoid cartilage pressure decreases lower esophageal sphincter tone. *Anesthesiology.* 1997;86:7-9.
138. Law JA, Broemling N, Cooper RM, et al. The difficult airway with recommendations for management—part 2--the anticipated difficult airway. *Can J Anaesth.* 2013;60:1119-1138.
139. Law JA, Duggan LV, Asselin M, et al. Canadian Airway Focus Group updated consensus-based recommendations for management of the difficult airway: part 2. Planning and implementing safe management of the patient with an anticipated difficult airway. *Can J Anaesth.* 2021;68:1405-1436.
140. Hein C, Owen H. The effective application of cricoid pressure. *J Emerg Prim Health Care.* 2005;3.
141. Vanner RG, O'Dwyer JP, Pryle BJ, Reynolds F. Upper oesophageal sphincter pressure and the effect of cricoid pressure. *Anaesthesia.* 1992;47:95-100.
142. Vanner RG, Pryle BJ. Regurgitation and oesophageal rupture with cricoid pressure: a cadaver study. *Anaesthesia.* 1992;47:732-735.
143. Meek T, Gittins N, Duggan JE. Cricoid pressure: knowledge and performance amongst anaesthetic assistants. *Anaesthesia.* 1999;54:59-62.
144. Meek T, Vincent A, Duggan JE. Cricoid pressure: can protective force be sustained? *Br J Anaesth.* 1998;80:672-674.
145. Crowley DS, Giesecke AH. Bimanual cricoid pressure. *Anaesthesia.* 1990;45:588-589.
146. Vanner RG, Clarke P, Moore WJ, Raftery S. The effect of cricoid pressure and neck support on the view at laryngoscopy. *Anaesthesia.* 1997;52:896-900.
147. Cook TM. Cricoid pressure: are two hands better than one? *Anaesthesia.* 1996;51:365-368.
148. Yentis SM. The effects of single-handed and bimanual cricoid pressure on the view at laryngoscopy. *Anaesthesia.* 1997;52:332-335.
149. Cook TM, Godfrey I, Rockett M, Vanner RG. Cricoid pressure: which hand? *Anaesthesia.* 2000;55:648-653.
150. Allman KG. The effect of cricoid pressure application on airway patency. *J Clin Anesth.* 1995;7:197-199.
151. Moynihan RJ, Brock-Utne JG, Archer JH, Feld LH, Kreitzman TR. The effect of cricoid pressure on preventing gastric insufflation in infants and children. *Anesthesiology.* 1993;78:652-656.
152. Vanner RG. Tolerance of cricoid pressure by conscious volunteers. *Int J Obstet Anesth.* 1992;1:195-198.
153. Hawthorne L, Wilson R, Lyons G, Dresner M. Failed intubation revisited: 17-yr experience in a teaching maternity unit. *Br J Anaesth.* 1996;76:680-684.
154. Lawes EG, Duncan PW, Bland B, Gemmel L, Downing JW. The cricoid yoke--a device for providing consistent and reproducible cricoid pressure. *Br J Anaesth.* 1986;58:925-931.
155. Hartsilver EL, Vanner RG. Airway obstruction with cricoid pressure. *Anaesthesia.* 2000;55:208-211.
156. Aoyama K, Takenaka I, Sata T, Shigematsu A. Cricoid pressure impedes positioning and ventilation through the laryngeal mask airway. *Can J Anaesth.* 1996;43:1035-1040.
157. Asai T, Barclay K, McBeth C, Vaughan RS. Cricoid pressure applied after placement of the laryngeal mask prevents gastric insufflation but inhibits ventilation. *Br J Anaesth.* 1996;76:772-776.
158. MacG Palmer JH, Ball DR. The effect of cricoid pressure on the cricoid cartilage and vocal cords: an endoscopic study in anaesthetised patients. *Anaesthesia.* 2000;55:263-268.
159. Levitan RM, Kinkle WC, Levin WJ, Everett WW. Laryngeal view during laryngoscopy: a randomized trial comparing cricoid pressure, backward-upward-rightward pressure, and bimanual laryngoscopy. *Ann Emerg Med.* 2006;47:548-555.
160. McNelis U, Syndercombe A, Harper I, Duggan J. The effect of cricoid pressure on intubation facilitated by the gum elastic bougie. *Anaesthesia.* 2007;62:456-459.
161. Turgeon AF, Nicole PC, Trepanier CA, Marcoux S, Lessard MR. Cricoid pressure does not increase the rate of failed intubation by direct laryngoscopy in adults. *Anesthesiology.* 2005;102:315-319.
162. Hodgson RE, Gopalan PD, Burrows RC, Zuma K. Effect of cricoid pressure on the success of endotracheal intubation with a lightwand. *Anesthesiology.* 2001;94:259-262.
163. Noguchi T, Koga K, Shiga Y, Shigematsu A. The gum elastic bougie eases tracheal intubation while applying cricoid pressure compared to a stylet. *Can J Anaesth.* 2003;50:712-717.
164. Harris T, Ellis DY, Foster L, Lockey D. Cricoid pressure and laryngeal manipulation in 402 pre-hospital emergency anaesthetics: essential safety measure or a hindrance to rapid safe intubation? *Resuscitation.* 2010;81:810-816.
165. Corda DM, Riutort KT, Leone AJ, Qureshi MK, Heckman MG, Brull SJ. Effect of jaw thrust and cricoid pressure maneuvers on glottic visualization during GlideScope videolaryngoscopy. *J Anesth.* 2012;26:362-368.
166. Apfelbaum JL, Hagberg CA, Connis RT, et al. 2022 American Society of Anesthesiologists Practice Guidelines for Management of the Difficult Airway. *Anesthesiology.* 2022;136:31-81.
167. Ovassapian A, Salem MR. Sellick's maneuver: to do or not do. *Anesth Analg.* 2009;109:1360-1362.
168. Gabbott DA. The effect of single-handed cricoid pressure on neck movement after applying manual in-line stabilisation. *Anaesthesia.* 1997;52:586-588.
169. Helliwell V, Gabbott DA. The effect of single-handed cricoid pressure on cervical spine movement after applying manual in-line stabilisation—a cadaver study. *Resuscitation.* 2001;49:53-57.
170. Wood PR. Direct laryngoscopy and cervical spine stabilisation. *Anaesthesia.* 1994;49:77-78.
171. Cook TM, Kelly FE. Time to abandon the 'vintage' laryngeal mask airway and adopt second-generation supraglottic airway devices as first choice. *Br J Anaesth.* 2015;115:497-499.
172. Roux M, Drolet P, Girard M, Grenier Y, Petit B. Effect of the laryngeal mask airway on oesophageal pH: influence of the volume and pressure inside the cuff. *Br J Anaesth.* 1999;82:566-569.
173. Joshi GP, Morrison SG, Okonkwo NA, White PF. Continuous hypopharyngeal pH measurements in spontaneously breathing anesthetized outpatients: laryngeal mask airway versus tracheal intubation. *Anesth Analg.* 1996;82:254-257.
174. Ho BY, Skinner HJ, Mahajan RP. Gastro-oesophageal reflux during day case gynaecological laparoscopy under positive pressure ventilation: laryngeal mask vs. tracheal intubation. *Anaesthesia.* 1998;53:921-924.
175. Hagberg CA, Vartazarian TN, Chelly JE, Ovassapian A. The incidence of gastroesophageal reflux and tracheal aspiration detected with pH electrodes is similar with the laryngeal mask airway and esophageal tracheal combitube—a pilot study. *Can J Anaesth.* 2004;51:243-249.
176. McCrory CR, McShane AJ. Gastroesophageal reflux during spontaneous respiration with the laryngeal mask airway. *Can J Anaesth.* 1999;46:268-270.

177. Cheong YP, Park SK, Son Y, et al. Comparison of incidence of gastroesophageal reflux and regurgitation associated with timing of removal of the laryngeal mask airway: on appearance of signs of rejection versus after recovery of consciousness. *J Clin Anesth.* 1999;11:657-662.
178. Evans NR, Gardner SV, James MF. ProSeal laryngeal mask protects against aspiration of fluid in the pharynx. *Br J Anaesth.* 2002;88:584-587.
179. Verghese C, Brimacombe JR. Survey of laryngeal mask airway usage in 11,910 patients: safety and efficacy for conventional and nonconventional usage. *Anesth Analg.* 1996;82:129-133.
180. Brimacombe JR, Berry A. The incidence of aspiration associated with the laryngeal mask airway: a meta-analysis of published literature. *J Clin Anesth.* 1995;7:297-305.
181. Keller C, Brimacombe J, Bittersohl J, Lirk P, von Goedecke A. Aspiration and the laryngeal mask airway: three cases and a review of the literature. *Br J Anaesth.* 2004;93:579-582.
182. Hung OR, Pytka S, Morris I, Murphy M, Stewart RD. Lightwand intubation: II--Clinical trial of a new lightwand for tracheal intubation in patients with difficult airways. *Can J Anaesth.* 1995;42:826-830.
183. Hung OR, Pytka S, Morris I, et al. Clinical trial of a new lightwand device (Trachlight) to intubate the trachea. *Anesthesiology.* 1995;83:509-514.
184. Bourke DL, Katz J, Tonneson A. Nebulized anesthesia for awake endotracheal intubation. *Anesthesiology.* 1985;63:690-692.
185. Ovassapian A, Krejcie TC, Yelich SJ, Dykes MH. Awake fibreoptic intubation in the patient at high risk of aspiration. *Br J Anaesth.* 1989;62:13-16.
186. Simmons ST, Schleich AR. Airway regional anesthesia for awake fiberoptic intubation. *Reg Anesth Pain Med.* 2002;27:180-192.
187. Walsh ME, Shorten GD. Preparing to perform an awake fiberoptic intubation. *Yale J Biol Med.* 1998;71:537-549.
188. Benumof JL. Management of the difficult adult airway. With special emphasis on awake tracheal intubation. *Anesthesiology.* 1991;75:1087-1110.
189. McCormick PW. Immediate care after aspiration of vomit. *Anaesthesia.* 1975;30:658-665.
190. Ambrosio AM, Luo R, Fantoni DT, et al. Effects of positive end-expiratory pressure titration and recruitment maneuver on lung inflammation and hyperinflation in experimental acid aspiration-induced lung injury. *Anesthesiology.* 2012;117:1322-1334.
191. Wynne JW, Modell JH. Respiratory aspiration of stomach contents. *Ann Intern Med.* 1977;87:466-474.
192. Lee M, Sukumaran M, Berger HW, Reilly TA. Influence of corticosteroid treatment on pulmonary function after recovery from aspiration of gastric contents. *Mt Sinai J Med.* 1980;47:341-346.
193. Sukumaran M, Granada MJ, Berger HW, Lee M, Reilly TA. Evaluation of corticosteroid treatment in aspiration of gastric contents: A controlled clinical trial. *Mt Sinai J Med.* 1980;47:335-340.
194. Wolfe JE, Bone RC, Ruth WE. Effects of corticosteroids in the treatment of patients with gastric aspiration. *Am J Med.* 1977;63:719-722.
195. Bone RC, Fisher CJ Jr, Clemmer TP, Slotman GJ, Metz CA, Balk RA. A controlled clinical trial of high-dose methylprednisolone in the treatment of severe sepsis and septic shock. *N Engl J Med.* 1987;317:653-658.
196. Johnson JL, Hirsch CS. Aspiration pneumonia. Recognizing and managing a potentially growing disorder. *Postgrad Med.* 2003;113:99-102, 5-6, 11-12.
197. El-Solh AA, Pietrantoni C, Bhat A, et al. Microbiology of severe aspiration pneumonia in institutionalized elderly. *Am J Respir Crit Care Med.* 2003;167:1650-1654.
198. Niederman MS, Bass JB Jr, Campbell GD, et al. Guidelines for the initial management of adults with community-acquired pneumonia: diagnosis, assessment of severity, and initial antimicrobial therapy. American Thoracic Society. Medical Section of the American Lung Association. *Am Rev Respir Dis.* 1993;148:1418-1426.
199. Bernstein JM. Treatment of community-acquired pneumonia—IDSA guidelines. Infectious Diseases Society of America. *Chest.* 1999;115:9S-13S.
200. Mandell LA, Marrie TJ, Grossman RF, Chow AW, Hyland RH. Canadian guidelines for the initial management of community-acquired pneumonia: an evidence-based update by the Canadian Infectious Diseases Society and the Canadian Thoracic Society. The Canadian Community-Acquired Pneumonia Working Group. *Clin Infect Dis.* 2000;31:383-421.

CHAPTER 6

Human Factors and Airway Management

Peter G. Brindley and Jocelyn Slemko

CASE PRESENTATION

A lady in her thirties presented for endoscopic sinus surgery and septoplasty. Preoperative assessment found only a congenitally fused neck vertebra and the need for nasal decongestant spray—given her long-standing sinusitis. Despite a slight restriction in neck movement, there was nothing to predict a problem with airway management. Specifically, there was minimal restriction in neck flexion, extension, or rotation. Mouth opening and thyromental distance were normal, and the Mallampati score was grade II.

An experienced and diligent anesthesia practitioner planned to avoid tracheal intubation by inserting a laryngeal mask airway (LMA). However, following induction with a remifentanil infusion (0.3 mcg·kg^{-1}·min^{-1}) and propofol (200 mg), the LMA could not be inserted. Fifty additional mg of propofol was given but repeated attempts (including two different sizes of LMA) were also unsuccessful. After 2 minutes, the patient's oxygen saturation had decreased to 75% and she looked cyanosed. By 5 minutes, her oxygen saturation deteriorated to below 40%. Administration of 100% oxygen using a face mask and oral airway failed to raise the oxygen saturation, and the heart rate decreased to the 40s.

The anesthesia practitioner then administered atropine and succinylcholine. He attempted tracheal intubation and was joined by a second anesthesia practitioner (who had additional airway training). Laryngoscopy provided a Cormack and Lehane grade IV view with no identifiable airway anatomy visible. Other staff entered the room, including the surgeon. Between attempts at laryngoscopy, patient ventilation was extremely difficult; despite use of a two-handed, two-person bag-mask-ventilation technique. At no point did anyone announce that this was a "failed airway" a "can't intubate, can't oxygenate" situation, or an "airway emergency."

Both anesthesia practitioners made further unsuccessful laryngoscopic intubation attempts. The second anesthesia practitioner attempted a flexible bronchoscopic intubation but without success, and other staff collected additional equipment including a tracheotomy set. Next, the surgeon attempted intubation by direct laryngoscopy with a bougie; he was also unsuccessful. By 20 minutes, an intubating laryngeal mask was inserted that allowed partial ventilation. The patient's blood pressure and heart rate increased; as did oxygen saturations: but not above 90%.

Blind attempts were made to insert a tracheal tube through the intubating laryngeal mask (as the device is intended to work) and then use a flexible bronchoscope. The surgeon failed to pass the bronchoscope through the end of the LMA (a recognized problem with this device). After more than 30 minutes, it was decided to abandon the procedure and let the patient wake up. The LMA was removed and an oral airway inserted. Oxygen saturation gradually improved to 95%. The anesthesia practitioners transferred her to the recovery room and told staff that they expected the patient to wake up. Both anesthesia practitioners carried on to their next cases.

While the patient did breathe on her own, her level of consciousness did not improve and her vital signs remained erratic. After at least an additional hour, a third anesthesia practitioner transferred the patient to an intensive care unit (ICU). On ICU admission, it was clear that the patient had marked brain damage. Finally, the ICU staff inserted a nasotracheal tube using a flexible bronchoscope. Her clinical course failed to improve and lead to her ultimate removal from the ventilator, and her death from anoxic brain damage.

INTRODUCTION

Why Focus on Human Factors in Medical Crises, such as the Difficult and Failed Airway?

This chapter—plus a subsequent chapter on airway management in the ICU patient (see Chapter 35)—offers a primer on human factors. Obviously, the focus is on the difficult and failed airway, but these insights could apply to a myriad of acute care situations. This is because nontechnical skills likely have the greatest impact upon patient safety and outcome.[1,2] Similarly, inadequate crisis resource management (which includes teamwork, leadership and followership, situational awareness, decision-making, resource utilization, and communication) appears to be the most common reason for preventable errors.[1–6] In short, there is far more to airway management than merely the ability to insert tracheal tubes.

To further illustrate the importance of nontechnical skills, it is worth emphasizing that the above case is not fictional: it is the infamous case of Elaine Bromiley.[7] Despite competent individuals, the team failed the patient and themselves,[7] and this contributed to the death of a 37-year-old woman, wife and mother of two. It was the wish of her husband Martin, a pilot and expert in Aviation Human Factors, that his wife did not die in vain. Our hope is to offer practical insights from this tragic case for those facing a difficult and failed airway. Given that this patient gave no reason to suspect difficulty with intubation, it follows that these lessons apply to all airway practitioners, and all intubating teams. In short, any practitioner (or any team) striving to be a true airway expert should understand that factual knowledge in isolation is not enough. Moreover, factual knowledge and nimble fingers are rarely enough to rescue the patient-in-peril. It is, therefore, time that "team dexterity" and "verbal dexterity" match individual manual dexterity.

Can Insights Be Learnt from Other High-Stakes Industries and Applied to the Difficult and Failed Airway?

These two chapters (Chapters 6 and 35)—the second of which specifically focuses on communication, given that it is likely the most important of the nontechnical skills—offer crisis management strategies from other high-stakes professions. While the idea of directly translating ideas from aviation to medicine can be oversimplified and trite, the prudent health care workers should be open to usable insights, no matter their origin. Moreover, health care has been a latecomer to the study of human factors and team dynamics.[1,2] For example, human factors training has been compulsory for pilots since the 1990s. Accordingly, aviation still offers many of the most readily available strategies regarding how to make a "science of reducing complexity" and a "science of team performance." The first lesson is that airway management, much like aviation, is increasingly a team sport. Second, teamwork is rarely innate and therefore should not be left to chance.

The largest aviation disaster (to date) occurred in 1977 when KLM 4805 and Pan Am 1736 collided. Investigators concluded that it was wholly preventable, and largely because the crew had "failed to take the time to become a team."[1] Eerily similar is our above clinical case.[7] As pointed out at the Bromiley inquest, she likely died not just because of difficulty intubating but because her team "lost control." Of note, the inquest concluded that there was nothing lacking in the staffing, training, facilities, preoperative assessment, anesthetic choice, initial use of an LMA, or with tracheal intubation once the LMA failed. Specifically, despite being senior anesthesia practitioners and nurses, they failed to identify (and verbalize) that they had a failed airway; they failed to expedite appropriate alternative strategies, and they failed to sound the alarm. In short, they failed the failed airway. Ultimately, it was the patient (and her husband, and children) who paid the price. Much like the summary from the KLM flight investigators: it may have been "preventable ... if they had taken time to become a team."[1]

TEAMWORK

Teamwork is commonly defined as "cooperative efforts to achieve a common goal." It is more than just subordinates blindly obeying an "all-knowing" leader.[2] Instead, it is about maximizing mental and physical problem-solving capabilities, such that the sum exceeds its parts.[2] Moreover, task demands (rescuing the patient) and social demands (running the team) work in parallel. This is why there are subtle but profound differences between taskwork and teamwork. Failure to appreciate the difference means once a crisis hits, we simply fall back on a "me versus the world" mentality. It also means that airway experts deliberately manage both taskwork and teamwork.[2,8] This means that leaders need to think about how to turn individuals into team players, and this starts with accepting that individual team members will not share their abilities unless they feel "safe" to do so.[2] This *does not* mean that we no longer need hierarchy and leadership, but does mean that we cannot create the teams that we want unless we create the culture that we need.[8]

Culture is complex, and may be easier to identify than define. Regardless, it includes the knowledge, beliefs, customs, and habits of a group and powerfully influences behaviors, attitudes, and actions.[8] Importantly, culture cannot be forced, but can be nudged and takes time to nurture. Moreover, culture typically matters more than the latest greatest manuscript or technical advance—as Peter Druker famously stated: "culture eats data for breakfast." All of this means that true airway experts invest time now in building a culture of safety in order to avert airway disasters later.

We should also understand the pros and cons of our medical culture. For example, acute care medicine has a laudable culture of patient-ownership and self-reliance. This needs to continue. However, like the western culture it mirrors, we typically over-focus on the individual agenda rather than the cohesion of the team.[2] This needs to change. Similarly, we typically presume that success results from individual efforts (and failure from individual shortcomings), rather than the team, environment, or culture.[2] This also means that we do not naturally ask for help, or naturally offer help. It also means that we commonly blame individuals and excuse systems.[2–6,9] This clearly needs to change.

Successful teams can be either lucky or good, and this chapter strives to be not only good but consciously competent. Teams that succeed know how to apportion their finite resources, and they know that their resources consist of more than just equipment and drugs. Moreover, team resources include more than just personnel who can perform tracheal intubation, but the greatest range of skills, opinions. Simply put, low-functioning teams are more likely to fail. Specifically, low-functioning teams are less likely to assign roles and responsibilities; to hold team members to account; to advocate a position or a corrective action; to use check-backs (i.e., "closed-loop communication"—see Chapter 35); to seek usable information (as opposed to just "data"); to prioritize tasks; and to cross-monitor other members of the team.[2] We also need to realize that a "team of experts is not necessarily an expert team."[2]

LEADERSHIP

Good leadership is also often much easier to recognize than to define. Regardless, in broad strokes, leadership provides structure to chaos, and maximizes the teams' outcome such that the sum exceeds individual parts.[8] A key strategy is the "shared mental model" (a common understanding, or, a sense that everyone is "on the same page").[2] This helps to form a task-focused (rather than power-focused or ego-focused) team and a structure to prioritize duties; manage information; establish roles; stabilize emotions; and build (appropriate) confidence.[2] If time allows, the team leader can invite members to suggest a mental model ("what should we do now?") offering diverse inputs that may provide a more comprehensive view.[2,8] However, under time-pressure, the leader has to be dexterous enough to rapidly establish a reasonable mental model that members will support ("this is a failed airway, please do the following").[3] Studies have shown that the best situational awareness and the shortest reaction time come from practice and prior exposure.[8] As a result, we should look to regular airway simulation not as a luxury, but as key to developing team "reflexes."[9]

The greater the overlap in mental models, the more likely that team members will predict, adapt, and coordinate, even if dealing with stress or novelty.[2] It is also essential to regularly update the mental model ("okay, so the airway is secured; our next priority is…") and to ensure that it still makes sense as new knowledge comes to light ("saturations are falling and we can't oxygenate: this is now a failed airway"). Task assignment is usually specified by profession (e.g., anesthesia practitioners intubate and surgeons operate).[2] Therefore, this does not usually need to be negotiated in the mental model. However, if there is confusion (i.e., two anesthesia practitioners are present; both surgeon and anesthesia practitioner could perform cricothyrotomy), then the leader's instructions need to be explicitly stated ("Dr Jones, you intubate, Dr Smith you get ready to insert an extraglottic device," "Dr Jones, you perform cricothyroidotomy and I will assist"). Without leadership, diffusion of responsibility can occur. Some tasks—typically the easiest—will be addressed by several people even though one would suffice. Other tasks—typically harder ones—remain undone.[2]

It may be tempting to scream out blunt instructions. It may even feel good, in the moment, to lambaste others. However, in order to engage other highly skilled individuals, we are best to employ a calm but credible approach.[8] This is because leadership cannot be claimed: it needs to be earned. In return, leaders are temporarily empowered by the team to be decisive, and, when necessary, to override others. The quid pro quo is, that in return, good leaders empower the team to speak up and make it clear that others' contributions are wanted.[8] In short, good leaders create a culture that focuses on "what" is right not "who" is right. In this way, the right leadership style promotes a culture of safety, and a culture that cares about the team.[2,4] Good leaders also routinely change the focus between clinical task completion and team coordination. This reduces fixation errors and prevents overtaxing individual members. Good leaders know that, typically, relationship conflicts should not be resolved during an emergency (which is why a debrief is so useful).[2] In contrast, task-related conflicts must be dealt with promptly (which is why we need to know how to speak up and to listen).[2]

Good leaders know that an inexperienced team can still function, but typically needs more direction. This usually means more hierarchy and centralizing control.[2,9,10] As the team matures, so should the team structure. The leader can now create a culture where members learn to volunteer relevant information, verbalize contingencies, and apportion responsibility (so-called "explicit coordination").[2] Mature teams also voice relevant concerns and ask critical questions. This "cross-monitoring," or "mutual-monitoring," is one way to gradually flatten the team's authority gradient.[2] As teams mature, they can anticipate each other's resource needs and actions, and can act with minimal talking (so-called "implicit coordination").[2] Typically, the more routine the task, the more experienced its members, and the more familiar they are with each other, the less explicit coordination is required. The more unfamiliar the task, or its members, the more explicit coordination is required.

FOLLOWERSHIP

Importantly, followership skills are no less important than leadership skills. In contrast, our obsession with "being in charge" is illustrated by the fact that, to date, there are approximately 60 publications on leadership for every one publication on followership.[11] Accordingly, there could still be a stigma associated with self-identifying as a follower (i.e., a relative subordinate), even though 85% of health care workers—including those who manage airways—are better understood to be followers. Airway management would be impossible without skilled followers, and once again these skills can and should be taught. Effective followers are able to step up when required and not take it personally when they need to step back. In short, followership is an advanced and dynamic airway skill. It can and should be taught, modeled, and valued.

Followers are able to self-manage and use their emotional intelligence to size up what they can and should contribute at any moment.[12] The binary ideas of all-knowing leader versus unquestioning follower are outdated. Instead, members of the airway team move in and out of leadership and followership roles. Therefore, it is better to simply talk about high-functioning airway team members, who, in turn, are those with the dexterity to adapt to *what* (rather than *who*) is right. As outlined, effective leaders and followers also cross-monitor. In other words, while we manage ourselves, we also remain vigilant to the needs of others. Part of being a good airway team member is having that "sixth sense," where you size up a situation and step up or step back in whatever way best serves the patient and team. It is also about removing the practitioner's ego and focusing on the patient's needs.

SITUATIONAL AWARENESS

Broadly defined, situational awareness encompasses how we perceive relevant cues (i.e., oxygen desaturation), how we comprehend their meaning (i.e., "the patient is worsening"), how we synthesize a mental model (i.e., "the patient needs to be reoxygenated"), and how we predict what should happen next (i.e., "we need to prepare for a possible surgical airway").[13,14] Situational awareness also requires "metacognition"—namely, an awareness and understanding of one's thought processes. For example, a technique used in counseling is to encourage people to "H.A.L.T.": that is, reflect upon whether your thinking/actions are impaired because you are Hungry, Angry, Late, or Tired? Similarly, during intubation, airway practitioners can learn to calm themselves in the moment using breathing exercises previously taught to soldiers: consciously slowing your own breathing rate (breath in for four; hold for four; out for four), or through mental rehearsal and cognitive imagery (i.e., thinking about the difficult airway during the night before, the drive to the hospital, or the elevator ride to the emergency room).[15–17]

The first level of situational awareness involves the perception of stimuli.[2] This requires focused attention, but by focusing "here," we risk missing "there." Because of the avalanche of stimuli, we must make conscious and unconscious decisions about where to prioritize, and what to ignore (or postpone). This can lead to fixation errors: where we focus our attention inappropriately and miss relevant cues (i.e., you are so focused on the airway that you miss the cardiac dysrhythmia). Fixation errors are especially likely during stress when we achieve a type of cognitive tunnel vision (i.e., the repeated attempts to intubate during the Bromiley case, rather than moving on to Plan B). Attention is like a searchlight—highlighting things that can either be perceived as an important cue or a distraction. As complexity increases, the number of possible cues also increases. Unfortunately, like the diameter of the searchlight's beam, our attention is limited. This can cause selection bias either because our attention is misdirected (toward irrelevant stimuli), or simply insufficient (not enough cues are collected).[2,13,14]

Fortunately, we can mitigate attention bias. For example, there are two main types of attention in nature, and we need both in an airway crisis. First, there is the scanning vigilance typified by prey (where focus is routinely refocused from one area to the next).[18] By constantly redirecting our attention and sampling different inputs, we reduce the likelihood of selection bias and fixation errors.[3,5,14] During airway management, we scan the patient and the monitors, looking for cues that suggest distress. Just like lifeguards who scan the beach, we avoid looking at just one spot. However, when danger strikes, we need the second type of attention: focus. This is typified by the focused gaze of a predator,[18] or the lifeguard who ignores others as he/she focuses on the person in distress. This is where nonessential stimuli are minimized and tunnel-vision takes over.[19] This second technique avoids wasting attention. However, as outlined, its potential downside is the fixation error and the illusion of centrality: that nothing outside of our immediate attention is properly seen or heard.

For those unconvinced about our cognitive fallibility, an excellent book by Chabris and Simons reviews their famous psychological experiment (also known as "the invisible gorilla").[20] In brief, viewers are asked to watch a video and simply count basketball passes between actors wearing white and black shirts. Given the complex things that most professions do, this may seem elementary. However, regardless of seniority, typically only half are correct when it comes to this experiment. This is because the others were distracted by an actor who walks into the video frame midway through. He is wearing a gorilla suit and spends eight seconds pounding his chest. Typically, viewers see either the gorilla or get the number of passes correct, but rarely both. What is equally insightful is when the video is replayed, many still refuse to believe that there was ever a gorilla in the original. In short, our attention is imperfect, but so is our insight. The video demonstrates how we have visual and judgment blind spots, where we only see what we are primed to see.[20]

MANAGING IMPENDING AIRWAY DISASTERS

■ What Are the Basics of Decision-Making and Action, and How Could They Apply to the Difficult and Failed Airway?

In disasters, whether medical or otherwise, a three-phase survival arc appears to exist: denial; deliberation; and decision.[8] Preparation (whether through simulation or cognitive imagery or experience) decreases denial, means you have already done the work of deliberation, and means you have a cognitive roadmap for decisive action. Expressed another way, how our brains respond depends greatly upon complexity and familiarity. So-called "automatic responses" occur immediately because responses are embedded due to simplicity or repetition.[14] For example, once the patient's oxygenation desaturates, the patient should be placed on "flush-oxygen" without much conscious thought. As such, our attention is freed up to contemplate the next steps.

"Simple decisions" (for example, which laryngoscope blade to request) occur when there are a few possibilities. Therefore, subconscious choosing usually takes a second or two. "Complex decisions" (for example, what airway rescue technique should you try while the complex patient's oxygen saturation is decreasing in front of you?) take longer because there is no appropriate response in the personal database. A response has to be created and this consumes additional precious time. Finally, there is the "inability to make decisions" where no behavioral schema exists, and no temporary schema can be created.[21] This typically causes stress, panic, or even paralysis, at exactly the wrong time.[2]

As each team member builds an individual awareness, they should report their findings and plans back to the team leader. The team leader then integrates these individual models into a shared mental model that summarizes the patient's current state (level two of situational awareness) and predicts their trajectory (level three of situational awareness). In this way, the team's awareness amplifies each individual's awareness. Most of this is done through verbal communication, which, as stated above, is discussed in more detail in Chapter 35.

What Are the Challenges when Teaching and Promoting Human Factors in Airway Management?

The "Semmelweis effect"[22]—named after the doctor who was ridiculed for promoting hand washing—is the reflex-like tendency to reject new approaches because they conflict with established practice (i.e., "I have always approached the airway this way: why change now?"). In a similar vein, the Dunning–Kruger[23] effect is a (complex) cognitive bias where (with the risk of oversimplification) unskilled individuals overestimate their ability, and highly-skilled individuals underestimate the complexity. This creates the potential risk where the inexperienced intubator assumes they will be fine, and the expert intubator also assumes that others will be fine. After all, for the nonexpert, most airways will still go well ... until they don't. For the expert, because this task is now relatively straightforward for them, they assume it will be for others. For all the above reasons, those promoting a greater need for teamwork, preparation, and caution are likely to encounter resistance. Be strong and tenacious, dear friends!

The Future of Human Factors and Complex Airway Management: Safety-I and Safety-II

Patient safety, and by extension airway safety, is often fallaciously understood as just the absence of failure. Similarly, an "error-is-everywhere" mindset has led to the idea that all we need is minimal variation and maximal (unthinking) compliance. This is overly simplistic and potentially dangerous. While standardization and predictability are definitely important, it has also meant that **S**afety (with a big S) has been largely defined by administrators, regulators, and external mandates, rather than frontline clinicians.[24,25] It has led to a "find and fix" strategy and relies on adverse events to guide safety, without acknowledging the irony of this approach (in other words, we rely on error to improve safety).[25] This approach—now known as Safety-I—largely assumes that systems are bimodal (i.e., things go right or wrong) and decomposable (i.e., complexity can be broken down into individual repairable parts). Safety-I is more likely to see humans as a liability because we introduce variability into a system that would work perfectly if we just followed the protocol.[25] This "scooby-doo principle"—namely, "it would be fine if it wasn't for those meddling kids"—is overly simplistic. Ironically, taken to an extreme, it could actually be dangerous.

Unfortunately, Safety-I can be highly attractive to some administrators and academics, especially those far from the frontlines. Complex health care is often so nuanced, and its components are so intertwined, that it cannot always be broken down or summarized on a one-page linear algorithm. This means that we may be better off looking at complexity theory (as attributed to Gloubermann and Zimmermann) or chaos theory (often attributed to Lorenz). Regardless, when things are unpredictable, it is hard to dictate a single way, or precisely define "ideal behavior"—except in the most basic cases. Achieving airway safety also means understanding how humans get things *right* most of the time. This in turn means empowering humans and respecting gestalt and experience. This study of "how most things go right" is known as Safety-II, and is a profound advance in terms of highlighting the importance of human factors. It could be a safer way of looking at safety.

Safety-II is the study of success rather than failure. It relies on the adaptation, improvisation, tenacity, and everyday problem-solving skills of practical people. Accordingly, "airway expertise" is recognized, rewarded, and encouraged. It means respecting intuition and accepting that some are better able to deal with unpredictability and chaos. Safety-II aims to learn how teams adapt, and see humans as an essential resource because of their practicality and experience.[25] Safety-II, does not forgive error, or human laziness, or human inexperience. It also does not give humans maverick license to do as they please. Instead, Safety-II matures our understanding of what humans bring to health care. It helps explain adverse events as transient phenomena at a specific time and place (the so-called Swiss Cheese model of error). It reinforces the idea that improvements come from numerous iterative everyday adjustments.[25]

Going forward, our understanding of human factors will need to combine the two paradigms: with Safety-I predominating for simple matters and Safety-II predominating for the more complex. Importantly, this updated understanding also adds extra nuance to why so many health care professionals report burnout and frustration.[24] Without oversimplifying complex ideas like well-being and resilience, most health care workers will be familiar with feeling despondent because a Safety-I solution (i.e., another unnecessary delay) was implemented without their input when a Safety-II solution would have been better (i.e., a senior airway practitioner could have been empowered). If we continue with a Safety-I focus, there is every likelihood that frontliners will be disproportionally blamed and disempowered, and forced to endure well-intentioned but wrong-headed solutions.

Examples of Safety-I versus Safety-II thinking abound. For example, doctors are (rightly) criticized because we frequently rely on workarounds. Sometimes these are cavalier, but sometimes they are inspired. Regardless, part of the reason for workarounds is that doctors and nurses sense they suffer from too much bureaucracy, not enough equipment, and too much work to blindly follow externally imposed rules. Safety-I means we often face numerous security stops when one, but done properly, would allow doctors to focus on immediate patient care. The erstwhile focus on Safety-I can mean we overly rely on one set of laboratory findings (i.e., the oxygen saturation level or systolic blood pressure) rather than a more comprehensive patient assessment.

Systems that obsess over Safety-I and ignore Safety-II may lead exhausted and frustrated health care workers to quit clinical work.[24] After all, anyone who understands even basic human factors appreciates that people can only take so much unnecessary bureaucratic burden. We want humans to do the right thing because of the system not despite it. A greater use of Safety-II thinking might help dedicated humans feel valued and able to craft systems that are not only safer but more human-focused. Keeping experienced people engaged means we keep their wisdom in the system, rather than just their anger and frustration. System-II could also mean a more nuanced understanding of the emotional and cognitive demands of airway management, and how tough it can be as a patient at the mercy of the system.

SUMMARY (SEE TABLE 6.1)

As outlined, human factors and nontechnical skills impact patient safety and outcome in the difficult and failed airway. Moreover, improving our crisis resource management skills (which include teamwork, leadership, situational awareness, decision-making, resource utilization, and communication) is key to making airway management safer for our patients. These skills should not—but fortunately need not—be left to chance. Practical strategies can be readily borrowed from other high-stakes professions. Our "team dexterity" and "verbal dexterity" should match our manual dexterity and factual know-how.

Teamwork is usually defined as "cooperative efforts to achieve a common goal." We need to understand that teamwork skills are neither innate nor typically promoted in the traditional medical education curriculum. As a result, a "team of experts is rarely an expert team." Leadership skills are needed to provide structure to chaos. A key strategy is having a "shared mental model," along with a credible but calm approach that appropriately prioritizes (actions), coordinates (data), and controls (emotions). Situational awareness requires mastery in three domains: (i) how we perceive relevant cues; (ii) how we comprehend their meaning; and (iii) how we synthesize a mental model in order to predict what might happen next.

Studies suggest that there are three Ds in disaster: denial; deliberation; and decision. Practice, whether through clinical experience, cognitive imagining (i.e., mental rehearsal), or through simulation are ways to reach the fourth D, namely "decisive action," faster and safer. Regarding human factors and airway management, the question is not whether they matter—they clearly do—and not whether practical strategies can be applied—they certainly can—but rather whether we have the humility and resolve to make the effort.

TABLE 6.1. Practical Crisis Resource Management Strategies for the Difficult and Failed Airway

Team Factor	Recommendation
Climate & culture	• More "we" less "me" • Mutual respect; calm and decisive • Hierarchy still has a role • "What" is right, not "who" is right
Establish structure	• Assign roles • Assign responsibilities • Establish priorities • Communicate throughout
Create a shared mental model	• Ensure all on "same page" • Invite input when possible • Outline priorities • Influence team emotions
Cross monitor	• Monitor performance • Monitor workload • Flatten the hierarchy • Encourage feedback
Maintain resilience	• Routine practice sessions • Request feedback • Encourage debrief • Provide time for casual interaction

SELF-EVALUATION QUESTIONS

6.1. The inquest following the death of Elaine Bromiley concluded that:

A. The anesthetist/anesthesiologist was grossly incompetent and should be sued for inability to intubate the patient.

B. The nursing staff were grossly incompetent and should be fired for failing to sound the alarm.

C. The surgeon was the best person to attempt intubation after the two anesthetists tried and failed to intubate.

D. Clearly, the patient would have lived if teamwork had been better.

E. The team "lost control" and failed to follow established guidelines for the failed airway.

6.2. Major categories in Crisis Resource Management Strategies include:

A. Leadership, communication, resource utilization, situational awareness

B. Hierarchy, obedience, implicit coordination, explicit coordination

C. Shared mental model, team dexterity, fixation error, communication

D. Focus, vigilance, deliberation, communication, cross-monitoring

E. None of the above

6.3. Which of the following is true?

A. Experienced teams need more explicit coordination; whereas inexperienced teams need more implicit coordination.

B. The Semmelweis reflex refers to the ability of people to learn new skills, but only once the rationale is properly explained.

C. The Dunning-Kruger effect is the effect of a medical error on subsequent team performance.

D. The three Ds of a disaster survival are denial, deliberation, and decision.

E. The **HALT** mnemonic means that you perform better if the team has hierarchy, aptitude, lots of resources, and training.

6.4. Which of the following is true?

A. Safety-I is all about teamwork, whereas Safety-II is about task work.

B. Taskwork and teamwork are the same thing.

C. Team culture is "owned" by the team leader, and good followers know to get in line.

D. The reality is that "error-is-everywhere" and what we need most is minimal variation and maximal compliance.

E. A Safety-I approach should predominate for simple matters, with Safety-II for the more complex.

REFERENCES

1. Gawande A. The checklist. In: Gawande A, ed. *The Checklist Manifesto*. New York, NY: Henry Holt and Company; 2009:32-48.
2. St Pierre M, Hofinger G, Buerschaper C. *Crisis Management in Acute Care Settings: Human Factors and Team Psychology in a High Stakes Environment*. New York, NY: Springer; 2008.
3. Brindley PG, Reynolds SF. Improving verbal communication in critical care medicine. *J Crit Care*. 2011;26:155-159.
4. Gaba DM, Fish KJ, Howard SK. *Crisis Management in Anesthesiology*. New York, NY: Churchill Livingstone; 1994.
5. Gaba DM. Dynamic decision-making in anesthesiology: cognitive models and training approaches. In: Evans DA, Patel VI, eds. *Advanced Models of Cognition for Medical Training and Practice*. Berlin: Springer-Verlag; 1992:123-147.
6. Aron D, Headrick L. Educating physicians prepared to improve care and safety is no accident: it requires a systematic approach. *Qual Saf Health Care*. 2002;11:168-173.
7. Bromiley, M. Just a routine operation (you tube). Available at http://www.youtube.com/watch?v=JzlvgtPIof4. Accessed July 2015.
8. Ripley A. *The Unthinkable: Who Survives When Disaster Strikes - and Why*. New York, NY: Crown publishers; 2008.
9. Brindley PG. Patient safety and acute care medicine: lessons for the future, insights from the past. *Crit Care*. 2010;14(2):217-222.
10. Heffernan, M. *Willful Blindness: Why We Ignore the Obvious at Our Peril*. New York, NY: Doubleday/Random House; 2011.
11. Leung C, Lucas A, Brindley P, et al. Followership: A review of the literature in healthcare and beyond. *J Crit Care*. [Internet]. 2018;46:99-104. Available at https://doi.org/10.1016/j.jcrc.2018.05.001.
12. Gillman LM, Brindley PG, Blaivas M, Widder S, Karakitsos D. Trauma team dynamics. *J Crit Care*. 2016;32:218-221.
13. Endsley MR. Toward a theory of situation awareness in dynamic systems. *Human Factors*. 1995;37(1):32-64.
14. Endsley MR. Theoretical underpinnings of situation awareness: A critical review. In: *Situation Awareness Analysis and Measurement*. Mahwah, NJ: Lawrence Erlbaum Associates; 2000;3-32.
15. What is tactical breathing. Available at http://www.breathmastery.com/what-is-tactical-breathing/Slow Breathing. Accessed July 2015.
16. Immenroth M, Burger T, Brenner J, Nagelschmidt M, Eberspacher H, Troide H. Mental training in surgical education: Randomized controlled trial. *Am J Surgery*. 2007;245(3):385-391.
17. Sanders C, Sadoski M, va Wlasum K, Bramson R, Wiprud R, Fossum TW. Learning basic surgical skills with mental imagery: using the simulation centre in the mind. *Med Educ*. 2008;42(6):607-612.
18. Proctor RN, Schiebinger L. *Agnotology: The Making and Unmaking of Ignorance*. Stanford University Press; 2008.
19. Stanton NA, Chambers PR, Piggott J. Review of situational awareness: concept, theory, and application. *Safety Sci*. 2001;39(39):189-204.
20. Chabris CF, Simons DJ. *The Invisible Gorilla: And Other Ways Our Intuitions Deceive Us*. New York, NY: Crown Publishers, Random House; 2010.
21. Leach J. Why people "freeze" in an emergency: temporal and cognitive constraints on survival responses. *Aviat Space Environ Med*. 2004.75(6):539-542.
22. Semmelweis Reflex. Wikipedia. Available at http://en.wikipedia.org/wiki/Semmelweis_reflex. Accessed July 2015.
23. Dunning-Kruger Effect. Available at https://en.wikipedia.org/wiki/Dunning–Kruger_effect. Accessed July 2015.
24. Smaggus A. Safety-I, Safety-II and burnout: how complexity science can help clinician wellness. *BMJ Qual Saf*. 2019;28(8):667-671.
25. Hollnagel E, Wears R, Braithwaite J. From Safety-I to Safety-II: a white paper. *Resilient Health Care Net*. 2015.

SECTION 2

AIRWAY TECHNIQUES

CHAPTER 7

Context-Sensitive Airway Management

Orlando R. Hung and Michael F. Murphy

CASE PRESENTATION

A 14-year-old female is scheduled to have an excision of a mandibular mass in a hospital in Kigali, Rwanda. She is otherwise healthy, takes no medications, and has no allergies. She weighs about 42 kg and is 144 cm tall (BMI 20.3 kg·m^{-2}). On examination, she appears to be nervous, but cooperative. She has a large right mandibular mass restricting her mouth opening (3 cm) (Figures 7.1 and 7.2). She has a Mallampati IV score and jaw protrusion is limited, but the range of motion of her cervical spine is normal. She agrees to have an awake intubation with some reluctance. Routine monitors (noninvasive blood pressure monitor, ECG, and pulse oximeter) are placed upon her arrival in the operating room (OR). Intravenous (IV) access is established and a judicious amount of IV ketamine (bolus of 10 mg) is administered for sedation. Topical anesthesia is achieved with lidocaine sprays. Since a flexible bronchoscope is unavailable, the following plans are prepared to secure her airway and communicated to everyone involved in her care. Plan A: awake blind nasal intubation using a BAAM (Beck Airway Airflow Monitor) whistle[1]; Plan B: orotracheal intubation using the only available videolaryngoscope (C-MAC Macintosh blade); and Plan C: a surgical airway. Unfortunately, blind nasal intubation is not successful after a number of attempts as the endotracheal tube (ETT) repeatedly enters the esophagus due to inadequate upper airway anesthesia. Tracheal intubation using the C-MAC is also difficult with poor visualization of the glottis, particularly when the posterior aspect of the tongue begins to bleed. With ongoing suction around the bleeding site, an attempt with direct laryngoscopic intubation also fails. It becomes obvious that the appropriate course of action is for the otorhinolaryngologist to perform an awake tracheotomy under ketamine sedation and local anesthesia. With oxygen supplementation through a facemask (8 L·min^{-1}) and repeated boluses of IV ketamine (10 mg per dose), tracheotomy is secured. Oxygen saturation remains above 90% during the procedure. Anesthesia is then induced with thiopental and is maintained with 1 to 1.5 MAC of halothane. The otorhinolaryngologist excises the

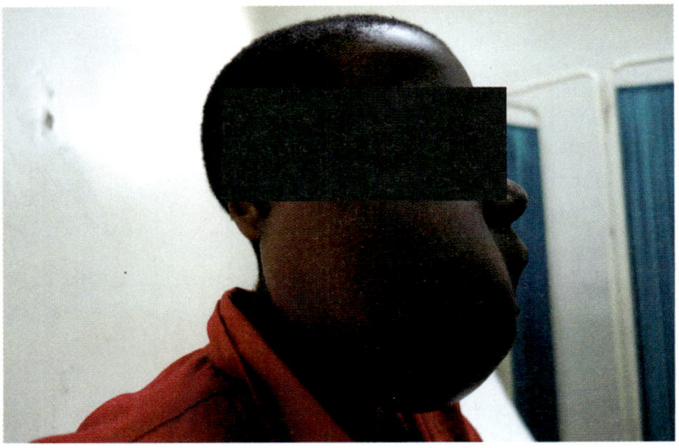

FIGURE 7.1. Lateral view of a 14-year-old patient with a large right mandibular mass.

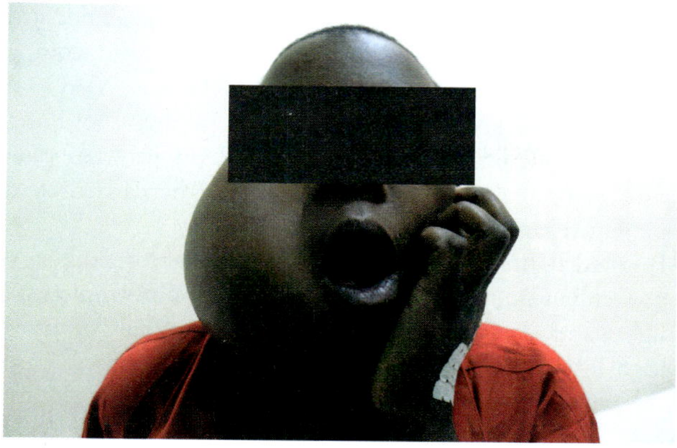

FIGURE 7.2. Front view of a 14-year-old patient with a large right mandibular mass restricting her mouth opening.

mandibular mass, and the patient is transferred to the intensive care unit (ICU) in stable condition at the conclusion of the surgical procedure. Ventilation is maintained through the tracheostomy tube.

INTRODUCTION

The fundamental goals of airway management are the maintenance of adequate ventilation, oxygenation, and protection from aspiration. In the majority of clinical settings, these three goals are achieved in tandem, usually during orotracheal intubation under direct laryngoscopy. As the location, time of day, skill set of the airway practitioner, and the devices available (i.e., the "context") change, the airway practitioner must be prepared to modify his or her approach and employ appropriate alternative techniques. Oxygenation by whatever method possibly takes precedence in all situations.

What Is Context-Sensitive Airway Management?

The concept of "context-sensitive" airway management represents a paradigm shift in the approach to airway management.[2] The seasoned practitioner is less focused on specific devices and techniques (e.g., video-laryngoscopic intubation), and is more aware of the *context* in which the patient presents and how that context influences the approach to airway management.

The "context-defining" questions can be conceptualized as the "who, what, when, where, why, and how," which are unique to each airway management encounter. These questions, or *context modifiers*, influence the decision-making of a skilled airway practitioner. In a more pragmatic sense, examples of these contextual factors might include:

- urgency factors of the case (e.g., the nothing by mouth status, a thorough airway assessment);
- availability of resources (in the case presented, the practitioner attempts blind nasal intubation because a flexible bronchoscope is unavailable);
- the expertise of an assistant or assistants;
- the time of day (influences the availability of additional skilled airway practitioners);
- the skill sets and personal experience of the practitioners (e.g., in the presented case, the skill set of the practitioner in blind nasal intubation, intubation using C-MAC, and the ability to perform front-of-neck access);
- the location in which the patient encounter occurs (in the presented case, resources such as airway equipment, atomizer for topicalization of the upper airway, drug availability, infusion pumps, etc., may be limited or unavailable).

Patient factors, such as anatomy and physiology, and the degree to which the patient can cooperate conspire to influence the context of the situation. In the case presented, the patient is anxious, but cooperative. If she had been uncooperative, an awake intubation may not have been possible and her airway management would be quite different. Although a facemask seal may be challenging in this patient, some practitioners might have considered inhalation induction of anesthesia and/or deep sedation using IV anesthetics, maintaining spontaneous ventilation while performing tracheal intubation or tracheotomy, although caution in choosing this technique was recommended by the 4th National Audit Project of the Royal College of Anaesthetists of Great Britain and Ireland and the Difficult Airway Society (NAP4).[3]

Does the Context of the Case Presented Suggest Which Technique Should Be Used to Provide Ventilation and Oxygenation to a Pediatric Patient with a Difficult Airway?

The case presentation demonstrates how airway management by its nature, is context-sensitive. "Who, what, when, where, why, and how" are all context-defining questions that affect the way airway management is best approached. The airway was successfully managed in this case by a surgical tracheotomy after several attempts of failed tracheal intubation, an option that may not have been considered by a similar team in a different environment. In other words, the context has changed.

Traditionally, face-mask ventilation (FMV) has been advocated as the initial approach to a patient unable to independently sustain adequate gas exchange. Indeed, among the four domains of airway management (FMV, extraglottic device use, tracheal intubation, and front-of-neck access [FONA]), FMV has been the most common initial maneuver employed by most airway practitioners. Unfortunately, mounting evidence and opinion suggest that FMV is a difficult skill to master, particularly in the hands of nonexpert practitioners.[4–7] In many cases, FMV is performed poorly with ineffective oxygenation and ventilation, and with gastric insufflation being the end result, particularly when high airway pressure is being employed. The use of FMV was predicted to be difficult in the case presented because of altered facial anatomy (large mandibular mass). As extraglottic devices (EGDs) continue to improve in design and ease of use, most experts agree that the placement of an EGD ought to supplant FMV as the initial technique of choice in an unconscious and apneic patient, particularly by nonexpert airway practitioners.[8] Difficulty seating and sealing an EGD is anticipated in this case due to the altered hypopharyngeal anatomy.

Clearly, a "one size fits all" approach does not work in airway management, and no single device or technique can be relied upon as the sole modality for airway management by *any* practitioner. The choice of device and technique depends on the context of the situation, recognizing that failing techniques need to be abandoned quickly for alternative techniques (from Plan A to Plan B, and then to Plan C if necessary).

The airway management encounter in the case presented was predicted to fail using FMV or EGD, or any oral intubation approach. The practitioner elected to employ a blind nasal intubation approach (in this case, using a BAAM whistle). A nasal bronchoscopic-assisted intubation, or nasal intubation, using a lightwand while at the same time preparing for a FONA might also have been considered had these devices been available. A blind nasal approach is therefore reasonable with FONA as an alternative plan.

How Has an Increasing Appreciation of the Context-Sensitive Nature of Airway Management Informed Technological Advances Leading to Improved Airway Management Tools?

Technological advances over the past two decades have dramatically improved the quality and clinical utility of many airway management tools, including:

1. The manufacturing and marketing of newer and improved EGDs for use in a variety of situations.[9,10] Gone are the days when the LMA-Classic™ was the only, or even the *preferred*, EGD for use in difficult or failed airways. In the United Kingdom, the i-gel® (Intersurgical Ltd) has been the EGD of choice for prehospital airway management since 2010.[11] The airway practitioner now has the option of choosing among devices that serve as tracheal intubation conduits in addition to those that have been shown to be effective rescue oxygenation devices in situations where intubation is not possible.[12]
2. Advances in video resolution and LCD monitor technology, producing high-quality color images, have led to the development of several video-camera endoscopic-based devices. These include the GlideScope® (Verathon Medical, Bothell WA), the Video Macintosh Intubating Laryngoscope System (C-MAC, Karl Storz Endoscopy Co., Culver City, CA), and the McGrath MAC Video-Laryngoscope (Aircraft Medical, Edinburgh, UK). Limitations due to fogging, and obscured glottic visualization in the presence of blood, vomitus, or secretions are issues.[13] Glidescope incorporates an antifog heating element in direct contact with a thin piece of glass covering the camera lens. The heating element of the disposable Cobalt GlideScope video-laryngoscope is on the video baton making it often less effective in transferring heat to the disposable plastic sheath so as to minimize lens fogging.[13] In other words, the utility of these video-laryngoscopes remains questionable in these contexts (see Chapter 11). Nonetheless, video-laryngoscopy continues to be an evolving field with intriguing possibilities in the absence of bodily fluids that may obscure their optics.
3. Devices are becoming more lightweight, portable, and robust in construction. These factors, coupled with the introduction of disposable variants, have broadened their utility. Battery-powered flexible endoscopes and compact video-laryngoscopes, such as the McGrath® MAC, the C-MAC® Pocket Monitor, and the GlideScope Ranger Video-Laryngoscopes, do not depend on external power sources or large video displays and can be carried to the patient regardless of location.
4. Boosted light intensity of some airway instruments in the past enhanced the transillumination capability employed by lightwand devices (Trachlight™).[14] Substantially improved high-intensity LED bulb devices are on the horizon[15] ensuring adequate transillumination under ambient lighting conditions obviating the need to dim the lights or darken the room when these devices are being used. One study involving 950 patients demonstrated that nearly 88% of Trachlight intubations were effectively accomplished under ambient light with or without simple shading of the neck.[16]
5. Reduction in the cost of some of the newer video-laryngoscopes and flexible bronchoscopes has improved access to these devices. While video-laryngoscopes and flexible bronchoscopes have been shown to improve the laryngoscopic view and tracheal intubation success rates in patients with a difficult airway, the cost of some of the devices is high and may be a barrier to their clinical use. With retail costs falling, some of the newer video-laryngoscopes (e.g., the King Vision and the AirTraq) and flexible bronchoscopes (e.g., the single-use flexible Ambu® aScope™ [Ambu A/S], Ballerup, Denmark) may become more affordable even for centers with limited resources (see Chapter 11).

In What Contexts Are Blind Intubating Techniques Indicated?

Over the years, direct laryngoscopic intubation has been shown to be an effective and safe technique that is relatively easy to perform. It has become the standard method of tracheal intubation in many clinical settings, and in the field. Unfortunately, even in the hands of experienced laryngoscopists, the rapid and accurate placement of an ETT remains a significant challenge in some patients. This is particularly true in *unprepared* patients, or in situations where resources are limited, such as "austere" environments (see Chapter 59) in which blind or nonvisual techniques *may* be more practical and successful.

Flexible bronchoscopic intubation has gained a measure of popularity as an alternative intubation technique over the past several decades. While effective and reliable, this technique requires expensive equipment, and special skill and training. Additionally, bronchoscopic intubation can be difficult in emergency situations in which *unprepared* or uncooperative patients may have copious secretions, blood, or vomitus in the upper airway. Nonetheless, one large study involving more than 1600 fiberoptic intubations recorded a success rate of approximately 94% in all comers.[17]

The limitations of laryngoscopic intubation under direct vision, particularly under emergency conditions, have fostered the development of blind techniques using a variety of devices such as intubating guides (e.g., the Eschmann tracheal introducer for tactile feel of the tracheal rings) and light-guided intubation using the principle of transillumination of the soft tissues of the anterior neck, which have proven to be effective, safe, and simple.

Would It Not Be Safer to Place a Tracheal Tube Using a Technique that Is Under Direct or Indirect Vision?

One would anticipate that the placement of an ETT into the trachea under direct or indirect vision using a laryngoscope or video-laryngoscope ought to be safer and achieve higher success rates than nonvisual techniques. Such is not the case: success and complication rates are *not* substantially different with blind techniques when performed by skilled practitioners,[16] as elaborated below. It is well recognized that the technique of direct or indirect vision intubation can be difficult or impossible in the face of difficult or distorted anatomy, as illustrated in the presented case. In addition, contextual factors influence the success rates and safety of indirect laryngoscopic intubation including the inability to visualize the passage of the ETT through the glottic opening in the presence of blood, secretions, and vomitus.

Many practitioners fail to understand that after having placed the flexible bronchoscope into the trachea under indirect vision, the actual passage of the ETT over the bronchoscope is done *blindly* employing the scope as a guide. In other words, during bronchoscopic intubation, after advancing the tip of the bronchoscope into the trachea, the bronchoscope functions only as a tracheal introducer to guide the ETT into the trachea, similar to an Eschmann Introducer.[18] The use of advanced airway devices to enable continuous glottic visualization during ETT exchange has been studied.[19] This intriguing application of these devices may be applied to primary intubation to further increase the safety of *blind* intubation techniques, such as intubation over a bronchoscope, although further research is required.

Define Blind Tracheal Tube Placement

We define "blindness" as the inability to directly or indirectly (e.g., VL or bronchoscope) visualize the glottic structures during tracheal tube placement. In the section above, we describe how intubation over a flexible bronchoscope is in fact a *blind* technique since the act of ETT passage through the glottis is not visualized. There are other airway management techniques that are similarly *blind*.

Even though direct visualization of the transilluminated light is employed to confirm placement of a lightwand into the trachea, neither the passage of the wand nor the passage of the ETT over the wand is visualized directly or indirectly. Blind nasal intubation is aided by the tactile sensation of expired gas against the cheek or the auditory assistance of a BAAM whistle, but the passage of the ETT is not visualized. Finally, tactile digital intubation uses fingers to guide the ETT into the trachea in which passage of the ETT through the glottis in a nonvisualized fashion. Even when a direct or indirect laryngoscopy technique is employed, the actual passage of the ETT through the glottis may be *blind* (e.g., a Cormack-Lehane grade 3 view in which the ETT is inserted under the epiglottis blindly into the trachea with or without a bougie; or blood, vomitus, or secretions in the airway).

Many other procedures performed in medicine are in fact *blind* techniques, including the placement of pulmonary arterial catheters, arterial cannulae, epidural catheters, and femoral nerve sheath catheters. All of these procedures demand placement blindly under the guidance of anatomical landmarks, and physiological responses, although the recent introduction of sonography has changed the landscape of the performance of some of these procedures.[20]

Blind intubating techniques have been shown to be effective and safe and are acceptable methods of airway management when employed in the appropriate contexts.

AIRWAY MANAGEMENT TOOLS

Which of the EGDs Has Been Shown to Provide Better Ventilation and Oxygenation and in What Contexts?

Implicit to any discussion about airway management tools and techniques is the realization that the *best* instrument for the situation depends entirely on the context. Unfortunately, there is no "one size fits all" device.

The context affects a variety of issues when one contemplates the use of an EGD. These include: patient anatomy and predicted ease of insertion, *full-stomach* precautions, need for airway protection from aspiration (e.g., Sellick's Maneuver), need for positive-pressure ventilation, and the presence or absence of obstructing airway pathology. These are just a few of the *factors* that shape the context of EGD use in airway management.

In general, EGDs are best reserved for fasted patients at low risk of aspiration, and those with acceptable airway resistance and pulmonary compliance should positive-pressure ventilation be desired. However, EGDs are invaluable *rescue* devices in the case of unexpected airway management difficulty or failure. They have proven to be valuable as primary airway management devices in Emergency Medical Services (EMS). In these contexts, placement of an EGD with intubation capabilities and a parallel lumen for gastroesophageal venting (second-generation EGDs) may be advisable. In clinical practice, the actual device is less important than the thoughtful consideration of all contextual factors. In the opinion of the authors, the EGDs currently available that best fulfill these objectives are the LMA-Supreme™ (nonintubating EGD), the LMA-Fastrach™ (intubating EGD), the LMA-Protector™, and the King LTS-D™.

What Extraglottic Devices Should I Incorporate into My Practice?

The most thoroughly studied EGDs currently in use are the Laryngeal Mask Airway (LMA) and the Combitube™. Many competing designs and variations of these devices have been released to market and are in use worldwide. We now have the option of using intubating LMAs and alternatives to the Combitube, such as the King Laryngeal Tube Airway (King LT™, King Systems), which are placed blindly into the oropharynx and seated in the hypopharynx, directing respiratory gases into the trachea. In addition, a new generation of disposable, single-use EGDs has entered the marketplace, including the LMA-Unique (Teleflex), Ambu LMA (Ambu USA), the i-gel (Intersurgical Ltd), and the Baska Mask (PROACT Medical Systems, Frenchs Forest NSW, Australia).

Of particular use in the difficult or failed airway scenario are the various models of intubating LMAs such as the LMA-Fastrach, LMA-Evo™, LMA-Protector, and Air-Q® Intubating Laryngeal Airway (Cookgas). Intubating LMA systems are fundamentally designed to permit the practitioner to ventilate the patient and to provide a conduit for tracheal intubation. This may be accomplished using a flexible bronchoscope, a lightwand, or even by blind insertion.

The final consideration to note when deciding on the best EGDs to purchase and implement in one's institution is the differentiation between disposable and reusable devices. Several high-quality disposable EGDs are now on the market. These were developed partially in response to concerns about potential transmission of prion-based infections, such as Creutzfeldt-Jakob disease (see Chapter 63). Disposable devices, such as the LMA-Supreme or i-gel, may be best suited to use in the prehospital context where a reusable device requiring sterilization may be discarded or lost. Environmental concerns with the routine use of disposable devices are worth noting.

What Tracheal Intubation Techniques Should I Incorporate into My Practice?

Recalling the principles of context-sensitive airway management, it is apparent that an expert practitioner should be comfortable with several techniques of tracheal intubation, including visual and nonvisual methods.

For most practitioners involved in airway management, tracheal intubation equates to direct laryngoscopy. It is true that the conventional laryngoscope, with interchangeable curved and straight blades, is likely the tool with the greatest recognition and use worldwide. Expertise with this tool is an essential skill for any airway practitioner. In addition, all practitioners should become familiar with the use of tracheal introducers, such as the Eschmann Tracheal Introducer or the Introes™ Pocket Bougie (BOMImed). This device should be kept readily at hand wherever airway management and direct laryngoscopy may be required, which includes the OR, emergency department, ICU, and in crash-carts throughout the hospital.

Beyond direct laryngoscopy, the best tracheal intubation tool for an individual's practice depends on the context of that practice. Specifically, what types of patients do you routinely expect to see? Does your institution deal with "difficult" airway situations on a regular basis? How will budgetary constraints dictate which tools may or may not be available for purchase?

While it is not possible to mandate a standard list of devices, it is reasonable to ensure access to a complementary armamentarium of tools to confront the challenges that might arise. This should include laryngoscopes with curve and straight blades, the Eschmann Introducer, a flexible bronchoscope, a video-laryngoscope, such as the Glidescope, Storz C-MAC, McGrath MAC, or King Vision video-laryngoscope (Ambu), a nonvisual technique, such as a lightwand and an EGD with intubating capacity. The remaining devices available should be considered on a case-by-case basis. A FONA kit, which should include a scalpel with a #20 blade, a tracheal introducer ("bougie"), and a tracheal tube is mandatory in all areas where airway management may occur.

CLINICAL APPLICATION OF AIRWAY MANAGEMENT TOOLS

There is a staggering array of airway management tools and techniques available today. For the average practitioner, it is unrealistic to expect proficiency with all devices. However, to be a competent airway management practitioner, one must be familiar with a number of airway management tools and techniques in order to be prepared for the inevitable challenges.

What Is the Most Appropriate Airway Management Tool for an Unconscious Patient?

The simple answer to this question is whichever device restores ventilation and oxygenation promptly! A subsidiary concern is that the device protects against gastric insufflation and aspiration. These goals suggest that tracheal intubation is the most-desired solution, currently most commonly achieved through direct laryngoscopy.

However, in reality, the context will define the "best" way to manage an airway. In the example given at the beginning of this chapter, blind nasal intubation, direct and indirect laryngoscopy, were not possible. A surgical airway as a planned alternative was performed.

Traditionally, individuals charged with emergency airway management have been taught that FMV ought to be the initial airway management strategy in the unconscious patient. This paradigm may be shifting, particularly as evidence supporting the ease of use and effectiveness of EGDs in the hands of those who infrequently manage the airway mounts. EGDs and FMV have similar drawbacks in that they leave the patient with an *unprotected* airway in terms of aspiration risk, and the ability to administer effective positive-pressure ventilation is variable. Overall, it is the authors' opinion that EGDs should be used to rescue a "failed" airway because they are *more* effective and successful than FMV in most cases. All airway management practitioners ought to be familiar with the use of EGDs in appropriate patients, or as rescue devices in the setting of an intubation failure.

How Would You Manage the Patient that Is Cyanotic and Uncooperative?

The situation (context) has changed. The management of the uncooperative patient is covered in detail in Chapters 25 and 40. In this case, the practitioner is faced with the unenviable decision as to whether or not to induce anesthesia with or without muscle relaxation in the face of a potentially difficult airway. In other words, should a rapid-sequence induction/intubation (RSI) be performed?

There is no simple answer to this question. In short, it is *always* desirable to have a controlled situation to permit examination and evaluation of the patient's anatomy prior to the induction of anesthesia or at the start of an airway management procedure. Due to patient factors, this may not always be possible. In this context, one must judge whether maneuvers or interventions to correct the patient's cyanosis without invasive intervention are likely to succeed. These include administration of supplemental oxygen or simple airway maneuvers, such as a chin lift or jaw thrust. If these are *unlikely* to succeed, or are impossible due to the underlying pathology or the behavior of the patient, an RSI may be the only course of action while preparing for an immediate FONA in the event of failure (a double setup). In Chapter 2, the "forced to act" dilemma was discussed and may be considered in this situation. No matter the course of action employed as Plan A, calling for help, meticulous preparation for the primary plan, and preparation for several backup plans is critical.

What Are the Most Appropriate Airway Management Strategies for COVID-19 Patients?

Securing the airway of a COVID patient provides the best example of context-sensitive airway management. At the beginning of the pandemic, more than 30 recommendations and guidelines for airway management were published but none reported methods for systematically searching or selecting evidence, and most guidelines were based extensively on expert opinion with little direct data.[21] These include the recommendations of avoiding awake intubation and the use of flexible bronchoscope (to minimize aerosol generation and aerosol exposure), avoidance of FMV and the use of EGDs (aerosol-generating procedures), the use of disposable devices (to minimize cross-contamination), the use of some "unneccesary" personal protective equipment (e.g., shoe overs, double gloves, and powered air-purifying respirators), and the use of negative pressure rooms. Many also recommended the use of an intubation barrier ("Aerosol" box) for tracheal intubation.[22] As more information became available, it became apparent that many of these recommendations were no longer valid or applicable.[21–25] For example, in a study using an optical particle sizer to record particle size, concentration, and mass (with size range 300 nm-10 μm in diameter), Shrimpton et al. showed that FMV in anesthetized patients, even with a leak, generated less aerosol than tidal breathing and far less aerosol than a cough.[24] Using the same study model, the same group of investigators also found that tracheal intubation, including FMV produced very low quantities of aerosolized particles.[23] In contrast, tracheal extubation, particularly when the patient coughed, produced a detectable aerosol, which was 15-fold greater than intubation but 35-fold less than a volitional (unstimulated) cough.[23] In other words, these findings do not support the designation of elective tracheal intubation as an aerosol-generating procedure. Even though extubation generates more detectable aerosol than intubation, it falls below the current criterion for designation as a high-risk aerosol-generating procedure.[23] The barrier enclosures or "aerosol boxes" are not recommended because secondary aerosolization may occur upon barrier removal.[22]

Because of these new findings, and the change in paradigm (change in context), strategies for managing the airways of COVID patients have been modified. If tracheal intubation is indicated (after a trial of noninvasive ventilation such as high-flow nasal oxygen [HFNO], and/or continuous positive airway pressure [CPAP]), it is prudent to take the following steps:

1. For COVID patients with an anticipated difficult anatomical airway: awake tracheal intubation using a video-laryngoscope or a flexible bronchoscope should be considered.
2. For COVID patients with a reassuring airway: tracheal intubation under general anesthesia with a modified rapid sequence induction and intubation should be considered using the following steps:
   a. Communicate airway management Plans A, B, and C in detail with the team, including equipment preparation prior to entering the patient's room (in the ICU or the operating room).
   b. Minimize the number of health care providers present in the room during airway management. The most experienced airway practitioner should secure the airway.
   c. Appropriate PPE and barrier precautions for health care providers emphasizing protection of the three entry points, the eyes, nose, and mouth. Less emphasis on shoe covers, double gloves, or waterproof gowns.
   d. Denitrogenation should be performed after placing all standard monitors.
   e. Perform a modified RSI without cricoid pressure. In the presence of severe hypoxemia, FMV can be performed with small tidal volumes with a Heat and Moisture Exchanger HME filter in place.
   f. While the use of intubation equipment most familiar to the airway practitioner is recommended, a video-laryngoscope with a hyperangulated blade is our preference as the primary intubating device. Use a stylet ETT to facilitate tracheal tube placement. A flexible bronchoscope is Plan B and the intubating LMA Plan C. Plan D is FONA cricothyrotomy.
   g. Inflate the ETT cuff before applying positive pressure ventilation. Confirm ETT placement with end-tidal CO_2 detection.
   h. Extubation produces more aerosol than intubation. It should be performed carefully with strict adherence to PPE, essential health care providers only in the room, and careful disposal of contaminated equipment.

What Other Factors Influence the Selection of an Airway Management Tool?

Successful context-sensitive airway management depends on the interplay between three general categories of modifiers. Each modifier demands a "*who, what, where, when, why, and how*" analysis. Consider the following:

1. **Practitioner factors.** These are factors unique to each airway practitioner and include, but are not limited to: degree of expertise, past experiences, ability to rapidly assess the needs of the situation, and the ability to modify or adapt one's approach to a dynamic and variable situation. In general, the

skilled practitioner will be able to quickly assess a given airway management situation and select the most appropriate technique from his or her personal arsenal of skills.

2. **Patient factors.** These factors are those unique to each individual patient including, but not limited to: degree of cooperation, anatomic and physiologic features pertinent to airway management (e.g., a parturient or a critical airway obstruction), size of the patient (children or morbidly obese patients), medical comorbidities and past medical/surgical history, full stomach considerations, presence of blood or vomitus in the airway, lung compliance, airways resistance, and the anticipated need for aggressive positive-pressure ventilation. In general, the patient factors are "what the patient brings to the table." They refer to those things the practitioner *may* be able to modify and individualize. There is no *one size fits all* in airway management!
3. **Situational factors.** This category refers to factors that are unique to the particular situation in which the airway must be managed. Situational factors include, but are not limited to: location of the encounter (e.g., prehospital vs. emergency department, etc.), ambient lighting, urgency (elective vs. emergency situations), availability of skilled assistants, the airway management tools and equipment available, presence of confounding/complicating factors such as C-spine immobilization collars, COVID-19 (coronavirus) precautions with personal protective equipment, and availability of expert backup in the event of difficulty. The situational factors present in the environment where one practices may be modifiable to some extent. For example, a practitioner can petition the hospital to purchase an airway management tool not currently available or advocate for higher standards of airway management training for prehospital care personnel.[21]

SUMMARY

The aim of this chapter is to introduce the concept of *context-sensitive* airway management. The most fundamental dilemma facing the practitioner wishing to improve his or her difficult or failed airway management skills is making logical, evidence-based, and clinically appropriate management decisions. The case at the beginning of this chapter is based on the author's (OH) encounter during his participation in a Global Outreach Program in Rwanda. It is used as an example of the principles involved in context-sensitive airway management. This case presented an airway management strategy for a patient with a difficult airway in a resource-challenged environment with limited resources.

Gaining familiarity and experience with a variety of airway management techniques and devices will best equip the practitioner for these inevitable and challenging situations. At the very least, a competent practitioner should be facile with the techniques of face-mask ventilation, direct laryngoscopy, and tracheal intubation, placement of an extraglottic device, and performance of an emergency cricothyrotomy. In addition, all practitioners should have predetermined plans "A," "B," and "C" when approaching any airway situation. The rare but extremely important *can't intubate, can't oxygenate* situation must be routinely considered.

SELF-EVALUATION QUESTIONS

7.1. A stridorous, mentally challenged patient was brought to the operating room for an urgent neck exploration because of a neck hematoma following a neck dissection 2 days prior. In the presence of hypoxemia with SaO_2 less than 80%, which of the following is a reasonable airway management option?

A. Face-mask ventilation
B. The use of an extraglottic device
C. Tracheal intubation using a Macintosh laryngoscope
D. Front-of-neck airway
E. All of the above

7.2. For the same patient, and in the absence of hypoxemia (with SaO_2 >95%), which of the following is a reasonable intubating technique?

A. Direct laryngoscopy using a Macintosh blade
B. Tracheal intubation using the intubating LMA (Fastrach)
C. Retrograde intubation
D. Intubation using a lightwand (Trachlight)
E. Digital intubation

7.3. For the same patient, in the presence of severe hypoxemia with SaO_2 less than 70%, while setting up for a cricothyrotomy, which of the following is a reasonable intubating technique?

A. Direct laryngoscopy using a Macintosh blade
B. Tracheal intubation using the intubating LMA (Fastrach)
C. Intubation using a lightwand (Trachlight)
D. Intubation using a GlideScope
E. All of the above

REFERENCES

1. Cook RTJr, Stene JK Jr. The BAAM and endotrol endotracheal tube for blind oral intubation. Beck Airway Air Flow Monitor. *J Clin Anesth*. 1993;5:431-432.
2. Hung O, Murphy M. Context-sensitive airway management. *Anesth Analg*. 2010;110:982-983.
3. Cook TM, Woodall N, Frerk C, Fourth National Audit P. Major complications of airway management in the UK: results of the Fourth National Audit Project of the Royal College of Anaesthetists and the Difficult Airway Society. Part 1: anaesthesia. *Br J Anaesth*. 2011;106:617-631.
4. Augustine JA, Seidel DR, McCabe JB. Ventilation performance using a self-inflating anesthesia bag: effect of operator characteristics. *Am J Emerg Med*. 1987;5:267-270.
5. Lawrence PJ, Sivaneswaran N. Ventilation during cardiopulmonary resuscitation: which method? *Med J Aust*. 1985;143:443-446.
6. Lee HM, Cho KH, Choi YH, Yoon SY, Choi YH. Can you deliver accurate tidal volume by manual resuscitator? *EMJ*. 2008;25:632-634.
7. Noordergraaf GJ, van Dun PJ, Kramer BP, et al. Airway management by first responders when using a bag-valve device and two oxygen-driven resuscitators in 104 patients. *Eur J Anaesth*. 2004;21:361-366.

8. Petrar S, Murphy M, Hung O. Is a seismic shift in EMS airway management coming? A closer look at oxygenation, ventilation, intubation & alternative airways. *JEMS.* 2009;34:54-59.
9. Bogetz MS. Using the laryngeal mask airway to manage the difficult airway. *Anesthesiol Clin North Am.* 2002;20:863-870, vii.
10. Cook TM. The classic laryngeal mask airway: a tried and tested airway. What now? *Br J Anaesth.* 2006;96:149-152.
11. Lockey D, Crewdson K, Weaver A, Davies G. Observational study of the success rates of intubation and failed intubation airway rescue techniques in 7256 attempted intubations of trauma patients by pre-hospital physicians. *Br J Anaesth.* 2014;113:220-225.
12. Gerstein NS, Braude DA, Hung O, Sanders JC, Murphy MF. The Fastrach Intubating Laryngeal Mask Airway: an overview and update. *Can J Anaesth.* 2010;57:588-601.
13. Sakles JC, Patanwala AE, Mosier J, Dicken J, Holman N. Comparison of the reusable standard GlideScope(R) video laryngoscope and the disposable cobalt GlideScope(R) video laryngoscope for tracheal intubation in an academic emergency department: a retrospective review. *Acad Emerg Med.* 2014;21:408-415.
14. Hung OR, Stewart RD. Lightwand intubation: I–a new lightwand device. *Can J Anaesth.* 1995;42:820-825.
15. Milne AD, d'Entremont MI, Hung OR. Optimum brightness of a new light-emitting diode lightwand device in a cadaveric model - a pilot study. *Can J Anaesth.* 2016;63:770-771.
16. Hung OR, Pytka S, Morris I, et al. Clinical trial of a new lightwand device (Trachlight) to intubate the trachea. *Anesthesiology.* 1995;83:509-514.
17. Heidegger T, Gerig HJ, Ulrich B, Schnider TW. Structure and process quality illustrated by fibreoptic intubation: analysis of 1612 cases. *Anaesthesia.* 2003;58:734-739.
18. Hung OR. Misconception of tracheal intubation using a fiberoptic bronchoscope. *Can J Anesth.* 1998;45:496.
19. Mort TC. Tracheal tube exchange: feasibility of continuous glottic viewing with advanced laryngoscopy assistance. *Anesth Analg.* 2009;108:1228-1231.
20. Mehta N, Valesky WW, Guy A, Sinert R. Systematic review: is real-time ultrasonic-guided central line placement by ED physicians more successful than the traditional landmark approach? *EMJ.* 2013;30:355-359.
21. Grudzinski AL, Sun B, Zhang M, et al. Airway recommendations for perioperative patients during the COVID-19 pandemic: a scoping review. *Can J Anaesth.* 2022;69:644-657.
22. Sorbello M, Rosenblatt W, Hofmeyr R, Greif R, Urdaneta F. Aerosol boxes and barrier enclosures for airway management in COVID-19 patients: a scoping review and narrative synthesis. *Brit J Anaesth.* 2020;125:880-894.
23. Brown J, Gregson FKA, Shrimpton A, et al. A quantitative evaluation of aerosol generation during tracheal intubation and extubation. *Anaesthesia.* 2021;76:1741-1781.
24. Shrimpton AJ, Brown JM, Gregson FKA, et al. Quantitative evaluation of aerosol generation during manual facemask ventilation. *Anaesthesia.* 2022;77:22-27.
25. Shrimpton AJ, Gregson FKA, Brown JM, et al. A quantitative evaluation of aerosol generation during supraglottic airway insertion and removal. *Anaesthesia.* 2021;76:1577-1584.

CHAPTER 8

Face-Mask Ventilation

Nicholas Sowers and George Kovacs

INTRODUCTION

Providing effective oxygenation and ventilation using a facemask is probably the single most important component of airway management. The ability to oxygenate and ventilate immediately, in almost any environment and potentially stabilize a critically ill patient makes face-mask ventilation (FMV) one of the cornerstone interventions with which all practitioners in the operating room, emergency department (ED), and prehospital environment must be proficient. FMV refers to the use of a bag-mask unit, most of which but not all have valves (in which case they are referred to as Bag-Valve-Mask units or BVMs) system/device to deliver gas rich in oxygen either passively or actively by manually ventilating the patient using a facemask interface. Examples of non-valved bag-mask devices include Mapleson E (Jackson Rees Modification of Ayres T-piece) and other t-piece occluding systems. Manual noninvasive ventilation also accurately describes the use of an FMV device to provide positive pressure ventilation (PPV). This should be differentiated from mechanical noninvasive ventilation, which also uses a facemask interface but provides respiratory effort assistance (PPV) delivered by specialized ventilator.

Is There Still a Role for Face-Mask Ventilation in This World of Advanced Difficult Airway Devices?

Definitive airway management has traditionally been defined as the secure placement of an endotracheal tube (ETT) in the trachea. Few would argue that there has been a philosophical and evidence-based shift away from defining airway management by the method of gas exchange to focus on the goals of resuscitation namely, maintaining patient's oxygenation and ventilation while preserving hemodynamic status. In other words, ETT doesn't save lives, whereas providing adequate perfusion and gas exchange does. Optimal oxygenation and ventilation may be provided using ETTs, extraglottic devices (EGDs), FMV devices, and surgical methods. Which method is most appropriately employed will depend on patient characteristics, the clinical situation, and practitioner's skill.

Face-mask ventilation, particularly in the prehospital setting, has been shown to be no less effective than endotracheal intubation (ETI) or EGD use.[1–4] In a large prospective population-based study of out-of-hospital cardiac arrest (OHCA) patients, survivors who received FMV had more favorable neurologic outcomes compared to those who had their airway managed by ETI or EGD.[5] With increasing controversy regarding the value of prehospital ETI, other means of maintaining oxygenation and ventilation including FMV are being reaffirmed as an airway management priority.[6–12]

For OHCA, ventilation has been deemphasized in the early phase of adult nonasphyxia-related resuscitation where oxygen delivery is more dependent on blood flow than on arterial oxygen content. There is consensus that advanced airway management should not be considered a priority over CPR/defibrillation and has the potential of causing harm by interrupting CPR, from complications of airway management, impairing cerebral perfusion, and perhaps inadvertent hyperventilation.[11] The use of EGDs in the context of cardiac arrest may theoretically provide benefit as they do not require an interruption in chest compressions for placement and use.

Three large, randomized control trials were published in 2018 comparing the use of noninvasive oxygenation techniques (EGD or FMV) as compared to ETI in patients sustaining nontraumatic OHCA.[13–15]

Benger and colleagues compared the use of an iGel to ETI in 9300 OHCA patients assessing improved neurologic outcome at 30 days (defined as a modified Rankin 0-3).[13] They showed that although the requirement of an advanced airway intervention was associated with an overall worse outcome, there was essentially no difference in those patients oxygenated with an iGel versus ETI. Wang and colleagues compared the use of a laryngeal tube (LT) to ETI in OHCA patients assessing for 72-hour survival, survival to hospital discharge, and assessment of neurologic outcomes using a modified Rankin score of 0 to 3. On posthoc analysis, there was no difference between an LT and an ETI for any of the examined outcomes.[15] Jabre and colleagues conducted a noninferiority trial comparing FMV to ETI in OHCA assessing for favorable neurologic outcome at 28 days. Statistically, this was an inconclusive study with FMV failing to show noninferiority or inferiority to ETI.[14]

Panchal et al. in the AHA 2020 Guidelines for cardiac arrest care have suggested that in the absence of clear evidence of superiority for OHCA patients, practitioners may use either FMV or an advanced airway (EGD or ETT) depending on the situation and practitioner skill set. When an advanced airway is performed, an EGD may be preferable in systems where intubation skills are difficult to maintain. Regardless of approach, continuous $EtCO_2$ waveform capnography should ideally always be used.[16]

Overall, recent literature would suggest that the use of an EGD or FMV may be a reasonable option as compared to ETI in OHCA, particularly in systems where exposure to ETI may be low, skill retention may be difficult, or objective measures of successful intubation (waveform $EtCO_2$ capnography) may not be available.

For non-OHCA patients, advanced airway management has not consistently shown to be of benefit when compared to a basic approach that includes FMV.[3,4,17] Many believe that prehospital airway management outcomes are less related to the device and more to do with the decisions and skills with which these airway devices are employed.[10,11] Worsening hypoxemia and inadvertent hyperventilation occurring during and postadvanced airway management placement are thought to be major contributors to the observed poor outcomes in the prehospital setting.[18] The technical imperative of succeeding in the placement of an advanced airway device may be distracting clinicians away from the homeostatic goal of improving and maintaining oxygen and ventilation status. This goal may often be best achieved with FMV. Most of the existing data comes from North American ground-based ambulance services.

Face-mask ventilation can be a challenging skill to learn and perform effectively.[19–21] Human factors research has found that when comparing inexperienced to experienced practitioners with FMV, inexperienced practitioners are typically overdependent on electronic vital signs (oxygen saturation) noting that inexperienced practitioners typically overventilate/hyperventilate, and potentially harm patients. Experienced practitioners were less likely to respond this way and more likely to use clinical parameters such as chest rise to ensure FMV was performed effectively.[22] Despite the advent of numerous alternative devices, just as direct laryngoscopy (DL) remains the current gold standard for ETT placement, FMV still remains the primary method of providing initial Basic Life Support (BLS) oxygenation and ventilation in most resuscitation settings.[23] Although this may change, there currently is no compelling evidence of superiority of advanced airway techniques over FMV.[24–30] Compared to FMV used by relatively inexperienced health care practitioners, LMAs have been reported to be rapidly placed, "easy to use," and effective ventilation devices.[31] Similar results have been shown with the LT.[27] Other reports of EGD "field use" have, however, demonstrated lower than expected success rates and worse outcomes when compared to FMV, despite self-reported ease of use.[25,30,32,33] In contrast, there is some evidence that for the neonatal population, EGD use is more effective than FMV during resuscitation efforts.[34]

Success and complications of any airway device are more often related to training and experience than the device itself. Despite its effectiveness in skilled hands, FMV is facing a growing competition from EGDs that even in unskilled hands, are relatively easy to teach, learn, and ultimately deliver as a primary method for oxygenation and ventilation.

What Are the Key Components of a Facemask System?

Also referred to as manual resuscitators, these devices usually employ a bag and an integrated one-way valve connected to an ETT, an EGD, or a mask to manually provide PPV. Despite there being various types of FMV systems, for the most part, they share common features (Figure 8.1).[35]

- Universal connector: with a 22-mm outside diameter (OD), which fits standard facemasks, and a 15-mm internal diameter (ID) that connects to standard ETTs, EGDs, and cricothyrotomy or tracheotomy cannulae.

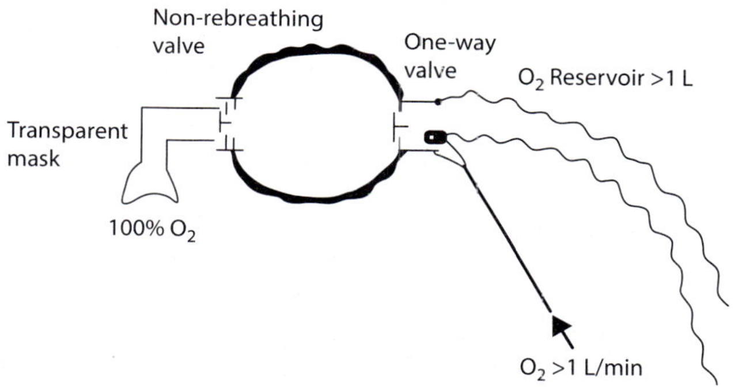

FIGURE 8.1. Facemask schematic (Reproduced with permission from Safer P. *Cardiopulmonary Cerebral Resuscitation*. Philadelphia, PA: WB Saunders; 1988.)

- Non-rebreathing patient valve: to prevent rebreathing while allowing exhalation.
- Self-inflating bag: supplied in adult (1600 mL); child (500 mL); and infant (240 mL) sizes that when manually compressed, deliver a corresponding tidal volume; or an oxygen reservoir bag, which is inflated by receiving high oxygen flow through an adjacent connector.
- Oxygen inlet valve: providing unidirectional flow from the oxygen reservoir to the self-inflating bag.
- Air intake valve (at reservoir end): a safety valve intended to allow entrainment of room air if the supplied oxygen source is disconnected.
- Safety outlet valve (at reservoir end): a flow-limiting valve.
- Other features of FMV systems may include Positive Pressure Relief or "Pop-off" valves located on the patient end of the system with the intent of limiting airway pressures to avoid barotrauma when the manual resuscitator is connected to an ETT.
- An expiratory port at the patient connector that allows attachment of a PEEP valve.
- Flow-limiting valve located at the patient end of the self-inflating bag, designed to limit inspiratory flow, decreasing the risk of both hyperventilation and excessive airway pressures (Smart Bag→).
- Manometer to measure inspiratory pressure generated by squeezing the bulb.

The facemasks used in conjunction with the manual resuscitator vary in material, size, seal type, and transparency. Traditionally, black/opaque rubber masks with an anatomically contoured seal were used in the operating room setting connected to an anesthetic circuit. These have been replaced to a large extent in most environments by transparent silicone, or plastic latex-free non-disposable and single-use masks that provide the added benefit of being able to visualize the mouth/nose-mask interface and therefore react to the presence of vomitus and other secretions. Rather than anatomically conforming to the patient's face, the seals in these disposable masks are either made of foam or an air-filled "cushion" that molds to the underlying facial anatomy.

While the unidirectional valves are similar among available FMV devices, it is important to appreciate whether the device has a dedicated expiratory valve. This valve provides a unidirectional flow for expired gases and will not allow room air entrainment for the spontaneously breathing patient. If there is an open expiratory port, it usually means there is no dedicated intrinsic expiratory valve and in the spontaneously breathing patient they may entrain room air.[36] This is easily dealt with by adding a PEEP valve.

BASIC PRINCIPLES

How Do You Accurately Anticipate Difficult Face-Mask Ventilation?

Perhaps the simple answer is you can never ensure 100% accuracy when you are trying to predict anything.[37] The safest approach is perhaps to "always anticipate the unexpected." In the anticipated difficult airway, proceeding depends on context. In an elective operating room setting, the predicted difficulty will often mean a very different course (including canceling the case) than in an emergency in which a choice of not proceeding is usually not an option. In trying to anticipate difficulty, the core two traditional questions that all practitioners should ask themselves prior to proceeding are:

- Will I be able to maintain oxygenation and ventilation by FMV if intubation attempts fail? If not, will I be able to oxygenate and ventilate rapidly using a rescue device or technique, such as an EGD or surgical airway?

Early literature on predicting the difficult airway focused on laryngoscopy and intubation.[38–40] Recognizing that maintenance of oxygenation and ventilation is the priority in airway management and that this is often best achieved rapidly and early by FMV, the identification of predictors of difficult FMV has also been a focus of research.[41–46] Most airway management decision algorithms require a "formal" patient assessment focused on identifying predictors of difficulty. This assessment is a major contributor in deciding whether neuromuscular blockade can safely be used to facilitate intubation. While it is important to assess all aspects of the difficult airway, FMV has been considered the most important as this intervention is usually the primary "go to" technique when tracheal intubation attempts fail. More recently, however, some guidelines suggest either FMV or an EGD following failed tracheal intubation or moving to an EGD instead of FMV at this stage.[47,48] At this point, oxygen desaturation has often already begun and clinical deterioration often follows rapidly. Despite there being numerous alternative rescue options available to the practitioner, FMV is universally available, familiar to most and very effective.

Earlier data estimated that "cannot intubate/cannot oxygenate" clinical situations occurred at a rate between 0.01 and 2 in 10,000 general anesthetic cases.[49] More recent data have reported that the incidence of difficult face-mask ventilation (DMV) in the operating room setting has varied from a low of 0.9% to a high of 7.8%.[42–50] This reported variation likely relates to differences in case definition, outcome criteria, and sample size. A large multicenter study of over 176,000 patients reported an incidence of DMV of 2.5% with an incidence of DMV with concurrent difficult intubation of 0.4%.[41] In a previous study of over 50,000 patients, "impossible" FMV defined as an inability to establish FMV using two-hand technique and "multiple airway adjuvants," occurred in 0.15% of the study population.[42]

Langeron et al. prospectively evaluated 1502 patients requiring routine general anesthesia to determine both the incidence and factors associated with DMV.[45] The reported incidence of DMV in this population was 5%. Five independent factors associated with DMV were identified: presence of a beard; age older than 55; body mass index (BMI) >26 kg.m^{-2}; lack of teeth; and a history of snoring. The presence of two of these factors in a patient was 72% sensitive and 73% specific for DMV.[45]

Despite established literature on predictors of difficult FMV, real-world application may be more difficult. Norskov et al. reviewed 94,000 OR patients in a retrospective database using a difficult FMV identification tool using 11 recognized predictors of difficulty as compared to usual practice. They found no difference in the incidence of unpredicted difficult FMV; however, the authors note that >85% of all difficult FMV were not predicted—either with the intervention tool or usual practice.[52]

Other studies involving large patient populations have validated the above findings and identified additional risk factors, including male gender, a history of neck radiation, high Mallampati grade (Grade III or IV), increased BMI >30 kg.m^{-2}, and limited jaw protrusion (Table 8.1).[41–44] In Kheterpal's study of patients with difficulty for both FMV and DL, Mallampati grade (III or IV), neck radiation or mass, male gender, limited thyromental distance, presence of teeth, and BMI >30 kg.m^{-2} were among the more significant risk factors (odds ratio >2).[41]

In the study by Kheterpal et al., the presence of three or more predictors (neck radiation, male, OSA, Mallampati III or IV, beard) significantly increased the risk of impossible mask ventilation (IMV) with an odds ratio of 8.9 compared to patients without these risk factors. Another important finding from this study is that of the IMV group, 25% were also difficult to intubate.[42] In a more recent follow-up study examining combined difficult FMV and difficult laryngoscopy, the odds of encountering difficulty increased significantly with the number of risks identified. However, these retrospective data are difficult to apply prospectively. While many airway practitioners may accept inadequacies in terms of positive predictive value, it would be unwise to apply these findings as a negative predictive tool.

Reports differentiating DMV from IMV recognize the fact that clinically FMV challenges are part of a continuum from easy to impossible.[50] A numeric representation of this DMV continuum has been proposed; however, it has not been consistently used or accepted to date in the literature.[53] The difference between DMV and IMV is simply that DMV is usually correctable (i.e., two-hand and two-person technique), whereas impossible mask ventilation represents a failure and the need to abandon FMV in favor of another intervention (DL, or video-laryngoscopy [VL] if not attempted, EGD or a surgical airway). Another important observation that has caused some degree of controversy is the value of "checking" for FMV difficulty prior to administering a neuromuscular blocking agent. Current evidence seems to support the use of muscle relaxants to facilitate both FMV and laryngoscopy.[51,54–56]

It is important to appreciate the fact that these studies did not examine the incidence of DMV in patients requiring emergency airway management. Although studies examining the incidence of difficult FMV outside of the OR are limited, Lee et al. noted an incidence of difficult FMV in 110 ED patients of 45.9%.[57] Levitan et al. examined the ability to assess for predictors of the difficult airway in ED patients requiring intubation and found that only 32% of this population would have been able to be assessed adequately for difficulty because of limitations such as an inability to follow commands or being immobilized for cervical spine (C-spine) precautions.[58]

TABLE 8.1. Studies Reporting Independent Predictors of Difficult FMV

Investigators	Design	Population	DMV Incidence	Risk Factors	Comments
Langeron et al. 2000	Prospective observational	1502, adult, routine GA[a] patients	5%	Age >55, BMI >26 kg.m^{-2}, beard, edentulous, snoring	First study evaluating independent risk factors
Yildiz et al., 2004	Prospective observational	576, adult, routine GA	7.8%, 15.5% of difficult intubations	Male, Mallampati IV, increasing age, snoring, increasing weight	Small sample size
Kheterpal et al., 2006	Prospective observational	22,660, adult, GA	1.4%	BMI >30 kg.m^{-2}, beard, Mallampati III IV, age >57, ↓ JP[c], snoring	Diverse clinician group
Kheterpal et al., 2009	Prospective observational	53,041, adult, GA	2.2%, 0.15%		
IMV[b]	IMV: neck radiation, male, OSA[d], Mallampati III IV, beard	Odds ratio 8.9 versus no risk factors			
Kheterpal et al., 2013	Prospective observational	176,679, adult, GA	2.5%, 0.4% both DMV & DDL	Combined DMV/DDL: Mallampati III IV, neck pathology/rads, male, limited thyromental distance, presence of teeth BMI >30 kg.m^{-2}	Odds ratio (OR) increase with # Risk factors (RF) 4 RF:OR 2.56 5 RF:OR 4.18 6 RF:OR 9.23 7-11 RF:OR 18.4

[a]General anesthesia.
[b]Impossible FMV.
[c]Jaw protrusion.
[d]Obstructive sleep apnea.

TABLE 8.2. Difficult FMV (DMV) Pathophysiology and Response

DMV Predictor	Pathophysiology	Response
Obesity	Rapid desaturation, ↓ compliance, ↑ upper airway soft tissues	Positioning: sitting denitrogenation, ramp
Snoring (airway sounds)	Snoring: ↑ upper airway collapse Sounds: stridor, wheezing ↑ resistance	OPA, 2-hand FMV, ↑ expiratory time
Age	↓ tissue elasticity, ↓ jaw & neck mobility, ↑ edentulous rate	Leave dentures in place
Beard	Mask seal	Apply ointment
Edentulous	Mask size, fit	Leave dentures in, OPA,
Neck radiation	Noncompliant, distorted tissues	OPA, 2-hand FMV, early SGA
Mallampati III or IV	Excess soft tissues, upper airway collapse	OPA, 2-hand FMV
Male	? associated comorbidities	
Diminished jaw protrusion	↓ ability to manage tongue, upper airway collapse	OPA, 2-hand FMV, early SGA
Difficult intubation	As per above, secondary injury from difficult laryngoscopy	

The incidence of DMV is not known in this population. However, emergency cricothyrotomy outside of the OR (as a marker for cannot intubate, cannot oxygenate) rates have fallen to between 0.1% and 0.5%, and may underrepresent the incidence DMV and are still much higher than that reported in the controlled operating room setting.[59–62] Table 8.2 summarizes the likely pathophysiology behind the various predictors of DMV.

What Anatomic Factors Need to Be Considered in Providing Safe and Effective FMV?

The primary goal of FMV is to facilitate oxygenation and ventilation by providing an unimpeded transfer of gas (oxygen/carbon dioxide) to and from the lungs. In the unconscious or anesthetized patient with normal anatomy, it has been traditionally thought that obstruction to the easy to-and-fro movement of gas with FMV was primarily related to the effect of a "relaxed" tongue falling back against the posterior pharyngeal wall. Data gathered during fluoroscopy in studies of obstructive sleep apnea (OSA) patients has improved our understanding of the pathophysiology of upper airway dynamics in the sleeping patient. In addition to obstruction caused by the tongue, there is also a loss of velopharyngeal and hypopharyngeal muscle tone.[63,64] This results in soft tissue collapse, leading to the posterior displacement of both the soft palate and epiglottis to oppose the posterior pharyngeal wall and contribute to obstruction (velopharyngeal and hypopharyngeal collapse).[63] The hypopharyngeal site of obstruction is clinically supported by the observation that placement of an OPA without performing an adequate jaw thrust may not alleviate obstruction caused by "normal" upper airway soft tissues.

When a patient is placed in the "sniffing" position, there is flexion in the cervico-thoracic region with extension occipito-cervical region. This position has been traditionally thought to facilitate "alignment" of the axes necessary to visualize the glottic inlet during DL. Although there has been some question as to whether this position provides any advantage over simple head extension, data do support the combination of neck flexion with head elevation in enabling glottic exposure during laryngoscopy.[65,66] It is less clear, however, if this position improves upper airway patency for FMV. There is some evidence that the retropalatal and retroglossal region is enlarged by placing anesthetized nonobese patients with OSA in the sniffing position and FMV may be improved.[67,68] Collectively, these pharyngeal dilator muscles lose their tone with anesthesia, thereby increasing the pharyngeal closing pressure. Pharyngeal patency is improved most significantly by maintaining a sitting position coupled with mandibular advancement, and less so by head and neck positioning.[69] In addition, it is well known that obese patients' oxygen desaturate quickly, a clinical factor, which can be delayed by denitrogenating in the sitting (as opposed to supine) position.[70] At this point, it is reasonable to state that head and neck repositioning from neutral to a position that involves a degree of neck flexion with head elevation may improve FMV and is appropriate in anticipation of performing DL, should it become necessary.

While head and neck positioning may be considered of vital importance for DL, the key anatomic manipulation that facilitates FMV is performing a jaw thrust.[71] The genioglossus muscle is attached to the mandible and the hyoepiglottic ligament attaches the tongue to the epiglottis. Therefore, translating the mandible anteriorly pulls the tongue, and in turn, the epiglottis anteriorly, and opens the airway. This maneuver originally described over a century ago (Esmarch-Heiberg's maneuver) has been demonstrated to be superior to "chin lift" and "head tilt" when performed alone, during observations made of anesthetized patients undergoing (preprocedure) head and neck fluoroscopy.[72,73] Recognizing that obstruction in the unconscious patient is related to more than the tongue falling posteriorly, the "triple airway" maneuver (open mouth, head tilt, jaw thrust) was suggested to be the best approach.[74,75] More recent evidence supports the jaw thrust alone as being equally effective to the triple airway maneuver in relieving obstruction.[73] Although numerous guidelines recommend a sniffing position for BMV,[48,76] references for this recommendation all lead back to a small study of 12 obese elective OR patients.[67] In addition to the sniffing position, Itagaki and colleagues demonstrated increased expiratory tidal volumes in a small series of anesthetized patients when FMV was provided in a sniffing position plus a 45-degree head turn to either side, as opposed to maintaining the head in the midline position.[77]

What Is the Role of FMV in Difficult Airway Algorithms?

Numerous algorithms have been published to guide practitioners in the management of the difficult airway[48,76,78,79] (see Chapter 2). Most of these guidelines or recommendations are generated using available evidence and expert opinion from specialized "working groups" and/or anesthesiology societies. Historically, algorithms have had limitations for being too complicated or impractical for application in emergency situations outside of the operating room, where it is not possible to "cancel" the case or "awaken" the patient.

A difficult airway may be any or all of difficult FMV, difficult laryngoscopy, difficult intubation, difficult EGD use, or difficult surgical airway placement. Most algorithms or approaches separate the *anticipated* from the *unanticipated* (or encountered) difficult airway. In the former scenario, predicted difficulty leads to a defined, usually more controlled path, whereas in the latter, whether predicted or not, "real-time" difficulty *is* being experienced and demands an immediate and specific course of action, depending on the type of difficulty encountered.

In approaching the difficult airway, the ability to successfully perform FMV is a critical management junction in most, if not all, algorithms. The most prominent place for FMV as part of any difficult airway algorithm is between failed intubation attempts. However, it is important to appreciate the role of FMV even before a first attempt at laryngoscopy and intubation. Assuming the patient can generate sufficient tidal volumes with an adequate respiratory rate, the bag portion of the FMV device does not have to be squeezed to deliver close to 100% oxygen. It is not uncommon (and in some situations, is potentially hazardous) that when switching from a nonrebreathing mask (or another mask type) to FMV, positive inspiratory pressure is often instinctively applied. If assisted FMV is applied without synchrony, gastric insufflation is much more likely to occur.

In the preintubation phase of airway management, the use of an FMV device to denitrogenate should be encouraged. This approach offers several advantages:

1. Passive delivery of a high concentration of oxygen (approaching 100%)
2. Opportunity to select a proper size of the mask
3. Provides "hands-on feel" for predicting DMV
4. Provides opportunity to improve gas exchange with assisted FMV

Various methods of denitrogenation have been suggested in an attempt to minimize desaturation during laryngoscopy and intubation. This is relatively easy to accomplish in healthy adults with normal pulmonary mechanics and oxygen consumption rates. It should be recognized that flow from the oxygen source will decay by as much as 50% through most BVM devices. While this is not an issue at normal minute ventilations, it can result in dilution of FiO_2 by room air entrainment, leaks around the mask, and an open expiratory port in BVMs without a dedicated expiratory valve.[36,80] In the physiologically normal patient (normal lungs, respiratory rate, and tidal volumes), the key to denitrogenation is having a closed delivery system (i.e., a bag-mask unit with an expiratory valve) attached to high-flow oxygen for a minimum of 3 minutes.[81,82]

In patients with shunt physiology and elevated minute ventilation, effective denitrogenation can be improved through the addition of a PEEP valve in the spontaneously breathing patient.[83] With the addition of a second high-flow oxygen source applied through nasal prongs (HFNO) under a well-fitted mask, the BVM/PEEP and HFNO combination will provide CPAP, and through alveolar recruitment, may provide for improved denitrogenation.[83] While the addition of manual-assisted ventilation synchronized with the patient's inspiration (PPV) may provide only marginal denitrogenation benefit, the addition of a PEEP valve to this sequence in an attempt to replicate ventilator-delivered BiPAP may be of value for denitrogenation in certain patient populations.[84] The use of continuous $EtCO_2$ waveform with FMV may facilitate practitioner-patient synchrony and ideally should be used whenever FMV is provided.[85]

Although ventilation of the apneic patient as part of a rapid sequence induction (RSI) has been met with controversy, this teaching, was based more on theory than science. In fact, Sellick's original paper stated that manual PPV in combination with cricoid pressure could be done without gastric distention risk.[86] Data have since supported active denitrogenation using a manual resuscitator with or without the application of cricoid pressure as long as "good" technique is used in avoiding high airway pressures.[87–89] FMV is in fact clinically indicated during RSI in certain patients (obese, hypoxemic, pediatric) who may have low baseline oxygen saturation, high oxygen consumption rates, and/or low functional residual capacity.[84,90,91] Finally, capnographic or clinical verification of adequate FMV soon after the drugs are given is reassuring, particularly in situations where difficult intubation may be encountered, and represents a common practice.[90]

Concerns about increased aspiration risk in patients with FMV during RSI are likely unfounded provided that practitioners are conscious of avoiding over-zealous inspiratory pressures. Casey et al. demonstrated that ventilating critically ill patients after induction with an FMV did not lead to any increased incidence of aspiration/aspiration pneumonia.[92]

TECHNIQUE

What Defines Optimal FMV Technique and How Do You Assess the Adequacy of Ventilation? (Video 12)

There are three important components to proper FMV technique: mask seal; airway opening; and ventilation.

Mask Seal: An appropriately sized facemask is attached to the bag-mask device and applied to the patient's face. The lower

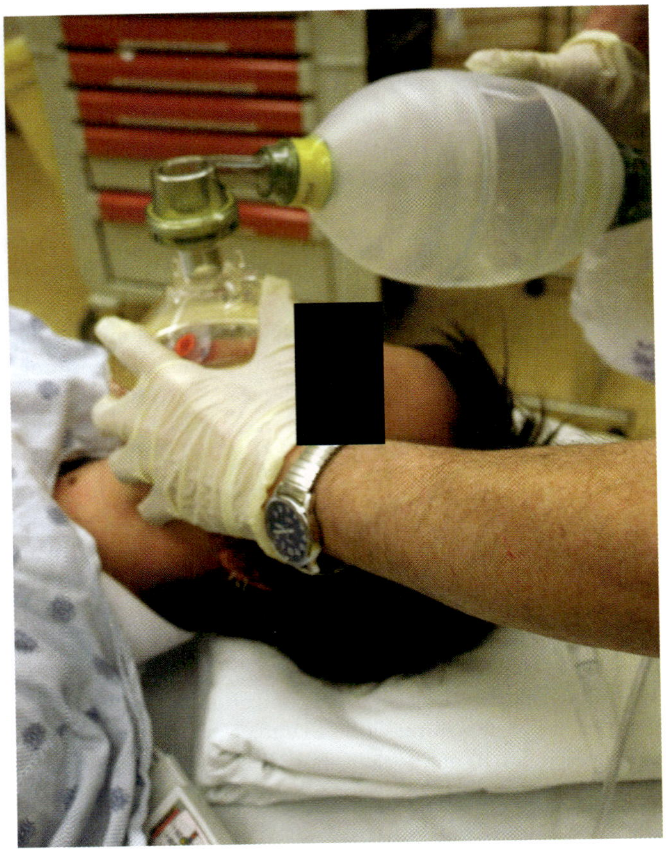

FIGURE 8.2. Proper face-mask ventilation technique: A good mask seal involves applying sufficient pressure on the facemask by the thumb and index finger of the practitioner's hand. The ring and long fingers of the nondominant hand grasp the bony ridge of the patient's mandible, and, if practical, the fifth finger hooks under the angle of the mandible to provide a jaw thrust.

border of the mask's cuff is first applied to the groove between the lower lip and the chin, then the mask can be placed down across the nasal bridge. The thumb and index finger of the airway practitioner's hand applies sufficient pressure on the facemask to achieve a good seal (Figure 8.2). Note, however, that sealing pressure must be achieved *without* excessive downward pressure on the patient's mandible, as this may aggravate functional obstruction. Rather, the mandible is *lifted* to meet the mask. Small adjustments to the position of the mask on the patient's face (e.g., with small movements to left or right) are made as needed to achieve a seal.

Airway Opening: When employing a one-person technique, the ring and long fingers of the nondominant hand grasp the bony ridge of the patient's mandible, and, if practical, the fifth finger hooks under the angle of the mandible to provide a jaw thrust (Figure 8.2). In the event, the airway practitioner has a small hand, the long finger is hooked under the mentum to provide a jaw pull. These three digits not only provide counter-pressure to the digits applying the mask to the face, but also apply an *upward lift* to the mandible to help perform an airway-opening jaw thrust. Note that these three fingers should *not* be placed directly under the patient's chin unless lifting it forward, as midline pressure under the chin can contribute to airway obstruction. This latter directive is particularly important in small children and infants. Concomitantly, the entire hand also attempts to keep the head extended (if no C-spine precautions).

Ventilation: The practitioner's dominant hand is free to gently squeeze the bag. Volumes should be delivered with attention to the inflating pressure and the patient's status: if apneic, the patient should be carefully ventilated (attached to high-flow oxygen) at a rate of 10 to 12 breaths per minute, at a tidal volume of 6 $mL.kg^{-1}$, or 500 to 600 mL in the average adult.[1] Smaller tidal volumes (e.g., 3-400 mL in the adult) at increased rates (15-18 breaths per minute) may lead to less gastric insufflation. Although adult (1.6 L) manual resuscitators may deliver varied volumes, excessive and rapid compression of the bag must be avoided. The goal, as stated previously, is to produce *visible* chest rise. In addition to the use of chest rise, we would encourage all practitioners to use continuous end-tidal CO_2 waveform capnography to monitor breath to breath efficacy of administered ventilation. In the patient still demonstrating respiratory effort, *assisted* FMV should be performed, synchronizing the positive pressure breath with the patient's inspiratory effort. If the patient is tachypneic, it will be appropriate to simply deliver assisted ventilation with every third or fourth breath. The use of a disposable inspiratory pressure manometer may facilitate avoiding overventilation and help practitioners reduce the risk of gastric insufflation and aspiration.

Defining Difficult FMV?

In a commentary by Lim and Nielsen,[93] the authors acknowledge that while "difficult mask ventilation may be easy to recognize, its definition remains subjective and overly complex. The American Society of Anesthesiologists (ASA) definition requires 114 words and includes lists of many clinical signs and potential causes. As a response they propose a grading system for difficult FMV using end-tidal capnography as an objective endpoint:

Grade A—plateau present
Grade B—no plateau, $EtCO_2$ >10 mmHg
Grade C—no plateau, $EtCO_2$ <10 mmHg
Grade D—no $EtCO_2$ trace

While this proposed grading system currently is without formal validation, we support the move towards more clear, objective measures of difficult FMV in an effort to enhance communication between practitioners and improve patient safety during airway management.

How to Respond to Difficult FMV Situations?

With optimal technique, significant difficulty with FMV is rarely encountered in the absence of airway pathology.[42,51] In the acute setting, FMV is often delegated to another health care practitioner while the primary practitioner prepares for definitive airway management. While this may be appropriate, it is important to accept that FMV is a difficult skill for those who perform it infrequently, and vigilance rather than inattention is recommended. Abandoning FMV in the uncommon scenario of failing FMV should only occur after the most experienced "set of hands" have failed.

Difficult mask ventilation is often defined as the inability to maintain an acceptable oxygen saturation despite using "good technique." However, it is the "dynamic" inability to maintain oxygen saturation that is important. Failure to maintain acceptable oxygen saturations or stall saturations that are falling demands a change in approach. Importantly, a latency in pulse oximetry display may lead to a delay in recognizing nonoptimized FMV technique resulting in unnecessary hypoxemic insult to the patient. Recognizing that a falling oxygen saturation during FMV indicates inadequate ventilation, the use of continuous $EtCO_2$ capnography during FMV allows practitioners to recognize difficulty and adjust technique before a critical decline in oxygenation occurs. Although one response to a DMV situation is to proceed to intubation, DMV may itself predict difficult laryngoscopy and/or intubation.[42,50,51] Good FMV skills and an approach to DMV are crucial skills in ensuring oxygenation of a patient prior to, or between laryngoscopy attempts.

In the setting of a failed airway in which one is not able to maintain acceptable oxygen saturations, immediate preparation for a cricothyrotomy is mandatory while one simultaneously attempts "better" FMV that may include the following:

A. Reposition the head by performing an exaggerated head tilt/chin lift (if not contraindicated);
B. Open cervical spine collars
C. Open the mouth to permit anterior translation of the mandible and tongue in concert with an aggressive jaw thrust;
D. Insert an appropriate size oropharyngeal airway (see Figure 8.3) and as many as two nasopharyngeal airways;
E. Perform two-person mask ventilation technique;
F. If cricoid pressure is being applied, ease up on, or release it;
G. Consider a mask change (size or type) if seal is an issue;
H. Rule out foreign body in the airway;
I. Consider a "rescue" ventilation device (e.g., an EGD, such as a laryngeal mask airway [LMA]);
J. Consider an early attempt at intubation;
K. Consider a primary surgical airway;

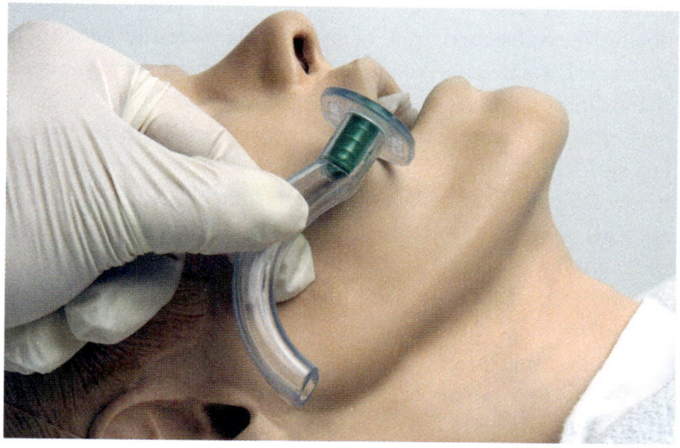

FIGURE 8.3. Insertion of an appropriate-size oropharyngeal airway is necessary to alleviate airway obstruction.

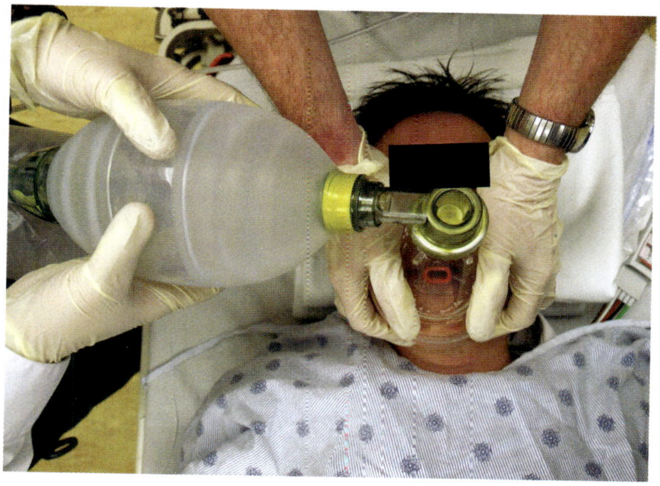

FIGURE 8.4. Two-hand and two-person face-mask ventilation.

Steps A, B, and C, as listed above, should occur almost simultaneously and very early in the DMV situation. DMV is often due simply to the failure to adequately open a functionally obstructed airway. Attempted ventilation against this obstruction results in a leak at the mask/face interface, often resulting in the practitioner's attempting to remedy the problem by pushing down harder on the mask to attain a seal, though this can aggravate an already obstructed airway. Rather, what must occur is a more pronounced jaw *lift or thrust*, with resultant airway opening occurring as anterior movement of the mandible elevates the tongue, epiglottis, and soft palate away from the posterior pharyngeal wall. This is best performed with the aid of a second person. Two-person FMV is easy to perform and is often much more effective than one-person FMV.[94,95] As shown in Figure 8.4, the two-person technique can be performed in a number of ways; however, the "thumbs forward thenar eminence" (T-E) grip appears to be more effective than the traditional C-E grip (place the thumb and first finger around the top of the mask, forming a "C," while using the third, fourth, and fifth fingers, forming an "E," to lift the angles of the jaw).[96–99]

Fei and colleagues compared these two techniques in a series of anesthetized, non-obese patients noting that the T-E technique resulted in higher measured tidal volumes and greater success in mask ventilation, noting that all patients who were difficult to ventilate with the C-E technique were successfully ventilated with the T-E approach.[100] The authors speculated that increased difficulty with the C-E technique was partly due to operator-introduced compression of tissue on the anterior neck and subsequent airway obstruction not seen with the T-E approach.[100]

Oropharyngeal airways (OPAs) help alleviate functional airway obstruction caused by relaxation of the tongue against the soft palate, and to a lesser extent, the posterior pharyngeal wall. They are most often used as an adjunct to FMV in an obtunded or unconscious patient. Made of plastic, the component parts are a curved hollow lumen (in the Guedel version) or side gutters (the Berman version) (Figure 8.5), both with a proximal flange, which abuts the patient's lips, and a proximal bite block, which may also be used as a color-coded size indicator.

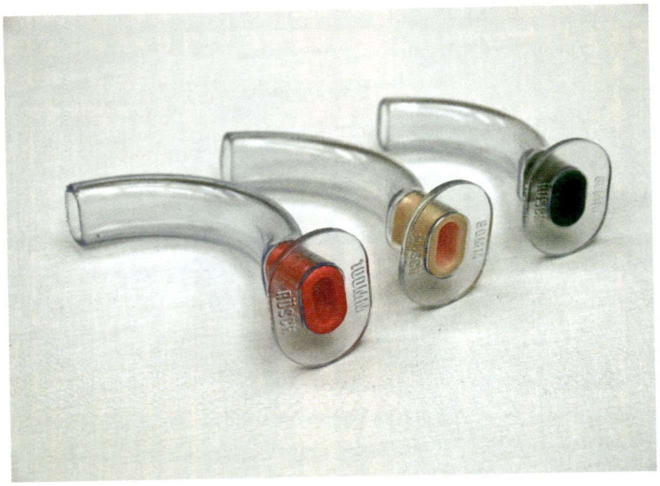

FIGURE 8.5. Different sizes of Guedel oropharyngeal airways.

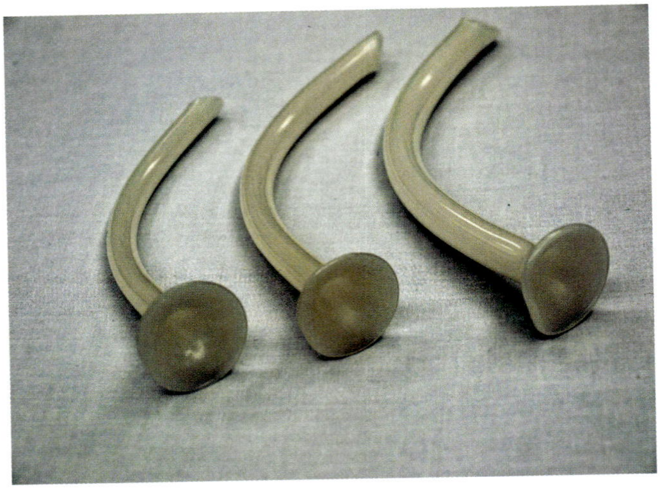

FIGURE 8.6. Different sizes of nasopharyngeal airways.

OPAs are sized by length in centimeters, and are available in sizes for all ages. Choosing the appropriate size is important, as an OPA that is too long may precipitate laryngospasm or create obstruction; and if too small, it may be ineffective. Although never formally validated, many airway practitioners approximate the correct OPA length by placing it alongside the patient's cheek:[71] from the corner of the mouth, the tip of the OPA should reach the angle of the mandible or the tragus of the ear (Figure 8.3). A typical adult female will take an 8-cm OPA, and an adult male, 9 or 10 cm.

The OPA should be inserted inverted (i.e., with its concave surface directed cephalad) and advanced until the distal tip will proceed no further in this inverted position. At that point, the OPA is rotated 180 degrees, so that the concavity faces caudad. Advancement continues around the curve of the tongue until fully inserted. Inverted insertion helps avoid aggravating obstruction due to posterior tongue displacement into the hypopharynx during OPA placement. Alternatively, it can be inserted noninverted with a tongue depressor to manage the tongue; this is the preferred technique in infants and younger children to help avoid trauma to delicate tissues and displace the relatively large tongue.

OPAs are not well tolerated in the awake or semiconscious patients with intact airway reflexes, where insertion may stimulate gagging, laryngospasm, or vomiting and aspiration. In addition, care must be taken to rule out a foreign body in the oropharynx prior to OPA insertion.

A nasopharyngeal airway (NPA) may be a useful option where trismus precludes OPA insertion (e.g., hypothermia, severe head injury), and may be better tolerated than an OPA in the awake or semiconscious patient with intact airway reflexes. While effective at alleviating functional airway obstruction, disadvantages of the NPA include transient patient discomfort during insertion and the potential to incite epistaxis. While application of a vasoconstrictor (e.g., xylometazoline, oxymetazoline) can minimize the risk of epistaxis, this may not be practical when an NPA is urgently needed. NPAs, also known as "nasal trumpets," are made from soft material (e.g., latex or silicon), have a hollow interior, beveled leading edge, and a proximal flange to abut the patient's nostril (Figure 8.6).

Adult NPAs are generally sized by their internal diameter (ID) in mm. Typical adult sizes for small, medium, and large NPAs are 6-, 7-, and 8-mm ID, respectively. One commonly used (but nonvalidated) sizing method is to use an NPA of a length corresponding to the distance from the nose tip to the tragus of the ear. Sizing based on patient height makes more anatomic sense, resulting in a recommendation for a 6-mm ID NPA for an average adult female and 7 mm for an average male.

The NPA is lubricated and advanced into the patient's nostril, perpendicular to the face, resulting in passage along the floor of the major nasal airway. Authorities vary in their recommendation as to whether the bevel of the NPA should face toward or away from the nasal septum. A slight twisting motion can be used during insertion. If significant resistance is encountered, insertion should be attempted through the other nostril. Insertion continues until the flange of the NPA abuts the nasal ala.

NPA use is *relatively* contraindicated in known bleeding diathesis, including heparinized, anticoagulated, or recently thrombolyzed patients, and in suspected cribriform plate fractures. In the head-injured patient, common sense dictates balancing the substantial risk of hypoxemia with the benefits of producing a patent NPA in the event an oral airway is ineffective or impossible.

Cricoid pressure can cause difficulty with both FMV and laryngoscopy, as previously discussed and mentioned again below. Excessive cricoid pressure (as may be applied during an RSI) may distort the airway and result in partial or complete airway obstruction. If significant difficulty with FMV is encountered during application of cricoid pressure, the assistant should momentarily ease (initially by 50%) or totally release the applied pressure.

It may become apparent once FMV is underway that the chosen mask size is incorrect requiring a size change. This is often the case if initial sizing occurred with a patient's dentures in place.

The decision to move to a rescue EGD, such as an LMA or laryngeal tube (King LT), will depend on the patient's clinical status and whether DL has yet been attempted. If there has been no initial attempt at DL, it may be appropriate to proceed to an intubation attempt. If, on the other hand, DMV is encountered in the setting of an already failed attempt at intubation, placement of a rescue ventilation device, such as an LMA, should be considered. Direct laryngoscopy is also the method of choice to rule out obstructing lesions, including foreign bodies and lingual tonsillar hypertrophy.

Is Cricoid Pressure Appropriate to Use with FMV?

Aspiration incidence rises with the number of attempts at intubation to a high of 22% in the emergency setting.[101] Mortality from aspiration has fallen but remains relatively high. Does the application of cricoid pressure prevent regurgitation, and, more importantly, does it reduce morbidity and mortality?

Since Sellick's description in 1961, cricoid pressure has been recommended as a safe and necessary airway maneuver meant to reduce the risk of aspiration during airway management.[86] However, based on accumulating evidence, this "standard" has been questioned.[89,102–105] Additionally, there is reasonable evidence for potential negative effects of cricoid pressure administered during FMV, which include reduced tidal volumes, increased peak inspiratory pressure, and difficult ventilation. Given that there is little evidence to support the widespread use of cricoid pressure to prevent aspiration and that there is evidence of potential harm in certain situations, many have suggested that the procedure should either be omitted or at least disengaged if a difficult airway is encountered.[88,102,103,106]

Anatomically, as studied by imaging, the value of cricoid pressure was also being questioned based on observations that the cricoid cartilage moves laterally with compression and causes incomplete luminal esophageal opposition.[107–109] More recent literature, however, has documented that with appropriate force applied, cricoid pressure occludes the esophageal entrance regardless of whether it is in midline or lateral position.[109]

A recent systematic review and meta-analysis by White et al. examining the efficacy of cricoid pressure in reducing pulmonary aspiration during RSI led the authors to conclude that cricoid pressure failed to demonstrate protection, while simultaneously increasing time to intubation and impeding laryngeal view on DL.[110] The clinical implication of these secondary effects is unclear.

The question of whether cricoid pressure reduces morbidity and mortality by preventing aspiration has not, and may not be answered. Aspiration has been documented to occur in cases where cricoid pressure has been applied, though it has been argued that this could have been from faulty technique.[105] The clinical risk/benefit debate over the use of cricoid pressure will likely continue. At this point, it can be said that when performed correctly, by occluding the hypopharynx and by preventing gastric inflation during FMV, cricoid pressure may reduce the risk associated with aspiration during airway management. In addition, during FMV, care should be taken to employ good technique by opening the airway, paying attention to inspiratory time, inflation pressure, and delivering appropriate tidal volumes to avoid gastric inflation using a disposable manometer attached to the FMV. If cricoid pressure is being applied, it should be done by an experienced assistant, and if FMV becomes difficult, cricoid pressure should be released to assess whether it may be impeding ventilation.

COMPLICATIONS

How to Maximize Gas Exchange While Minimizing the Risk of Gastric Inflation and Regurgitation During FMV?

With an unprotected airway, the risks of gastric inflation and subsequent aspiration are a real risk during FMV. In autopsies of patients having failed resuscitation, the incidence of aspiration has been reported to be 29%.[111] Delivering an intended tidal volume and avoiding gastric inflation during FMV depends on various factors, such as lung compliance, airway resistance, and lower esophageal sphincter pressure (LESP).[112,113] In healthy adults, the LESP is 20 to 25 cm H_2O.[87,113]

The risk of gastric inflation is finely balanced with the need to generate sufficient upper airway pressures to achieve ventilation, while maintaining airway pressures low enough to avoid gastric insufflation. Traditionally, it has been taught that peak airway pressures below 20 cm H_2O would minimize the risk of gastric insufflation. However, Bouvet et al. have shown using ultrasound examination of the stomach of nonobese elective surgical patients that airway pressures of 15 cm H_2O caused gastric inflation in 35% of patients. A 15 cm H_2O peak airway pressure was shown to generate sufficient ventilation.[114] This information led the authors to conclude that airway practitioners performing FMV ought to employ smaller tidal volumes at higher rates to minimize inflation pressures and the risk of gastric insufflation.

Recognizing that the risk of aspiration and its related potential morbidity is related to high airway pressure during FMV, every attempt should be made to provide effective ventilation at minimum peak airway pressures. Conditions that reduce compliance or increase resistance require higher peak pressures, which would increase the risk of gastric insufflation, and aspiration. Meticulous attention to technique, such as the use of oral or nasal airways, maximum airway opening maneuvers, and reduced tidal volumes, may attenuate this risk. The breathing patient who is receiving "assisted" manual PPV using an FMV device is at particularly high risk. In this situation, the airway practitioner must pay close attention to the timing and delivery of a positive pressure breath at the end of the patient's expiratory phase to prevent higher airway pressures more likely to result in gastric inflation. A vicious cycle of "gastric insufflation," reduced compliance requiring higher airway pressures that diverts even more gas to the stomach ensues.[113] In extreme circumstances, this can lead to decreased cardiac output from increased intrathoracic pressure and a "can't ventilate" scenario.

Previous studies in the prehospital setting have documented that stress and an excited state may contribute to "overzealous" ventilation with large tidal volumes and rapid respiratory rates.[11,18,115] The practitioners in these studies perceived feedback of inadequate oxygenation and/or ventilation (which is often from inadequate relief of upper airway soft tissue obstruction), generating a response of pushing "harder" on the facemask while at the same time generating more forceful and frequent ventilations. This response led to further gastric insufflation, breath stacking, and the cycle described above. The result is worsening oxygenation and ventilation and a further decrease in cardiac output. The other consequence of increased minute ventilation is the development of respiratory alkalosis, gaining attention recently as a contributor to poor patient outcomes in certain acute care settings.[11,116,117]

Research related to the delivery of appropriate tidal volumes when using an FMV device has yielded different results depending on the clinical situation.[118] The American Heart Association recommends the delivery of sufficient tidal volumes to produce a *visible* chest rise.[1] This recommendation is based on evidence that in an unprotected airway, smaller tidal volumes producing chest rise (approximately 500 mL) result in less gastric insufflation. Secondly, it is reasoned that during CPR, perfusion approximates 30% of normal, meaning that less oxygen is needed and less CO_2 produced, and lower tidal volumes and respiratory rates are needed.

Concurrently, practitioners should consider the use of continuous waveform capnography to ensure adequate BMV and monitor the efficacy of ongoing efforts. This objective measure of ventilation is an invaluable resource, particularly when airway management occurs as part of a loud and/or chaotic resuscitation.

In patients with a sudden dysrhythmic cardiac arrest (e.g., ventricular fibrillation), hypoxemia and acidosis develop over several minutes.[118] In the very early phases of resuscitation, oxygen delivery is more dependent on tissue perfusion than arterial oxygen content. These findings are in part behind the recommendations that prioritize early CPR in advance of ventilation in this subgroup of patients.[119] On the other hand, the asphyxiated, respiratory arrest patient has maximal oxygen consumption associated with a lactic acidosis and CO_2 accumulation such that delays in oxygenation and ventilation should not occur during resuscitation efforts.

HIGH-FLOW NASAL OXYGENATION

What Is High-Flow Nasal Oxygenation?

High-flow nasal cannula (HFNC) systems, sold under brand names such as Optiflow or Vapotherm, are simple systems that consist of a flow generator, a heated circuit, and a humidifier that allow the delivery of oxygen up to 60 L min^{-1} at an FiO_2 of 95% to 100% via nasal cannula. The proposed benefits of HFNC include: with high flow rates, the ability to match or exceed the minute ventilation requirements of critically ill patients (and therefore prevent dilution of supplemental oxygen with room air), reduced anatomic dead space, and washout of CO_2 and improved work of breathing by increasing the effectiveness of efforts and reducing minute ventilation requirements. They also produce CPAP (5-6 cm H_2O) when the patient's mouth is closed as high flow rates produce impedance to expiratory.[120] Additionally, humidification of gas facilitates secretion clearance, decreases bronchospasm, and maintains mucosal integrity.[121]

High-flow nasal cannula systems have become increasingly used for oxygenation of patients with acute respiratory failure in the ICU, the ED, and in postoperative surgical patients. Available evidence for the use of HFNC in patients with acute hypoxemic respiratory failure is somewhat contradictory with some studies showing that HFNC, as compared to conventional oxygen therapy, decreases intubation rates in ICU/ED patients,[121–123] whereas other meta-analyses have concluded HFNC did not reduce the risk of critically ill patients requiring intubation in the ED[124] or in the ICU.[125]

The use of HFNC has been shown to reduce the rate of re-intubation in both critically ill ICU patients[126] and postoperative surgical patients.[127]

Limited evidence exists as to the effect of HFNC in patients with hypercapnic respiratory failure; however, one meta-analysis has suggested that HFNC may be considered noninferior to the use of NIV in this patient population.[128]

No studies have shown a mortality benefit of HFNC as compared to conventional oxygen therapy or NIV in patients with acute respiratory failure.[121–123,125,128]

Can HFNC Be Used as a Denitrogenation Technique Prior to Intubation?

A number of studies have examined the use of HFNC as a denitrogenation technique, comparing it to standard facemask or NIV in populations that include healthy volunteers, surgical patients, and ICU patients with acute respiratory failure. Collectively, the available evidence comparing HFNC versus FM in ICU or operating room patients shows that there is either no difference in oxygen desaturation during intubation or that the evidence slightly favors HFNC.[129–132]

HFNC has been shown to be less effective than NIV in preventing oxygen desaturation during intubation in ICU patients with PaO_2/FiO_2 <200[133] or in those with reduced FRC due to obesity or pregnancy.[134,135]

A small single-center study has looked at the combination of HFNC and NIV for denitrogenation in ICU patients with acute respiratory failure showing higher oxygen saturation with a combination approach;[136] however, given the small size of this single study, more evidence is required before any valid conclusions can be drawn.

One benefit of HFNC noted across a number of studies is that although initially used for denitrogenation, either as a lone technique or combined with NIV, HFNC has the additional benefit of supporting apneic oxygenation during intubation attempts or may be a continued source of oxygenation in patients chosen for an awake intubation on the basis of apnea intolerance.

Overall, HFNC is an appealing option to provide high flow rate oxygen that is often more tolerable for patients than NIV either as a standalone oxygen therapy or as step in escalating resuscitation.

SUMMARY

Face-mask ventilation remains an important, potentially life-saving airway management skill. However, it can be a difficult skill to teach, learn, and perform adequately unless one does so on a regular basis. The advent of extraglottic devices that are easy to teach, learn, and use may supplant FMV as a first-line airway management technique.

Difficult mask ventilation will usually respond to corrective measures and impossible mask ventilation is uncommon in experienced hands. Predicting difficult or impossible FMV is never foolproof but is fundamental to the practice of advanced airway management, influencing decision-making as to how to proceed.

SELF-EVALUATION QUESTIONS

8.1. Functional upper airway obstruction in the unconscious patient involves soft tissue collapse between:

A. The tongue and the posterior pharynx
B. The epiglottis and the posterior pharynx
C. The soft palate and the posterior pharynx
D. The tongue and the palate
E. All of the above

8.2. The most effective means of relieving a nonpathologic upper airway obstruction in the unconscious patient is:

A. Placing the patient in sniffing position
B. Placing a nasopharyngeal airway
C. Simple extension of the neck
D. Performing a jaw thrust
E. Placing an extraglottic device

8.3. Difficult mask-ventilation is associated with:

A. Increasing age
B. Mallampati II or III
C. Difficult laryngoscopy
D. The presence of dentures
E. A and C

REFERENCES

1. Link MS, Berkow LC, Kudenchuk PJ, et al. Part 7: Adult advanced cardiovascular life support: 2015 American Heart Association Guidelines Update for Cardiopulmonary Resuscitation and Emergency Cardiovascular Care. *Circulation.* 2015;132(18 Suppl 2):S444-S464.
2. Studnek JR, Thestrup L, Vandeventer S, et al. The association between prehospital endotracheal intubation attempts and survival to hospital discharge among out-of-hospital cardiac arrest patients. *Acad Emerg Med.* 2010;17(9):918-925.
3. Gausche M, Lewis RJ, Stratton SJ, et al. Effect of out-of-hospital pediatric endotracheal intubation on survival and neurological outcome: a controlled clinical trial. *JAMA.* 2000;283(6):783-790.
4. Stockinger ZT, McSwain NE Jr. Prehospital endotracheal intubation for trauma does not improve survival over bag-valve-mask ventilation. *J Trauma.* 2004;56(3):531-536.
5. Hasegawa K, Hiraide A, Chang Y, Brown DFM. Association of prehospital advanced airway management with neurologic outcome and survival in patients with out-of-hospital cardiac arrest. *JAMA.* 2013;309(3):257-266.
6. Fouche PF, Simpson PM, Bendall J, Thomas RE, Cone DC, Doi SA. Airways in out-of-hospital cardiac arrest: systematic review and meta-analysis. *Prehospital Emerg Care.* 2014;18(2):244-256.
7. Tiah L, Kajino K, Alsakaf O, et al. Does pre-hospital endotracheal intubation improve survival in adults with non-traumatic out-of-hospital cardiac arrest? A systematic review. *West J Emerg Med.* 2014;15(7):749-757.
8. Carlson JN, Wang HE. Does intubation improve outcomes over supraglottic airways in adult out-of-hospital cardiac arrest? *Ann Emerg Med.* 2015;67(3):396-398.
9. Wang HE, Yealy DM. Managing the airway during cardiac arrest. *JAMA.* 2013;309(3):285-286.
10. Pepe PE, Roppolo LP, Fowler RL. Prehospital endotracheal intubation: elemental or detrimental? *Crit Care.* 2015;19(1):1-7.
11. Benoit JL, Prince DK, Wang HE. Mechanisms linking advanced airway management and cardiac arrest outcomes. *Resuscitation.* 2015;93:124-127.
12. Benoit JL, Gerecht RB, Steuerwald MT, McMullan JT. Endotracheal intubation versus supraglottic airway placement in out-of-hospital cardiac arrest: A meta-analysis. *Resuscitation.* 2015;93:20-26.
13. Benger J, Kirby K, Black S, et al. Effect of a strategy of a supraglottic airway device vs tracheal intubation during out of hospital cardiac arrest on functional outcome. *JAMA.* 2018;320(8):779-791.
14. Jabre P, Penaloza A, Pinero D, et al. Effect of bag mask ventilation vs endotracheal intubation during cardiopulmonary resuscitation on neurological outcome after out of hospital cardiorespiratory arrest. *JAMA.* 2018;319(8):779-787.
15. Wang H, Schmicker RH, Daya MR, et al. Effect of a strategy of initial laryngeal tube insertion vs endotracheal intubation on 72-hour survival in adults with out of hospital cardiac arrest. *JAMA.* 2018;320(8):769-778.
16. Panchal A, Bartos JA, Cabañas JG, et al. AHA guidelines for cardiopulmonary resuscitation and emergency cardiovascular care. Part 3: adult basic and advanced life support. *Circulation.* 2020;142(sup 2):S366-S468.
17. Stiell IG, Nesbitt LP, Pickett W, et al. The OPALS Major Trauma Study: impact of advanced life-support on survival and morbidity. *CMAJ.* 2008;178(9):1141-1152.
18. Davis DP, Dunford JV, Poste JC, et al. The impact of hypoxia and hyperventilation on outcome after paramedic rapid sequence intubation of severely head-injured patients. *J Trauma.* 2004;57(1):1-10.
19. Alexander R, Hodgson P, Lomax D, Bullen C. A comparison of the laryngeal mask airway and Guedel airway, bag and facemask for manual ventilation following formal training. *Anaesthesia.* 1993;48(3):231-234.
20. Cummins RO, Austin D, Graves JR, Litwin PE, Pierce J. Ventilation skills of emergency medical technicians: a teaching challenge for emergency medicine. *Ann Emerg Med.* 1986;15(10):1187-1192.
21. Elling R, Politis J. An evaluation of emergency medical technicians' ability to use manual ventilation devices. *Ann Emerg Med.* 1983;12(12):765-768.
22. Mumma J. Bag valve mask ventilation as a perceptual cognitive skill. *Human Factors.* 2018;60(2):212-221.
23. Voss S, Rhys M, Coates D, et al. How do paramedics manage the airway during out of hospital cardiac arrest? *Resuscitation.* 2014;85(12):1662-1666.
24. Nagao T, Kinoshita K, Sakurai A, et al. Effects of bag-mask versus advanced airway ventilation for patients undergoing prolonged cardiopulmonary resuscitation in pre-hospital setting. *J Emerg Med.* 2012;42(2):162-170.
25. Shin S Do, Ahn KO, Song KJ, Park CB, Lee EJ. Out-of-hospital airway management and cardiac arrest outcomes: a propensity score matched analysis. *Resuscitation.* 2012;83(3):313-319.
26. Grein AJ, Weiner GM. Laryngeal mask airway versus bag-mask ventilation or endotracheal intubation for neonatal resuscitation. *Cochrane Database Syst Rev.* 2005;(2):CD003314.
27. Kurola JO, Turunen MJ, Laakso JP, Gorski JT, Paakkonen HJ, Silfvast TO. A comparison of the laryngeal tube and bag-valve mask ventilation by emergency medical technicians: a feasibility study in anesthetized patients. *Anesth Analg.* 2005;101(5):1477-1481.
28. Dörges V, Wenzel V, Knacke P, Gerlach K. Comparison of different airway management strategies to ventilate apneic, nonpreoxygenated patients. *Crit Care Med.* 2003;31(3):800-804.
29. Murray MJ, Vermeulen MJ, Morrison LJ, Waite T. Evaluation of prehospital insertion of the laryngeal mask airway by primary care paramedics with only classroom mannequin training. *CJEM Can J Emerg Med Care.* 2002;4(5):338-343.
30. Hasegawa K, Hiraide A, Chang Y, Brown DFM. Association of prehospital advanced airway management with neurologic outcome and survival in patients with out-of-hospital cardiac arrest. *JAMA.* 2013;309(3):257-266.
31. Dörges V, Wenzel V, Knacke P, Gerlach K. Comparison of different airway management strategies to ventilate apneic, nonpreoxygenated patients. *Crit Care Med.* 2003;31(3):800-804.
32. Murray MJ, Vermeulen MJ, Morrison LJ, Waite T. Evaluation of prehospital insertion of the laryngeal mask airway by primary care paramedics with only classroom mannequin training. *CJEM.* 2002;4(5):338-343.

33. Müller J-U, Semmel T, Stepan R, et al. The use of the laryngeal tube disposable by paramedics during out-of-hospital cardiac arrest: a prospectively observational study (2008-2012). *Emerg Med J.* 2013;30(12):1012-1016.
34. Trevisanuto D, Cavallin F, Nguyen LN, et al. Supreme laryngeal mask airway versus face mask during neonatal resuscitation: a randomized controlled trial. *J Pediatr.* 2015:1-7.
35. Khoury A, Hugonnot S, Cossus J, et al. From mouth-to-mouth to bag-valve-mask ventilation: evolution and characteristics of actual devices — a review of the literature. *Biomed Res Int.* 2014:1-7.
36. Chrimes N. Not all bag-valva-mask devices are created equal: beware a possible lower FiO2 during spontaneous vetilation. *Anaesth Intensive Care.* 2014;42(2):276.
37. Priebe H-J. Assessment of anaesthetists' ability to predict difficulty of bag-mask ventilation. *Br J Anaesth.* 2014;112(4):769-770.
38. Benumof JL. Management of the difficult adult airway. With special emphasis on awake tracheal intubation. *Anesthesiology.* 1991;75(6):1087-1110.
39. Cormack RS, Lehane J. Difficult tracheal intubation in obstetrics. *Anaesthesia.* 1984;39(11):1105-1111.
40. Mallampati SR, Gatt SP, Gugino LD, et al. A clinical sign to predict difficult tracheal intubation: a prospective study. *Can Anaesth Soc J.* 1985;32(4):429-434.
41. Kheterpal S, Healy D, Aziz MF, et al. Incidence, predictors, and outcome of difficult mask ventilation combined with difficult laryngoscopy: a report from the multicenter perioperative outcomes group. *Anesthesiology.* 2013;119(6):1360-1369.
42. Kheterpal S, Martin L, Shanks AM, Tremper KK. Prediction and outcomes of impossible mask ventilation: a review of 50,000 anesthetics. *Anesthesiology.* 2009;110(4):891-897.
43. Kheterpal S, Han R, Tremper KK, et al. Incidence and predictors of difficult and impossible mask ventilation. *Anesthesiology.* 2006;105(5):885-891.
44. Yildiz TS, Solak M, Toker K. The incidence and risk factors of difficult mask ventilation. *J Anesth.* 2005;19(1):7-11.
45. Langeron O, Masso E, Huraux C, et al. Prediction of difficult mask ventilation. *Anesthesiology.* 2000;92(5):1229-1236.
46. Valois-Gõmez T, Oofuvong M, Auer G, Coffin D, Loetwiriyakul W, Correa JA. Incidence of difficult bag-mask ventilation in children: a prospective observational study. *Paediatr Anaesth.* 2013;23(10):920-926.
47. Law JA, Broemling N, Cooper RM, et al. The difficult airway with recommendations for management - Part 1 - Intubation encountered in an unconscious/induced patient. *Can J Anesth.* 2013;60(11):1089-1118.
48. Frerk C, Mitchell VS, McNarry AF, et al. Difficult Airway Society 2015 guidelines for management of unanticipated difficult intubation in adults. *Br J Anaesth.* 2015;115(6):827-848.
49. Benumof JL. Management of the difficult adult airway. With special emphasis on awake tracheal intubation. *Anesthesiology.* 1991;75(6):1087-1110.
50. El-Orbany M, Woehlck HJ. Difficult mask ventilation. *Anesth Analg.* 2009;109(6):1870-1880.
51. Kheterpal S, Healy D, Aziz MF, et al. Incidence, predictors, and outcome of difficult mask ventilation combined with difficult laryngoscopy: a report from the multicenter perioperative outcomes group. *Anesthesiology.* 2013;119(6):1360-1369.
52. Norskov A. 2017. Prediction of difficult mask ventilation using a systematic assessment of risk factors vs existing practice – a cluster randomized clinical trial in 94,006 patients. *Anaesthesia.* 2017;72:296-308.
53. Han R, Tremper KK, Kheterpal S, O'Reilly M. Grading scale for mask ventilation. *Anesthesiology.* 2004;101(1):267.
54. Priebe H-J. Should anesthesiologists have to confirm effective face-mask ventilation before administering the muscle relaxant? *J Anesth.* 2016;30(1):132-137.
55. Joffe AM, Ramaiah R, Donahue E, et al. Ventilation by mask before and after the administration of neuromuscular blockade: a pragmatic non-inferiority trial. *BMC Anesthesiol.* 2015:1-9.
56. Ramachandran SK, Kheterpal S. Difficult mask ventilation: does it matter? *Anaesthesia.* 2011;66(Suppl. 2):40-44.
57. Lee S. Patient specific factors associated with difficult mask ventilation in the emergency department. *Int J Gerontol.* 2017;11:263-266.
58. Levitan RM, Everett WW, Ochroch EA. Limitations of difficult airway prediction in patients intubated in the emergency department. *Ann Emerg Med.* 2004;44(4):307-313.
59. Brown CA, Bair AE, Pallin DJ, Walls RM. NEAR III Investigators. Techniques, success, and adverse events of emergency department adult intubations. *Ann Emerg Med.* 2015;65(4):363-370.e1.
60. Brown CA 3rd, Cox K, Hurwitz S, Walls RM. 4,871 Emergency Airway Encounters by Air Medical Providers: A Report of the Air Transport Emergency Airway Management (NEAR VI: "A-TEAM") Project. *West J Emerg Med.* 2014;15(2):188-193.
61. Kerslake D, Oglesby AJ, Di Rollo N, et al. Tracheal intubation in an urban emergency department in Scotland: a prospective, observational study of 3738 intubations. *Resuscitation.* 2015;89:20-24.
62. Calvin A. Brown III, Cox K, Hurwitz WR. 4,871 Emergency Airway Encounters by Air Medical Providers: A Report of the Air Transport Emergency Airway Management (NEAR VI: "A-TEAM") Project. *West J Emerg Med.* 2013;26(1):217-220.
63. Hillman DR, Platt PR, Eastwood PR. The upper airway during anaesthesia. *Br J Anaesth.* 2003;91(1):31-39.
64. McGee JP II, Vender JS. Chapter 14 - Nonintubation management of the airway: mask ventilation. 2007:345-370.
65. Adnet F, Baillard C, Borron SW, et al. Randomized study comparing the "sniffing position" with simple head extension for laryngoscopic view in elective surgery patients. *Anesthesiology.* 2001;95(4):836-841.
66. Levitan RM, Mechem CC, Ochroch EA, Shofer FS, Hollander JE. Head-elevated laryngoscopy position: improving laryngeal exposure during laryngoscopy by increasing head elevation. *Ann Emerg Med.* 2003;41(3):322-330.
67. Isono S, Tanaka A, Ishikawa T, Tagaito Y, Nishino T. Sniffing position improves pharyngeal airway patency in anesthetized patients with obstructive sleep apnea. *Anesthesiology.* 2005;103(3):489-494.
68. Mitterlechner T, Paal P, Kuehnelt-Leddhin L, et al. Head position angles to open the upper airway differ less with the head positioned on a support. *Am J Emerg Med.* 2013;31(1):80-85.
69. Sato Y, Ikeda A, Ishikawa T, Isono S. How can we improve mask ventilation in patients with obstructive sleep apnea during anesthesia induction? *J Anesth.* 2013;27(1):152-156.
70. Altermatt FR, Muñoz HR, Delfino AE, Cortínez LI. Pre-oxygenation in the obese patient: effects of position on tolerance to apnoea. *Br J Anaesth.* 2005;95(5):706-709.
71. Davies JD, Costa BK, Asciutto a. J. Approaches to manual ventilation. *Respir Care.* 2014;59(6):810-824.
72. Kovacs G, Law JA, eds. *Airway Management in Emergencies.* 1st ed. New York, NY: McGraw Hill; 2007.
73. Uzun L, Ugur MB, Altunkaya H, Ozer Y, Ozkocak I, Demirel CB. Effectiveness of the jaw-thrust maneuver in opening the airway: a flexible fiberoptic endoscopic study. *ORL J Otorhinolaryngol Relat Spec.* 2005;67(1):39-44.
74. Boidin MP. Airway patency in the unconscious patient. *Br J Anaesth.* 1985;57(3):306-310.
75. Morikawa S, Safar P, Decarlo J. Influence of the headjaw position upon upper airway patency. *Anesthesiology.* 1961;22:265-270.
76. Law A, Duggan L, Asselin M. Canadian Airway Focus Group updated consensus-based recommendations for management of the difficult airway: Part 1. Difficult airway management encountered in an unconscious patient. *Can J Anaesthesiol.* 2021:68(9):1373-1404.
77. Itagaki T, Ota J, Burns S, Jiang Y, Kacmarek R, Mountjoy J. The effect of head rotation on efficiency of face mask ventilation in anaesthetized apneic patients. *Eur J Anesthesiol.* 2017;34:432-440.
78. Apfelbaum JL, Hagberg CA, Caplan RA, et al. Practice guidelines for management of the difficult airway: an updated report by the American Society of Anesthesiologists Task Force on Management of the Difficult Airway. *Anesthesiology.* 2013;118(2):251-270.
79. Piepho T, Cavus E, Noppens R, et al. S1 guidelines on airway management. *Anaesthesist.* 2015;64(S1):27-40.
80. Sim M a B, Dean P, Kinsella J, Black R, Carter R, Hughes M. Performance of oxygen delivery devices when the breathing pattern of respiratory failure is simulated. *Anaesthesia.* 2008;63(9):938-940.
81. Pandit JJ, Duncan T, Robbins PA. Total oxygen uptake with two maximal breathing techniques and the tidal volume breathing technique: a physiologic study of preoxygenation. *Anesthesiology.* 2003;99(4):841-846.
82. Groombridge C, Chin CW, Hanrahan B, Holdgate A. Assessment of common preoxygenation strategies outside of the operating room environment. *Acad Emerg Med.* 2016;23(3):342-346.
83. Weingart SD, Levitan RM. Preoxygenation and prevention of desaturation during emergency airway management. *Ann Emerg Med.* 2012;59(3):165-175.
84. Harbut P, Gozdzik W, Stjernfalt E, Marsk R, Hesselvik JF. Continuous positive airway pressure/pressure support pre-oxygenation of morbidly obese patients. *Acta Anaesthesiol Scand.* 2014;58(6):675-680.
85. Bradley W, Lyons C. Facemask ventilation. *BJA Education.* 2022;22(1):5-11.
86. Sellick BA. Cricoid pressure to control regurgitation of stomach contents during induction of anaesthesia. *Lancet.* 1961;2(7199):404-406.
87. Isono S. Facemask ventilation during induction of anesthesia how "gentle" is "gentle" enough? *Anesthesiology.* 2014;(2):2013-2015.
88. El-Orbany M, Connolly LA. Rapid sequence induction and intubation: current controversy. *Anesth Analg.* 2010;110(5):1318-1325.

89. Algie CM, Mahar RK, Tan HB, Wilson G, Mahar PD, Wasiak J. Effectiveness and risks of cricoid pressure during rapid sequence induction for endotracheal intubation. *Cochrane Database Syst Rev.* 2015;11(4):CD011656.
90. Brown P, Werret G. Bag-mask ventilation in rapid sequence induction: a survey of current practice among members of the UK Difficult Airway Society. *Eur J Anaesthesiol.* 2015;32(6):446-448.
91. Brown JPR, Werrett G. Bag-mask ventilation in rapid sequence induction. *Anaesthesia.* 2009;64(7):784-785.
92. Casey J, Janz, D, Russell, D. Bag mask ventilation during tracheal intubation of critically ill adults. *N Engl J Med.* 2019;380:811-821.
93. Lim K, Neilsen J. Objective description of mask ventilation. *BJA.* 2017;117(6):P828-829.
94. Otten D, Liao MM, Wolken R, et al. Comparison of bag-valve-mask hand-sealing techniques in a simulated model. *Ann Emerg Med.* 2014;63(1):6-12.e3.
95. Hart D, Reardon R, Ward C, Miner J. Face mask ventilation: a comparison of three techniques. *J Emerg Med.* 2013;44(5):1028-1033.
96. Davidovic L, LaCovey D, Pitetti RD. Comparison of 1- versus 2-person bag-valve-mask techniques for manikin ventilation of infants and children. *Ann Emerg Med.* 2005;46(1):37-42.
97. Gerstein NS, Carey MC, Braude DA, et al. Efficacy of facemask ventilation techniques in novice providers. *J Clin Anesth.* 2013;25(3):193-197.
98. Braude DA, Tawil I, Gerstein NS, Carey MC, Petersen TR. Comparison of bag-valve-mask hand-sealing techniques in a simulated model. *Ann Emerg Med.* 2014;63(6):784-785.
99. Joffe AM, Hetzel S, Liew EC. A two-handed jaw-thrust technique is superior to the one-handed "EC-clamp" technique for mask ventilation in the apneic unconscious person. *Anesthesiology.* 2010;113(4):873-879.
100. Fei M, Blair JL, Rice MJ. Comparison of effectiveness of two commonly used two handed mask ventilation techniques on unconscious apneic obese adults. *BJA.* 2018;118(4):618-624.
101. Mort TC. Emergency tracheal intubation: complications associated with repeated laryngoscopic attempts. *Anesth Analg.* 2004;99(2):607-613.
102. Ellis DY, Harris T, Zideman D. Cricoid pressure in emergency department rapid sequence tracheal intubations: a risk-benefit analysis. *Ann Emerg Med.* 2007;50(6):653-665.
103. Butler J, Sen A. Towards evidence-based emergency medicine: best BETs from the Manchester Royal Infirmary. BET 1: Cricoid pressure in emergency rapid sequence induction. *Emerg Med J.* 2013;30(2):163-165.
104. Stewart JC, Bhananker S, Ramaiah R. Rapid-sequence intubation and cricoid pressure. *Int J Crit Illn Inj Sci.* 2014;4(1):42-49.
105. Ovassapian A, Salem MR. Sellick's maneuver: to do or not do. *Anesth Analg.* 2009;109(5):1360-1362.
106. Joshi S, Prakash S, Mullick P, et al. Clinical evaluation of the cricoid pressure effect on bag mask ventilation, ProSeal laryngeal mask airway placement and ventilation. *Turk J Anesthesiol.* 2018;46(5):381-387.
107. Boet S, Duttchen K, Chan J, et al. Cricoid pressure provides incomplete esophageal occlusion associated with lateral deviation: a magnetic resonance imaging study. *J Emerg Med.* 2012;42(5):606-611.
108. Smith KJ, Dobranowski J, Yip G, Dauphin A, Choi PT-L. Cricoid pressure displaces the esophagus: an observational study using magnetic resonance imaging. *Anesthesiology.* 2003;99(1):60-64.
109. Zeidan AM, Salem MR, Mazoit JX, Abdullah MA, Ghattas T, Crystal GJ. The effectiveness of cricoid pressure for occluding the esophageal entrance in anesthetized and paralyzed patients: an experimental and observational glidescope study. *Anesth Analg.* 2014;118(3):580-586.
110. White L, Thang C, Hodsdon A, et al. Cricoid pressure during intubation: a systematic review and meta-analysis of randomized controlled trials. *Heart Lung.* 2020;49(2):175-180.
111. Lawes EG, Campbell I, Mercer D. Inflation pressure, gastric insufflation and rapid sequence induction. *Br J Anaesth.* 1987;59(3):315-318.
112. Saddawi-Konefka D, Hung SL, Kacmarek RM, Jiang Y. Optimizing Mask Ventilation: Literature Review and Development of a Conceptual Framework. *Respir Care.* 2015;60(12):1834-1840.
113. Wenzel V, Idris AH, Dörges V, et al. The respiratory system during resuscitation: a review of the history, risk of infection during assisted ventilation, respiratory mechanics, and ventilation strategies for patients with an unprotected airway. *Resuscitation.* 2001;49(2):123-134.
114. Bouvet L, Albert M-L, Augris C, et al. Real-time detection of gastric insufflation related to facemask pressure-controlled ventilation using ultrasonography of the antrum and epigastric auscultation in nonparalyzed patients: a prospective, randomized, double-blind study. *Anesthesiology.* 2014;120(2):326-334.
115. Davis DP, Douglas DJ, Koenig W, Carrison D, Buono C, Dunford JV. Hyperventilation following aero-medical rapid sequence intubation may be a deliberate response to hypoxemia. *Resuscitation.* 2007;73(3):354-361.
116. Davis DP. Early ventilation in traumatic brain injury. *Resuscitation.* 2008;76(3):333-340.
117. Davis DP, Heister R, Poste JC, Hoyt DB, Ochs M, Dunford JV. Ventilation patterns in patients with severe traumatic brain injury following paramedic rapid sequence intubation. *Neurocrit Care.* 2005;2(2):165-171.
118. Gabrielli A, Layon AJ, Wenzel V, Dorges V, Idris AH. Alternative ventilation strategies in cardiopulmonary resuscitation. *Curr Opin Crit Care.* 2002;8(3):199-211.
119. Kleinman ME, Brennan EE, Goldberger ZD, et al. Part 5: Adult Basic Life Support and Cardiopulmonary Resuscitation Quality. *Circulation.* 2015;132(18 suppl 2):S414-S435.
120. Nishimura M. High flow nasal cannula oxygen therapy in adults: physiological benefits, indication, clinical benefits and adverse effects. *Resp Care.* 2016;61(4):529-541.
121. Lee CC, Mankodi D, Shaharyar S, et al. High flow nasal cannula versus conventional oxygen therapy and non-invasive ventilation in adults with acute hypoxemic respiratory failure: a systematic review. *Resp Med.* 2016;121:100-108.
122. Rochwerg B, Granton D, Wang DX, et al. High flow nasal cannula compared with conventional oxygen therapy for acute hypoxemic respiratory failure: a systematic review and meta-analysis. *Intensive Care Med.* 2019;45:563-572.
123. Zhao H, Wang H, Sun F, et al. High flow nasal cannula oxygen therapy is superior to conventional oxygen therapy but not to noninvasive mechanical ventilation on intubation rate: a systematic review and meta-analysis. *Critical Care.* 2017;21:184.
124. Tinelli V, Cabrini L, Fominskiy E, et al. High flow nasal cannula oxygen vs conventional oxygen therapy and non-invasive ventilation in emergency department patients: a systematic review and meta-analysis. *J Emerg Med.* 2019;57(3):322-328.
125. Nedel W, Deutschendorf C, Filho EMR, et al. High flow nasal cannula in critically ill subjects with or at risk of respiratory failure: a systematic review and meta-analysis. *Resp Care.* 2017;62(1):123-132.
126. Huang H, Sun XM, Shi ZH, et al. Effect of high flow nasal cannula oxygen therapy versus conventional oxygen therapy and noninvasive ventilation on reintubation rate in adult patients after extubation: a systematic review and meta-analysis of randomized controlled trials. *J Intensive Care Med.* 2019;33(11):609-623.
127. Chang Z, Meng SS, Zhang X, et al. Effect of high flow nasal cannula oxygen therapy compared with conventional oxygen therapy in post-operative patients: a systematic review and meta-analysis. *BMJ Open.* 2019;9:e027523.
128. Huang Y, Lei W, Zhang W, Huang J. High flow nasal cannula in hypercapnic respiratory failure: a systematic review and meta-analysis. *Can Resp J.* 2020;7406457.
129. Simon M, Wachs C, Braune S, de Heer G, et al. High flow nasal cannula versus bag valve mask for preoxygenation before intubation in subjects with hypoxemic respiratory failure. *Resp Care.* 2016;61(9):1160-1167.
130. Vourc'h M, Asfar P, Voltreau C, et al. High flow nasal cannula oxygen during endotracheal intubation in hypoxemic patients: a randomized controlled clinical trial. *Intensive Care Med.* 2015;41:1538-1548.
131. Guitton C, Ehrmann S, Volteau C, et al. Nasal high flow preoxygenation for endotracheal intubation in the critically ill patient: a randomized clinical trial. *Intensive Care Med.* 2019;45:447-458.
132. Lodenius A, Piehl J, Ostlund A, et al. Transnasal humidified rapid insufflation ventilatory exchange (THRIVE) vs facemask breathing preoxygenation for rapid sequence induction in adults: a prospective randomized non-blinded clinical trial. *Anesthesia.* 2018;73:564-571.
133. Frat JP, Ricard JD, Quenot JP, et al. Non-invasive ventilation versus high-flow nasal cannula oxygen therapy with apnoeic oxygenation for preoxygenation before intubation of patients with acute hypoxaemic respiratory failure: a randomized, multicentre, open-label trial. *Lancet Resp Med.* 2019;7(4):303-312.
134. Vourc'h M, Baud G, Feuillet F, et al. High-flow nasal cannulae versus non-invasive ventilation for preoxygenation of obese patients: the PREOPTIPOP randomized trail. *E Clin Med.* 2019;5(13):112-119.
135. Shippam W, Preston R, Douglas J, et al. High flow nasal oxygen vs standard flow rate facemask pre-oxygenation in pregnant patients: a randomized physiological study. *Anesthesia.* 2019;74:450-456.
136. Jaber S, Monnin M, Girard M, et al. Apneic oxygenation via high flow nasal cannula oxygen combined with non-invasive ventilation preoxygenation for intubation in hypoxemic patients in the intensive care unit: the single centre blinded, randomized, controlled OPTINIV trial. *Intensive Care Med.* 2016;42:1877-1887.

CHAPTER 9

Direct Laryngoscopy

Samuel G. Campbell and George Kovacs

INTRODUCTION

In this day and age with video laryngoscopy (VL) rapidly becoming more freely available for orotracheal intubation (OTI) one might ask if there is still a need for a chapter on direct laryngoscopy (DL). However, while VL is gaining ground on DL, particularly in countries with developed economies, VL has yet to replace DL as the most common device employed worldwide to facilitate OTI. Proficiency with DL remains a vitally important skill for difficult and failed intubation rescue, and in parts of the world that cannot afford or do not have access to VL.[1]

What Is the History and Evolution of Direct Laryngoscopy?

In the modern era, DL is usually associated with tracheal intubation, even though the procedure was initially developed for diagnosing and treating laryngeal pathology. Following the development of mirror laryngoscopy in the 1800s by Garcia, Tuerck, and Czermak,[2] Kirstein reported the first use of DL in 1895.[3] Over the next twenty years, the basic tenets of the procedure were refined by surgeons interested in laryngeal examination and surgical exposure.

A step-wise approach, the focus on epiglottoscopy, recognition of posterior laryngeal landmarks, optimal positioning for laryngeal exposure, and the benefits of external laryngeal manipulation and head elevation, etc. were all detailed by Chevalier Jackson in his 1922 text, "Bronchoscopy and Esophagoscopy, a Manual for Peroral Endoscopy and Laryngeal Surgery."[4]

With the evolution of modern anesthesia, the straight laryngoscope designs developed by ear, nose, and throat (ENT) surgeons gave way to instruments specifically designed for tracheal intubation, such as the straight Magill (1930),[5] Miller blades (1941),[6] and the curved Macintosh blade (1943).[7] It was also during this time that the design of a detachable blade and battery handle became commonplace.

Between the 1930s and 1970s many different laryngoscope blades were designed to facilitate intubation (e.g., Wisconsin, Phillips, Guedel, etc.), but the Magill, Miller, and Macintosh models (albeit with some modifications) remain universally used, and in most settings, are the only laryngoscope blades available.

The development of flexible fiberoptics, with subsequent attachment of fiberoptics to rigid blades (Bullard laryngoscope,[8] WuScope,[9] etc.), and more recently video laryngoscopes (GlideScope, McGrath, Storz Video MAC, etc.)[10] have spawned a wide array of indirect visual devices for both diagnostic imaging of the larynx and tracheal intubation, leaving a narrowed clinical role for standard, line-of-sight (LOS), DL. Alternative devices are being increasingly deployed for both routine and anticipated "difficult laryngoscopy."

EQUIPMENT

What Are the Principal Design Components and Function of Laryngoscopy Blades?

Laryngoscope blade design, light, and battery systems affect procedural performance due to their impact on illumination, laryngeal exposure, and endotracheal tube (ETT) delivery. Laryngeal exposure is achieved by managing the oral opening and teeth, the tongue and epiglottis, all of which interpose between the operator's eye and the larynx. The blade and flange are tasked with removing the tongue from blocking the field of view, while the distal end of the blade is used to manage the epiglottis. The flange of the laryngoscope remains a threat to dentition and should never be levered backward against the teeth. Straight and curved blades differ in the strategy that each shape uses to expose the larynx.

The concept of "submandibular space volume" as a determinant of "space" into which the tongue can be pushed during laryngoscopy is particularly important in clinical practice as the practitioner evaluates for difficult curved blade laryngoscopy and intubation (see Chapter 1).

Early pioneers, such as Magill,[5] employing straight blades recognized that tongue displacement to one side facilitated laryngeal visualization, particularly if the blade of the laryngoscope was inserted in the corner of the mouth and along the paraglossal gutter. Importantly, it was recognized that this "paraglossal" or "retromolar" technique optimized the laryngeal view mostly because it shortened the distance between the teeth and the larynx (i.e., the molars are closer to the larynx than the incisors). The other benefit of right paraglossal laryngoscopy is that the rigid laryngoscope blade impacts the molar teeth rather than the relatively more fragile central incisors, decreasing the risk of dental trauma and bypassing any obstruction to the laryngeal view by prominent incisors. This paraglossal technique remains the preferred initial approach to blade DL.

The straight blade laryngoscope, such as the Magill blade functions to pass lateral to the tongue, moving it to the left side of the mouth. Not conforming to the curve of the dorsum of the tongue, the tip of the straight blade does not naturally point into the vallecula, but under the epiglottis itself, which the tip is used to lift up directly.

Straight laryngoscope blades tend to have smaller displacement volumes (defined by the dimensions of the spatula and flange) than curved designs. The paraglossal approach is useful in patients who have a large or swollen tongue and/or a small submandibular volume both of which might restrict the ability to displace the tongue anteriorly during DL. Examples of such patients are small children (below the age of 8, but especially below age 5) and adults who have a receding chin or a lesion occupying the submandibular space.

It should be mentioned that, although it is important to recognize the strengths and weaknesses with each shape of the blade, either technique may work on the other shaped blade, for example a curved blade may be used to lift the epiglottis, or a straight blade may engage the hyoepiglottic ligament.

Because laryngoscopy was originally an operative technique where the practitioner needed their dominant right hand (85% of the population is right-hand dominant) to be free to operate, the laryngoscope became by default a left-handed instrument, fortuitously allowing the practitioner (or at least 85% of them) to manipulate an intubation aid (e.g., Eschmann Tracheal Introducer, [ETI]) or a styletted ETT with their dominant hand.

As discussed, laryngoscopy and intubation are performed through the right side of the mouth. The left hand is used to insert the laryngoscope blade into the mouth to expose the glottis. The right hand is thus free to perform a variety of tasks including manipulation of the larynx, lifting of the head, suctioning of the airway, and ultimately the placement of the ETI or ETT.

What Are the Distinguishing Features of Commonly Used Curved (Macintosh) Blade Designs? (Video 3)

The term "Macintosh blade" is generally used to mean any curved blade. However, since Macintosh's original description in 1943[7] several modifications have been produced that are distinguishable by their flange height, flange shape, light position, and light type. These designs are commonly designated by their geographic manufacturing origin, i.e., American (also referred to as "Standard"), English (also known as "Classic"), and German designs. The common features are a gently curved spatula and a large reverse Z-shaped flange (Figure 9.1).

American blades most closely follow Macintosh's original description, i.e., a large vertical, square-shaped, proximal flange that does not extend to the distal tip, coupled with a bulb-on-blade illumination system. The English design has a smaller, curvilinear proximal flange that runs all the way to the distal tip, and, like its American counterpart, uses a conventional light. Heine of Germany developed a fiber-lit blade that follows the English contour in terms of a short proximal flange, into which is incorporated a large rectangular-shaped 5-mm glass fiber bundle. The English and German designs have a much shorter light-to-tip distance (Figure 9.2), providing greater illumination than the American design. While most American designs use a frosted bulb, most English designs have a clear lens. Both American and English designs now offer fiber illumination options. Numerous manufacturers around the world now offer "American," "English," and "German" curved blades and many blades have mixed features.

It is interesting to note that Macintosh envisioned one adult size for his blade (corresponding to approximately a Macintosh size 3). Market demand has led to the current variety of pediatric and adult sizes. Size selection is largely a matter of the patient's size and the practitioner's choice. Whatever the size chosen, it should be noted that the most common error committed by novice practitioners is the insertion of the blade too deeply and into the upper esophagus before the visualization is performed.

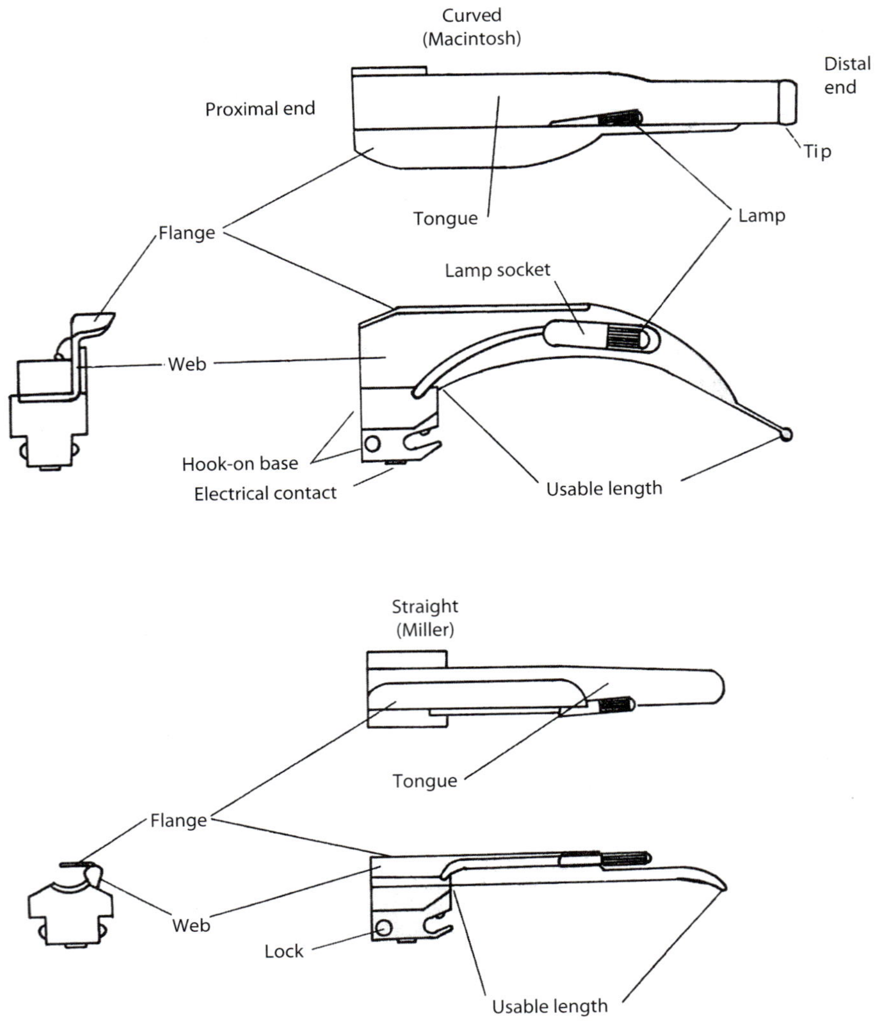

FIGURE 9.1. Design of the laryngoscope blades.

An adjustable variation of the Macintosh design, the McCoy blade (also known as Corazelli-London-McCoy [CLM]) levering laryngoscope blade (Figure 9.3 and Video 16), is a Macintosh shaped blade with an articulating distal tip that when activated is intended to elevate the tissue at the base of the tongue (improving epiglottis lift and laryngeal exposure). This blade has become quite popular in the United Kingdom (where it originated) but published clinical investigations have reported mixed results.[11–16]

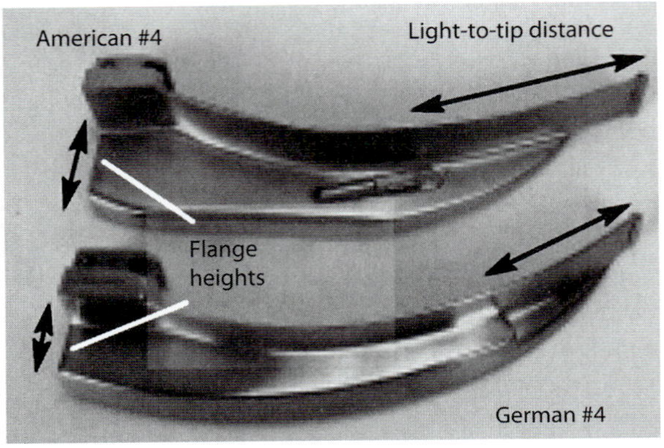

FIGURE 9.2. Design of the curved Macintosh laryngoscope blades: the German design has a much shorter light-to-tip distance than the American design.

What Are the Features of Different Straight Blade Laryngoscope Designs?

Robert Miller's straight blade design in 1941 adapted the straight shape of early laryngoscopes, in particular that of Magill (see Figure 1.1), adding a slightly upturned distal tip and a narrower flange.[6] The flange had a compressed D-shape (when viewed longitudinally) with a height large enough to accept a 37 French Argyle tube. Compared to tubular-shaped blades (Jackson-Wisconsin, for example)[17,18] the much shallower proximal flange was intended to minimize dental injury (Figure 9.4). The light was situated at the distal tip on the right side of the spatula, opposite the flange side and tilted toward midline (Figure 9.1).

Since Miller's original description, various manufacturers have compressed the flange height, and some have changed the

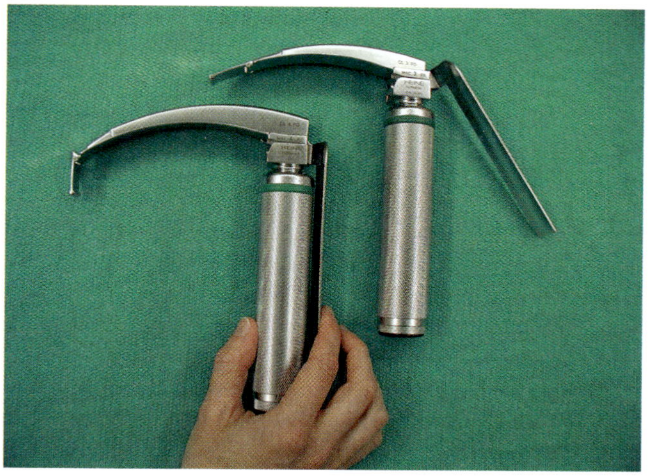

FIGURE 9.3. The McCoy (also known as Corazelli-London-McCoy [CLM]) levering laryngoscope blade.

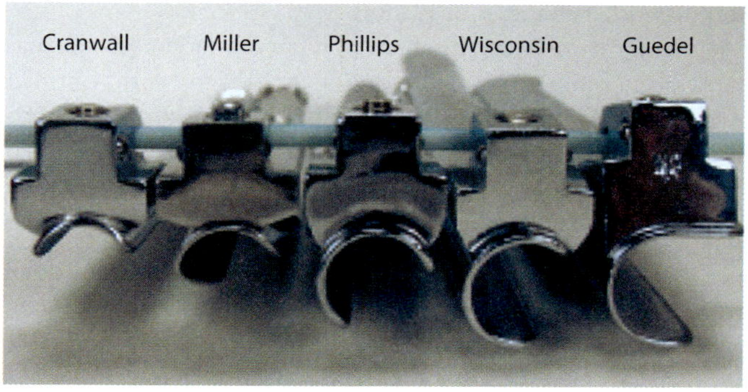

FIGURE 9.4. Different design of the straight laryngoscope blades with different tubular shapes.

bulb location (to the left flange edge or recessed within the flange). Designs with light sources located on the exposed edge of the left flange have the challenge that the light at this location can become embedded in the tongue decreasing illumination. The very narrow design of modern Miller blades necessitates careful paraglossal placement (the small flange cannot sweep the tongue) and tube (or ETI) delivery from the extreme right corner of the mouth (which often requires manual retraction by an assistant). The narrow channel of most Miller blades makes landmark recognition difficult, and the barrel is usually too narrow to accommodate an adult-sized cuffed ETT. Tube passage down the barrel can also obstruct the LOS to the target.

Landmark recognition and ease of tube delivery improve as the flange height and spatula size of a straight blade are increased, although this comes at the cost of increased difficulty in introducing the blade alongside the tongue, and reaching the larynx, as the displacement volume of the blade increases. To address this paradox, Miller shortened his flange height but left the resulting D-shaped barrel large enough to accept an ETT.

Straight blade designs with larger flanges (and spatulas) than the Miller design include the Phillips (a 2/3 small "C" shape flange), Wisconsin (a higher, nearly full "C" shaped flange), and the Guedel (a very large, sideways "U" shaped flange and spatula) (Video 6; Figure 9.4).[18]

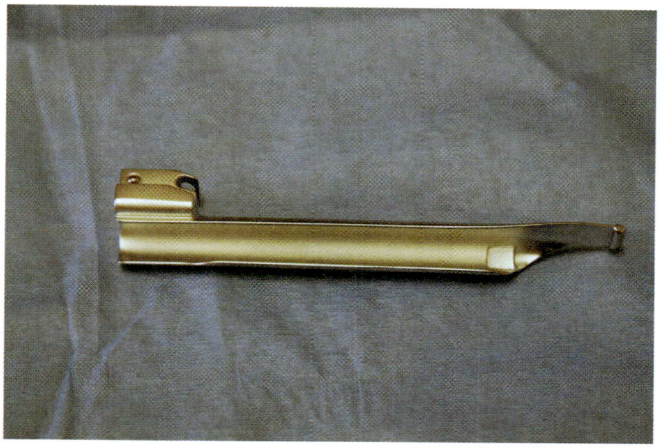

FIGURE 9.5. The Henderson laryngoscope.

The Henderson straight blade has a small incomplete 2/3 "C" shaped flange that is large enough for tube delivery. It also has a uniquely visible distal tip (a curled edge at the distal blade tip is visible when viewed down the barrel), and a large, recessed, fiber bundle light source (Figure 9.5).

Apart from the Pre-Mentioned Blades, What Other Blade Designs Are Likely to Be Encountered?

The Dorges universal blade has been designed to replace Macintosh size 2-4 blades with one blade for all patients from age 1 to adult.[19] The curve is reduced, the spatula is tapered from the proximal end to the distal tip, and the proximal flange height is very short (15 mm), allowing it to be used with children and those with limited mouth opening, while at the same time permitting deeper insertion in larger adults owing to its length (Figure 9.6).

The Grandview blade is an emergency blade for adult patients that is available in two sizes.[20] It combines a very wide spatula with a slight overall curve and a narrow proximal flange (Figure 9.7). The resulting blade can be used to lift the epiglottis directly or indirectly.

What Are the Variables that Determine the Degree of Illumination of the Laryngoscope?

Light Sources

Adequate illumination of the glottis and surrounding tissue during DL is critically important and may be inadequate in equipment that is not well maintained.[21] Bright light is

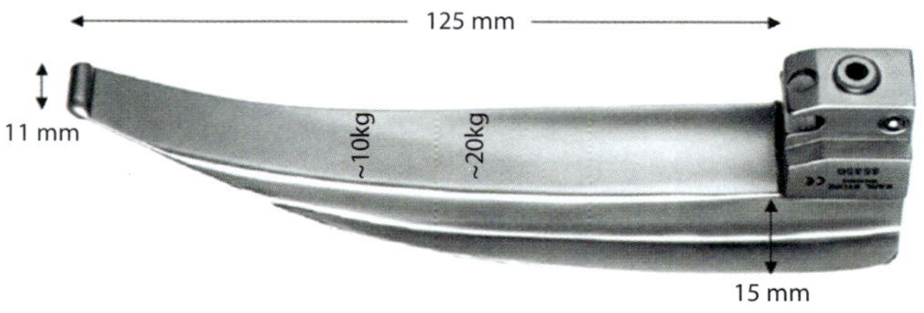

FIGURE 9.6. The Dorges universal laryngoscope blade.

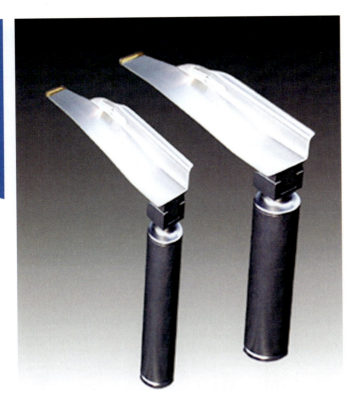

FIGURE 9.7. The Grandview universal laryngoscope blade.

necessary for tissue edge and color discrimination, and the identification of tissues and structures[22] is particularly important in preterm infants where the appreciation of subtle color differences is critical to intubation success, although too much light has also been reported as sub-optimal.[23] In the presence of blood, secretions, and vomitus, common to emergency airways, more light is needed to discriminate landmarks.

Laryngoscope lighting systems can be divided into those with a light source mounted directly on the blade (bulb-on-blade), and those in which the light source is in the handle with the light conducted down to the distal end of the blade via a light-conducting fiber made of glass or plastic (bulb-on-handle). Although these fibers are often called "fiber-optic," they have no actual optical "fibers," so a more appropriate term would be "fiber-lit." Glass fibers conduct light more efficiently but cost significantly more than bulb-on-blade light sources.

Bulb-on-blade designs (sometimes referred to as conventional blades) have a simple "screw on" electrical connection between the bulb socket on the blade and the handle (with enclosed batteries). This connection is very robust and less subject to malfunction than the spring-loaded, on-off lights used with bulb-on-handle systems. The removable bulbs can usually be replaced if they fail. This feature confers the risk that the bulb can become loose and may flicker during operation, or worse yet, become dislodged and lost into the patient.[24,25] To eliminate this risk, some manufacturers fuse the bulb to the blade rendering the bulb nonreplaceable.

Laryngoscope bulbs for both designs are of several types: incandescent filament (tungsten with halogen gas), xenon gas, and light-emitting diodes (LED). The bulb itself can have either a frosted or clear lens and may incorporate a reflector (common with bulb-on-handle designs).

Compared to other light-producing systems, LED bulbs produce brilliant light while using very little energy, operate with less heat, and have a much longer life span, thereby eliminating bulb replacement as a major concern. The light from LED bulbs tends to be whiter and bluer than traditional bulbs. LED lights can now be produced at a lower cost than other bulbs and have become the predominant mode of light on contemporary intubation devices (VLs, mirror laryngoscopes, chip-on-stick complementary metal oxide semiconductor imaging devices, etc.).

Disposable blades commonly use a light-conducting bundle made of plastic, whereas in nondisposable fiber-lit blades fiber bundles are usually made of glass. In the United States, any blade or handle that uses fiber illumination has a green dot on the blade base and a green circle at the top of the handle (commonly referred to as a "green-line handle"). These fiber-lit blades and handles are not interchangeable with conventional bulb-on-blade handles or blades.

The light intensity produced by curved laryngoscopes has also been found to vary according to design, with German fiber-illuminated blades producing the highest luminance, followed by English and then American bulb-on-blade designs. In one study of emergency department laryngoscopes, there was a 500-fold difference in light output between the best and worst blade-handle combinations.[26]

Regardless of the type of light, the intensity of light reaching the point of view depends on the distance the light must travel. This phenomenon is governed by the inverse square law of physics: if the distance from the light source to an object is doubled, the resultant amount of light energy reaching the object is reduced to one-quarter of the original amount. Thus saying, blade designs with shorter light-to-tip distances create more intense light at the point of interest. This distance produces substantial variability in the amount of light emitted by different laryngoscopes. The light-to-tip distances of German and English blades (median 51 mm and 47 mm, respectively) are significantly shorter than that of American blades (65 mm).[27]

Power Sources

Every laryngoscope requires a power source to activate the light. Direct laryngoscopes are generally self-contained and comprise batteries in the handle to store electrical energy. Traditional alkaline batteries are inexpensive and freely available but have a gradually declining discharge curve which, as illumination declines below a certain level, will result in compromised or ineffective laryngoscopy. Lithium batteries have a much flatter, higher discharge curve than alkaline batteries, but fail precipitously once the energy output falls below a certain threshold. Lithium batteries are much more expensive and tend to generate more heat than alkaline batteries.

Some manufacturers, especially those producing high quality fiber-lit blades, offer nickel-metal-hydride rechargeable battery systems, which produce very intense light when combined with a xenon bulb and glass fibers. While the light output from these high-end fiber-lit systems is impressive, they are very expensive.

Newer LED technology with low energy requirements has the potential to rival the light output of the aforementioned systems at a fraction of their cost and is offered in a single-use, disposable, bulb-on-blade design.

Few clinical settings monitor the light output objectively. Lighting standards in dentistry or surgery recommend 5000 lux.[28] While there is no well-accepted standard for the laryngoscopes, the International Organization for Standardization has suggested 700 lux as a minimum light output for laryngoscopes.[29]

BIOMECHANICS AND OPTICS

■ What Optical and Biomechanical Considerations Are Important for Direct Laryngoscopy?

DL is a procedure designed to overcome inherent visual and biomechanical restrictions. The visual restrictions include the variable ability of mouth opening, the teeth, the tongue, the long axis view down a laryngoscope blade, and the structures about the laryngeal inlet that surround the glottic opening. Biomechanical challenges involve employing the best way to move each visual restriction, and an awareness of how different anatomic elements react to the movement of adjacent structures. Each element of the anatomy of the airway between the mouth and glottis must be recognized sequentially as they are exposed along this restricted visual space. In many instances, only a small posterior portion, if any, of the glottic opening may be visible. The ETT itself may add to the visual challenge if it obstructs the view of the glottis, so must be manipulated with this in mind. A high level of comfort and familiarity with laryngeal and surrounding anatomy, and all of its variations, is of utmost importance for the practitioner in order to recognize the sequence and appearance of structures as they come into view, and to be aware of how visual obstructions and biomechanics impact on laryngeal exposure and tube delivery.

■ How Can I Best Maximize Mouth Opening and Jaw Distraction During Direct Laryngoscopy?

Mouth opening in the anesthetized or unresponsive patient (although it often occurs with the head and neck positioning described in the following text), can be achieved by simply pushing the chin in a caudad direction or by employing the cross-fingered or "scissors" technique, with the thumb of the right hand pushing the mandible or lower teeth downward, while the crossed index finger pushes against the upper teeth. As previously mentioned, optimal laryngoscopy requires the introduction of the laryngoscope blade into the right corner of the mouth. While a paraglossal approach is absolutely essential with a straight blade, with little if any part of the tongue visible to the right of the blade, even with a curved blade, midline placement of the blade must be avoided to prevent "tongue flop" on each side of the blade.

The amount of mouth opening possible is a function of jaw distraction, and head and neck positioning. Positioning that facilitates jaw distraction and mouth opening is important in all patients, but especially so in the obese. Supine patients without cervical spine (c-spine) immobilization or known cervical pathology are optimally positioned for laryngoscopy when the external auditory meatus and sternal notch are horizontally aligned when viewed from the patient's side (see Figure 52.2 in Chapter 52). This is called "ear-to-sternal notch" or "ramped position"

The traditional "sniffing position" is created by a combination of neck flexion and head extension at the atlanto-occipital joint a position that a person would assume leaning forward to sniff at a rose. Although the "sniffing position" if often espoused, ear-to-sternal notch positioning usually requires of 8 to 10 cm of elevation under the occiput, generally far more head elevation than that produced by the standard "sniffing" position. Ear-to-sternal notch positioning also forces one to objectively, using external landmarks, manipulate variations in the anatomy of the head and neck. These anatomical variations are most frequently encountered in individuals who are obese, in which case a ramp may need to be several feet high and incorporate support under the upper torso and shoulders as well as the head to align the ear with the sternum. While achieving this position optimizes laryngoscopy, it also improves gas exchange mechanics.

When performing laryngoscopy with the patient supine, along with ear-to-sternal notch positioning, the face plane of the patient should be parallel to the ceiling (see Figure 52.2 in Chapter 52). A common error is over-extending or tilting the head backward.[4] Atlanto-occipital extension alone may push the base of tongue and epiglottis against the posterior hypopharyngeal wall, making recognition of the epiglottis more difficult upon blade insertion narrowing the space available to pass the laryngoscope and restricting laryngeal exposure. Extension alone may also create tension on the anterior neck muscles opposing simultaneous efforts to open the mouth and distract the jaw.

Successful laryngoscopy requires that the patient's head be below the practitioner's xiphoid process. so that the practitioner can still increase head elevation dynamically during laryngoscopy if laryngeal exposure is inadequate.[30] Dynamic head elevation can be very difficult in the morbidly obese, so these patients must be ramped into a proper "ear-sternum" position in advance (see Figure 52.2 in Chapter 52). A well ramped patient may, after correct positioning, slide down the ramp slightly, flexing the atlanto-occipital joint and decreasing the sniffing position, so the position should be rechecked before introduction of the laryngoscope.

■ What Is the Optimal Position for Laryngoscopy in Patients with Known or Suspected Cervical Spine Injury?

DL has been shown to be safe in patients with known or suspected c-spine injury, There has been considerable attention and controversy regarding airway management in the known or presumed c-spine injured patient;[31–34] randomized controlled trials are generally absent, and documented evidence in support of cervical immobilization is limited, while there is a growing body of evidence and opinion against the practice.[34] The benefit of cervical collars in trauma has recently been questioned[35] and arguments have been made that manual in-line stabilization (MILS) leads to unnecessary delay in managing the trauma airway, a decision which in some cases could result in increased morbidity and mortality (e.g., hypoxemia and/or hypercarbia in head injured patients).[34] Concerns about a potential delay in appropriate management of trauma victims has caused advanced trauma life support to back away from an earlier recommendation that C-spine imaging should precede airway management. Furthermore, there is little evidence to support secondary spinal cord injury directly attributable to airway management.[31,32,36] The major priority in managing suspected c-spine injured patients is to safely optimize view on laryngoscopy. Indicated airway management should not be delayed in fear of causing secondary spinal cord injury.

Despite evidence that MILS does not completely prevent c-spine motion, and may increase intubation failure rates,[33] it remains a recommendation at this time. So saying, the current "standard of care" suggests that in this scenario laryngoscopy should preferably be performed with MILS after the removal of a cervical collar (see Chapter 17).[37,38] Ear-to-sternal notch positioning should be avoided in patients in whom c-spine injury might be suspected. Properly performed MILS will reduce the incidence of an epiglottis only view to 22%.[39] When applying MILS, care should be taken to ensure application of MILS in a manner that mouth opening is not limited this is achieved by the assistant performing stabilization placing the hands over the patient's ears (ear-muff approach) and away from the mandible.[40,41] Mouth opening is markedly limited with a collar in place where epiglottis only views (or worse) can occur in more than 60% of cases,[42] so the front of a cervical collar should be removed in order to permit jaw distraction. It is also helpful to drop the foot end the stretcher while keeping the stretcher straight (i.e., "Reverse Trendelenberg"), which improves pulmonary mechanics and positions the airway higher than the stomach so may prevent passive regurgitation. An assistant should maintain MILS throughout the process of laryngoscopy and intubation, with the collar replaced until unstable c-spine injury has been excluded.

Research comparing intubation devices have revealed no convincing superiority of any device over well-performed DL in terms of limiting c-spine motion[37] or success with intubation in patients with suspected c-spine injury receiving MILS (although direct Macintosh laryngoscopy was found to be inferior to seven other devices when methods other than MILS—usually cervical collars, were employed).[43] The use of alternative devices, such as flexible bronchoscope devices, optical stylets or VL may help overcome a challenging view,[44] although simple maneuvers, such as the application of optimal external laryngeal manipulation[45] (OELM or BURP, backwards upwards rightwards pressure[46]) and the use of an ETI (commonly referred to as a "gum elastic bougie") are equally effective in managing the airway in a trauma patient with a suspected c-spine injury.[37]

How Should the Laryngoscope Be Gripped to Minimize Effort and Maximize Fine Control of the Blade Tip?

The mechanics of laryngoscopic technique differ between curved and straight blades. The curved blade tip is guided into vallecula to depress the underlying hyoepiglottic ligament,

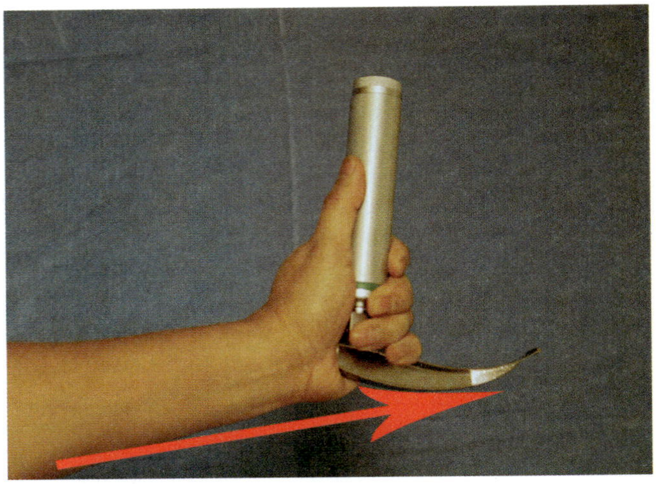

FIGURE 9.8. Laryngoscope grip: Both curved and straight blade handles should be gripped with the tips of the fingers where the handle meets the proximal blade. The handle should be gripped low enough that the blade is essentially an extension of the forearm.

lifting the epiglottis forward, and pulling it toward the blade and away from the glottic inlet. The tip of the straight blade classically lifts the epiglottis directly, closing the vallecula. Both curved and straight blade handles should be gripped with the tips of the fingers where the handle meets the proximal blade. (Figure 9.8). The handle should be gripped low enough so that the blade is essentially an extension of the forearm. Holding the handle higher (as one would hold a hammer) increases the length of the lever arm requiring significantly more muscular effort. When properly gripped with the thumb pointing upward on the handle, fine control and effective mechanical advantage are achieved, and levering on the upper incisors is less likely to occur. Laryngoscopy is a delicate procedure, dependent on the gentle positioning of vector forces at the blade tip. When properly positioned, the amount of force required for most patients is minimal and can be achieved by a light grip. When the blade tip is not correctly positioned, excessively forceful lifting is unlikely to correct the problem.

Another way to maximize lifting efficacy with minimal muscular effort is to keep the left elbow adducted to your side (roughly the anterior axillary line), rather than pointing outward. With the elbow in, the handle gripped down low, the forearm is kept straight, and body weight can be applied to the arm by tightening axillary muscles used to rock forward slightly so that minimal arm strain occurs. Force is efficiently transferred along the forearm and down the long axis of the blade.

How Do We Visualize the Larynx During Direct Laryngoscopy and Optimize Ocular-Laryngeal Distance?

Contrary to popular belief and traditional instruction, even with the arm extended, it is not possible to see the larynx during laryngoscopy with both eyes.[47] This is due to the inherent visual restrictions of DL, created by the opening of the mouth, the teeth, the tongue, the laryngoscope blade itself, and the structures of the laryngeal inlet. Visually, DL can be compared to looking down a narrow pipe at a target the size of a quarter, from a distance of 14 to 16 in.

Both eyes can be opened during the procedure but sighting of the larynx is performed with the dominant eye only; the brain subconsciously blocks out the nondominant image through a process called "binocular suppression." The same phenomenon occurs when looking through a peep-hole in a door, or when sighting during target sports. In situations without visual restriction, the right and left eyes have slightly different perspectives on an object, due to the distance separating the eyes in the skull. These slightly disparate views are fused into a single stereoscopic image. The visual restrictions encountered during laryngoscopy make it that this stereoscopic sight cannot be achieved. Because binocular suppression occurs subconsciously, even experienced practitioners may not be aware of which eye they use to sight the larynx.

The monocularity of laryngeal sight during laryngoscopy is evident when viewing novice practitioners attempting laryngoscopy for the first time by noting a subtle side-to-side head rotation, intermittently sighting the target with one eye and then the other.

The old adage that "experienced practitioners maintain a distance from the target, while novices climb into the mouth" is due not to experience but rather restrictions on accommodation that occur with age. By the mid-forties, the near visual accommodation point begins to move out approximately 2 to 3 cm per year, by the mid-fifties regardless of your underlying acuity, presbyopia results in the near focus point being at about arm's length. Accommodation in younger practitioners is more flexible to focus on near objects. Age related accommodation changes are exacerbated by low light conditions. The amount of light needed for laryngoscopy by the same practitioner is different at age 40 versus age 50 or 60; more light improves the near focus ability significantly and is another reason for using laryngoscope systems with good light output.

Is It Beneficial to Identify Ocular Dominance, Acuity, and Accommodation Distance in Trainees and How Is This Done?

Ocular dominance, visual acuity, and accommodation are important elements of laryngoscopy, and an awareness of our limitations (and, if needed, correction) in this regard can be useful for the laryngoscopist. It is a good idea to assess these at the start of procedure training and in practitioners on the steep curve of presbyopia (mid-forties).

Ocular dominance is tested by having the practitioner perform DL on a training mannequin. After the practitioner confirms that the larynx is sighted, instruct them to keep their head still. Selectively cover each eye, individually. When the nondominant eye is covered the laryngeal view is not compromised; when the dominant eye gets covered the larynx will no longer be sighted (or it will be seen partially, off angle). One cannot change one's natural ocular dominance. Eyedness tends to follow handedness assuming there is equal acuity, and since majority of the population is right-handed, most practitioners are also right-eyed. Persons who have a difference in visual acuity (wear lenses), or are left-handed, have a greater likelihood of being left-eyed when it comes to laryngoscopy.

Identification of ocular dominance, formal visual acuity, and accommodation testing is valuable to the trainee to proactively prevent procedural performance problems. Notwithstanding severe visual acuity problems, most accommodation issues can be addressed by corrective lenses. Many practitioners have corrective lenses made for driving, or reading, and not designed for the procedural distance of laryngoscopy. The proper procedural distance for a given practitioner is between their reach at full extension, and forearm reach with the elbow flexed at 90 degrees. For most practitioners this is about 14 to 16 in (35-40 cm). Corrective lenses become a valuable aid to DL in most practitioners by their mid- to late-forties.

DIFFICULT DIRECT LARYNGOSCOPY—ASSESSMENT AND PREDICTION

What Factors Contribute to Difficult Direct Laryngoscopy?

Difficult DL can result from two different issues: (1) problems with landmark recognition; and (2) mechanical problems that prevent laryngeal exposure.

Landmark recognition is made more difficult in the presence of blood, secretions, vomitus, or distorted anatomy from a number of pathologies. Successful laryngoscopy requires recognition of the epiglottis, the structures of the laryngeal inlet and the vocal cords, and glottic openings. The epiglottic mucosa is very similar to that of the posterior hypopharynx even without the additional distraction of fluids, vomitus, or distorted anatomy. Fluids from the oropharynx and hypopharynx may collect above the epiglottis when a patient is positioned in a supine position with poor muscular tone (or after the use of muscle relaxants), which can easily cause failure to recognize the edges of the epiglottis as the blade is inserted. Elevation of the epiglottis out of the fluids by proper jaw distraction during the first phase of laryngoscopy, which is, in turn, a function of proper head and neck position, and avoidance of over-extension is important. Because fluids are often present in the airway, an effective suction (Yankauer or other) should always be immediately available.

Mechanical problems that can limit laryngeal exposure often result from sub-optimal patient positioning as discussed above. Even with good positioning, causes of mechanical difficulties include limited mouth opening, prominent dentition and overbite, a large tongue relative to the pharynx (i.e., the Mallampati score), short thyromental distance (a small displacement volume for the tongue), and limitations of neck mobility. Although great effort has been put into devising scoring systems for predicting difficult laryngoscopy, the clinical utility of such screening tests remains very limited, particularly in emergency situations. Only about one in three emergency patients about to undergo intubation can follow simple commands permitting even a basic screening assessment. Emergency patients with the poor muscular tone, lying in a supine position, will almost universally have a poor Mallampati score and a short thyromental distance. Compounding theses are those with suspected c-spine injury because they cannot undergo neck mobility testing.

As reviewed by Yentis,[48] it is statistically challenging to devise an effective screening test, or combination of tests, for detecting a rare outcome (failed laryngoscopy), and a systematic review of over 20,000 patients concluded that current bedside tests have limited and inconsistent capacity to discriminate between patients with difficult and easy airways.[49] The trachea of a vast majority of patients can be successfully intubated with DL, and unless a screening test has extremely high specificity (which will be more likely to "miss" cases), most predicted failures will be false positives. Conversely, some patients who would be predicted to be easy may be difficult or impossible because laryngoscopy primarily involves interaction with tissue not visible to external inspection (the base of the tongue and epiglottis, for example lingual tonsillar hypertrophy).

While it is important to be attentive to factors that can contribute to difficulty screening performs poorly, so regardless of the difficulty predicted, practitioners should always prepare for difficulty, planning a means of rescue gas exchange and rescue technique should DL and/or face-mask ventilation prove difficult or impossible.[50] Fortunately, newer developments in alternative effective options for intubation, and rescue ventilation (especially the laryngeal mask airway [LMA]) have quieted much of the historic concern about difficult laryngoscopy.

Given the effectiveness of these rescue options, and evidence of an association between poor outcomes and the number of intubation attempts,[51] failures of the first two to three attempts should be considered an indication that the patient is "difficult" to intubate, and alternate methods of ensuring oxygenation should be employed. Thus saying, efforts at DL should be limited to a maximum of three or fewer attempts, depending on the practitioner's experience.

How Is Direct Laryngoscopic View Articulated and How Is This Clinically Relevant?

Laryngeal exposure is only one step in the sequence leading to successful intubation. It is possible to have an excellent laryngeal view and still be unable to intubate the trachea as can occur, for example, with tracheal stenosis. Conversely, an epiglottis-only view can sometimes be easily intubated with an ETI on the first attempt without a direct view of the glottis.

To assist with laryngoscopy research and documentation, different systems have been created for reporting the laryngeal view achieved. The original system of grading laryngeal view was developed by Cormack and Lehane (CL).[52] The CL categorizes laryngeal exposure into 4 grades, each describing the laryngeal components visualized (Table 9.1).

Grade 1 describes a view where all of the vocal cords/glottic openings are visible; a grade 2 view reveals only part of the glottis (depending on external laryngeal pressure, part of the vocal cords and/or arytenoids may be in view). A grade 3 view only demonstrates the superior surface of the epiglottis, while in a grade 4 view no landmarks are recognized.[52] Some researchers have subdivided grades 2 and 3 of the CL system into 2A and 2B, and 3A and 3B, respectively. A 2A view reveals at least a portion of the vocal cords, while 2B shows the arytenoid cartilages only. A 3A view is one where the epiglottis is able to be lifted off the posterior hypopharynx, compared to a 3B view where the epiglottis remains touching the posterior wall (Figure 9.9).[53] This difference in the position of the epiglottis in grade three views is important; a posteriorly directed epiglottis creates a relatively more anterior glottic inlet that will not be easily accessed using an adjunct such as an ETI. A moderate degree of interobserver and intra-observer variability with this scoring system is known to exist.

A more statistically useful method of reporting laryngeal view is the Percentage of Glottic Opening (POGO) Score, which is a numerical value from 0% to 100%.[54] A full 100% POGO score would be a full view of the glottic opening from the anterior commissure of the vocal cords to the interarytenoid notch between the posterior cartilages. This system better distinguishes between CL grades 1 and 2, which make up the vast majority of cases, but makes no distinction between CL 3 and 4, both of which have a POGO score of 0.

Adnet et al.[55] proposed an Intubation Difficulty Scale (IDS) (Table 9.2), which retrospectively incorporates laryngeal view as well as other aspects of intubation. They proposed an IDS score that is a function of seven parameters, resulting in a progressive, quantitative retrospective determination of intubation complexity. The score was intended to be used to compare the difficulty of intubation under varying circumstances by isolating variables of interest.

There are numerous challenges when applying grading systems of laryngoscopy or intubation to patients. Fundamentally, the effectiveness of the procedure relies heavily on the skill and ability of the practitioner. A grade 3 CL view or difficult intubation employing Adnet's scoring system may be a grade 1

TABLE 9.1. Cormack and Lehane Grading System

Cormack and Lehane Grade	Description of Grade View	Sub-Grade Description of View (and Notes)
Grade 1	All of the vocal cords/glottic opening	(POGO 100%)
Grade 2	Only the posterior aspect of the glottis including the arytenoid cartilages	2A view—at least some of the vocal cord (POGO > 0%) 2B view—the arytenoid cartilages only (POGO = 0%)
Grade 3	Epiglottis-only	3A view—epiglottis is able to be lifted off the posterior hypopharynx 3B view—epiglottis remains touching the posterior wall
Grade 4	No landmarks recognized	Most commonly an esophageal view

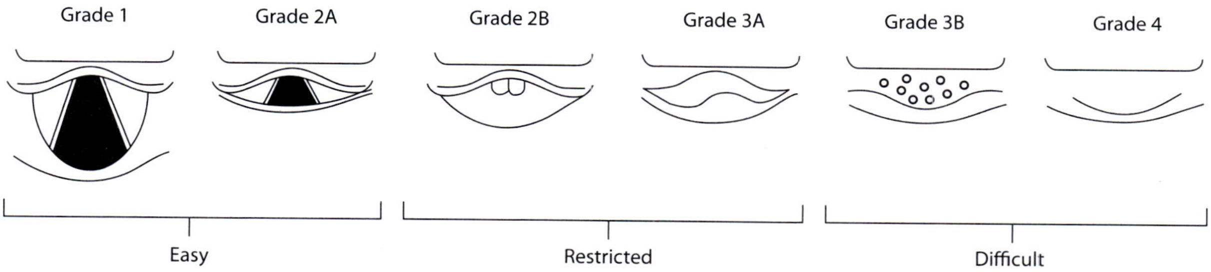

FIGURE 9.9. Modified Cormack and Lehane grading system of laryngoscopic view. (Reproduced with permission from Cook TM. A new practical classification of laryngeal view. *Anaesthesia*. 2000;55(3):274-279.)

view and an easy intubation, respectively, in a different practitioner's hands.

Direct laryngoscopic view and endotracheal intubation is not an objective, easily graded diagnostic 'test', such as Blood pressure measurement or cancer staging. Not only does the practitioner's technique impact dramatically on the result, but the performance is routinely graded from the practitioner's unique perspective, and therefore cannot be objectively assessed by other persons. DL is dynamic, with the larynx transiently visualized for 5 to 15 seconds, and sighted by only one eye of the practitioner. Even if it was possible to capture what the practitioner was or is actually seeing during DL and evaluate the performance, this would still only capture the procedural performance of one practitioner and one event.

PREPARING FOR LARYNGOSCOPY—OPTIMIZING CONDITIONS

What Is "Optimal Laryngoscopy" and How Should the Practitioner Prepare to Achieve This?

"Optimal laryngoscopy" refers to a combination of the proper equipment, a preplanned laryngoscopy strategy, and ideal patient conditions that collectively create optimal conditions for laryngeal exposure and first-pass intubation success (Table 9.3).

Available equipment must include functioning suction (e.g., Yankauer), oxygen delivery devices, and a well-functioning laryngoscope with optimal illumination. Tube delivery requires stylets and appropriately sized tubes, along with a means of managing an epiglottis-only view (e.g., ETI). Optimal laryngoscopy includes preparation for failure, thus oral and nasal airways, and an appropriately sized extraglottic rescue device (e.g., LMA®), as well as an alternative device for intubation, should all be immediately available.

The importance of proper positioning of the patient, as described, for both ventilation and DL, cannot be overstated. Not only will ventilation be more effective in the ear-to-sternal notch position, but it will lengthen the time to oxygen desaturation.[57–59] Different methods of denitrogenation have been suggested to extend apnea time,[60] including having a cooperative patient take eight vital capacity breaths, or tidal volume breathing for 3 to 4 minutes using high flow oxygen via a bag-mask device. It must be remembered that in some patients, such as younger pediatric patients, and patients with morbid obesity or critical illness, oxygen utilization is increased while reserves may be diminished.[61] Oxygen desaturation will occur rapidly following apnea in these patients, requiring early mechanical ventilation, often before adequate intubation conditions (muscle relaxation) are achieved.[62] Assisted ventilation in patients with low baseline saturation is indicated during the preintubation phase, as the risk of aspiration following gastric insufflation in carefully applied face-mask ventilation (FMV) is much less than the risk of oxygen desaturation in the critically ill patient. Denitrogenation will maximize safe apnea times to allow maximally achievable time for laryngoscopy and intubation.

While historically there has been debate about the indications for muscle relaxants outside of the operating room, there is no doubt that laryngoscopy is easier, more successful, and performed more quickly, and with fewer attempts when relaxants are used. The use of muscle relaxants offers two other very significant advantages. It eliminates the risk of active vomiting during laryngoscopy, and it permits the use of rescue ventilation

TABLE 9.2. The Seven Parameters of the Intubation Difficulty Scale[55]

Intubation Difficulty Scale
• The number of attempts
• The number of operators
• The number of techniques (or devices)
• Cormack Lehane view grade
• Lifting force
• Need for external laryngeal manipulation
• Position of the vocal cords (abducted/adducted)

TABLE 9.3. The "Optimum Laryngoscopic Attempt" Was Characterized by Benumof as Possessing 6 Factor"[56]

Characteristics of an "Optimum Laryngoscopic Attempt"
Most skilled individual
Best paralysis
Best position
Best laryngeal manipulation
Best laryngoscope blade type
Best laryngoscope blade length

devices (i.e., LMA) should laryngoscopy fail. In emergency patients with full stomachs and short apnea times, these advantages may be important.

Is There a Role for Decompression of the Stomach Prior to Emergency Laryngoscopy, and What Should We Do When a Nasogastric Tube Is Already in Place?

Patients with known bowel obstruction, significant GI bleeding, and perhaps patients who have received prolonged assisted FMV (e.g., long prehospital course), are at significant risk of passive regurgitation (see Chapter 5). For these reasons, it may be helpful to decompress the bowel as much as possible before muscle relaxation and laryngoscopy.

Sellick recommended evacuating the stomach with a gastric tube and then removing the tube before induction of anesthesia.[63] Others demonstrated no difference in the incidence of regurgitation with or without a nasogastric tube.[64] It is the opinion of the authors that the nasogastric tubes should if placed, remain *in situ* for the intubation.

ANATOMIC CONSIDERATIONS, LARYNGOSCOPY TECHNIQUE, AND TROUBLESHOOTING (VIDEO 22)

What Is "Epiglottoscopy" and Why Is It Important When Performing Laryngoscopy?

"Epiglottoscopy" emphasizes the importance of visualizing the epiglottis prior to exposing the larynx and was one of Chevalier Jackson's basic rules of laryngoscopy.[4] As an anatomic landmark the epiglottis has a unique importance to laryngoscopy for numerous reasons.

As the organ that closes the laryngeal opening to protect the lungs from aspiration during routine swallowing, the epiglottis is a prominent indicator of the position of the glottis and, attaching to both the tongue and the larynx, forms the bridge between the first anatomic landmark (the tongue) and the goal (the larynx). The "relational anatomy," between the tongue, epiglottis, and larynx remains a constant despite person-to-person anatomic and pathologic variations. The epiglottis is connected to the base of the tongue at the vallecula. It also forms the most superior aspect of the laryngeal inlet, the ring of structures that encircles the glottic opening, which comprises the epiglottis, the paired aryepiglottic folds, the paired posterior cartilages, and the interarytenoid notch. Within the laryngeal inlet lies the glottic opening and vocal cords. The epiglottis also acts as a marker for the midline.

What Can Make the Epiglottis Hard to Visualize?

As stated earlier, the mucosa of the epiglottis is identical to that of the posterior pharyngeal wall. In a supine position, with poor muscular tone, or after the administration of muscle relaxants, the jaw and base of the tongue falling backward and the epiglottis lies against the posterior pharynx. Depending upon head and neck position, and the manner in which the laryngoscope is directed, it is easy to advance past the epiglottis as it is camouflaged against the pharynx. Over-extension of the head at the atlanto-occipital joint moves the base of the tongue and epiglottis backward, making the situation worse, as do secretions, blood, and vomitus.

To overcome the camouflage of the epiglottis and make the epiglottis edge distinctly visible, it is necessary to distract the jaw effectively and lift the base of the tongue. Keeping the face plane horizontal to the floor and elevating the head to achieve an ear-to-sternal notch position (if possible), permits optimal jaw distraction.

What Is the Best Method for Controlling the Tongue and How Does Tongue Control Integrate with Epiglottoscopy?

Effective control of the tongue is probably the most important factor in DL, with subtle, yet important differences in technique when using a curved or straight blade.

Tongue Management: Curved Blade Laryngoscopy

When managing the tongue with a curved blade, the curve of the blade conforms to the shape of the superior aspect of the tongue, while the large reverse Z-shaped flange allows the tongue to be swept to the left. To avoid the thick chest or breasts, particularly in patients with a short neck, many practitioners prefer to insert the blade with the handle tilted sideways toward the right and insert the blade into the mouth in a slight right lateral position. A potential problem with this approach is that the epiglottis and the larynx are then approached "off angle" and, depending upon the depth of insertion, this can create landmark confusion. The aryepiglottic fold can be misinterpreted as the epiglottis edge, and if inserted too deeply the tip of the blade will pass under the posterior cartilages into the esophagus.

With the patient's face plane parallel to the ceiling, the authors prefer to follow the curve of the blade down the curve of the tongue, slightly to the right of the midline, with early compression/lift of the tongue as necessary to visualize the epiglottis edge. In this first stage of laryngoscopy, only a gentle force is required to distract the jaw caudad, lifting the epiglottis edge off the posterior pharyngeal wall. The direction of the handle upon insertion and with initial jaw distraction is toward the patient's feet, and at a very shallow angle as the blade is advanced down the tongue (perhaps only ~20 degrees up from horizontal). Inexperienced practitioners will commonly place the blade tip too far, before looking for landmarks. This is particularly common when using a longer blade (e.g., #4 Macintosh blade). After the epiglottis has been recognized, and before the tissue is engaged with greater force, the practitioner should check tongue position and move the blade rightward as necessary to effectively control the tongue. In practice, epiglottoscopy and tongue control happen simultaneously.

Tongue Management: Straight Blade Laryngoscopy

As mentioned earlier, when using a straight blade, any amount of tongue positioned to the right of the blade will make target visualization and tube delivery difficult. The small flange height, especially of some Miller designs, prevents any ability to sweep the tongue, and practitioners should resist the attempt to do so. Proper position of a straight blade is achieved by deliberately directing the blade into the right paraglossal space,[36] with the proximal portion of the blade lateral to the patient's right nostril and the entire tongue to the left of the blade. The distal blade may then be directed medially, although the proximal blade should never be brought back toward the upper incisors or midline. The blade should be inserted adjacent to the right lateral oral commissure and over the molar dentition. The medially directed distal blade may then engage the epiglottis, with the proximal blade being kept close to the lateral oral commissure, away from the midline. Helpful techniques include directing the patient's nose about 20 degrees to the left and/or asking an assistant to retract the lateral oral commissure slightly using their little finger.

How Can Sequential Recognition of Landmarks Make Direct Laryngoscopy More Predictable?

From the insertion of the blade until visualization of the larynx the practitioner should visualize a predictable, sequential series of landmarks that results from the progressive advancement of the LOS. As a laryngoscope blade is advanced over and down the surface of the tongue, into the pharynx and then the hypopharynx, the LOS moves from the uvula to the posterior pharynx, and then at the base of the tongue, to the epiglottis.

With the curved blade, the epiglottis is indirectly elevated (suspended by the blade tip), while with the straight blade, the epiglottis is directly lifted. Once the epiglottis is visualized, the practitioner knows where the larynx is located. Effective epiglottis control (either indirectly with a curved blade, or directly with a straight blade) will then permit progressive exposure of the anticipated laryngeal landmarks.

The structures of the larynx become visible from the most posterior to the most anterior. The most posterior laryngeal structures, and the first visible under the epiglottis edge, are the interarytenoid notch and the accompanying right and left arytenoid cartilages. Above the interarytenoid notch, and just medial to the arytenoid cartilages, is the posterior aspect of the glottic opening. Moving more anteriorly, the aryepiglottic folds are visible laterally, and the true and false vocal cords medially. Finally, the most anterior and farthest within the laryngeal inlet, is the anterior commissure of the vocal cords.

What Are the Subtleties and Troubleshooting Tips of Curved Blade Laryngoscopy?

The effectiveness of indirect epiglottis elevation hinges on the proper placement of the blade tip in the vallecula as well as correctly directing force down the blade. Following epiglottoscopy, the tip of the blade needs to be fully advanced into the vallecula and the lifting force increased compared to that which was needed for distracting the jaw to visualize the epiglottis. The force is directed along the forearm and down the blade, in a manner that the practitioner's arm and forearm are extended away from their torso. The handle should not be tilted

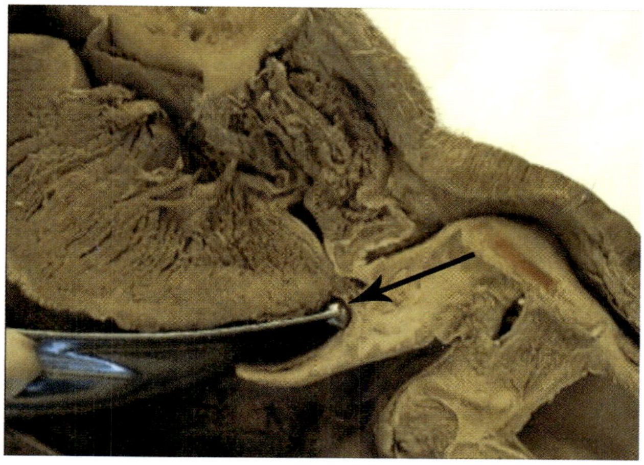

FIGURE 9.10. Direct laryngoscopy with a curved Macintosh laryngoscope in a sagittal section of a cadaver: the tip of the blade should be placed into the vallecula and the resulting pressure on the hyoepiglottic ligament (arrow) will cause the epiglottis to indirectly elevate.

backward, lest the tip of the blade rise out of the vallecula resulting in inadequate engagement of the underlying hyoepiglottic ligament. With the force directed down the blade (i.e., the force vector approximately perpendicular to the practitioner) the tip of the blade can be gently driven into the vallecula and the resulting pressure on the hyoepiglottic ligament will cause the epiglottis to be indirectly lifted (Figure 9.10).

If the tip of the blade is not fully seated into the vallecula engaging the hyoepiglottic ligament (which essentially suspends the epiglottis), no amount of lifting force will correctly elevate the epiglottis. Even a few millimeters difference in blade tip placement will affect the degree of epiglottic control. Fine control of the tip is one of the primary causes of skill/experience-based variations in the ability to attain a laryngoscopic view. One way to help seat the blade tip correctly is the performance of bimanual laryngoscopy.[65] The free right hand of the practitioner can reach around to the anterior neck of the patient and apply external manipulation to the thyroid cartilage with a downward (backward, posterior) force.

It may help to think of the tip of the blade as a key being inserted into the lock of the vallecula. Bimanual laryngoscopy serves to fully insert the key all the way into the lock, which will then allow turning (elevating the epiglottis) and "opening" the larynx. In some cases, bimanual laryngoscopy may be best at the cricoid cartilage, or even the hyoid, although Benumof found that optimal manipulation was at the thyroid cartilage in almost 90% of cases.[45] The practitioner needs not to be concerned about the exact position of the right hand. There is instantaneous visual feedback about the effectiveness of epiglottis elevation, and it is easy to move the right hand slightly up or down on the patient's neck to optimize the view.

Bimanual laryngoscopy improves laryngeal view in two ways. First, it changes the mechanics as described, correctly sitting the blade tip where it needs to be. Second, it helps to move the larynx downward (backward) into the practitioner's LOS. The mobility of the larynx and the ability of the practitioner to move it backward into view during the procedure was something known even to Czermark in the mid-nineteen century when mirror laryngoscopy was first developed. Early wood block prints of Czermark performing mirror laryngoscopy show one hand on the patient's neck while his other hand holds the mirror within the mouth.[4]

A critical component of bimanual laryngoscopy is the direct practitioner connection between neck manipulation and the immediately observed effect on the laryngeal view. Cricoid pressure (as discussed in the following text) and BURP[46] involve an assistant applying pressure to the neck. Given the subtlety of laryngoscopy, and that minor changes in blade tip position or force can significantly alter exposure and epiglottis control, bimanual laryngoscopy performed by the practitioner him/herself (referred to by some as OELM) is the most effective means of optimizing laryngeal view.[45] An assistant can be taught to maintain pressure at this location while the practitioner uses the right hand to pass the ETT.

The term "bimanual laryngoscopy" has also been used to describe two other techniques whereby the right had can be used to improve laryngeal visualization; one is a technique where the left hand manipulates the laryngoscope while the right hand is placed behind the occiput to manipulate the head and neck position to obtain the best view of the glottis, and the other is using the right hand to assist the left hand called "two handed laryngoscopy." For the latter, once a view has been attained, it can normally be sustained by wedging the left elbow into the lower left abdomen, while the right hand is freed to manipulate the tube or ETI.

How Do "Optimal External Laryngeal Manipulation" and Cricoid Pressure (the "Sellick Maneuver") Differ (See Chapter 5)?

In 1961, Sellick described backward pressure on the cricoid ring done by an assistant as a method of preventing passive regurgitation of stomach contents during elective anesthesia.[63] It has become a standard part of emergency laryngoscopy and rapid sequence induction and intubation (RSI). It seemed logical that pressure on the cricoid could occlude the esophagus and that this is advantageous in full stomach or aspiration prone patients.

Recent evidence regarding the ability of cricoid pressure to reduce the risk of aspiration and whether it should be a standard part of emergency laryngoscopy has cast doubt on the utility of the procedure (see a detailed discussion in Chapter 5). Smith and colleagues, imaging the neck with CT and MRI, established that although some compression of the esophagus occurred with Sellick's maneuver,[66,67] lateral displacement of the esophagus occurred in 91% of patients when cricoid pressure was applied. In a study with awake adult volunteers using MRI, Rice et al.[68], however, found that the mean anteroposterior diameter of the hypopharynx was reduced by 35% and the lumen likely obliterated with cricoid pressure, and this compression was maintained even when the cricoid ring was lateral to the vertebral body. These findings suggest that the location of the esophagus is not relevant to the efficacy of the cricoid pressure with regard to the prevention of gastric regurgitation into the pharynx and that there is no reason to suggest that traditional practice be abandoned.

Even considering the findings of Rice et al.,[68] another reason for re-evaluating the need for cricoid pressure is the knowledge that ventilation parameters and patient positioning have changed dramatically since Sellick conceived his technique. With regard to patient positioning, Sellick believed that cricoid pressure would only work if the head and neck were placed in hyperextension in order to pin the esophagus between the cricoid and the vertebrae.[63] He further advocated that the head be in a head-down position, so that should any regurgitation recur, the material could drain out and not into the lungs.[63] These hyperextended head and neck positions, with the head down, are antithetical to what we now know is optimal for effective ventilation and maximizing upper airway patency.

Regarding the risk of regurgitation as a result of insufflation of the stomach, ventilation volumes in Sellick's time averaged 10 to 15 $mL \cdot kg^{-1}$ with ventilation rates of 12 to 15 breaths per minute, which would be expected to cause frequent and significant diversion of air delivered under positive pressure into the stomach. Current practice is to use much smaller ventilation volumes (6-7 $mL \cdot kg^{-1}$) and higher ventilation rates to reduce the risk of exceeding esophageal opening pressure (25-30 cm H_2O), reducing the baseline risk of gastric insufflation and regurgitation.

Laryngeal manipulation (BURP or bimanual laryngoscopy) should not be confused with cricoid pressure. Cricoid pressure is usually done by an assistant rather than the practitioner and it is not primarily intended to improve laryngeal exposure. It is also applied lower on the neck than laryngeal manipulation. If initiated upon induction (before blade insertion), cricoid pressure may prevent the blade tip from being correctly seated in the vallecula. Recent evidence has identified that the application of cricoid pressure may increase the incidence of a difficult emergency laryngoscopy (grade 3 or 4 Cormack and Lehane view)[52]. A growing body of literature has highlighted the detrimental effects of cricoid pressure on laryngoscopy, face-mask ventilation, and LMA placement although it has yet to demonstrate an increased problem with gas exchange or intubation failure rates.[69,70]

In summary, recognizing the paucity of definitive data, the question of whether Sellick's maneuver should be used has not been definitively answered. It seems reasonable to continue with the practice of applying cricoid pressure in patients where the benefit of an attempt to prevent aspiration is considered higher than the risk of that effort hindering laryngoscopy.

Apart from Paraglossal Placement, What Are the Specifics of Correctly Performing Straight Blade Laryngoscopy?

Many of the specifics of straight blade laryngoscopy have already been discussed, i.e., paraglossal placement, and use of the extreme right corner of the mouth for blade positioning, tilting, and tube delivery. However, there is a critical aspect of straight blade laryngoscopy that needs to be addressed which is the direct lifting of the epiglottis.

After the epiglottis edge is identified, the handle must be tilted forward (e.g., the tip backward, toward the posterior hypopharynx), the blade inserted slightly (approximately 1-2 cm), and the tip passed under the epiglottis. Once the epiglottis is "trapped" under the blade tip, the blade is rocked slightly backward (handle brought slightly more upright) and then the lifting force increases. Jackson described the lifting direction as suspending the patient's head with the flat section of the blade, at a point underneath the hyoid bone.[4]

Miller blades have an upturned distal tip that varies among manufacturers. This renders the distal blade tip invisible to the practitioner when viewed down the channel of the blade. A potential problem with this design is that the practitioner does not know if the blade has been advanced far enough to trap the epiglottis until the blade is rocked backward; frequently the tip of the epiglottis is not trapped and the advancement and tilting maneuver needs to be repeated.

The Henderson blade is a novel straight blade design that has a deliberately visible distal tip. Underneath, within the barrel of the distal tip is a curled edge that is easily seen when the practitioner looks down at the blade (Figure 9.5). This allows the practitioner to place the tip under the epiglottis and know with certainty that the epiglottis is trapped.

OELM is helpful with straight blades because the posterior laryngeal pressure displaces the target into view.

In Addition to OELM, What Other Maneuvers Can Be Done During Laryngoscopy to Improve a Poor Laryngeal View?

Practitioners should understand and be ready to respond to poor laryngeal view within their first laryngoscopy attempt. There should be a specific planned approached to find the epiglottis and optimize blade tip position. In addition to OELM, and making sure that the curved tip is driven fully into the vallecula, another technique for improving an epiglottis-only view is to dynamically lift the patient's head higher. This technique, which the author has called "Head Elevated Laryngoscopy Positioning" (HELP and others have called "bimanual laryngoscopy"), was first described by Richard Johnston in 1909 and later adopted by Jackson and included in his subsequent textbooks.[3,4,71] As already noted, head elevation permits greater jaw distraction because of its mechanically favorable effect on mouth opening. It enlarges the area beneath the base of the tongue and epiglottis improving visualization. According to Jackson, exaggerated head elevation also better aligned the blade axis with the axis of the upper trachea and larynx.

The practitioner can perform head elevation by using their right hand to lift the patient's occiput, or an assistant can help by using two hands to lift the head from the patient's side. Some practitioners describe using their abdomen to lean forward and prop up and elevate the patient's head. In the morbidly obese patient, dynamic lifting is often not feasible given the weight involved, so a large ramp is required extending from under the occiput, to the upper shoulders, then tapering to the mid-low back, in order to provide proper positioning (see Figure 52.2 in Chapter 52). An inflatable ramp has been designed for this purpose for airway management in the morbidly obese, called the Rapid Airway Management Positioner.[72] A noninflatable version is called the Troop Pillow.

Regardless of which lifting technique is used, the patient's stretcher height must be kept low enough to permit head elevation and yet still provide a good perspective for the practitioner to look down the mouth into a patient whose face plane is parallel to the ceiling. For some practitioners, especially when dealing with larger patients, this may require a footstool for the practitioner to be at the proper height.

What Are the Most Common Errors of Direct Laryngoscopy by Novices?

The three most common errors that novice practitioners make during laryngoscopy include:

1. Placing the blade too deep before looking (not performing sequence-directed epiglottoscopy)
2. Entering the vallecula and lifting without engaging the hyoepiglottic ligament
3. Not using their right hand (bimanual laryngoscopy, OELM, BURP, HELP) to optimize the view

Novice practitioners move right past the epiglottis, insert the blade tip too deep, and then cannot recognize any laryngeal structures. Instead of recognizing that a grade 4 view is usually a view of the esophagus, and slowly withdrawing the blade under vision, they persist in looking around at that depth, and then give up at once, pulling out before realizing their position. Novices typically try to transfer their practice experience from an intubation trainer to an actual patient and find recognition of structures very difficult. This occurs because of unrecognized visual restrictions, epiglottis camouflage, and insufficient understanding of the nuances of laryngeal anatomy. They also may not appreciate how minor manipulative adjustments of the blade tip affects laryngeal exposure, instead resorting to extra lifting effort or levering. Their response to a poor laryngeal view is to move the blade in and out with large movements, leading to edema, tissue trauma, bleeding, and possibly perforation of the upper esophagus or hypopharynx. The best way to avoid landmark confusion is to be meticulous about anatomy recognition and epiglottoscopy.

Novice practitioners should carefully study video imaging of DL prior to practicing on real patients paying particular attention to the nuances of anatomy and technique. The visual restrictions inherent to DL make targeted feedback and supervision during the procedure impossible. With intensive video training, novice practitioners can achieve a 90% success rate on their first ten attempts, while initial success rates with standard mannequin-only training are low (50%).[73] Following mannequin-only practice, a statistical modeling showed that the number of laryngoscopic intubations required to achieve a 90% success rate in anesthetized patients with a normal airway in an operating room environment was 47.[74]

Are There Specific Patients, Apart from Small Children, in Whom Curved Blades Perform Poorly or in Whom a Straight Blade Would Be the First Choice?

Patients who have lingual tonsillar hyperplasia have excess tissue at the base of the tongue often blocking the vallecula from vision or from blade placement, making epiglottoscopy very difficult. This is a rare condition, but can lead to unexpected failed laryngoscopy, since the base of the tongue and epiglottis are not visible during preprocedural assessment. There are case reports of such patients being able to be intubated using a paraglossal straight blade technique.[75] If the condition was known in advance, it would be prudent to avoid DL altogether since it could prevent laryngeal exposure with a laryngoscope and potentially also lead to very difficult face-mask and LMA ventilation.

Laryngoscopy of patients with large central dental gaps may be complicated by the large flange on the curved blade locking into the gap creating a very restricted space for tube delivery. In such instances, an ETI can be very helpful, or alternatively, a straight blade can be used with a paraglossal approach.

Large or protruding incisors may make curved blade laryngoscopy difficult because of the restricted space between the upper and lower incisors to introduce the blade. Vulnerable incisors as a result of poor dentition, are also more likely to sustain damage from a curved blade. A straight blade, introduced over the molars as described above, may help avoid this problem.[36]

ENDOTRACHEAL TUBE PLACEMENT

What's the Role of Placing a Stylet Inside an Endotracheal Tube to Assist Placement?

Tube delivery is a separate and distinct challenge from laryngeal exposure as the tube has to travel from the mouth to the glottis and may need manipulation to enter the trachea. Polyvinyl chloride (PVC) ETTs are produced with a gentle arcuate shape, as prescribed by the American Society of Testing of Materials standards. The standard tube also has an asymmetric tip, with the bevel of the tube facing leftward when viewed from the practitioner's perspective ("Magill bevel"), down the long axis of the tube, as the tube is inserted into a patient.

The optical challenges of DL have already been described. When there is favorable laryngeal exposure, tube delivery is rarely problematic. Conversely, when only a small portion of the glottic opening is visible, or even just the interarytenoid notch can be seen, tube delivery may obscure simultaneous visualization of the target.

The large curvature of standard PVC ETTs (or those prepackaged with a matching arcuate-shaped stylet) is difficult to maneuver in the mouth and hypopharynx. They have a wide side-to-side dimension when viewed down the long axis, increasing the likelihood of the tube contacting the sides of the mouth, tongue, and teeth. As efforts are made to direct the tip upward, for example, the mid-section of the tube will contact the teeth, causing bending of the mid-section of the tube. The other problem with an arcuate-shaped tube is that minor rotational change will cause the distal tip to move substantially. When this occurs at the last moment of insertion toward the target, the mid-section of the tube may visually block the target itself, leading to the inadvertent and unseen passage of the tube into the esophagus. The "floppiness" of the PVC may be corrected to a large extent by a malleable stylet, which increases the ability for the end of the tube to be manipulated. Simply maintaining the standard curvature, however, will not fix the problems of wide dimension and rotational tip movement mentioned above.

Many instruments designed to be passed into narrow body cavities have a narrow long-axis dimension and an upward distal turn. Instruments that adhere to this shape include alligator forceps, laryngeal mirrors, and ETI. The optical benefit of this shape is that the long straight section allows good maneuverability toward a target, while the upturned distal tip makes the tip of the device visible. For this reason, it is recommended that the stylet is manipulated to provide a straight tube with a distal upturn at the proximal edge of the cuff. This "straight-to-cuff" shaped tube -stylet combination has a narrow long axis and offers significant visual advantages over the natural curve of the tube, or a tube with an arcuate-shaped stylet.[26,76] When viewed down the long axis it has a narrower dimension, and can be passed into the mouth and easily maneuvered without obscuring the target as it is advanced. The ideal method of inserting an ETT is to always pass the tube from beneath the LOS, and bring the distal tube tip up from below, passing over the interarytenoid notch under direct vision without obscuring the glottic target itself. Many practitioners prefer using a styletted tube for all tracheal intubations because of this maneuverability and visualization advantage. When the tube is first inserted in the extreme right corner of the mouth, the tube is placed visually behind the maxilla and the distal tip is not even seen. By rocking the proximal tube backward, the distal tip moves posteriorly from behind the maxilla, up into the LOS, and anteriorly, until it is placed above the posterior landmarks of the larynx and into the trachea.

What Is the Ideal "Straight to Cuff" Position?

The historic approach to stylet shaping was to use a "hockey stick," with the optimal bending point, and the proper angle not being clearly defined. A more precisely termed "straight-to-cuff" stylet shape recommends that the stylet should hold the tube in a straight line up to the proximal end of the cuff, where it should be bent at an angle not exceeding 35 degrees, from where it runs straight to the tip.[77] This narrow long-axis shape is ideal for tube delivery toward the glottis, without blocking the LOS, providing enough of a bend upward to allow the distal tube tip to be easily seen. The end of the stylet should not protrude beyond the distal end of the cuff, allowing the distal tip to retain some softness.

Angles beyond 35 degrees confer no visual advantage and hinder maneuverability within the mouth and hypopharynx, and can cause the tip of the tube to impact on the anterior tracheal rings after the tip has passed the glottis.[77] This phenomenon explains why it is possible to have a correctly sized tube between the vocal cords yet the tube resists passing down into the trachea, even though the trachea itself is large enough to accept it.

What Should the Practitioner Do if the Tube Tip Catches in the Cricothyroid Space or on the Tracheal Rings After Insertion?

If the tip of the tube gets lodged in the anterior tracheal rings or cricothyroid space, several maneuvers can help facilitate its advancement. One option is to ask an assistant to withdraw the stylet a few inches without withdrawing the tube itself, while the practitioner continues to hold the tube and laryngoscope, maintaining the view of the glottis. The reduction of the stiffness of the distal tube will usually allow it to advance down the trachea. This maneuver can result in dislodgement of the tube with resultant esophageal intubation on advancement, so control of the tube and view of the glottis should be protected as far as possible.

Another option to rectify this mechanical hang-up on the anterior tracheal wall is to rotate the tube clockwise (anterior side to the right) when resistance is felt. By turning the tube 90 degrees clockwise the left-facing bevel of the ETT moves from facing leftward to facing upward. The leading edge of the tube rotates downward, away from the rings, and the flat bevel will slide along the anterior trachea, disengaging the hang-up.[26]

If time permits, Hung et al.[78] have suggested the combination of softening of the ETT by immersing the ETT in warm saline solution and "reverse loading" of the ETT onto the stylet may potentially overcome the problems with the "hang up" during intubation. With the reverse loading, (bending the angle on the tube in the opposite direction to the natural curve of the tube) the tip of the ETT is more likely to be directed down the trajectory of the trachea, as it recovers its natural curve during the retraction of the stylet, which pulls it away from the anterior tracheal rings, making it easier to advance.

What Are the Options for an Epiglottis-Only View?

Assuming every effort has been made to maximize laryngeal view with the laryngoscope, there are several options for intubation. The first of these is to slide the tip of the tube along the undersurface of the epiglottis with the straight-to-cuff styletted tube, and being mindful of the tip orientation (keeping it upright), to insert the tube blindly into the area where, anatomically speaking, the glottis should be. In general, however, this is not consistently reliable, so blind insertion should be avoided.

Another excellent option for intubation in epiglottis-only views is to use an ETT introducer (ETI) can be used. Several inexpensive disposable ETI are available. The ETI is approximately 60 cm long, straight over its entire length, except for its distal end, which has a slight upward bend (Coude tip). The original Portex product (made of resin covered fiberglass) has a bend angle of 38 degrees and this angle has been copied in the many disposable tracheal introducers now produced.

When compared with the use of a stylet in simulated Cormack and Lehane grade 3 views, the success rate using this device is as high as 98% with the ETI and 87% using a stylet.[79]

In the true epiglottis-only view, the tip of the ETI is directed upward stroking the undersurface of the epiglottis. Practitioners should be aware that minor rotational changes will cause the tip to move laterally to the aryepiglottic fold (missing the larynx). After the tracheal introducer has passed into the trachea, the anterior tracheal rings may be felt (clicks) as the rounded tip passes over them. This occurs in 60% to 95% of cases, but it is practitioner and situation dependent, and also a function of the orientation of the distal tip. If the tip rotates downward after insertion, the tip will ride along the posterior membranous portion of the trachea and not pass over the rings (i.e., no tactile feedback of tracheal placement). In the trachea, as the tip passes beyond the mainstem bronchus, the narrowing diameter will cause it to stop after advancing between 30 and 35 cm. This distinct endpoint is more reliable in assessing tracheal placement. On reaching this endpoint, the tracheal introducer should be pulled back by 2 to 3 cm. When the tracheal introducer is placed into the esophagus, no rings are felt, and there should be no limit to advancement as it curls up in the stomach.

After tracheal introducer placement, the ETT is placed over the proximally stabilized tracheal introducer (by an assistant) and slid down ("railroaded") its length into the mouth and ultimately the trachea. The laryngoscope should be maintained in the same position as was achieved during the initial laryngoscopy attempt. This promotes a long axis slide of the ETT over the tracheal introducer, and protects the advancing tube from obstruction by the tongue. Without the laryngoscope, the tracheal introducer will bend in the pharynx and be surrounded and pushed on by adjacent soft tissues which can cause difficulties with tube advancement. The gap between the beveled leading edge of the larger diameter ETT and the ETI can "holdup" at the laryngeal inlet (right aryepiglottic fold, right arytenoid cartilage, or right vocal cord) as the tube is advanced over the tracheal introducer. This is less likely when a smaller ETT is used. This holdup is easily managed by turning (quarter turn) the ETT counter clockwise as it approaches the laryngeal inlet. This maneuver positions the bevel facing inferiorly, allowing uninhibited passage into the trachea.

It is important to note that there is a major difference between the Cormack and Lehane grade 3A and 3B—the latter being the situation where the epiglottis is visible but lies against the posterior hypopharyngeal wall. In this situation the tracheal introducer is not likely to be stiff enough to lift the epiglottis and it becomes more difficult to direct it into the glottis. The true incidence of this view is not known, and as stated earlier, may relate to improper blade tip placement deflecting the epiglottis posteriorly, so the first maneuver when encountering a 3B view is to ensure that the blade tip is correctly placed in the vallecula; too far can push the epiglottis down, while too proximal will not suspend the epiglottis enough.

SUMMARY

Placement of a tracheal tube under direct vision using a laryngoscope remains one of the most important skills to master for all airway practitioners. Many types of laryngoscopes with curved and straight blades have been developed over the years with the objectives to improve visualization of the glottis and easy passage of the tracheal tube. While these devices are highly effective and safe, they all have limitations that require troubleshooting, and in certain situations specific tools should be avoided. Overall, the successful and safe use of DL requires attention to basic principles and techniques.

SELF-EVALUATION QUESTIONS

9.1. Regarding the mechanics of laryngoscopy all are true **EXCEPT**:

A. A fully extended arm position permits binocular sighting of the larynx for most practitioners.

B. A low grip, i.e., where the blade meets the handle, provides greater control with less muscular effort.

C. Morbidly obese patients require proper ear-to-sternal notch positioning before laryngoscope insertion, since dynamic lifting of the head during the procedure may be impossible.

D. The degree of lifting force applied during laryngoscopy is minimal when advancing the curved blade down the tongue and maximal after the blade is correctly positioned in the vallecula.

9.2. Bimanual laryngoscopy is:

A. Distinct from cricoid pressure because it is applied by the practitioner

B. Distinct from cricoid pressure because it is done to improve laryngeal view

C. Distinct from Backward Upward Rightward Pressure (BURP) because it is done by the practitioner, not an assistant

D. Distinct from cricoid pressure because it is generally applied at the thyroid cartilage, not the cricoid ring

E. All of the above

9.3. The mechanical problem rail-roading an endotracheal tube over a tube introducer (or a flexible bronchoscope):

A. Can be overcome by rotating the tracheal tube counterclockwise (leftward) 90 degrees at 14 to 16 cm of insertion

B. Is a consequence of the asymmetric left-facing bevel of a standard tracheal tube

C. Is due to the gap between the outer diameter of the introducer (or scope) and the inner diameter of the tracheal tube

D. Occurs at the laryngeal inlet, specifically at the right aryepiglottic fold and right posterior cartilages

E. All of the above

REFERENCES

1. de Carvalho CC, da Silva DM, Lemos VM, et al. Videolaryngoscopy vs. direct Macintosh laryngoscopy in tracheal intubation in adults: a ranking systematic review and network meta-analysis. *Anaesthesia*. 2022;77:326-338.
2. Brodnitz FS. One hundred years of laryngoscopy: to the memory of Garcia, Tuerck and Czermak. Trans Am Acad. *Ophthalmol Otolaryngol*. 1954;58:663-669.
3. Zeitels SM. Universal modular glottiscope system: the evolution of a century of design and technique for direct laryngoscopy. *Ann Otol Rhinol Laryngol Suppl*. 1999;179:2-24.
4. Jackson C. *Bronchoscopy and esophagoscopy. A manual of peroral endoscopy and laryngeal surgery*. Philadelphia, PA: W. B. Saunders;1922.
5. Magill IW. Technique in Endotracheal Anaesthesia. *Br Med J*. 1930;2:817-819.
6. Miller RA. A new laryngoscope. *Anesthesiology*. 1941;2:318-320.
7. Macintosh RR. A new laryngoscope. *Lancet*. 1943;1:205.
8. Borland LM, Casselbrant M. The Bullard laryngoscope. A new indirect oral laryngoscope (pediatric version). *Anesth Analg*. 1990;70:105-108.
9. Smith CE, Sidhu TS, Lever J, Pinchak AB. The complexity of tracheal intubation using rigid fiberoptic laryngoscopy (WuScope). *Anesth Analg*. 1999;89:236-239.
10. Niforopoulou P, Pantazopoulos I, Demestiha T, Koudouna E, Xanthos T. Video-laryngoscopes in the adult airway management: a topical review of the literature. *Acta Anaesthesiol Scand*. 2010;54:1050-1061.
11. Chisholm DG, Calder I. Experience with the McCoy laryngoscope in difficult laryngoscopy. *Anaesthesia*. 1997;52:906-908.
12. Haridas RP. The McCoy levering laryngoscope blade. *Anaesthesia*. 1996;51:91.
13. Johnston HM, Rao U. The McCoy levering laryngoscope blade. *Anaesthesia*. 1994;49:358.
14. Laurent SC, de Melo AE, Alexander-Williams JM. The use of the McCoy laryngoscope in patients with simulated cervical spine injuries. *Anaesthesia*. 1996;51:74-75.
15. Uchida T, Hikawa Y, Saito Y, Yasuda K. The McCoy levering laryngoscope in patients with limited neck extension. *Can J Anaesth*. 1997;44:674-676.
16. Ward M. The McCoy levering laryngoscope blade. *Anaesthesia*. 1994;49:357-358.
17. Burkle CM, Zepeda FA, Bacon DR, Rose SH. A historical perspective on use of the laryngoscope as a tool in anesthesiology. *Anesthesiology*. 2004;100:1003-1006.
18. McIntyre JW. Laryngoscope design and the difficult adult tracheal intubation. *Can J Anaesth*. 1989;36:94-98.
19. Gerlach K, Wenzel V, von Knobelsdorff G, Steinfath M, Dorges V. A new universal laryngoscope blade: a preliminary comparison with Macintosh laryngoscope blades. *Resuscitation*. 2003;57:63-67.
20. Kelley MA, Boskovich S, Allegretti PJ. Laryngoscope blade review. *Am J Emerg Med*. 2008;26:952-955.
21. Cheung KW, Kovacs G, Law JA, Brousseau P, Hill W. Illumination of bulb-on-blade laryngoscopes in the out-of-hospital setting. *Acad Emerg Med*. 2007;14:496-499.
22. Harlow M, Kovacs G, Brousseau P, Law JA. An in vitro assessment of light intensity provided during direct laryngeal visualization by videolaryngoscopes with Macintosh geometry blades. *Can J Anaesth*. 2021;68:1779-1788.
23. Malan CA, Scholz A, Wilkes AR, Hampson MA, Hall JE. Minimum and optimum light requirements for laryngoscopy in paediatric anaesthesia: a manikin study. *Anaesthesia*. 2008;63:65-70.
24. Delport SD, Gibson BH. Ingestion of a laryngoscope light bulb during tracheal intubation. *S Afr Med J*. 1992;81:579.
25. Naumovski L, Schaffer K, Fleisher B. Ingestion of a laryngoscope light bulb during delivery room resuscitation. *Pediatrics*. 1991;87:581-582.
26. Levitan RM, Kinkle WC. *The Airway Cam Pocket Guide to Intubation*. 2nd ed. Wayne, PA: Airway Cam Technologies; 2007.
27. Levitan RM, Kelly JJ, Kinkle WC, Fasano C. Light intensity of curved laryngoscope blades in Philadelphia emergency departments. *Ann Emerg Med*. 2007;50:253-257.
28. America IESoN. *Recommended Practice: Lighting Hospital and Healthcare Facilities*. New York, NY: IES; 2020.
29. Standardization. ECf. Anaesthetic and Respiratory Equipment – Laryngoscopes for Tracheal Intubation. 2020. Available at https://www.iso.org/obp/ui/#iso:std:iso:7376:ed-3:v1:en
30. Levitan RM, Mechem CC, Ochroch EA, Shofer FS, Hollander JE. Head-elevated laryngoscopy position: improving laryngeal exposure during laryngoscopy by increasing head elevation. *Ann Emerg Med*. 2003;41:322-330.
31. Manoach S, Paladino L. Manual in-line stabilization for acute airway management of suspected cervical spine injury: historical review and current questions. *Ann Emerg Med*. 2007;50:236-245.
32. Manoach S, Paladino L. Laryngoscopy force, visualization, and intubation failure in acute trauma: should we modify the practice of manual in-line stabilization? *Anesthesiology*. 2009;110:6-7.
33. Thiboutot F, Nicole PC, Trepanier CA, Turgeon AF, Lessard MR. Effect of manual in-line stabilization of the cervical spine in adults on the rate of difficult orotracheal intubation by direct laryngoscopy: a randomized controlled trial. *Can J Anaesth*. 2009;56:412-418.
34. Wiles MD. Manual in-line stabilisation during tracheal intubation: effective protection or harmful dogma? *Anaesthesia*. 2021;76:850-853.
35. Sundstrom T, Asbjornsen H, Habiba S, Sunde GA, Wester K. Prehospital use of cervical collars in trauma patients: a critical review. *J Neurotrauma*. 2014;31:531-540.
36. Henderson JJ. The use of paraglossal straight blade laryngoscopy in difficult tracheal intubation. *Anaesthesia*. 1997;52:552-560.
37. Crosby ET. Airway management in adults after cervical spine trauma. *Anesthesiology*. 2006;104:1293-318.

38. Gerling MC, Davis DP, Hamilton RS, et al. Effects of cervical spine immobilization technique and laryngoscope blade selection on an unstable cervical spine in a cadaver model of intubation. *Ann Emerg Med.* 2000;36:293-300.
39. Robitaille A, Williams SR, Tremblay MH, Guilbert F, Theriault M, Drolet P. Cervical spine motion during tracheal intubation with manual in-line stabilization: direct laryngoscopy versus GlideScope videolaryngoscopy. *Anesth Analg.* 2008;106:935-941.
40. Kovacs G, Sowers N. Airway management in trauma. *Emerg Med Clin North Am.* 2018;36:61-84.
41. Ollerton JE, Parr MJ, Harrison K, Hanrahan B, Sugrue M. Potential cervical spine injury and difficult airway management for emergency intubation of trauma adults in the emergency department—a systematic review. *Emerg Med J.* 2006;23:3-11.
42. Heath KJ. The effect of laryngoscopy of different cervical spine immobilisation techniques. *Anaesthesia.* 1994;49:843-845.
43. Singleton BN, Morris FK, Yet B, Buggy DJ, Perkins ZB. Effectiveness of intubation devices in patients with cervical spine immobilisation: a systematic review and network meta-analysis. *Br J Anaesth.* 2021;126:1055-1066.
44. Aziz M. Use of video-assisted intubation devices in the management of patients with trauma. *Anesthesiol Clin.* 2013;31:157-166.
45. Benumof JL, Cooper SD. Quantitative improvement in laryngoscopic view by optimal external laryngeal manipulation. *J Clin Anesth.* 1996;8:136-140.
46. Knill RL. Difficult laryngoscopy made easy with a "BURP." *Can J Anaesth.* 1993;40:279-282.
47. Levitan RM, Higgins MS, Ochroch EA. Contrary to popular belief and traditional instruction, the larynx is sighted one eye at a time during direct laryngoscopy. *Acad Emerg Med.* 1998;5:844-846.
48. Yentis SM. Predicting difficult intubation—worthwhile exercise or pointless ritual? *Anaesthesia.* 2002;57:105-109.
49. Vannucci A, Cavallone LF. Bedside predictors of difficult intubation: a systematic review. *Minerva Anestesiol.* 2016;82:69-83.
50. Shiga T, Wajima Z, Inoue T, Sakamoto A. Predicting difficult intubation in apparently normal patients: a meta-analysis of bedside screening test performance. *Anesthesiology.* 2005;103:429-437.
51. Mort TC. Emergency tracheal intubation: complications associated with repeated laryngoscopic attempts. *Anesth Analg.* 2004;99:607-613.
52. Cormack RS, Lehane J. Difficult tracheal intubation in obstetrics. *Anaesthesia.* 1984;39:1105-1111.
53. Cook TM. A new practical classification of laryngeal view. *Anaesthesia.* 2000;55:274-249.
54. Ochroch EA, Hollander JE, Kush S, Shofer FS, Levitan RM. Assessment of laryngeal view: percentage of glottic opening score vs Cormack and Lehane grading. *Can J Anaesth.* 1999;46:987-990.
55. Adnet F, Borron SW, Racine SX, et al. The intubation difficulty scale (IDS): proposal and evaluation of a new score characterizing the complexity of endotracheal intubation. *Anesthesiology.* 1997;87:1290-1297.
56. Benumof JL. Difficult laryngoscopy: obtaining the best view. *Can J Anaesth.* 1994;41:361-365.
57. Boyce JR, Ness T, Castroman P, Gleysteen JJ. A preliminary study of the optimal anesthesia positioning for the morbidly obese patient. *Obes Surg.* 2003;13:4-9.
58. Dixon BJ, Dixon JB, Carden JR, et al. Preoxygenation is more effective in the 25 degrees head-up position than in the supine position in severely obese patients: a randomized controlled study. *Anesthesiology.* 2005;102:1110-1115.
59. Lane S, Saunders D, Schofield A, Padmanabhan R, Hildreth A, Laws D. A prospective, randomised controlled trial comparing the efficacy of pre-oxygenation in the 20 degrees head-up vs supine position. *Anaesthesia.* 2005;60:1064-1067.
60. Benumof JL. Preoxygenation: best method for both efficacy and efficiency. *Anesthesiology.* 1999;91:603-605.
61. Benumof JL, Dagg R, Benumof R. Critical hemoglobin desaturation will occur before return to an unparalyzed state following 1 mg/kg intravenous succinylcholine. *Anesthesiology.* 1997;87:979-982.
62. Mort TC. Preoxygenation in critically ill patients requiring emergency tracheal intubation. *Crit Care Med.* 2005;33:2672-675.
63. Sellick BA. Cricoid pressure to control regurgitation of stomach contents during induction of anaesthesia. *Lancet.* 1961;2:404-406.
64. Satiani B, Bonner JT, Stone HH. Factors influencing intraoperative gastric regurgitation: a prospective random study of nasogastric tube drainage. *Arch Surg.* 1978;113:721-723.
65. Levitan RM, Kinkle WC, Levin WJ, Everett WW. Laryngeal view during laryngoscopy: a randomized trial comparing cricoid pressure, backward-upward-rightward pressure, and bimanual laryngoscopy. *Ann Emerg Med.* 2006;47:548-555.
66. Smith KJ, Dobranowski J, Yip G, Dauphin A, Choi PT. Cricoid pressure displaces the esophagus: an observational study using magnetic resonance imaging. *Anesthesiology.* 2003;99:60-64.
67. Smith KJ, Ladak S, Choi PT, Dobranowski J. The cricoid cartilage and the esophagus are not aligned in close to half of adult patients. *Can J Anaesth.* 2002;49:503-507.
68. Rice MJ, Mancuso AA, Gibbs C, Morey TE, Gravenstein N, Deitte LA. Cricoid pressure results in compression of the postcricoid hypopharynx: the esophageal position is irrelevant. *Anesth Analg.* 2009;109:1546-1552.
69. Ellis DY, Harris T, Zideman D. Cricoid pressure in emergency department rapid sequence tracheal intubations: a risk-benefit analysis. *Ann Emerg Med.* 2007;50:653-665.
70. Neilipovitz DT, Crosby ET. No evidence for decreased incidence of aspiration after rapid sequence induction. *Can J Anaesth.* 2007;54:748-764.
71. Johnston RH. Extension and flexion in direct laryngoscopy: A comparative study. *Ann Oto Rhino Laryn.* 1910;19:19-24.
72. Cattano D, Melnikov V, Khalil Y, Sridhar S, Hagberg CA. An evaluation of the rapid airway management positioner in obese patients undergoing gastric bypass or laparoscopic gastric banding surgery. *Obes Surg.* 2010;20:1436-1441.
73. Levitan RM, Goldman TS, Bryan DA, Shofer F, Herlich A. Training with video imaging improves the initial intubation success rates of paramedic trainees in an operating room setting. *Ann Emerg Med.* 2001;37:46-50.
74. Mulcaster JT, Mills J, Hung OR, et al. Laryngoscopic intubation: learning and performance. *Anesthesiology.* 2003;98:23-27.
75. Ovassapian A, Glassenberg R, Randel GI, Klock A, Mesnick PS, Klafta JM. The unexpected difficult airway and lingual tonsil hyperplasia: a case series and a review of the literature. *Anesthesiology.* 2002;97:124-132.
76. Levitan RM. *The Airway Cam Guide to Intubation and Practical Emergency Airway Management.* Wayne, PA: Airway Cam Technologies; 2004.
77. Levitan RM. Design rationale and intended use of a short optical stylet for routine fiberoptic augmentation of emergency laryngoscopy. *Am J Emerg Med.* 2006;24:490-495.
78. Hung OR, Tibbet JS, Cheng R, Law JA. Proper preparation of the Trachlight and endotracheal tube to facilitate intubation. *Can J Anaesth.* 2006;53:107-108.
79. Gataure PS, Vaughan RS, Latto IP. Simulated difficult intubation. Comparison of the gum elastic bougie and the stylet. *Anaesthesia.* 1996;51:935-938.

CHAPTER 10

Flexible Bronchoscopic Intubation

Jinbin Zhang

CASE PRESENTATION

A 78-year-old male presents for surgical fixation of an unstable cervical spine fracture. He weighs 50 kg and is 157 cm tall (BMI 20.3 $kg \cdot m^{-2}$). He has a history of ankylosing spondylitis and hypertension. On airway examination, his neck is immobilized in a hard cervical collar, but it is apparent that he has a significant fixed neck flexion; Mallampati III score; 2 cm mouth opening, full dentition and a receding mandible. He has predictors of difficult face-mask ventilation, difficult direct laryngoscopy, difficult video laryngoscopy, and difficult EGD use. Due to the presence of an unstable cervical spine injury and multiple predictors of a difficult airway, an awake bronchoscopic intubation was performed which was uneventful as was his subsequent surgery.

INTRODUCTION

How Did Bronchoscopic Intubation Develop?

The first recorded endoscopic tracheal intubation was reported by Murphy in 1967.[1] In that case report, the trachea of a patient with Still's disease was successfully intubated through the nose using a flexible choledochoscope.[1] The flexible bronchoscope using fiberoptic technology was first introduced into clinical practice in 1964 and although it was not developed for the purpose of airway management, its value as a device to facilitate endotracheal intubation was soon appreciated.[2,3] A series of 100 tracheal intubations using the flexible bronchoscope was reported in 1972, with a success rate of 96%.[4] However, utilization of flexible fiberoptic technology for endotracheal intubation remained limited among health care providers throughout the 1970s and 1980s.[5] Following the publication of the ASA Guidelines on Difficult Airway Management in 1993,[6] the use of flexible bronchoscopic intubation (FBI) among anesthesia practitioners greatly increased[7] and the technique has come to play a pivotal role in the management of patients with a difficult airway.[8] In a review of general anesthetics administered at a Canadian tertiary care center between 2002 and 2013, 1554 of the 146,252 (1.06%) intubations were performed awake and a flexible bronchoscope was used in 99.2% of these awake intubations.[9]

Surveys from the United States, France, and Denmark published between 1998 and 2003 confirm the widespread use of flexible bronchoscopes particularly for the management of the anticipated difficult airway.[10–14] A Canadian survey in 2013 revealed that 98% of respondents had performed awake FBI and 93% were comfortable with the technique. In addition, 91% had performed asleep FBI and 88% were comfortable with the technique. When presented with an unanticipated difficult intubation with failed direct laryngoscopy, 41% chose FBI as the first-choice alternative, whereas 90% chose a video laryngoscope.[15] Although it has been advocated as the technique of choice in the management of difficult intubation,[16–19] this view is not universally shared and a reluctance to perform awake bronchoscopic intubation continues to occur.[20,21] An American study reported a decreasing use of bronchoscopic intubation over 12 years ending in February 2013.[22] In 2011, the 4th National Audit Project (NAP 4) of the Royal College of Anesthetists and the Difficult Airway Society (DAS)[23] reported a failure to consider or employ awake bronchoscopic intubation as a first choice in difficult airway management when it was clinically indicated and that harm occurred as a result.

When Is Bronchoscopic Intubation Indicated?

The primary indication for awake bronchoscopic intubation is in the elective (or at least nonemergency) management of the anticipated difficult airway (Table 10.1). The difficult airway can be defined as one in which an experienced practitioner anticipates or encounters difficulty with any or all face-mask ventilation, direct or indirect (e.g., video) laryngoscopy and tracheal intubation, extraglottic device (EGD) use, or front-of-neck airway (FONA).[24] If difficult intubation after induction of general anesthesia (GA) is predicted with the practitioner's chosen device(s) and ventilation by face-mask or EGD is also predicted to be difficult, awake intubation should be strongly considered.[24,25] Contextual issues such as a predicted short safe apnea time, aspiration risk, and lack of skilled help may also favor an awake technique.[24] Although awake intubation can be performed using other devices or a combination of devices, awake intubation of the elective surgical patient will most often be performed using a flexible bronchoscope.[24] FBI continues to be the accepted standard in elective airway management of the awake spontaneously breathing patient with an anticipated difficult airway[25] and maintains a wide margin of safety.[26–28]

Radiation treatment for head and neck cancers can cause edema and fibrosis which can limit mouth opening and neck mobility and distort the submandibular space making direct laryngoscopy difficult or impossible.[29,30] Neck radiation is also a predictor of difficult video laryngoscopy, face-mask ventilation, EGD use, and FONA[24,31]; it is the most significant clinical predictor of impossible mask ventilation.[32] In a patient who has had neck radiation, awake bronchoscopic intubation can be an invaluable option.

Ludwig's Angina is a rapidly progressive cellulitis of the floor of the mouth usually caused by odontogenic infection.[33,34] Spread of the infection into the submandibular space produces edema and swelling which causes superior and posterior displacement of the tongue.[33] Infection in the submandibular space can extend into the lateral and retropharyngeal spaces and thus encircle the airway.[33,35] Pus accumulation can occur.[33] The swelling can involve the larynx and the infection can reach the mediastinum.[33] Neck movement can be restricted[33]; trismus can be severe and may not improve with neuromuscular blockade.[36] Although less advanced deep neck infection can be managed by antibiotics alone, true Ludwig's Angina typically requires definitive airway control and surgical drainage. Face-mask ventilation, EGD use, direct laryngoscopy, video laryngoscopy, and FONA can all be difficult.[36] Awake tracheotomy under local anesthesia has been considered the gold standard airway management in this setting, however awake FBI has also been used with a high success rate[37] and can be a feasible alternative.[35]

In the presence of airway trauma, FBI can permit precise evaluation of the injury, facilitate placement of an endotracheal tube (ETT) beyond the level of the injury, and has been said to be the method of choice for airway management in this setting.[29,38]

In the presence of potential cervical spine instability, no intubation technique has been shown to be clearly superior.[26,27,39–43] However, movement of the cervical spine must be minimized during intubation if neurologic injury is to be avoided. FBI can be a valuable alternative in this setting and has been extensively utilized.[40,44]

FBI can also be used in the unanticipated difficult airway as an alternative technique when intubation by a primary technique has failed but ventilation by face-mask or EGD is successful (can't intubate, but can oxygenate).[45–47] The flexible bronchoscope may also be the preferred device for intubation after induction of GA by practitioners who are

TABLE 10.1. Indications and Contraindications for Flexible Bronchoscopic Intubation

Indications	Contraindications
Anticipated difficult airway, such as: - History of difficult airway - History of neck irradiation for head and neck cancers - Head and neck infection, e.g., Ludwig's angina, - Airway trauma and burns Minimize neck movement in view of potential cervical spine instability	Absolute: - Patient refusal - Documented allergy to local anesthetics if awake intubation is planned Relative: - Uncooperative patient - Active bleeding and vomiting - Massive tissue disruption from trauma - High-grade airway obstruction - Immediate airway control is required
Unanticipated difficult airway: - Failed intubation, but able to oxygenate	

experts in its use.[46] However, NAP4 reported that bronchoscopic intubation under GA a was technically more difficult than in an awake cooperative patient due to loss of muscle tone leading to upper airway obstruction.[23] Bronchoscopic intubation was attempted in seven patients reported to the audit after induction of GA either as the primary technique or after failed direct laryngoscopy. The asleep bronchoscopic intubation failed in all seven patients and all seven required an emergency surgical airway.

In general, if airway compromise or respiratory distress exists, awake intubation maintains the widest margin of safety.[26] However, in this circumstance, the urgency with which airway control must be achieved and the extent of the airway compromise may limit the choice of technique, and bronchoscopic intubation may not be feasible or appropriate. In addition, incomplete topical anesthesia of the upper airway makes bronchoscopic intubation more difficult, as does the presence of blood and secretions in the airway. A decrease caliber in the upper airway following local anesthesia of the airway has been demonstrated even in normal subjects,[48–50] while complete airway obstruction has been reported following the topical application of local anesthesia to the airway in awake patients with a compromised airway.[20,51] As such, patients with severe airway obstruction due to edema or tumor must be approached with extreme caution if completion airway obstruction is to be avoided[3] and due consideration must be given to awake tracheotomy in this setting.[47]

When Is Flexible Bronchoscopic Intubation Best Avoided?

Contraindications to FBI must be considered relative and weighed against the risks associated with alternative airway management techniques (Table 10.1).[26] Some measure of patient cooperation is required for awake FBI, and the total absence of cooperation may preclude this technique, as can bleeding in the airway and massive tissue disruption.[3,26,47] Fixed laryngeal obstruction with stridor at rest implies a reduction in the caliber of the airway to 4.0 mm or less in diameter.[52] FBI is unlikely to be successful in this setting and at best will produce a higher grade of obstruction when the scope is passed through the involved area. In this setting, a surgical airway (e.g., awake tracheotomy) performed under local anesthesia is a better alternative.[53] FBI is contraindicated when immediate airway control is necessary and the time required to complete the procedure is not available.[7]

Patient refusal in the adult population without mental disorder is exceedingly rare if an appropriate explanation of the procedure has been provided.

EQUIPMENT

How Do Flexible Bronchoscopes Work? What Is the Best Instrument for Flexible Bronchoscopic Intubation?

The standard "adult" flexible bronchoscope remains unsurpassed as an instrument with which to perform bronchoscopic intubation in the vast majority of circumstances in the adult population. These bronchoscopes have a sufficient length (about 60 cm) to accommodate an ETT ensleeved proximally while leaving an adequate distal segment for maneuverability. A bronchoscope with an outside diameter of 5.9 to 6.0 mm will readily accommodate a 7-mm internal diameter (ID) ETT and has adequate stiffness to function well as a stylet over which to advance the ETT (see Figure 10.1).[26,54] Bronchoscopes with thinner insertion cords tend to be more flexible and form a floppy stylet that is easily buckled away from the glottis as the ensleeved ETT is advanced into the airway (see Figure 10.2).[27]

The flexible bronchoscope consists of a proximal handle and a distal insertion cord or shaft. An umbilical or universal cord is attached to the side of the handle and connects the bronchoscope to an external light source (see Figure 10.3). Modern flexible bronchoscopes include fiberoptic bronchoscopes, video bronchoscopes, and hybrid designs. Flexible bronchoscopes are also available with a battery-operated light source, which greatly

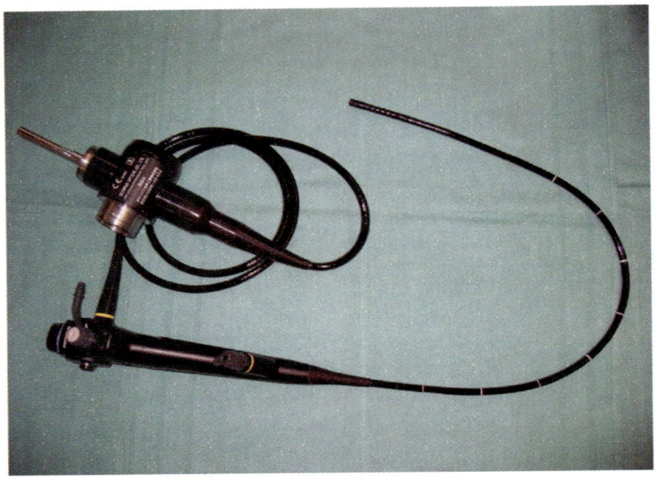

FIGURE 10.1. The adult flexible bronchoscope. An Olympus BF-XT160 is shown here with an insertion cord diameter of 6.3 mm and a length of 60 cm.

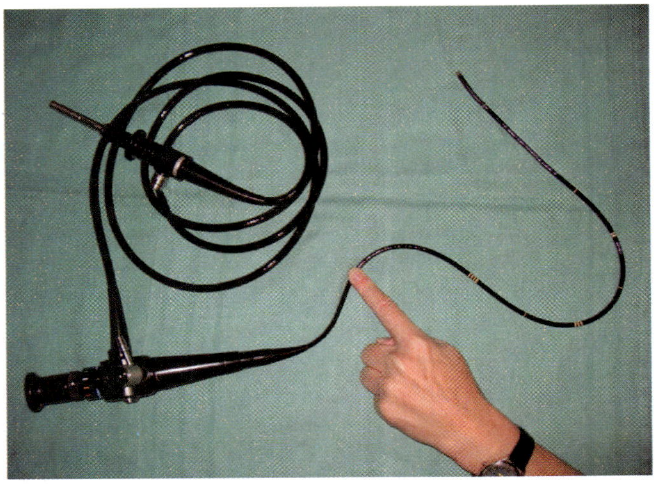

FIGURE 10.2. The "pediatric" flexible bronchoscope. An Olympus LF2 is shown here with an insertion cord diameter of 4 mm and a length of 60 cm. Note the increased flexibility of the thinner insertion cord.

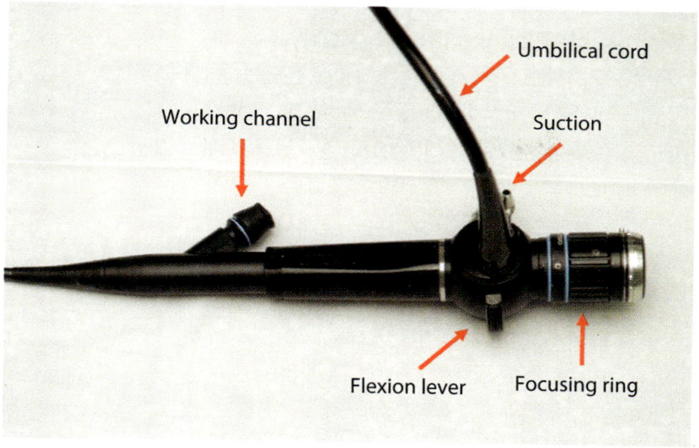

FIGURE 10.3. Features of the flexible bronchoscope: it consists of a proximal handle and a distal insertion cord or shaft. An umbilical or universal cord is attached to the side of the handle and connects the bronchoscope to an external light source. The handle also contains the proximal port of the working channel, a suction port, and the flexion lever.

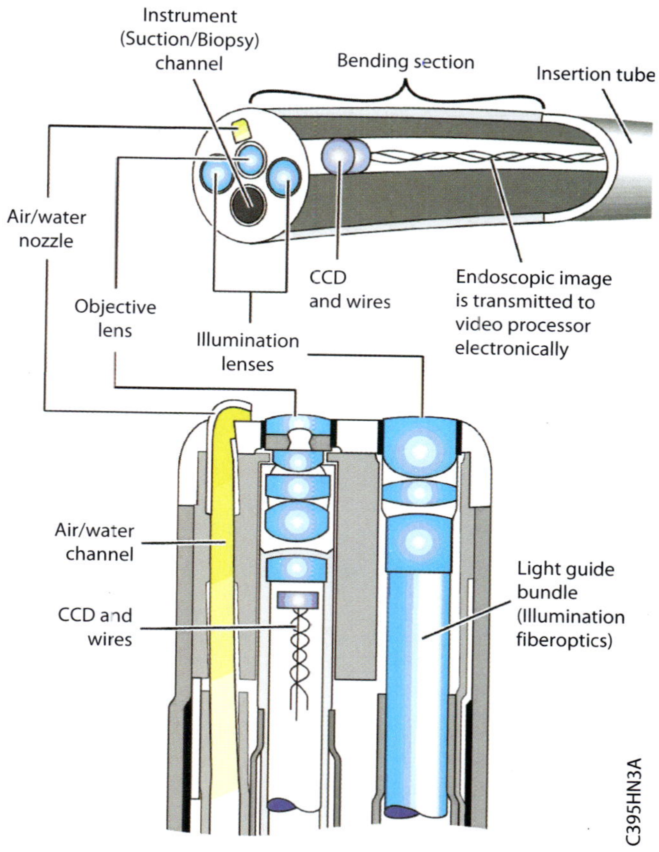

FIGURE 10.4. Schematic diagram of the insertion cord of a flexible videobronchoscope. (Reprinted with permission, Copyright 2017, ECRI Institute. Www.ecri.org. 5200 Butler Pike, Plymouth Meeting, PA 19462 610-825-6000.)

improves portability. The handle of the bronchoscope is fitted with a lever that controls the flexion of the tip of the scope (the bending section)[18] in a single plane (see Figure 10.3). The handle also contains the proximal port of the working channel which extends distally to the tip of the scope. This channel can be used to pass various instruments into the airway and can be used for irrigation, administration of medications, and suction. Over the years, fiberoptic bronchoscopes have been gradually replaced by video bronchoscopes which have superior optical quality. Readers interested in the mechanics of fiberoptic bronchoscopes can refer to the following references[18,55] for details. In the video bronchoscope, a charged coupled device or silicone chip is located at the distal tip of the insertion cord and is used to sense and transmit the image (see Figure 10.4). The image data are transmitted electronically through the bronchoscope to an external video processing unit. The image is then displayed on a screen and can be printed, stored electronically, or transmitted to a remote location. A video camera can be coupled to the eye piece of a conventional fiberoptic bronchoscope, however, the image obtained is inferior to that provided by the video bronchoscope.

Bronchoscopes are produced by a number of different manufacturers and are available with insertion cord diameters ranging from 2.2 to 6.3 mm. In general, minimizing the discrepancy between the outer diameter (OD) of the bronchoscope and the ID of the ensleeved ETT facilitates the passage of the tube through the larynx over the scope.[2,3,27,56–62] Bronchoscopes with smaller diameter insertion cords have allowed FBI to be performed in the pediatric population, and very thin scopes such as the Olympus BF-N_2O with a shaft diameter of 2.2 mm can be used in infants. However, the use of "pediatric" bronchoscopes to perform FBI of the adult, in general, makes the procedure more difficult.[27] The use of a pediatric bronchoscope to perform awake intubation in an adult with severe upper airway obstruction may be complicated by complete obstruction and must be approached with great caution.[3,20,53,63]

Flexible bronchoscopes with shaft diameters of 3.5 to 4.0 mm can readily be passed through the lumen of a #35-Fr or larger double-lumen tube and are invaluable for the precise tube placement required for lung isolation.

Bronchoscopes are delicate instruments and must be handled with care. Damage to the bronchoscope is not only costly to repair but it also means that the scope is unavailable for clinical use for a period of time. Striking the distal tip of the insertion cord against a hard surface or excessive bending or twisting of the shaft of the scope can damage the lens and fiberoptic bundles, respectively. If the external shaft of the insertion cord or the working channel wall is punctured, fluids can enter the inside of the scope and lead to a degradation or loss of the image transmitted.

Single-use flexible bronchoscopes are gaining popularity in recent years and their use is encouraged during global pandemics involving respiratory viruses.[64,65] Commonly used single-use bronchoscopes include the AMBU® aScope™ (Ballerup, Denmark), the C-MAC® Flexible Intubation Video Endoscope and Rhino-laryngoscope (FIVE S) (Karl Storz, Tuttlingen, Germany), and the GlideScope® Bflex™ (Verathon Inc, USA). The range of bronchoscopes includes a selection of channel diameters. The specifications of commonly used reusable and disposable flexible bronchoscopes are tabulated in Table 10.2. Much of the literature on single-use flexible bronchoscopes is

TABLE 10.2. Specifications of Commonly Used Reusable and Disposable Flexible Bronchoscopes

Bronchoscope	Distal Tip Outer Diameter (mm)	Working Length (cm)	Working Channel Inner Diameter (mm)	Angle of View (°)	Deflection Up/Down
REUSABLE					
Pediatric					
Olympus BF XP190	3.1 (tapered part distal tip 2.9 mm)	60	1.2	110	210° /130°
Karl Storz ABXK	2.85	52	NIL	100	140° /140°
Adult					
Olympus BF P190	4.2	60	2.0	110	210° /130°
Olympus LF Type V	4.1	60	1.2	120	120° /120°
Karl Storz BDXK	4.1	65	1.5	100	140° /140°
Karl Storz BNXK	5.5	65	2.1	100	140° /140°
Karl Storz BCXK	6.5	65	3.0	100	180°/140°
SINGLE-USE					
Karl Storz single-use FIVE S					
091361-06	3.5	65			
091261-06	2.9	65	1.2	90	180°/180°
091251-06	2.9	52			
AMBU aScope 4					
Slim	3.8		1.2	85	180°/180°
Regular	5.0		2.2		180°/180°
Large	5.8	60	2.8		180°/160°
GlideScope Bflex	3.8		1.2	85 (horizontal/ vertical)	175°/180°
	5.0		2.2	120 (diagonal)	165°/160°
	5.8	61	2.8		140°/135°

based on the AMBU aScope; now in the fourth generation since its launch in 2010, the AMBU aScope demonstrates comparable performance to reusable flexible bronchoscopes in anesthetic settings and for bronchoalveolar lavage.[26,66,67]

The cost of a bronchoscopic intubation using reusable bronchoscopes includes the purchase cost of the scopes, repairs, maintenance, and labor.[68] In addition, certain procedures such as percutaneous tracheotomy might be associated with a greater risk of damage to the bronchoscope, compared to bronchoalveolar lavage.[69,70] An adequate number of scopes must be purchased to ensure availability when clinically needed. Cost analysis comparing traditional reusable bronchoscopes and single-use bronchoscopes concluded that costs are approximately the same per procedure in a department performing a high volume of bronchoscopic intubations, whereas in departments that perform bronchoscopic intubation occasionally, costs associated with the use of the disposable scope may be lower.[26] It is hence suggested that units performing a smaller amount of bronchoscopic procedures could manage solely with single-use bronchoscopes, whereby reusable bronchoscopes make more economical sense to institutions with increased demand while concurrently having a small subset of single-use bronchoscopes available for emergency use.[71,72] Tvede et al. determined that the break-even point at which the cost of using disposable and nondisposable flexible scopes was identical at their institution was 22.5 intubations per month.[73]

Additional advantages of single-use bronchoscopes include the option for parallel as opposed to linear use of bronchoscopes, which can potentially decrease delays between procedures, as well as the elimination of the possibility of infection transmission that is associated with the use of nondisposable bronchoscopes.[69] In developing countries, adherence to recommendations for reprocessing and disinfecting reusable bronchoscopes may impose prohibitively high costs. Single-use bronchoscopes may alleviate this problem, depending on the anticipated usage and demand.

How Are Reusable Flexible Bronchoscopes Disinfected?

In general, the issue of sterilization of bronchoscopes is addressed by infection control and risk management personnel in each health care facility. Specific recommendations for sterilization are also provided by the individual manufacturer. Accurate reprocessing of flexible endoscopes is a multistep procedure that includes manual cleaning followed by high-level disinfection (HLD), rinsing, drying, and appropriate storage.[74] Reprocessing can be performed using automated endoscope reprocessors (AERs) and manual methods according to a strict protocol. Most flexible endoscopes are classified as semicritical devices which come into contact with intact mucous membranes and should undergo at least HLD. Reusable flexible endoscopes used for therapeutic procedures, and reusable accessories such as biopsy forceps, are classified as critical devices and must be sterilized after each procedure.[74] Ethylene oxide and hydrogen peroxide plasma sterilization have reliable efficacy as compared to HLD but can damage the flexible endoscopes. Gas sterilization with ethylene oxide may fail in the presence of organic debris or biofilm. Manual cleaning precedes sterilization or HLD and includes brushing of the external surfaces of the scope, including the channels, ports, and removable parts, and immersion in a detergent solution.[74,75] This is followed by irrigation of internal channels with a detergent, inspection for damage, and a leak test. HLD is then preformed manually or by using an AER. The use of an AER is recommended. Agents appropriate for HLD include 2% to 4% glutaraldehyde, peracetic acid, orthophthaldehyde, and superoxidized and electrolyzed acid water. Glutaraldehyde can however coagulate and fix proteins and fail to eliminate atypical bacteria within standard contact times.[74] Peracetic acid is the agent usually used for HLD of flexible scopes in AERs. After disinfection, the disinfectant must be removed from the exterior and the internal channels of the scope by rinsing with bacterium-free water. This is followed by the flushing of the channels with ethyl or isopropyl alcohol. The flexible scope should then be dried with filtered compressed air manually or in an AER between procedures (short drying cycle) and at the end of the day (intensive final drying). The scope is then stored and hung vertically in a dust-free drying cabinet with laminar airflow (Figure 10.5).

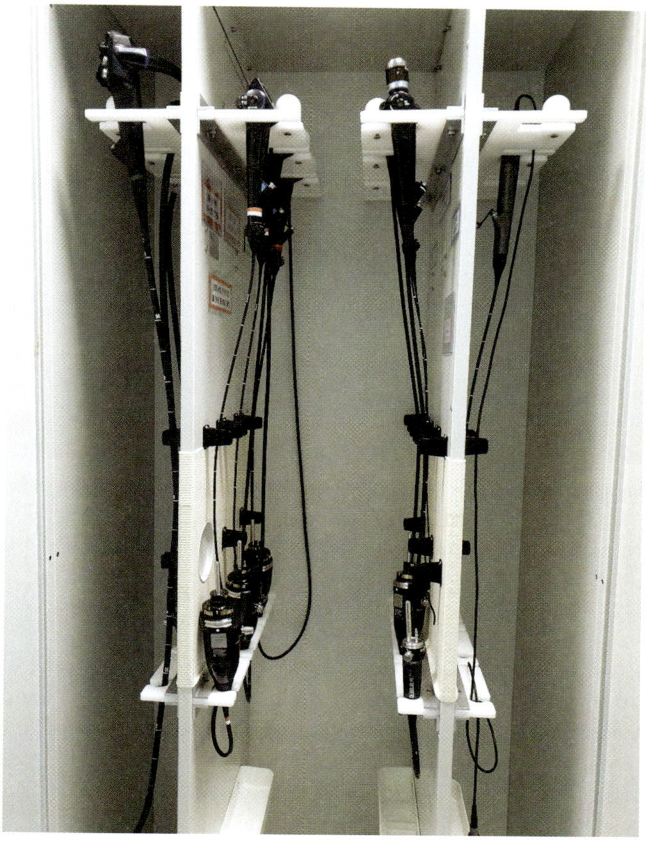

FIGURE 10.5. Storing processed bronchoscopes vertically in a dust-free drying cabinet.

How Can the Risk of Pathogen Transmission with Reusable Bronchoscopes Be Reduced?

Reprocessing aims to prevent exogenous pathogen transmission to patients. The American College of Chest Physicians and the American Association for Bronchology issued a consensus statement in 2005 on principles related to the specific maintenance and disinfection of bronchoscopes.[75] However, outbreaks of bacterial infection associated with reusable bronchoscopes have occurred when reprocessing protocols were breached.[74,76,77] Pseudoinfection or transmission (cultural evidence of transmission of organisms without evidence of patient infection) has also been reported. In 2016, a possible pseudotransmission of gentamicin-resistant *Enterobacter cloacae* was discovered between two patients during an investigation of positive environmental cultures with *Enterobacter cloacae* from an endobronchial ultrasound bronchoscope.[78] This has occurred in spite of adherence to reprocessing steps. A recent study in 2018 demonstrated contamination and microbial growth (*Pseudomonas aeruginosa, Sternotrophomonus maltophila, E.coli/Shigella* species) on bronchoscopes that were fully reprocessed with complete adherence to protocols.[79] The high level of bio-burden was found to be unacceptably high, leading to the authors concluding that a move toward sterilization might be warranted. They also went on to recommend that when sterilization methods are not readily available or practical, institutions could separate bronchoscope from gastrointestinal endoscope reprocessing for risk reduction. If this is not possible or if high levels of reprocessing quality cannot be maintained, sterile single-use bronchoscopes should be used to ensure patient safety.[79]

It has been shown that routine cleaning and autoclaving do not remove protein material, including prions (protein particles without nucleic acid), from reusable airway devices,[80] and concern has been expressed with respect to the possible transmission of infection with subsequent usage.[81] The true incidence of bronchoscopy-associated infections is unknown in part due to inadequate surveillance and episodic reporting.[74,75] Although the risk of infection transmission in gastrointestinal endoscopy has been quoted to be 1 in 1.8 million.[74,75] Others have suggested that the true incidence of infection transmission is impossible to determine.[68,74,82] The emergence of variant Creutzfeldt Jakob Disease (vCJD) which is transmitted by prions as an important pathogen in humans has further complicated the issue of decontamination.[68,74] Prions are highly resistant to routine methods of sterilization and decontamination. Dry heat, glutaraldehyde, and ethylene oxide are ineffective, and recommended chemical methods include a decontamination step with concentrated sodium hydroxide, sodium hypochlorite, or formic acid, and prolonged steam sterilization.[74] Most contemporary flexible endoscopes cannot withstand heat sterilization and disinfection with high concentrations of disinfectants without sustaining severe damage.[74] A 2013 review has suggested that flexible endoscopes that have been used in patients with CJD should be discarded.[74]

Transmission of viral respiratory pathogens such as severe acute respiratory syndrome coronavirus 2 (SARS-CoV-2) via reusable bronchoscopes has not been reported to date. Nonetheless, bronchoscopy is an aerosol-generating procedure and is hence relatively contraindicated in patients who are suspected of or confirmed with SARS-CoV-2 infection to reduce disease transmission and to protect health care personnel.[83] Single-use bronchoscopes should be used first-line in addition to proper personal protective equipment and safe management measures if bronchoscopic intubation cannot be avoided.[65,83]

TECHNIQUE

How Is the Flexible Bronchoscope Maneuvered? What Are the Key Aspects of the Technique for Fast, Successful Bronchoscopic Intubation? (Video 10)

The bronchoscope is most easily maneuvered by holding the handle of the scope in the palm of the dominant (usually right) hand with the **thumb** placed on the **flexion** lever (see Figure 10.6). The fingers should comfortably encircle the handle of the scope and the index finger can be used to activate the suction mechanism. When the scope is held such that the flexion lever is in the 6 o'clock position, moving the lever downward (toward the shaft of the scope) flexes the tip of the scope upward toward the 12 o'clock position. Conversely, moving the lever up toward the proximal aspect of the handle flexes the tip downward toward the 6 o'clock position (see Figure 10.7). Movement of the flexion lever (thumb flexion) then flexes the tip of the scope *in a single plane*. To flex the tip in any other plane, *the entire instrument must be rotated* clockwise or counterclockwise using the wrist and hand holding the handle of the scope. This **wrist rotation** is the second important and perhaps not intuitively obvious movement required when manipulating the bronchoscope during FBI (see Figures 10.8A and B). The tip of the bronchoscope can then be manipulated to view objects in any plane within the scope's field of vision by a combination of **wrist rotation** and **thumb flexion**. Some bronchoscopes have a triangular marker or divot located at the 12 o'clock position at the periphery of the scope's field of vision (see Figure 10.9). This marker helps the practitioner maintain spatial orientation

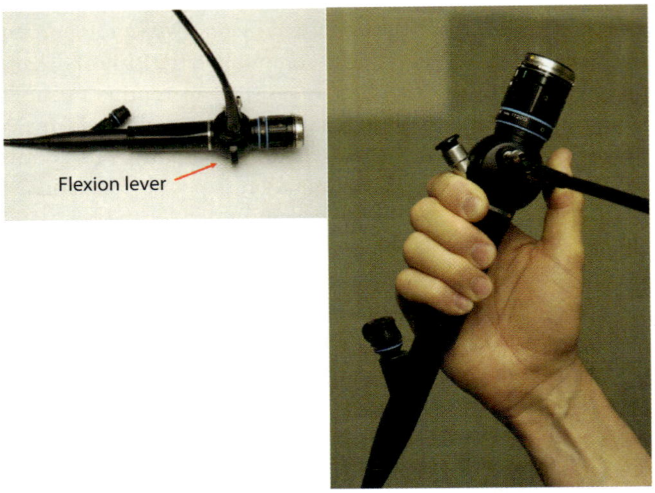

FIGURE 10.6. Holding the bronchoscope. The fingers comfortably encircle the handle. The thumb is placed on the flexion lever.

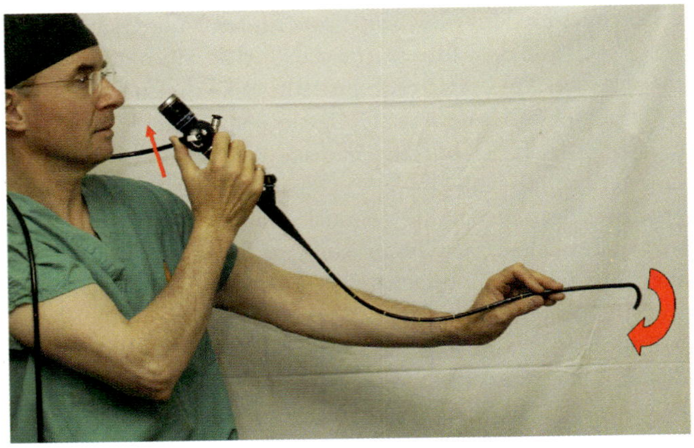

FIGURE 10.7. Movement of the flexion lever flexes the tip of the insertion cord in a single plane.

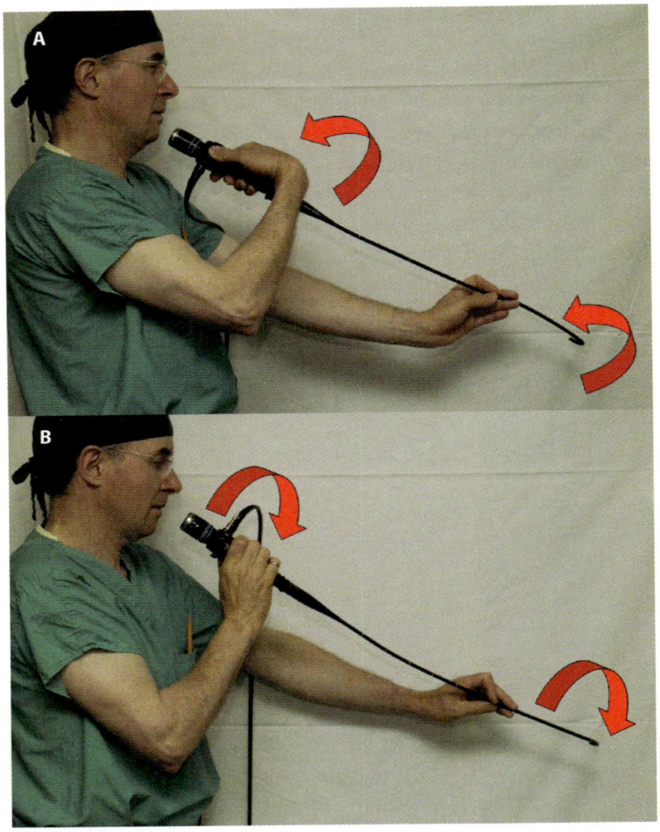

FIGURE 10.8. **(A)** Rotation of the bronchoscope counterclockwise. **(B)** Rotation of the bronchoscope clockwise. The entire instrument is rotated using the wrist at the handle of the scope. The hand holding the shaft allows the instrument to rotate.

as the tip of the scope always flexes in the diametrical plane of the marker. The practitioner's nondominant (usually left) hand holds the shaft or insertion cord of the bronchoscope a few centimeters proximal to the tip with the forearm pronated (see Figure 10.10). The shaft should be held *lightly* between the tips of the thumb and index finger and can be stabilized between the ring and middle finger or some other combination of digits if desired. The hand holding the distal shaft of the scope must

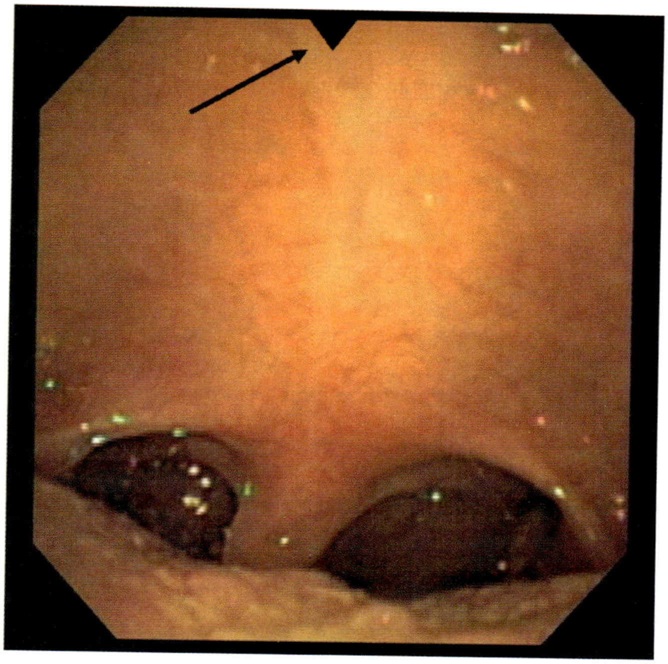

FIGURE 10.9. The marker or "divot" located at 12 o'clock (arrow) in the scope's field of vision.

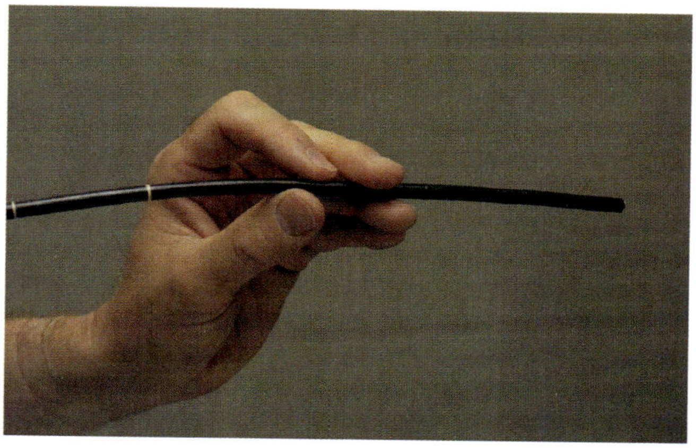

FIGURE 10.10. Holding the insertion cord of the bronchoscope. With the forearm pronated, the nondominant hand holds the insertion cord a few centimeters proximal to the tip of the bronchoscope.

feed the scope forward into the airway in a controlled manner without excessive (shaky) movement that can make visualization difficult. During FBI, the scope must travel about 21 cm from the incisors to the mid-trachea. If the shaft is held at about 20 cm proximal from the tip, then feeding can be minimized.

Generally, it is easier to rotate the bronchoscope using the dominant (usually right) hand positioned at the handle. The nondominant hand holding the distal aspect of the shaft ***must allow the shaft to rotate as a single unit***, and therefore the shaft cannot be gripped tightly. If the distal aspect of the shaft is held tightly, rotation at the handle twists the insertion cord, the scope fails to go in the desired direction (see Figures 10.8A and B), and the components in the shaft, particularly with the ones using fiberoptic technology, can be damaged. As experience is gained in the handling of the scope, the shaft does not need to be held taut to maneuver the tip. However, holding the shaft of the scope relatively straight can be useful to maintain orientation and control movement. The most important concepts to master are **thumb flexion** and **wrist rotation**. During FBI, movements of the scope (flexion, rotation, and forward feeding) should be small, slow, and deliberate. Over steering of the scope is a common error.

The ETT can be precut to a desired length (usually about 28 cm) to maximize the length of the insertion cord beyond the tube and thereby optimize maneuverability.[26] The inside of the tube can be lubricated using a water-based lubricant. The tube is then ensleeved proximally and fixed to the handle with tape or an elastic band. Lubricant jelly placed on the cuff of the tube may facilitate glottic entry. Lubricating the shaft of the scope may not be necessary and sometimes makes it difficult to handle.

Is Bronchoscopic Intubation More Easily Performed from the Head of the Bed or from the Front on the Patient's Right Side?

Awake FBI can be performed with the practitioner standing at the head of the bed, and for those who are most familiar with visualization of the airway by direct laryngoscopy, this position preserves the spatial orientation of the airway structures as they are viewed through the scope.[26,27] However, this position requires the practitioner to negotiate an S-shaped curve to the trachea (see Figure 10.11) and the patient to be supine or nearly supine. Standing at the patient's right side facing the patient facilitates negotiation of the natural C-shaped curve of the airway (see Figure 10.12), permits easy visualization of patient monitors, and as eye contact can be readily maintained this position may be less intimidating for the patient.[26,27] The patient may be supine or in the semi-sitting or sitting position.[27]

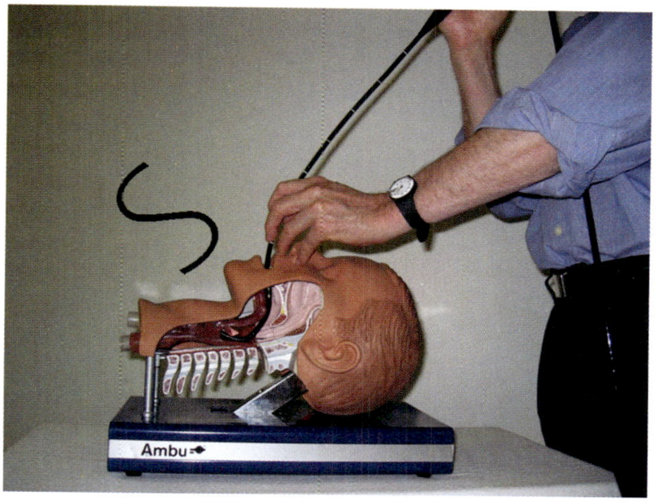

FIGURE 10.11. Flexible bronchoscopic intubation performed from the head of the bed requires the insertion cord to negotiate an S-shaped curve and the patient must be supine or nearly supine.

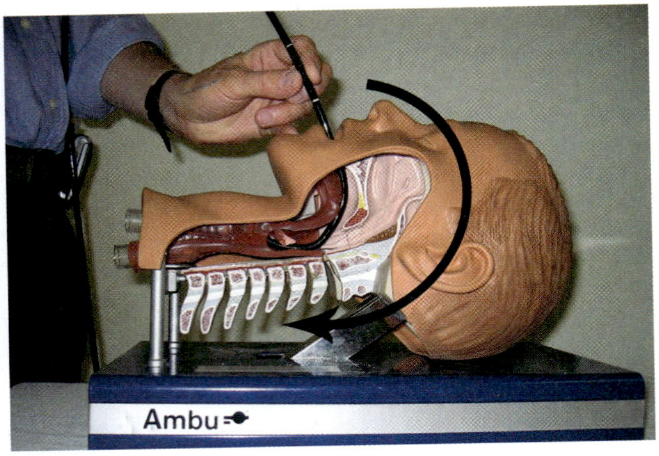

FIGURE 10.12. Flexible bronchoscopic intubation from the patient's right side requires the scope to negotiate a C-shaped curve.

The semi-seated or sitting position may also be less intimidating for the awake patient, better maintain the patency of the pharyngeal lumen[27,84] and confer a superior view during bronchoscopic intubation.[85] Extension at the atlanto-occipital joint moves the epiglottis anteriorly away from the posterior pharyngeal wall and facilitates passage of the bronchoscope through the pharynx.[3,27,62,86,87] Neck flexion, however, tends to produce pharyngeal obstruction and can make FBI more difficult.[27,86–88]

How Is Awake Oral Bronchoscopic Intubation Performed? What Instructions Should Be Given to the Patient During the Procedure?

For awake oral FBI, the author prefers to stand facing the patient on the patient's right side, with the patient in the semi-seated or sitting position (see Figure 10.13). The video bronchoscope system is located in front of or slightly to the left of the practitioner. Oxygen can be administered by nasal prongs or high-flow nasal cannula.[89] An assistant is positioned at the patient's left side and provides gentle tongue traction using a piece of gauze. Use of a bite block tends to push the tongue posteriorly and cephalad into the oropharyngeal isthmus, can make passage of the scope into the oropharynx more difficult, and is not necessary if adequate local anesthesia has been achieved.[27] Intubating oral airway adjuncts can be used in place of manual tongue traction.

The scope should be inserted into the oral cavity over the dorsum of the tongue following the midline groove toward **the first midline landmark, the uvula**, seen in the superior aspect of the scope's field of vision (see Figure 10.9). Gently resting the hand holding the shaft of the scope on the patient's chin may help keep the scope in the midline but requires the shaft to be held close to the tip and necessitates more feeding as compared to holding the shaft at about 20 cm from the tip. If the uvula is in contact with the dorsal aspect of the tongue, the patient can be instructed to take a deep breath, thereby elevating the uvula and opening the oropharyngeal isthmus.[26,27] The scope is then advanced slowly forward just past the uvula and flexed caudally to visualize **the second midline landmark, the epiglottis**, seen inferiorly in the scope's field of vision (see Figure 10.14). If the epiglottis is oriented posteriorly or is in contact with the posterior pharyngeal wall, the awake patient can again be instructed to take a deep breath and thereby move the epiglottis anteriorly to create an air space through which to pass the scope. The scope is then passed, posterior to the epiglottis to visualize **the third midline landmark, the vocal cords** (see Figure 10.15). If the bronchoscope is passed behind the epiglottis in the midline, then it is naturally lined up for the approach to the larynx. Conversely, if the bronchoscope is off-midline at the level of

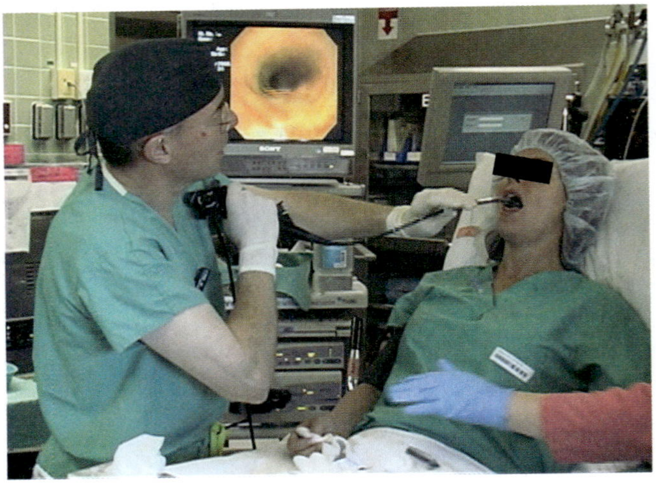

FIGURE 10.13. Flexible bronchoscopic intubation with the practitioner on the patient's right side facing the patient: the ETT is advanced in the midline during a deep inspiration while following the natural C-shaped curve of the airway.

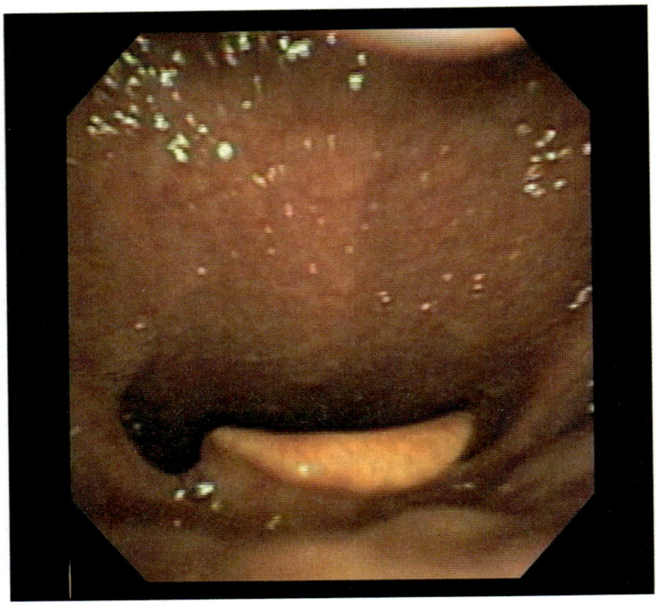

FIGURE 10.14. Bronchoscopic view of the second midline landmark (the epiglottis) during flexible bronchoscopic intubation with the practitioner on the patient's right side facing the patient.

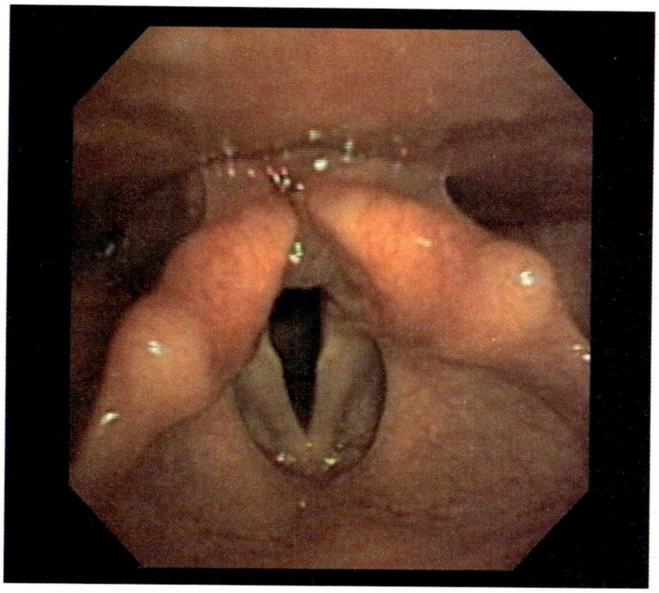

FIGURE 10.15. Bronchoscopic view of the third midline landmark (the vocal cords) during flexible bronchoscopic intubation with the practitioner on the patient's right side facing the patient.

the epiglottis, the approach to the larynx can be much more difficult.

The scope is then advanced in the midline through the glottis and positioned proximal to the carina. As the scope is advanced through the larynx, the patient is again instructed to take a deep breath to maximally abduct the vocal cords and thereby facilitate passage of the scope. As the bronchoscope is passed from the level of the dental arches to the trachea, flexion and rotation movements should be small and deliberate such that the scope can be kept in the midline and advanced along the C-shaped curve of the airway, analogous to staying in a given lane during highway driving using small movements of the steering wheel. Unnecessary touching of the mucosa by the bronchoscope should be avoided.

Having positioned the tip of the bronchoscope in the mid to distal trachea, the practitioner should then look directly at the patient and advance the ETT over the scope being careful to aim for the midline and to follow the natural curve of the airway (see Figure 10.13).[26,27] The bronchoscope must be kept stationary as the tube is advanced[16] in order to avoid inadvertent contact with the carina, cannulation of a mainstem bronchus, or premature removal of the scope from the trachea. Again, as the tube is advanced, the patient should be instructed to take a deep breath to move the epiglottis anteriorly away from the advancing tube and to maximally abduct the vocal cords.

The correct intratracheal position of the ETT can be confirmed endoscopically before the scope is removed. However, the presence of both the bronchoscope and ETT in the trachea produces a degree of airway obstruction that can be distressing for the awake patient, and the bronchoscope should be removed expeditiously once the ETT is in a proper position. The correct position can be further confirmed by capnography and lung auscultation.

Is Nasal Bronchoscopic Intubation Easier? Which Nostril Is the More Appropriate for Intubation?

Nasotracheal intubation produces less stimulation of the gag reflex[3,7,90] and requires less patient cooperation, but is generally more uncomfortable for the awake patient. If the nasal cavity can be readily cannulated, nasotracheal intubation using a flexible bronchoscope is technically somewhat easier than oral FBI.

If the nasal route is chosen for FBI, an attempt to identify the more patent nostril can be made by asking the patient to assess airflow through each nasal cavity in turn during exhalation, and by feeling airflow from the nostril.[91] However, these simple diagnostic tests have been shown to have a failure rate of about 45%.[91] Some degree of nasal obstruction can be present in the absence of a history of nasal trauma, surgery, or obstruction and can interfere with the attempted passage of a nasal tube. The mucosa over the turbinates is easily traumatized.[91] Endoscopic examination of the nasal cavity may help to identify the more appropriate nostril for intubation.[91] Administration of a nasal vasoconstrictor may also increase the caliber of the nasal airway. In the absence of a history of nasal obstruction, it is controversial whether the left or right nostril should be used for nasal intubation as it is not known whether the bevel or the tip of the tube is more responsible for potential damage to the nasal mucosa (see also "Blind Nasal Intubation" in Chapter 12).

During nasal FBI, either the ETT or the bronchoscope can be passed initially through the nasal cavity.[2,26,27,55] If the tube is passed first, it can be advanced along the floor of the nose using a gentle alternating clockwise-counterclockwise motion to facilitate its passage until the tip of the tube exits the choana and enters the nasopharynx.[2,27] The scope can then be passed through the lubricated tube and as it exits the distal aspect of the tube, the glottis is usually in view (see Figure 10.16). If on exiting the tip of the ETT the view is obstructed, the tube may be in contact with the pharyngeal mucosa or the tip of the scope may be covered with blood or debris. The scope can

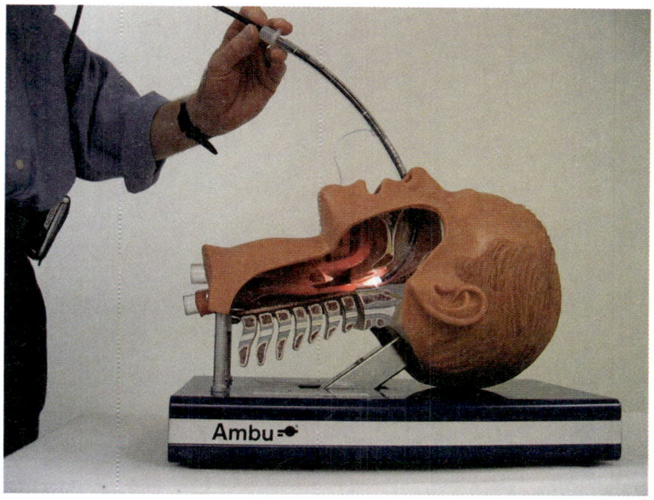

FIGURE 10.16. Nasal intubation using a flexible bronchoscope in a manikin: the bronchoscope is passed through the ETT which was initially positioned in the pharynx.

SECTION 2

be removed, the tip cleaned and warmed, and then reinserted into the tube. If on exiting the distal aspect of the tube, still no recognizable structures are visualized, then the scope and tube should be slowly retracted together until pharyngeal or laryngeal landmarks (the uvula, epiglottis, or vocal cords) are identified.[26] If the epiglottis is oriented posteriorly against the posterior pharyngeal wall, the patient can be instructed to take a deep breath and thereby move the epiglottis anteriorly and create an adequate airspace for the scope to pass behind it, without touching mucosa and losing the visual field.[27] The flexible bronchoscope is then advanced into the trachea and the ETT advanced over the scope as for oral intubation during a deep inspiration, optimally with the patient in the semi-sitting or sitting position.[26,27]

Alternatively, the flexible bronchoscope can be passed first through the nasal cavity and on into the trachea under endoscopic vision and then the ensleeved ETT passed over the scope (see Figure 10.17). On advancing the ETT over the flexible bronchoscope, the leading edge of the tube may impact on the laryngeal structures and resist further advancement.[92] The most likely site of impingement during nasal FBI is controversial.[93,94] Rotating the tube such that the bevel faces anteriorly,[95] or posteriorly,[92] or advancing with a twisting motion[27,57,93] may facilitate glottic entry. Serial dilatation of the nostril with lubricated, incremental sizes of nasopharyngeal airways can be performed before subsequent insertion of the ETT to explore the nasal cavity such that an appropriately sized ETT can be chosen. Further decompression of the nasal mucosa may also be thereby achieved[96] and trauma due to the more rigid ETT may be reduced. Alternatively, a nasopharyngeal airway split longitudinally can be inserted into the nasopharynx and used as a guide through which to pass the bronchoscope.[27,96] The split nasopharyngeal airway can then be removed before the subsequent passage of the ETT.

On occasion, the caliber of the nasal cavity may be such that it will permit passage of the ETT or nasopharyngeal airway but not the bronchoscope through the tube or airway due to external compression.[26,27] Conversely, the nasal cavity may permit initial passage of the scope but not the tube over the scope.[26,27] In this circumstance, it may be necessary to use a smaller scope, a smaller tube, the other nostril, oral intubation, or another means of airway management.

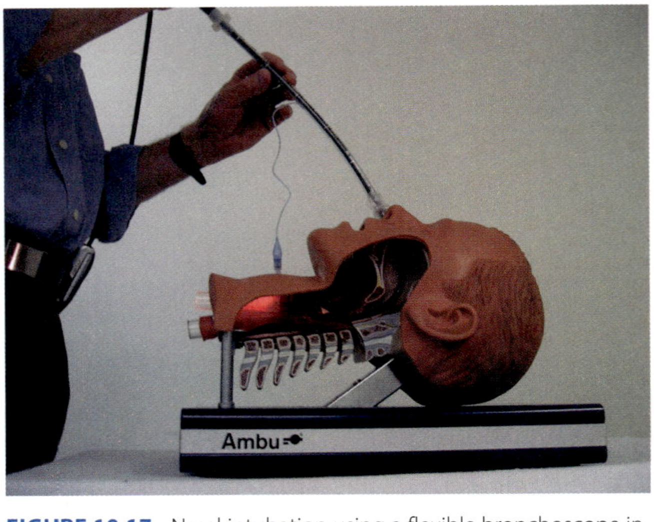

FIGURE 10.17. Nasal intubation using a flexible bronchoscope in a manikin: the bronchoscope can be passed first into pharynx and trachea. The ETT is then advanced over the bronchoscope.

Nasotracheal intubation has been considered to be contraindicated in the presence of coagulopathy, intranasal abnormalities, paranasal sinusitis, extensive facial fractures, and basal skull fracture.[97–100] Conversely, basal skull fracture has been said not to be a contraindication to nasotracheal intubation,[97] which has been performed safely as reported in the literature with no documented intracranial passage of the ETT or associated infections.[97,101,102] If nasal intubation cannot be avoided in patients with base of skull fracture, cannulation of the trachea can be done under indirect vision with a flexible bronchoscope[101] before railroading the ETT over to prevent intracranial misplacement of the ETT. Complications peculiar to nasotracheal intubation include epistaxis,[41,96,98,100,103,104] damage to the nasal or nasopharyngeal mucosa with creation of a false passage,[103] and potential abscess formation[98] bacteremia,[41,100] damage to nasal polyps or adenoidal tissue with possible dislodgement and aspiration, nasal necrosis,[41,98,100] sinusitis,[41,98,100] and otitis.[41,100] Minimal epistaxis has been reported in 11% to 40% of emergency nasotracheal intubations[103,104] and moderate to severe bleeding in 7%,[104] whereas the reported incidence of minor bleeding from nasotracheal bronchoscopic intubation under elective conditions was 5% to 11%.[96,105]

When Is Bronchoscopic Intubation Under GA Indicated? What Are the Problems Associated with This Technique?

Oral FBI has been successfully performed following simulated rapid sequence induction (RSI),[106] and FBI under GA has been used for training purposes.[27,107] FBI of the anticipated and unanticipated difficult intubation under GA, has also been reported, although some intubation failures did occur.[17,108] This technique may be particularly useful in uncooperative adult and pediatric patients.[109,110]

As consciousness is lost, loss of tone in the submandibular muscles allows the tongue and epiglottis to move posteriorly and potentially obstruct the airway at the level of the pharynx and larynx, respectively.[91,111] The soft palate also approximates the posterior pharyngeal wall.[111] The degree of airway obstruction produced is influenced by variations in airway anatomy, body habitus, and depth of anesthesia.[27,87] In the unconscious individual, this reduction in the caliber of the pharyngeal lumen can make endoscopic visualization more difficult.[27,112] Contact of the bronchoscope lens with the mucosa results in loss of the visual field, and the practitioner's ability to maneuver past an epiglottis in contact with the posterior pharyngeal wall is limited.[27,54,57,112]

In the supine individual under GA, lingual traction with Duval's forceps has been shown to move the tongue away from the uvula and soft palate better than the jaw thrust maneuver, whereas jaw thrust (Figure 10.18) moved the epiglottis away from the posterior pharyngeal wall more effectively than tongue traction.[91] Jaw thrust and tongue traction applied

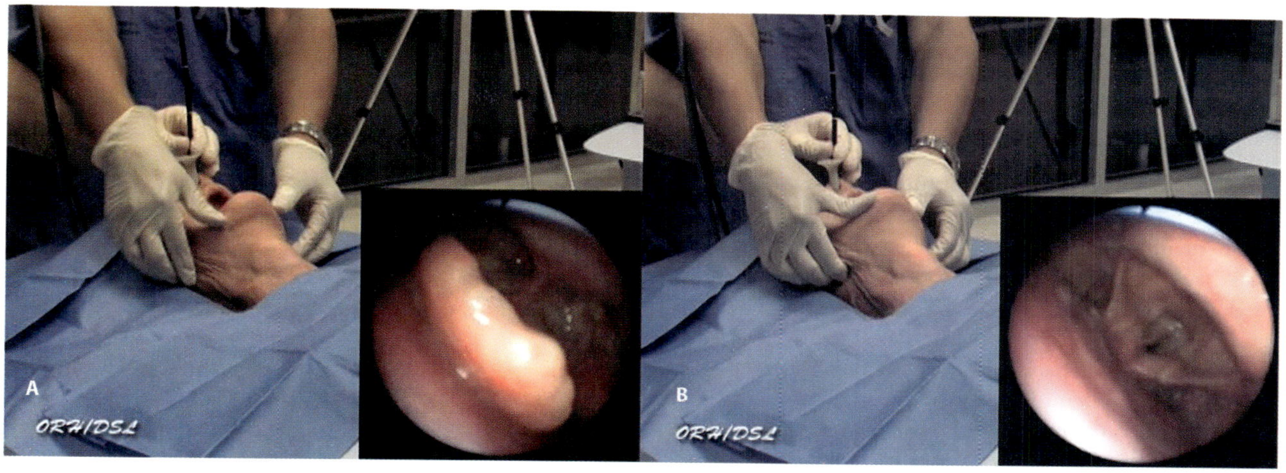

FIGURE 10.18. A flexible nasopharyngoscope was used to show the effectiveness of jaw thrust to lift the epiglottis away from the posterior pharyngeal wall, exposing the glottic inlet for flexible bronchoscopic intubation: **(A)** without jaw thrust and **(B)** jaw thrust applied.

simultaneously opened the airway at the soft palate and epiglottic level in all patients studied.[91] These combined maneuvers require two assistants.[91] While intubating oral airways such as the Berman or Ovassapian airway can also be used to keep the pharyngeal airway open as well as to direct the flexible bronchoscope toward the larynx, jaw thrust is of paramount importance to open up the glottic inlet and facilitate tube passage under GA.[113] Anterior displacement of the tongue base using the rigid laryngoscope may also improve visualization.[27,54] An endoscopy mask fitted with a diaphragm permits endoscopy during positive pressure-mask ventilation,[114] and can be used in conjunction with an intubating airway.[7,18,114] The nasotracheal route can also be used in the unconscious individual.[112]

In the presence of apnea or suboptimal ventilation, arterial desaturation imposes a time limit on bronchoscopic techniques.[26,27] Denitrogenation creates an oxygen reservoir in the lungs and in healthy adults can extend the duration of apnea before oxygen desaturation occurs from 1-2 minutes to 8 minutes.[46,115] Denitrogenation in the 20° head-up position has been shown to increase the apnea time before oxygen desaturation to 95% as compared to the supine position.[116] The apnea time before oxygen desaturation to 92% in severely obese patients was similarly shown to be increased after denitrogenation in the 25° head up position as compared to the supine position.[117] Passive oxygenation during the apneic period (apneic oxygenation) can also prolong the duration of apnea before oxygen desaturation occurs.[46] Oxygen can be delivered to the pharynx during apnea using a nasal cannula at flow rates of 5 to 15 $L \cdot min^{-1}$ or specialized high-flow nasal cannulas that humidify the oxygen allow flow rates up to 60 $L \cdot min^{-1}$.[46,118]

FBI of a patient under GA can be difficult[119] and arterial oxygen desaturation can occur. Although the technique has been used with high levels of success,[106,108,113,120] failure of FBI following induction of GA has also been reported.[113] If FBI is planned under GA, denitrogenation and administration of oxygen by nasal cannula during the procedure can extend the apnea time before oxygen desaturation occurs. Tongue traction and jaw thrust can open the pharyngeal airway and improve visualization.

How Can Difficulty in Passing the Ensleeved Endotracheal Tube into the Trachea over the Flexible Bronchoscope Be Minimized?

Difficulty in passing the ensleeved ETT through the larynx has been variously reported to occur in 0% to 90% of FBIs,[56,59,90,92,121–123] and has occurred in awake patients, as well as those under GA, and with both the nasal and oral routes of tracheal intubation. During oral FBI, as the tube is advanced with the concave aspect of the tube facing anteriorly and the bevel facing toward the patient's left, the leading edge of the tube may meet resistance at the right arytenoids, aryepiglottic fold, or interarytenoid soft tissue (see Figure 10.19).[92,93,124–126] After a slight retraction of the ETT, rotation of the tube 90 degrees counterclockwise orients the bevel posteriorly and the leading edge into the 12 o'clock position and has been advocated to improve the passage of the ETT through the larynx.[93,125,127–130] Rotation of the

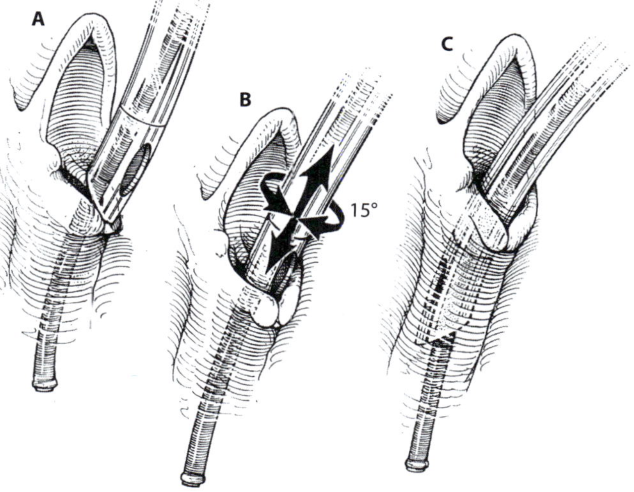

FIGURE 10.19. Impingement of ETT at the right arytenoid or right epiglottic fold. (Reproduced with permission from Dellinger RP. Fiberoptic bronchoscopy in adult airway management. *Crit Care Med.* 1990;18(8):882-887.)

tube counterclockwise may also keep the leading edge in closer contact with the bronchoscope and provide less of a gap between the two with which to catch a laryngeal structure.[56,94]

During nasal FBI, it has been postulated that the tube tends to impinge on the epiglottis.[92–94] However the usual point of obstruction during nasal tracheal intubation may also be the right arytenoid.[94] In addition, impingement can occur at the posterior pharyngeal wall or other laryngeal structures.[123] Improved success rates have been reported for glottic cannulation during nasal FBI, using a 90-degree counterclockwise rotation of the tube.[92]

The larger the discrepancy between the outside diameter of the bronchoscopic insertion cord and the internal diameter of the ensleeved ETT, the greater is the chance that the tube may impinge on laryngeal structures and resist entry into the trachea (see Figure 10.20).[2,3,27,58,59,124] Therefore, this discrepancy should be minimized by choosing the largest bronchoscope which will easily fit into the ETT to be used.[62] In the adult, a bronchoscope with an outer diameter of 5.9 to 6.0 mm works well when used with a 7.5- to 8.5-mm ID ETT. When the combination of a relatively large bronchoscope and an ETT are both present in the trachea, the practitioner must be aware that a degree of airway obstruction has been produced[57] and the bronchoscope should be removed without delay following tube placement and confirmation. If the bronchoscope must remain inside the tube positioned in the trachea for a relatively long period as during diagnostic or therapeutic bronchoscopy, then the concentric airway remaining must be adequate to permit ventilation to occur.[27,57,131]

Wire-reinforced spiral tubes are more flexible than polyvinyl chloride (PVC) tubes and may more easily follow the curve of the bronchoscope as it passes through the larynx.[27,124,131–133] Although flexible wire-reinforced tubes were reported to be associated with a lower rate of impingement in the larynx than a standard tube,[132] subsequent studies reported frequent laryngeal impaction with spiral tubes.[121,122] Preformed PVC ETTs can also be warmed to increase flexibility although the effect of warming on ease of insertion is unclear.[18,26,27,56] Laryngeal cannulation with the ensleeved ETT may also be facilitated by using a tube with a modified tip design.[26,27,124,127] The silicone wire-reinforced tube for the intubating laryngeal mask airway (LMA-Fastrach™) is reusable and has a soft hemispherical bevel that has a leading edge in the midline (see Figure 10.21),[124] making ETT passage easier than conventional tracheal tubes during both oral and nasal tracheal intubation.[121,124]

The Parker Flex-tip tube (see Figure 10.22) has a flexible tip that points toward the center of the distal lumen and the convex side of the tube and a bevel that faces posteriorly,[56,59] which theoretically reduces the risk of impingement on laryngeal structures.[134] A greater incidence of success with the passage of the tracheal tube through the larynx was reported in earlier studies comparing the Parker Flex-tip tube with a standard PVC or wire-reinforced tracheal tube during oral FBI under GA.[59,135] However, there is no significant difference in the success rate and time to intubation and ease of intubation was demonstrated in studies comparing the Parker Flexi-tip

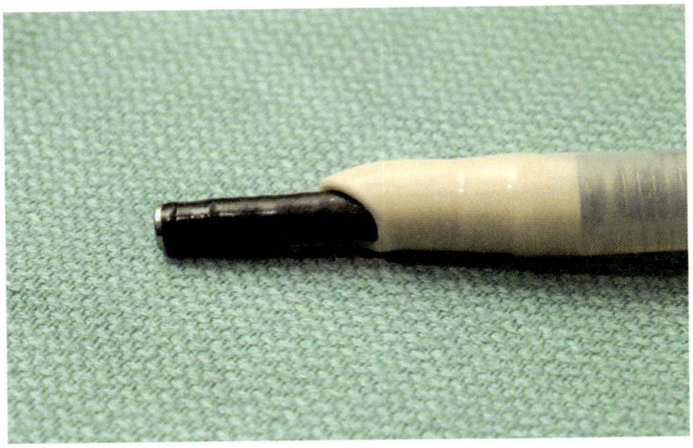

FIGURE 10.21. The ILMA (LMA-Fastrach) reusable silicone endotracheal tube ensleeved over a standard adult bronchoscope; note the hemispherical bevel with a leading edge in the midline of the tube.

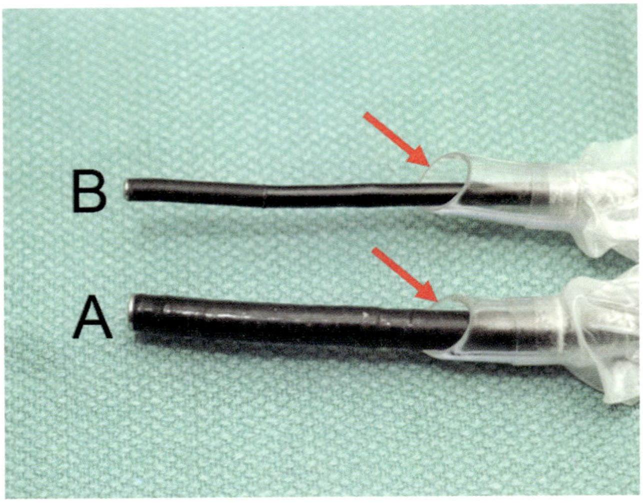

FIGURE 10.20. A 7.5-mm ID PVC ETT ensleeved over **(A)** a standard adult bronchoscope and **(B)** a pediatric bronchoscope. Note the discrepancy between the external diameters of the scopes and the internal diameters of the ETTs (arrows).

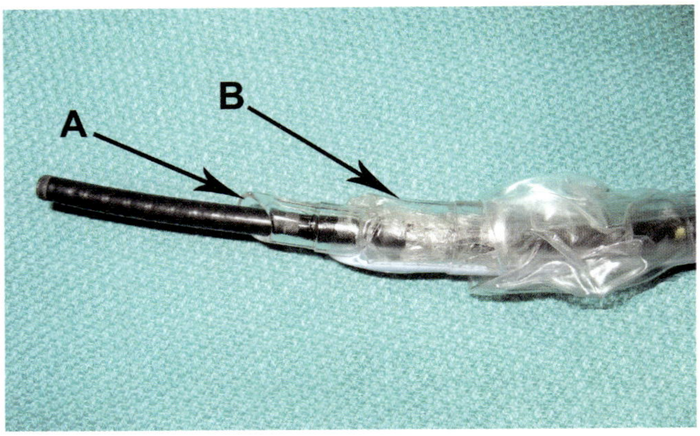

FIGURE 10.22. The Parker flex-tip tube: a 7-mm ID PVC endotracheal tube ensleeved over a standard pediatric bronchoscope **(A)**, and a 7-mm ID Parker flex-tip tube ensleeved over a pediatric bronchoscope **(B)**. Note the discrepancy between the leading edge of the two different types of endotracheal tubes (arrows).

with standard or reinforced tracheal tubes during oral FBI in patients with predicted or simulated difficult airways, unstable cervical spines and obesity.[136–138]

Difficulty in advancing the ETT through the larynx may be encountered as well in the awake patient without obtunded laryngeal reflexes.[3] However, difficulty with passage of the ETT through the larynx is exceedingly rare *in the awake cooperative patient in the sitting position with adequate topical anesthesia of the airway, when an optimally sized bronchoscope is used relative to the ETT, and the tube is advanced during a deep inspiration.*

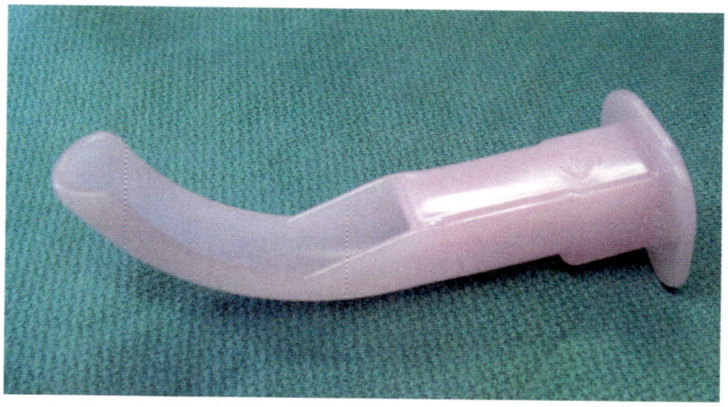

FIGURE 10.24. The Williams Airway Intubator: the Williams Airway Intubator has a cylindrical proximal half whereas the distal half of the device has an open lingual surface.

ADJUNCTS TO FACILITATE BRONCHOSCOPIC INTUBATION

Are Oral Intubating Airways Useful or Necessary?

Various oral intubating airways are available and can be used during FBI. The purpose of these airways is to displace the tongue anteriorly and the soft palate superiorly thus opening the pharyngeal space, keeping the bronchoscope in the midline and aligning it with the glottic opening, and protecting the scope from bite damage.[3,139]

The Berman Intubating Pharyngeal Airway, also known as the Berman Breakaway Airway (see Figure 10.23), is cylindrical and has a longitudinal opening along its side which permits its disengagement ("breakaway") from the bronchoscope loaded with the ETT.[18] It is available in numerous sizes suitable for use in neonates to adults. The maneuverability of the bronchoscope is limited when inside the airway, and if the airway is not in line with the glottis, visualization requires manipulation of the device.[18]

The Williams Airway Intubator has a cylindrical proximal half, whereas the distal half of the device has an open lingual surface (see Figure 10.24).[18,139] The airway is available in two sizes (90 and 100 mm ID) which admit 8.0- and 8.5-mm ID ETTs, respectively.[18,139] However, damage to the trachea tube cuff can occur if a large tracheal tube is used without proper lubrication. As such, smaller caliber tracheal tubes (7.0-7.5 mm ID) should be considered.[3] Manipulation of the bronchoscope inside the airway is limited.[18] If the distal aspect of the airway is not aligned with the glottis, visualization of the vocal cords can be difficult.[18,139] Another drawback of the Williams Airway is that the ETT connector must be removed to allow for extrication of the airway following intubation, which may result in tracheal tube dislodgement.

The Ovassapian Fiberoptic Intubating Airway has a flat lingual surface at the proximal half of the device which minimizes its movement (see Figure 10.25).[18,139] The distal half of the airway has a wide curve designed to prevent the tissues of the anterior pharyngeal wall from moving posteriorly. The posterior distal aspect of the airway is open. As the airway is available only in a single size, variable performance of the airway might be observed in patients with varying airway anatomy. Studies found that both the Berman and Williams airways achieved better glottic views than the Ovassapian airway and were superior in directing the bronchoscope toward the glottis.[3,140] The cylindrical shape of the former two airways produces a conduit

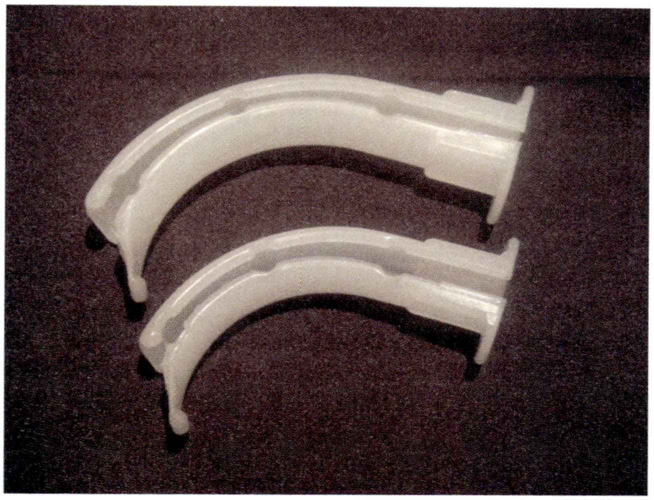

FIGURE 10.23. The Berman Intubating Pharyngeal Airway: the Berman Intubating Pharyngeal Airway is cylindrical and has a longitudinal opening along its side which permits its disengagement from the endotracheal tube following intubation.

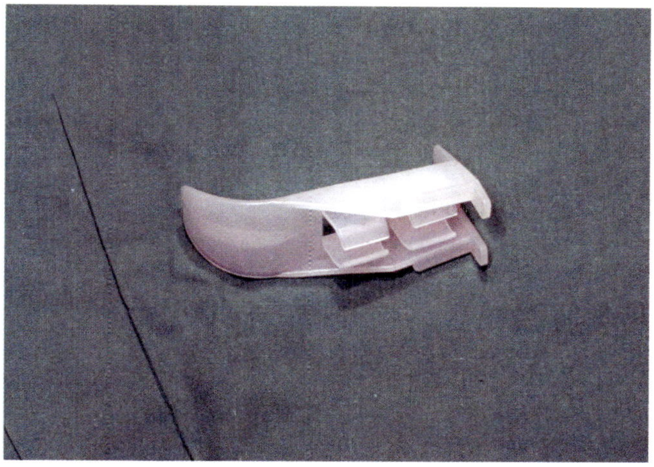

FIGURE 10.25. The Ovassapian intubating airway: the Ovassapian Fiberoptic Intubating Airway has a flat lingual surface at the proximal half of the device which minimizes its movement.

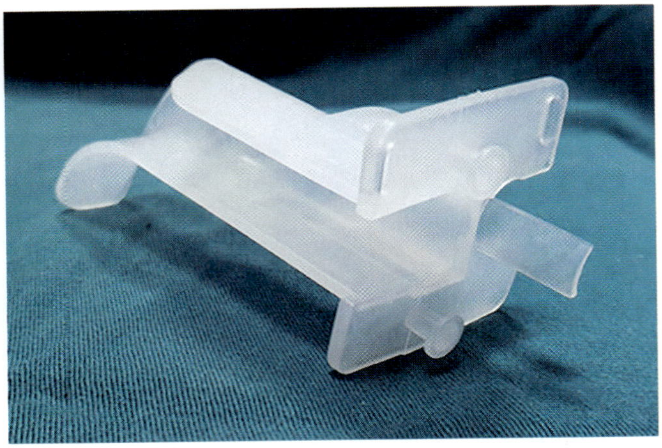

FIGURE 10.26. The Bronchoscope Airway: the Bronchoscope Airway is cylindrical in the proximal half with a lateral opening for easy removal following intubation.

in the retrolingual area for tube passage, which is not achieved by the spatula-shaped Ovassapian Airway.[3]

The Bronchoscope Airway (VBM Medizintechnik GmbH, Germany) is cylindrical in the proximal half and has a lateral opening for easy removal following intubation (Figure 10.26). The airway is available in three sizes of varying lengths and its integrated bite block protects the bronchoscope from damage.

Intubating oral airways can be used to facilitate FBI. However, several deficiencies still exist in their construction. The airways must be kept midline, which might be difficult in patients with missing incisors to keep the airway in place. The inner surface of the oral airways must be well lubricated to facilitate easy tracheal tube passage and minimize the risk of tracheal cuff damage. All airways are unable to provide a clear passage to the glottic opening under GA without extra assistance from a jaw thrust,[3] which lifts the epiglottis away from the posterior pharyngeal wall. The cylindrical shape often limits the maneuverability of the bronchoscope within the intubating oral airway. Asai and Shingu[56] suggested that it may be better to remove the airway after the bronchoscope has been positioned in the trachea as it may interfere with the advancement of the ETT. However, this also leads to the loss of the retrolingual and pharyngeal conduit created by the oral airway and may result in impingement on laryngeal structures during ETT advancement. The great advantage of FBI is that the instrument is flexible and restricting its flexibility seems counter intuitive. FBI can be rapidly achieved without the use of these devices and the emphasis should be on the development of skill with bronchoscopic manipulation and topical anesthesia of the airway.

UTILIZATION OF BRONCHOSCOPIC INTUBATION IN DIFFERENT SETTINGS

How Useful Is Bronchoscopic Intubation in the Emergency Setting?

Success rates of emergency FBI have been reported by various authors to be 72% to 82%.[141–145] Visualization can be improved by pharyngeal suctioning.[142] While Desjardins and Varon[146] have reported the use of awake FBI in a "large proportion" of their trauma patients, as well as the use of the rapid sequence bronchoscopic technique, the flexible bronchoscope was rarely used in many emergency departments.[144,147,148] Immediate airway control in the emergency setting can be difficult using bronchoscopic techniques due to the presence of blood, emesis, or secretions in the airway.[27,141,144,149] Poor preparation of the patient and lack of patient cooperation can also be problematic.[27,141,142] FBI can nevertheless be a valuable option in selected patients, such as those with confirmed or suspected cervical spine injury,[144] those with anticipated difficult direct laryngoscopic intubation due to variant anatomy,[144] and in the presence of airway pathology such as Ludwig's angina,[35,100], burn injury[100] or angioedema.[149] Its use as part of a rapid sequence intubation technique has also been described.[146] Complete airway obstruction has however been reported during attempted FBI in the presence of upper-airway compromise.[20,44,51]

Awake FBI has been advocated in the management of penetrating neck injuries.[146] However, this technique may only be feasible in cooperative stable patients who do not require immediate airway control.[143,146] The optimal initial airway management approach in a patient with a penetrating neck injury remains controversial.[150,151] A high success with laryngoscopy coupled with the technical and time constraints of FBI results in airway management practitioners preferring to perform RSI and direct laryngoscopy, or a primary surgical airway when an emergency airway was required.[150,151]

FBI has also been advocated for the emergency management of blunt injury to the airway, although reported experience is limited.[152,153] Awake nasal FBI is challenging in such circumstances due to various factors, such as intolerance of supine position from airway obstruction,[154] significant oropharyngeal bleeding,[155] and the risk of further airway disruption during blind ETT passage over the bronchoscope. In the presence of significant laryngotracheal injury, tracheotomy under local anesthesia may be required.[156]

Emergency FBI has also been performed successfully in patients with respiratory failure, congestive heart failure, altered consciousness due to stroke, overdose, head trauma, status asthmaticus, hematemesis, partial upper-airway obstruction,[141,142,144] obstructing tracheal blood clot,[157] and following inadvertent extubation in the prone position with the neck in fixed flexion.[158]

Can Flexible Bronchoscopic Intubation Be Performed Through Extraglottic Devices?

The 2013 American Society of Anesthesiologists Practice Guidelines for Management of the Difficult Airway include the use of an EGD as an intubation conduit with or without bronchoscopic guidance in the alternative approaches to intubation.[45] Similarly, the Canadian Airway Focus Group (CAFG) included bronchoscopy-aided intubation via an EGD as an exit strategy in the presence of adequate oxygenation following failed intubation.[24] In the DAS guidelines for the management of the unanticipated difficult intubation in adults, FBI through an EGD is in Plan B (Maintaining oxygenation: EGD insertion).[46] Plan B is implemented when tracheal intubation by

TABLE 10.3. Bronchoscopic 4-Point Brimacombe Score Assessing the Anatomic Placement of a Laryngeal Mask. The Score Can Be Used to Objectively Determine If the Laryngeal Mask Is a Suitable Intubation Conduit

Brimacombe Score			Suitability as Intubation Conduit
4	Only vocal cords visible	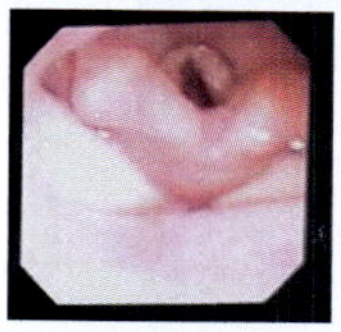	Yes
3	Vocal cords and posterior epiglottis visible	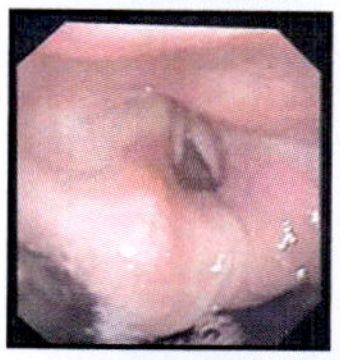	Yes
2	Vocal cords and anterior epiglottis visible	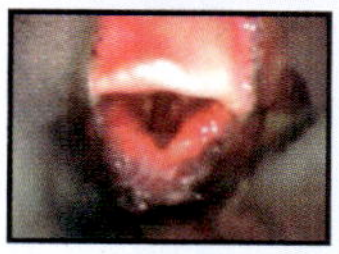	Likely yes. Additional jaw thrust may be required to further lift the epiglottis away from the glottic inlet to facilitate ETT passage
1	Vocal cords not seen	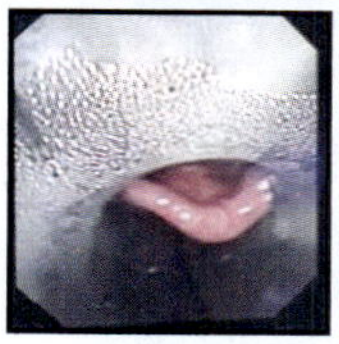	No. The laryngeal mask must be repositioned

direct laryngoscopy or an alternate technique of proven value in experienced hands has failed. The choice of EGD as a rescue device should have been made before the induction of GA and is determined by the clinical situation, device availability, and the practitioner's experience.[46] The availability of second-generation EGDs has been recommended. Intubation through the EGD is only appropriate in this setting if the clinical situation is stable, oxygenation through the EGD is possible, and the anesthesia practitioner is trained in the technique.[46]

Brimacombe and Berry proposed a bronchoscopic scoring system to assess the anatomic placement of the LMA.[159] The modified 4-point scale: Grade 4, only vocal cord seen; Grade 3, vocal cord and posterior epiglottis seen; Grade 2, vocal cords and anterior epiglottis seen; Grade 1, vocal cords not seen[160] also provides the operator with objective information on the suitability of the laryngeal mask or EGD as an intubating conduit (Table 10.3).

How Do I Intubate Through EGDs that Do Not Permit the Passage of a Full-Sized ETT?

A 7-mm ID ETT can be passed through a #5 LMA-Classic™, and a 6-mm ID ETT through a #3 or #4 LMA-Classic.[24,55] However, the long and relatively narrow airway tube requires the use of a longer ETT such as the 6-mm ID (40 cm in length) microlaryngoscopy tube (MLT) or the 6- or 7-mm ID nasal Ring-Adair-Elwyn (RAE) tube.[161] The LMA can be removed over the ETT using a second tube as a stabilizer to exert counter pressure on the ETT in the trachea to prevent its inadvertent dislodgement during the removal of the LMA.[162] In addition, the passage of an adult full-sized ETT through EGDs, such as the LMA-ProSeal™ and LMA-Supreme™, is also not possible due to the narrow internal diameter of the airway tube.

Several techniques have been reported to facilitate FBI via these EGDs. FBI through the LMA-Classic using a pediatric flexible bronchoscope with an ensleeved Aintree Intubation Catheter (AIC, Cook Medical Inc Bloomington, IN) has been referred to as a "low skill bronchoscopic intubation,"[163] and is regarded as a core skill that should be within the ability of all anesthesia practitioners after minimal training.[163,164] This technique can also be applied to intubation through LMA-Unique™, LMA-ProSeal, and AuraOnce™.[165] The AIC has an internal diameter of 4.8 mm, an external diameter of 6.5 mm, and a length of 56 cm with depth markings along the shaft to guide insertion. Introduced in 1996, it was designed to facilitate FBI through the aperture bars of the LMA-Classic.[166] The AIC can be ensleeved proximally over a 4.0-mm flexible bronchoscope (Figure 10.27A) such that the distal 3 cm of the shaft, the bending section, of the scope is free (Figure 10.27B). The scope with the ensleeved catheter can then be passed through the LMA-Classic aperture bars into the trachea (Figure 10.28A) under indirect vision. The scope can then be removed leaving the AIC in the trachea, paying attention to the depth of insertion to prevent endobronchial placement (Figure 10.28B). The LMA can then be removed and a cut (around 26 cm) ETT ≥ 7.0 mm ID passed into the trachea over the AIC. The AIC is then removed. A Rapi-Fit adapter supplied with the AIC (Figure 10.27A) permits ventilation through the catheter if this becomes necessary,[166] but the risk of barotrauma with ventilation through an airway exchange catheter must be appreciated.

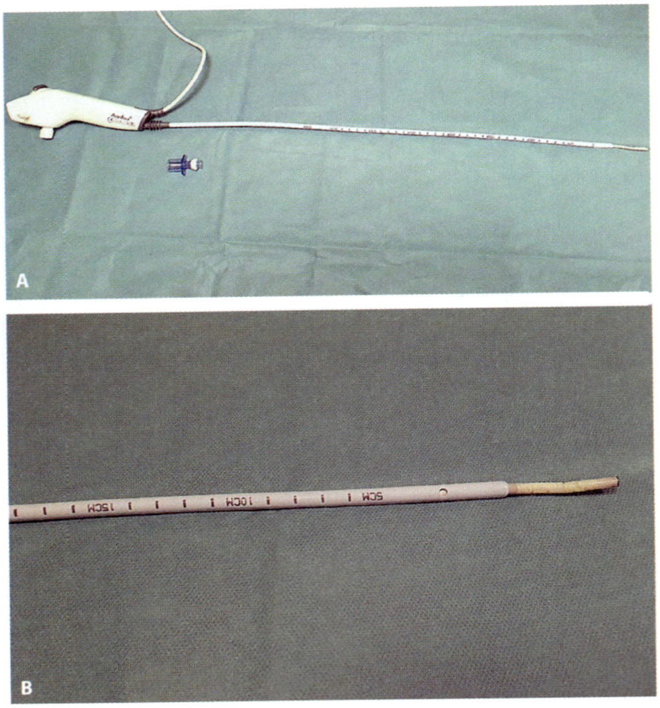

FIGURE 10.27. (A) The Aintree Intubating Catheter loaded over an AMBU aScope Broncho Slim. The accompanying Rapi-Fit adaptor permits ventilation through the catheter if necessary. **(B)** Distal shaft of the bronchoscope is exposed for maneuverability.

Atherton et al.[166] reported that the experienced endoscopist could master the AIC-FBI technique after 4 intubations and those inexperienced in FBI after 6 intubations. AIC-guided FBI through EGDs has been used successfully in patients requiring rescue EGD insertion following failed intubation.[163,167,168] Berkow et al.[169] reviewed 500 patients who had been entered into a difficult airway database at their institution between 2006 and 2009. The LMA-Classic-AIC-FBI technique for intubation had been utilized in 128 patients and was successful in 119 (93%).[169] A 2012 review of the use of AIC through extraglottic airways demonstrated an overall success rate of 88% when the AIC was used with the LMA-Classic or LMA-Unique.[165] However, with the LMA-Supreme, the epiglottic fins on the LMA-Supreme restricted the maneuverability of the bronchoscope with the ensleeved AIC, impeding its insertion through the glottis.[170] Directing the bronchoscope above these fins was frequently difficult.[170] In summary, the use of an AIC over a flexible bronchoscope has permitted bronchoscopic intubation through an EGD when direct bronchoscopic intubation was not possible.[46] Moreover, the use of the AIC through various EGDs has a high success rate in both elective and emergency situations, although the efficacy of the AIC combined with the LMA-Proseal, LMA-Supreme, and i-gel® in normal and difficult airway scenarios will require more research to ascertain.[165] AIC-facilitated intubation through an LMA-Supreme is not reliable and is not recommended in the 2015 DAS guidelines.[46]

A bronchoscope and a tracheal introducer (also known as "bougie") can also be passed in parallel through an EGD and advanced in tandem. The bougie is then manipulated into the trachea under bronchoscope guidance.[165] Allison and McCrory reported success in 22/25 patients using this technique.[171] The technique requires the coordinated efforts of two skilled practitioners.[165]

How Do I Intubate Through EGDs that Allow the Passage of a Full-Sized ETT?

In addition to the recommendation of using second-generation EGDs for airway rescue after failed intubation, we further support the use of EGDs that permit the passage of a full-sized ETT. While the use of adjuncts such as the AIC is no doubt, useful, the need for multiple exchanges (e.g., LMA over AIC, ETT over AIC) presents numerous opportunities for device dislodgement and technique failure. Previously, the Intubating LMA (ILMA or LMA-Fastrach) was the only EGD that allowed the insertion of an adult full-sized ETT. Unfortunately, it was considered a specialized piece of equipment and was not universally available in all areas where anesthetics are administered or airway management occurs; it also required a distinct skill with its learning curve.[163] The airway tube of the LMA-Fastrach has a minimal ID of 13 mm and can accommodate any cuffed

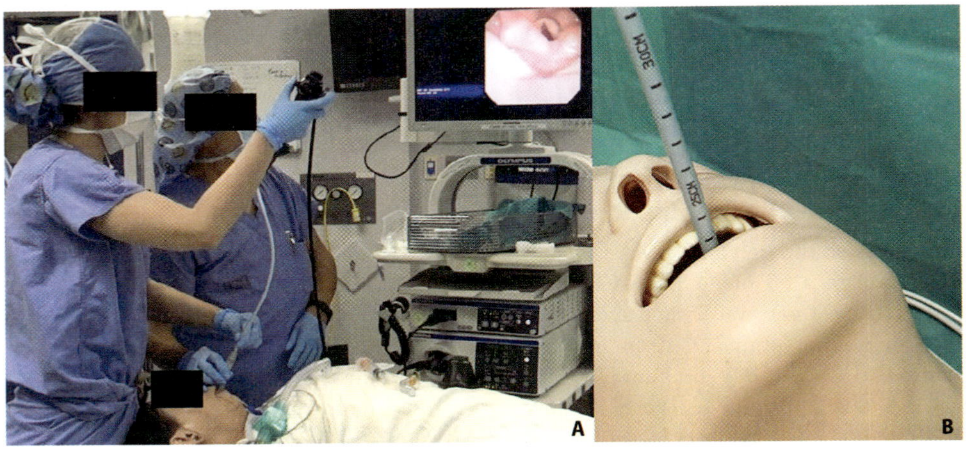

FIGURE 10.28. (A) Passage of the Aintree Intubating Catheter under indirect vision using the flexible bronchoscope. **(B)** Markings along the shaft of the Aintree Intubating Catheter help guide the depth of insertion.

TABLE 10.4. Maximum ETT Size to Be Used with the AMBU AuraGain, i-gel, and LMA-Protector for Bronchoscopic-Aided Intubation

	AMBU AuraGain			i-gel			LMA-Protector		
	#3	#4	#5	#3	#4	#5	#3	#4	#5
Maximum ETT size (mm ID)	6.5	7.5	8.0	6.0	7.0	8.0	6.5	7.5	7.5

ETT size up to an 8 mm ID.[172] Although blind intubation through the Intubating LMA has been reported with a high success rate, first-attempt success rates are higher using bronchoscopic guidance.[46]

Presently, second-generation EGDs with direct intubating capabilities such as the AMBU AuraGain, i-gel, and LMA-Protector, are now widely available and should be considered for use as a first-line airway rescue device. The maximum ETT size that can be used with the AMBU AuraGain, i-gel, and LMA-Protector are summarized in Table 10.4. Following proper placement of the EGD, a well-lubricated and appropriately-sized ETT is loaded over an adult bronchoscope as per usual practice for FBI. The bronchoscope is passed into the tracheal lumen before advancing the ETT over the bronchoscope, through the EGD (Figure 10.29). The ETT cuff must be well lubricated to avoid damage during its passage through the EGD. In elective situations, the inner surface of the EGD's airway tube should also be lubricated prior to insertion, to facilitate subsequent ETT passage. Once tracheal intubation has been established, the EGD may be left in-situ in short surgical procedures. However, the EGD will need to be removed in most circumstances and the ETT must be stabilized to prevent inadvertent dislodgement. ETT stabilization may be achieved by several methods, such as using the LMA-Fastrach stabilizing rod, a second ETT to exert counter pressure on the ETT in the trachea,[162] or a Magill forceps.[173–175] Success rates of 98% to 100% have been reported for bronchoscopic intubation through the AMBU AuraGain, i-gel, and LMA-Protector.[176,177]

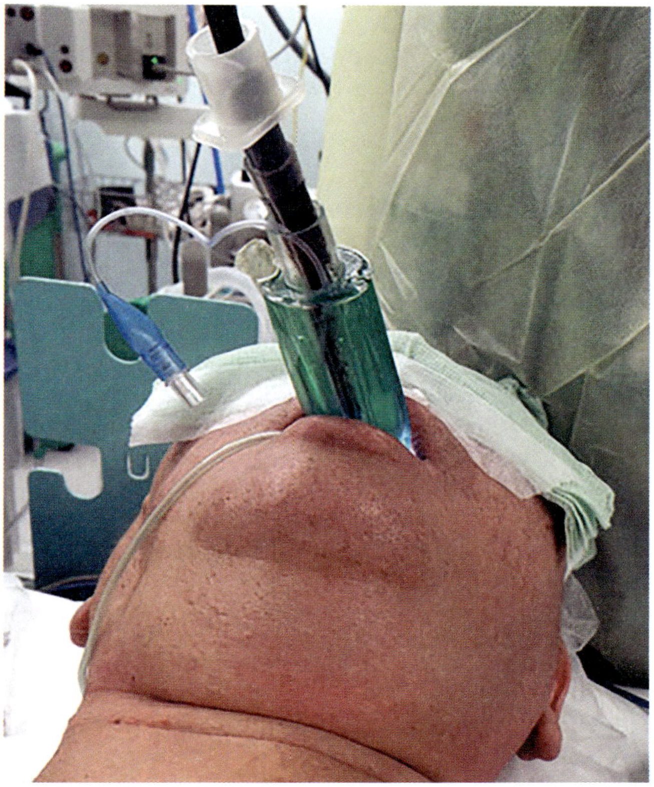

FIGURE 10.29. Direct intubation through the i-gel using a 7.5-mm ID ETT with the aid of a 4.2-mm flexible bronchoscope.

Can the Flexible Bronchoscope Be Combined with Laryngoscopy?

The flexible bronchoscope can be used in combination with a direct laryngoscopy.[11,178]. In the recent two decades, the increased use of video laryngoscopy led to more reports of video laryngoscopy-assisted FBI, using the GlideScope[179–183] and CMAC[184] video laryngoscopes as well as the Airtraq optical laryngoscope.[185–187]

The combined use of the video laryngoscope (VL) and the flexible bronchoscope can utilize the strengths of both techniques[184] and compensate for their respective limitations.[185] The laryngoscope can be utilized to lift the tongue, mandible, and soft palate, thereby increasing the caliber of the pharyngeal lumen and facilitating the identification of landmarks as seen through the bronchoscope.[178,183,184,188] The view on the VL screen allows both bronchoscope and VL operators to simultaneously observe and coordinate each step of the procedure,[187] facilitating the advancement of the bronchoscope toward the larynx (Figure 10.30). This approach is particularly useful in

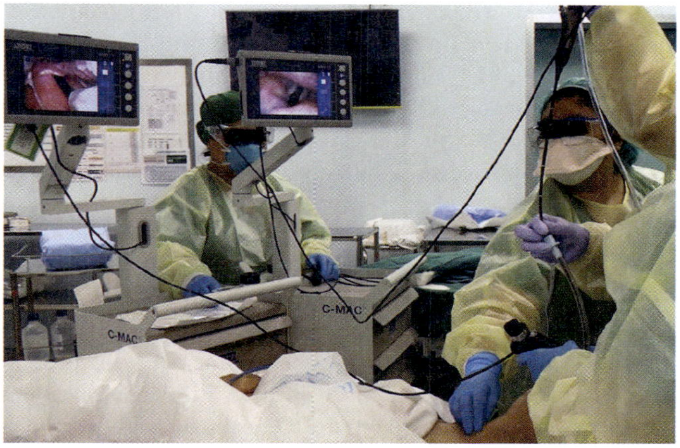

FIGURE 10.30. Combined video laryngoscope (CMAC) and flexible bronchoscopic intubation. The VL screen allows both videolaryngoscope and bronchoscope operators as well as anesthesia assistants to simultaneously observe and coordinate each step of the intubation procedure.

situations where the glottis cannot be visualized adequately by the VL, e.g., in a Cormack & Lehane grade 3 or 4 view.[187] The video-laryngoscopist can also manually guide the bronchoscope as desired[184] and the bronchoscope has been described as a controllable stylet in this setting.[180] After the bronchoscope has been positioned in the trachea, the combined technique permits passage of the tube over the scope to be visualized on the VL monitor such that any maneuvering or rotation of the tube can be done under indirect visual control.[181,183,184] The combined VL and FBI technique was reportedly more useful than VL alone in the intubation of patients with cervical spine pathology.[189] The technique was also successful in facilitating the passage of a 6-mm ID electromyographic tracheal tube past a stenotic tracheal segment as a result of external compression by a goiter.[179] One limitation of the combined VL and FBI technique is that it requires two practitioners.[184]

OTHER CONSIDERATIONS

What Are the Limitations and Complications of Bronchoscopic Intubation?

Bronchoscopes are delicate, expensive instruments and require careful use if the damage is to be avoided. The sterilization process is complex and requires time and resources. FBI in the presence of secretions, emesis, or blood in the airway is difficult and the applicability of the technique in an emergency situation is limited. Some measure of patient cooperation is also necessary for awake intubation. When both the bronchoscope and the ensleeved ETT are in the larynx or trachea, significant airway obstruction can be produced,[18,57] and can cause respiratory distress.

Although they are rare, complications associated with FBI can occur. These include laryngospasm,[2,3] complete airway obstruction,[20,44,51] local anesthetic toxicity,[190] respiratory depression secondary to sedative overdose,[3] loss of the endoscopy mask diaphragm into the airway,[2,3], laryngeal trauma[191] pyrexia and rigors,[192] and respiratory infection.[105] The ETT is advanced blindly over the bronchoscope and may impinge on laryngeal or pharyngeal structures. Supraglottic swelling, pharyngeal hematoma, and vocal cord immobility and bruising have been reported after FBI.[191] A markedly displaced arytenoid cartilage has also been reported.[193] The ETT should be advanced gently over the bronchoscope, the gap between the ETT and scope diameters minimized, and the use of tubes with modified bevels may be considered.

There is little information on the specific incidence and scope of complications attributable to the FBI. Heidegger et al. reported that 8.5% (11/130) of patients who underwent nasal bronchoscopic intubation experienced vocal cord sequelae (erythema, 8; hematoma, 5) and a 4% incidence of postoperative hoarseness.[194] In a series of 2031 FBIs, complications were limited to laryngospasm in 51, pain or hematoma secondary to cricothyroid injection in 33, gagging or vomiting in 8, and mild epistaxis in 70 who were nasally intubated.[3] None of the cases of epistaxis required packing. A retrospective electronic database review of 146,252 intubations performed at a Canadian tertiary care center between 2002 and 2013 revealed 1554 awake intubations, of which all but 12 were performed with a flexible bronchoscope.[9] There were 31 failed attempted awake intubations (2%). Of the 1523 successful awake intubations, complications were reported in 239 (15.7%) and included cough or gag, 54; tube hang up in larynx, 42; change to smaller or parker tube required, 29; blood or secretions, 16; airway compromise with application of local anesthetic, 12; patient uncooperative, 7; cuff leak after intubation, 5; change of nasal/oral route required, 5; excess sedation, 4; inadvertent immediate extubation, 1.[9]

How Much Training Is Required to Develop Proficiency in BronchoscopicIntubation? How Can the Training Be Acquired?

FBI is not a difficult skill to master; however, it requires familiarity with the anatomy of the upper airway, and dexterity with bronchoscopic manipulation. *Awake* FBI requires skill in regional anesthesia of the airway as well as gentleness on the part of the practitioner. Each step of the procedure must be planned in advance and methodically carried out. The ability to quickly and reliably maneuver the bronchoscope in a given direction is an absolute requirement for a fast, successful, and safe FBI. Surveys done in North America and the United Kingdom revealed that most trainees did not meet the minimum targets (set arbitrarily in the surveys to define competency) of supervised bronchoscopic intubations.[195–197]

Proficiency in scope handling and dexterity can be developed using various methods (see also Chapter 67, "Teaching and Simulation for Airway Management"):

A) **Nonanatomic Models**

Marsland et al.[198] have described a nonanatomical modular endoscopic training system called the Dexter endoscopic dexterity trainer. This system consists of a manikin, an image chart, a series of maps, and a structured training module. The objective is to endoscopically explore the manikin and find the images placed inside it. Novice endoscopists took about 3.5 hours to complete the Dexter training modules and were then able to perform clinical endoscopy on awake subjects from mouth to carina in a mean time of 32.5 seconds.[198] Training on the Dexter endoscopic dexterity trainer was found to improve proficiency in bronchoscopy in manikins[199] and clinical volunteers from mouth to carina[200]; it was also more effective than a nonanatomic choose-the-hole model.[201]

Video systems permit ongoing guidance and immediate feedback by an expert instructor who shares the view of the airway and appears to enhance the acquisition of bronchoscopic skills.[19,202] Smith et al.[203] and Wheeler et al.[202] both reported improved bronchoscopic intubation performance in randomized studies that compared video and eyepiece endoscopes.

B) **Virtual Reality Simulators**

More complex systems for bronchoscopic intubation training include Virtual Reality Simulators and Virtual Reality Simulation software. Simulation-based bronchoscopy training is associated with benefits on skills, behavior, and time.[204]

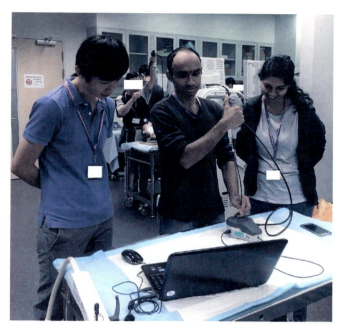

FIGURE 10.31. Anesthesia residents practicing bronchoscopy using the ORSIM bronchoscopy simulator at an airway workshop.

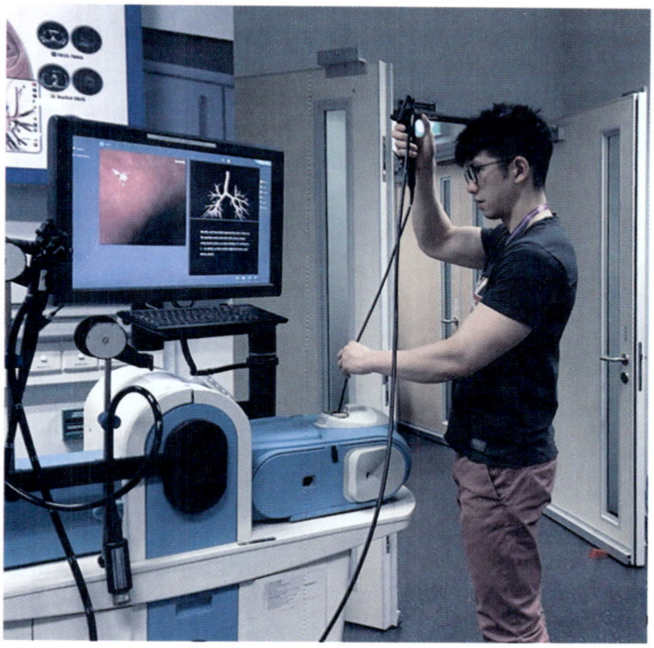

FIGURE 10.32. An anesthesia resident practicing bronchoscopy using the Simbionix Bronch Mentor at an airway workshop.

The Accutouch flexible bronchoscopy simulator was suggested to be effective in teaching psychomotor skills as it improved performance indicators (such as time to intubation, and the number of mucosal hits) by novice operators during clinical bronchoscopy in children[205] and cadavers.[206] Skills decay was noted 2 months after training but required a shorter time and fewer attempts to retrain.[207]

The Virtual Fiberoptic Intubation (VFI) software can be used for self-directed deliberate practice on any computer, without additional materials or instructors. Self-directed learning using the VFI software improved the acquisition of bronchoscopic skills[208] and bronchoscopy success rates.[209]

The ORSIM bronchoscopic simulator (Figure 10.31) incorporates a replica video-bronchoscope that interacts with software components to create a variety of high-fidelity, virtual reality difficult airway scenarios.[207] Wong et al.[24] demonstrated improved clinical bronchoscopy performance and intubation times by novice operators after training on the ORSIM for 60 minutes.

The Simbionix Bronch Mentor (Figure 10.32) demonstrated validity in differentiating skills in scope manipulation and airway anatomy between novice and experienced operators.[210]

The use of a low-cost mobile gaming application, Airway Ex App (Level Ex, Inc), was associated with better scope manipulation in emergency medicine physicians who performed self-directed learning after receiving conventional training,[211]

C) **Anatomic Models**

Chandra et al.[212] compared bronchoscopic intubation skill acquisition using low and high-fidelity models and found no difference in median intubation times and intubation success rates. Interestingly, a 2013 systematic review noted that animal models or manikins may be superior to and possibly less expensive than virtual reality simulators.[204] Latif et al.[213] used didactic instruction, a Virtual Reality simulator (VRS), and a Human Anatomy Airway Simulator (HAAS, consisting of a manikin-like face, head, neck, and upper chest that can be intubated with a flexible bronchoscope) with expert guidance to train novices in bronchoscopic intubation. On retesting after 2 months, skills decay was noted on the VRS but no skill decay was found with the HAAS.

With the advent of three-dimensional (3D) printing technology, creating low-cost anatomical models for bronchoscopy training may resolve the limitations of acquiring expensive virtual reality simulators.[214] Training with 3D printed models has been shown to improve novices' standards of task performance,[215] procedural completion time[175,215,216], and retention of bronchoscopic skills.[217]

D) **Patients with Normal Airways**

FBI has been advocated as an alternate technique that may be used whenever tracheal intubation is indicated.[3] FBI of normal airways under GA may be beneficial in learning to manipulate the bronchoscope and to advance the ETT over the scope,[3,27,218] hence improving intubation time and success.[107,219] However, the use of "non-routine" techniques may require discussion with the patient beforehand and the issue of consent has been raised.[220] Furthermore, the FBI of patients with normal airways under GA may not extrapolate well to the intubation of the difficult airway in the awake patient.[218,221]

In addition to learning FBI in patients under GA, in the author's institution, fourth and final-year anesthesia residents are rostered to the ENT clinic to perform nasoendoscopy in awake patients under the guidance of an ENT surgeon. This arrangement provides them the opportunity to improve endoscopy skills and builds confidence in performing endoscopy facing the patient who is in a sitting position, one that is most commonly adopted by patients who are in respiratory distress in an emergency setting. As part of the anesthesia-ENT collaboration, the residents are further allowed to perform drug-induced sleep endoscopy under the supervision of an ENT surgeon, to further advance their endoscopy skills in obstructed airways.

Ideally, FBI should be demonstrated by a knowledgeable and skilled instructor.[5] The learner should then be supervised until the principles of bronchoscopic manipulation are mastered. The availability of video bronchoscopes permits the instructor to easily coach the learner in the flexion and rotation movements required to properly steer the bronchoscope and appears to facilitate bronchoscopic skill acquisition.[19] Practice is then required to further develop and improve psychomotor skills. A reasonable level of dexterity in manipulating the bronchoscope can be achieved within 3 to 4 hours of independent manikin practice.[5]

An acceptable level of technical expertise may be achievable after 10 FBIs in anesthetized patients[222] and 15 to 20 awake FBIs in patients with normal anatomy.[5] Smith and Jackson[223] reported that trainees were "becoming reasonably proficient" after performing 20 FBIs in anesthetized patients with predicted difficult intubation. It has also been suggested that 30 FBIs in conscious and anesthetized patients be performed before a practitioner is ready to handle the difficult intubation.[54] A survey of New Zealand anesthesia practitioners reported that those who had performed 100 bronchoscopic intubations considered themselves to be experienced or experts.[196,224]

The amount of experience and training required for safe and effective use of the flexible bronchoscope in the difficult airway is unknown[18,224]; however, an experience of 100 or more bronchoscopic procedures may be necessary to acquire expertise in this setting.[5,18,224] How best to facilitate bronchoscopic skill development and to determine when an acceptable level of expertise is achieved remains unknown.

SUMMARY

After direct laryngoscopy, videolaryngoscopy and flexible bronchoscopy are the most common techniques for tracheal intubation,[197] and awake bronchoscopic intubation continues to be the gold standard for the management of the anticipated difficult airway.[225] In most situations, in the presence of significant predictors of difficult intubation *and* difficult face-mask or EGD ventilation, awake intubation should be strongly considered.[24,25] Bronchoscopic intubation can also be a valuable alternative technique in the "can't intubate, can oxygenate situation,"[45] and may be the preferred Plan A choice for practitioners who are experts in the technique.[46] Over the 12 years till 2013, the incidence of awake bronchoscopic intubation did not decrease at a Canadian tertiary care center despite the increasing use of video laryngoscopy.[9] Predictors of difficult VL include neck pathology and limited mandibular protrusion and limited mouth opening may preclude introduction of the scope. The ability to perform awake FBI continues to be an absolute vital skill for anesthesia practitioners and its importance cannot be overemphasized. It should be mastered by all anesthesia practitioners and other practitioners responsible for airway management.

SELF-EVALUATION QUESTIONS

10.1. Complications associated with bronchoscopic intubation include:

A. Laryngospasm

B. Complete airway obstruction

C. Local anesthesia toxicity

D. Laryngeal trauma

E. All of the above

10.2. What is the appropriate management following the insertion of a rescue extraglottic device (EGD) for a "Can't intubate, can't oxygenate" situation?

A. The EGD should be removed to allow video laryngoscopy by an expert airway practitioner.

B. A size 7.0-mm ID ETT should be loaded onto a pediatric flexible bronchoscope for intubation through the EGD.

C. An Aintree intubation catheter should be loaded onto an adult flexible bronchoscope for intubation through the EGD.

D. A size 6.0-mm ID or larger ETT should be loaded over an adult flexible bronchoscope for intubation through the EGD, if the EGD used permits the passage of a large ETT.

E. A surgical airway should be performed while oxygenation and ventilation are maintained via the EGD.

10.3. During bronchoscopic intubation, which of the following can facilitate the advancement of the ensleeved endotracheal tube to advance into the trachea over the bronchoscopic bronchoscope?

A. Profound regional anesthesia of the airway.

B. Rotation of the tube 90 degree counterclockwise may be necessary to orient the bevel posteriorly.

C. Minimize the discrepancy between the outside diameter of the bronchoscope and the internal diameter of the endotracheal tube.

D. The use of the ILMA tube which has a soft hemispherical bevel and a leading edge in the midline.

E. All of the above.

REFERENCES

1. Murphy P. A fibre-optic endoscope used for nasal intubation. *Anaesthesia.* 1967;22:489-491.
2. Ovassapian A. The flexible bronchoscope. A tool for anesthesiologists. *Clin Chest Med.* 2001;22:281-299.
3. Greenland KB, Irwin MG. The Williams Airway Intubator, the Ovassapian Airway and the Berman Airway as upper airway conduits for fibreoptic bronchoscopy in patients with difficult airways. *Curr Opin Anaesthesiol.* 2004;17:505-510.
4. Stiles CM, Stiles QR, Denson JS. A flexible fiber optic laryngoscope. *JAMA.* 1972;221:1246-1247.
5. Ovassapian A, Yelich SJ. Learning fiberoptic intubation. *Anesth Clin N Amer.* 1991;9:175-186.
6. Practice guidelines for management of the difficult airway. A report by the American Society of Anesthesiologists Task Force on Management of the Difficult Airway. *Anesthesiology.* 1993;78:597-602.

7. Stackhouse RA. Fiberoptic airway management. *Anesthesiol Clin North America*. 2002;20:933-951.
8. Weiss YG, Deutschman CS. The role of fiberoptic bronchoscopy in airway management of the critically ill patient. *Crit Care Clin*. 2000;16:445-451.
9. Law JA, Morris IR, Brousseau PA, de la Ronde S, Milne AD. The incidence, success rate, and complications of awake tracheal intubation in 1,554 patients over 12 years: an historical cohort study. *Can J Anaesth*. 2015;62:736-744.
10. Avargues P, Cros AM, Daucourt V, Michel P, Maurette P. Procedures use by French anesthetists in cases of difficult intubation and the impact of a conference of experts. *Ann Fr Anesth Reanim*. 1999;18:719-724.
11. Ezri T, Szmuk P, Warters RD, Katz J, Hagberg CA. Difficult airway management practice patterns among anesthesiologists practicing in the United States: have we made any progress? *J Clin Anesth*. 2003;15:418-422.
12. Heidegger T, Gerig H. Anticipated difficult airway: the role of fiberoptics. *Anesth Analg*. 2002;95:1124.
13. Kristensen MS, Moller J. Airway management behaviour, experience and knowledge among Danish anaesthesiologists—room for improvement. *Acta Anaesthesiol Scand*. 2001;45:1181-1185.
14. Rosenblatt WH, Wagner PJ, Ovassapian A, Kain ZN. Practice patterns in managing the difficult airway by anesthesiologists in the United States. *Anesth Analg*. 1998;87:153-157.
15. Wong DT, Mehta A, Tam AD, Yau B, Wong J. A survey of Canadian anesthesiologists' preferences in difficult intubation and "cannot intubate, cannot ventilate" situations. *Can J Anaesth*. 2014;61:717-726.
16. Benumof JL. Management of the difficult adult airway. With special emphasis on awake tracheal intubation. *Anesthesiology*. 1991;75:1087-110.
17. Heidegger T, Gerig HJ, Ulrich B, Kreienbuhl G. Validation of a simple algorithm for tracheal intubation: daily practice is the key to success in emergencies—an analysis of 13,248 intubations. *Anesth Analg*. 2001;92:517-522.
18. Ovassapian A, Wheeler M. Fiberoptic Endoscopy-aided techniques. In: Benumof JL, ed. *Airway Management Principles and Practice*. St. Louis, MO: Mosby, Inc; 1996:282-319.
19. Sidhu VS, Whitehead EM, Ainsworth QP, Smith M, Calder I. A technique of awake fibreoptic intubation. Experience in patients with cervical spine disease. *Anaesthesia*. 1993;48:910-913.
20. Allan AG. Reluctance of anaesthetists to perform awake intubation. *Anaesthesia*. 2004;59:413.
21. Basi SK, Cooper M, Ahmed FB, Clarke SG, Mitchell V. Reluctance of anaesthetists to perform awake intubation. *Anaesthesia*. 2004;59:918.
22. Wanderer JP, Ehrenfeld JM, Sandberg WS, Epstein RH. The changing scope of difficult airway management. *Can J Anaesth*. 2013;60:1022-1024.
23. Popat MT, Woodall NM. Chapter 14: Fiberoptic intubation: Uses and omissions. *NAP4 Report and finfings of the 4th National Audit Project of the Royal College of Anaesthetists*. 2011;4:114.
24. Law JA, Duggan LV, Asselin M, et al. Canadian Airway Focus Group updated consensus-based recommendations for management of the difficult airway: part 1. Difficult airway management encountered in an unconscious patient. *Can J Anaesth*. 2021;68:1373-1404.
25. Ahmad I, El-Boghdadly K, Bhagrath R, et al. Difficult Airway Society guidelines for awake tracheal intubation (ATI) in adults. *Anaesthesia*. 2020;75:509-528.
26. Chan JK, Ng I, Ang JP, et al. Randomised controlled trial comparing the Ambu(R) aScope2 with a conventional fibreoptic bronchoscope in orotracheal intubation of anaesthetised adult patients. *Anaesth Intensive Care*. 2015;43:479-484.
27. Hartley M, Morris S, Vaughan RS. Teaching fibreoptic intubation. Effect of alfentanil on the haemodynamic response. *Anaesthesia*. 1994;49:335-337.
28. Reed AP. Preparation for intubation of the awake patient. *Mt Sinai J Med*. 1995;62:10-20.
29. Collins SR, Blank RS. Fiberoptic intubation: an overview and update. *Respir Care*. 2014;59:865-878; discussion 78-80.
30. Iseli TA, Iseli CE, Golden JB, et al. Outcomes of intubation in difficult airways due to head and neck pathology. *Ear Nose Throat J*. 2012;91:E1-E5.
31. Langeron O, Semjen F, Bourgain JL, Marsac A, Cros AM. Comparison of the intubating laryngeal mask airway with the fiberoptic intubation in anticipated difficult airway management. *Anesthesiology*. 2001;94:968-972.
32. Kheterpal S, Martin L, Shanks AM, Tremper KK. Prediction and outcomes of impossible mask ventilation: a review of 50,000 anesthetics. *Anesthesiology*. 2009;110:891-897.
33. Marcus BJ, Kaplan J, Collins KA. A case of Ludwig angina: a case report and review of the literature. *Am J Forensic Med Pathol*. 2008;29:255-259.
34. Saifeldeen K, Evans R. Ludwig's angina. *Emerg Med J*. 2004;21:242-243.
35. Candamourty R, Venkatachalam S, Babu MR, Kumar GS. Ludwig's Angina – An emergency: a case report with literature review. *J Nat Sci Biol Med*. 2012;3:206-208.
36. Schumann M, Biesler I, Borgers A, Pfortner R, Mohr C, Groeben H. Tracheal intubation in patients with odentogenous abscesses and reduced mouth opening. *Br J Anaesth*. 2014;112:348-354.
37. Ovassapian A, Tuncbilek M, Weitzel EK, Joshi CW. Airway management in adult patients with deep neck infections: a case series and review of the literature. *Anesth Analg*. 2005;100:585-589.
38. Abernathy JH 3rd, Reeves ST. Airway catastrophes. *Curr Opin Anaesthesiol*. 2010;23:41-46.
39. Crosby ET. Airway management in adults after cervical spine trauma. *Anesthesiology*. 2006;104:1293-1318.
40. Meschino A, Devitt JH, Koch JP, Szalai JP, Schwartz ML. The safety of awake tracheal intubation in cervical spine injury. *Can J Anaesth*. 1992;39:114-117.
41. Morris IR. Airway management. In: Rosen P, et al, eds. *Emergency Medicine: Concepts and Clinical Practice*. St. Louis, MO: Mosby Yearbook; 1992:79-105.
42. Suderman VS, Crosby ET, Lui A. Elective oral tracheal intubation in cervical spine-injured adults. *Can J Anaesth*. 1991;38:785-789.
43. Walls RM. Airway management. In: Rose P, et al, eds. *Emergency Medicine: Concepts and Clinical Practice*. St. Louis, MO: Mosby Yearbook; 1998:2-24.
44. McGuire G, el-Beheiry H. Complete upper airway obstruction during awake fibreoptic intubation in patients with unstable cervical spine fractures. *Can J Anaesth*. 1999;46:176-178.
45. Apfelbaum JL, Hagberg CA, Caplan RA, et al. Practice guidelines for management of the difficult airway: an updated report by the American Society of Anesthesiologists Task Force on Management of the Difficult Airway. *Anesthesiology*. 2013;118:251-270.
46. Frerk C, Mitchell VS, McNarry AF, et al. Difficult Airway Society 2015 guidelines for management of unanticipated difficult intubation in adults. *Br J Anaesth*. 2015;115:827-848.
47. Law JA, Broemling N, Cooper RM, et al. The difficult airway with recommendations for management–part 1–difficult tracheal intubation encountered in an unconscious/induced patient. *Can J Anaesth*. 2013;60:1089-1118.
48. Liistro G, Stanescu DC, Veriter C, Rodenstein DO, D'Odemont JP. Upper airway anesthesia induces airflow limitation in awake humans. *Am Rev Respir Dis*. 1992;146:581-585.
49. Beydon L, Lorino AM, Verra F, et al. Topical upper airway anaesthesia with lidocaine increases airway resistance by impairing glottic function. *Intensive Care Med*. 1995;21:920-926.
50. Kuna ST, Woodson GE, Sant'Ambrogio G. Effect of laryngeal anesthesia on pulmonary function testing in normal subjects. *Am Rev Respir Dis*. 1988;137:656-661.
51. Shaw IC, Welchew EA, Harrison BJ, Michael S. Complete airway obstruction during awake fibreoptic intubation. *Anaesthesia*. 1997;52:582-585.
52. Donlon JVJ. Anesthetic management of patients with compromised airways. *Anesth Rev*. 1980;7:22-31.
53. Wong DT, McGuire GP. Management choices for the difficult airway (Author reply). *Can J Anaesth*. 2003;50:624.
54. Edens ET, Sia RL. Flexible fiberoptic endoscopy in difficult intubations. *Ann Otol Rhinol Laryngol*. 1981;90:307-309.
55. Fulling PD, Roberts JT. Fiberoptic intubation. *Int Anesthesiol Clin*. 2000;38:189-217.
56. Asai T, Shingu K. Difficulty in advancing a tracheal tube over a fibreoptic bronchoscope: incidence, causes and solutions. *Br J Anaesth*. 2004;92:870-881.
57. Dellinger RP. Fiberoptic bronchoscopy in adult airway management. *Crit Care Med*. 1990;18:882-887.
58. El-Orbany MI, Salem MR, Joseph NJ. Tracheal tube advancement over the fiberoptic bronchoscope: size does matter. *Anesth Analg*. 2003;97:301.
59. Kristensen MS. The Parker Flex-Tip tube versus a standard tube for fiberoptic orotracheal intubation: a randomized double-blind study. *Anesthesiology*. 2003;98:354-358.
60. Marsh NJ. Easier fiberoptic intubations. *Anesthesiology*. 1992;76:860-861.
61. Sutherland AD, Sale JP. Fibreoptic awake intubation—a method of topical anaesthesia and orotracheal intubation. *Can Anaesth Soc J*. 1986;33:502-504.
62. Witton TH. An introduction to the fiberoptic laryngoscope. *Can Anaesth Soc J*. 1981;28:475-478.
63. Deam R, McCutcheon C. Management choices for the difficult airway. *Can J Anaesth*. 2003;50:62362-62364.
64. Coccolini F, Perrone G, Chiarugi M, et al. Surgery in COVID-19 patients: operational directives. World *J Emerg Surg*. 2020;15:25.
65. Wahidi MM, Lamb C, Murgu S, et al. American Association for Bronchology and Interventional Pulmonology (AABIP) Statement on the Use of Bronchoscopy and Respiratory Specimen Collection in Patients With Suspected or Confirmed COVID-19 Infection. *J Bronchology Interv Pulmonol*. 2020;27:e52-e54.

66. Kristensen MS, Fredensborg BB. The disposable Ambu aScope vs. a conventional flexible videoscope for awake intubation – a randomised study. *Acta Anaesthesiol Scand.* 2013;57:888-895.
67. Zaidi SR, Collins AM, Mitsi E, et al. Single use and conventional bronchoscopes for Broncho alveolar lavage (BAL) in research: a comparative study (NCT 02515591). *BMC Pulm Med.* 2017;17:83.
68. Gupta D, Wang H. Cost-effectiveness analysis of flexible optical scopes for tracheal intubation: a descriptive comparative study of reusable and single-use scopes. *J Clin Anesth.* 2011;23:632-635.
69. Barron SP, Kennedy MP. Single-Use (Disposable) Flexible Bronchoscopes: The Future of Bronchoscopy? *Adv Ther.* 2020;37:4538-4548.
70. Perbet S, Blanquet M, Mourgues C, et al. Cost analysis of single-use (Ambu((R)) aScope) and reusable bronchoscopes in the ICU. *Ann Intensive Care.* 2017;7:3.
71. Edenharter GM, Gartner D, Pforringer D. Decision Support for the Capacity Management of Bronchoscopy Devices: Optimizing the Cost-Efficient Mix of Reusable and Single-Use Devices Through Mathematical Modeling. *Anesth Analg.* 2017;124:1963-1967.
72. Mouritsen JM, Ehlers L, Kovaleva J, Ahmad I, El-Boghdadly K. A systematic review and cost effectiveness analysis of reusable vs. single-use flexible bronchoscopes. *Anaesthesia.* 2020;75:529-540.
73. Tvede MF, Kristensen MS, Nyhus-Andreasen M. A cost analysis of reusable and disposable flexible optical scopes for intubation. *Acta Anaesthesiol Scand.* 2012;56:577-584.
74. Kovaleva J, Peters FT, van der Mei HC, Degener JE. Transmission of infection by flexible gastrointestinal endoscopy and bronchoscopy. *Clin Microbiol Rev.* 2013;26:231-254.
75. Mehta AC, Prakash UB, Garland R, et al. American College of Chest Physicians and American Association for Bronchology [corrected] consensus statement: prevention of flexible bronchoscopy-associated infection. *Chest.* 2005;128:1742-1755.
76. Bou R, Aguilar A, Perpinan J, et al. Nosocomial outbreak of Pseudomonas aeruginosa infections related to a flexible bronchoscope. *J Hosp Infect.* 2006;64:129-135.
77. Shimono N, Takuma T, Tsuchimochi N, et al. An outbreak of Pseudomonas aeruginosa infections following thoracic surgeries occurring via the contamination of bronchoscopes and an automatic endoscope reprocessor. *J Infect Chemother.* 2008;14:418-423.
78. Dickson A, Kondal P, Hilken L, Helgesen M, Sjolin W, Jensen D. Possible pseudotransmission of Enterobacter cloacae associated with an endobronchial ultrasound scope. *Am J Infect Control.* 2018;46:1296-1298.
79. Ofstead CL, Quick MR, Wetzler HP, et al. Effectiveness of Reprocessing for Flexible Bronchoscopes and Endobronchial Ultrasound Bronchoscopes. *Chest.* 2018;154:1024-1034.
80. Taylor DM, Brimacomb J, Stone T. Inactivation of prions by physical and chemical means. *J Hosp Infect.* 1999;43(Suppl):S69-S76.
81. Walsh EM. Reducing the risk of prion transmission in anaesthesia. *Anaesthesia.* 2006;61:64-65.
82. Spach DH, Silverstein FE, Stamm WE. Transmission of infection by gastrointestinal endoscopy and bronchoscopy. *Ann Intern Med.* 1993;118:117-128.
83. Lentz RJ, Colt H. Summarizing societal guidelines regarding bronchoscopy during the COVID-19 pandemic. *Respirology.* 2020;25:574-577.
84. Telford RJ, Liban JB. Awake fibreoptic intubation. *Br J Hosp Med.* 1991;46:182-184.
85. Lai YY, Chien JT, Huang SJ. Fiberoptic intubation with patients in sitting position. *Acta Anaesthesiol Taiwan.* 2007;45:169-173.
86. Morikawa S, Safar P, Decarlo J. Influence of the headjaw position upon upper airway patency. *Anesthesiology.* 1961;22:265-270.
87. Safar P. Ventilatory efficacy of mouth-to-mouth artificial respiration; airway obstruction during manual and mouth-to-mouth artificial respiration. *J Am Med Assoc.* 1958;167:335-341.
88. Boyson PG. Fiberoptic Instrumentation for Airway Management. *ASA Refresher Course Lectures.* 1993;266:1-5.
89. Badiger S, John M, Fearnley RA, Ahmad I. Optimizing oxygenation and intubation conditions during awake fibre-optic intubation using a high-flow nasal oxygen-delivery system. *Br J Anaesth.* 2015;115:629-632.
90. Ovassapian A. Flexible bronchoscopic intubation of awake patients. *J Bronchology.* 1994;1:240-245.
91. Durga VK, Millns JP, Smith JE. Manoeuvres used to clear the airway during fibreoptic intubation. *Br J Anaesth.* 2001;87:207-211.
92. Hughes S, Smith JE. Nasotracheal tube placement over the fibreoptic laryngoscope. *Anaesthesia.* 1996;51:1026-1028.
93. Katsnelson T, Frost EA, Farcon E, Goldiner PL. When the endotracheal tube will not pass over the flexible fiberoptic bronchoscope. *Anesthesiology.* 1992;76:151-152.
94. Nakayama M, Kataoka N, Usui Y, Inase N, Takayama S, Miura H. Techniques of nasotracheal intubation with the fiberoptic bronchoscope. *J Emerg Med.* 1992;10:729-734.
95. Wheeler M, Dsida RM. Fiberoptic intubation: troubles with the "Tube"? *Anesthesiology.* 2003;99:1236-1237.
96. Latorre F, Otter W, Kleemann PP, Dick W, Jage J. Cocaine or phenylephrine/lignocaine for nasal fibreoptic intubation? *Eur J Anaesthesiol.* 1996;13:577-781.
97. Arrowsmith JE, Robertshaw HJ, Boyd JD. Nasotracheal intubation in the presence of frontobasal skull fracture. *Can J Anaesth.* 1998;45:71-75.
98. Bainton CR. Complications of managing the airway. In: *Airway Management Principles and Practice.* St. Louis: Mosby; 1996:886-899.
99. Dauphinee K. Nasotracheal intubation. *Emerg Med Clin North Am.* 1988;6:715-723.
100. Doyle DJ, Arellano R. Medical Conditions Affecting the airway: a Synopsis. In: Hagberg CA, ed. *Handbook of Difficult Airway Management.* Philadelphia, PA: Churchill Livingstone; 2000:227-256.
101. Greenland KB, Lam MC, Irwin MG. Comparison of the Williams Airway Intubator and Ovassapian Fibreoptic Intubating Airway for fibreoptic orotracheal intubation. *Anaesthesia.* 2004;59:173-176.
102. Mittal G, Mittal RK, Katyal S, Uppal S, Mittal V. Airway management in maxillofacial trauma: do we really need tracheostomy/submental intubation. *J Clin Diagn Res.* 2014;8:77-79.
103. Iserson KV. Blind nasotracheal intubation. *Ann Emerg Med.* 1981;10:468-471.
104. Tintinalli JE, Claffey J. Complications of nasotracheal intubation. *Ann Emerg Med.* 1981;10:142-144.
105. Woodall NM, Harwood RJ, Barker GL. Complications of awake fibreoptic intubation without sedation in 200 healthy anaesthetists attending a training course. *Br J Anaesth.* 2008;100:850-855.
106. Pandit JJ, Dravid RM, Iyer R, Popat MT. Orotracheal fibreoptic intubation for rapid sequence induction of anaesthesia. *Anaesthesia.* 2002;57:123-127.
107. Cole AF, Mallon JS, Rolbin SH, Ananthanarayan C. Fiberoptic intubation using anesthetized, paralyzed, apneic patients. Results of a resident training program. *Anesthesiology.* 1996;84:1101-1106.
108. Heidegger T, Gerig HJ, Ulrich B, Schnider TW. Structure and process quality illustrated by fibreoptic intubation: analysis of 1612 cases. *Anaesthesia.* 2003;58:734-749.
109. Nakazawa K, Ikeda D, Ishikawa S, Makita K. A case of difficult airway due to lingual tonsillar hypertrophy in a patient with Down's syndrome. *Anesth Analg.* 2003;97:704-705.
110. Walker RW, Ellwood J. The management of difficult intubation in children. *Paediatr Anaesth.* 2009;19(Suppl 1):77-87.
111. Albanon-Sofelo R, Atkins JM, Broom RS, et al. *Textbook of Advanced Cardiac Life Support.* American Heart Association; 1987.
112. Coe PA, King TA, Towey RM. Teaching guided fibreoptic nasotracheal intubation. An assessment of an anaesthetic technique to aid training. *Anaesthesia.* 1988;43:410-413.
113. Ajay S, Singhania A, Akkara AG, Shah A, Adalja M. A study of flexible fiberoptic bronchoscopy aided tracheal intubation for patients undergoing elective surgery under general anesthesia. *Indian J Otolaryngol Head Neck Surg.* 2013;65:116-119.
114. Patil V, Stehling LC, Zauder HL, Koch JP. Mechanical aids for fiberoptic endoscopy. *Anesthesiology.* 1982;57:69-70.
115. Tanoubi I, Drolet P, Donati F. Optimizing preoxygenation in adults. *Can J Anaesth.* 2009;56:449-466.
116. Lane S, Saunders D, Schofield A, Padmanabhan R, Hildreth A, Laws D. A prospective, randomised controlled trial comparing the efficacy of pre-oxygenation in the 20 degrees head-up vs supine position. *Anaesthesia.* 2005;60:1064-1067.
117. Dixon BJ, Dixon JB, Carden JR, et al. Preoxygenation is more effective in the 25 degrees head-up position than in the supine position in severely obese patients: a randomized controlled study. *Anesthesiology.* 2005;102:1110-1115.
118. Weingart SD, Levitan RM. Preoxygenation and prevention of desaturation during emergency airway management. *Ann Emerg Med.* 2012;59:165-175 e1.
119. Rewari V, Ramachandran R, Trikha A. Lingual traction: a useful manoeuvre to lift the epiglottis in a difficult oral fibreoptic intubation. *Acta Anaesthesiol Scand.* 2009;53:695-696.
120. Ching YH, Karlnoski RA, Chen H, et al. Lingual traction to facilitate fiber-optic intubation of difficult airways: a single-anesthesiologist randomized trial. *J Anesth.* 2015;29:263-268.
121. Barker KF, Bolton P, Cole S, Coe PA. Ease of laryngeal passage during fibreoptic intubation: a comparison of three endotracheal tubes. *Acta Anaesthesiol Scand.* 2001;45:624-646.

122. Hakala P, Randall T, Valli H. Comparison between tracheal tubes for orotracheal fibreoptic intubation. *Br J Anaesth*. 1999;82:135-136.
123. Randell T. Fibreoptic orotracheal intubation – Reply (correspondence). *Br J Anaesth*. 1999;83:683-684.
124. Greer JR, Smith SP, Strang T. A comparison of tracheal tube tip designs on the passage of an endotracheal tube during oral fiberoptic intubation. *Anesthesiology*. 2001;94:729-731.
125. Johnson DM, From AM, Smith RB, From RP, Maktabi MA. Endoscopic study of mechanisms of failure of endotracheal tube advancement into the trachea during awake fiberoptic orotracheal intubation. *Anesthesiology*. 2005;102:910-914.
126. Preis CA, Preis IS. Oversize endotracheal tubes and intubation via laryngeal mask airway. *Anesthesiology*. 1997;87:187.
127. Jones HE, Pearce AC, Moore P. Fiberoptic intubatin: influence of tracheal tube tip design. *Anaesthesia*. 1993;48:672-674.
128. Schwartz D, Johnson C, Roberts J. A maneuver to facilitate flexible fiberoptic intubation. *Anesthesiology*. 1989;71:470-471.
129. Wilhelm W, Biedler A, Hammadeh ME, Fleser R, Gruness V. Remifentanil for oocyte retrieval: A new single-agent monitored anaesthesia care technique. *Anaesthesist*. 1999;48:698-704.
130. Sharma D, Bithal PK, Rath GP, Pandia MP. Effect of orientation of a standard polyvinyl chloride tracheal tube on success rates during awake flexible fibreoptic intubation. *Anaesthesia*. 2006;61:845-848.
131. Raj PP, Forestner J, Watson TD, Morris RE, Jenkins MT. Technics for fiberoptic laryngoscopy in anesthesia. *Anesth Analg*. 1974;53:708-714.
132. Brull SJ, Wiklund R, Ferris C, Connelly NR, Ehrenwerth J, Silverman DG. Facilitation of fiberoptic orotracheal intubation with a flexible tracheal tube. *Anesth Analg*. 1994;78:746-748.
133. Calder I. When the endotracheal tube will not pass over the flexible fiberoptic bronchoscope. *Anesthesiology*. 1992;77:398.
134. Baraka A, Rizk M, Muallem M, Bizri SH, Ayoub C. Posterior-beveled vs lateral-beveled tracheal tube for fibreoptic intubation. *Can J Anaesth*. 2002;49:889-890.
135. Jafari A, Gharaei B, Kamranmanesh MR, et al. Wire reinforced endotracheal tube compared with Parker Flex-Tip tube for oral fiberoptic intubation: a randomized clinical trial. *Minerva Anestesiol*. 2014;80:324-329.
136. Chang LC, Lee SC, Ding AL, Rajagopalan S. Fibreoptic Orotracheal intubation of obese patients using Parker flex-tip vs. standard endotracheal tube. *Turk J Anaesthesiol Reanim*. 2019;47:387-391.
137. Joo HS, Naik VN, Savoldelli GL. Parker Flex-Tip are not superior to polyvinylchloride tracheal tubes for awake fibreoptic intubations. *Can J Anaesth*. 2005;52:297-301.
138. Narhari R, Nazaruddin Wan Hassan WM, Mohamad Zaini RH, Che Omar S, Abdullah Nik Mohamad N, Seevaunnamtum P. Comparison of the Parker flex tip and the unoflex reinforced endotracheal tube for orotracheal fibreoptic intubation in simulated difficult intubation patients. *Anaesthesiol Intensive Ther*. 2020;52:377-382.
139. Walsh ME, Shorten GD. Preparing to perform an awake fiberoptic intubation. *Yale J Biol Med*. 1998;71:537-549.
140. Randell T, Valli H, Hakala P. Comparison between the Ovassapian intubating airway and the Berman intubating airway in fibreoptic intubation. *Eur J Anaesthesiol*. 1997;14:380-384.
141. Afilalo M, Guttman A, Stern E, et al. Fiberoptic intubation in the emergency department: a case series. *J Emerg Med*. 1993;11:387-391.
142. Delaney KA, Hessler R. Emergency flexible fiberoptic nasotracheal intubation: a report of 60 cases. *Ann Emerg Med*. 1988;17:919-926.
143. Demetriades D, Velmahos GG, Asensio JA. Cervical pharyngoesophageal and laryngotracheal injuries. *World J Surg*. 2001;25:1044-1048.
144. Mlinek EJ Jr, Clinton JE, Plummer D, Ruiz E. Fiberoptic intubation in the emergency department. *Ann Emerg Med*. 1990;19:359-362.
145. Schafermeyer RW. Fiberoptic laryngoscopy in the emergency department. *Am J Emerg Med*. 1984;2:160-163.
146. Desjardins G, Varon AJ. Airway management for penetrating neck injuries: the Miami experience. *Resuscitation*. 2001;48:71-75.
147. Levitan RM, Kush S, Hollander JE. Devices for difficult airway management in academic emergency departments: results of a national survey. *Ann Emerg Med*. 1999;33:694-698.
148. Reeder TJ, Brown CK, Norris DL. Managing the difficult airway: a survey of residency directors and a call for change. *J Emerg Med*. 2005;28:473-478.
149. Hamilton PH, Kang JJ. Emergency airway management. *Mt Sinai J Med*. 1997;64:292-301.
150. Mandavia DP, Qualls S, Rokos I. Emergency airway management in penetrating neck injury. *Ann Emerg Med*. 2000;35:221-225.
151. Shearer VE, Giesecke AH. Airway management for patients with penetrating neck trauma: a retrospective study. *Anesth Analg*. 1993;77:1135-1138.
152. Morris IR. Anaesthesia and airway management of laryngoscopy and bronchoscopy. In: Hagberg CA, ed. *Benumof's Airway management Principles and Practice*. 2nd ed. Elsevier; 2006.
153. Walls RM, Vissers RJ. The traumatized airway. In: Hagberg C, ed. *Benumof's Airway Management*. 2nd ed. Philadelphia, PA: Mosby Elsevier; 2007:939-960.
154. Neal MR, Groves J, Gell IR. Awake fibreoptic intubation in the semi-prone position following facial trauma. *Anaesthesia*. 1996;51:1053-1054.
155. Preis CA, Hartmann T, Zimpfer M. Laryngeal mask airway facilitates awake fiberoptic intubation in a patient with severe oropharyngeal bleeding. *Anesth Analg*. 1998;87:728-729.
156. Nelson LA. Airway trauma. *Int Anesthesiol Clin*. 2007;45:99-118.
157. Strand J, Maktabi M. The fiberoptic bronchoscope in emergent management of acute lower airway obstruction. *Int Anesthesiol Clin*. 2011;49:15-19.
158. Hung MH, Fan SZ, Lin CP, Hsu YC, Shih PY, Lee TS. Emergency airway management with fiberoptic intubation in the prone position with a fixed flexed neck. *Anesth Analg*. 2008;107:1704-1706.
159. Brimacombe J, Berry A. A proposed fiber-optic scoring system to standardize the assessment of laryngeal mask airway position. *Anesth Analg*. 1993;76:457.
160. Joshi S, Sciacca RR, Solanki DR, Young WL, Mathru MM. A prospective evaluation of clinical tests for placement of laryngeal mask airways. *Anesthesiology*. 1998;89:1141-1146.
161. Takenaka I, Aoyama K. Optimizing endotracheal tube size and length for tracheal intubation through single-use supraglottic airway devices. *Can J Anaesth*. 2010;57:389-390.
162. Watson NC, Hokanson M, Maltby JR, Todesco JM. The intubating laryngeal mask airway in failed fibreoptic intubation. *Can J Anaesth*. 1999;46:376-378.
163. Higgs A, Clark E, Premraj K. Low-skill fibreoptic intubation: use of the Aintree Catheter with the classic LMA. *Anaesthesia*. 2005;60:915-9220.
164. Pearce AC. Airway Strategy. *Curr Anaesth Crit Care*. 2001;12:207-212.
165. Wong DT, Yang JJ, Mak HY, Jagannathan N. Use of intubation introducers through a supraglottic airway to facilitate tracheal intubation: a brief review. *Can J Anaesth*. 2012;59:704-715.
166. Atherton DP, O'Sullivan E, Lowe D, Charters P. A ventilation-exchange bougie for fibreoptic intubations with the laryngeal mask airway. *Anaesthesia*. 1996;51:1123-1126.
167. Zura A, Doyle DJ, Avitsian R, DeUngria M. More on intubation using the Aintree catheter. *Anesth Analg*. 2006;103:785.
168. Zura A, Doyle DJ, Orlandi M. Use of the Aintree intubation catheter in a patient with an unexpected difficult airway. *Can J Anaesth*. 2005;52:646-649.
169. Berkow LC, Schwartz JM, Kan K, Corridore M, Heitmiller ES. Use of the Laryngeal Mask Airway-Aintree Intubating Catheter-fiberoptic bronchoscope technique for difficult intubation. *J Clin Anesth*. 2011;23:534-539.
170. Greenland KB, Tan H, Edwards M. Intubation via a laryngeal mask airway with an Aintree catheter—not all laryngeal masks are the same. *Anaesthesia*. 2007;62:966-967.
171. Allison A, McCrory J. Tracheal placement of a gum elastic bougie using the laryngeal mask airways. *Anaesthesia*. 1990;45:419-420.
172. Brain AI, Verghese C, Addy EV, Kapila A. The intubating laryngeal mask. I: development of a new device for intubation of the trachea. *Br J Anaesth*. 1997;79:699-703.
173. Ludena JA, Alameda LEM. Use of the Magill forceps as an aid for i-gel® removal after endotracheal intubation: A safe and simple technique. *J Anaesthesiol Clin Pharmacol*. 2017;33:551-552.
174. Russo S, Timmermann A. The Magill forceps for removing the intubating laryngeal mask airway after tracheal intubation. *J Clin Anesth*. 2006;18:477-479.
175. Parotto M, Jiansen JQ, AboTaiban A, et al. Evaluation of a low-cost, 3D-printed model for bronchoscopy training. *Anaesthesiol Intensive Ther*. 2017;49:189-197.
176. Mendonca C, Tourville CC, Jefferson H, Nowicka A, Patteril M, Athanassoglou V. Fibreoptic-guided tracheal intubation through i-gel® and LMA® Protector™ supraglottic airway devices – a randomised comparison. *Anaesthesia*. 2019;74:203-210.
177. Moser B, Audige L, Keller C, Brimacombe J, Gasteiger L, Bruppacher HR. A prospective, randomized trial of the Ambu AuraGain laryngeal mask versus the LMA® protector airway in paralyzed, anesthetized adult men. *Minerva Anestesiol*. 2018;84:684-892.
178. Stacey MR, Rassam S, Sivasankar R, Hall JE, Latto IP. A comparison of direct laryngoscopy and jaw thrust to aid fibreoptic intubation. *Anaesthesia*. 2005;60:445-448.

179. Kim SM, Kim HJ. Successful advancement of endotracheal tube with combined fiberoptic bronchoscopy and videolaryngoscopy in a patient with a huge goiter. *SAGE Open Med Case Rep*. 2020;8:2050313X20923232.
180. Moore MS, Wong AB. GlideScope intubation assisted by fiberoptic scope. *Anesthesiology*. 2007;106:885.
181. Sharma D, Kim LJ, Ghodke B. Successful airway management with combined use of Glidescope videolaryngoscope and fiberoptic bronchoscope in a patient with Cowden syndrome. *Anesthesiology*. 2010;113:253-255.
182. Vitin AA, Erdman JE. A difficult airway case with GlideScope-assisted fiberoptic intubation. *J Clin Anesth*. 2007;19:564-565.
183. Xue FS, Li CW, Zhang GH, et al. GlideScope-assisted awake fibreoptic intubation: initial experience in 13 patients. *Anaesthesia*. 2006;61:1014-1015.
184. Greib N, Stojeba N, Dow WA, Henderson J, Diemunsch PA. A combined rigid videolaryngoscopy-flexible fibrescopy intubation technique under general anesthesia. *Can J Anaesth*. 2007;54:492-493.
185. Gomez-Rios MA, Nieto Serradilla L. Combined use of an Airtraq® optical laryngoscope, Airtraq video camera, Airtraq wireless monitor, and a fibreoptic bronchoscope after failed tracheal intubation. *Can J Anaesth*. 2011;58:411-412.
186. Matioc AA. Use of the Airtraq with a fibreoptic bronchoscope in a difficult intubation outside the operating room. *Can J Anaesth*. 2008;55:561-562.
187. Yuan YJ, Xue FS, Liao X, Liu JH, Wang Q. Facilitating combined use of an Airtraq® optical laryngoscope and a fiberoptic bronchoscope in patients with a difficult airway. *Can J Anaesth*. 2011;58:584-585.
188. Doyle DJ. GlideScope-assisted fiberoptic intubation: a new airway teaching method. *Anesthesiology*. 2004;101:1252.
189. Lenhardt R, Burkhart MT, Brock GN, Kanchi-Kandadai S, Sharma R, Akca O. Is video laryngoscope-assisted flexible tracheoscope intubation feasible for patients with predicted difficult airway? A prospective, randomized clinical trial. *Anesth Analg*. 2014;118:1259-1265.
190. Wu FL, Razzaghi A, Souney PF. Seizure after lidocaine for bronchoscopy: case report and review of the use of lidocaine in airway anesthesia. *Pharmacotherapy*. 1993;13:72-78.
191. Maktabi MA, Hoffman H, Funk G, From RP. Laryngeal trauma during awake fiberoptic intubation. *Anesth Analg*. 2002;95:1112-1114.
192. Patil AA, Barker GL, Woodall NM, Harwood RJ. Pyrexia and rigors following fiberoptic intubation in a delegate attending an awake fiberoptic intubation training course. *Anaesthesia*. 2004;59:1045-1046.
193. Aoyama K, Takenaka I. Markedly displaced arytenoid cartilage during fiberoptic orotracheal intubation. *Anesthesiology*. 2006;104:378-389.
194. Heidegger T, Starzyk L, Villiger CR, et al. Fiberoptic intubation and laryngeal morbidity: a randomized controlled trial. *Anesthesiology*. 2007;107:585-590.
195. Joffe AM, Liew EC, Olivar H, et al. A national survey of airway management training in United States internal medicine-based critical care fellowship programs. *Respir Care*. 2012;57:1084-1088.
196. McNarry AF, Dovell T, Dancey FM, Pead ME. Perception of training needs and opportunities in advanced airway skills: a survey of British and Irish trainees. *Eur J Anaesthesiol*. 2007;24:498-504.
197. Pott LM, Randel GI, Straker T, Becker KD, Cooper RM. A survey of airway training among U.S. and Canadian anesthesiology residency programs. *J Clin Anesth*. 2011;23:15-26.
198. Marsland CP, Robinson BJ, Chitty CH, Guy BJ. Acquisition and maintenance of endoscopic skills: developing an endoscopic dexterity training system for anesthesiologists. *J Clin Anesth*. 2002;14:615-619.
199. Agro F, Sena F, Lobo E, Scarlata S, Dardes N, Barzoi G. The Dexter Endoscopic Dexterity Trainer improves fibreoptic bronchoscopy skills: preliminary observations. *Can J Anaesth*. 2005;52:215-216.
200. Marsland C, Larsen P, Segal R, et al. Proficient manipulation of fibreoptic bronchoscope to carina by novices on first clinical attempt after specialized bench practice. *Br J Anaesth*. 2010;104:375-381.
201. Martin KM, Larsen PD, Segal R, Marsland CP. Effective nonanatomical endoscopy training produces clinical airway endoscopy proficiency. *Anesth Analg*. 2004;99:938-944.
202. Wheeler M, Roth AG, Dsida RM, et al. Teaching residents pediatric fiberoptic intubation of the trachea: traditional fiberscope with an eyepiece versus a video-assisted technique using a fiberscope with an integrated camera. *Anesthesiology*. 2004;101:842-846.
203. Smith JE, Fenner SG, King MJ. Teaching fibreoptic nasotracheal intubation with and without closed circuit television. *Br J Anaesth*. 1993;71:206-211.
204. Kennedy CC, Maldonado F, Cook DA. Simulation-based bronchoscopy training: systematic review and meta-analysis. *Chest*. 2013;144:183-192.
205. Rowe R, Cohen RA. An evaluation of a virtual reality airway simulator. *Anesth Analg*. 2002;95:62-66.
206. Goldmann K, Steinfeldt T. Acquisition of basic fiberoptic intubation skills with a virtual reality airway simulator. *J Clin Anesth*. 2006;18:173-178.
207. Baker PA, Weller JM, Baker MJ, et al. Evaluating the ORSIM® simulator for assessment of anaesthetists' skills in flexible bronchoscopy: aspects of validity and reliability. *Br J Anaesth*. 2016;117(Suppl 1):i87-i91.
208. Giglioli S, Boet S, De Gaudio AR, et al. Self-directed deliberate practice with virtual fiberoptic intubation improves initial skills for anesthesia residents. *Minerva Anestesiol*. 2012;78:456-461.
209. Boet S, Bould MD, Schaeffer R, et al. Learning fibreoptic intubation with a virtual computer program transfers to "hands on" improvement. *Eur J Anaesthesiol*. 2010;27:31-35.
210. Pastis NJ, Vanderbilt AA, Tanner NT, et al. Construct validity of the Simbionix bronch mentor simulator for essential bronchoscopic skills. *J Bronchology Interv Pulmonol*. 2014;21:314-321.
211. Yau YW, Li Z, Chua MT, Kuan WS, Chan GWH. Virtual reality mobile application to improve videoscopic airway training: A randomised trial. *Ann Acad Med Singap*. 2021;50:141-148.
212. Chandra DB, Savoldelli GL, Joo HS, Weiss ID, Naik VN. Fiberoptic oral intubation: the effect of model fidelity on training for transfer to patient care. *Anesthesiology*. 2008;109:1007-1013.
213. Latif R, Bautista A, Duan X, et al. Teaching basic fiberoptic intubation skills in a simulator: initial learning and skills decay. *J Anesth*. 2016;30:12-19.
214. Leong TL, Li J. 3D printed airway simulators: Adding a dimension to bronchoscopy training. *Respirology*. 2020;25:1126-1128.
215. DeBoer EM, Wagner J, Kroehl ME, et al. Three-Dimensional Printed Pediatric Airway Model Improves Novice Learners' Flexible Bronchoscopy Skills With Minimal Direct Teaching From Faculty. *Simul Healthc*. 2018;13:284-288.
216. Ghazy A, Chaban R, Vahl CF, Dorweiler B. Development and evaluation of 3-dimensional printed models of the human tracheobronchial system for training in flexible bronchoscopy. *Interact Cardiovasc Thorac Surg*. 2019;28:137-143.
217. Feng DB, Yong YH, Byrnes T, et al. Learning gain and skill retention following unstructured bronchoscopy simulation in a low-fidelity airway model. *J Bronchology Interv Pulmonol*. 2020;27:280-285.
218. Ball DR. Awake versus asleep fibreoptic intubation. *Anaesthesia*. 1994;49:921.
219. Schaefer HG, Marsch SC, Keller HL, Strebel S, Anselmi L, Drewe J. Teaching fibreoptic intubation in anaesthetised patients. *Anaesthesia*. 1994;49:331-334.
220. Bray JK, Yentis SM. Attitudes of patients and anaesthetists to informed consent for specialist airway techniques. *Anaesthesia*. 2002;57:1012-1015.
221. Mason RA. Learning fibreoptic intubation: fundamental problems. *Anaesthesia*. 1992;47:729-731.
222. Johnson C, Roberts JT. Clinical competence in the performance of fiberoptic laryngoscopy and endotracheal intubation: a study of resident instruction. *J Clin Anesth*. 1989;1:344-349.
223. Smith JE, Jackson AP. Learning fibreoptic endoscopy. Nasotracheal or orotracheal intubations first? *Anaesthesia*. 2000;55:1072-1075.
224. Dawson AJ, Marsland C, Baker P, Anderson BJ. Fibreoptic intubation skills among anaesthetists in New Zealand. *Anaesth Intensive Care*. 2005;33:777-783.
225. Agro FE, Cataldo R. Teaching fiberoptic intubation in Italy: state of the art. *Minerva Anestesiol*. 2010;76:684-685.

CHAPTER 11

Rigid Fiberoptic and Video Laryngoscopes

James R. McAlpine, Alexander Poulton, and Orlando R. Hung

INTRODUCTION

■ Why Were Rigid and Semirigid Fiberoptic and Video Laryngoscopes Developed?

Macewan originally performed endotracheal intubation with his fingers.[1] In 1913 Janeway used a speculum very similar to the laryngoscopes introduced by Miller and Macintosh in 1941 and 1942, respectively.[2] And until recently, we've remained largely dependent upon the line-of-sight technique exemplified by direct laryngoscopy (DL). It was proposed that "the sniffing position" aligns the axes of the mouth, pharynx, and trachea, yet the incisors, the tongue, the epiglottis, and occasionally the position of the larynx itself, often conspire against a clear line-of-sight view. Studies on conscious adults with normal airway features, in neutral, sniffing, and simple extension demonstrate that positioning alone does not align the axes[3] and there was little difference between the sniffing position and simple extension in a large series of patients undergoing DL.[4] If positioning does not align these axes, how do we accomplish intubation by DL? We apply force, displacing and compressing the tongue, mandible, and frequently the larynx itself. Yet even among adults with seemingly normal airways, it is not possible to view the larynx by direct means in approximately 6% to 10%.[5–7] Despite attempts to do so, we frequently fail to identify patients in whom DL will prove difficult or worse.[8] Studies suggest that when DL fails, all too frequently we try harder and have more attempts,[9] sometimes with adverse consequences.[9–11]

Instruments that are more or less anatomically shaped can overcome the anatomical barriers that may make DL difficult or impossible. Rigid and semirigid fiberoptic, optical, and video laryngoscopes are designed specifically for this purpose.

Another significant limitation of DL is that the experience is difficult to share.[12,13] Since only the laryngoscopist can visualize the glottis during the laryngoscopy, this reduces the ability of an assistant in anticipating the laryngoscopist's needs, complicates the teaching and recording of laryngoscopy, limits clinical documentation and the possibilities for quality improvement as well as the conduct of airway research. Video laryngoscopy circumvents many of these limitations but generally relies upon alternative devices.

Flexible endoscopes have greatly expanded our ability to diagnose and manage problems in previously inaccessible body parts. These devices are versatile but complex. For tracheal intubation, flexible fiberoptic and video endoscopes demand a different skill set than DL. Nonetheless, practitioners must master these devices since they remain to play an important role in some situations. Unfortunately, their complexity and versatility also add to their cost and fragility. As well, blood, secretions, vomitus, or fogging may significantly interfere with visualization.

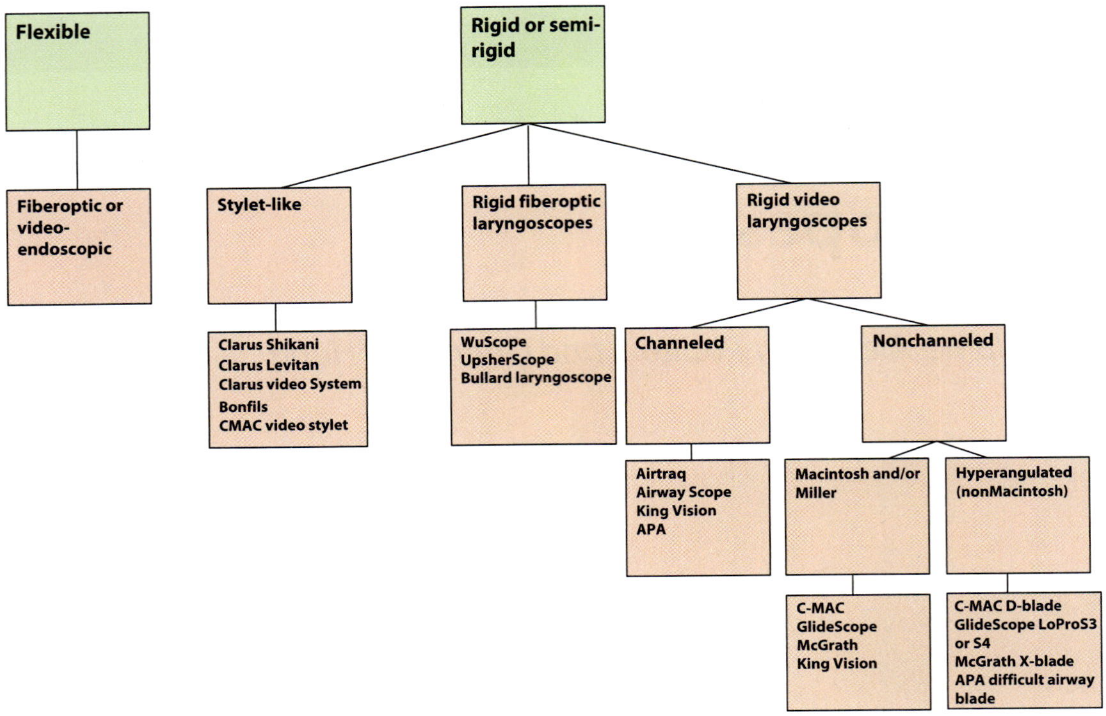

FIGURE 11.1. Example of classification system for rigid fiberoptic and video laryngoscopes.

Fiberoptic and video technology have been incorporated into flexible, semi-rigid, or rigid devices, designed specifically for tracheal intubation. Flexible fiberoptic and video endoscopic intubation will be discussed in Chapter 10. Rigid and semi-rigid devices may be stylet-like, channeled, or nonchanneled and blade-like (see Figure 11.1). All provide illumination and enable non-line-of-sight viewing of the glottis.

With ongoing advances in technology, laryngoscopy is an evolving field, and new devices will likely appear and disappear by the time of the publication of this textbook. The knowledge and use of video laryngoscopy in particular have rapidly increased since the introduction of the GlideScope (Verathon Inc, Bothell, WA) in the early 2000s. This chapter is not intended as a comprehensive review of all currently available devices, but rather as an overview of the common concepts that underpin the design of these devices. As such, the authors have endeavored to include supporting clinical evidence related to these devices.

What Are the Challenges Inherent in Evaluating the Literature Regarding Alternative Devices?

Evaluating the literature relating to the devices described herein is challenging. Many of the published reports involve practitioners with a variable experience in airway management; more often they are unfamiliar with or poorly trained on the device being evaluated. The reader must be cautious when drawing conclusions based upon such studies. Comparisons too must be treated with caution. It is unlikely that the laryngoscopist will be as familiar with a new device as they are with a standard tool such as a Macintosh laryngoscope. Using the conventional definition, a failed intubation is uncommon, and studies aimed at demonstrating the superiority of one technique over another require a very large sample size. A selected population of patients known to be a difficult DL is more likely to give rise to meaningful data but may be difficult to justify ethically. Thus many of the studies have been done on a "standardized patient" (i.e., a manikin), a simulated difficult airway (e.g., with an applied cervical collar), in patients with features predictive of difficulty (which will undoubtedly include many false positives) or with surrogate outcomes (e.g., time-to-intubation, Cormack-Lehane [C-L] view[14] or the number of attempts).

Caution should also be used with respect to nomenclature and categorization of devices. While DL blades such as Macintosh and Miller are standardized, video laryngoscopy (VL) blades are not so. Often the catch-all term "video laryngoscope" is used in the literature (see Figure 11.1), but there is no attempt to separate out exactly what is being discussed or studied (i.e., Macintosh vs. hyperangulated blades, channeled vs. nonchanneled). Within any classification system, there will be variations in the blade design (e.g., shape, curvature and camera position) that will affect the performance of the devices and as such attempts to determine the efficacy of these devices will depend on the studies being cited.

Finally, the reader should critically assess whether the studies involve subjects that match the patients they encounter in their practice. The reader is invited to refer to a recent review[15] in which the investigators found statistically significant differences between the laryngoscopes for time-to-intubation, but these differences were not considered clinically relevant. They concluded that different video laryngoscopes have differential intubation performance and some may be currently preferred among the available devices. In addition, there is insufficient evidence to ensure the significant superiority of one device over the others for intubation-related outcomes. The same author subsequently re-analyzed the data using a pairwise meta-analysis comparing only hyperangulated versus Macintosh video laryngoscopes for the efficacy of orotracheal intubation in adults.[16] Again, the author concluded that there was no evidence to suggest that there is any difference or equivalence between the hyperangulated versus Macintosh video laryngoscopes for most tracheal intubation outcomes. In the future, well-designed comparative studies are necessary to clarify whether any specific set of devices is better than another.[17]

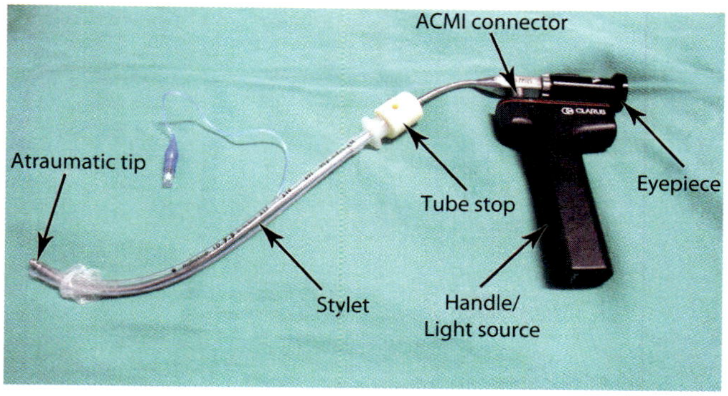

FIGURE 11.3. The Clarus Shikani optical stylet.

OPTICAL STYLETS

What Are Optical Stylets?

Optical stylets have a metal exterior containing fiberoptic bundles or a camera and light source. When inserted within an endotracheal tube (ETT), the practitioner can view ETT advancement through a proximal eyepiece or from a video monitor display. The instruments vary in their external diameter, image resolution, source of illumination, and flexibility of the tip of the stylet. Some examples of commercially available optical stylets include:

(1) **The Bonfils Intubation Endoscope** (Bonfils, KARL STORZ Endoscopy Canada Ltd, Mississauga, Canada): The Bonfils fiberscope (see Figure 11.2) has a straight, nonmalleable shaft with a distal 40 degree anterior bend, a movable tube holder and an integrated luer-lock connector for oxygen insufflation down the ETT. The adult version accommodates an ETT of 5.5 mm or greater internal diameter (ID). Smaller pediatric versions are available. Light is provided remotely via cable or by attachable battery-powered light-emitting diode (LED). It is compatible with the Storz C-MAC system display screen for video image transfer.

(2) **The Clarus Shikani stylet** (Clarus Medical LLC, Minneapolis, MN) (Video 8): The Clarus Shikani optical stylet (SOS; see Figure 11.3) is semi-malleable and can accommodate an arc of up to 120°. It can accept ETTs > 5.5-mm ID. A pediatric version is available. It has a "Tube Stop" adapter for ETT fixation and oxygen delivery down the ETT. It has a fixed-focus, proximal eyepiece that is compatible with proximally-attached camera adapters. Illumination is via a standard Green specification fiberoptic laryngoscope handle or a small battery-powered LED source.

(3) **The Clarus Levitan stylet** (Clarus Medical LLC, Minneapolis, MN) (Video 1): The Clarus Levitan Stylet (see Figure 11.4) has a malleable shaft, a fixed-location ETT connector adapter (ETT must be cut to an appropriate length to ensure that the stylet is within but close to the distal end of the ETT) and a proximal connector for oxygen insufflation down the ETT. The light source is supplied via an adapter from a standard Greenline handle or a dedicated portable LED.

(4) **The Clarus Video System** (Clarus Medical LLC, Minneapolis, MN) (Video 25): The Clarus Video System (see Figure 11.5) is a video-based optical stylet with a handle-mounted liquid crystal display (LCD) screen, the viewing angle of which can be adjusted using a thumb control. The shaft is semi-malleable and has an adjustable "Tube Stop" adapter for ETT fixation. It has two light sources: two white light LEDs, and one red LED, the latter being for anterior neck transillumination. It is compatible with the Clarus Medical ClearSCOPE adapter to enable video capture using a smart phone.

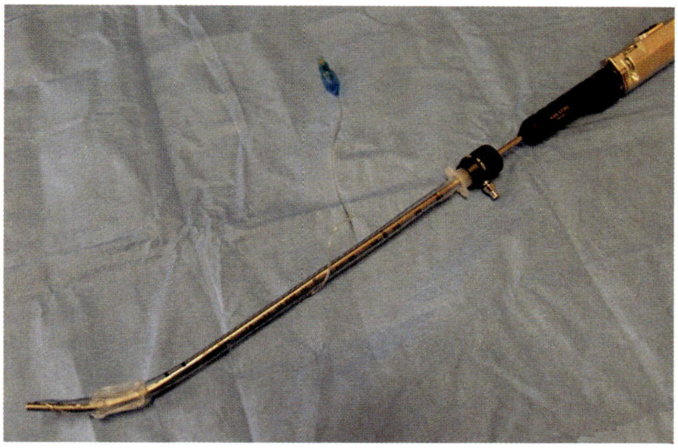
FIGURE 11.2. The Bonfils Retromolar Intubation Fiberscope loaded with an ETT.

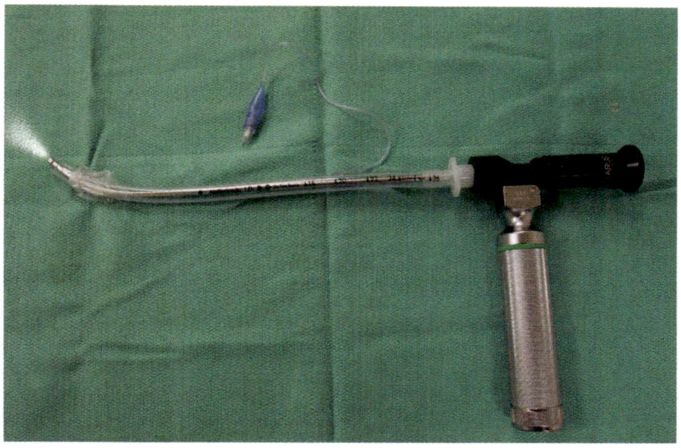
FIGURE 11.4. The Clarus Levitan stylet.

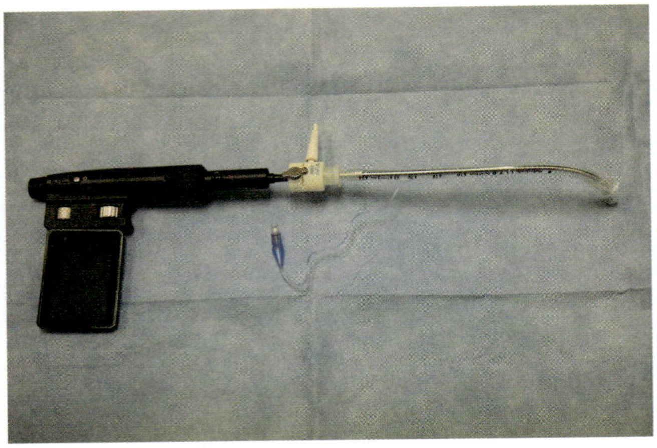

FIGURE 11.5. The Clarus video system.

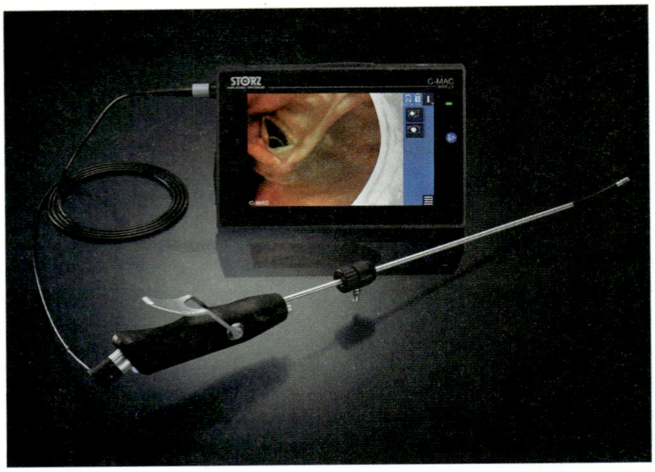

FIGURE 11.6. The C-MAC video stylet connecting to a C-MAC monitor for image display. (© KARL STORZ SE & Co. KG, Germany)

(5) **The C-MAC® Video Stylet** (KARL STORZ Endoscopy Canada Ltd, Mississauga, Canada): The C-MAC video stylet (see Figure 11.6) is a new video-endoscope with a semi-flexible sheath and deflectable tip that can angle up to 60 degrees via a lever on the handle, with passive return. It has a moveable ETT adaptor for ETT fixation and oxygen insufflation. It connects to a C-MAC monitor for image display.

What Are the Unique Characteristics of Optical Stylets?

Common to all optical stylets is a rigid or semi-rigid shaft and a proximal tube holder compatible with a 15-mm ETT connector. The tube holders can, on most devices (except the Clarus Levitan stylet), be adjusted on the stylet shaft, enabling appropriate positioning of the tip of the endoscope just within the distal tip of the ETT. Most optical stylets transmit light distally and the image proximally to an eyepiece or a display with variable resolution. The distal viewing angle varies from 50 to 90 degrees. Light is generally powered from a battery source to enhance portability, although some scopes can be attached via a cable to a remote light source. None of the optical stylets have a hollow working channel. All of the optical stylets are susceptible to fogging and should be prepared with an antifogging solution or warmed prior to use. The C-MAC Video Stylet is slightly different in that it has a deflectable tip that allows the distal end of the stylet to be actively bent via a proximal lever with passive return (see Figure 11.6).

How Are Optical Stylets Prepared for Tracheal Intubation?

An ETT should be preloaded on the optical stylet, and the proximal ETT connector is stabilized within the tube holder on the stylet's shaft. The tube holder and ETT are then positioned on the stylet's shaft such that the scope tip is located just proximal to the ETT bevel. The tube holder is then fixed to the stylet shaft by tightening a locking screw. For semi-rigid devices, the desired degree of distal stylet angulation will depend on the technique of use: stand-alone use generally requires more angulation (e.g., 40-90 degrees), while optical stylet use as an adjunct to DL should require a distal curvature of 30 to 40 degrees.

How Are Optical Stylets Used to Perform Tracheal Intubation?

Although optical stylets can also be used as an adjunct to DL, most practitioners opt for stand-alone use. A jaw lift, jaw thrust, tongue pull, or combination thereof[18,19] should be performed to enlarge the pharyngeal space by elevating the tongue and epiglottis away from the posterior pharyngeal wall. The jaw thrust may also be beneficial by expanding the laryngeal aperture.[20] Following suctioning, the stylet-ETT assembly is inserted from the side of the mouth (i.e., advanced over or behind the molars) and slowly rotated upright and toward the midline during advancement,[19] or alternatively, it can be inserted and advanced via a midline approach. For the midline approach, the stylet should generally be bent at a more acute angle, and during advancement, identification of the uvula and epiglottis will help maintain orientation to the midline position of the tip of the device. Once the tip of the stylet-ETT assembly is at the laryngeal aperture, the ETT can be advanced off the stylet through the glottis and into the trachea.

For optical stylet use as an adjunct to DL, the best laryngoscopic view is obtained. Faced with a poor view, e.g., Cormack/Lehane (C-L)[14] Grade 3, an optical stylet loaded with an ETT is carefully placed just beneath the epiglottis, under direct vision. With the ETT tip under, but no more than 0.5 cm beyond the tip of the epiglottis, the practitioner then seeks a view through the stylet's eyepiece (or on-screen display): the vocal cords should be immediately visible, facilitating the advancement of the ETT through the cords. If stand-alone optical stylet use has failed, using DL[19,21,22] or VL[23] in this fashion helps control the tongue and create space in the oropharynx for optical stylet manipulation. Concomitant use of DL with an optical stylet appears to be as effective as stand-alone use.[24]

Optical stylets have also been used in a similar fashion to lighted stylets. Using only transillumination of the anterior neck to suggest successful tracheal access, secondary confirmation of correct placement can then follow by indirect visualization of the trachea through the eyepiece. This is particularly useful in soiled airways or in the presence of blood when visualization of the airway is compromised. This has been described with adult and pediatric optical stylets[25] with a success rate that rivals the traditional visual advancement techniques.

What Is the Clinical Utility of Optical Stylets?

The use of the optical stylet has been described to facilitate postinduction and awake[26–28] intubations of adult and pediatric patients, with and without predicted difficult airway anatomy. Successful use has been reported with both single- and double-lumened tubes.[29]

How Effective Are Optical Stylets for Intubation in a Patient with a Difficult Airway?

Rudolph et al.[21] in 1996 reported on the use of the Bonfils stylet in a series of 107 patients, of whom 18 presented C-L Grade 3 or 4 views at DL. Tracheal intubation was successful in 16 out of 18 difficult cases with the Bonfils, including all four patients with DL-C-L Grade 4 views. Twenty-one percent of the total series required concomitant use of DL.[21] Shikani, in his initial study of the SOS,[22] looked at 120 patients, 74 of them children, including seven patients with DL-C-L Grade 3 or 4 views. All patients in the series, including five awake patients, were successfully intubated with the scope, 88% on the first-attempt. Five of the seven C-L Grade 3 and 4 patients required concomitant use of DL. Rudolph et al.[30] followed this study up with the 2007 publication of a 4-year observational study of 116 patients presenting unanticipated difficult DL (defined as C-L Grade 3 or 4, or more than two attempts). Patients were randomized to use the Bonfils or a flexible bronchoscope (with sizes varying between 2.3- and 6-mm diameter). Concomitant use of DL, jaw thrust, an intubating oral airway, and size of ETT were not standardized. Total time-to-intubation was shorter with the Bonfils, with no difference in complications. Number of attempts was not separately reported. Later, Bein et al.[18] compared the use of the Bonfils with the LMA-Fastrach™ in 80 patients with predictors of difficult DL. Thirty-nine of 40 patients randomized to Bonfils use were intubated on the first-attempt with a median time of 40 seconds, in contrast to a 28/40 first-attempt success rate for the "blind" tracheal intubation technique through the LMA-Fastrach. Bein et al.[31] conducted another study that evaluated the Bonfils use after failed DL. In 25 patients recruited following two failed DL attempts, 88% were successfully intubated with the Bonfils at the first-attempt, and all but one (96%) by the second attempt, with a median time of 47.5 seconds. In Falcetta's learning curve study involving 216 patients using the Bonfils, 15 patients presented a C-L grade 3 or 4 view during prior DL. All were intubated successfully with stand-alone use of the Bonfils in a median time comparable to patients who presented a C-L grade 1 or 2 by DL.[32] Finally, in a similar study, Kim and colleagues randomized 40 elective adult surgical patients presenting DL-C-L grade 3 view to use of the Bonfils or a 3.8 mm flexible bronchoscope.[33] Both devices were used with concomitant DL. First-attempt success rate was comparable at about 50%, while times to ultimate success was shorter in the Bonfils group. Two cases failed with the Bonfils and succeeded with the flexible bronchoscope.

Case reports document the successful use of the Bonfils in patients with limited mouth opening (7 and 15mm).[34]

How Effective Are Optical Stylets for the Awake Tracheal Intubation of the Patient with Anticipated Difficult Airway Management?

Several series and reports have documented the successful use of Bonfils optical stylet for awake tracheal intubation (ATI), for a variety of indications, and in some cases after the failure of flexible bronchoscopic intubation.[26,27,35,36] The Clarus Video System was described in one case report to facilitate awake intubation with a double-lumen tube (DLT) in a topically anesthetized patient with a large epiglottic cyst,[37] and for awake intubation of a patient immobilized in a halo jacket.[38]

How Effective Are Optical Stylets for Tracheal Intubation in the Simulated Difficult Airway?

Greenland et al.[39] compared the Levitan FPS (first pass success) scope with the single-use Portex tracheal introducer in a randomized cross-over study of 34 adult patients. They found equal success and a shorter time-to-intubation with the tracheal introducer under conditions where only a C-L Grade 3A view was deliberately obtained during DL.

The Bonfils stylet was compared with Macintosh blade DL in a population of elective surgical patients in whom difficulty was simulated by the application of a cervical collar. Tube placement was successful in 81.6% of patients randomized to the Bonfils stylet versus 39.5% of the Macintosh DL patients.[40] More recently, in a study of 120 elective surgical patients wearing cervical collars randomized to use of left molar laryngoscopy with adjunctive used of a tracheal tube introducer (TTI) or intubation with the Bonfils, the Bonfils resulted in a significantly shorter total time-to-intubation, with a comparable overall success rate.[41] Another study performed under similar conditions compared the GlideScope® with the SOS. Comparable overall and first-attempt success rates and time-to-intubation occurred.[42]

What Is the Role of the Optical Stylet for Intubation of the Patient with Known or Possible Cervical Spine Instability?

Two studies have compared Bonfils-aided with Macintosh blade (attempted full view exposure of cords) DL, one using noncontinuous radiographs[43] and the other using external markers as a surrogate of cervical spine movement.[44] Subjects in the two studies started with the head and neck in a neutral position, but had no application of in-line cervical immobilization. Both studies documented significantly less upper cervical spine movement with the Bonfils. Using the SOS with in-line cervical immobilization and continuous fluoroscopy, another study similarly concluded that less movement occurred with the SOS than with Macintosh blade DL.[45] The clinical significance of these studies is unknown.

What Is the Utility of Optical Stylets in the Placement of Double-Lumen Tubes?

Successful use of optical stylets for DLT placement has been described in case reports with both the Bonfils[29,46] and the OptiScope (Pacific Medical, Seoul, South Korea), a modified version of the Trachway video-based optical stylet. This device, also semi-malleable, is 40.5-cm long and has an outer diameter of 5 mm, meaning that it can be used in 35-Fr or larger DLs.[47] Yang et al.[47] conducted a study of 400 patients randomized to 35- and 37 French DLT insertion with Macintosh blade DL or stand-alone use of the OptiScope. OptiScope-facilitated intubation was faster, and succeeded on the first-attempt significantly more often than Macintosh-blade facilitated intubation. Overall success rate was similar, although the incidence of mucosal or dental injury was significantly less with OptiScope use.

The Clarus Video System/Trachway was used in a study of 60 patients,[48] similarly randomized to Macintosh blade DL or the Trachway for placement of a DLT. Intubation occurred on the first-attempt in all 60 patients, but more quickly (mean of 48 vs. 28 seconds) with the Trachway, and with less postoperative hoarseness on the first of 4 days of observation for such complications.

Can Optical Stylets Be Used for Nasal Intubations?

Semi-malleable optical stylets have been described for nasotracheal intubations. Hsu and colleagues studied 100 patients, allocating 50 to the use of the Trachway stylet through the nose, or nasotracheal intubation facilitated by oral Macintosh DL. All Trachway intubations succeeded on the first-attempt in less time than those facilitated by DL, with less need for corrective maneuvers during the procedure and comparable complications such as bleeding.[49] Lee et al.[50] studied 80 patients with limited mouth opening and an average body mass index (BMI) <25 kg·m^{-2}, randomizing them to nasotracheal intubation with the Trachway or a flexible bronchoscope. Intubation with the Trachway occurred significantly faster and with less difficulty on a modified intubation difficulty scale. Success rates within two attempts were comparable, as were bleeding complications.

What Is the Pediatric Experience with Optical Stylet Use?

Case reports have been published documenting successful tracheal intubation using optical stylets in pediatric patients with actual or predicted difficulty due to Pierre Robin sequence;[51,52] Hurler syndrome;[53] Goldenhar syndrome;[51] Treacher Collins syndrome;[51] restricted mouth opening with popliteal pterygium syndrome;[54] and small for gestational age conditions.[55] In all of these cases, either a Brambrink or Shikani stylet was used as a stand-alone technique. However, unlike the foregoing successes, Bein et al.[56] published a series of 55 uses of the Bonfils and Brambrink optical stylet in elective pediatric surgery patients without predictors of difficult airway anatomy. Although performed by an investigator experienced in adult use of the Bonfils, this study reported a relatively poor success rate with the device, with many of the failures due to secretions. In the series, the tracheas of only 40 of 55 (73%) patients were intubated on the first-attempt, and after 3 attempts there was a failure rate of 9%. Houston et al.[57] randomized 50 healthy children to intubation with the Bonfils or DL with prior laryngoscopy with the alternate device: although the Bonfils resulted in more Grade 1 views, four patients required two attempts, and two patients failed after two attempts; compared with two patients requiring two attempts with DL and no failures with DL.

More recently, Kaufmann et al.[58] compared the Bonfils with the GlideScope Cobalt AVL video laryngoscope in 100 children. Visualization of the larynx was better with the Bonfils, and time needed for intubation was significantly less. All cases were successfully intubated with both devices. Subsequently, the same group compared the use of the Bonfils with the flexible bronchoscope for intubation of 26 pediatric patients with anticipated or actual difficult airway anatomy.[59] All 26 patients were intubated successfully on the first-attempt with either device, although the time required, image quality and ease of the procedure were significantly improved with the Bonfils. Successful use of the semi-malleable SOS has been described to facilitate intubation through an air-Q extraglottic device in seven pediatric patients.[60]

One interesting case report documents the successful use of the Bonfils in "parallel" with an in situ extraglottic device (air-Q): the loaded Bonfils was successfully advanced via the retromolar approach around the right side of the cuff of the air-Q, to and through the glottic opening.[61]

OPTICAL STYLET—OTHER CONSIDERATIONS

What Is the Learning Curve for Optical Stylet Use?

Using time to successful tracheal intubation as a marker for proficiency, published learning curve data on the Bonfils fiberoptic stylet suggest that 20 to 25 uses are needed to achieve competence.[19,27,32] Other published reports of experience with optical stylets detail most of the failures at the beginning of their respective series (i.e., within the first 10 uses).[22] In one series,[19] the most commonly encountered preventable difficulties included secretions, fogging (avoidable by suctioning and antifogging maneuvers, respectively), and difficulty getting under the epiglottis (aided by additional jaw lift, concomitant DL or VL, or deliberate scope placement in the upper esophagus, then slowly withdrawing it until the larynx is visualized).

What Are the Potential Complications Associated with the Use of Optical Stylets?

To date, most complications reported in the literature due to optical stylets have been limited to failures to intubate[56]: airway trauma has been reported only infrequently.[19] One case report has appeared documenting extensive facial and neck edema after an intubation attempt during which O_2 was insufflated at 10 L·min^{-1} via the tube holder adapter on a Bonfils stylet.[62] Otherwise, failure to intubate has sometimes resulted from a view being obscured by fog or secretions, often a preventable complication.

What Are the Potential Advantages of Optical Stylets?

As a class, optical stylets are portable, and, relative to flexible bronchoscopes, can be less expensive and possibly more robust. Their rigidity may make them easier to navigate to the laryngeal inlet than flexible devices. As outlined above, published studies and case series suggest that at least in the hands of experienced practitioners, optical stylets enable a high success rate of tracheal intubation in patients presenting with predicted or actual difficult DL. Compared to DL with the Macintosh blade, tracheal intubation with both the Bonfils[63,64] and the StyletScope[65,66] have been associated with a lower incidence of adverse hemodynamic responses, although in another study comparing DL by a left molar approach to use of the Bonfils, hemodynamic responses (although a secondary outcome in this study) were no different.[41] In a study comparing the Bonfils (using a midline approach) with tracheal intubation using a flexible bronchoscope in anesthetized patients, a comparable hemodynamic response was noted.[67]

What Are the Disadvantages of Optical Stylets?

Prior antifogging preparation and suctioning are recommended for optical stylet use. Some optical stylets (e.g., the Levitan FPS) require the ETT to be cut to a specific length. During advancement toward the glottic opening, orientation within the upper airway can be difficult unless soft tissues are well controlled with a jaw lift or by concomitant use of a direct- or video laryngoscope. It follows that poor jaw protrusion, as well as significant blood or secretions in the airway may create difficulties. It is also probable that intubation using optical stylets will be more successful in the hands of practitioners already experienced in the use of flexible bronchoscopes. Nonmalleable versions of optical stylet (i.e., the Bonfils) are not suitable for nasotracheal intubation.

RIGID FIBEROPTIC LARYNGOSCOPES

What Are Rigid Fiberoptic Laryngoscopes?

This section is included predominantly for historical purposes as these devices are no longer in widespread routine clinical use. For further detail on these devices, please refer to Chapter 11 in the previous edition of this textbook. The interested reader can also find additional details about these devices elsewhere.[68,69]

Three devices typified this class of laryngoscopes: the WuScope, the UpsherScope, and the Bullard Laryngoscopes (see Figure 11.7). They have several features in common—a rigid, anatomically-shaped blade, a fiberoptic bundle, a viewing port, and the decision by their respective manufacturers to discontinue the products. They will be discussed briefly because of their relationship to VL, and the fact that they still have their adherents and are referred to in the literature. These devices lacked angulation controllers making them less versatile and less expensive but easier to use. The rigid fiberoptic laryngoscope is inserted into the mouth and positioned around the base of the tongue, providing the practitioner with an excellent glottic view. Unlike the flexible fiberoptic device, these laryngoscopes remained above the larynx allowing the laryngoscopist to observe the insertion and advancement of the ETT. This differs fundamentally from flexible endoscopes that are generally advanced well into the trachea, thereafter serving as an introducer over which the ETT is blindly advanced.[70]

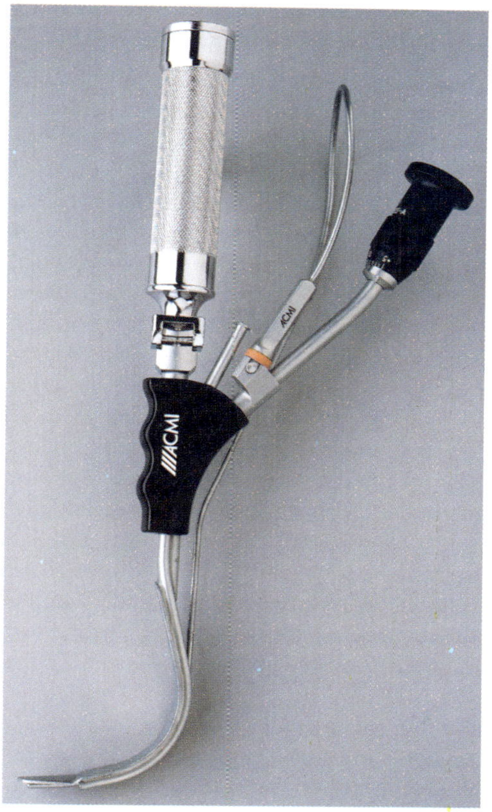

FIGURE 11.7. The Bullard laryngoscope (Reproduced with permission from Wackett A, Anderson K, Thode H. Bullard laryngoscopy by naïve operators in the cervical spine immobilized patient. *J Emerg Med*. 2005;29(3):253-257.).

While some practitioners were frustrated by fogging, secretions, and the need to elevate the epiglottis, a greater obstacle to clinical and marketing success was the relatively flat learning curve and limited number of experienced practitioners to serve as mentors. Practitioners had presumably found the transition to VL easier because of the similarity of VL to conventional Macintosh blades and the clinical use of the rigid fiberoptic laryngoscopes all but disappeared.

Other rigid fiberoptic devices have come and gone. None of these enjoyed popularity in North America and there are limited clinical studies demonstrating their effectiveness.

RIGID VIDEO LARYNGOSCOPES

What Are the Characteristic Features of Rigid Video Laryngoscopes?

Earlier rigid fiberoptic laryngoscopes conveyed their image along a bundle of glass fibers to an eyepiece. If the eyepiece was connected to a video camera, the benefits of VL were achieved, albeit with somewhat greater complexity. The optical stylets and rigid fiberoptic laryngoscopes (e.g., the Bullard Laryngoscope, UpsherScope, and WuScope) as well as the Truview-EVO can all be connected to a video camera in this way. More recent video laryngoscopes incorporate a video camera, or more precisely a video chip (complementary metal oxide semiconductor [CMOS] or charged couple device [CCD]) into the stylet or blade. They use LEDs for illumination and a LCD for monitoring the image. This system allows an image of the glottic view to be projected to the screen, enabling the practitioner to look past the curvature of the tongue and into the larynx without the need to align the pharyngeal, laryngeal, and tracheal axes as is required with DL. There are several ways of classifying these devices: single-use versus reusable blades; traditional Macintosh-style versus more angulated blades (or "hyperangulated" blades) and channeled versus nonchanneled blades. Each category has advantages and disadvantages. For example, single-use products permit a faster turn-over between use since reprocessing is not required. Other considerations relating to the single-use versus reusable products include the environmental impact of packaging, disposal and potentially hazardous reprocessing, the cost-per-use, the design, strength, and performance of single-use versus reusable devices. In some jurisdictions, the practitioner may have no choice in that single-use products are mandated in the interests of infection control (e.g., during the COVID-19 pandemic).

There have been several glottic view scoring systems developed for use with VL. The Cormack and Lehane system developed for DL is often used, however, this can be misleading. With DL the line-of-sight view achieved directly relates to the ease of tracheal intubation.[71,72] This is not the case with the indirect view obtained with VL where the view may be good, but intubation difficult. Hence other systems have been developed in an attempt to provide a more informative way to describe glottic views obtained with VL, using qualitative and quantitative measures. The percentage of glottic opening (POGO) score described by Levitan et al.[73] estimates percentage of glottis visualized. The Freemantle Score uses 3 elements to record view information: view (full/partial/none), ease (1/2/3), and device.[74] The intubation difficulty scale uses a seven-point system (number of attempts, additional operators, alternative techniques, glottic exposure, lifting force, external laryngeal manipulation [ELM], and cord position) and is used mainly in research studies due to its complexity.[75]

VIDEO LARYNGOSCOPES WITH CHANNELED BLADES

Although indirect VL blades are effective in obtaining a view of the larynx, on occasion, advancement of the ETT through the glottis may be problematic. To help address this issue, a number of VL blades incorporate a channel designed to help guide the ETT through the oropharynx to and beyond the larynx.

■ What Are the Common Features of the Video Laryngoscopes with Channeled Blades?

These devices consist of a blade with the incorporated channel, handle, and visualization component (prism or blade-mounted camera) which displays the image via an eye piece, handle-mounted video screen, or cable-connected screen.

Airtraq Avant (Prodol Meditec, Biscay, Spain) (Video 24)

The Airtraq Avant (see Figure 11.8) is a J-shaped laryngoscope with a re-usable, rechargeable optical unit that slides into a single-use channeled blade. It can be used either with its standard integrated optical viewer or with attachable video-enabling technology. A series of mirrors optically delivers an indirect image to a proximal eyepiece. It is available in many sizes. Illumination is supplied from a distal LED bulb, and a heating element heats up the distal viewing lens as an antifogging measure.

Pentax AirwayScope (AWS) (Nihon Kohden America Inc, Irvine, CA, USA)

The Pentax AirwayScope (see Figure 11.9) has a video display incorporated into the proximal handle and a distal cable that houses an LED light and CMOS sensor which drops into a single-use blade ("PBlade"), available in various sizes. The blade has separate channels for an ETT and a suction catheter. Its unique feature is an aiming reticle (i.e., "cross-hairs") that can be optionally activated on the video display and is designed to help line up the scope with the glottic opening to optimize ease of ETT passage.

APA™ (previously called Venner A.P. Advance, AAM Healthcare, Jersey, England)

The APA (see https://www.red-dot.org/project/venner-ap-advance-video-laryngoscope-10436) consists of a video viewer, the camera module, the handle, and the anti-fog coated single-use

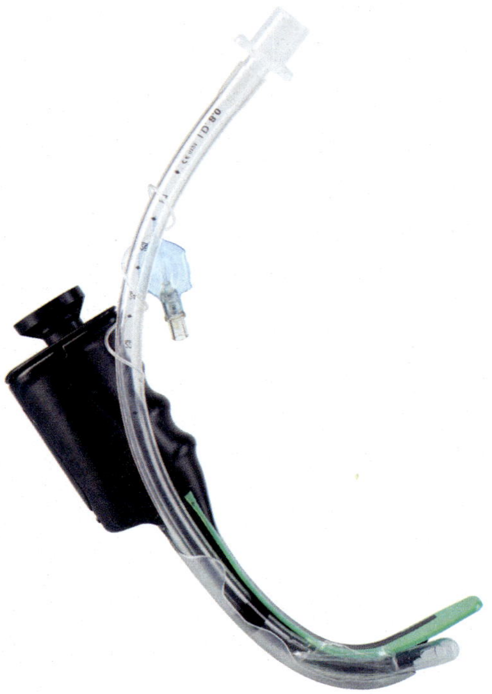

FIGURE 11.8. The Airtraq AVANT with a loaded endotracheal tube. (Reproduced with permission from Prodol Meditec.)

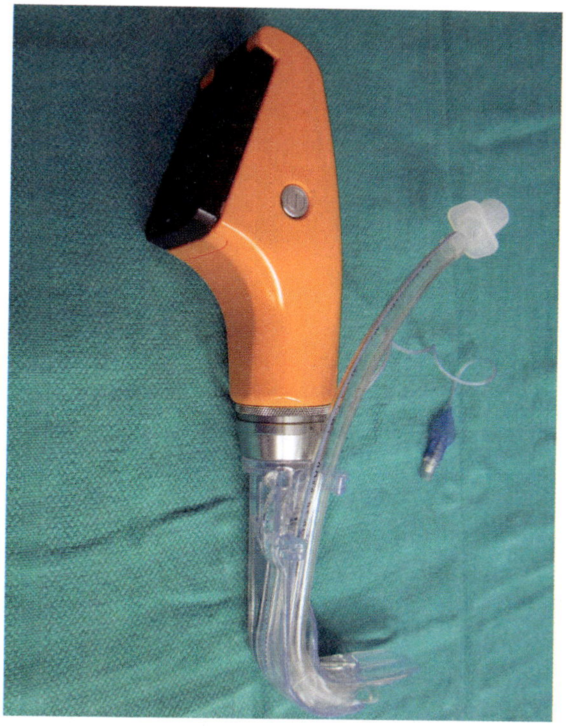

FIGURE 11.9. Pentax AirwayScope with a single-use blade ("PBlade").

blade. The camera module incorporates a high-intensity LED light source and CMOS camera sensor. The blade is available in multiple options including Macintosh, hyperangulated (channeled and nonchanneled), and Miller.

King Vision® (Ambu Inc, Columbia, MD, USA)

The King Vision aBlade™ video laryngoscope (see Figure 11.10) features a reusable display and video adaptor that includes the LED light and CMOS camera in its distal tip. The adaptor is placed within a single-use blade that is clear, antifog coated and has channeled and nonchanneled versions. For more details about these devices please refer to the previous edition of this textbook.

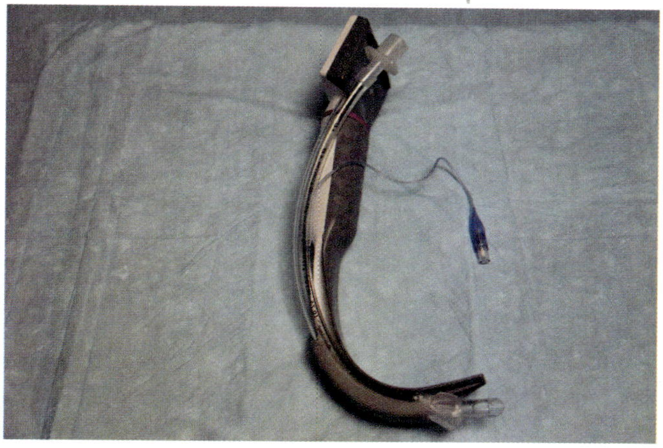

FIGURE 11.10. The King Vision laryngoscope with channeled blade aBlade.

■ What Are the Steps for Use of Channeled VL?

The following steps are helpful to facilitate tracheal intubation using the channeled VL (common to all devices):

- Choose an appropriately sized device/blade (e.g., it would be difficult to use some high-profile channeled blades in patients with a small mouth opening)
- Lubricate within the channel and the outer surface of the ETT
- Preload ETT within the channel but not beyond the tip of the blade (e.g., see the AirTraq Avant, Figure 11.8)
- Insert the device into the mouth in the midline
- Advance the tip of the blade into the vallecula (Airtraq), or directly lift the epiglottis (Pentax-AWS)
- An appropriate blade position is indicated by the view of the glottis being centered in the viewfinder
- Advance the ETT through the channel into the glottis and then trachea
- After successful intubation, rotate the device forward out of the patient's mouth, whilst separating the ETT laterally from the channel.

By design, channeled video laryngoscopes require a C-L grade 1 view with the glottis centralized on the video screen. The outer diameter of the ETT must be matched with the internal diameter of the channel to ensure ease of passage.

Most channeled blades are wider or thicker than their nonchanneled counterparts. This may be a limitation, particularly for patients with a small mouth opening or inter-incisor distance. A technical comparison of several channeled devices may be found elsewhere.[76]

VIDEO LARYNGOSCOPES WITH NONCHANNELED BLADES

■ What Are the Common Features of Nonchanneled VL?

Similar to channeled blades, nonchanneled video laryngoscopes are made up of a blade with mounted camera, a handle, and a screen for visualization (mounted on the handle or cable-connected to a screen display). Examples of commonly used nonchanneled video laryngoscopes include: GlideScope; C-MAC; and McGRATH™ MAC.

GlideScope (Verathon Inc Bothell, WA, USA) (Video 27)

GlideScope Video Laryngoscope Titanium (see Figure 11.11) is the reusable version of the hyperangulated and Macintosh blade. The GlideScope is available in various configurations: the handle and blade can be reusable titanium ("Titanium") or single-use plastic ("Spectrum™") which can be connected to a handle-mounted screen (GlideScope Go) or mobile workstation (GlideScope Video Monitor or the newer GlideScope Core™). A range of blades are available (Macintosh, Miller and angulated configurations and in a variety of sizes) and contain a high-resolution CMOS video camera and integrated LED light source. Snapshots or video recordings can be captured on

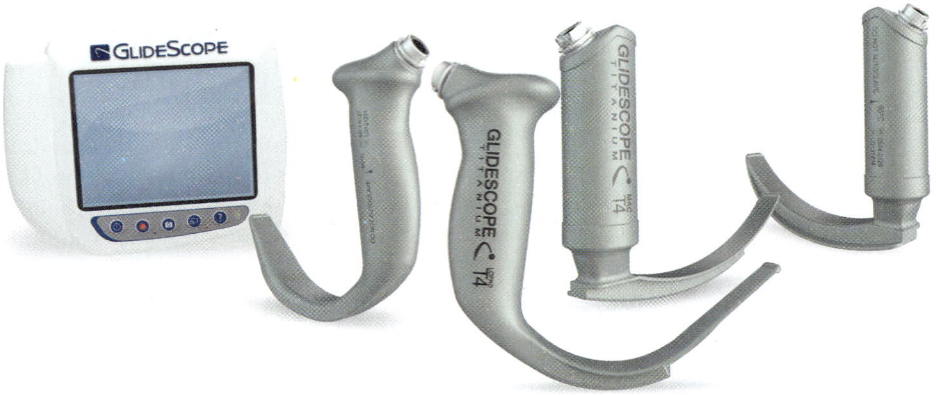

FIGURE 11.11. GlideScope video laryngoscope (titanium). This photo shows the reusable version in the angulated and Macintosh styles. (Reproduced with permission, ©Verathon Inc.)

a USB flashdrive, and the screen image can also be exported to an external monitor via a video-out port (HDMI-DVI). The GlideScope AVL Single Use system are video batons used with a single-use plastic blade cover ("GVL Stats") that interface with the Core™, Go™, and/or Video Monitor. The GlideScope Ranger is a portable, self-contained monitor intended for EMS and military use that uses the same blades as the AVL Single use system.

C-MAC (KARL STORZ Endoscopy Canada Ltd, Mississauga, ON, Canada) (Video 11)

The C-MAC (see Figure 11.12) is a reusable video laryngoscope with a handle and blade component that connects directly to a LCD monitor, and is capable of recording snapshots and video. There are a number of re-useable blades available (Macintosh, Miller and the hyperangulated Dörges blade (known as the D-blade)).

The 7-inch C-MAC video monitor can also be used with the C-MAC Video Stylet, the Storz Bonfils stylet, and the Flexible Intubation Video Endoscope (FIVE). A 3.5-inch portable Pocket Monitor is also available.

The C-MAC S is a portable video baton-style system that utilizes single-use plastic blades.

McGRATH MAC (Medtronic, Dublin, Ireland) (Videos 17 and 23)

The McGRATH MAC (see Figure 11.13) has a fixed-position camera stick with a handle-mounted 2.5-in LCD display in portrait orientation with a single plane swivel. It uses single-use

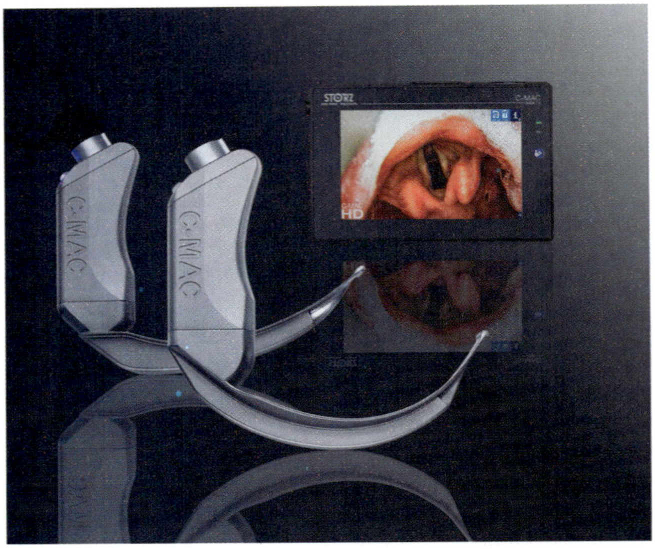

FIGURE 11.12. The Storz C-MAC video laryngoscope. (© KARL STORZ SE & Co. KG, Germany.)

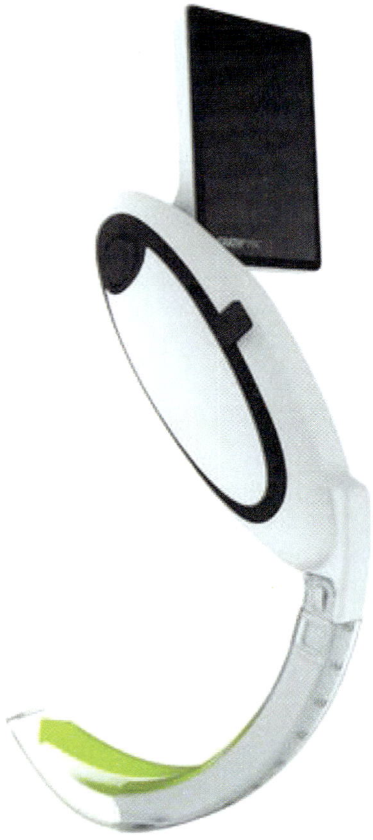

FIGURE 11.13. McGRATH MAC video laryngoscope. (Reproduced with permission from Medtronic, Boulder, Colorado.)

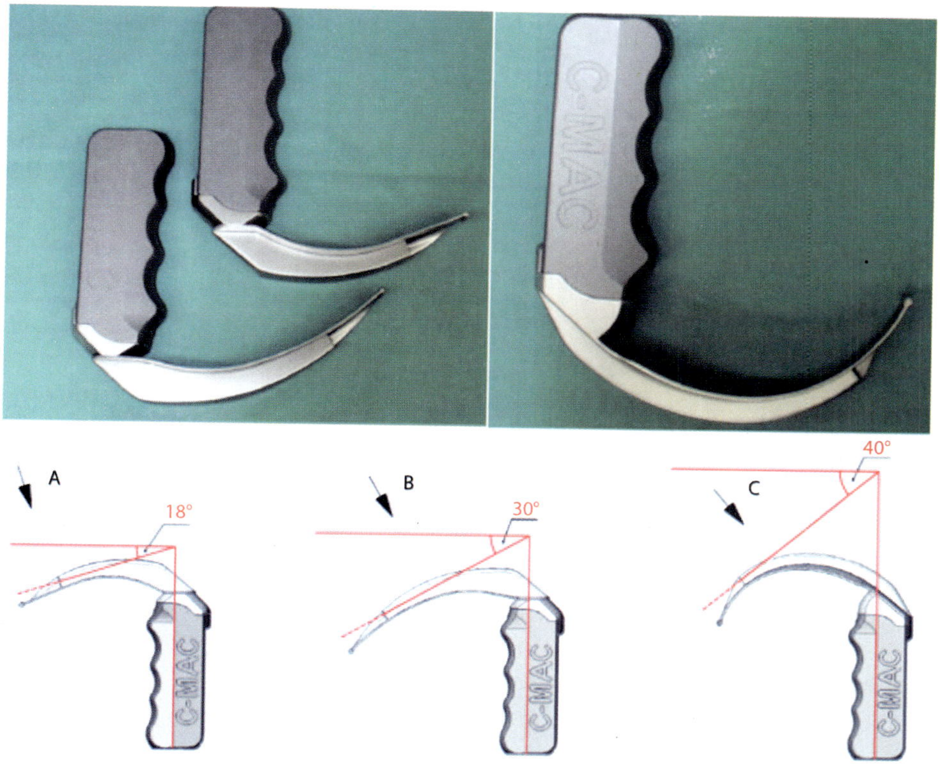

FIGURE 11.14. Comparison of the conventional C-MAC video laryngoscope blades (Macintosh sizes 3 and 4; left panel, **A, B**) with the hyperangulated blade C-MAC D-Blade (right panel, **C**). (Reproduced with permission from Cavus E, Neumann T, Doerges V, et al. First clinical evaluation of the C-MAC D-Blade videolaryngoscope during routine and difficult intubation. *Anesth Analg.* 2011;112(2):382-385.)

polycarbonate blade covers that are available in Macintosh and hyperangulated (X3 blade) format. It does not have recording capability.

For more details on these devices and other VLs, please refer to the previous edition of this textbook.

Nonchanneled video laryngoscopes can have a Macintosh or a non-Macintosh blade. The VL Macintosh blade has the same geometry as a DL Macintosh blade. By comparison, the nonMacintosh blade, or hyperangulated blade, has a more acute angle (e.g., 40 degree with the CMAC Dblade [HA blade] compared to 18 degree [size 3] and 30 degree [size 4] with the CMAC Macintosh blade)[77] which allows for indirect visualization of the glottis in patients in whom it is difficult to align the pharyngeal, laryngeal, and tracheal axes (see Figure 11.14). There may be slight variations in shape of the hyperangulated blade between the different manufacturers of video laryngoscopes.

How Are Nonchanneled Video Laryngoscopes Used for Tracheal Intubation? (Video 29)

The following steps are helpful to facilitate tracheal intubation using a VL: (1) ETT preparation; (2) laryngeal visualization; (3) ETT delivery; and (4) ETT advancement.

ETT Preparation

Special attention should be paid to preparing the ETT prior to laryngoscopy. The ETT can be softened in warm water to help with malleability and smooth delivery as well as minimize trauma to the upper airway. Use of a straight ETT may make molding easier and avoid the tendency of the tip of the curved ETT to abut the anterior trachea as it is inserted past the glottis.[78] This can also be avoided by reverse-loading of a curved ETT onto the stylet (ETT is rotated 180 degree to normal so that when the stylet is removed the ETT tip curves posteriorly in the same orientation as the trachea) (see Figure 11.15).[79,80] To avoid the ETT cuff obscuring the glottic view during insertion, the cuff can be pulled to one side or wrapped around the ETT as it is deflated during the cuff check (Figure 11.16).

A well-lubricated stylet is strongly recommended. A malleable (or dedicated rigid) stylet is recommended particularly for the hyperangulated blade VL when the larynx is not in the line-of-sight. Alternatively, a "dynamic stylet" such as the Parker Flex-it™ (Parker Medical, Englewood, CO), the Truflex™ (Truphatek, Netanya, Israel), or the Rapid Positioning Intubation Stylet "RPiS" (AME, Wellesdley MA), can be used. Various stylet shapes have been described but Cooper et al.[81] suggested that it resemble the distal aspect of the blade. Essentially, the curve should be shaped so that the ETT can be easily rotated around the tongue base. This should be individualized depending on patient- and device-dependent factors. Excessive bending may make intubation more complicated than it need be.

Laryngeal Visualization

Fogging and a soiled airway can affect the visualization of the glottis during tracheal intubation using the VL.[82,83] The

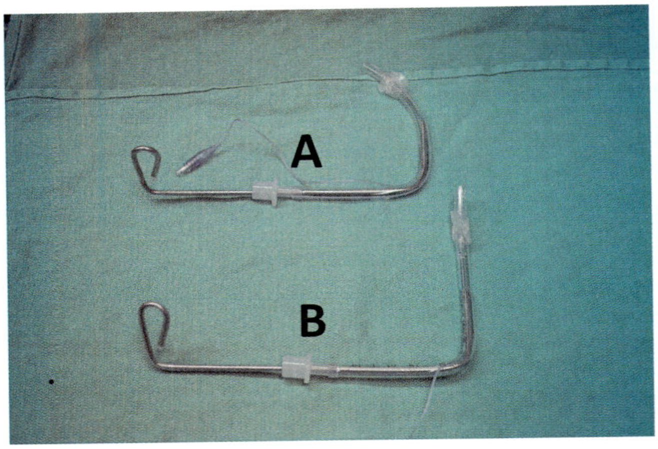

FIGURE 11.15. The degree of anterior bending of the endotracheal tube (ETT) following the retraction of the stylet. The tip of the ETT has a tendency to bend more anteriorly if the stylet is bend along the natural curvature ETT **(A)** as compared to the reverse loading of the ETT onto the stylet **(B)**.

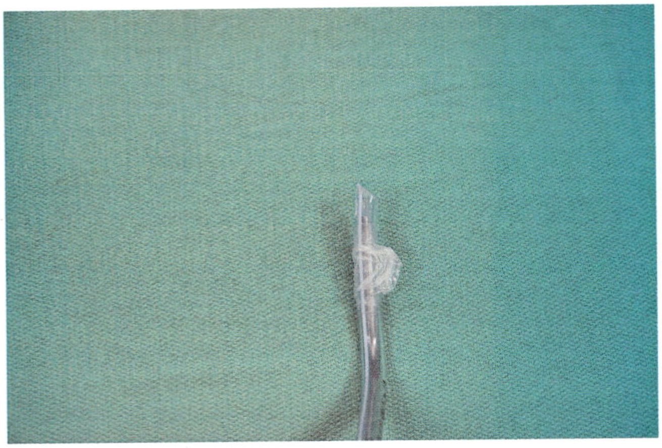

FIGURE 11.16. The ETT cuff pulls to one side (away from the camera of the VL).

GlideScope is the only video laryngoscope with the antifog heating element in direct contact with a thin piece of glass covering the camera lens. However, to fully optimize the antifog feature, the device must be turned on 1 to 2 minutes prior to intubation.[84] To decrease fogging when using other VLs, it may be helpful to apply an antifog agent (e.g., Fred™ Anti-Fog Solution, Medtronic Limited, Watford, UK) or warming the device (e.g., placed in warm water) before use.[85] In patients with a soiled airway, it is recommended to thoroughly suction the airway with a Yankauer suction catheter before initiating laryngoscopy.[83]

Special head and neck positioning is not required. Anatomical alignment of the three axes is not required; optical alignment is provided by the video camera and the hyperangulation of the device may make blade insertion difficult in patients with short or rigid necks, large chests or if cricoid pressure is being applied. Ramping is still recommended for patients with morbid obesity both for intubation and to optimize the effectiveness of face-mask ventilation should it become necessary (see Chapter 52 and Figure 52.2).

The laryngoscope should be carefully inserted into the mouth under visual control, in the midline and maintained in the midline as it is rotated around the tongue base for the hyperangulated VL. The application of a water-soluble lubricant on the tongue blade may facilitate smooth insertion. Care should be taken to avoid injury to the lips and teeth during laryngoscope insertion. There is a tendency to introduce the blade too deeply which has several disadvantages: (i) by reducing the distance between the camera and the larynx, narrowing the visual field; (ii) the more distal location of the camera increases the distance between the lips and the point at which the ETT first appears on the monitor and if ETT insertion and passage through this "blind spot" is not observed directly, it increases the risk of soft tissue injuries — particularly vulnerable is the right palatopharyngeal fold;[86,87] and (iii) it elevates the larynx, making ETT delivery to the larynx and the subsequent advancement of the ETT more challenging.[88,89] The laryngoscopist should resist the temptation to deeply engage the vallecula thereby maximizing glottic exposure as this will frustrate efforts to intubate. It is worth checking the orientation of the laryngoscope handle; the more vertical the handle, the less favorable the angle of incidence between the approaching ETT and the trachea. If the epiglottis blocks laryngeal exposure, the angulated blade can be used like a straight blade, directly elevating the epiglottis.

The video laryngoscope with a Macintosh blade is introduced from the right corner of the mouth and displaces the tongue while engaging the vallecula, in a similar fashion to DL with a Macintosh blade. Once appropriately positioned, the practitioner has the ability to visualize the larynx both directly (line-of-sight) through the mouth and indirectly on the video screen (see Chapter 9, "Direct Laryngoscopy").

ETT Delivery

When DL is performed using a video laryngoscope with a Macintosh blade, the ETT insertion is directly observed as it passes through the oropharynx and therefore an adjunct such as a stylet is seldom needed. During intubation using the videolaryngoscope, particularly with a hyperangulated blade, there is a temptation to focus attention on the monitor while the styletted-ETT is being introduced into the mouth.

It is also necessary to insert the ETT with care to avoid patient injury or damage to the ETT cuff.

Some practitioners prefer to introduce the ETT into the mouth prior to the laryngoscope. This is particularly helpful in patients with a small mouth or when a DLT is being placed. (It has the additional advantage of ensuring that the insertion of the tube is performed under visual control.) The uvula, base of tongue and epiglottis should be seen in succession to ensure proper midline orientation. The blade is preferentially advanced toward but not deeply into the vallecula. It is important to introduce the laryngoscope blade under direct vision to ensure that the lips and teeth are not injured.

The vector of force applied to the laryngoscope is very similar to DL, namely along the same axis as a handle. Lifting with the left hand, rather than levering will create space to allow

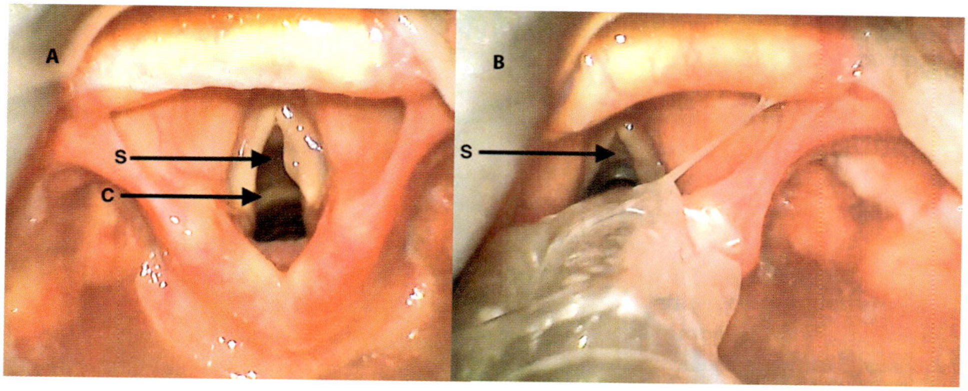

FIGURE 11.17. Indirect laryngoscopy using a C-MAC Dblade showing the cricoid cartilage (C) and the space above it (S) in panel **(A)**. To avoid trapping the tip of the ETT in the space (S), it is best to place the tip of the reverse loaded styletted-ETT in the middle of the glottis during intubation as shown in panel **(B)**.

simple lifting (rather than levering) of the styletted ETT. The practitioner essentially wraps the ETT around the base of the tongue and lifts it as if retracting the tongue. This maneuver is subtle but quite effective.

When the tip of the ETT is positioned beyond the vocal folds, care should be taken not to insert the tip of the ETT into the space above the cricoid cartilage. (Figure 11.17) as this can cause the ETT to hold-up. The stylet should be partially withdrawn which will generally straighten the ETT and facilitate its advancement down the trachea.

If advancement is not easily achieved, the ETT can be slowly rotated until its tip is disengaged from the anterior tracheal wall. This should result in a "loss of resistance." No increased force should be required to advance the ETT.

Further tips for overcoming commonly encountered difficulties with nonchanneled VL intubation use can be found in Table 11.1.

What Are the Predictors of Difficult and Failed Tracheal Intubation Using Video Laryngoscopes?

Compared with DL, few studies have been published on the anatomic predictors of difficulty in performing tracheal intubation using VL. Tremblay et al.[96] prospectively studied 400 elective surgical patients. A detailed airway evaluation was done, followed by the induction of general anesthesia and pharmacologic muscle paralysis. DL was performed initially, and the C-L grade determined. Thereafter, another laryngoscopy using the GlideScope (Verathon, Bothell, WA) with a hyperangulated blade was performed, the view again graded and tracheal intubation performed. After multiple regression analysis, a C-L grade 3 or 4 view at DL, poor mandibular protrusion (as reflected by a high upper lip bite test[97]), and a short sternothyroid distance were significantly correlated with both longer time-to-intubation and a higher number of intubation attempts.

Aziz et al.[98] retrospectively evaluated the records of 2004 uses of the GlideScope in two institutions, most (81%) of which were performed on patients with preoperative predictors of difficult DL. Used as a primary or rescue device, failure to intubate occurred in 60 cases. Three anatomic predictors were significantly associated with GlideScope failure: altered neck anatomy (including mass, surgical scar, or radiation); decreased (<6 cm) thyromental distance and reduced cervical motion. In this study, patient age, gender, BMI, Mallampati classification, and reduced mouth opening (<3 cm) were not significantly correlated with difficult intubation using the GlideScope.

Siu et al.[99] reported a prospective observational study of GlideScope intubations with a hyperangulated blade in 742 patients. The probability of successful first-attempt tracheal intubation dropped from 81% in patients with normal airways to 73% in those with predicted or documented difficult DL.

Aziz and colleagues[100] performed a secondary analysis of data obtained during a randomized controlled trial (RCT) comparing the GlideScope hyperangulated blade with the Storz C-MAC D-blade for tracheal intubation of patients with predicted difficult DL. In this analysis, characteristics associated with greater risk for difficult VL were head and neck positioning in the "supine sniffing" versus "supine neutral" position, surgery type (otolaryngology and cardiac vs. general), intubation performed by an attending anesthesiologist versus an anesthesiology trainee, and small mouth opening.

Joshi et al.[101] studied 906 consecutive intubations of ICU patients to identify the characteristics associated with first-attempt failed intubation when using VL with both hyperangulated VL (HA-VL) and Macintosh (Mac-VL) blades in the ICU setting. They found an association with blood in the airway, airway oedema, obesity, and cervical immobility.

Whether these anatomic predictors would also predict difficulty with video laryngoscopes other than the GlideScope or C-MAC with D-blade is unknown.

Predictors of difficult tracheal intubation using nonchanneled hyperangulated VL are summarized in Table 11.2.

What Is the Learning Curve for VL Intubation?

Skills in traditional DL are not necessarily fully transferable to VL, particularly when a hyperangulated blade is used. There are a number of subtle differences in technique, as well as variations

TABLE 11.1. Some Potential Solutions to Commonly Encountered Problems While Performing Nonchanneled Hyperangulated VL Intubation

Problem	Potential Solutions
Laryngeal visualization	
Can't insert blade into mouth	Scissor grip to open mouth further; insert blade in right of mouth like DL;[90] insert blade at 90 or 180 degree angle (as with an oropharyngeal airway) before rotating to normal position once in mouth.[90]
Can't insert ETT into mouth	Shift blade to left;[91] Try inserting styletted ETT before or concomitant with video laryngoscope blade.
Best view, but too close	Back up; rotate blade handle toward patient feet; try "good enough" view.[90,91]
ETT obscures view of glottis	Move blade to left, ETT to right, or slight left rotation of video laryngoscope handle to create more room for ETT; When preparing/checking ETT cuff, wrap or pull to side while deflating to create lower profile.
ETT delivery	
Difficulty manipulating ETT	Hold ETT closer to the connector for more maneuverability.[91]
ETT advancement	
ETT keeps passing posterior to glottis	Use a stylet or bougie;[90] inflate cuff whilst advancing toward glottis to direct anteriorly;[90] withdraw laryngoscope for wider angle of view;[90] try "good enough" view to lessen anterior angle.[91,92]
Can't advance ETT into the trachea	If ETT catches on cricoid ring, try to place ETT in mid-glottis as advancing (see Figure 11.17); withdraw stylet a few centimeters, then advance ETT into trachea before removing stylet completely;[91,92] rotate ETT 45-90 degree clockwise once tip is in trachea to overcome impingement on cricoid cartilage or tracheal ring;[92] reverse load ETT on stylet;[80,90,93,94] try using a bougie;[90] try slight flexion of the head and neck;[90] apply cricoid pressure;[90] use a straight tracheal tube.[52,78,79,95]

TABLE 11.2. Predictors of Difficult Tracheal Intubation Using Indirect Video Laryngoscopy

- Predicted[99] or actual[96,99] difficult direct laryngoscopy (e.g., Cormack-Lehane Grade 3 or 4 view)
- High upper lip bite test (i.e., reduced mandibular protrusion)[96]
- Reduced mouth opening[100]
- Short sternothyroid distance[96]
- Altered neck anatomy (mass, surgical scar, radiation)[98]
- Decreased (<6 cm) thyromental distance[98]
- Reduced cervical motion[98,101]
- Positioning in sniffing position (vs. neutral)[100]
- Inexperience with technique[98,100]
- Surgery type (e.g., otolaryngology; cardiac)[100]
- Blood in the airway[101]
- Airway edema[101]

in positioning, blade insertion, and use of stylets, or other ETT introducers that may increase the time it takes to learn and master the use of VL. Of note, obtaining an adequate view of the glottis may be easier to master than the skill of endotracheal intubation once the view has been obtained.

As discussed in a recent editorial, the change from DL to VL requires a perspective shift in terms of utilizing an indirect view of the glottis on a screen to deliver an ETT.[79] It can be likened to performing a laparoscopic procedure or playing a video game, a skill that requires visuospatial coordination different to DL. The subtle differences between devices also means that a practitioner must identify and understand such differences and how a device will respond in challenging scenarios. The editorial notes that successful VL intubation *likely depends on a complex and dynamic interplay of innate visuospatial co-ordination abilities, coupled with skills acquired from training and repeated learning experience.*[79]

The need for specific VL training and experience was highlighted in the previously mentioned study by Aziz et al.[98] involving 2004 patients in which one nonanatomic predictor of failed GlideScope-facilitated intubation was intubation occurring in one of the two participating institutions. Over the study period, in the institution with the higher rate of failed intubation, practitioners had performed a median of only 6 intubations each, compared with a median of 19 at the second institution. This emphasizes the significance of the learning curve and maintenance of competence issues applicable to indirect VL.

Cortellazzi et al.[102] studied the development of expertise in GlideScope VL in trainee anesthesia practitioners experienced with Macintosh blade (DL), but naïve to indirect VL. As expertise was the study endpoint, an "optimal" attempt was defined by successful first-attempt intubation within 60 seconds, obtaining a C-L 1 laryngeal view and "no significant defect in technique". Using these parameters, 76 intubations were required to predict a >90% probability of an optimal intubation. Another study of VL performed in the operating room environment also implies a significant learning curve: in a large observational cohort, Siu et al.[99] reported that the first-attempt success rate increased from 69% for those with 0 to 9 previous uses of the GlideScope to 90% for those with 20 to 29 previous uses.

In the Emergency Department setting, Sakles et al.[103] compared the first-pass success rate of emergency medicine residents using the GlideScope (HA-VL blade) in each of their 3 years of training with the corresponding rates for DL. For the GlideScope, success rates progressively improved, at 74.4%, 83.6%, and 90% through training years 1, 2, and 3 years respectively. In contrast, the corresponding figures for DL were 69.9%, 71.7%, and 72.9%, respectively, indicating no significant improvement beyond the first year. In the same institution, first-pass success with the GlideScope used by attending staff physicians increased from 75.6% to 95.6% from the first to the last of 7 years studied.[104]

Baciarello et al.[105] conducted a learning curve study of the Airtraq, comparing it to Macintosh DL skills acquisition in a group of 10 novice medical students. After a practice phase, clinical experience was observed in elective surgical patients. Over the course of ten intubations with each device, 7 students achieved a ≥90% success rate with the Airtraq, compared with only one for Macintosh DL. Differences in success rate were significant from the fourth attempt onward.

Learning curve studies are difficult to directly compare given varying study designs, definitions of success, and participating practitioner experience. Notwithstanding, the available evidence indicates a significant learning curve for indirect VL in human subjects, particularly for the nonchanneled hyperangulated blades. This implies that when planning the approach to a patient with predictors of difficult airway management, the practitioner should be confident that they have ascended the learning curve for the technique, before relying on VL for tracheal intubation.

How Effective Is Indirect Video Laryngoscopy Following Failed Direct Laryngoscopy?

In their study of 2004 GlideScope intubations, Aziz et al.[98] reported a 94% success rate (224 of 239) for GlideScope-facilitated tracheal intubations in the subset of patients who had failed DL compared to their overall success rate of 98%.

Amathieu et al.[106] reported on the efficacy of an airway algorithm applied to anesthetized, pharmacologically paralyzed patients. The algorithm called for use of the Airtraq after failed intubation by Macintosh DL with or without adjunctive use of a TTI. Of 12,225 patients included, 98% were successfully intubated with DL on its own; 207 of 236 were successfully intubated with DL/TTI, and of the remaining 29 patients, 27 were successfully intubated with the Airtraq. Malin et al.[107] reported an 80% success rate of Airtraq-facilitated intubation in a series of 47 patients after failed intubation with a Macintosh blade. A TTI was used to facilitate the Airtraq intubation in a third of these cases. Earlier, Maharaj et al.[108] had reported a case series of 7 patients successfully intubated with the Airtraq after failed intubation using Macintosh laryngoscopy.

On the Flip Side, How Effective Is Direct Laryngoscopy Following Failed Tracheal Intubation by Indirect Video Laryngoscopy?

No studies were identified that specifically addressed the success of DL in facilitating tracheal intubation after failed intubation using VL. In Tremblay's study[96] of predictors of difficult use of the GlideScope, one patient in the series of 400 could not be intubated with the GlideScope despite 3 attempts and a C-L Grade 1 view: DL allowed successful intubation on the first-attempt. Aziz et al.[98] witnessed failures in 60 of 2004 GlideScope attempted intubations: DL was used to successfully intubate 28 (47%) of these patients, while various other techniques were used for the remainder.

In a study by Cavus et al.[109] comparing VL (APA with Macintosh blade, C-MAC D-blade and King Vision channeled size 3 blade) in physician-based prehospital emergency intubation, 19 of the 168 included patients (2 in APA group, 1 in C-MAC, 16 on King Vision group) were unable to be intubated with VL, but were successfully intubated with traditional Macintosh DL. There were also a number of patients intubated in the APA and C-MAC groups in which the device was used as direct instead of indirect laryngoscopy.

Why Might Tracheal Intubation Fail Despite a Good View of the Larynx Obtained by Indirect VL?

Direct and indirect laryngoscopy are different techniques, requiring different skills. The specific differences depend upon the device. In general, with DL the objective is to optimize the glottis view and to the extent it can be achieved and placement of the ETT is relatively straight forward. When this can't be achieved, head elevation, ELM or backward-upward-rightward-pressure (BURP) or use of a TTI might be attempted in an effort to bring the larynx into view or intubate blindly. With indirect techniques, a good laryngeal view does not assure ETT placement. There are specific techniques that may increase the success of tracheal intubation. A general discussion may be found elsewhere.[91,110]

Efficacy of Video Laryngoscopy

What Is the Clinical Utility of VL in the Operating Room Setting?

Since their introduction in the early 2000s, the availability and use of video laryngoscopes have increased dramatically. There is increasing evidence that video laryngoscopy can improve aspects of intubation within certain settings, however no one device has been shown to be superior. As discussed previously, there is often heterogeneity in study design, outcomes, and devices used, therefore caution is needed when drawing conclusions from the literature. It is most likely that the device with which an airway practitioner is most familiar and skilled will provide the best outcomes.

Of the channeled blades, there is evidence to support the use of Airtraq, Pentax-AWS, King Vision, and APA. The Airtraq has been shown to improve laryngeal view compared to Macintosh DL, but there is sometimes disagreement with respect to first-attempt intubation success rate, time-to-intubation, and results in expert versus novice hands. In their systematic review and meta-analysis of RCTs comparing the Airtraq with Macintosh blade DL, Lu et al.[111] found that the Airtraq reduced intubation time in both experienced and novice hands, but increased first-attempt success only for novices. Esophageal intubation was reduced, but other complications were no different. Intubation Difficulty Scale[75] scores when reported were reduced by the Airtraq, and the percentage of glottic opening (POGO)[73] was improved.[111]

In another systematic review and meta-analysis, RCTs of patients undergoing cervical spine immobilization were pooled to compare multiple indirect VL devices with Macintosh blade DL.[112] The Airtraq alone was associated with improved glottic visualization and a significant reduction in the risk of first-attempt intubation failure, time-to-intubation, and oropharyngeal complications. Other devices, including the Pentax-AWS, GlideScope, C-MAC (blade type not stated), and McGRATH (type and blade not stated) were associated only with improved glottic visualization.

The Pentax-AWS has also been shown to have a high first-attempt success rate (≥95%)[5,113,114] in elective surgical patients, largely without anatomic predictors of difficult tracheal intubation. A similar first-attempt success rate was reported in a later observational study in which the AWS was used in 293 patients with known or predicted difficult DL.[115] A systematic review of 16 RCTs comparing the AWS to Macintosh blade DL in adult patients with "normal" and "difficult" airways concluded that while the AWS permits a superior laryngeal view to that obtained with DL, there was no difference between the devices in first-attempt success, intubation time, or oral/pharyngeal injury.[116] A second systematic review assessed the efficacy of alternatives to DL in the patient undergoing cervical spine immobilization and confirmed the significantly better view afforded by the AWS compared with Macintosh DL but did not report improved first-attempt success or time-to-intubation.[112]

The channeled hyperangulated King Vision was included in a multi-center RCT of video laryngoscopes used in 720 patients without predictors of difficult laryngoscopy but wearing cervical collars. Under these study conditions, the first-attempt success rate was 87% on the first-attempt, rising to 92% after two attempts.[117] In a study using lightly preserved clinical grade cadavers also wearing a cervical collar, 32 participants were uniformly successful in intubating using the King Vision, in contrast to the 10 failures with DL, the latter facilitated at will by stylet or the TTI.[118]

To date, few clinical trials and limited case reports[119–122] have appeared on the APA DAB (Difficult Airway Blade). One published study randomized elective surgical patients without predictors of difficult airway management but with an applied cervical collar to the use of one of six video laryngoscopes for tracheal intubation, 1 of which was the APA DAB.[117] Under these study conditions, for the primary study outcome, the DAB enabled a first-attempt success rate of 37%, contrasting with 85% for the channeled Airtraq and 87% for the channeled King Vision.

Many studies had assessed the efficacy of nonchanneled video laryngoscopes. A 2012 meta-analysis and systematic review of GlideScope versus DL identified 17 trials involving nearly 2000 patients.[123] The conclusions were that compared with DL, GlideScope provided better laryngeal views but no difference in first-attempt intubation success among experienced practitioners. This was not true of those with less experience in which GlideScope was favored and accomplished in a much shorter time.

As previously mentioned, Aziz et al.[98] assessed 2004 tracheal intubations using the GlideScope as either the primary or rescue device. When used as the primary device, most of the patients had features predictive of a difficult DL. Nonetheless, the success rate was 98%. As a rescue device when DL failed, the overall success rate was 94%. Although the success rates differed significantly in the two participating institutions, neither center had a very high usage rate (median experience: 19 and 6 uses respectively). Using propensity scores, Ibinson and colleagues[124] attempted to compare two cohorts each with 313 intubations using GlideScope or DL performed by a range of practitioners (from medical, nursing, and respiratory therapy students to experienced faculty anesthesiologists) at a single tertiary care facility. The patients were matched using propensity scores based upon seven predictors of DL difficulty such as Mallamapati score, cervical range of motion, and decreased mouth opening. Their primary outcome, first-attempt success with the GlideScope was 93.6% versus 80.8% for DL ($p < 0.001$). As a rescue device, GlideScope was used successfully 98.8% of the time.

Choi and colleagues[125] used propensity scores to match patients in 13 Korean metropolitan Emergency Departments intubated using GlideScope or DL (Macintosh), though the "prediction" of difficulty was assessed after intubations were attempted. Their propensity scores were derived from 11 intubators and patient-related variables. Their primary outcome was the first-attempt success which did not differ (GlideScope 85.7% vs. Mac 82.3% $p=0.05$) overall even though the GlideScope outperformed DL in the hands of junior residents while the opposite was true for more experienced practitioners. These findings are comparable to those studies from Sakles et al.[126] and Mosier et al.[127] Both of those studies demonstrated higher first-attempt success rates with GlideScope. Reasons for the differences between these studies is speculative and there may be unknown confounders.

Kaplan and co-workers[128] evaluated the Storz Macintosh Video laryngoscope (MVL), an earlier device, on 235 patients, 18 of whom had features suggesting a difficult conventional DL. In 22 of the 217 (10%) patients in whom no difficulties were anticipated, ELM was required and the video system enabled the assistant to evaluate its effect and make the appropriate adjustments. All but one of these intubations was successful. ELM was required in the patients predicted to be difficult and all these intubations were also successful. The authors concluded that the MVL had a very short learning curve and provided a larger, brighter image that could be viewed by the practitioner and instructor. It was therefore a useful device for teaching. Unfortunately, they did not compare the laryngeal views with DL, making it difficult to determine whether this device provides a different view or simply a bigger, brighter one. While it is useful for an assistant to be able to make adjustments to the location, direction and force of ELM, the need to apply it in 40/238 (17%) cases suggests that the MVL does not provide better glottic exposure in challenging airways. A subsequent multicentered study[129] compared direct and indirect laryngeal views in 865 patients using the MVL. Direct viewing resulted in poor laryngeal exposure (C-L 3) in 100 patients which improved by indirect viewing. A poor laryngeal view (C-L 3) was seen with both methods, direct and indirect, in 21 patients.

Cavus and coworkers[130] performed crossover laryngoscopies comparing three attempts on each of 150 patients without regard to the anticipated ease or difficulty, using Macintosh DL and C-MAC Macintosh blade VL. They concluded that the C-MAC provided better C-L scores. Aziz and colleagues[131] randomized 300 elective surgical patients with one or more features associated with difficult DL to either C-MAC Macintosh blade VL or DL attempted by suitably trained anesthesia practitioners. First-attempt intubation success was more common in the C-MAC group (93%, 95% CI, 87%-96% vs. 84%, 78%-90%; $p=0.026$); it was associated with better laryngeal views and required the use of a bougie and/or ELM less frequently but intubation time was longer (45 [40-51] vs. 33 [29-36] seconds). Although the study involved patients with anticipated difficult DL, the need for a bougie, ELM and reduced laryngeal views was nonetheless rather high in the C-MAC group. This suggests that while a video laryngoscope configured with a Macintosh blade does facilitate laryngoscopy well, a hyperangulated blade may be more beneficial in achieving a better view of the glottis when challenging anatomy is encountered.

The McGRATH MAC has been used successfully after a failed attempt with a Pentax-AWS in a patient with a halo vest,[132] in a child with Treacher Collins Syndrome in whom a C-L 4 view by Macintosh-DL was converted to a C-L 1,[133] as well as better laryngeal views requiring fewer intubation attempts using a DLT.[134] In a study of 158 patients, Wallace and coworkers[135] compared Macintosh-DL with McGRATH direct and indirect views. The three groups had similar airway characteristics, however the investigators observed lower Intubation Difficulty Scores[75] and utilized the least effort when indirect viewing was used. Interestingly, although the laryngeal view was best with indirect viewing and the intubation difficulty scale (IDS) was lower in the indirect group, all three groups were easily intubated. They also observed poorer performance using the McGRATH MAC as a direct device compared with indirect viewing or a conventional Macintosh DL.

In a large recent Cochrane Systematic Review by Lewis et al.,[136] 64 RCTs were analyzed to assess whether VL for adult intubation reduces the risk of complications and failure when compared to DL. The devices used in these studies included GlideScope, Pentax-AWS, C-MAC with Macintosh blade, McGRATH series 5, X-lite, C-MAC D-blade, Airtraq, Truview, and CEL-100. As to be expected, there was differential performance between the different video laryngoscope designs. Overall, the authors reported that there was evidence to suggest that VL reduced failed intubations, including in patients with a predicted difficult airway. They found no evidence of reduced hypoxemia or mortality, but there was evidence of reduced laryngeal/airway trauma and hoarseness. VL resulted in less difficulty obtaining better laryngeal views and less intubation difficulty. There was no evidence that VL reduces the number of intubation attempts nor affects the time required for intubation. In experienced practitioners there were less failed intubations, but not in inexperienced practitioners.

As a result of increasing evidence to support video laryngoscope use, there are advocates for its use in situations when difficulty with laryngoscopy is anticipated, as a rescue device when those difficulties are in fact encountered and for its routine use in place of DL.[137,138] Most studies have confirmed that hyperangulated blades such as the GlideScope provide better laryngeal visualization than DL, but this may be at the expense of additional time to accomplish intubation. Likewise, as discussed previously, a good laryngeal view is desirable but does not ensure intubation success. Many of the earlier studies were hampered by nonstandardized outcomes, comparisons and extrapolations from manikins, inhomogeneous patient populations and inadequate training of the practitioners using the devices being compared.[139,140] VL is now part of the American Society of Anesthesiologists (ASA), Difficult Airway Society (DAS) and the Canadian Airway Focus Group (CAFG) Guidelines[92,141–143] for difficult and failed airways. Its role in the management of oral and nasal intubations, rapid sequence intubations,[144] patients with at-risk cervical spines,[112] morbidly obese patients,[145] obstetrical patients,[146] and critical care and emergency patients[126,147–149] continues to be a source of investigation and discussion.

The CAFG and DAS Guidelines[92,142,143] emphasize the importance of maximizing the likelihood of successful intubation on the first attempt. Suboptimal attempts are squandered, wasting time and risking additional complications. VL increases the probability that laryngoscopy will allow visually-controlled intubation and not be reliant upon blind techniques or tactile feedback. Other potential advantages include sharing the view with those who may be able to provide assistance, less force being applied by the laryngoscope, and less cervical manipulation. There is also the potential to record the intubation for clinical documentation, teaching, research, quality control, and remote supervision.[150] Experience with DL does not confer expertise with indirect techniques. This comes only with practice and experience using indirect techniques. If practice is reserved for situations when DL repeatedly fails, it is unlikely that a practitioner will acquire the necessary experience to perform successfully under stressful conditions. VL is now an essential part of the airway practitioner's armamentarium and it is important to be appropriately trained on the devices available at one's facility. Furthermore, it is important to acquire a sufficient volume of experience to maintain the skills and appreciate the limitations of a device in one's own hands.

What Is the Clinical Utility of VL in the Emergency or ICU Settings?

Griesdale et al.[151] conducted a small prospective trial of critically ill patients randomized to intubation by GlideScope nonchanneled hyperangulated VL or DL. Although VL produced better laryngeal views and a higher first-attempt success rate, this was at the cost of longer intubations times and lower SpO_2. The intubation times in both groups were uncommonly long (221 [IRQ 103-291] seconds vs. 156 [67-220] seconds for VL and DL, respectively), suggesting either very difficult patients, poor conditions, or inadequate practitioner experience. The laryngoscopists were internal medicine trainees and medical students. Hypes and coworkers[152] used propensity scores to compare first-attempt success with DL and VL in the ICU. The VL group, included patients in whom laryngoscopy was attempted using the GlideScope (150), C-MAC (507), King Vision (2), and McGRATH MAC (14) while the DL group included both Macintosh (131) and Miller (5) blades. They prospectively collected data on 809 consecutive intubations over a 36-month period in a single tertiary care ICU. Overall, the first-attempt success rates were 90.4% (95% CI, 77.2%-83.3%) and 65.4% (95% CI, 56.8%-73.4%) for VL and DL respectively. The odds ratio for first-attempt success was 2.81 (95% CI, 2.34-3.45) favoring VL. In addition, they demonstrated less oxygen desaturation and fewer esophageal intubations in the VL group. Griesdale et al.[151] did not show superior first-attempt success in an ICU study using comparing the GlideScope and DL whereas Silverberg et al.[153] did. Of note, in the latter study the failure rate with DL was 40% which raises questions about patient selection or practitioner skill. A systematic review and meta-analysis of prospective randomized controlled and observational trials of adult ICU intubations comparing VL and DL was conducted by De Jong and colleagues.[154] This yielded 9 studies involving a total of 2133 patients with both hyperangulated VL and Macintosh blade VL included in the VL group. These studies demonstrated the superiority of VL with respect to "difficult orotracheal intubation," first-attempt success (pooled OR 2.07, 95% CI, 1.35-3.15), fewer C-L III/IV views (OR 0.26, 95% CI, 0.17-0.41), and lower rates of esophageal intubation (OR 0.14, 95% CI, 0.02-0.81).

More recently, Arulkumaran et al.[155] performed a systematic review and meta-analysis to compare the success of VL versus DL for emergency intubation outside the operating room. They included 32 studies and had a mixture of hyperangulated, Macintosh type blade, channeled, and nonchanneled blade variations in their VL group. They found no difference in first-pass intubation with VL compared to DL in the emergency or prehospital setting, but increased first-pass intubation in ICU. There was greater first-pass intubation amongst novice/trainee clinicians, but this was not seen in experienced practitioners. VL was associated with fewer esophageal intubations, but also with more arterial hypotension. This was in contrast to two preview meta-analyses which concluded that VL did not increase first-attempt intubation success rates in ICU, nor improve outcomes compared to DL.[156,157]

The MACMAN2 trial[158] compared the use of four channeled videolaryngoscopes with Macintosh DL when used by residents to intubate the trachea of a simulated ICU patient with acute respiratory distress with some features of a difficult airway (inflated tongue). They demonstrated a 97.5% first-attempt intubation success with Airtraq, Pentax-AWS, and King Vision, along with improved glottic visualization and faster intubation times when compared with Macintosh DL. The VividTrac was also included in this trial and was not found to be as beneficial as the other devices studied, the authors reporting a first-attempt success rate of 92.4%.[158]

In the 2018 published guidelines for the management of intubation in critically ill adults, Higgs et al. suggested that a video laryngoscope be available and considered for all intubations of critically ill patients, and that practitioners involved in tracheal intubation in the critical care setting should be trained in the use of VL.[159] In addition, they suggested that VL use should be considered from the outset if laryngoscopy is predicted to be difficult, and that it should be used for subsequent intubation attempts if an initial DL attempt is unsuccessful.

What Is the Clinical Utility of VL in the Prehospital Setting?

In a German RCT looking at emergency prehospital intubations performed by emergency practitioners (predominantly anesthesiologists), King Vision (channeled blade) had lower intubation success rate and lower overall handling scores compared to C-MAC and APA, despite no difference in the best achievable glottis visualization.[109] The main reported problem with the King Vision was guidance difficulty passing the ETT through the device channel. The authors concluded that achieving expertise in use of the device is necessary before using it for emergency intubations.

Another study in Austria involving more than 500 prehospital emergency patients requiring tracheal intubation compared McGRATH MAC VL (Macintosh blade) to traditional DL.[160] They reported an equivalent intubation success rate and no significant difference in intubation times, number of attempts, or difficulty. While the glottic view was better with VL, there were more technical problems noted (with fogging, monitor reflexes, and ambient light).

Can the Video Laryngoscope Be Used in Awake Tracheal Intubation?

With increasing availability and use, VL is now being used in ATI as an alternative to flexible bronchoscopic intubation. It is also included as a technique in the DAS Guidelines for Awake Tracheal Intubation in adults.[161]

Recent reviews suggest that awake video laryngoscopic intubation is faster than flexible bronchoscopic intubation with similar rates of success and similar patient and practitioner satisfaction.[162]

A systematic review of 8 studies in 2018 assessed VL versus flexible bronchoscopy for ATI, including a mixture of device and blade types in their VL group.[163] They reported that intubation time was shorter when VL was used. There was no difference in failure rates, first-attempt success rate, patient satisfaction, or adverse events (hoarseness/sore throat and low oxygen saturations), leading them to conclude that VL for ATI seems to have comparable success and safety profile to ATI with flexible bronchoscopy.

A small RCT from Mendonca et al.[164] compared ATI with the channeled Pentax-AWS video laryngoscope to flexible bronchoscopy and found faster intubation and total procedure time, but no difference in procedure difficulty or patient discomfort.

There is also a small study that reported successful awake intubations using the channeled King Vision in a number of elective patients with peri-glottic tumors.[165]

Can VL Be Used in the Placement of Double-Lumen Tube?

A study published in 2017 concluded no difference in the success rate of DLT insertion in patients with predicted or known difficult airway when using either Airtraq or GlideScope.[166] However, a 2018 study concluded that in mixed-experience practitioners, the use of Airtraq required less time for DLT intubation and was easier to use compared to GlideScope. However failures did occur with Airtraq, but not with other systems used in the study (GlideScope, King Vision, Macintosh laryngoscope).[167]

In a systematic review looking at DL versus VL (multiple device and blade types included) in DLT placement, Liu et al.[168] reported higher first-attempt success rates, lower rates of oral, mucosal or dental injury, and less postoperative sore throat for DLT intubation using VL compared to DL. While there was no difference in intubation time, VL appeared to have a higher incidence of malpositioned DLT.

What Is the Efficacy in Nasal Intubation Using VL?

A systematic review that synthesized 14 RCTs comparing DL versus VL (multiple device and blade types included) in nasal intubations reported similar overall success rates in adult patients.[169] They reported that VL was associated with a higher first-attempt success rate, shorter intubation time, higher rate of CL-1 views, and less use of Magill forceps. In a subgroup analysis however, the higher overall success and first-attempt success was only shown in those with difficult airways.

What Is the Efficacy of VL Intubation in a Pediatric Population?

The use of VL in children has not seen the same rapid uptake as in adults, with many early studies showing no benefit when used in the pediatric population. This is thought to be due to both anatomical and physiological differences.

In a 2017 study, GlideScope VL was compared to DL in children with difficult airways using data from the pediatric difficult intubation registry, Park et al.[82] concluded that the use of GlideScope was associated with a higher chance of successful intubation and no increased risk of complications.

In a paper published in 2018 using data from the APRICOT trial (designed primarily to look at severe critical events during and immediately after anesthesia or sedation), a secondary analysis was performed in order to assess European airway management practices.[170] The use of VL was very low which was thought to reflect either poor availability of video laryngoscopes or their principal use as a rescue tool during unexpected difficulty with intubation. This contrasted with the results of the PeDI study.[171]

In a recent meta-analysis by Hu et al.,[172] 27 RCTs were analyzed to compare the efficacy and safety of VL to DL in pediatric patients. They included a mixture of video laryngoscope blade types in their VL group. The study found that intubation with VL required a longer time to intubation in children, but similar time in infants compared to DL. There was no difference in intubation failure at first-attempt, however VL did improve POGO and reduce intubation trauma.

Peyton and colleagues[173] reported a study using cases entered in the Paediatric Difficulty Intubation Registry between March 2017 and January 2020 comparing the intubation success rates between the standard geometry VL blades (those with a similar design to blades used in DL) and nonstandard geometry blades. They found that in children weighting less than 5 kg, standard blades had significantly greater success at initial and eventual attempts at tracheal intubation. There was no difference in children weighing more than 5 kg.

What Are the Other Potential Uses of VL? (Video 30)

Combining VL and flexible bronchoscopic intubation has become a technique which has gained popularity. Case reports have detailed the successful use of the combination of the channeled King Vision with a flexible bronchoscope in patients with difficult airway anatomy.[174–177]

Koopman et al.[178] performed a cadaver study to compare the use of VL alone with video-assisted flexible bronchoscopic intubation. They found that in their difficult cadaver airway model, the combined technique resulted in significantly better glottis visualization along with a higher success rate of tracheal intubation. But, there was no difference in the time to successful intubation.

Lenhardt et al.[179] undertook an RCT to evaluate the feasibility of a combined VL and flexible bronchoscopic approach to patients with a predicted difficulty airway. They compared patients intubated with the combined technique versus with VL and a stylet. Results showed no difference in number of intubation attempts or time-to-intubation between groups. However, they did note that for cervical spine pathology specifically the combined technique outperformed the VL and stylet technique, leading them to conclude the technique to be not only feasible but potentially preferable in patients with cervical-spine immobility.

There have also been recent articles published describing the use of VL to guide the re-positioning of sub-optimally placed extraglottic devices (EGDs),[180] and to aid in the insertion of transesophageal echocardiography probes to improve success and reduce associated trauma.[56]

What Are the Other Potential Benefits of Using VL for Tracheal Intubation?

Schieren et al.[181] assessed the force applied to teeth during intubation in a mannikin model. They found that the use of King Vision aBlade resulted in significantly less force on the incisors during intubation in manikins with both normal and difficult airway conditions when compared with Macintosh DL. Interestingly, they also reported that more experienced anesthesia practitioners generated greater peak force than less experienced practitioners.

In 2019, Cordovani et al.[182] reported that GlideScope laryngoscopy had a lower peak and average forces in patients with predictors of difficult laryngoscopy when compared with DL. As laryngoscopy duration increased, however, the product of force and time was similar. While the clinical significance of these results is unknown, the data suggested that if force is a surrogate measure for physiological stress and soft tissue trauma, the use of GlideScope may be associated with less intubation stress and complications.

What Are the Potential Complications of VL Intubation?

Perforation of the right anterior tonsillar pillar (or palatopharyngeal fold) has been described with the GlideScope.[86,87] This complication is not a consequence of the stylet or introducer, but results from the practitioner blindly introducing the styletted-ETT into the oropharynx while observing the monitor. This is not limited to the GlideScope and has occurred with other indirect techniques since the camera is located toward the distal end of the laryngoscope blade. Thus the monitor is blind to the ETT advancement between the lips and the camera. Aziz et al.[98] observed complications in 21 of 2004 GlideScope uses, 13 of which were minor including lip and gum lacerations. This is probably comparable to that observed with DL though this study was not designed to enable such a conclusion. Perforation of the tonsillar pillar occurred in one patient.[98] Such perforation has generally been managed conservatively, with vigilance to ensure the absence of a delayed infection. When comparing the C-MAC used with Macintosh geometry blade to DL in patients with features suggesting a difficult airway, there was no difference in the complication rate between the devices.[131] It is the opinion of the authors of this chapter that a reduction in the incidence of blind, esophageal, and multiple attempts at intubation is a greater benefit than the risk of airway trauma, especially if the practitioner directly observes ETT insertion into the mouth until it passes the camera on the VL blade.

SUMMARY

Video laryngoscopes enjoy growing acceptance in prehospital care as well as many clinical settings[183] and are advocated by some as a new standard of care for facilitating tracheal intubation.[137,138,150,184,185] Our inability to reliably predict patients with a difficult direct laryngoscopic intubation suggest that many DL intubation will require multiple attempts with increasing force and may ultimately be intubated blindly or unsuccessfully. Even when features suggest that DL will not be difficult, it proves to be otherwise at least 6% to 10% of the time.[7,9,186] Multiple and blind attempts are associated with an increased risk of complications, particularly in critically ill patients.[187] Video laryngoscopes provide a more predictable laryngeal view, even in less experienced hands but do not always ensure that intubation can be accomplished despite a good laryngeal view. Increased success comes with a better understanding that the skills required for DL and VL are related but different. Given the differences in VL device type and blade geometry, familiarization with the specific device or devices available to the airway practitioner is critical. Proficiency is best acquired and maintained by practicing with these devices when they are not thought to be necessary and incorporating selected devices into routine practice. This does not compromise patient safety; if the less familiar device fails, the practitioner can revert to the more familiar. This strategy will better equip the practitioner with the judgment required to identify situations that are within or beyond his/her skill level. It is unlikely that a single device or even a class of devices will emerge as a solution to every airway challenge. Thus, it is important to retain a range of airway management skills that include ventilation using a face-mask or extraglottic device, direct and indirect laryngoscopy, and flexible bronchoscopic intubation and if all these fail, the ability to quickly perform an emergency front-of-neck access.

SELF-EVALUATION QUESTIONS

11.1. Which of the following statements about video laryngoscopes is **TRUE**?

A. Video laryngoscopes can facilitate the recording of the laryngoscopy.

B. The technique for using the hyperangulated GlideScope makes it well suited for teaching direct laryngoscopy.

C. The laryngeal view obtained using the Storz Video Macintosh makes it well-suited for managing the known difficult airway.

D. The laryngeal view is essentially the same as the line-of-sight view with hyperangulated video laryngoscopes.

E. The images obtained using any of the video laryngoscopes are equally hampered by fogging.

11.2. Which of the following statements about optical/fiberoptic stylets (e.g., the Bonfils, Shikani Optical Stylet, or Levitan FPS scope) is **TRUE**?

A. Fiberoptic stylets should generally be used as standalone tools.

B. Once the tube is loaded, fiberoptic stylets have the advantage of requiring no other preparation of the patient or instrument.

C. Fiberoptic stylets have been proven to be effective in awake intubations.

D. Fiberoptic stylets can be used as an adjunct to direct laryngoscopy.

E. The learning curve of these devices is such that novices can be expected to have a good chance at a successful intubation using a fiberoptic stylet.

11.3. Which of the following regarding rigid fiberoptic laryngoscopes is **FALSE**?

A. The rigid fiberoptic laryngoscopes are delicate and are easily damaged.

B. The laryngeal view may be obscured by fogging or the presence of blood and secretions.

C. Advancement of the endotracheal tube can be observed.

D. All of these devices require wider mouth opening than is required for direct laryngoscopy.

E. These devices are well suited for managing difficult airways.

REFERENCES

1. James CDT. Sir William Macewen and anaesthesia. *Anaesthesia*. 1974;29:743-753.
2. Cooper RM. Laryngoscopy – its past and future. *Can J Anaesth*. 2004;51:R6.
3. Adnet F, Borron SW, Dumas JL, Lapostolle F, Cupa M, Lapandry C. Study of the "sniffing position" by magnetic resonance imaging. *Anesthesiology*. 2001;94:83-86.
4. Adnet F, Baillard C, Borron SW, et al. Randomized study comparing the "sniffing position" with simple head extension for laryngoscopic view in elective surgery patients. *Anesthesiology*. 2001;95:836-841.
5. Asai T, Enomoto Y, Shimizu K, Shingu K, Okuda Y. The Pentax-AWS video-laryngoscope: the first experience in one hundred patients. *Anesth Analg*. 2008;106:257-259.
6. Rose DK, Cohen MM. The incidence of airway problems depends on the definition used. *Can J Anaesth*. 1996;43:30-34.
7. Shiga T. Predicting difficult intubation in apparently normal patients: a meta-analysis of bedside screening test performance. *Anesthesiology*. 2005;103:429-437.
8. Norskov AK, Rosenstock CV, Wetterslev J, Astrup G, Afshari A, Lundstrom LH. Diagnostic accuracy of anaesthesiologists' prediction of difficult airway management in daily clinical practice: a cohort study of 188 064 patients registered in the Danish Anaesthesia Database. *Anaesthesia*. 2015;70:272-281.
9. Rose DK, Cohen MM. The airway: problems and predictions in 18,500 patients. *Can J Anaesth*. 1994;41:372-383.
10. Mort TC. Emergency tracheal intubation: complications associated with repeated laryngoscopic attempts. *Anesth Analg*. 2004;99:607-613.
11. Sakles JC, Chiu S, Mosier J, Walker C, Stolz U, Reardon RF. The importance of first pass success when performing orotracheal intubation in the emergency department. *Acad Emerg Med*. 2013;20:71-78.
12. Kaplan MB, Ward D, Hagberg CA, Berci G, Hagiike M. Seeing is believing: the importance of video laryngoscopy in teaching and in managing the difficult airway. *Surg Endosc*. 2006;20(Suppl 2):S479-S483.
13. Weiss M, Schwarz U, Dillier CM, Gerber AC. Teaching and supervising tracheal intubation in paediatric patients using videolaryngoscopy. *Paediatr Anaesth*. 2001;11:343-348.
14. Cormack RS, Lehane J. Difficult tracheal intubation in obstetrics. *Anaesthesia*. 1984;39:1105-1111.
15. de Carvalho CC, da Silva DM, Lemos VM, et al. Videolaryngoscopy vs. direct Macintosh laryngoscopy in tracheal intubation in adults: a ranking systematic review and network meta-analysis. *Anaesthesia*. 2022;77:326-338.
16. de Carvalho CC. Hyperangulated vs. Macintosh videolaryngoscopes for efficacy of orotracheal intubation in adults: a pairwise meta-analysis of randomised clinical trials. *Anaesthesia*. 2022;77(10):1172-1174.
17. Lewis SR, Nicholson A, Cook TM, Smith AF, Lewis SR. Videolaryngoscopy versus direct laryngoscopy for adult surgical patients requiring tracheal intubation for general anaesthesia. *Cochrane Database Syst Rev*. 2014;(1):CD010320.
18. Bein B, Worthmann F, Scholz J, et al. A comparison of the intubating laryngeal mask airway and the Bonfils intubation fibrescope in patients with predicted difficult airways. *Anaesthesia*. 2004;59:668-664.
19. Halligan M, Charters P. A clinical evaluation of the Bonfils Intubation Fibrescope. *Anaesthesia*. 2003;58:1087-1091.
20. Takenaka I, Aoyama K, Kadoya T, Sata T, Shigematsu A. Fibreoptic assessment of laryngeal aperture in patients with difficult laryngoscopy. *Can J Anaesth*. 1999;46:226-231.
21. Rudolph C, Schlender M. Clinical experiences with fiber optic intubation with the Bonfils intubation fiberscope. *Anaesthesiol Reanim*. 1996;21:127-130.
22. Shikani AH. New "seeing" stylet-scope and method for the management of the difficult airway. *Otolaryngol Head Neck Surg*. 1999;120:113-116.
23. Van Zundert AAJ, Pieters BMA. Combined technique using videolaryngoscopy and Bonfils for a difficult airway intubation. *Br J Anaesth*. 2012;108:327-328.
24. Young C, Vadivelu N. Can the Shikani Optical Stylet facilitate intubation in simulated difficult direct laryngoscopy. *Anesthesiology*. 2006;105:A1281.
25. Xue FS, Liao X, Zhang YM, Luo MP. More maneuvers to facilitate endotracheal intubation using the Bonfils fiberscope in children with difficult airways. *Pediatric Anesthesia*. 2009;19:418-419.
26. Abramson SIM, Holmes AAM, Hagberg CAM. Awake insertion of the Bonfils Retromolar Intubation FiberscopeTM in five patients with anticipated difficult airways. [Report]. *Anesth Analg*. 2008;106:1215-1217.
27. Corbanese U, Morossi M. The Bonfils intubation fibrescope: clinical evaluation and consideration of the learning curve. *Eur J Anaesthesiol*. 2009;26:622-624.
28. Kovacs G, Law AJ, Petrie D. Awake fiberoptic intubation using an optical stylet in an anticipated difficult airway. *Ann Emerg Med*. 2007;49:81-83.
29. Bein B, Caliebe D, Römer T, Scholz J, Dörges V. Using the Bonfils intubation fiberscope with a double-lumen tracheal tube. *Anesthesiology*. 2005;102:1290-1291.
30. Rudolph C, Henn-Beilharz A, Gottschall R, Wallenborn J, Schaffranietz L. The unanticipated difficult intubation: rigid or flexible endoscope? *Minerva Anestesiol*. 2007;73:567-574.
31. Bein B, Yan M, Tonner PH, Scholz J, Steinfath M, Dorges V. Tracheal intubation using the Bonfils intubation fibrescope after failed direct laryngoscopy. *Anaesthesia*. 2004;59:1207-1209.
32. Falcetta S, Pecora L, Orsetti G, et al. The Bonfils fiberscope: a clinical evaluation of its learning curve and efficacy in difficult airway management. *Minerva Anestesiol*. 2012;78:176-184.
33. Kim SH, Woo SJ, Kim JH. A comparison of Bonfils intubation fiberscopy and fiberoptic bronchoscopy in difficult airways assisted with direct laryngoscopy. *Korean J Anesthesiol*. 2010;58:249-255.
34. Shollik NA, Ibrahim SM, Ismael A, Agnoletti V, Piraccini E, Corso RM. Use of the bonfils intubation fiberscope in patients with limited mouth opening. *Case Rep Anesthesiol*. 2012;2012:297306.
35. Liew G, Leong XF, Wong T. Awake tracheal intubation in a patient with a supraglottic mass with the Bonfils fibrescope after failed attempts with a flexible fibrescope. *Singapore Med J*. 2015;56:e139-e141.
36. Mazères JE, Lefranc A, Cropet C, et al. Evaluation of the Bonfils intubating fibrescope for predicted difficult intubation in awake patients with ear, nose and throat cancer. *Eur J Anaesthesiol*. 2011;28:646-650.
37. Seo H, Lee G, Ha S-i, Song J-G. An awake double lumen endotracheal tube intubation using the Clarus Video System in a patient with an epiglottic cyst: a case report. *Korean J Anesthesiol*. 2014;66:157-159.
38. Cheng WC, Lan CH, Lai HY. The Clarus Video System (Trachway) intubating stylet for awake intubation. *Anaesthesia*. 2011;66:1178-1180.
39. Greenland KB, Liu G, Tan H, Edwards M, Irwin MG. Comparison of the Levitan FPS ScopeTM and the single-use bougie for simulated difficult intubation in anaesthetised patients. *Anaesthesia*. 2007;62:509-515.
40. Byhahn C, Nemetz S, Breitkreutz R, Zwissler B, Kaufmann M, Meininger D. Brief report: Tracheal intubation using the Bonfils intubation fibrescope or direct laryngoscopy for patients with a simulated difficult airway. *Can J Anesth*. 2008;55:232-237.
41. Gupta A, Thukral S, Lakra A, Kumar S. A comparison between left molar direct laryngoscopy and the use of a Bonfils intubation fibrescope for tracheal intubation in a simulated difficult airway. *Can J Anaesth*. 2015;62:609-617.
42. Phua DS, Mah CL, Wang CF. The Shikani optical stylet as an alternative to the GlideScope® videolaryngoscope in simulated difficult intubations – a randomised controlled trial. *Anaesthesia*. 2012;67:402-406.
43. Rudolph C, Schneider JP, Wallenborn J, Schaffranietz L. Movement of the upper cervical spine during laryngoscopy: a comparison of the Bonfils intubation fibrescope and the Macintosh laryngoscope. *Anaesthesia*. 2005;60:668-672.
44. Wahlen BM, Gercek E. Three-dimensional cervical spine movement during intubation using the Macintosh and Bullard laryngoscopes, the bonfils fibrescope and the intubating laryngeal mask airway. *EurJ Anaesthesiol*. 2004;21:907-913.
45. Turkstra TP, Pelz DM, Shaikh AA, Craen RA. Cervical spine motion: a fluoroscopic comparison of Shikani Optical Stylet® vs Macintosh laryngoscope. *Can J Anesth*. 2007;54:441-447.
46. Subramani S, Poopalalingam R. Bonfils assisted double lumen endobronchial tube placement in an anticipated difficult airway. *J Anaesthesiol Clin Pharmacol*. 2014;30:568-570.
47. Yang M, Kim J, Ahn H, Choi J, Kim D, Cho E. Double-lumen tube tracheal intubation using a rigid video-stylet: a randomized controlled comparison with the Macintosh laryngoscope. *Br J Anaesth*. 2013;111:990-995.

48. Hsu HT, Chou SH, Chen CL, et al. Left endobronchial intubation with a double-lumen tube using direct laryngoscopy or the Trachway® video stylet. *Anaesthesia*. 2013;68:851-855.
49. Hsu H-T, Lin C-H, Tseng K-Y, et al. Trachway in assistance of nasotracheal intubation with a preformed nasotracheal tube in patients undergoing oral maxillofacial surgery. *Br J Anaesth*. 2014;113:720-721.
50. Lee MC, Tseng KY, Shen YC, et al. Nasotracheal intubation in patients with limited mouth opening: a comparison between fibreoptic intubation and Trachway. *Anaesthesia*. 2016;71:31-38.
51. Shukry M, Hanson RD, Koveleskie JR, Ramadhyani U. Management of the difficult pediatric airway with Shikani Optical StyletTM. *Paediatr Anaesth*. 2005;15:342-345.
52. Su K, Gao X, Xue FS, Ding GN, Zhang Y, Tian M. Difficult tracheal tube passage and subglottic airway injury during intubation with the GlideScope® videolaryngoscope: a randomised, controlled comparison of three tracheal tubes. *Anaesthesia*. 2017;72:504-511.
53. Aucoin S, Vlatten A, Hackmann T. Difficult airway management with the Bonfils fiberscope in a child with Hurler syndrome. *Paediatr Anaesth*. 2009;19:421-422.
54. Jansen AH, Johnston G. The Shikani Optical Stylet: a useful adjunct to airway management in a neonate with popliteal pterygium syndrome. *Paediatr Anaesth*. 2008;18:188-190.
55. Caruselli M, Zannini R, Giretti R, et al. Difficult intubation in a small for gestational age newborn by bonfils fiberscope. *Paediatr Anaesth*. 2008;18:990-991.
56. Bein B, Wortmann F, Meybohm P, Steinfath M, Scholz J, Doerges V. Evaluation of the pediatric Bonfils fiberscope for elective endotracheal intubation. *Paediatr Anaesth*. 2008;18:1040-1044.
57. Houston G, Bourke P, Wilson G, Engelhardt T. Bonfils intubating fibrescope in normal paediatric airways. *Br J Anaesth*. 2010;105:546-547.
58. Kaufmann J, Laschat M, Hellmich M, Wappler F. A randomized controlled comparison of the Bonfils fiberscope and the GlideScope Cobalt AVL video laryngoscope for visualization of the larynx and intubation of the trachea in infants and small children with normal airways. *Paediatr Anaesth*. 2013;23:913-919.
59. Kaufmann J, Laschat M, Engelhardt T, Hellmich M, Wappler F. Tracheal intubation with the Bonfils fiberscope in the difficult pediatric airway: a comparison with fiberoptic intubation. *Paediatr Anaesth*. 2015;25:372-378.
60. Jagannathan N, Kho MF, Kozlowski RJ, Sohn LE, Siddiqui A, Wong DT. Retrospective audit of the air-Q intubating laryngeal airway as a conduit for tracheal intubation in pediatric patients with a difficult airway. *Paediatr Anaesth*. 2011;21:422-427.
61. Drolet S, Michaud S. Bonfils intubation in parallel with a supraglottic air-Q® intubating laryngeal airway. *Can J Anaesth*. 2016;63:501-502.
62. Hemmerling TM, Bracco D. Subcutaneous cervical and facial emphysema with the use of the Bonfils fiberscope and high-flow oxygen insufflation. *Anesth Analg*. 2008;106:260-262.
63. Boker A, Almarakbi WA, Arab AA, Almazrooa A. Reduced hemodynamic responses to tracheal intubation by the Bonfils retromolar fiberscope: a randomized controlled study. *Middle East J Anaesthesiol*. 2011;21:385-390.
64. Najafi A, Rahimi E, Moharari RS, Khan ZH. Bonfils fiberscope: Intubating conditions and hemodynamic changes without neuromuscular blockade. *Acta Medica Iranica*. 2011;49:201-207.
65. Kimura A, Yamakage M, Chen X, Kamada Y, Namiki A. Use of the fibreoptic stylet scope (Styletscope) reduces the hemodynamic response to intubation in normotensive and hypertensive patients. *Can J Anaesth*. 2001;48:919-923.
66. Kitamura T, Yamada Y, Chinzei M, Du HL, Hanaoka K. Attenuation of haemodynamic responses to tracheal intubation by the styletscope. *Br J Anaesth*. 2001;86:275-277.
67. Gupta K, Girdhar KK, Anand R, Majgi SM, Gupta SP, Gupta PB. Comparison of haemodynamic responses to intubation: flexible fibreoptic bronchoscope versus bonfils rigid intubation endoscope. *Indian J Anaesth*. 2012;56:353.
68. Cooper RM. The role of rigid fiberoptic laryngoscopes. In: Glick DB, Cooper RM, Ovassapian A, eds. *The Difficult Airway: An Atlas of Tools and Techniques for Clinical Management*. Springer; 2013:65-76.
69. Cooper RM, Law JA. Rigid fiberoptic and video laryngoscopes. In: Hung O, Murphy MF, eds. *Management of the Difficult and Failed Airway*. 2nd ed. McGraw Hill; 2011:159-185.
70. Hung OR. Misconception of tracheal intubation using a fibreoptic bronchoscope. *Can J Anaesth*. 1998;45:496.
71. Koh LK, Kong CE, Ip-Yam PC. The modified Cormack-Lehane score for the grading of direct laryngoscopy: evaluation in the Asian population. *Anaesth Intensive Care*. 2002;30:48-51.
72. Yentis SM, Lee DJ. Evaluation of an improved scoring system for the grading of direct laryngoscopy. *Anaesthesia*. 1998;53:1041-1044.
73. Levitan RM, Ochroch EA, Kush S, Shofer FS, Hollander JE. Assessment of airway visualization: validation of the percentage of glottic opening (POGO) scale. *Acad Emerg Med*. 1998;5:919-923.
74. Swann AD, English JD, O'Loughlin EJ. The development and preliminary evaluation of a proposed new scoring system for videolaryngoscopy. *Anaesth Intensive Care*. 2012;40:697-701.
75. Adnet F, Borron SW, Racine SX, et al. The intubation difficulty scale (IDS): proposal and evaluation of a new score characterizing the complexity of endotracheal intubation. *Anesthesiology*. 1997;87:1290-1297.
76. Cierniak M, Timler D, Wieczorek A, Sekalski P, Borkowska N, Gaszynski T. The comparison of the technical parameters in endotracheal intubation devices: the Cmac, the Vividtrac, the McGrath Mac and the Kingvision. *J Clin Monit Comput*. 2015:1-9.
77. Cavus E, Neumann T, Doerges V, et al. First clinical evaluation of the C-MAC D-Blade videolaryngoscope during routine and difficult intubation. *Anesth Analg*. 2011;112:382-385.
78. Emsley JG, Hung OR. A "VL tube" for endotracheal intubation using video laryngoscopy. *Can J Anaesth*. 2016;63:782-783.
79. Hung O. Can't see for looking: tracheal intubation using video laryngoscopes. *Can J Anaesth*. 2020;67:505-510.
80. Hung OR, Tibbet JS, Cheng R, Law JA. Proper preparation of the Trachlight and endotracheal tube to facilitate intubation. *Can J Anaesth*. 2006;53:107-108.
81. Cooper RM, Pacey JA, Bishop MJ, McCluskey SA. Early clinical experience with a new videolaryngoscope (GlideScope). *Can J Anaesth*. 2005;52:191-198.
82. Park R, Peyton JM, Fiadjoe JE, et al. The efficacy of GlideScope® videolaryngoscopy compared with direct laryngoscopy in children who are difficult to intubate: an analysis from the paediatric difficult intubation registry. *Br J Anaesth*. 2017;119:984-992.
83. Sakles JC, Corn GJ, Hollinger P, Arcaris B, Patanwala AE, Mosier JM. The impact of a soiled airway on intubation success in the emergency department when using the glidescope or the direct laryngoscope. *Acad Emerg Med*. 2017;24:628-636.
84. Glidescope Video-laryngoscopes: Operations & Maintenance Manual. Bothell, WA, USA: Verathon Inc.; 2020.
85. Karalapillai D, Darvall J, Mandeville J, Ellard L, Graham J, Weinberg L. A review of video laryngoscopes relevant to the intensive care unit. *Indian J Crit Care Med*. 2014;18:442-452.
86. Choo MKF, Yeo VST, See JJ. Another complication associated with videolaryngoscopy. *Can J Anaesth*. 2007;54:322-324.
87. Cooper RM. Complications associated with the use of the glidescope videolaryngoscope. *Can J Anaesth*. 2007;54:54-57.
88. Goodine C, Sparrow K, Asselin M, Hung D, Hung O. The alignment approach to nasotracheal intubation. *Can J Anaesth*. 2016;63:991-992.
89. Gu Y, Robert J, Kovacs G, et al. A deliberately restricted laryngeal view with the GlideScope® video laryngoscope is associated with faster and easier tracheal intubation when compared with a full glottic view: a randomized clinical trial. *Can J Anaesth*. 2016;63:928-937.
90. Jain D, Kumar R, Kumar S, A. J. Tips and tricks to improve videolaryngoscopy skills. *Airway*. 2021;4.
91. Bacon ER, Phelan MP, Doyle DJ. Tips and troubleshooting for use of the glidescope video laryngoscope for emergency endotracheal intubation. *Am J Emerg Med*. 2015;33:1273-1277.
92. Law JA, Duggan LV, Asselin M, et al. Canadian Airway Focus Group updated consensus-based recommendations for management of the difficult airway: part 1. Difficult airway management encountered in an unconscious patient. *Can J Anaesth*. 2021;68:1373-1404.
93. Dow WA, Parsons DG. "Reverse loading" to facilitate Glidescope intubation. *Can J Anaesth*. 2007;54:161-162.
94. Dupanovic M, Isaacson SA, Borovcanin Z, et al. Clinical comparison of two stylet angles for orotracheal intubation with the GlideScope video laryngoscope. *J Clin Anesth*. 2010;22:352-359.
95. Minonishi T, Kinoshita H, Tange K, et al. Tracheal intubation with the AirwayScope videolaryngoscope using straight vs curved reinforced tubes. *Can J Anaesth*. 2010;57:92-93.
96. Tremblay M-H, Williams S, Robitaille A, Drolet P. Poor visualization during direct laryngoscopy and high upper lip bite test score are predictors of difficult intubation with the GlideScope® videolaryngoscope. *Anesth Analg*. 2008;106:1495-1500.
97. Khan ZH, Kashfi A, Ebrahimkhani E. A comparison of the upper lip bite test (a simple new technique) with modified Mallampati classification in predicting difficulty in endotracheal intubation: a prospective blinded study. *Anesth Analg*. 2003;96:595-599.
98. Aziz MF, Healy D, Kheterpal S, Fu RF, Dillman D, Brambrink A. Routine clinical practice effectiveness of the glidescope in difficult airway management: an analysis of 2,004 glidescope intubations, complications, and failures from two institutions. *Anesthesiology*. 2011;114:34-41.

99. Siu LW, Mathieson E, Naik VN, Chandra D, Joo HS. Patient- and operator-related factors associated with successful Glidescope intubations: a prospective observational study in 742 patients. *Anaesth Intensive Care.* 2010;38:70-75.
100. Aziz MF, Bayman EO, Van TMM, Todd MM, Brambrink AM. Predictors of difficult videolaryngoscopy with GlideScope® or C-MAC® with D-blade: secondary analysis from a large comparative videolaryngoscopy trial. *Br J Anaesth.* 2016;117:118-123.
101. Joshi R, Hypes CD, Greenberg J, et al. Difficult Airway Characteristics Associated with First-Attempt Failure at Intubation Using Video Laryngoscopy in the Intensive Care Unit. *Ann Am Thorac Soc.* 2017;14:368-375.
102. Cortellazzi P, Caldiroli D, Byrne A, Sommariva A, Orena EF, Tramacere I. Defining and developing expertise in tracheal intubation using a GlideScope® for anaesthetists with expertise in Macintosh direct laryngoscopy: an in-vivo longitudinal study. *Anaesthesia.* 2015;70:290-295.
103. Sakles JC, Mosier J, Patanwala AE, Dicken J. The learning curves for direct laryngoscopy and GlideScope video laryngoscopy in an emergency medicine residency training program. *West J of Emerg Med.* 2014;15:930-937.
104. Sakles JC, Mosier J, Patanwala AE, Dicken J. Improvement in GlideScope® video laryngoscopy performance over a seven-year period in an academic emergency department. *Intern Emerg Med.* 2014;9:789-794.
105. Baciarello M, Zasa M, Manferdini ME, Tosi M, Berti M, Fanelli G. The learning curve for laryngoscopy: Airtraq versus Macintosh laryngoscopes. *J Anesth.* 2012;26:516-524.
106. Amathieu R, Combes X, Abdi W, et al. An algorithm for difficult airway management, modified for modern optical devices (Airtraq laryngoscope; LMA CTrach): a 2-Year prospective validation in patients for elective abdominal, gynecologic, and thyroid surgery. *Anesthesiology.* 2011;114:25-33.
107. Malin E, Montblanc Jd, Ynineb Y, Marret E, Bonnet F. Performance of the Airtraq™ laryngoscope after failed conventional tracheal intubation: a case series. *Acta Anaesthesiologica Scandinavica.* 2009;53:858-863.
108. Maharaj CH, Costello JF, McDonnell JG, Harte BH, Laffey JG. The Airtraq as a rescue airway device following failed direct laryngoscopy: a case series. *Anaesthesia.* 2007;62:598-601.
109. Cavus E, Janssen S, Reifferscheid F, et al. Videolaryngoscopy for physician-based, prehospital emergency intubation: a prospective, randomized, multicenter comparison of different blade types using A.P. Advance, C-MAC System, and KingVision. *Anesth Analg.* 2018;126:1565-1574.
110. Levitan RM, Heitz JW, Sweeney M, Cooper RM. The complexities of tracheal intubation with direct laryngoscopy and alternative intubation devices. *Ann Emerg Med.* 2011;57:240-247.
111. Lu Y, Jiang H, Zhu YS. Airtraq laryngoscope versus conventional Macintosh laryngoscope: a systematic review and meta-analysis. *Anaesthesia.* 2011;66:1160-1167.
112. Suppan L, Tramer MR, Niquille M, Grosgurin O, Marti C. Alternative intubation techniques vs Macintosh laryngoscopy in patients with cervical spine immobilization: systematic review and meta-analysis of randomized controlled trials. *Br J Anaesth.* 2016;116:27-36.
113. Hirabayashi Y, Seo N. Airway Scope: early clinical experience in 405 patients. *J Anesth.* 2008;22:81-85.
114. Suzuki A, Abe N, Sasakawa T, Kunisawa T, Takahata O, Iwasaki H. Pentax-AWS (Airway Scope) and Airtraq: big difference between two similar devices. *J Anesth.* 2008;22:191-192.
115. Asai T, Liu EH, Matsumoto S, et al. Use of the Pentax-AWS(R) in 293 patients with difficult airways. *Anesthesiology.* 2009;110:898-904.
116. Hoshijima H, Kuratani N, Hirabayashi Y, Takeuchi R, Shiga T, Masaki E. Pentax Airway Scope® vs Macintosh laryngoscope for tracheal intubation in adult patients: a systematic review and meta-analysis. *Anaesthesia.* 2014;69:911-918.
117. Kleine-Brueggeney M, Greif R, Schoettker P, Savoldelli GL, Nabecker S, Theiler LG. Evaluation of six videolaryngoscopes in 720 patients with a simulated difficult airway: a multicentre randomized controlled trial. *Br J Anaesth.* 2016;116:670-679.
118. Murphy LD, Kovacs GJ, Reardon PM, Law JA. Comparison of the king vision video laryngoscope with the macintosh laryngoscope. *J Emerg Med.* 2014;47:239-246.
119. Butchart A, Young P. Correspondence: Use of a Venner A.P. Advance videolaryngoscope in a patient with potential cervical spine injury. *Anaesthesia.* 2010;65:953-954.
120. Butchart AG, Tjen C, Garg A, Young P. Paramedic laryngoscopy in the simulated difficult airway: comparison of the Venner A.P. Advance and GlideScope Ranger Video laryngoscopes. *Acad Emerg Med.* 2011;18:692-698.
121. Hughes J, Paul R, O'Flynn P. Use of the Venner A.P. Advance video laryngoscope for biopsy examination of the base of the tongue. *Br J Oral Maxillofac Surg.* 2013;51(2):e22-e23.
122. Zampone S, Corso RM, Parrinello L, Gambale G, Sorbello M. The A.P. Advance video laryngoscope as a rescue airway device in an unpredicted difficult airway. *J Anaesthesiol Clin Pharmacol.* 2015;31:134-136.
123. Griesdale DE, Liu D, McKinney J, Choi PT. Glidescope® video-laryngoscopy versus direct laryngoscopy for endotracheal intubation: a systematic review and meta-analysis. *Can J Anaesth.* 2012;59:41-52.
124. Ibinson JW, Ezaru CS, Cormican DS, Mangione MP. GlideScope use improves intubation success rates: an observational study using propensity score matching. *BMC Anesthesiol.* 2014;14:101.
125. Choi HJ, Kim YM, Oh YM, Kang HG, Yim HW, Jeong SH. GlideScope video laryngoscopy versus direct laryngoscopy in the emergency department: a propensity score-matched analysis. *BMJ open.* 2015;5:e007884.
126. Sakles JC, Mosier JM, Chiu S, Keim SM. Tracheal intubation in the emergency department: a comparison of GlideScope® video laryngoscopy to direct laryngoscopy in 822 intubations. *J Emerg Med.* 2012;42:400-405.
127. Mosier JM, Stolz U, Chiu S, Sakles JC. Difficult airway management in the emergency department: GlideScope videolaryngoscopy compared to direct laryngoscopy. *J Emerg Med.* 2012;42:629-634.
128. Kaplan MB, Ward DS, Berci G. A new videolaryngoscope – an aid in intubation and teaching. *J Educ of Perioper Med.* 2003;5:E025.
129. Kaplan MB, Hagberg CA, Ward DS, et al. Comparison of direct and video-assisted views of the larynx during routine intubation. *J Clin Anesth.* 2006;18:357-362.
130. Cavus E, Thee C, Moeller T, Kieckhaefer J, Doerges V, Wagner K. A randomised, controlled crossover comparison of the C-MAC videolaryngoscope with direct laryngoscopy in 150 patients during routine induction of anaesthesia. *BMC Anesthesiol.* 2011;11:6.
131. Aziz MF, Dillman D, Fu R, Brambrink AM. Comparative effectiveness of the C-MAC® video laryngoscope versus direct laryngoscopy in the setting of the predicted difficult airway. *Anesthesiology.* 2012;116:629-636.
132. Hyuga S, Sekiguchi T, Ishida T, Yamamoto K, Sugiyama Y, Kawamata M. Successful tracheal intubation with the McGrath® MAC video laryngoscope after failure with the Pentax-AWS in a patient with cervical spine immobilization. *Can J Anaesth.* 2012;59:1154-1155.
133. Tsujimoto T, Tanaka S, Yoshiyama Y, Sugiyama Y, Kawamata M. Successful intubation using McGRATH MAC in a patient with Treacher Collins syndrome. *Middle East J Anaesthesiol.* 2014;22:523-525.
134. Kido H, Komasawa N, Matsunami S, Kusaka Y, Minami T. Comparison of McGRATH MAC and Macintosh laryngoscopes for double-lumen endotracheal tube intubation by anesthesia residents: a prospective randomized clinical trial. *J Clin Anesth.* 2015;27:476-480.
135. Wallace CD, Foulds LT, McLeod GA, Younger RA, McGuire BE. A comparison of the ease of tracheal intubation using a McGrath MAC® laryngoscope and a standard Macintosh laryngoscope. *Anaesthesia.* 2015;70:1281-1285.
136. Lewis SR, Butler AR, Parker J, Cook TM, Schofield-Robinson OJ, Smith AF. Videolaryngoscopy versus direct laryngoscopy for adult patients requiring tracheal intubation: a Cochrane Systematic Review. *Br J Anaesth.* 2017;119:369-383.
137. Cook TM, Boniface NJ, Seller C, et al. Universal videolaryngoscopy: a structured approach to conversion to videolaryngoscopy for all intubations in an anaesthetic and intensive care department. *Br J Anaesth.* 2018;120:173-180.
138. Hemmerling TM, Zaouter C. Videolaryngoscopy: is there a path to becoming a standard of care for intubation? *Anesth Analg.* 2020;131:1313-1316.
139. Frerk C, Lee G. Laryngoscopy: time to change our view. *Anaesthesia.* 2009;64:351-354.
140. Mihai R, Blair E, Kay H, Cook TM. A quantitative review and meta-analysis of performance of non-standard laryngoscopes and rigid fibreoptic intubation aids. *Anaesthesia.* 2008;63:745-760.
141. Apfelbaum JL, Hagberg CA, Connis RT, et al. 2022 American Society of Anesthesiologists practice guidelines for management of the difficult airway. *Anesthesiology.* 2022;136:31-81.
142. Frerk C, Mitchell VS, McNarry AF, et al. Difficult Airway Society 2015 guidelines for management of unanticipated difficult intubation in adults. *Br J Anaesth.* 2015;115:827-848.
143. Law JA, Duggan LV, Asselin M, et al. Canadian Airway Focus Group updated consensus-based recommendations for management of the difficult airway: part 2. Planning and implementing safe management of the patient with an anticipated difficult airway. *Can J Anaesth.* 2021;68:1405-1436.
144. Asai T. Videolaryngoscopes: do they have role during rapid-sequence induction of anaesthesia? *Br J Anaesth.* 2016;116:317-319.
145. Andersen LH, Rovsing L, Olsen KS. GlideScope videolaryngoscope vs. Macintosh direct laryngoscope for intubation of morbidly obese patients: a randomized trial. *Acta Anaesthesiologica Scandinavica.* 2011;55:1090-1097.

146. Aziz MF, Kim D, Mako J, Hand K, Brambrink AM. A retrospective study of the performance of video laryngoscopy in an obstetric unit. *Anesth Analg*. 2012;115:904-906.
147. Hinkelbein J, Cirillo F, De Robertis E, Spelten O. Update on video laryngoscopy in the emergency environment: the most important publications of the last 12 months. *Trends in Anaesthesia and Critical Care*. 2015;5:188-194.
148. Mosier J, Chiu S, Patanwala AE, Sakles JC. A comparison of the GlideScope video laryngoscope to the C-MAC video laryngoscope for intubation in the emergency department. *Ann Emerg Med*. 2013;61(4):414-420.e1.
149. Mosier J, Whitmore SP, Bloom JW, et al. Video laryngoscopy improves intubation success and reduces esophageal intubations compared to direct laryngoscopy in the medical intensive care unit. *Critical Care*. 2013;17:R237.
150. Kelly FE, Cook TM. Seeing is believing: getting the best out of videolaryngoscopy. *Br J Anaesth*. 2016;117(Suppl 1):i9-i13. doi:10.1093/bja/aew052.
151. Griesdale DE, Chau A, Isac G, et al. Video-laryngoscopy versus direct laryngoscopy in critically ill patients: a pilot randomized trial. *Can J Anaesth*. 2012;59:1032-1039.
152. Hypes CD, Stolz U, Sakles JC, et al. Video laryngoscopy improves odds of first-attempt success at intubation in the intensive care unit. a propensity-matched analysis. *Ann Am Thorac Soc*. 2015;13:382-390.
153. Silverberg MJ, Li N, Acquah SO, Kory PD. Comparison of video laryngoscopy versus direct laryngoscopy during urgent endotracheal intubation: a randomized controlled trial. *Crit Care Med*. 2015;43:636-641.
154. De Jong A, Molinari N, Conseil M, et al. Video laryngoscopy versus direct laryngoscopy for orotracheal intubation in the intensive care unit: a systematic review and meta-analysis. *Intensive Care Med*. 2014;40:629-639.
155. Arulkumaran N, Lowe J, Ions R, Mendoza M, Bennett V, Dunser MW. Videolaryngoscopy versus direct laryngoscopy for emergency orotracheal intubation outside the operating room: a systematic review and meta-analysis. *Br J Anaesth*. 2018;120:712-724.
156. Huang S, Hua FZ, Xu GH. GlideScope-assisted insertion of a transesophageal echocardiography probe. *J Cardiothorac Vasc Anesth*. 2017;31:e51.
157. Jiang J, Ma D, Li B, Yue Y, Xue F. Video laryngoscopy does not improve the intubation outcomes in emergency and critical patients – a systematic review and meta-analysis of randomized controlled trials. *Crit Care*. 2017;21:288.
158. Decamps P, Grillot N, Le Thuaut A, et al. Comparison of four channelled videolaryngoscopes to Macintosh laryngoscope for simulated intubation of critically ill patients: the randomized MACMAN2 trial. *Ann Intensive Care*. 2021;11:126.
159. Higgs A, McGrath BA, Goddard C, et al. Guidelines for the management of tracheal intubation in critically ill adults. *Br J Anaesth*. 2018;120:323-352.
160. Kreutziger J, Hornung S, Harrer C, et al. Comparing the McGrath Mac video laryngoscope and direct laryngoscopy for prehospital emergency intubation in air rescue patients: a multicenter, randomized, controlled trial. *Crit Care Med*. 2019;47:1362-1370.
161. Ahmad I, El-Boghdadly K, Bhagrath R, et al. Difficult Airway Society guidelines for awake tracheal intubation (ATI) in adults. *Anaesthesia*. 2020;75:509-528.
162. Moore A, Schricker T. Awake videolaryngoscopy versus fiberoptic bronchoscopy. *Curr Opin Anaesthesiol*. 2019;32:764-768.
163. Alhomary M, Ramadan E, Curran E, Walsh SR. Videolaryngoscopy vs. fibreoptic bronchoscopy for awake tracheal intubation: a systematic review and meta-analysis. *Anaesthesia*. 2018;73:1151-1161.
164. Mendonca C, Mesbah A, Velayudhan A, Danha R. A randomised clinical trial comparing the flexible fibrescope and the Pentax Airway Scope (AWS)® for awake oral tracheal intubation. *Anaesthesia*. 2016;71:908-914.
165. Markova L, Stopar-Pintaric T, Luzar T, Benedik J, Hodzovic I. A feasibility study of awake videolaryngoscope-assisted intubation in patients with periglottic tumour using the channelled King Vision® videolaryngoscope. *Anaesthesia*. 2017;72:51251-51258.
166. Belze O, Lepage E, Bazin Y, et al. Glidescope versus Airtraq DL for double-lumen tracheal tube insertion in patients with a predicted or known difficult airway: a randomised study. *Eur J Anaesthesiol*. 2017;34:456-463.
167. El-Tahan MR, Khidr AM, Gaarour IS, Alshadwi SA, Alghamdi TM, Al'ghamdi A. A comparison of 3 videolaryngoscopes for double-lumen tube intubation in humans by users with mixed experience: a randomized controlled study. *J Cardiothorac Vasc Anesth*. 2018;32:277-286.
168. Liu TT, Li L, Wan L, Zhang CH, Yao WL. Videolaryngoscopy vs. Macintosh laryngoscopy for double-lumen tube intubation in thoracic surgery: a systematic review and meta-analysis. *Anaesthesia*. 2018;73:997-1007.
169. Jiang J, Ma DX, Li B, Wu AS, Xue FS. Videolaryngoscopy versus direct laryngoscopy for nasotracheal intubation: A systematic review and meta-analysis of randomised controlled trials. *J Clin Anesth*. 2019;52:6-16.
170. Engelhardt T, Virag K, Veyckemans F, Habre W, Network AGotESoACT. Airway management in paediatric anaesthesia in Europe-insights from APRICOT (Anaesthesia Practice In Children Observational Trial): a prospective multicentre observational study in 261 hospitals in Europe. *Br J Anaesth*. 2018;121:66-75.
171. Fiadjoe JE, Nishisaki A, Jagannathan N, et al. Airway management complications in children with difficult tracheal intubation from the Pediatric Difficult Intubation (PeDI) registry: a prospective cohort analysis. *Lancet Respir Med*. 2016;4:37-48.
172. Hu X, Jin Y, Li J, Xin J, Yang Z. Efficacy and safety of videolaryngoscopy versus direct laryngoscopy in paediatric intubation: A meta-analysis of 27 randomized controlled trials. *J Clin Anesth*. 2020;66:109968.
173. Peyton J, Park R, Staffa SJ, et al. A comparison of videolaryngoscopy using standard blades or non-standard blades in children in the Paediatric Difficult Intubation Registry. *Br J Anaesth*. 2021;126:331-339.
174. El-Tahan MR, Doyle DJ, Khidr AM, Abdulshafi M, Regal MA, Othman MS. Use of the King Vision video laryngoscope to facilitate fibreoptic intubation in critical tracheal stenosis proves superior to the GlideScope®. *Can J Anaesth*. 2014;61:213-214.
175. El-Tahan MR, Doyle DJ, Khidr AM, Regal MA, El Morsy AB, El Mahdy M. Awake tracheal intubation with combined use of King Vision videolaryngoscope and a fiberoptic bronchoscope in a patient with giant lymphocele. *Middle East J Anaesthesiol*. 2014;22:609-612.
176. Gaszyński T. A combination of KingVision video-laryngoscope and flexible fibroscope for awake intubation in patient with laryngeal tumor—case report and literature review. *Anaesthesiol Intensive Ther*. 2015;47:433-435.
177. Sowers N, Kovacs G. Use of a flexible intubating scope in combination with a channeled video laryngoscope for managing a difficult airway in the emergency department. *J Emerg Med*. 2016;50:315-319.
178. Koopman EM, van Emden MW, Geurts JJG, Schwarte LA, Schober P. Comparison of videolaryngoscopy alone with video-assisted fibreoptic intubation in a difficult cadaver airway model. *Eur J Anaesthesiol*. 2021;38:318-319.
179. Lenhardt R, Burkhart MT, Brock GN, Kanchi-Kandadai S, Sharma R, Akca O. Is video laryngoscope-assisted flexible tracheoscope intubation feasible for patients with predicted difficult airway? A prospective, randomized clinical trial. *Anesth Analg*. 2014;118:1259-1265.
180. Van Zundert AAJ, Gatt SP, Kumar CM, Van Zundert T, Pandit JJ. "Failed supraglottic airway": an algorithm for suboptimally placed supraglottic airway devices based on videolaryngoscopy. *Br J Anaesth*. 2017;118:645-649.
181. Schieren M, Kleinschmidt J, Schmutz A, et al. Comparison of forces acting on maxillary incisors during tracheal intubation with different laryngoscopy techniques: a blinded manikin study. *Anaesthesia*. 2019;74:1563-1571.
182. Cordovani D, Russell T, Wee W, Suen A, Cooper RM. Measurement of forces applied using a Macintosh direct laryngoscope compared with a Glidescope video laryngoscope in patients with predictors of difficult laryngoscopy: a randomised controlled trial. *Eur J Anaesthesiol*. 2019;36:221-226.
183. Pott LM, Randel GI, Straker T, Cooper RM. A Survey of Airway Training among US and Canadian Anesthesiology Residency Programs. *J Clin Anesth*. 2011;23:15-26.
184. Bulatovic R, Taneja R. Videolaryngoscopy – for all intubations? *Br J Anaesth*. 2015;115:135-136.
185. Zaouter C, Calderon J, Hemmerling TM. Videolaryngoscopy as a new standard of care. *Br J Anaesth*. 2014;114:181-183.
186. Adnet F, Racine SX, Borron SW, et al. A survey of tracheal intubation difficulty in the operating room: a prospective observational study. *Acta Anaesthesiol Scand*. 2001;45:327-332.
187. Mosier J, Joshi R, Hypes C, Pacheco G, Valenzuela T, Sakles J. The physiologically difficult airway. *West J Emerg Med*. 2015;16:1109-1117.

CHAPTER 12

Nonvisual Intubation Techniques

Loran T. Morrison, Orlando R. Hung, and Chris C. Christodoulou

INTRODUCTION

Do We Still Need Nonvisual Intubating Techniques?

For many decades, tracheal intubation under direct vision using a laryngoscope has been considered the standard technique of intubation. Unfortunately, this approach to intubation has limitations. Difficult and failed intubation employing this technique can be as high as 21%, particularly in emergency situations.[1] Not surprisingly, studies have shown that considerable experience is required before a trainee becomes proficient in laryngoscopic intubation. Konrad[2] and Mulcaster[3] have constructed learning curves showing that a 90% probability of success requires between 47 and 57 laryngoscopic intubations.

The high incidence of difficulty and failure, coupled with these kinds of learning curves for laryngoscopic intubation have driven the development of many alternative intubation devices and techniques, such as rigid and flexible endoscopes, videolaryngoscopes, and optical intubating stylets. All of these devices have gained a measure of popularity. Unfortunately, these devices are substantially more expensive than the Macintosh laryngoscope. Furthermore, the cleaning and sterilization processes of some of the reusable devices, such as the flexible bronchoscope, require an average of 50 to 60 minutes to complete, hindering their availability and practicality in emergency airway management and in prehospital care (i.e., they may be "context" driven).

The challenge of visual techniques employing optical stylets and video scopes is visualization of laryngeal anatomy and the passage of the ETT through the glottic opening in the face of fogging or the presence of blood, secretions, and vomitus in the upper airway. It is precisely these kinds of difficulties that have motivated the search for nonvisual techniques using a variety of devices, such as intubating guides, light-guided intubation using the principle of transillumination, blind nasal intubation, digital intubation, and retrograde intubation, all of which have proven to be effective, safe, and simple techniques when employed by a skilled and experienced practitioner in the appropriate clinical setting.

INTUBATING STYLETS OR GUIDES

What Is the Eschmann Tracheal Tube Introducer? How Does It Facilitate the Placement of an Endotracheal Tube?

In 1949, Macintosh reported the use of an introducer (gum-elastic bougie) to facilitate orotracheal intubation under direct laryngoscopy.[4] Using the concept of the introducer, Venn designed the Eschmann Introducer (Eschmann Tracheal Tube Introducer, Portex Limited, Hythe, UK), a tube-like core woven from polyester threads and covered with a resin layer.[5] The Eschmann Introducer (EI) is 60 cm long, with a J (coudé) tip (a 35-degree angle bend) at the distal end to facilitate advancement anteriorly underneath the epiglottis into the trachea and to provide tactile tracheal confirmation (Figure 12.1A). Centimeter markings designate the distance from the tip. The EI is often referred to as the "gum-elastic bougie" or "bougie." However, to avoid confusion, historically the "gum-elastic bougie" has been used to refer to a shorter urinary catheter made of different material and without a curved tip.[6]

The EI is particularly useful when the glottic opening cannot be clearly seen using a laryngoscope (e.g., Grade 3 laryngoscopic view as described by Cormack/Lehane [C/L]).[7] Under these circumstances, the EI can be "hooked" underneath the epiglottis and advanced into the trachea. If it is correctly placed in the trachea, a subtle tactile "clicking" sensation can be felt as the tip of the EI slides over the tracheal rings while advancing it into the trachea. Furthermore, if the EI correctly enters the trachea, as it is gently advanced, it will eventually be lodged (or "holdup") in a distal airway and cannot advance beyond the 30- to 35-cm mark. In contrast, if it is placed in the esophagus, the entire EI can be advanced without encountering resistance. With the EI in place and positioned at 20 to 25 cm at the teeth, the ETT can then be advanced over the EI into the trachea. To facilitate the advancement of the ETT over the EI, the tongue and epiglottis must be elevated by a gentle jaw lift, a jaw thrust, or preferably, by the laryngoscope already in place. If difficulty persists while advancing the ETT, rotating the ETT 90 degrees counterclockwise will turn the ETT bevel posteriorly and minimize the risk of catching on glottic structures.[8] Following intubation, the position of the ETT is confirmed using conventional methods, such as end-tidal CO_2 and auscultation. The EI has also been used to facilitate retrograde intubation in a trauma patient,[9] and placement of a tracheostomy device during the performance of a difficult or emergency surgical airway (e.g., cricothyrotomy).[10,11]

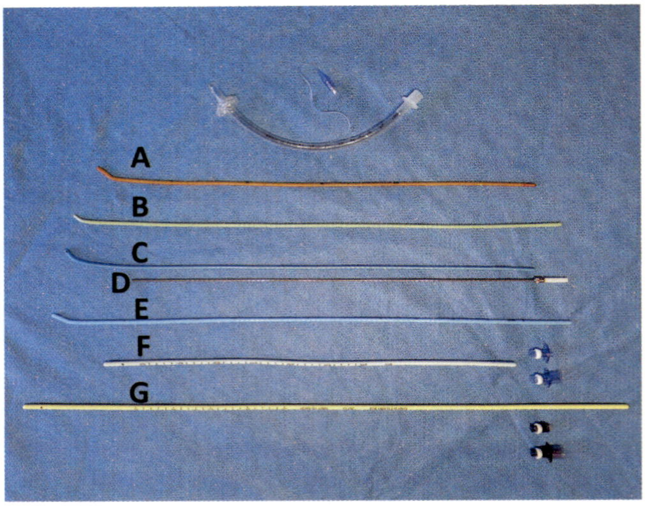

FIGURE 12.1. Intubating Guides: **(A)** The Eschmann Introducer (EI) with a coudé tip at the distal end; **(B)** the Muallem Stylet is a single-use 65 cm long tracheal introducer with a soft distal coudé tip; **(C)** Frova Intubation Introducer is an intubating catheter with a hollow lumen and a coudé tip at the distal end; **(D)** a removable internal metal stylet for the Frova Intubation Introducer. The stylet is designed to increase the stiffness of the Frova Intubation Introducer to facilitate ETT passage over the introducer; **(E)** the Endotracheal Tube Introducer is similar to the EI in size and shape with a coudé tip, but it is 10 cm longer; **(F)** the Aintree Catheter is also a hollow flexible straight tube designed for tracheal intubation together with a pediatric bronchoscope through an extraglottic device (EGD) such as the LMA-Classic or LMA-Unique; and **(G)** the Cook Airway Exchange Catheter with an inner lumen, distal ports, and an adapter at the proximal end.

What Other Intubating Guides or Introducers Are Commercially Available?

Since the introduction of the EI, many intubating guides of different sizes, shapes, lengths, and materials have been developed. All of the designs serve a function similar to the EI, but many have some additional features.

(a) The Flex-Guide ET Tube Introducer (Green Field Medical Sourcing Inc, Northborough, MA) is a single-use 60-cm length of flexible polyethylene tubing (5.0 mm in diameter) with a similar distal coudé tip as the Eschmann Tracheal introducer.[12]

(b) The Muallem Stylet (VBM Medizintechnik, Sulz am Neckar, Germany) (Figure 12.1B) is a single-use 65 cm long tracheal introducer with a soft distal coudé tip. Unfortunately, there is no published data comparing this device to other intubating guides.

(c) Frova Intubation Introducer (Cook® Critical Care Inc, Bloomington, IN) is an intubating catheter with a coudé tip at the distal end (Figure 12.1C).[13] It has a hollow lumen with side ports distally; Rapi-Fit® adapters (luer lock and standard 15/22 mm) come with the device to permit oxygen insufflation in the event intubation cannot be achieved. It also has a removable internal rigid metal stylet (Figure 12.1D) to prevent kinking and damage during shipping and to increase stiffness, facilitating tracheal placement and ETT passage. The Frova introducer has two sizes: the adult version for ETTs with greater than 5.5-mm internal diameter (ID) and the pediatric version for ETTs 3- to 5-mm ID.

(d) Endotracheal Tube Introducer (Sun Med, Largo, FL) is similar to the EI in size and shape, but it is 10 cm longer (Figure 12.1E). This confers some advantage in employing the device as more of the device protrudes from the mouth making it easier to thread a standard 30-cm adult-sized ETT and capture the proximal end of the introducer. It is stiffer than the EI, conferring an advantage in guiding the ETT, but at the same time serving to emphasize the importance of gentle maneuvers to prevent airway injury. There is a single marking at 20 cm on the device to indicate the depth of insertion. It is a single-use disposable device, though resterilization is possible.

(e) The Aintree Catheter (Cook Critical Care Inc, Bloomington, IN) is also a hollow flexible straight tube designed for tracheal intubation together with a pediatric bronchoscope through an extraglottic device (EGD) such as the LMA®-Classic™ or LMA-Unique™. The Aintree Catheter can be advanced over a pediatric tube exchanger to obtain additional stiffness to facilitate advancement of

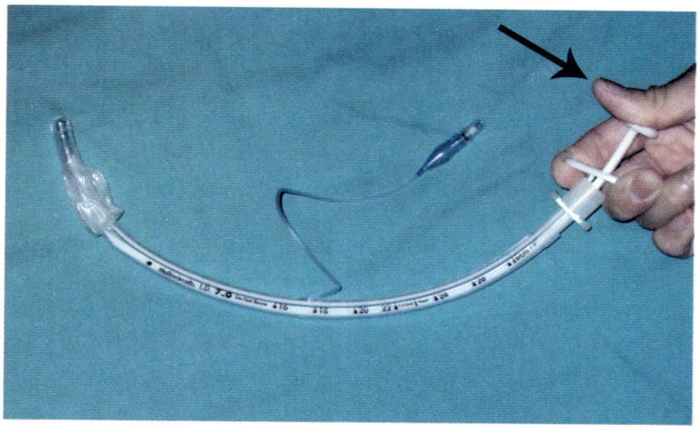

FIGURE 12.2. The Schroeder (Parker Flex-It Directional Stylet) Oral/Nasal Directional Stylet. Elevation of the tip of the ETT can be achieved by wrapping the index and middle fingers around the proximal tracheal tube and using the thumb to depress the proximal end of the stylet (arrow).

an ETT over the pliable tube changer. Because of the hollow tube, it can also be used to oxygenate patients under difficult circumstances through the inner lumen and the distal ports after fitting the provided adaptor at the proximal end (Figure 12.1F).

(f) The Cook Airway Exchange Catheter (Cook Critical Care Inc, Bloomington, IN) is a hollow flexible straight tube (with no coudé tip bend at the distal end) designed as a tube exchanger for patients with difficult airways (Figure 12.1G). It can be used to oxygenate patients under difficult circumstances through the inner lumen, distal ports, and an adapter at the proximal end.

(g) The Sheridan Tube Exchanger (Sheridan Catheter Corp., Oregon, NY) serves a similar function as the Cook Airway Exchange Catheter.

(h) The Schroeder (Parker Flex-It™ Directional Stylet) Oral/Nasal Directional Stylet (Parker Medical, Englewood, CO) is a disposable articulating stylet that requires no bending prior to intubation (Figure 12.2). Inserting the stylet into an ETT allows the practitioner to elevate the tip of the ETT by wrapping the index and middle fingers around the proximal tracheal tube and using the thumb to depress the proximal end of the stylet. Although the stylet is suitable for both oral and nasal intubation, it has been reported to be somewhat awkward to use and the curvature created is not at the tip, but rather over the distal half of the tube.[14] However, it has been reported to be effective for difficult and blind intubations.[15]

(i) Portex intubation stylet (SIMS Portex Ltd, Hythe, Kent, UK) is available in outer diameter sizes ranging from 2.2 mm to 5.0 mm. These stylets can be inserted into a variety of endotracheal tubes. Blind awake orotracheal intubation has been successfully performed utilizing a stylet loaded into an ETT, in a patient with a laryngeal carcinoma and ankylosing spondylitis.[16] Guided tactile probing is used to direct the ETT-stylet unit into the trachea.

(j) Flexible Tip Bougie™ (PerSys Medical, Houston, TX) is a disposable articulating bougie (Figure 12.3) for use with an adult oral ETT with an inner diameter of 7 mm and higher. Operated with one hand, the tip of the bougie is maneuvered up and down by manipulating the device's slider tabs while inserting the fluorescent tip through the vocal cords. The graduating centimeter marks along the device guide (10 cm to 50 cm, 65 cm overall length) the depth of placement into the trachea for subsequent advancement of the loaded ETT. The overall performance of the Flexible Tip Bougie (FTB) is comparable to that of the standard bougie.[17]

Is There Any Clinical Evidence to Support the Widespread Use of These Intubating Introducers?

Over the last several decades, numerous studies have reported the effectiveness and safety of employing an EI to facilitate tracheal intubation in patients with difficult laryngoscopy.[18–21] The EI has been well accepted by most practitioners in the United Kingdom, and it continues to play an important role in the management of the difficult laryngoscopic intubation. According to a survey in the United Kingdom, 100% of the respondents

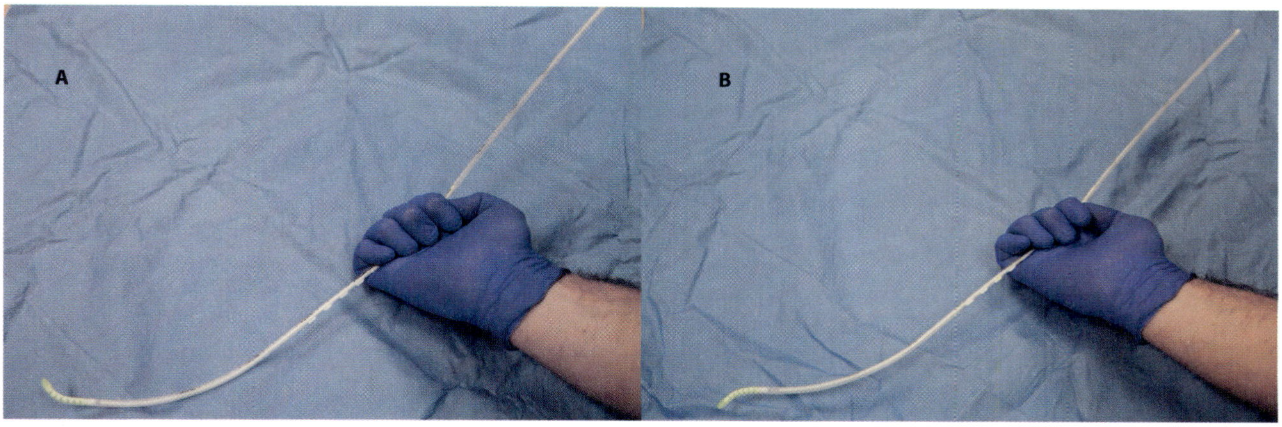

FIGURE 12.3. The Flexible Tip Bougie. The tip of the bougie can be maneuvered up (Panel **A**) and down (Panel **B**) by manipulating the device's slider tabs using the thumb as shown.

reported the use of the EI as their technique of choice when faced with an unanticipated difficult laryngoscopic intubation.[22] Though primarily a device used by anesthesia practitioners in the past, over the past decade, this relatively inexpensive and simple device has found its way to the hands of emergency practitioners and prehospital health care practitioners as a standard airway management adjunct.[23–25] A telephone survey of emergency departments in England revealed that 99% of respondents stocked the EI on their difficult airway carts.[26]

Following a review of the evidence, the Difficult Airway Society Guidelines for Management of the Unanticipated Difficult Intubation in the United Kingdom recommend the use of the EI as the initial device to facilitate a difficult laryngoscopy.[27] Many authorities recommend that this device be a standard piece of equipment for every laryngoscopic intubation.

While the EI has been widely accepted as a useful tracheal intubation adjunct, other types of introducers bearing similar features do not share the same popularity. This may be due to a paucity of clinical evidence supporting their use compared to the EI. In addition, most of these new intubating guides and stylets are disposable devices intended for single use and perhaps less cost-effective than the reusable EI.

What Are the Potential Limitations of These Intubating Guides and Introducers?

The popularity of the EI rests on its simplicity, ease of use, high success rates, and relatively few complications. However, it does have limitations.

The much-anticipated "clicks" and the "holdup" as described by many may prove elusive. The appreciation of clicks is particularly subtle in many patients. In 1988, Kidd et al.[28] studied the reliability of these signs. They found that "holdup" was observed in 100% of tracheal EI placement, whereas "clicks" were appreciated in only 90%. Importantly, however, neither was observed in any of the 22 esophageal placements. It is also possible that "holdup" might occur with esophageal placement of the EI in cases of esophageal stenosis, pharyngeal pouch or diverticulum, or with cricoid pressure, although one would anticipate these occurrences would be rare. Practitioners should be aware of these limitations, particularly where "holdup" can occur without the presence of "clicks." It is the opinion of the author (ORH) that the probability of feeling the "clicks" with EI placement into the trachea depends largely on the angle of insertion of the EI relative to the trachea. It is unlikely that the tip of the EI will "rub" against the tracheal rings if the EI is advancing into the trachea from a more vertical position. It is also related to the degree to which the EI contacts other soft tissues in the airway (e.g., tongue or lip) insulating against the transmission of the subtle tactile sensation.

Although complications are rare with these devices, they tend to occur when they are used improperly. Soft tissue lacerations, esophageal perforation, and tracheo-bronchial tree injuries have been reported with aggressive insertion of the EI and forceful "railroading" of the ETT over the EI.[29–31] The incidence of these complications can be minimized by employing a gentle advancement technique, and using the laryngoscope to move soft tissues out of the way to improve the angle of insertion of the ETT over the EI. Tip detachment has also been reported. Gardner et al.[32] reported a detachment of the tip of the EI following its withdrawal. The tip was initially identified just above the bifurcation of the trachea, although it was later documented to have moved into the right middle lobe bronchus. Manually checking the integrity of the tip of the EI prior to use is recommended.

Are There Any Clinical Differences Between the EI and Other Introducers with Identical Features?

Inspired by the simplicity and effectiveness of the EI, many newer introducers (e.g., the Frova Intubation Introducer, and the Sun Med Endotracheal Tube Introducer) share similar characteristics such as the J (coudé) tip at the distal end. By and large, these newer devices are made of different materials and are designed for single use. The Frova Intubation Introducer and the Cook Airway Exchange Catheter are hollow intubating introducers that permit urgent oxygenation and ventilation should the tracheal tube fail to advance into the trachea over the introducer. In addition to the "tracheal clicks" and "holdup" of the introducers during the insertion into the trachea, an aspiration test using a self-inflating bulb (SIB; also known as an Esophageal Detection Device [EDD]) can also be used with the hollow intubating introducers to further confirm tracheal placement. Tuzzo et al.[33] recently reported that a prompt and complete reinflation of the SIB failed to occur when the hollow intubating introducer was placed accidentally into the esophagus with 100% sensitivity and at a 3.5% false positive rate. While these newer devices appear to function similarly to the EI in facilitating tracheal intubation, they may not have comparable success rates. Using a simulated C/L Grade 3 laryngoscopic view in a manikin, a recent comparative study showed that successful placement of the Frova Introducer (65%) and the EI (60%) was significantly higher than with the Portex Introducer (8%).[12] A separate experiment also revealed that the peak force exerted by the Frova and Portex introducers was two to three times greater than that which could be exerted by the EI, suggesting that placement of the single-use introducers may be more traumatic.

Is There Any Evidence to Suggest that the Flexible Tip Bougie Performs Better than the Tracheal Introducer?

In 2020, Ruetzler et al.[17] conducted a study to compare the new FTB catheter with the standard bougie for tracheal intubation. In this simulation study of normal and difficult airways managed by anesthesiologists, they found that the overall success rate was similar between the two devices. However, they found that, especially in more difficult airway scenarios, the FTB had less intubation attempts, and required fewer optimization maneuvers. A similar prospective, randomized, cross-over study by Mahli et al.[34] also compared the FTB and standard bougie in intubating a simulated difficult airway model. This study found that the FTB offered a higher first-pass success rate with a faster time-to-intubation and less required attempts when compared to the standard bougie. In a recent study with a simulated difficult airway in cadavers, Hung et al.[35] showed that the time-to-intubation using GlideScope performed by anesthesiologists was similar between the standard bougie and the FTB. However, despite lack of prior experience with the FTB by study participants, there was a trend (but no statistical significance) that the participants preferred the FTB over the regular bougie with a higher subjective ratings of intubation ease.

LIGHTWANDS

What Is a Lightwand? How Does It Help with the Placement of an Endotracheal Tube?

The technique of transillumination using a lightwand (lighted-stylet) was first described by Yamamura et al. in 1959 with nasotracheal intubation.[36] The lightwand (LW) employs the principle of transillumination of the soft tissues of the anterior neck to guide the tip of the LW, and the mounted ETT, into the trachea. It also takes advantage of the anterior (superficial) location of the trachea relative to the esophagus.

When the tip of the ETT/LW combination enters the glottic opening, a well-defined circumscribed glow can be readily seen slightly below the thyroid prominence (Figure 12.4A). However, if the tip of the ETT/LW is in the esophagus, the transmitted glow is diffuse and cannot be readily detected under ambient lighting conditions (Figure 12.4B). If the tip of the ETT/LW is placed in the vallecula, the light glow is diffuse and appears slightly above the thyroid prominence. Using these landmarks and principles, the practitioner can guide the tip of the ETT easily and safely into the trachea without the use of a laryngoscope.

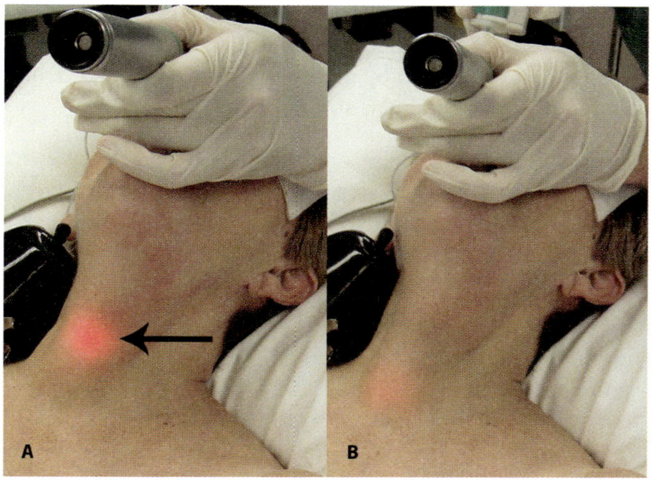

FIGURE 12.4. **(A)** When the tip of the ETT with the lightwand is placed at the glottic opening under direct laryngoscopy, a well-defined circumscribed glow (arrow) in the anterior neck just below the thyroid prominence can be readily seen. **(B)** When the tip of the endotracheal tube is placed in the esophagus under direct laryngoscopy, transillumination is poor and the transmitted glow is diffuse in the anterior neck and cannot be seen easily under ambient lighting condition.

Are All Lightwands the Same?

Through the 1970s and 1980s, many versions of a lighted stylet had been introduced, including the Fiberoptic Lighted-Intubation Stylette (Anesthesia Medical Specialties, Santa Fe, CA), Lighted Intubation Stylet (Aaron Medical, St. Peterborough, FL), Flexilum™ (Concept Corporation, Clearwater, FL) (Figure 12.5A), Tubestat™ (Xomed, Jacksonville, FL) (Figure 12.5B), Fiberoptic Malleable Lighted Stylette (Metropolitan Medical Inc, Winchester, VA) (Figure 12.5C), and Imagica Fiberoptic Lighted Stylet (Fiberoptic Medical Products Inc, Allentown, PA). Some of these devices have proven to be effective and safe in placing an ETT both orally and nasally.[37–39] Even though favorable results have been reported with these devices, substantial limitations have been identified: (1) poor light intensity; (2) short length, limiting the use of the LW device to a short or cut ETT; (3) absence of a connector to secure the ETT to the LW device; (4) rigidity of the LW, hampering use of the devices with other techniques, such as light-guided nasal intubation; and (5) most LWs were designed for single use, increasing the cost per intubation. For these reasons and others, intubation using a LW did not receive widespread popularity until the introduction of the Trachlight™ (Laerdal Medical, Wappingers Falls, NY) device in 1995.

What Are Some of the Unique Characteristics of the Trachlight Compared to Other Lightwand Devices?

The Trachlight (TL) has a long and flexible wand with a retractable metal wire stylet and an improved light source. These features add flexibility, broaden the utility of the device for both oral and nasal intubation, make intubation easier, and permit the evaluation of the position of the tip of the ETT after intubation. To date, the TL has been the most popular and well-studied of the LWs. Although the TL is no longer manufactured, a new version of the LW with similar features of the TL is being developed.[40,41] One of the authors (OH) of this chapter was involved in the original design and development of the TL. For these reasons, much of the following discussion reflects this experience and bias toward the TL.

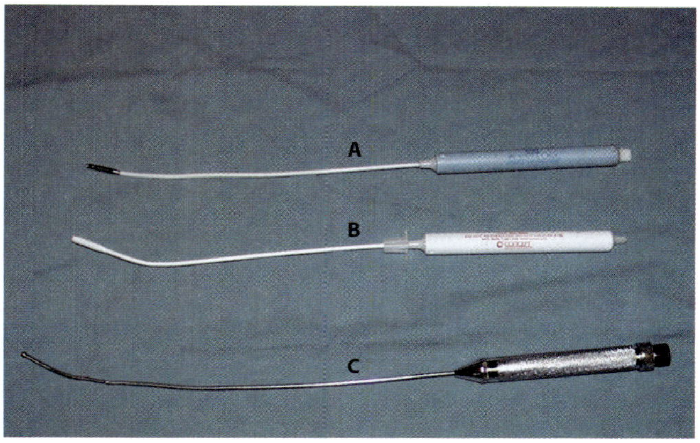

FIGURE 12.5. Commercially available lightwands: **(A)** Flexilum, **(B)** Tubestat, and **(C)** Fiberoptic Malleable Lighted Stylette.

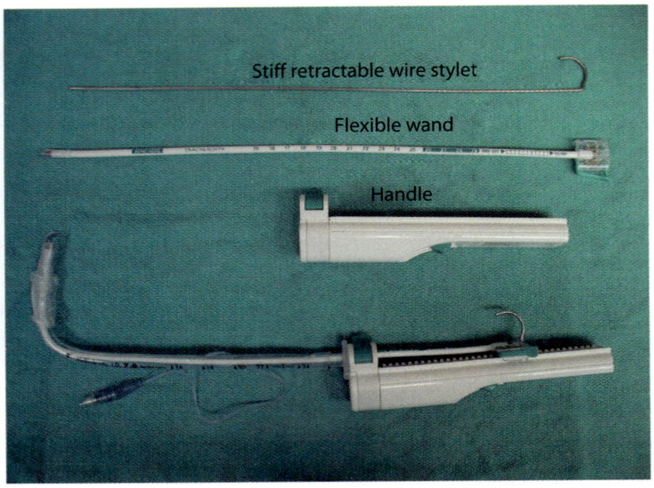

FIGURE 12.6. The Trachlight consists of three parts: a handle, a flexib e wand, and a stiff retractable stylet wire. With the TL in place, the ETT-TL unit is bent at a 90-degree angle just proximal to the cuff of the tube in the shape of a "field-hockey stick."

Nevertheless, the concept and principles of intubation using transillumination are applicable to all other LWs.

The TL consists of three parts: a reusable handle, a flexible wand, and a stiff retractable wire stylet (Figure 12.6). The power control circuitry and three triple "A" alkaline batteries are encased in the handle. A locking clamp located on the handle accepts and secures a standard 15-mm ETT connector. The stylet or "wand" consists of a durable, flexible plastic shaft with a bright light bulb affixed at the distal end, permitting intubation under ambient lighting conditions. After 30 seconds of illumination, the light bulb blinks to minimize heat production and provide a convenient reminder of elapsed time. Ensuring that the tip of the stylet is inside the distal tip of ETT enhances its heat safety profile. A animal study confirmed an absence of heat-related tissue histopathological changes, suggesting that thermal injury following the use of the TL is unlikely.[42]

A rigid plastic connector with a release arm at the proximal end of the TL handle allows adjustment of the wand along the handle and into the ETT when the release arm is depressed. Enclosed within the wand is a stiff but malleable, retractable wire stylet. When the stiff wire stylet is retracted, the wand becomes pliable, permitting the ETT to advance easily into the trachea. This may well be the most important feature of this LW device, since it significantly improves its ease of use and intubation success rate.

The retractable wire stylet stiffens the wand sufficiently so that it can be shaped in the form of a "field-hockey stick" (Figure 12.6). This configuration directs the bright light of the bulb against the anterior wall of the larynx and trachea. In addition, the "hockey stick" configuration enhances maneuverability during intubation and facilitates the placement of the ETT through the glottic opening. However, once through the glottis, the "field hockey stick" configuration can impede further advancement of the tube into the trachea. Retraction of the stiff wire stylet produces a pliable ETT-TL unit, permitting its advancement into the trachea until the transilluminated glow reaches the sternal notch, a point known to be at the level of the mid-trachea.

How Do You Prepare the Trachlight Device? (Video 2)

As with any intubation technique, regular use of an LW improves the practitioner's performance and intubation success rates and reduces the risk of complications.

Lubrication of the internal wire stylet of the wand using silicone fluid (Endoscopic Instrument Fluid, ACMI, Southborough, MA) ensures its easy retraction during intubation. The wand should also be lubricated with the same silicone fluid to facilitate retraction of the wand following the ETT placement. The rail gear of the TL handle should always be inspected for missing fragments (prior to loading of the stylet, after retraction of the stylet).[43] Cutting the ETT to a length of 26 cm is recommended to facilitate maneuverability of the ETT-TL during oral tracheal intubation. The wand is then inserted into the ETT and the tube attached to the handle. The length of the wand is adjusted by sliding the wand along the handle to position the light bulb close to, but not protruding beyond, the tip of the ETT. With the TL in place, the ETT-TL unit is bent to a 90-degree angle just proximal to the cuff of the tube in the shape of a "field hockey stick" (Figure 12.6). Even though the degree of bend should be individualized to the patient, a 90-degree angle generally makes the intubation considerably easier and projects the maximum light intensity toward the surface of the skin as the device traverses the glottis and trachea, producing a well-defined exterior circumscribed glow. If the TL is bent to 45 degrees, the maximum light intensity will be directed down the trachea. For obese patients or patients with short necks, a more acute bend (greater than 90 degrees) provides better transillumination. Although it is the author's experience that the recommended length of the TL from bend to tip of 6.5 to 8.5 cm is suitable for most patients, some investigators have suggested that the length from bend to tip is best established by matching it to the patient's thyroid prominence-to-mandibular angle distance.[44]

How Do You Use the Trachlight to Perform Tracheal Intubation?

Although the practitioner usually stands at the head of the table or bed during LW intubation, it is possible to employ this technique from the front or side of the patient, in the prehospital environment, for instance. When the head is in the sniffing position, the epiglottis is in close contact with the posterior pharyngeal wall making it more difficult for the ETT-TL unit to advance behind the epiglottis. It is preferable that the patient's head and neck be positioned in a neutral or slightly extended position.

In most cases, patients can be intubated easily under ambient lighting conditions.[45] In very thin patients, the light intensity is so bright that it is possible to mistakenly interpret an esophageal intubation as an intratracheal placement. It is therefore recommended that intubations using the TL in otherwise normal individuals be carried out under ambient light.

Dimming room lights may be advantageous in obese patients, patients with thick necks or dark skin, or when the technique is being learned. In settings where controlling the ambient lighting is not possible (e.g., prehospital), it may be helpful to shade the neck with a towel or a hand.

Denitrogenation of the patient should precede all light-guided intubations. In an unconscious patient lying supine, the tongue falls posteriorly, pushing the epiglottis against the posterior pharyngeal wall (Figure 12.7). In order to have clear access to the glottic opening during intubation, it is necessary for the practitioner to grasp the jaw and lift it upward using the thumb and index finger of the non-dominant hand. This lifts the tongue and epiglottis away from the posterior pharyngeal wall to facilitate placement of the tip of the ETT posterior to the epiglottis and into the glottic opening (Figure 12.8). The ETT-TL unit is then inserted into the midline of the oropharynx. The midline position of the ETT-TL is maintained while the device is advanced gently in a rocking motion along an imaginary anterior–posterior arc. When resistance to cephalad rocking of the handle is felt, the ETT-TL handle should be "rocked" forward (toward the feet) and the tip redirected toward the laryngeal prominence using the glow of the light as a guide. A faint glow seen above the laryngeal prominence indicates that the tip of the ETT-TL is located in the vallecula. When the tip of ETT-TL enters the glottic opening, a well-defined circumscribed glow can be seen in the anterior neck slightly below the laryngeal prominence (Figure 12.9). Retracting the inner stiff wire stylet approximately 10 cm makes the ETT-TL tip more pliable, permitting advancement into the trachea with reduced risk of trauma. The ETT-TL is then advanced until the glow begins to disappear at the sternal notch indicating that the tip of the ETT is approximately 5 cm above the carina in the average adult.[46] Following release of the locking clamp, the TL can be removed from the ETT.

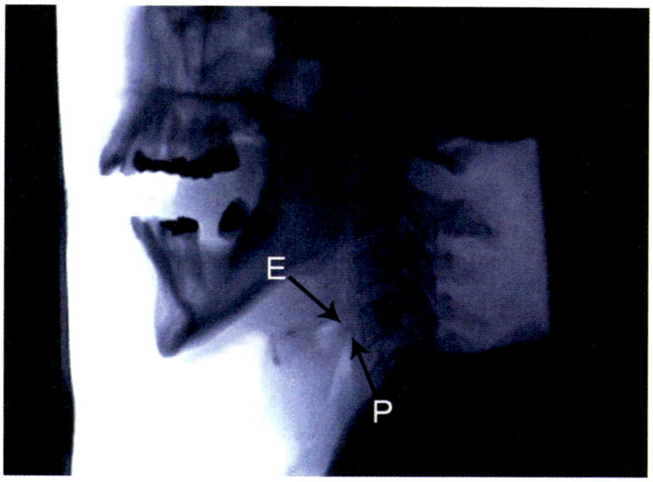

FIGURE 12.7. This radiological film of the upper airway shows that under anesthesia and with the patient lying supine, the tongue falls posteriorly, pushing the epiglottis (E) against the posterior pharyngeal wall (P).

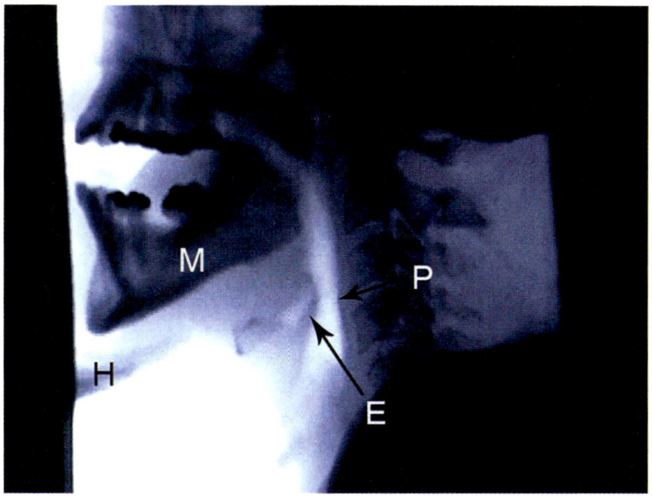

FIGURE 12.8. This radiological film of the upper airway shows that the jaw or mandibular (M) lift by the non-dominant hand (H) can elevate the tongue and epiglottis (E) off the posterior pharyngeal wall (P), thus providing a clear passage for the endotracheal tube to enter the glottic opening.

Occasionally, the circumscribed glow cannot be readily seen in the anterior neck due to anatomical features such as morbid obesity or a short neck. Neck extension as described above may be helpful. Retraction of the breast or chest wall tissues together with "spreading" of the tissues around the trachea by an assistant enhances transillumination of the soft tissues in the anterior neck. Dimming the ambient light is seldom required.

Occasionally, following retraction of the stiff wire stylet, the tip of the tube and LW can "hang up" on laryngeal structures, the cricoid ring, or a tracheal ring and cannot be advanced into the trachea readily. This is likely due to the fact that when an ETT is loaded along its natural curvature onto the TL, the tip of the ETT has a tendency to bend anteriorly upon retraction of the stiff internal stylet. While maintaining tube tip contact with the anterior airway, the practitioner should rotate the ETT-TL 90 degrees or more to the right or the left side permitting the tip of the ETT to alter the orientation of the tube tip perhaps enhancing the chance that

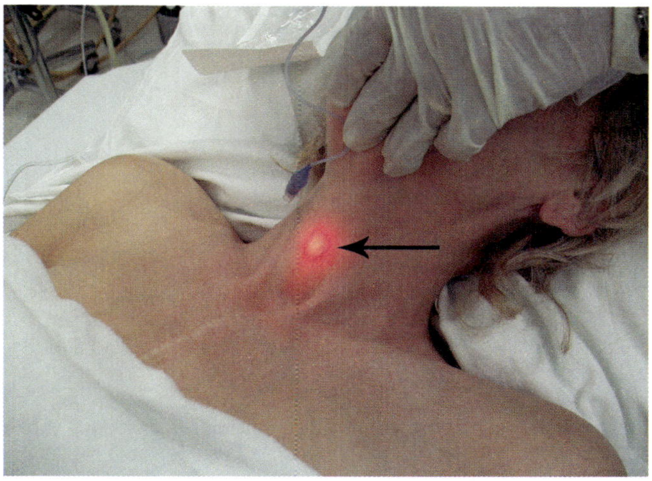

FIGURE 12.9. A bright, well-defined, circumscribed glow (arrow) is seen below the thyroid prominence when the ETT-TL enters the glottic opening.

the ETT will enter the trachea. Alternatively, immersing the ETT in warm saline solution prior to tracheal intubation will reduce its stiffness and the memory of its natural curvature. In addition, reverse loading of the ETT onto the TL may minimize the tendency of the ETT tip to bend anteriorly while retracting the internal stiff stylet of the TL. The combination of softening and reverse loading of the ETT has been shown to overcome the problem of "hang up" during intubation with the TL.[47]

Can the Trachlight Be Used for Nasotracheal Intubation? How Do You Use the Trachlight to Perform a Nasotracheal Intubation?

In contrast to other commercially available lighted stylets, once the stiff internal wire stylet is removed, the wand of the TL becomes pliable and able to facilitate a light-guided nasotracheal intubation. When used with a nasal RAE (Ring, Aldair, & Elwyn) ETT, the inner wire stylet should be inserted halfway (about 15 cm) to allow unbending of the proximal curvature of the nasal RAE tube (Figure 12.10). Application of a vasoconstricting nasal spray to the nasal mucosa prior to intubation may help to minimize bleeding. The ETT-TL should be immersed in a bottle of warm sterile water or saline to soften the ETT and reduce the risk of mucosal damage during nasal intubation. Water-soluble lubricant is applied to the nostril to facilitate entry of the ETT-TL through the nose. As with oral intubation, a jaw lift during intubation will elevate the tongue and epiglottis away from the posterior wall of the pharynx (see Figure 12.8), facilitating the placement of the tip of the ETT behind the epiglottis and into the glottic opening. The TL is switched on once the tip of the ETT-TL has advanced into the oropharynx, positioned in the midline, and advanced gently using the light glow as a guide. A faint glow seen above the laryngeal prominence indicates that the tip of the ETT-TL is located in the vallecula. A jaw lift and slight withdrawal of the ETT-TL will help to elevate the epiglottis and enhance the passage of the ETT-TL under it. When the ETT-TL enters the glottic opening, a well-defined circumscribed glow is seen in the anterior neck just below the thyroid prominence (Figure 12.11). Following the release of the locking clamp, the TL is withdrawn from the ETT. Correct tube placement should be confirmed using end-tidal CO_2 and auscultation.

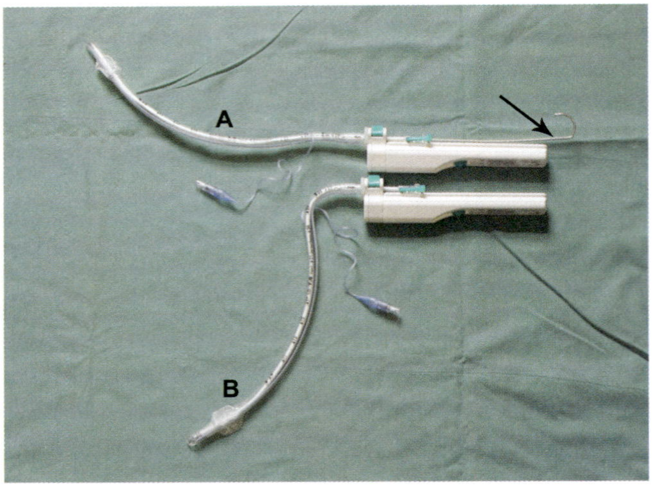

FIGURE 12.10. For light-guided nasal intubation using the Trachlight, the internal wire stylet is generally removed so that the wand of the TL becomes pliable to facilitate nasotracheal intubation. However, if a nasal RAE tube is used, the proximal curvature of the nasal RAE Tracheal Tube will bend the pliable wand of the TL (B), making it difficult to control the tip of the tracheal tube during intubation. When the TL is used with a nasal RAE ETT, the wire stylet (arrow) should be retracted only halfway (about 15 cm) to allow unbending of the proximal curvature of the nasal RAE tube (A) to facilitate light-guided nasal intubation.

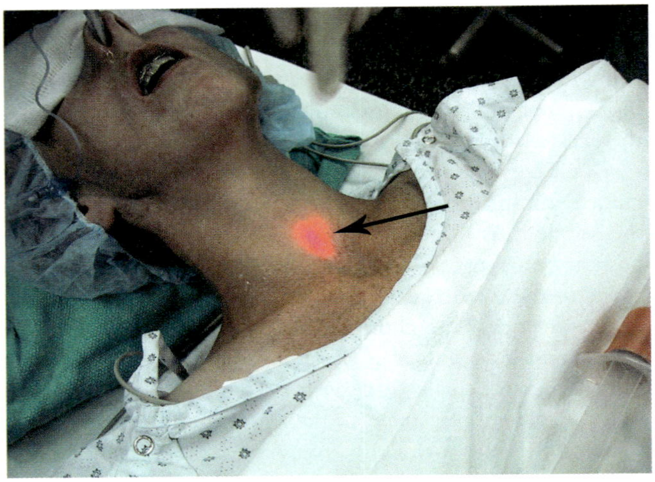

FIGURE 12.11. During nasotracheal intubation, when the ETT-TL enters the glottic opening, a well-defined circumscribed glow (arrow) is seen in the anterior neck just below the thyroid prominence.

What Are the Common Problems with a Blind or Light-Guided Nasotracheal Intubation? How Do You Overcome These Problems?

Due to the natural curvature of the ETT, the tip of the tube often goes posteriorly into the esophagus during a "blind" or light-guided nasal intubation, despite external posterior pressure on the thyroid cartilage. To elevate the tip of the ETT anteriorly during intubation, it is sometimes necessary to flex the neck of the patient while advancing the ETT-TL slowly. In the event that flexing the neck of the patient is contraindicated, inflating the ETT cuff with 15 to 20 mL of air will help to elevate the ETT tip and align it with the glottis during intubation.[48,49] Alternatively, the use of a directional-tip tube, such as an Endotrol™ tube (Mallinckrodt Critical Care, Inc, St. Louis, MO), flexes the tube tip anteriorly and into the glottis.[50] In certain circumstances (e.g., tube tip impingement in the posterior nasopharynx), nasotracheal intubation using the TL can be performed safely with the stiff, internal stylet in place.[51] This technique may be associated with fewer head and neck manipulations and deliver better control of the tip of the ETT.

What Are the Limitations of the Lightwand Intubating Technique?

The LW intubating technique requires transillumination of the soft tissues of the anterior neck without visualization of the laryngeal structures. Therefore, LW should not be used in patients with known abnormalities of the upper airway, such as tumors, polyps, infection (e.g., epiglottitis, retropharyngeal abscess), and trauma to the upper airway, or if there is a foreign body in the upper airway. In these cases, alternate intubating techniques using direct or indirect vision, such as bronchoscopic intubation, should be considered. Lightwand should also be used with caution in patients in whom transillumination of the anterior neck may not be adequate, such as patients with a large anterior neck mass (goiter, or tumor) or who are severely obese or with a limited neck extension. However, these contraindications and precautions must be weighed in light of the urgency of achieving a patent airway in any patient whose ventilation may be compromised and urgent intubation is required. Clearly, this light-guided technique should not be attempted with an awake uncooperative patient unless a bite block is used to prevent damage to the device or injury to the practitioner.

Since its introduction in 1995, the TL has been used extensively in many countries. While the potential risks of damage to the glottic opening during tracheal intubation using a "nonvisual" intubating technique is real, there have been no serious complications reported. Aoyama et al.[52] used a nasally placed bronchoscope to visualize the airway during TL intubation. They reported that the epiglottis may be pushed into the laryngeal inlet by the ETT-TL during a TL intubation. Fortunately, the epiglottis usually spontaneously returned to its correct position. They also reported that structures around the glottic opening, including the epiglottis and the arytenoids, were transiently displaced during the placement of the ETT using the TL. The investigators concluded that there are potential risks of laryngeal damage in addition to the down folding of the epiglottis during the ETT placement using the TL, but such occurrences do not appear to cause permanent damage. Other investigators have identified a reduced incidence of sore throat in patients intubated using the TL compared to laryngoscopic intubation.[45]

Intubation using an LW device has other potential risks. Stone et al.[53] reported disconnection of the light bulb from an LW requiring retrieval from a major bronchus. However, the LW device employed in this instance (Flexilum) (Figure 12.5A) was not designed or recommended for tracheal intubation. A later version of the same device solved the problem of bulb loss into the trachea by encasing stylet and bulb in a tough plastic sheath (Tubestat). In contrast to the older LW devices, it is extremely unlikely that the light bulb will be detached from the TL, since the light bulb is firmly attached to the durable plastic sheath of TL. In fact, since its introduction in 1995, there have been no reported cases of detached light bulb from the TL. Although rare, subluxation of the cricoarytenoid cartilage has been reported in a study using an older version of an LW (Tubestat).[54] However, with the retractable wire stylet, the risk of damaging the arytenoid cartilage during TL intubation should be low.

Is There Any Clinical Evidence to Suggest that the Lightwand Is an Effective and Safe Intubating Device?

A large clinical study involving 950 elective surgical patients conducted to determine the effectiveness and safety of orotracheal intubation using either the TL or direct-vision intubation using a laryngoscope[45] showed a statistically significant difference in the total intubation time between the groups (15.7 ± 10.8 vs. 19.6 ± 23.7 s for TL and laryngoscopy, respectively). However, such a small difference is probably of little clinical importance. There was a 1% failure rate with the TL and 92% success rate on the first attempt, compared with a 3% failure rate and an 89% success rate on the first attempt using the laryngoscope. There were significantly fewer traumatic events and sore throats in the TL group compared to laryngoscopy patients. Tsutsui et al.[55] reported similar findings in a study with 511 patients. Trachlight intubation was highly successful (99%) with the majority of the successful intubations (93%) being accomplished after one attempt. Unsuccessful intubation even at the third attempt occurred in only three patients (1%).

In 1995, Hung et al.[56] reported the effectiveness of TL intubation in 265 patients with a "difficult" airway (206 patients with a documented history of difficult intubation or anticipated difficult airways and 59 anesthetized patients with an unanticipated failed laryngoscopic intubation). Tracheal intubation was successful in all patients except two (obesity Class III) in the anticipated difficult laryngoscopic intubation group. Apart from minor mucosal bleeding (mostly from nasal intubation), no serious complications were observed in any of the study patients. The results of this study indicate that TL is an effective technique for placement of ETTs (nasally and orally) for patients with both anticipated and unanticipated difficult airways. Other investigators have reported successful use of the TL in patients with a difficult airway. These include patients with a history of limited mouth opening,[57] cervical spine abnormality,[58] Pierre-Robin Syndrome,[59] and cardiac patients with a difficult airway.[60]

The ASA 2022 Difficult Airway Guidelines continue to include intubation with the use of the LW as part of its difficult airway algorithm when considering alternative intubation approaches.[61] These guidelines present evidence for higher frequency of successful intubations and shorter intubation times using an LW when compared to blind intubation in patients with anticipated difficult airways.

What Are Some of the Potential Uses of the Trachlight?

Tracheal intubation can fail with TL and with the laryngoscope. However, one study of 950 patients showed that all TL failures were resolved with direct laryngoscopy.[45] Similarly, all failures of direct laryngoscopy were resolved with TL. These results suggest that a tracheal intubation success rate approaching 100% can be achieved by combining the techniques. This combined approach may be particularly useful when an unanticipated Cormack/Lehane (C/L) Grade 3 laryngoscopic view is encountered.[7] Instead of using a styletted ETT with a

90-degree bend, one might employ an ETT-TL with the same bend. Under direct laryngoscopy, the tip of the ETT-TL can be "hooked" under the epiglottis. A well-defined circumscribed glow seen in the anterior neck slightly below the laryngeal prominence indicates that the tip of the ETT is placed at the glottic opening. If such a glow is not seen, the ETT-TL can be repositioned until it can be seen. In 2002, Agro et al.[62] reported the effectiveness of this combined technique. In this study, the investigators successfully performed tracheal intubation in all 350 surgical patients studied with a simulated difficult airway using a combined laryngoscope/TL approach.

The TL has been combined successfully with other intubating techniques, including intubation through the LMA-Classic,[63,64] used in conjunction with the intubating LMA (LMA-Fastrach™),[65] with the Bullard laryngoscope,[66,67] and with a retrograde intubating technique.[68]

The TL has been shown to be useful in identifying the intratracheal position of the ETT tip during percutaneous dilational tracheotomy.[69] The TL wand without the stiffening wire is passed through the in situ ETT matching the length numbers on the ETT to position the TL tip at the ETT tip. This simple technique may help to prevent inadvertent punctures of the ETT and/or its cuff ensuring that adequate ventilation and oxygenation can be reinstituted during the percutaneous procedure if required. This technique is inexpensive and minimizes the risk of damaging expensive equipment ordinarily used during such procedures such as the flexible bronchoscope. Used properly, it is possible that this simple light-guided technique can also be used to accurately determine when the tip of the ETT is above the surgical tracheotomy site as the tube is pulled back during surgical tracheotomy.

DIGITAL INTUBATION

What Is Digital Intubation? When Was It Introduced?

Airway management has been revolutionized by the abundance of extraglottic devices that not only facilitate effective ventilation but also aid tracheal intubation. Despite these advances, certain situations may make the blind insertion of an ETT into the trachea using the digits of the hand (digital intubation or tactile orotracheal intubation) a suitable alternative method of securing an airway.

It is believed that this technique was first described by Herholt and Rafn in 1796 in drowning victims. It surfaced as a viable method of intubation in the emergency medicine literature in the mid-1980s.[70,71] Blind digital intubation has also been used to establish an airway during neonatal resuscitation[72] and as an adjunct in blind nasotracheal intubation.[73]

What Are the Indications for Digital Intubation?

The skill levels of the practitioner, coupled with previous experience in using the technique of blind digital intubation are important prerequisites for success. The importance of practicing this technique in non-emergency situations cannot be overemphasized. The risk of infectious disease transmission must always be borne in mind. Awake patients with an intact gag reflex are not suitable for this technique. Muscle paralysis may be helpful in certain situations. The following list briefly describes the clinical situations where blind digital intubation may be used to establish a patent airway:

(a) Inadequate access to a patient's airway that prevents standard laryngoscopic techniques from being used (e.g., a patient trapped in a motor vehicle after a crash).
(b) Lack or failure of other airway management devices.
(c) Inability to secure an airway with laryngoscopic techniques or extraglottic devices.
(d) In the setting of cervical spine instability in an unconscious patient.
(e) When blood, secretions, or vomitus make adequate visualization of the glottis impossible.

How Do You Perform Digital Intubation? (Video 14)

The skilled practitioner ensures that an oxygen source, rescue airway devices, suction, and emergency drugs are immediately at hand. In-line immobilization should be performed in the setting of cervical spine instability. Cricoid pressure should be applied where clinically indicated. Although digital intubation can usually be performed without other adjuncts (Figure 12.12), the classic description of blind digital intubation requires a malleable stylet to be inserted into the ETT.[74] The ETT is then bent into a shape such that it can elevate the epiglottis and enter the trachea. Alternatively, as the authors believe, an intubating guide (e.g., the EI) together with an appropriately sized ETT is a simpler technique. The advantage of this latter technique is that it is easier to guide an EI

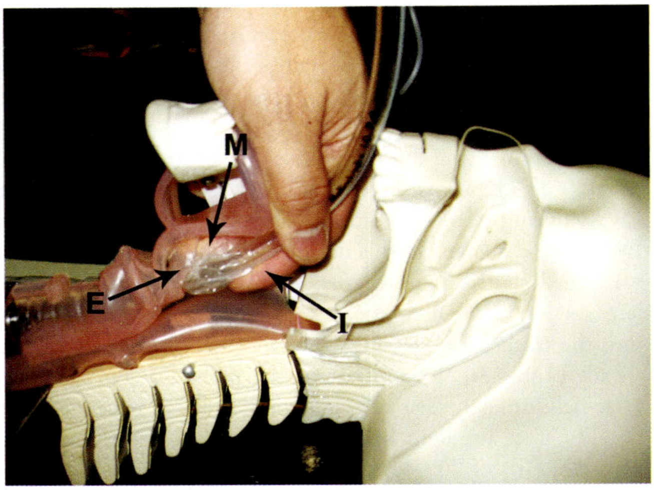

FIGURE 12.12. Manikin demonstration of digital intubation without using a stylet or intubating guide: the index and middle fingers of the non-dominant hand are inserted into the mouth. Once the epiglottis (E) is palpated by the middle finger (M), it is lifted in an anterior direction. The index finger (I) of the non-dominant hand is then flexed to guide the tracheal tube under the epiglottis and into the trachea.

through the glottic opening, and then railroad the ETT into the trachea than it is to place a stylet-ETT combination in the trachea. The intubating guide has a small external diameter and is easily manipulated with the fingers to enable passage through the vocal cords. In addition, the clicks felt as the intubating guide (e.g., EI) advances over the tracheal rings combined with "holdup" will assist in confirmation that the EI has entered the trachea. The ETT with the malleable stylet is rigid and perhaps more likely to cause blunt trauma to the airway structures, especially if repeated manipulation is necessary for successful entry into the trachea.

To perform the procedure:

(a) The patient's head should be placed in the sniffing position as for standard laryngoscopic intubation except in situations where cervical instability exists.
(b) The practitioner stands or kneels adjacent to the patient (facing the patient's head) so that the non-dominant side of the practitioner is closest to the patient (Figure 12.13).
(c) If available, an assistant can grasp and pull the tongue forward using gauze. This maneuver helps to lift the epiglottis anteriorly and makes palpation of the structures of the upper airway easier.
(d) The practitioner then places the index and middle fingers of the non-dominant hand into the patient's mouth. Once the epiglottis is palpated by the middle finger, it is lifted in an anterior direction.
(e) The intubating guide is then guided into the mouth along the palmar surface of the index finger of the non-dominant hand.
(f) The index finger of the non-dominant hand is then flexed to steer the intubating guide under the epiglottis and into the trachea (Figure 12.13). Occasionally the middle finger of the non-dominant hand lifting the epiglottis must be moved slightly laterally to allow successful passage of the intubating guide.
(g) The clicks on the tracheal rings and holdup of the intubating guide on the lower bronchial tree serve as indicators of correct tracheal placement.
(h) The ETT is then railroaded over the intubating guide into the trachea. Maintaining anterior displacement of the epiglottis facilitates ETT passage.
(i) Confirmation of successful tracheal intubation should be determined by end-tidal CO_2 detection.

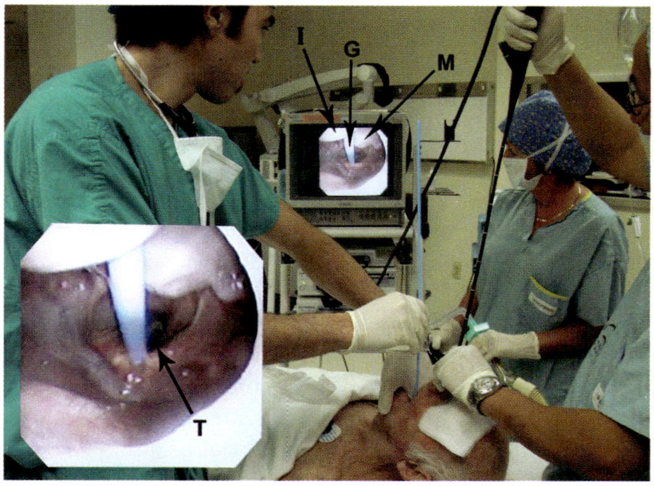

FIGURE 12.13. Digital intubation using an intubating guide: to visualize the technique of digital intubation, a flexible bronchoscope was placed through the right nostril into the nasopharynx of the patient. During the digital intubation, the index and middle fingers of the non-dominant hand are inserted into the mouth. As shown in the monitor (and the enlarged insert), once the epiglottis is palpated by the middle finger (M), it is lifted in an anterior direction. The index finger (I) is then flexed to guide the Intubating Guide (G) under the epiglottis and into the trachea (T).

Should Digital Intubation Always Be Performed from the Left Side of the Patient?

Although digital intubation can be performed on either side of the patient, approaching the patient from the left side is ergonomically more favorable. In other standard intubation procedures, the endotracheal tube is inserted into the oropharynx and advanced into the trachea using the right hand, while the left hand is responsible for opening the airway and displacing relevant tissue and structures to create a more favorable path for intubation. Therefore, the most familiar approach for digital intubation will be the one in which the right hand introduces the endotracheal tube while the left displaces the structures and tissue. Approaching the patient from the left side is more ergonomically favorable for insertion of the left-hand's digits into the oropharynx and is therefore preferred.

Highlighting the clinical relevance of the left-sided approach, digital intubation is a technique that may be considered in the prehospital setting for an unresponsive patient who is trapped in the seat of a crashed motor vehicle. This is an environment where the patient is likely to be in a sitting position making traditional laryngoscopy challenging. The airway is likely to be bloody, which can impair glottic visualization with videolaryngoscopy, and more advanced airway equipment may not be available. Digital intubation is a simple technique that allows the practitioner to manage the airway while facing the patient or standing at the opening of the driver's door. The location of the driver's seat may influence which hand the practitioner uses to palpate the epiglottis versus deliver the ETT. The driver sits on the left side of the car in North America, making it easier for the practitioner to place the fingers of the left hand into the oropharynx and deliver the ETT with the right hand (Figure 12.14). This approach would be ergonomically awkward in countries where drivers are seated on the right side of the car, and reversing the roles of the hands should be considered (Figure 12.15).

Can Digital Intubation Be Performed on a Child?

Although the principles and techniques of digital intubation are similar, digital intubation can readily be performed without the use of a stylet or the EI in children. Hancock et al.[72] have employed this technique during neonatal resuscitation and accidental extubation scenarios. Digital intubation of neonates and infants can be considered in situations where direct

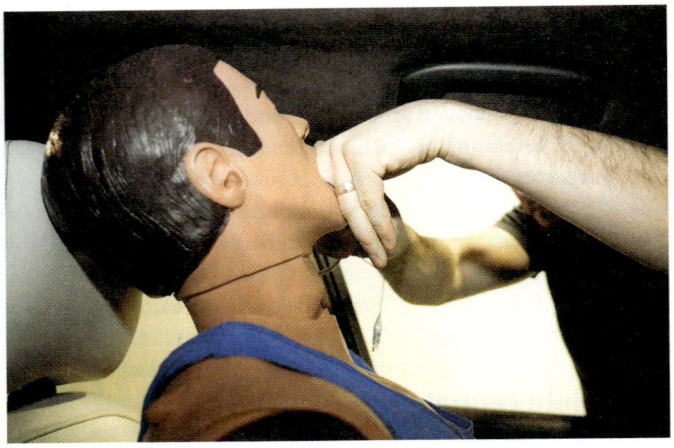

FIGURE 12.14. Digital intubation of a trapped driver (manikin) on the left side of the vehicle. The left hand of the practitioner palpates the epiglottis while the right hand delivers the ETT.

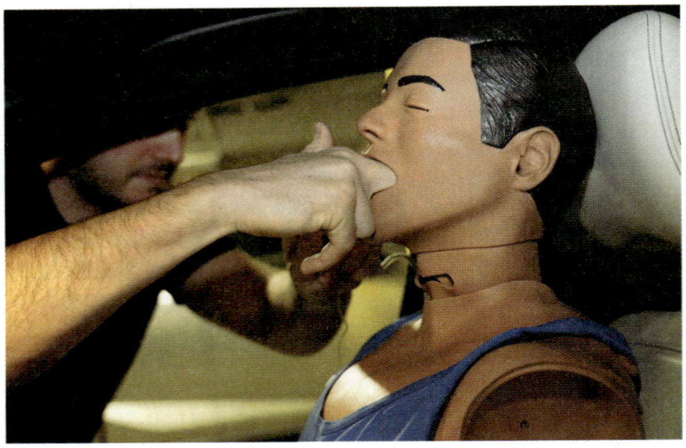

FIGURE 12.15. Digital intubation of a trapped driver (manikin) on the right side of the vehicle. The right hand of the practitioner palpates the epiglottis while the left hand delivers the ETT.

laryngoscopic techniques have failed, airway equipment failure has occurred, for meconium aspiration in the neonate, or during transport when inadequate access may preclude conventional techniques.

What Are the Limitations of Digital Intubation?

Although digital intubation is a simple and easy-to-learn technique, it is difficult to perform when the epiglottis cannot be identified or felt during intubation. This is particularly true for the patients who are excessively tall or with a full set of maxillary incisors and a small mouth opening. The procedure can also be difficult to perform if the practitioner has short or large fingers in relation to the patient's anatomy.

To minimize the risk of injury to the practitioner's fingers, digital intubation is generally contraindicated for patients who are awake and uncooperative. However, in emergency situations when limited equipment is available, a digital intubation may be an option with a bite block in place.

BLIND NASAL INTUBATION

What Are the Indications for Blind Nasal Intubation?

The technique of blind nasal intubation was first popularized by Sir Ivan Magill and Stanley Rowbotham in the 1920s. This method of tracheal intubation has proved life-saving in many difficult airway situations, and continues to be a useful adjunct in the difficult airway armamentarium.[61,75,76] It can be performed in patients who are unable to lie flat, and maintenance of spontaneous ventilation facilitates blind nasal intubation requiring minimal neck manipulation. The experience and skill of the practitioner are key determinants for success with this technique. Indications for blind nasal intubation include:

(a) elective oral, pharyngeal, and dental surgery
(b) when the oral route is difficult or impossible (e.g., limited mouth opening, temporomandibular joint diseases, or severe masseter spasm)
(c) difficult airway—elective or unanticipated

What Are the Contraindications of Blind Nasal Intubation?

The following may contraindicate blind nasal intubation:

(a) inadequate experience or skill of the practitioner
(b) base of the skull cranial fractures
(c) severe maxillofacial fractures with distorted nasal or midface anatomy
(d) known or suspected nasal obstruction secondary to pathology (e.g., massive nasal polyps or tumors)
(e) bleeding diathesis secondary to hematological disease or anticoagulant medication
(f) severe laryngeal trauma or infection

Which Nostril Should Be Used for Blind Nasal Intubation?

As most practitioners are right-handed, naturally, most would favor the use of the right hand to advance the ETT through the right nostril while using the left hand to feel the anterior neck to assess the position of the tip of the ETT during blind nasal intubation. In the absence of a septal abnormality (e.g., a septal deviation), traditional teaching also suggests the right nostril over the left for nasal intubation.[77] It is generally felt that the left-facing bevel of the tracheal tube is the main cause of nasal trauma. The nasal mucosa over the turbinates is highly vascular and can be easily traumatized. It is likely that the mucosa over the left turbinate is particularly at risk during left-sided intubation since the bevel tends to impact directly against it. So, to minimize trauma, most practitioners would insert the ETT with the bevel facing the flat nasal septum rather than facing the irregularly shaped turbinates along the lateral wall of the nasal cavity. However, others consider that the tip of the tracheal tube is more likely to cause nasal trauma than the bevel and therefore it is more reasonable to have the tip of the ETT advance alongside the septal mucosa during intubation. Hence, some practitioners choose to advance the ETT through the left nostril during nasal intubation. Unfortunately, no scientific evidence currently exists to suggest that one nostril is safer than the other for nasal intubation in patients with a normal nasal anatomy.[78] Instead of debating which is the preferred nostril to minimize the risk of injury, it is perhaps more important to properly prepare the ETT (e.g., selecting an appropriate size ETT and softening the ETT in warm saline or water) and the patient (e.g., apply vasoconstrictor to the nostrils prior to performing the nasal intubation), resist excessive force during intubation, and change to a different nostril or use a smaller ETT when necessary.

How Do You Perform a Blind Nasal Tracheal Intubation? (Video 13)

The answer to this question is largely determined by the indication for tracheal intubation. In elective situations, the nares are best prepared with a vasoconstrictor (although there is little evidence that this maneuver reduces bleeding or enhances success rates) and the upper airway topicalized with local anesthetic. Light sedation using drugs such as short-acting opioids, ketamine or benzodiazepines may be required to improve patient cooperation and for anxiolysis. However, in emergency situations with life-threatening hypoxemia, this may not be possible. The potential for severe epistaxis with airway hemorrhage must always be kept in mind. Rescue airway equipment including extraglottic devices and surgical airway kits should be available. Vital sign monitors are attached and the patient is fully denitrogenated if practical prior to the procedure being undertaken. Cervical spine precautions and cricoid pressure should be instituted as indicated. Maintenance of spontaneous ventilation is preferred to assist with successful tracheal intubation. Confirmation of tracheal tube placement is obtained by the usual clinical criteria and CO_2 detection methods. Some practitioners insert an appropriately sized nasopharyngeal airway, or fully insert their little finger to gently dilate the nostril to minimize bleeding on tube insertion. In addition, this maneuver may help to identify mid or posterior nares anatomical abnormalities that would preclude use of that nostril.

To perform the procedure:

(a) Insert the appropriate size ETT into the naris.
(b) Gently advance the ETT. Do not use excessive force if there is resistance during insertion. This may mean that the tip of the ETT has entered the depression in the nasopharynx where the Eustachian Tube enters (see **Chapter 3**). Consider extending the patient's neck if not contraindicated, or switching to the alternative nostril. Do not use excessive force, which might result in retropharyngeal perforation.
(c) Listen for breath sounds as you advance the ETT. The use of whistle devices such as the BAAM Whistle[79] (***B****eck* ***A****irway* ***A****irflow* ***M****onitor*, Great Plains Ballistics, Inc, Lubbock, TX) (Figure 12.16) or the Patil Audible Intubation Guide (Mercury Medical, Clearwater, FL) (Figure 12.17) to provide an auditory cue in the form of a to-and-fro whistle to facilitate nasotracheal intubation may be useful. Other adjuncts such as the light-guided devices, capnography, and endotracheal tube stethoscopes have also been described.[80–83]

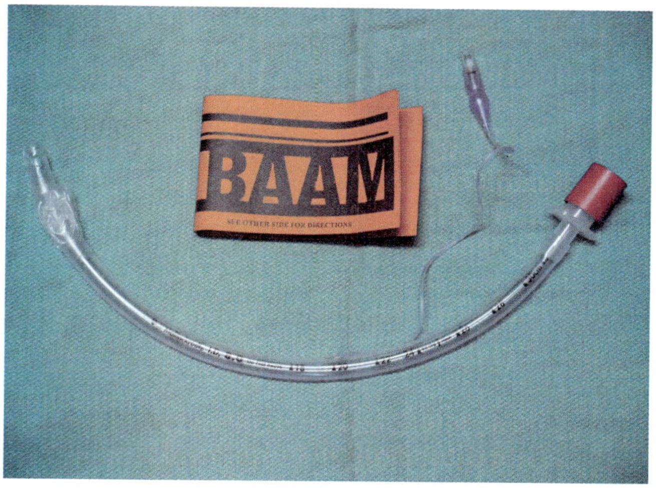

FIGURE 12.16. The BAAM (Beck Airway Airflow Monitor) Whistle.

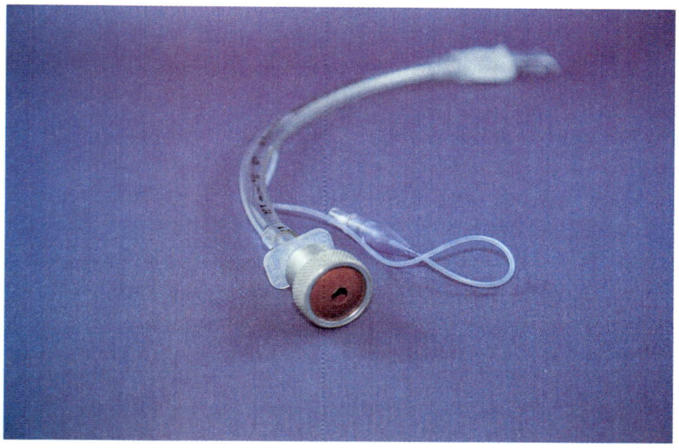

FIGURE 12.17. The Patil Audible Intubation Guide.

Careful inspection and palpation of the neck can also provide useful clues to the location of the tip of the ETT.

(d) Neck flexion is a commonly used maneuver to aid in passage of the ETT into the trachea if the ETT repeatedly impinges anterior to the epiglottis. If esophageal entry occurs repeatedly, neck extension is employed. Clearly, this maneuver should not be performed in patients with known or suspected cervical pathology. Alternatively, the ETT can be withdrawn to the hypopharynx and the cuff of the ETT inflated with 20 mL of air to produce anterior displacement of the ETT tip toward the glottic opening.[49] An Endotrol® ETT (Mallinckrodt Medical Inc Argyle, NY) may increase the success of the technique.[50,84–86] Table 12.1 summarizes the recommended maneuvers for tube manipulation.
(e) Advance the ETT past the vocal cords during inspiration. Confirm ETT placement once tracheal entry is suspected.

Is Blind Nasal Intubation Still Relevant?

The popularity of blind nasal intubation has declined greatly since the advent of paralyzing agents and visual

TABLE 12.1. Recommended Maneuvers for Troubleshooting of Blind Nasal Intubation

Position of the ETT	Recommended Maneuvers
In the pyriform fossa Bulge in lateral neck	• Withdraw ETT into hypopharynx until breath sounds are heard, redirect and rotate ETT away from the bulge. • Turn patient's head to ipsilateral side if no contraindications.
In the esophagus	• Withdraw ETT into hypopharynx, advance ETT after inflating cuff with 20 mL air. ETT will be displaced anteriorly toward glottic opening. Once ETT tip is intralaryngeal, deflate cuff before advancing ETT into trachea. • Slight extension of the neck if not contraindicated. • Use an Endotrol ETT.
Anterior to epiglottis – Supralaryngeal bulge at level of hyoid bone	• Slight flexion of the neck facilitates passage.
Impinging the arytenoid cartilage and vocal cord	• Withdraw ETT and rotate tube gently to realign bevel with vocal cords.

intubating devices. However, blind nasal intubation may be useful in clinical situations where fogging, blood, secretions, and vomitus in the upper airway has rendered visual techniques impossible, or when oral intubation is difficult due to a limited mouth opening and advanced intubating devices are not readily available. Average success rates of blind nasal intubation vary between 57% and 71% with conventional tracheal tubes, and 72% and 86% using directional tip control tubes.[86–89] In under-resourced countries, where expensive video and fiberoptic equipment is lacking, blind nasal intubation may be life-saving in emergency airway management.

Practitioner competence is the most important determinant of success of blind nasal intubation. Teaching this technique does not require special equipment. A simple manikin model (Figure 12.18) can be used to teach blind nasal intubation in a safe and effective manner without jeopardizing patient safety.[90,91] This allows novice practitioners to practice the technique in a controlled environment before bringing blind nasal intubations into real clinical situations.

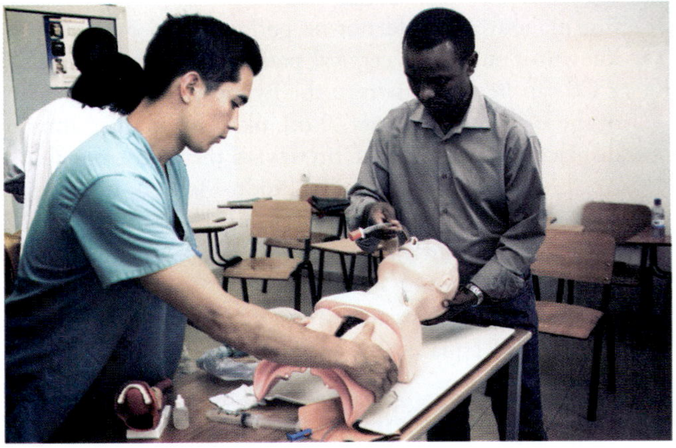

FIGURE 12.18. Teaching blind nasal intubation using a BAAM Whistle in a manakin in Rwanda.

RETROGRADE INTUBATION

What Is Retrograde Intubation and When Was It Introduced?

In 1960, two surgeons, Butler and Cirillo[92] reported the first retrograde intubation in surgical patients through an existing tracheostomy opening. The technique was subsequently modified by Waters[93] who performed a cricothyroid membrane puncture using a Touhy needle. Waters inserted an epidural catheter through the Touhy needle and advanced it cephalad so that the catheter was brought out through the mouth. An ETT was then advanced over the epidural catheter into the trachea while pulling both ends of the catheter taut. After the ETT entered the trachea, the epidural catheter was pulled out through the oral cavity.

How Do You Perform a Retrograde Intubation? (Video 7)

To improve success rates for this technique, many modifications have been suggested since its introduction. For instance, the use of a guidewire rather than an epidural catheter, even though the authors continue to prefer an epidural catheter because it is substantially cheaper, more pliable, and perhaps less traumatic.

(1) Equipment:

Although a preassembled kit is commercially available, the list of equipment necessary for the retrograde intubation is summarized in Table 12.2.

(2) Patient preparation:

In contrast to the sniffing position advocated for laryngoscopic intubation, the patient's head and neck should be in a neutral or relatively extended position to favor an epiglottic position that is off the posterior pharyngeal wall. The epiglottis is almost in contact with the posterior pharyngeal wall when the head is in the sniffing position, making it difficult for the ETT to go underneath the epiglottis. In obese patients or patients with an extremely short neck, placing a pillow under the shoulders and neck may be useful.

TABLE 12.2. Equipment Necessary to Facilitate Light-Guided Retrograde Intubation

Equipment	Function
Chlorhexidine or other antiseptic solutions	To minimize risk of infection
An appropriately sized tracheal tube	For tracheal intubation
An 18-gauge needle or intravenous angiocath	Cricothyroid membrane puncture
A 5-mL fluid-filled syringe	Aspiration of free air
21-gauge epidural catheter (Portex) or a 110 cm long guidewire (0.038-in diameter)	To guide the ETT into the trachea
A tapered anterograde guide catheter is required for the guidewire technique 70 cm	To facilitate the ETT into the trachea
Magill forceps and a laryngoscope	To retrieve the epidural catheter from the oral cavity
Two hemostats	To hold the epidural catheter or guidewire
4 × 4 gauze	To hold the tongue forward during intubation
Water-soluble lubricant	To lubricate the tip of the ETT

(3) The "Classic" Technique:

This technique can be used in patients who are awake under topical anesthesia with sedation or under general anesthesia.[68,94] Although a cricothyroid membrane puncture can be performed using a blunt-tip Touhy needle, the angiocath is less traumatic and substantially easier to use. The cricothyroid membrane is punctured at an angle 90 degree to the skin using the 18-gauge angiocath (or needle) in the midline position. Correct tracheal placement can be confirmed by aspirating a free stream of air bubbles in a fluid-filled syringe. Once the tracheal lumen is entered, the angiocath needle is removed, leaving the catheter behind. The angiocath catheter is then angled at 45 degree in a cephalad direction through which a 21-gauge epidural catheter (or a guidewire) can be inserted and advanced cephalad into the oropharynx. The epidural catheter can be readily retrieved from the mouth using the Magill forceps. After the removal of the angiocath catheter from the anterior neck, and to avoid accidentally pulling the epidural catheter (or the guidewire) through, a hemostat is attached to the distal end of the epidural catheter or guidewire at the skin entry point. Similarly, a hemostat is attached to the epidural catheter or wire where it emerges from the mouth. The epidural catheter or guidewire is then inserted into the ETT. Lubrication of the tip of the ETT will facilitate its entry into the glottic opening. To elevate the tongue and epiglottis away from the posterior pharyngeal wall, the tongue of the patient is then gently pulled forward by an assistant if the procedure is performed under general anesthesia. While pulling the epidural catheter or the guidewire taut from both ends by an assistant, the ETT is inserted into the oropharynx in the midline position. When the tip of the ETT enters the glottic opening, the tension of the epidural catheter at the distal end should be relaxed and the ETT can be advanced gently into the trachea. (For the guidewire technique, the guidewire should be removed before advancing the ETT into the trachea.) While leaving the epidural catheter in place, the correct placement of ETT is confirmed using end-tidal CO_2. The epidural catheter is then removed through the mouth end of the ETT.

What Other Techniques Can Be Used to Improve the Success Rate of the Retrograde Intubation?

While retrograde intubation is a simple technique, the success rate of tracheal intubation is unacceptably low. A study involving 35 cadavers, Lenfant et al.[95] reported a success rate of 69% using the conventional guidewire technique. The investigators suggested that failures were likely due to incorrect positioning of the endotracheal tube. In addition, because of the short distance between the cricothyroid membrane and the vocal cords, the depth of insertion of the ETT is not deep (<10 mm in adults[94]), and accidental extubation can easily occur during the removal of the guidewire with this technique.

A number of technique modifications have been suggested to improve the success rate of the retrograde intubation. These include the insertion of the epidural catheter (or guidewire) through the "Murphy's" eye of the endotracheal tube[96] from "outside" to "inside" to increase the length of ETT actually in the trachea, the use of a subcricoid puncture[97] for the same reason, pulling rather than guided technique,[98] and employing a multi-lumen catheter guide.[99] To increase the stiffness and allow easier negotiation of the ETT through the oropharynx into the trachea, a tapered tip anterograde guide catheter (e.g., pediatric tube changer) placed over the guidewire has been suggested to improve the effectiveness of retrograde intubation.[94,100] Although these modifications are useful, they do not overcome the difficulty of determining the location of the tip of the ETT during intubation. Simultaneous visualization of the ETT passage can be achieved if a flexible endoscope is placed through the nose beforehand.

Retrograde intubation using a guidewire-passed retrograde through the working channel of a flexible bronchoscope has also been shown to be effective as the tip of the ETT can be guided into the glottis under indirect vision.[101–103] However, the bronchoscope is expensive and the retrograde passage of the guidewire through the working channel of the bronchoscope can potentially damage the internal lining of the channel.[104] In addition, visualization of the laryngeal structures through a bronchoscope can also be difficult in the presence of blood and secretions.

The tip of the ETT can also be guided into the trachea using transillumination. The placement of the bulb of an LW at the tip of the ETT during retrograde intubation may assist ETT advancement. A bright circumscribed glow can be readily seen in the anterior neck when the tip of the ETT enters the glottic opening and advances to the cricothyroid membrane puncture site potentially improving the success rate of the technique. The light-guided retrograde intubating technique using the flexible TL (without the stiff internal stylet) has been shown to be an effective and safe in patients with cervical spine instability.[68]

What Is the Clinical Utility of the Retrograde Intubation?

While retrograde intubation is not often considered to be a technique of choice, it remains a useful and effective technique. The technique can be performed either under general anesthesia or awake with skin infiltration and topical anesthesia.[68,94] In the original[105] and the revised American Society of Anesthesiologists Difficult Airway Algorithms,[61,106,107] retrograde intubation is recommended as an alternative method of intubation when encountering a difficult tracheal intubation if the patient's lungs can still be ventilated. In other words, retrograde intubation can play an important role in the management of a "cannot intubate, but can oxygenate" failed airway. It can also be used in patients with a predicted difficult laryngoscopic intubation but no anticipated difficulties in face-mask ventilation, such as patients with cervical spine instability.[68]

What Are the Complications of the Retrograde Intubation?

While the retrograde intubation is an effective intubating technique, it has some potential complications. Although rare, complications, such as sore throat, hoarseness, bleeding (puncture site, and peritracheal hematomas), subcutaneous emphysema, upper airway obstruction (secondary to subcutaneous emphysema), pneumothorax, pneumomediastinum, pre-tracheal abscess, and trigeminal nerve trauma have been reported with retrograde intubation.[94] Fortunately, most of these complications are minor and self-limiting. It should be emphasized that, compared to the Touhy needle, the use of an 18-gauge angiocath or needle has made the cricothyroid membrane puncture substantially easier to perform and less traumatic compared to the Touhy needle. In addition, to avoid wound contamination by oral bacterial flora, the epidural catheter or guidewire should be removed from the cephalad end wherever possible following intubation.

SUMMARY

Although tracheal intubation under direct vision using a laryngoscope remains the conventional method of tracheal intubation, there remains a small percentage of patients and scenarios in which this technique is particularly challenging or even impossible. Many alternative techniques have been developed over the last several decades to improve the success rate of tracheal intubation. However, these techniques often require expensive equipment, specialized skills, and are sometimes not particularly useful for patients in an emergency situation with limited resources or in the presence of a bloody or soiled airway.

Nonvisual intubating techniques play an important role in airway management. Over the last several decades, these nonvisual techniques have been shown to be effective and safe in securing an airway. However, as with all technical skills, one must recognize that there is a learning curve and a skill maintenance requirement for each of these individual techniques to play an important clinical role.

SELF-EVALUATION QUESTIONS

12.1. Which of the following conditions does **NOT** impact the effectiveness of light-guided intubation using a lightwand?

A. Patients with Obesity Class III

B. Foreign body in the upper airway

C. Retropharyngeal abscess

D. Blood and secretion in the oropharynx

E. Large goiter in the anterior neck

12.2. Which of the following modifications has **NOT** been shown to improve the success rate of the retrograde intubation?

A. The use of a subcricoid puncture

B. The use of a guidewire passing through the working channel of a flexible bronchoscope

C. The use of a flexible lightwand

D. The use of a guidewire instead of an epidural catheter

E. The insertion of the guidewire through the "Murphy's" eye of the endotracheal tube during intubation

12.3. Which of the following is **NOT** a characteristic feature of the Eschmann Tracheal Tube Introducer ("gum-elastic bougie")?

A. The Eschmann Introducer is 60 cm long.

B. The Eschmann Introducer has a J (coudé) tip (a 35-degree angle bend) at the distal end.

C. The Eschmann Introducer has a hollow lumen with two side ports.

D. The Eschmann Introducer is a reusable device.

E. The Eschmann Introducer consists of a core of tube woven from polyester threads covered with a resin layer.

REFERENCES

1. Bair AE, Filbin MR, Kulkarni RG, Walls RM. The failed intubation attempt in the emergency department: analysis of prevalence, rescue techniques, and personnel. *J Emerg Med.* 2002;23:131-140.
2. Konrad C, Schupfer G, Wietlisbach M, Gerber H. Learning manual skills in anesthesiology: is there a recommended number of cases for anesthetic procedures? *Anesth Analg.* 1998;86:635-639.
3. Mulcaster JT, Mills J, Hung OR, et al. Laryngoscopic intubation: learning and performance. *Anesthesiology.* 2003;98:23-27.
4. Macintosh RR. An aid to oral intubation (letter). *BMJ.* 1949;1:28.
5. Venn PH. The gum elastic bougie. *Anaesthesia.* 1993;48.
6. El-Orbany MI, Salem MR, Joseph NJ. The Eschmann tracheal tube introducer is not gum, elastic, or a bougie. *Anesthesiology.* 2004;101:1240.
7. Cormack RS, Lehane J. Difficult tracheal intubation in obstetrics. *Anaesthesia.* 1984;39:1105-1111.

8. Hagberg CA. Special devices and techniques. *Anesthesiol Clin North Am.* 2002;20:907-932.
9. Marciniak D, Smith CE. Emergent retrograde tracheal intubation with a gum-elastic bougie in a trauma patient. *Anesth Analg.* 2007;105:1720-1721, table of contents.
10. Braude D, Webb H, Stafford J, et al. The bougie-aided cricothyrotomy. *Air Med J.* 2009;28:191-194.
11. Reardon R, Joing S, Hill C. Bougie-guided cricothyrotomy technique. *Acad Emerg Med.* 2010;17:225.
12. Moscati R, Jehle D, Christiansen G, et al. Endotracheal tube introducer for failed intubations: a variant of the gum elastic bougie. *Ann Emerg Med.* 2000;36:52-56.
13. Hodzovic I, Latto IP, Wilkes AR, Hall JE, Mapleson WW. Evaluation of Frova, single-use intubation introducer, in a manikin. Comparison with Eschmann multiple-use introducer and Portex single-use introducer. *Anaesthesia.* 2004;59:811-816.
14. Levitan R, Ochroch EA. Airway management and direct laryngoscopy a review and update. *Crit Care Clin.* 2000;16:373-388.
15. Weiss M. Management of difficult tracheal intubation with a video-optically modified schroeder intubation stylet. *Anesth Analg.* 1997;85:1181-1182.
16. Dutta A, Kumra VP, Sood J, Swaroop A. Guided tactile probing: a modified blind orotracheal intubation technique for the problem-oriented difficult airway. *Acta Anaesthesiol Scand.* 2005;49:106-109.
17. Ruetzler K, Smereka J, Abelairas-Gomez C, et al. Comparison of the new flexible tip bougie catheter and standard bougie stylet for tracheal intubation by anesthesiologists in different difficult airway scenarios: a randomized crossover trial. *BMC Anesthesiol.* 2020;20:90.
18. Bokhari A, Benham SW, Popat MT. Management of unanticipated difficult intubation: a survey of current practice in the Oxford region. *Eur J Anaesthesiol.* 2004;21:123-127.
19. Combes X, Le Roux B, Suen P, et al. Unanticipated difficult airway in anesthetized patients: prospective validation of a management algorithm. *Anesthesiology.* 2004;100:1146-1150.
20. Nolan JP, Wilson ME. Evaluation of the gum elastic bougie. *Anaesthesia.* 1992;47:878-881.
21. Nolan JP, Wilson ME. Orotracheal intubation patients with potential cervical spine injury. *Anaesthesia.* 1993;48:630-633.
22. Annamaneni R, Hodzovic I, Wilkes AR, Latto IP. A comparison of simulated difficult intubation with multiple-use and single-use bougies in a manikin. *Anaesthesia.* 2003;58:45-49.
23. Jones I, Roberts K. Towards evidence based emergency medicine: best BETs from the Manchester Royal Infirmary. Difficult intubation, the bougie and the stylet. *Emerg Med J.* 2002;19:433-434.
24. Nocera A. A flexible solution for emergency intubation difficulties. *Ann Emerg Med.* 1996;27:665-667.
25. Phelan MP. Use of the endotracheal bougie introducer for difficult intubations. *Am J Emerg Med.* 2004;22:479-482.
26. Morton T, Brady S, Clancy M. Difficult airway management in English emergency departments. *Anaesthesia.* 2000;55:485-488.
27. Henderson JJ, Popat MT, Latto IP, Pearce AC. Difficult Airway Society guidelines for management of the unanticipated difficult intubation. *Anaesthesia.* 2004;59:675-694.
28. Kidd JF, Dyson A, Latto IP. Successful difficult intubation. Use of the gum elastic bougie. *Anaesthesia.* 1988;43.
29. Arndt GA, Cambray AJ, Tomasson J. Intubation bougie dissection of tracheal mucosa and intratracheal airway obstruction. *Anesth Analg.* 2008;107:603-604.
30. Kadry M, Popat M. Pharangeal wall perforation—an unusual complication of blind intubation with a gum elastic bougie. *Anaesthesia.* 1999;54: 393-408.
31. Smith BL. Haemopneumothorax following bougie-assisted tracheal intubation. *Anaesthesia.* 1994;48:91.
32. Gardner M, Janokwski S. Detachment of the tip of a gum-elastic bougie. *Anaesthesia.* 2002;57:88-89.
33. Tuzzo DM, Frova G. Application of the self-inflating bulb to a hollow intubating introducer. *Minerva Anestesiol.* 2001;67:127-132.
34. Mahli N, Md Zain J, Mahdi SNM, et al. The performance of flexible tip bougie in intubating simulated difficult airway model. *Front Med.* (Lausanne) 2021;8:677626.
35. Hung D, McAlpine J, Poulton A, Tsai M, Morrison L, Hung O. A comparative study of airway adjuncts used with a hyperangulated videolaryngoscope to intubate cadavers with a simulated difficult airway. Society of Airway Management Meeting, Tuscan, AR; 2022.
36. Yamamura H, Yamamoto T, Kamiyama M. Device for blind nasal intubation. *Anesthesiology.* 1959;20:221.
37. Ainsworth QP, Howells TH. Transilluminated tracheal intubation. *Br J Anaesth.* 1989;62:494-497.
38. Ellis DG, Stewart RD, Kaplan RM, Jakymec A, Freeman JA, Bleyaert A. Success rates of blind orotracheal intubation using a transillumination technique with a lighted stylet. *Ann Emerg Med.* 1986;15:138-142.
39. Vollmer TP, Stewart RD, Paris PM, Ellis D, Berkebile PE. Use of a lighted stylet for guided orotracheal intubation in the prehospital setting. *Ann Emerg Med.* 1985;14:324-328.
40. Hung OR, Milne A, D'Entremont M, inventors; Scoita MD Engineering Inc, assignee. Tracheal Intubation Device. USA patent US 10,456,025 B2; October 29, 2019.
41. Milne AD, d'Entremont MI, Hung OR. Optimum brightness of a new light-emitting diode lightwand device in a cadaveric model - a pilot study. *Can J Anaesth.* 2016;63:770-771.
42. Nishiyama T, Matsukawa T, Hanaoka K. Safety of a new lightwand device (Trachlight): temperature and histopathological study. *Anesth Analg.* 1998;87:717-718.
43. Hosokawa K, Nakajima Y, Hashimoto S. Chipped rail gear of a lightwand device: a potential complication of tracheal intubation. *Anesthesiology.* 2008;109:355; discussion 6.
44. Chen TH, Tsai SK, Lin CJ, et al. Does the suggested lightwand bent length fit every patient? The relation between bent length and patient's thyroid prominence–to–mandibular angle distance. *Anesthesiology.* 2003;98:1070-1076.
45. Hung OR, Pytka S, Morris I, et al. Clinical trial of a new lightwand (Trachlight™) to intubate the trachea. *Anesthesiology.* 1995;83:509-514.
46. Stewart RD, LaRosee A, Kaplan RM, Ilkhanipour K. Correct positioning of an endotracheal tube using a flexible lighted stylet. *Crit Care Med.* 1990;18:97-99.
47. Hung OR, Tibbet JS, Cheng R, Law JA. Proper preparation of the Trachlight and endotracheal tube to facilitate intubation. *Can J Anaesth.* 2006;53:107-108.
48. Chung YT, Sun MS, Wu HS. Blind nasotracheal intubation is facilitated by neutral head position and endotracheal tube cuff inflation in spontaneously breathing patients. *Can J Anaesth.* 2003;50:511-513.
49. Gorback MS. Inflation of the endotracheal tube cuff as an aid to blind nasal endotracheal intubation [letter]. *Anesth Analg.* 1987;66:913.
50. Asai T. Endotrol tube for blind nasotracheal intubation (Letter). *Anaesthesia.* 1996;50:507.
51. Agro F, Brimacombe J, Marchionni L, Carassiti M, Cataldo R. Nasal intubation with the Trachlight. *Can J Anaesth.* 1999;46:907-908.
52. Aoyama K, Takenaka I, Nagaoka E, et al. Potential damage to the larynx associated with light-guided intubation: a case and series of fiberoptic examinations. *Anesthesiology.* 2001;94:165-167.
53. Stone DJ, Stirt JA, Kaplan MJ, McLean WC. A complication of lightwand-guided nasotracheal intubation. *Anesthesiology.* 1984;61:780-781.
54. Debo RF, Colonna D, Dewerd G, Gonzalez C. Cricoarytenoid subluxation: complication of blind intubation with a lighted stylet. *Ear Nose Throat J.* 1989;68:517-520.
55. Tsutsui T, Setoyama K. A clinical evaluation of blind orotracheal intubation using Trachlight in 511 patients. *Masui.* 2001;50:854-858.
56. Hung OR, Pytka S, Morris I, Murphy M, Stewart RD. Lightwand intubation: II. Clinical trail of a new lightwand to intubate patients with difficult airways. *Can J Anaesth.* 1995;42:826-830.
57. Favaro R, Tordiglione P, Di Lascio F, et al. Effective nasotracheal intubation using a modified transillumination technique. *Can J Anaesth.* 2002;49:91-95.
58. Inoue Y, Koga K, Shigematsu A. A comparison of two tracheal intubation techniques with Trachlight and Fastrach in patients with cervical spine disorders. *Anesth Analg.* 2002;94:667-671; table of contents.
59. Iseki K, Watanabe K, Iwama H. Use of the Trachlight for intubation in the Pierre-Robin syndrome. *Anaesthesia.* 1997;52:801-802.
60. Gille A, Komar K, Schmidt E, Alexander T. Transillumination technique in difficult intubations in heart surgery. *Anasthesiol Intensivmed Notfallmed Schmerzther.* 2002;37:604-608.
61. Apfelbaum JL, Hagberg CA, Connis RT, et al. 2022 American Society of Anesthesiologists Practice Guidelines for Management of the Difficult Airway. *Anesthesiology.* 2022;136:31-81.
62. Agro F, Benumof JL, Carassiti M, Cataldo R, Gherardi S, Barzoi G. Efficacy of a combined technique using the Trachlight together with direct laryngoscopy under simulated difficult airway conditions in 350 anesthetized patients. *Can J Anaesth.* 2002;49:525-526.
63. Asai T, Latto IP. Use of the lighted stylet for tracheal intubation via the laryngeal mask airway. *Br J Anaesth.* 1995;75:503-504.
64. Asai T, Latto IP. Unexpected difficulty in the lighted stylet-aided tracheal intubation via the laryngeal mask. *Br J Anaesth.* 1996;76:111-112.
65. Fan KH, Hung OR, Agro F. A comparative study of tracheal intubation using an intubating laryngeal mask (Fastrach) alone, or together with a lightwand (Trachlight). *J Clin Anesth.* 2000;12:581-585.

66. Gutstein HB. Use of the bullard laryngoscope and lightwand in pediatric patients. *Anesthesiol Clin North Am*. 1998;16:795-812.
67. McGuire G, Krestow M. Bullard assisted trachlight technique. *Can J Anaesth*. 1999;46:907.
68. Hung OR, Al-Qatari M. Light-guided retrograde intubation. *Can J Anaesth*. 1997;44:877-882.
69. Addas BM, Howes WJ, Hung OR. Light-guided tracheal puncture for percutaneous tracheostomy. *Can J Anaesth*. 2000;47:919-922.
70. Stewart RD. Tactile orotracheal intubation. *Ann Emerg Med*. 1984;13:175.
71. Stewart RD. Digital intubation. In: Dailey RH, Simon B, Young GP, Stewart RD, et al., eds. *The Airway: Emergency Management*. St. Louis, MO: Mosby; 1992.
72. Hancock PJ, Peterson G. Finger intubation of the trachea in newborns. *Pediatrics*. 1992;89:325-327.
73. Korber TE, Henneman PL. Digital nasotracheal intubation. *J Emerg Med*. 1989;7.
74. Murphy MF, Hung O. Blind digital intubation. In: Benumof JL, ed. *Airway Management: Principles and Practice*. 1st ed. Philadelphia, PA: Mosby-Year Book Inc; 1996:277-281.
75. Law JA, Broemling N, Cooper RM, et al. The difficult airway with recommendations for management–part 1–difficult tracheal intubation encountered in an unconscious/induced patient. *Can J Anaesth*. 2013;60:1089-1118.
76. Law JA, Duggan LV, Asselin M, et al. Canadian Airway Focus Group updated consensus-based recommendations for management of the difficult airway: part 2. Planning and implementing safe management of the patient with an anticipated difficult airway. *Can J Anaesth*. 2021;68:1405-1436.
77. Aitkenhead AR, Smith G. *Textbook of Anaesthesia*. Edinburg: Churchill Livingstone; 1998.
78. Smith JE, Reid AP. Identifying the more patent nostril before nasotracheal intubation. *Anaesthesia*. 2001;56:258-262.
79. Cook RT Jr, Stene JK, Marcolina B Jr. Use of a Beck Airway Airflow Monitor and controllable-tip endotracheal tube in two cases of nonlaryngoscopic oral intubation. *Am J Emerg Med*. 1995;13:180-183.
80. Dong Y, Li G, Wu W, Su R, Shao Y. Lightwand-guided nasotracheal intubation in oromaxillofacial surgery patients with anticipated difficult airways: a comparison with blind nasal intubation. *Int J Oral Maxillofac Surg*. 2013;42:1049-1053.
81. Harris RD, Gillett MJ, Joseph AP, Vinen JD. An aid to blind nasal intubation. *J Emerg Med*. 1998;16:93-95.
82. King HK, Wooten JD. Blind nasal intubation by monitoring end-tidal CO2. *Anesth Analg*. 1989;69:412-413.
83. Nofal O. Awake light-aided blind nasal intubation: prototype device. *Br J Anaesth*. 2010;104:254-259.
84. Asai T. Use of the endotrol endotracheal tube and a light wand for blind nasotracheal intubation. *Anesthesiology*. 1999;91:1557.
85. Cook RT Jr, Stene JK Jr. The BAAM and endotrol endotracheal tube for blind oral intubation. Beck airway air flow monitor. *J Clin Anesth*. 1993;5:431-432.
86. Hooker EA, Hagan S, Coleman R, Heine MF, Greenwood P. Directional-tip endotracheal tubes for blind nasotracheal intubation. *Acad Emerg Med*. 1996;3:586-589.
87. Dronen SC, Merigian KS, Hedges JR, Hoekstra JW, Borron SW. A comparison of blind nasotracheal and succinylcholine-assisted intubation in the poisoned patient. *Ann Emerg Med*. 1987;16:650-652.
88. O'Brien DJ, Danzl DF, Hooker EA, Daniel LM, Dolan MC. Prehospital blind nasotracheal intubation by paramedics. *Ann Emerg Med*. 1989;18:612-617.
89. O'Connor R E, Megargel RE, Schnyder ME, Madden JF, Bitner M, Ross R. Paramedic success rate for blind nasotracheal intubation is improved with the use of an endotracheal tube with directional tip control. *Ann Emerg Med*. 2000;36:328-332.
90. Iserson KV. Blind nasotracheal intubation: a model for instruction. *Ann Emerg Med*. 1984;13:601-602.
91. Zhang J, Lamb A, Hung O, Hung C, Hung D. Blind nasal intubation: teaching a dying art. *Can J Anaesth*. 2014;61:1055-1056.
92. Butler FS, Circillo AA. Retrograde tracheal intubation. *Anesth Analg*. 1960;39:333-338.
93. Waters DJ. Guided blind endotracheal intubation. *Anaesthesia*. 1963; 18:159.
94. Dhara SS. Retrograde tracheal intubation. *Anaesthesia*. 2009;64: 1094-1104.
95. Lenfant F, Benkhadra M, Trouilloud P, Freysz M. Comparison of two techniques for retrograde tracheal intubation in human fresh cadavers. *Anesthesiology*. 2006;104:48-51.
96. Bourke D. Modification of retrograde guide for endotracheal intubation. *Anesth Analg*. 1974;53:1013-1014.
97. Shantha TR. Retrograde intubation using the subcricoid region. *Br J Anaesth*. 1992;68:109-112.
98. Abdou-Madi MN, Trop D. Pulling versus guiding: a modification of retrograde guided intubation. *Can J Anaesth*. 1989;36:336-339.
99. Dhara SS. Retrograde intubation - a facilitated approach. *Br J Anaesth*. 1992;69:631-633.
100. Tobias R. Increased success with retrograde guide for endotracheal intubation. *Anesth Analg*. 1983;62:366-367.
101. Carlson CA, Perkins HM. Solving a difficult intubation. *Anesthesiology*. 1986;64:537.
102. Przybylo HJ, Stevenson GW, Vicari FA, Horn B, Hall SC. Retrograde fibreoptic intubation in a child with Nager's syndrome. *Can J Anaesth*. 1996;43:697-699.
103. Rosenblatt WH, Angood PB, Maranets I, Kaklamanos IG, Garwood S. Retrograde fiberoptic intubation. *Anesth Analg*. 1997;84:1142-1144.
104. Ovassapian A, Mesnick PS. The art of fiberoptic intubation. *Anesthesiol Clinic North America*. 1995;13:391-409.
105. American Society of Anesthesiologists Task Force on Management of the Difficult Airway. Practice guidelines for the difficult airway. *Anesthesiology*. 1993;78:597-602.
106. American Society of Anesthesiologists Task Force on Management of the Difficult Airway. Practice guidelines for management of the difficult airway: an updated report by the American Society of Anesthesiologists Task Force on Management of the Difficult Airway. *Anesthesiology*. 2003;98:1269-1277.
107. Apfelbaum JL, Hagberg CA, Caplan RA, et al. Practice guidelines for management of the difficult airway: an updated report by the American Society of Anesthesiologists Task Force on Management of the Difficult Airway. *Anesthesiology*. 2013;118:251-270.

CHAPTER 13

Extraglottic Devices for Ventilation and Oxygenation

Matthew Mackin, Orlando R. Hung, and Thomas J. Coonan

CASE PRESENTATION

A 57-year-old male was admitted for laparoscopic appendectomy for acute appendicitis. He was otherwise healthy, apart from essential hypertension, for which he took hydrochlorothiazide. He had fasted for more than 12 hours.

On examination, he was lying on a stretcher in a moderate amount of pain. He was hemodynamically stable. His height was 183 cm and his weight was 80 kg, with a BMI 23.9 kg·m^{-2}. His airway examination demonstrated a Mallampati score of II, mouth opening of 4.5 cm, thyromental distance of 6 cm, and good jaw protrusion. He had a full set of teeth, was not obese, and was estimated to be easy to ventilate. His cardiac and respiratory examinations were normal.

The patient was premedicated with intravenous midazolam 1 mg, fentanyl 200 μg, and this was followed by denitrogenation with 100% oxygen by face mask. As he did not have any indicators of a difficult airway, a decision was made to induce anesthesia with propofol 200 mg and rocuronium 50 mg. Face-mask ventilation (FMV) was established with an oral airway. Initial evaluation with direct laryngoscopy (DL), using a Macintosh laryngoscope, showed a Cormack-Lehane (C/L) grade 3 view. The first attempt with DL and an Eschmann Tracheal Introducer (ETI) resulted in an esophageal intubation. FMV was re-established and a GlideScope® was prepared. When the GlideScope was inserted, only the posterior arytenoids could be visualized, and two attempts with an endotracheal tube (ETT) stylet and a tracheal tube introducer were unsuccessful (and were associated with a small amount of bleeding in the oropharynx).

At this point, the decision was made to attempt flexible bronchoscopy (FB). Unfortunately, FMV became more difficult, the patient's oxygen saturation dropped into the low 80s, and it became necessary to insert nasal and oral pharyngeal airways and begin a two-hand and two-person FMV technique. A #4 Laryngeal Mask Airway® (LMA®-Classic™) was rapidly prepared and inserted without complication, at which point it became possible to easily ventilate the patient. Sevoflurane was selected to maintain anesthesia, and to manage escalating tachycardia and hypertension. A pediatric bronchoscope with an ensleeved Aintree Intubation Catheter (AIC, Cook Medical Inc, Bloomington, IN) was then inserted through the LMA-Classic into the trachea. Both the bronchoscope and the LMA-Classic were then removed leaving the AIC in the trachea. An ETT was advanced into the trachea over the AIC. Correct tracheal placement was confirmed by auscultation and capnograph recording.

The surgery was uneventful, and the patient emerged from anesthesia fully awake, warm, with adequate analgesia, and with no residual neuromuscular blockade. The difficult airway cart was brought to the room. Tracheal extubation was uneventful, although he did complain of a sore throat in the postanesthetic care unit, which gradually improved. He was later informed of the difficulty and provided with a notice to inform any subsequent anesthesia practitioner of his difficult airway.

INTRODUCTION

What Are Extraglottic Devices (EGDs)? Why Do We Need These Devices?

Difficulties in airway management are associated with significant morbidity and mortality,[1] and it is crucial that practitioners responsible for airway management continue to refine existing skills and acquire new knowledge and skills as they become available. Two decades ago, ventilation and oxygenation were achieved primarily via a face mask or an ETT.

While FMV is seemingly simple to perform, it has limitations.[2,3] Tracheal intubation has been considered the "gold standard" for providing effective ventilation, while at the same time providing protection from the aspiration of gastric contents. However, tracheal intubation is a skill that is not easily mastered[4] and requires regular practice. Employing an EGD to successfully facilitate gas exchange may be a more easily acquired skill for the nonexpert airway practitioner.

In contrast to a mask placed on the face to provide FMV, an EGD establishes a direct conduit for air to flow when placed in the periglottic area. Although the terms EGD and "supraglottic airway devices" (SGA) are often used interchangeably, we do not feel this is correct. The classification of these devices has never been formally established. Previously, it was recommended that they be classified based upon the sequence in development.[5] To date, the American Society of Anesthesiologists (ASA) continues to use this categorization of devices.[6] Due to the increasing confusion associated with this terminology, as this does not always indicate superior devices, alternative classifications have been suggested.

It has been suggested that EGDs should be classified on the basis of the presence of the following features: a high seal pressure, gastric access, and ability to intubate.[7] Based upon these criteria, EGDs with these features would be considered advanced extraglottic airway devices (EADs). It is our opinion that EGDs be categorized into two groups: supraglottic and infraglottic. Infraglottic devices have components that extend infraglottically (e.g., the Combitube®, the Laryngeal Tube® [King LT in North America], and the EasyTube®).[8] Supraglottic airway devices, such as the LMA-Classic, i-gel® (Intersurgical Ltd, UK), and the AuraGain™ (Ambu, Ballerup, Denmark), would sit superiorly to the glottic opening. The terminology around these latter devices has been somewhat confusing since some have referred to these devices as "supraglottic airway devices," or SGAs. Hence, we agree with Brimacombe that the term "extraglottic devices," or EGDs, is the more appropriate terminology.[8]

EGDs vary in size, shape, and material. Most have balloons, or cuffs, that upon inflation can provide a reasonably tight seal in the upper airway. As illustrated in the case presentation, these EGDs (including the LMA-Classic) have been used successfully as rescue airway devices. There is clear evidence of their effectiveness and safety in providing ventilation and oxygenation. These devices have changed the landscape of contemporary airway management and they are part of the Difficult Airway Management Algorithm recommended by the ASA,[6] the Canadian Airway Focus Group,[9,10] and the Difficult Airway Society[11] in managing unanticipated difficult intubations in adults.

Do Manufacturing Standards Exist for EGDs to Ensure Patient Safety?

The American Society for Testing and Materials Standards (ASTM) Committee F29 on Anesthetic and Respiratory Equipment has proposed the establishment of standards related to EGDs used in human subjects. A task group has proposed the standardization of terminology, design, production, manufacturing, testing, labeling, and promotion. Devices produced according to the proposed ASTM standards will:

- Facilitate unobstructed access of respiratory gases to the glottic inlet by displacing tissue.
- Not require a (external) facial seal to maintain airway patency.
- Terminate in a 15/22 mm connector to facilitate positive pressure ventilation (PPV) via an anesthetic breathing system.
- Be capable of maintaining airway patency when the (15/22 mm) airway connector is open to ambient atmosphere.
- Minimize the escape of airway gases to the atmosphere.

What EGDs Are Commercially Available?

Many EGDs have been introduced.[8] The best known are the LMA-Classic, LMA®-ProSeal™ (PLMA), LMA-Fastrach™ (or Intubating LMA [ILMA]), LMA®-Supreme™ (LMAS), LMA®-Protector™ (LMAP), and Combitube (CBT). Other EGDs include the Laryngeal Tube (LT), CobraPLA® (CPLA), Airway Management Device® (AMD), LaryVent® (LV), Air-Q® device, Ambu AuraGain Laryngeal Mask, Portex® Soft Seal® Laryngeal Mask, Streamlined Liner of the Pharynx Airway (SLIPA®), i-gel, and Baska® Mask.

At least 25 different types of EGDs are available.[12] There is sufficient information available on these EGDs in the literature. This chapter will review the commonly used EGDs, but it will not be an exhaustive review. Some devices (e.g., the COPA, LaryVent, Airway Management Device, and PAxpress®) are no longer manufactured, and so they would not be discussed in this chapter. For clarity, we have divided the EGDs into two separate groups: the Inflatable Cuff EGDs and Noninflatable Cuff EGDs.

NONINFLATABLE CUFF EXTRAGLOTTIC DEVICE: LARYNGEAL MASK AIRWAY, LMA-CLASSIC

What Is the LMA? When Was It Introduced?

The LMA (Teleflex®, Morrisville, NC [Figure 13.1]) was designed in 1981 by Dr. Archie Brain, as he searched for a device that was easier to use and more effective than the face mask and less invasive than an ETT. The LMA is designed to cover the periglottic area and provide continuity of airflow between the environment and the lungs. The device has a wide-bore tube connecting to an oval inflatable cuff that seals around the larynx. It is currently available in eight different sizes for use in patients ranging from neonates to large adults. For simplicity reasons and to avoid confusion, the LMA will be used to refer to the original laryngeal mask airway designed by Dr. Brain (i.e., the LMA-Classic) throughout this chapter unless otherwise specified. Typically, a #3 LMA is used in teenagers and small adult females, while #4, #5, and #6 are used in average and large size adults.

The use of LMAs has transformed the practice of anesthesiology and airway management.[13,14] The LMA is specified in the ASA's Difficult Airway Management Algorithm.[6,15,16] Moreover, the LMA has a role in emergency airway management during cardiopulmonary resuscitation (CPR), the transport of critically ill patients, and in the intensive care unit.[17,18] Although the LMA is a potentially useful device in situations in which tracheal intubation and mask ventilation are not possible (e.g., "can't intubate, can't ventilate" [CICV], or more appropriately "can't intubate, can't oxygenate" [CICO]),[6,15,16,19,20] it should never be used as a substitute for a front-of-neck airway (see Chapter 2). While this device can provide adequate ventilation and oxygenation, it does not protect the airway from aspiration, and it does not easily allow for the removal of pulmonary secretions. Therefore, when employed as a rescue airway device, the LMA can only be considered a temporizing measure until a more definitive and protective airway is secured.

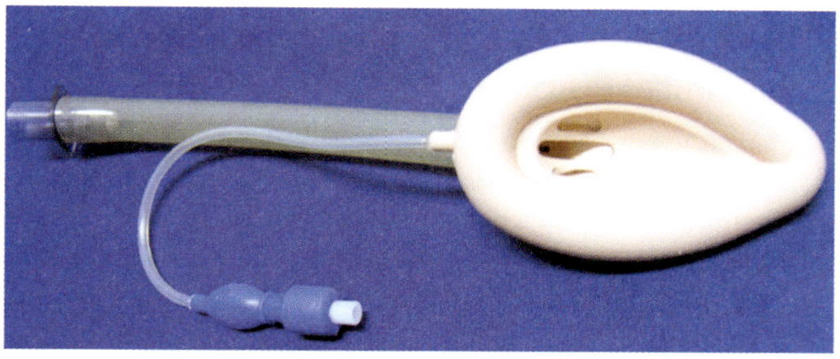

FIGURE 13.1. The LMA-Classic has a wide-bore tube connected to an oval inflatable cuff that seals around the larynx and the aperture bars.

What Is the Proper Way to Insert the LMA?

While many techniques have been suggested for the insertion of the device, including the midline approach, the lateral approach, and the thumb technique,[21] the authors recommend the following steps:

1. To minimize the risk of downfolding the epiglottis, it is recommended that the cuff be completely deflated.
2. The LMA cuff should be well lubricated with a water-soluble lubricant.
3. Provided that there is no contraindication to moving the cervical spine, the patient's head and neck should be placed in a sniffing position. A head tilt will help to open the mouth.
4. In order to have clear access to the glottic opening and minimize downfolding of the epiglottis, it is recommended that the practitioner perform a jaw lift using the thumb and index finger of the nondominant hand. This lifts the tongue and epiglottis away from the posterior pharyngeal wall to facilitate placement of the LMA. The LMA should be inserted into the mouth with the index finger placed at the mask-tube junction, pressing the cuff against the hard palate and advancing the LMA into the oropharynx following the natural curve of the posterior pharyngeal wall. The dimensions and design of the device allow the tip of the LMA to wedge into the hypopharynx. A definite resistance should be felt when the tip of the LMA enters the hypopharynx. Occasionally, resistance is encountered during insertion because of backward folding of the cuff (also called "tip roll"). Sweeping a finger behind the cuff to redirect it inferiorly into the laryngopharynx can usually overcome this problem.[22]
5. Following placement, the cuff should be inflated with the minimal volume of air necessary to achieve an adequate seal. However, this "just-seal" volume may not be adequate to seal the hypopharynx from the esophagus.[21] Therefore, most practitioners commonly inflate the cuff with more volume. In general, approximately 20 mL is required for #3, 30 mL for #4, and 40 mL for #5 LMA. Seal characteristics may be improved by ensuring that the LMA is secured in the midline of the mouth, and the head and neck placed in a neutral position.
6. The LMA should be fixed in position by taping it to the face, or by attaching it to the anesthesia breathing circuit.[23]

Since blind insertion technique of EGD is easy and simple with a good success rate, it is generally the preferred method to place EGD. Recently, a number of studies have shown that both direct laryngoscopy and indirect laryngoscopy can facilitate the EGD placement when encountering difficulties.[9,24,25] More clinical data are needed before visually guided EGD placement using either a direct or an indirect laryngoscope can be recommended for routine use (Videos 9 and 20).

What Is the Proper Way to Remove the LMA?

In its normal position, the LMA is less stimulating than an ETT and is generally well tolerated by most patients on emergence. Many studies have compared removal under deep anesthesia versus while awake. Although airway obstruction appears to be less frequent if the device is removed with the patient awake, this technique is associated with more coughing, laryngospasm, biting, and hypersalivation.[26] While much controversy remains, it is the opinion of the authors that, in adults, the LMA should be removed awake. This is particularly true if FMV is expected to be difficult. However, many pediatric airway practitioners prefer removal under deep anesthesia, as children are more prone to laryngospasm.

It is unclear whether the LMA should be removed with the cuff deflated or inflated. Some recommend an inflated cuff because of its capacity to remove secretions that accumulate above the device from the oral cavity.[27] Others argue that the cuff should be deflated to minimize trauma and damage to the cuff itself. Brimacombe recommends the removal of the LMA with the cuff partially deflated.[26]

What Are the Advantages and Disadvantages of Using the LMA as Opposed to an Endotracheal Tube?

Brimacombe conducted a meta-analysis of randomized prospective trials involving 2440 patients comparing the LMA with other forms of airway management, including tracheal intubation.[28] He reported many advantages of the LMA including rapidity and ease of placement (particularly for inexperienced practitioners), improved hemodynamic stability on induction and during emergence, minimal rise in intraocular pressure following insertion, reduced anesthetic requirements for airway tolerance, lower frequency of coughing during emergence, improved oxygen saturation during emergence, and a lower incidence of sore throat in adults.

An additional advantage of the LMA is its utility as a rescue device and during resuscitation.[29] Furthermore, studies have shown that the LMA has less impact on mucociliary clearance than an ETT, and may reduce the risk of retention of secretions, atelectasis, and pulmonary infection.[30]

The major disadvantage of the LMA is its inability to seal the larynx and protect against aspiration, gastric insufflation, and air leak with PPV.[28] The mask is designed in such a way that the distal end of the device is intended to become wedged into the upper esophageal sphincter. However, in reality, the distal end may lie anywhere from the nasopharynx to the hypopharynx.

The magnitude of potential gastric insufflation probably depends on the airway pressure generated and the position of the LMA. However, a very large study has shown that PPV with the LMA is both safe and effective, with no episodes of gastric dilatation in 11,910 patients on LMA anesthetics under both spontaneous ventilation and PPV.[31]

According to a meta-analysis involving 547 LMA publications, the incidence of gastric aspiration associated with the use of laryngeal mask airway is rare (0.02%),[28] and most of these cases had predisposing risk factors for pulmonary aspiration. However, fatal aspiration of gastric content has been reported,[32] and so proper assessment for aspiration risk prior to the use of the LMA is imperative. Of note, LMA use during prehospital care in patients who did not fast was found to have no significant difference in rates of aspiration with LMA versus ETT.[33] Most airway practitioners hesitate to use the LMA in patients with a history of symptomatic hiatal hernia, gastroesophageal reflux, in obstetrical patients, or in patients with a bowel obstruction. Careful placement of the device, and vigilance at emergence from anesthesia, may attenuate the risk of gastric aspiration.

Is It Safe to Use the LMA for Positive Pressure Ventilation?

Over the past two decades, the use of a face mask to facilitate the administration of anesthesia has largely been replaced by the LMA. While a few studies have reported the successful use of the LMA for PPV in a variety of patient populations and procedures,[34–36] they involved mostly small numbers of patients, with few large prospective randomized trials.[37] In a study involving 65,712 patients, Bernardini and Natalini[38] compared the risk of pulmonary aspiration with PPV via an ETT (30,082 procedures) to PPV with an LMA (35,630 procedures). Although three pulmonary aspirations occurred in the LMA group compared to seven with the ETT, there were no deaths related to these pulmonary aspirations. The investigators concluded that while there was a selection bias related to contraindications and exclusions to the use of the LMA in their study group, the use of a laryngeal mask airway was not associated with an increased risk of pulmonary aspiration compared with an ETT in this selected population.

Based on the current evidence, the LMA appears to be effective and probably safe for PPV in patients with normal airway resistance and compliance and normal tidal volumes. However, gastroesophageal insufflation may occur when the LMA is used in conjunction with, and in the presence of, decreased pulmonary or chest wall compliance.[39,40]

Pressure-controlled ventilation (PCV), rather than volume-controlled ventilation (VCV), may provide effective mechanical ventilation in patients with high airway pressure, or reduced lung compliance, while at the same time minimizing the risk of gastric insufflation with the LMA.[41] It must be re-emphasized that, although rare, cases of serious and even fatal gastric aspiration associated with the use of LMA have been reported.[32,42–46] Because of the potential for serious complications, more evidence with studies involving a large number of patients may be needed to confirm the safety of the use of the LMA for PPV.

How Are LMAs Used Appropriately in Clinical Practice?

Since its introduction in 1988, the LMA has been used in more than 200 million patients worldwide,[14] and it has largely replaced the ETT and face mask for patients undergoing simple and uncomplicated surgical procedures. The extensive use of the LMA is a reflection of its overwhelming effectiveness and safety in a variety of age groups and surgical procedures. The LMA has also been shown to be effective and safe for elective cesarean section in nonobese parturients, though its use for this indication is controversial.[47]

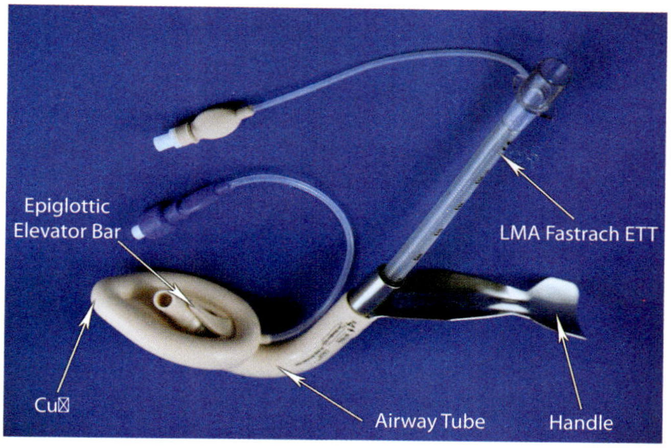

FIGURE 13.2. The LMA-Fastrach or Intubating LMA (ILMA) has a rigid curved metal airway tube with a manipulating handle, an epiglottic elevating bar, a deeper bowl, and a ramp that directs an endotracheal tube (ETT) up and into the larynx, enhancing the success rate of blind intubation. In this figure, a dedicated wire-reinforced silicone-tipped ETT is inserted into the metal lumen of the ILMA. When the horizontal black line on the ETT meets the proximal end of the ILMA, the tip of the ETT will emerge from beneath the epiglottic elevating bar.

A meta-analysis of currently available data shows that the LMA is safe and effective for pediatric airway management.[48] Furthermore, the LMA has been used successfully in the management of large numbers of difficult pediatric airways associated with a variety of congenital anomalies. In 2010, Weiss and Engelhardt[49] proposed the use of LMA in the management of the unexpected difficult pediatric airway algorithm.

The LMA was approved for resuscitation by the European Resuscitation Council in 1996,[50] and the American Heart Association (AHA) in 2000.[51] However, the possibility of gastric insufflation, related to high peak airway pressure, continues to be a concern in these patient populations, similar to those managed with FMV.

Brimacombe summarized the available evidence with respect to the use of the LMA in the management of the difficult and failed airway.[52] With the exception of airway pathology that may interfere with the LMA placement or seal, there is a considerable body of evidence to support the use of the LMA in both predicted and unpredicted difficult airways.[6,9–11]

The LMA also provides a conduit for tracheal intubation using either a blind technique, a transillumination technique (using the Trachlight® without the stiff wire stylet),[53,54] or an FB together with an AIC.[55,56] Intubation success rates through the LMA have been found to be similar for patients with both normal and abnormal airways.[57]

The Flexible Laryngeal Mask Airway™ (FLMA) was specifically designed for use in ear, nose and throat, head and neck, and dental surgery. It has been used for adenotonsillectomy,[58] laser pharyngoplasty,[59] and dental extraction.[60] The device consists of an LMA bowl connected to a floppy, wire-reinforced tube with a slightly narrower bore than the LMA. The long, flexible, narrow-bore tube provides better surgical access to the oropharyngeal cavity than the standard laryngeal mask airway. The technique for placement of the FLMA is similar to that for the LMA.

The reusable LMA is the *original* LMA-Classic. Variations on the original include:

- LMA-Fastrach, also known as the Intubating LMA (ILMA), and also available in a disposable form (Figure 13.2).
- LMA®-Flexible™, similar in design to the Classic, but incorporating a nonkinkable, wire-reinforced tube.
- LMA-ProSeal (PLMA), a second-generation EGD that has improved seal characteristics and incorporates a gastric drainage capability (Figures 13.3 and 13.4).

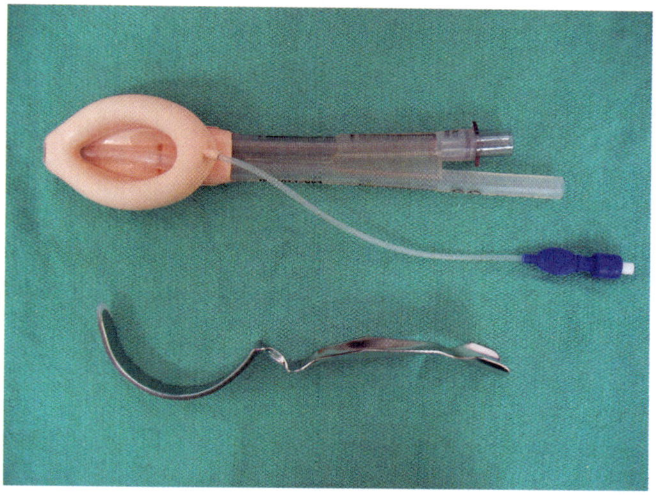

FIGURE 13.3. The LMA-ProSeal (PLMA) incorporates a drainage tube placed lateral to the airway tube and a second dorsal cuff. The drainage tube travels from the proximal end of the device through the bowl opening into the upper esophagus. It permits the insertion of standard nasogastric tubes to facilitate the drainage of gastric contents. Also shown is the metal introducer employed to facilitate placement of the PLMA.

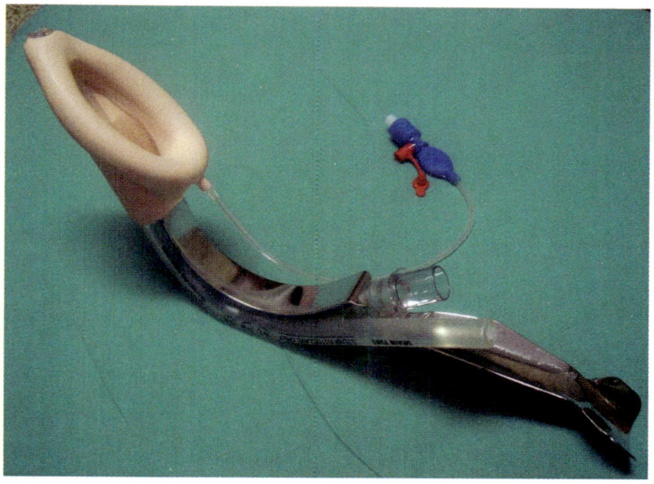

FIGURE 13.4. The LMA-ProSeal (PLMA) loaded onto the introducer. The distal end of the metal introducer is placed in an "insertion strap" on the PLMA and the airway tube is folded around the introducer and "clipped" into a proximal matching slot.

- LMA®-Unique™, a single-use device virtually identical to the Classic (Figure 13.5).
- LMA-Supreme (LMAS), a disposable second-generation EGD that incorporates the insertion advantages of the Fastrach, with the seal and drainage characteristics of the PLMA (Figure 13.6).
- LMA-Protector (LMAP), a new disposable second-generation silicone EGD that also incorporates the insertion advantages of the LMA-Fastrach. It has two drainage channels that emerge as separate ports proximally. It also has a built-in bite block to reduce the risk of obstruction of the airway tube in the event of biting (Figure 13.7).

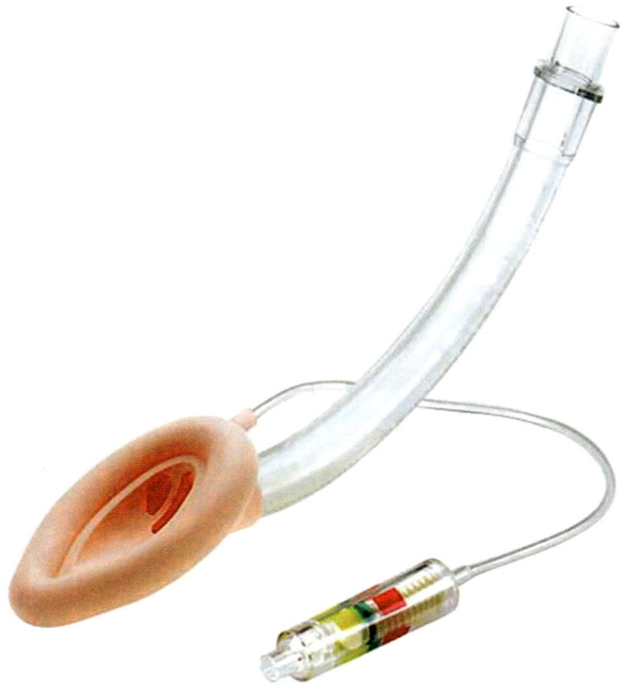

FIGURE 13.5. The LMA-Unique is a single-use device virtually identical to the LMA-Classic with aperture bars.

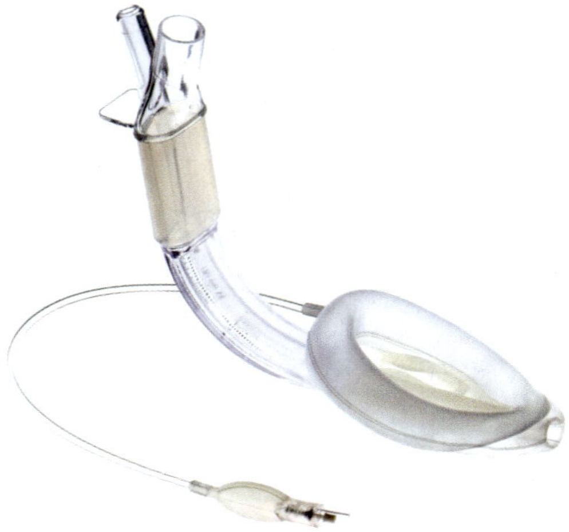

FIGURE 13.6. The LMA-Supreme is a new disposable device that incorporates the insertion advantages of the LMA-Fastrach and the seal characteristics of the LMA-ProSeal.

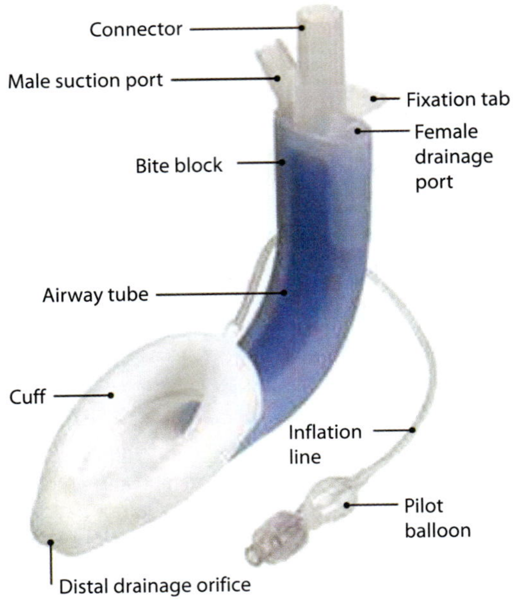

FIGURE 13.7. The LMA-Protector is a new disposable silicone extraglottic device that incorporates the seal and drainage characteristics of the LMA-ProSeal. It has two separate proximal drainage ports (a male suction port and a female drainage port) which have drainage channels that run distally into a chamber behind the cuff bowl. The chamber then narrows distally into the orifice at the tip of the cuff which communicates closely with the upper esophageal sphincter. It also has an anatomically shaped airway tube similar to that of the LMA-Unique and a built-in bite block.

INTUBATING LARYNGEAL MASK AIRWAY: LMA-FASTRACH (ILMA)

What Is the LMA-Fastrach, or Intubating LMA (ILMA), and Why Was It Developed?

While it is possible to intubate the trachea through an LMA, success rates are variable. The Intubating LMA (LMA-Fastrach [ILMA], Teleflex [Figure 13.2]) was designed by Dr. Brain. The device has a rigid metal curved airway tube with a guiding handle, an epiglottic elevating bar, a deeper bowl, and ramp that directs an ETT up and into the larynx. The device is easy to use, is associated with high success rates of intubation, and has received widespread acceptance. The ILMA is a reusable device which can be cleaned and sterilized using an autoclave. Single-use ILMAs are also available.

How Is Tracheal Intubation Performed Using the ILMA? (Video 26)

Tracheal intubation through the ILMA can be achieved blindly. To facilitate the insertion of an ETT through the ILMA, the following steps are recommended:

1. Lubricate the ILMA and the ETT (including the connector of the tracheal tube) with a water-soluble lubricant. Ensure that the ETT slides easily through the ILMA.
2. With the patient in a sniffing position, open the airway by using a head tilt. It should be emphasized that the insertion

of an ILMA may be difficult if the interincisor gap is less than 20 mm.

3. Grasp the metal handle of the ILMA and insert the device straight back over the tongue to the back of the oropharynx. Then, advance the cuff into the hypopharynx, following the palatopharyngeal curve by rotating the device using the metal handle and maintaining gentle pressure against the palate. Once in place, inflate the cuff to achieve a seal for manual ventilation. The metal handle may be used to manipulate the device to achieve a seal to ensure adequate ventilation and oxygenation. The device should be gently rotated in the sagittal plane (commonly known as the "first" Chandy maneuver) to establish optimally unobstructed ventilation.[61]
4. While a number of ETTs, including the Mallinckrodt Hi-Lo PVC tube®, can be used for tracheal intubation, the dedicated wire-reinforced silicone-tipped ETT supplied with the ILMA has been shown to give the highest success rates.[62] With the black vertical line on the tube facing the practitioner, insert the tube into the metal lumen of the ILMA until the horizontal black line on the tracheal tube meets the proximal end of the ILMA metal tube (see Figure 13.2). At this point, the tip of the silicone-tipped ETT is just emerging from beneath the epiglottic elevating bar. Resistance will be felt as the silicone-tipped ETT elevates this bar exiting the distal end of the ILMA and entering the patient's glottis (see Figure 13.2).
5. Tracheal placement is confirmed in the usual manner. Manipulation of the ILMA by lifting the device from the posterior pharyngeal wall using the metal handle (the "second" Chandy maneuver) may enhance successful passage of the ETT in the event of failure. This maneuver helps to prevent the silicone-tipped ETT from colliding with the arytenoids and minimizes the angle between the aperture of the ILMA and the glottis.[63]

Some evidence suggests that the ILMA in situ produces sufficient pressure on the posterior hypopharyngeal wall to potentially compromise mucosal blood flow.[64] For this reason, except perhaps in an airway rescue or resuscitation situation, it is recommended that the device be removed over the ETT. A stabilizing rod is provided with the ILMA to hold the ETT in position while the ILMA is withdrawn.

Many investigators have studied the effectiveness of the blind intubating technique through the ILMA. The reported mean (range) first-time and overall success rate is 73% (53-100) and 90% (44-100), respectively.[64] Several factors that *decrease* success rates of blind intubation through the ILMA technique have been identified: the use of a #3 ILMA, instead of #4 or #5 ILMA, for adult male patients; the application of cricoid pressure; lifting the ILMA handle; the use of a collar; and an inexperienced practitioner.

What Other Techniques Have Been Described to Enhance Success Rates for Tracheal Intubation Through the ILMA?

Several studies have been published evaluating the effectiveness of airway devices to assist ILMA intubation. The overall success rate appears to be better than the blind technique. Light-guided techniques employing a flexible lightwand (Trachlight) have also been investigated, and have demonstrated improved success rates.[65] Lightwand-guided intubation through the ILMA has a first-time and overall success rate of 84% and 99%, respectively.[64] Several researchers have shown high success rates with a lightwand-guided tracheal intubation through an ILMA.[66,67]

Pandit et al.[68] found that bronchoscopic-guided intubation had a higher success rate (95%) through the ILMA than through the LMA (80%), although the time to intubation was longer with the FB-assisted technique, compared to the blind technique (74 vs. 49 seconds). Overall, in a range of studies, FB-guided intubation through the ILMA has a first-time and overall success rate of 87% and 96%, respectively. However, following a failed blind technique, flexible FB-guided intubation through the ILMA has a success rate of only 86%.[64] Agro et al.[69] reported the use of a shorter semirigid fiberoptic device, the Shikani Seeing Eye Stylet® (Clarus Medical, Minneapolis, MN, USA), to facilitate an ILMA intubation. Although tracheal intubation was successful, the investigators commented that the major limitation of the Shikani device was its inability to control the direction of the tip of the device.

Using the Patil Intubation Guide® (Anesthesia Associates Inc, San Marcos, CA, USA), a whistle diaphragm to detect breath sounds, Osborn successfully intubated the trachea through the ILMA under topical anesthesia in a patient with a recent cervical spine fusion.[70] In 2005, a case series was published describing the successful use of the airway whistle with the ILMA in four patients with known difficult airways.[71]

What Are the Indications for the ILMA?

The ILMA alone does not prevent the aspiration of gastric contents and may produce hypopharyngeal mucosal ischemia if it is left in place for a prolonged duration. Therefore, its role in routine airway management may be limited. However, when used as a temporizing measure, it is a highly effective device in the emergency environment, as an adjunct to a failed or difficult FMV, and as a rescue device in a failed airway. Brain has suggested that the ILMA may not be indicated when the patient is anticipated to be an easy intubation (easy DL), but may be of considerable benefit when the glottis is high and anterior (difficult DL). Furthermore, studies have confirmed earlier findings that ventilation and intubation through the ILMA can be successfully achieved in obese patients.[72,73]

With respect to Emergency Medical Services (EMS) and prehospital care, the importance of early and effective airway control is universally acknowledged. Tracheal intubation under DL is associated with a number of practical problems in prehospital trauma, and there is evidence to suggest that the ILMA may play an important role, in the prehospital setting, in securing the airway of trauma patients with a head injury.[74,75]

Gercek et al.[76] compared the degree of cervical spine movement of three common methods of tracheal intubation in patients with c-spine injuries (DL, ILMA, and FB) using real-time, three-dimensional ultrasonography in healthy elective surgical patients with manual in-line immobilization. They showed that manual in-line immobilization reduced the cervical spine range of motion during different intubation procedures to a limited extent. The least diminution (i.e., the greatest c-spine movement) occurred with DL (with an overall flexion/extension range of 17.57 degrees) versus significantly less c-spine movement with ILMA (overall flexion/extension range of 4.60 degrees), and FB use (overall flexion/extension range of 3.61 degrees—oral, 5.88 degrees—nasal). Furthermore, the mean (±SD) total time required for intubation was shortest for the ILMA (16.5 ± 9.76 s), followed by DL (27.25 ± 8.56 s), and the longest for both FB techniques (oral: 52.91 ± 56.27 s, nasal: 82.32 ± 54.06 s).

The prime role of the ILMA lies in managing the airway of patients with a difficult or a failed airway. From a retrospective study involving 254 patients with difficult airways (including patients with Cormack-Lehane (C/L) Grade 4 views, immobilized cervical spines, stereotactic frames, or airways distorted by surgery or radiation therapy), the clinical experience with the ILMA (both elective and emergency use) has been largely positive.[63]

The Difficult Airway Society (UK) guidelines for management of the unanticipated difficult tracheal intubation in the nonobstetric adult patient without upper airway obstruction include the ILMA.[11,77]

LMA-PROSEAL (PLMA)

What Is the PLMA? How Does It Differ from the LMA?

The PLMA (Teleflex [Figure 13.3]) is a "second-generation" laryngeal mask airway that incorporates several modifications to the LMA:

- An esophageal conduit is incorporated to provide access to the esophagus and the gastrointestinal tract in order to minimize the risk of aspiration. This incorporated conduit renders a "dual-tube" look to the device.
- A second cuff on the "dorsal" aspect of the PLMA is intended to enhance the seal characteristics of the device.
- The PLMA lacks mask aperture bars, and (like the ILMA) has a deeper bowl which makes the migration of the epiglottis into the distal lumen of the device less likely.
- The PLMA also has a flexible wire-reinforced airway tube to improve flexibility and minimize kinking, and a bite-block to reduce the danger of bite-induced airway obstruction, or tube damage.

The drainage conduit traverses the bowl of the cuff on its way to the upper esophagus in an effort to reduce the risk of gastric insufflation when positive pressure is applied to the airway. Standard gastric tubes (≤18 French [Fr] gauge) can be accommodated by the conduit to facilitate gastric decompression. An accessory vent under the drain tube is intended to prevent the pooling of secretions and can act as an accessory ventilation port.[78]

Employing moderate force to advance the laryngeal cuff forward into the periglottic tissues may improve the airway seal. The dual-tube arrangement seems to reduce the incidence of accidental device rotation during anesthesia. This feature enhances the ability to secure the device in position, giving greater confidence for use in longer procedures.

How Is the PLMA Placed?

The technique of insertion of the PLMA is similar to that of the LMA. While there is no randomized controlled study comparing the placement technique of the PLMA (with or without a muscle relaxant), it has been shown that successful placement of the PLMA requires deeper anesthesia when compared with the LMA (Videos 9 and 21).[79]

Three insertion techniques for the PLMA have been advocated:

1. The Introducer-Assisted Insertion Technique. Prior to its placement, the PLMA is loaded onto an introducer by placing the distal end of a metal introducer in an "insertion strap" on the PLMA (Figure 13.4). The airway tube is folded around the introducer and "fitted" into a proximal matching slot. The head and neck of the patient should be placed in a sniffing position. Following the placement of the PLMA, the introducer is removed as the PLMA is held in position.
2. The Digital Technique. Similar to the LMA, the digital technique involves the placement of the index finger under the insertion strap during the insertion of the PLMA. Rotating the PLMA 90 degrees in the mouth until resistance is felt at the hypopharynx was found to be more successful and associated with a decrease in blood staining on the device, and in the incidence of sore throat.[80]
3. The Tracheal Introducer-Guided Insertion Technique. This is probably the most reliable technique to optimally place the tip of the PLMA cuff in the hypopharynx.[81] A well-lubricated tracheal introducer (e.g., an ETI) is placed into the esophagus under direct vision with a laryngoscope. The PLMA is guided into position by placing the tracheal introducer through the esophageal conduit. While this technique enjoys a high success rate, it is time-consuming, and probably more stimulating and traumatic.

In a study by Eschertzhuber et al.,[82] these three insertion techniques were compared in patients with simulated difficult laryngoscopy using a rigid neck collar. Insertion was more frequently successful with the ETI technique at the first attempt (ETI—100%, Digital—64%, Introducer-Assisted Technique—61%). The time taken for successful placement was similar among groups on the first attempt. However, it was shorter for the ETI technique after three attempts (ETI 31 ± 8 s, Digital 49 ± 28 s, Introducer-Assisted Technique 54 ± 37 s).

Proper placement of the PLMA can be confirmed by a number of techniques. Air leak through the drainage tube at low airway pressures suggests malposition of the PLMA. Although air leaks are ordinarily easily detected by auscultation, or by feeling air exiting the drainage tube, a small volume leak is probably best detected by the soap bubble test.[83] Three other tests have been suggested to check the patency of the drainage tube, including: passing a gastric tube though the drainage tube; passing an FB through the drainage tube; and performing a suprasternal notch tap while observing a soap bubble, or lubricant, at the proximal end of the drainage tube.[83]

What Are the Advantages of the PLMA, Compared to the LMA?

In principle, the PLMA would be expected to reduce the aspiration risk when compared to the LMA. Laboratory (and cadaver) evidence is supportive of the theoretical efficacy of the PLMA.[84] However, clinical evidence is lacking, largely because the incidence of aspiration of gastric contents with the LMA is so low (0.02%), and a randomized controlled clinical trial with a large patient population is needed. Aspiration of gastric contents has been reported with the PLMA, and malposition of the PLMA has been identified as a cause of the aspiration.[85]

The design of the PLMA cuff significantly improves airway seal when compared to the LMA. The larger, softer, wedge-shaped PLMA cuff enables the anterior cuff to better adapt to the shape of the pharynx.[84] Most believe that pressure exerted on the pharyngeal mucosa by the cuffs of LMAs is the cause of sore throat seen with the device. Compared to the LMA, PLMA intracuff pressures are lower and airway seal pressure higher for any given intracuff volume.[86] Moreover, pressure exerted on the hypopharyngeal mucosa has been found to be below that considered critical for mucosal perfusion. In a Cochrane review by Hoda et al.,[87] PLMA appears to provide a better seal than LMA for PPV in adults undergoing elective surgery.

Perhaps the greatest limitation of the use of the LMA in small children is that the seal is often inadequate for PPV, even at high intracuff pressures. This does not appear to be as significant a limitation when the PLMA is used in these patients. Multiple studies comparing PLMA and LMA in children showed first-time insertions of PLMA were more successful, had less gastric insufflation, and produced a better seal to allow for PPV compared to the LMA.[88–94]

What Are the Disadvantages of the PLMA?

It is generally felt that the PLMA is more difficult to place than the LMA. The success rate for first-time PLMA insertion is lower than the first-time insertion success rate for the LMA (average success rate of 85% with a range of 81-100% for the PLMA vs. average success rate of 93% with a range of 89-100% for LMA).[95] It is possible that the insertion difficulty may in part be related to the larger, deeper, and softer cuff of the PLMA. It has been suggested that 20 to 30 insertions of the PLMA are required before competency is achieved.[95] A recent Cochrane review did not suggest there was adequate quality of evidence to suggest clinical significant differences between PLMA and LMA with regard to insertion failure, coughing, excessive leak, mucosal injury, sore throat, or bronchospasm.[87]

What Are the Potential Clinical Uses of the PLMA?

The improved airway seal characteristics and touted lower risk of gastric aspiration with the PLMA, compared to the LMA, has expanded its applicability to surgical procedures that would not have been considered safe had an LMA been employed. These procedures include laparoscopy,[87] open abdominal surgery, surgery in patients with obesity, and in patients with gastroesophageal reflux.[95] A study by Hohlrieder et al.[96] demonstrated less postoperative nausea, vomiting, airway morbidity, and analgesic requirements for the PLMA than the tracheal tube in females undergoing breast and gynecological surgery.

The PLMA has been used to provide ventilation and oxygenation in patients with a history of difficult laryngoscopic intubation.[97] A number of investigators reported the successful use of the PLMA to rescue a failed airway in obstetrical patients after a failed intubation.[84,98–100]

LARYNGEAL MASK AIRWAY-SUPREME (LMAS)

What Is the LMA-Supreme (LMAS) and What Is Its Clinical Utility Compared to the PLMA?

The LMAS (Teleflex) is a disposable, latex-free, LMA device with a drainage tube (Figure 13.6). It was designed to combine the desirable features of both the ILMA (ease of insertion, because of the rigid anatomically shaped airway tube made of medical-grade polyvinyl chloride) and the PLMA (higher seal pressures and gastric access).[101] The cuff of the LMAS is designed to provide higher seal pressures than the LMA or the single-use (disposable) LMA-Classic (LMA-Unique [LMAU]). In an early clinical study involving 70 patients, Ali et al.[102] reported that the LMAS is superior to the LMA because of its ease of insertion, with low cuff pressure and high oropharyngeal leakage pressure. However, several clinical studies comparing the LMAS and PLMA reported conflicting findings.[101,103,104] While both Verghese's[101] and Hosten's[103] studies reported that both LMAS and PLMA had similar leak pressures, Lee et al.[104] found that the oropharyngeal leak pressure and the maximum achievable tidal volume are lower with the LMAS than with the PLMA. However, there was no difference in the efficacy of ventilation and safety between the LMAS and PLMA in these studies.

Because of the ease and speed of successful insertion, higher glottic seal pressures, and ability to access gastric contents, Verghese et al.[101] suggested that the LMAS may have a role in airway management in CPR, and in the CICV (more recently called CICO[9]) scenario, the ASA Practice Guidelines had previously recommended for the LMA.[15,16]

LARYNGEAL MASK AIRWAY-PROTECTOR (LMAP)

What Is the LMAP? How Does It Differ from the PLMA?

The LMA-Protector (LMAP) is a newly introduced single-use, silicone second-generation EGD (Figure 13.7).[105] Similar to the PLMA, the LMAP provides access to, and functional separation of, the respiratory and digestive tracts. The LMAP has two separate proximal drainage ports (a male suction port and a female drainage port), which have drainage channels that run distally into a chamber behind the cuff bowl. The chamber then narrows distally into the opening located at the tip of the cuff, which communicates closely with the upper esophageal sphincter. While a suction tube may be attached to the male suction port, a well-lubricated gastric tube may be passed through the female drainage port to the stomach. The manufacturer claimed that the drainage channel can be used as a monitor of correct positioning of the device following insertion, and providing continuous monitoring of mask displacement during use.

It has an anatomically shaped airway tube similar to that of the LMAU. Therefore, unlike the PLMA, the LMAP provides easy insertion without the need for digital or introducer tool guidance as discussed above. It also has a built-in bite block to minimize the risk of airway tube occlusion in the event of biting.

What Is the Clinical Utility of the LMAP?

Since it shares many characteristics of the PLMA and LMAU, the clinical applications of the LMAP are expected to be similar to these two second-generation EGDs. Unfortunately, at the time of writing of this chapter, no large clinical studies are presently available. However, Tan et al.[106,107] reported positive experiences (e.g., ease of insertion, and minimal dislodgement of the device) with the LMAP in providing PPV and oxygenation in patients under general anesthesia for shoulder surgeries and laparoscopic cholecystectomies in a small number of patients. In a comparative study involving 110 anesthetized and paralyzed adult patients, Chang et al.[108] reported that while the insertion time was longer with the LMAP than with the i-gel, the airway leak pressure was higher with the LMAP. Unfortunately, there is not much clinical information available regarding the feasibility of tracheal intubation via the LMAP, other than a case report using the LMAP as a conduit for successful tracheal intubation in three patients undergoing thyroid surgeries.[109]

THE COMBITUBE (CBT)

What Is CBT and How Does It Differ from the LMA?

The CBT (Tyco-Healthcare-Kendall-Sheridan, Mansfield, MA [Figure 13.8]) is an easily inserted and highly efficacious EGD. While this device has been historically included in the ASA Difficult Airway Algorithm[15,110] as a primary rescue device in CICO situations, it is no longer a part of the most recent iterations of the guidelines.[6,16] It also has been used successfully during CPR and in trauma patients.[111–117]

The CBT is a double-lumen airway, one of which is open at both ends, as with a normal ETT. The other consists of an open proximal lumen and a distal blocked lumen, which resembles an esophageal obturator airway. The device has two balloons designed to trap the glottis between them. An oropharyngeal balloon is designed to be positioned just behind the posterior part of the hard palate. Once inflated, this balloon presses the base of the tongue in a ventrocaudal direction and the soft palate in a dorsocranial direction, sealing the oral and nasal airways from behind. Another smaller cuff seals the esophagus once inflated. Perforations between the two balloons in the distally blocked lumen permit the egress of air or oxygen when PPV is applied to a proximal port. Two circumferential rings printed on the proximal end of the tube indicate that the device has

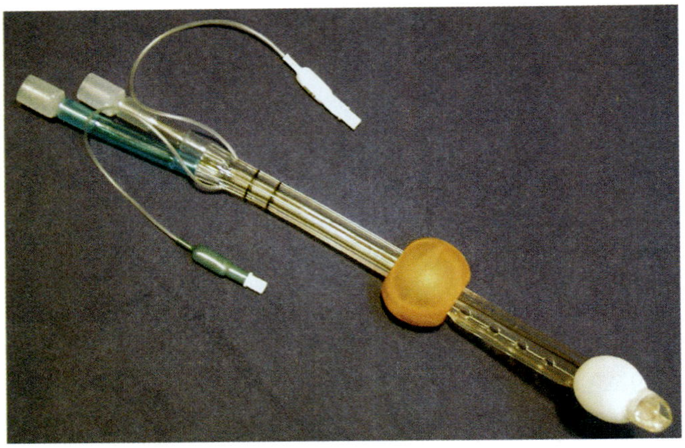

FIGURE 13.8. The Combitube is a double-lumen airway, with one lumen for ventilation and the other for access to the GI tract. The oropharyngeal balloon is designed to be positioned just behind the posterior part of the hard palate sealing both the mouth and the nose. A smaller cuff seals the esophagus. Two printed ring marks at the proximal end of the tube indicate appropriate depth of insertion when the upper teeth or alveolar ridges are situated between these two marks.

been inserted to the proper depth, when the upper teeth or alveolar ridges are situated between these two marks. The CBT is available in two sizes: the CBT 37F SA (small adult) to be used in patients 4 to 6 feet in height (approximately 120 to 180 cm); and the CBT 41F, for patients taller than 6 feet (approximately >180 cm).

How Is the CBT Inserted?

Insertion is facilitated by bending the CBT between the balloons for a few seconds before insertion to mimic the curvature of the pharynx. It is made more pliable if heated to body temperature, perhaps attenuating its blunt trauma potential. Placement of the CBT is most readily performed with the patient's head placed in a neutral position,[116] although some practitioners prefer slight extension or flexion. The classical sniffing position is usually not helpful. In the fully awake patient, sedation and topical anesthesia are necessary to ensure that the patient does not react to the insertion. To elevate the tongue and epiglottis, a jaw lift is performed by grasping the lower jaw with the thumb and forefinger. The CBT is inserted blindly along the surface of the tongue with initial gentle downward, curved, dorsocaudal movement, and then directed parallel to the patient's horizontal plane until the printed ring marks lie between the upper and lower teeth, or alveolar ridges in edentulous patients. After insertion, the oropharyngeal balloon of the CBT 37F is inflated with 85 mL of air through a blue pilot balloon. The corresponding filling volume for the CBT 41F is 100 mL. Then, the distal balloon is inflated with approximately 10 mL of air (Videos 9 and 19).

With blind insertion, the CBT is successfully placed in the esophagus in more than 95% of cases. Ventilation is achieved via the longer blue connector (No. 1), leading to the blocked lumen which contains perforations at the level of the larynx, between the two balloons. The trachea is effectively ventilated because the nose, mouth, and esophagus are sealed by the two balloons. The second "tracheoesophageal" lumen of the CBT can be used for decompression of the esophagus and stomach, thereby minimizing the risk of aspiration.

Auscultation of breath sounds over the chest, the absence of gastric insufflation, end-tidal CO_2 detection, and esophageal detection devices can all assist in the confirmation of correct positioning.[118,119]

Should the CBT enter the trachea on blind insertion, it can function like a standard ETT and there will be no need for inflation of the pharyngeal cuff. Ventilation can be achieved through the shorter, unobstructed clear tube (No. 2) leading to the tracheal lumen.

Although it is rare, ventilation may be impossible through either the proximal or distal lumen. This usually signifies that the CBT has been placed too deeply, with the obturator lumen positioned in the esophagus and the oropharyngeal balloon obstructing the entrance to the larynx. After deflation of the balloons, the CBT should be withdrawn approximately 2.0 to 3.0 cm. While the CBT may be inserted blindly, the use of a laryngoscope is recommended whenever possible.

What Are the Advantages of the CBT Compared to the LMA?

The CBT was designed primarily for use in CPR,[113,114] even by nonmedical personnel. It has been demonstrated to permit effective ventilation during routine surgery, and in the ICU.[112] Most believe that the principal role of the CBT is in emergency airway control when tracheal intubation is not immediately possible.[120–123] The CBT may be kept in situ for up to 8 hours and allows controlled mechanical ventilation at inflating pressures as high as 50 cm H_2O. The CBT can be replaced by deflation of the oropharyngeal balloon and insertion of an ETT either under DL, or by indirect view using an FB placed anterior, or lateral to the CBT.

Several case reports describe the successful use of the CBT in cases of unanticipated difficult airways.[124–126] Thus, it is not surprising that the ASA task force on difficult airway management lists the CBT, along with the LMA and transtracheal jet ventilation, as CICO (formerly called CICV) rescue methods.[15,110]

A major advantage of CBT over conventional tracheal intubation is that the device can be inserted with the head and neck in a neutral position. Additionally, it requires only modest mouth opening for insertion, and its tubular profile permits insertion in situations that cannot be negotiated by more bulky devices. The CBT can be inserted from a variety of angles, making it useful in awkward environments (e.g., a patient who is trapped in a vehicle). The CBT may be of special benefit in patients with massive bleeding or regurgitation, when visualization of the vocal cords is impossible. While protection from aspiration is not absolute, the CBT may be more effective than the LMA in this regard, due to much higher sealing pressures.[127]

What Are the Disadvantages of the CBT?

The CBT was not designed to replace other devices for routine surgery. While the esophageal cuff offers some protection against the reflux of gastric contents into the periglottic area, the level of protection against aspiration does not approach that of a cuffed ETT.

The suctioning of tracheal secretions is very difficult when the CBT is in the esophageal position. To address the issue of secretions and suctioning, Krafft et al.[128] proposed a modification in the CBT, in which the two anterior, proximal perforations of the CBT are replaced by a single, larger, ellipsoid-shaped hole that allows for fiberoptic access of the trachea, tracheal suctioning, and tube exchange over a guidewire. It should be noted that FBs with a small outer diameter (3.0-mm OD) allow passage through the unmodified pharyngeal perforations.

Contraindications to the use of the CBT include an intact gag reflex, airway obstruction by foreign bodies, tumors, or swelling, the presence of known esophageal disease, and the prior ingestion of caustic substances.

Complications associated with the use of CBT have been reported.[129,130] In a retrospective study of 1139 patients requiring resuscitation using the CBT, four cases of subcutaneous emphysema, pneumomediastinum, and pneumoperitoneum associated with the CBT during prehospital management were reported.[130] The reason for these complications appeared to be hyperinflation of the distal balloon (20-40 mL), although external chest compression and continuous PPV may also have been factors. Other rare complications include transient cranial nerve dysfunction,[131] esophageal rupture,[132] and tongue engorgement.[133]

What Are the Potential Clinical Uses of the CBT?

The CBT is an easy-to-use, rapidly inserted emergency airway device that has performed satisfactorily in many circumstances. It is accepted as a primary rescue device in CICO situations, for CPR, and in trauma patients. The CBT was previously recommended in the "Practice Guidelines for Management of the Difficult Airway" of the ASA.[15,110] It has also been recommended in the "Guidelines for Cardiopulmonary Resuscitation and Emergency Cardiac Care" of the AHA. In 2000, the CBT was upgraded by the AHA as a class IIa device. Furthermore, the CBT may provide an element of protection in patients at risk for aspiration, and it may be of benefit for patients in whom manipulation of the cervical spine is hazardous or impossible. Successfully placed, the device is capable of facilitating adequate ventilation and oxygenation, and in most instances, it is as effective as endotracheal intubation.[115]

LARYNGEAL TUBE (KING LT AIRWAY [LT])

What Is the LT and How Does It Differ from the LMA?

The Laryngeal Tube Airway® (VBM Medizintechnik, Sulz am Neckar, Germany [Figure 13.9]), also known as the King LT Airway in North America, is an EGD that was introduced to the European market in 1999.[134] It is similar in appearance and function to the CBT, and is available in three configurations (refer to the last paragraph in this section). The fundamental

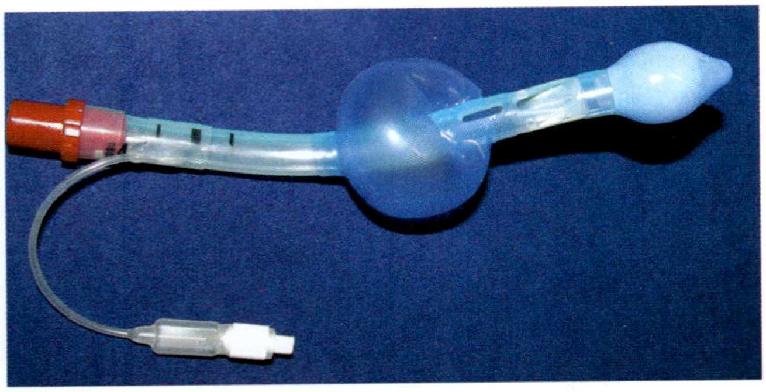

FIGURE 13.9. The Laryngeal Tube Airway consists of a silicone airway tube with two ventilation outlet perforations lying between two cuffs, a single pilot balloon, and a 15-mm male adapter.

configuration of the LT is a silicone airway tube with ventilation outlet perforations lying between two cuffs, pharyngeal and esophageal. As opposed to the CBT, the LT has a single pilot balloon connected to both cuffs, and a single 15-mm standard male adapter. The airway tube is short, and "J" shaped with an average diameter of 1.5 cm, leading to a blind tip. The device requires a mouth opening of at least 23 mm for its insertion. After device placement, the proximal cuff should lie in the hypopharynx and the distal cuff in the upper esophagus. Both cuffs are high volume-low pressure in design to establish an adequate seal while minimizing the risk for ischemic mucosal damage. Two ventilation outlets are located between the two cuffs in the anterior aspect of the tube. The proximal outlet is "protected" by a "V"-shaped deflection in the pharyngeal cuff, such that when the cuff is inflated, soft tissue is deflected from this opening, helping to maintain patency. There are two side holes near the distal outlet.

Even though the two cuffs are supplied by a single-inflation pilot balloon apparatus, the design of the inflation system allows the pharyngeal cuff to fill first, stabilizing the position of the tube.[134] Once the pharyngeal cuff has molded to the anatomy of the patient, the esophageal cuff inflates. The amount of air for cuff inflation is specific to tube size and is indicated on a syringe that is included in the package. Six sizes, suitable for neonates up to large adults, are available.[135] Safe inflation of the dual cuffs may be enhanced with the aid of a cuff pressure gauge and ought to be limited to 60 cm H_2O. In a recent report, an overinflation of the LT in a difficult prehospital airway management of a patient with Down syndrome resulted in a clinical misdiagnosis of Ludwig's angina in the Emergency Department, necessitating an emergency tracheotomy.[136]

There are several versions of the laryngeal tube: Standard Laryngeal Tube®, Disposable Laryngeal Tube® (LT-D), Laryngeal Tube-Suction II® (LTS), and Disposable Laryngeal Tube-Suction II® (LTS-D).[135] Similar to the PLMA, the LTS-D has two lumens: one for ventilation, and the other serves as a conduit to the esophagus and stomach.

How Is an LT Inserted?

An appropriately sized LT should be selected based on the patient's weight and height. Prior to insertion, the cuffs should be completely deflated and well lubricated. The device should be inserted with the patient's head and neck in a "sniffing" position.[135] The head is extended on the neck with the nondominant hand, to open the mouth. The LT is then inserted blindly in the midline, with the tip pressed against the hard palate and then advanced along the palate into the hypopharynx until resistance is felt, at which point a proximal horizontal black line should be aligned with the front teeth. The device is usually easily inserted with insertion times comparable to those reported for the LMA.[137]

The device provides a patent airway in the majority of patients following the first insertion attempt, and success does not require extensive training.[138,139] Indicators of correct placement include end-tidal carbon dioxide detection, auscultation of bilateral breath sounds, absence of gastric insufflation, and adequate chest movement. Capnographic waveform analysis may be of particular use in confirming proper position of the LT. A brief period of PPV may also confirm proper alignment of the LT and the absence of obstruction.

The LT should be removed with the patient either deeply anesthetized or totally awake. In an awake patient, the LT should be removed only when airway protective reflexes have completely returned.

What Are the Advantages of the LT, Compared to the LMA and the CBT?

Insertion of this device is relatively easy and successful in most patients on the first attempt. The soft tip minimizes mechanical trauma on insertion and high-volume/low-pressure cuffs provide a good seal and protection against mucosal ischemic damage. A single pilot balloon confers an element of simplicity and speed in emergency situations. Other advantages of LT include:

1. The adequacy of ventilation with the LT is comparable to that obtained with other EGDs. The ease of insertion and high quality of the seal achieved may confer a preferred role for the LT in airway management during CPR.[138]
2. The LT can be used successfully in children as young as 2-years old, with superior seal pressures and equivalent ease of insertion.[140]
3. The esophageal cuff of the laryngeal tube may provide an element of protection against the reflux of gastric contents into the periglottic area and the tube-suction options permit gastric decompression. Both of these features may reduce the risk of aspiration, relative to the LMA.[141,142]
4. Due to the form and length of the device, unintended tracheal intubation should not occur.

What Are the Disadvantages of the LT?

Disadvantages include:

1. Protection from aspiration is less than that offered by a cuffed ETT, and in high aspiration risk situations, tracheal intubation remains necessary. While the newer Laryngeal Tube-Suction II (LTS) and the Disposable Laryngeal Tube-Suction II (LTS-D) may have the potential to provide some protection from aspiration, presently there are no clinical data available.

2. The intracuff pressure may increase by as much as 15 cm H_2O within 30 minutes after its insertion if nitrous oxide is employed, due to the diffusion of this gas into the cuff. Manometric monitoring of the cuff pressure has been suggested.[143]
3. Position adjustments to ensure airflow continuity may be required more frequently in obese patients.[144]
4. PPV through the LT may provide inadequate ventilation in patients who require high pulmonary inflation pressures.
5. The mouth opening required for LT insertion is at least 23 mm.
6. As with any EGD, the LT may not be effective in the presence of anatomic distortion of the upper airway, such as lesions of the epiglottis or laryngopharynx.
7. The LT is less effective than the LMA in children younger than 10 with respect to ease of ventilation and endoscopic view through the device.[145]
8. The insert time for LT was slower than i-gel in prehospital use, even though first-attempt success rates were the same.[146]

What Are the Potential Clinical Uses of the LT?

In anesthetic practice, the LT can be used in patients who are candidates for face mask or LMA-delivered anesthesia. It may also play a role in the failed airway, similar to that of the LMA and the CBT.

The dimension and position of the ventilation holes and the protection offered by the overhanging cuff block permit the insertion of a suction catheter, ETT exchange device, FB, or an ETI, over which an ETT may be advanced.[147]

PERILARYNGEAL AIRWAY (COBRAPLA [CPLA])

What Is the CPLA and How Does It Differ from the LMA?

The CPLA (Engineered Medical Systems, Inc, Indianapolis, IN [Figure 13.10]) consists of a breathing tube with a circumferential inflatable cuff proximal to a ventilation outlet, a 15-mm standard adapter, and a distal-widened cobra-shaped head designed to separate soft tissues and to allow ventilation of the trachea. Once in place, the cobra head lies in front of the laryngeal inlet. Internal to the cobra head, a ramp directs ventilation into the trachea. A soft grill shields the inferior aperture of the device in an attempt to deflect the epiglottis anteriorly. The bars of the grill are sufficiently flexible to permit an ETT to pass easily. The cuff is shaped such that it resides in the hypopharynx at the base of the tongue and, when inflated, raises the base of the tongue exposing the laryngeal inlet and effects an airway seal. The unique shape of the distal part of the device allows it to slide easily along the hard palate during insertion and to move soft tissues away from the laryngeal inlet once in place.

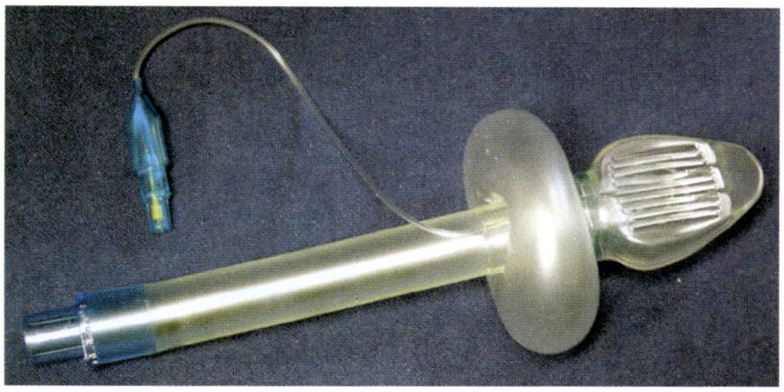

FIGURE 13.10. The CobraPLA consists of a breathing tube with a circumferential inflatable cuff proximal to the ventilation outlet portion, a 15-mm standard adapter, and a distal widened "Cobra head" designed to separate the soft tissues of the hypopharynx and permit ventilation.

The CPLA is available in eight sizes and it can be used in small children, including neonates.[148] Size selection is governed by the weight of the patient. Generally, #3 is used in most female patients, #4 for most men, and #5 for larger men. When one is unsure which size is best, or when learning placement technique, selecting the lower size is recommended. In general, larger sizes required considerably higher cuff pressures to produce an acceptable seal compared to the smaller sizes.[149]

Several modifications of the original design of the CPLA have been introduced.[148] The second-generation CPLA has a distal curve in the breathing tube to avoid kinking, and softer material to facilitate insertion and minimize trauma. The Cobra PLUS® has a temperature probe to measure core temperature, and a gas sampling line for the three smallest pediatric sizes.

How Do You Insert the CPLA?

The CPLA is simple to insert, but difficulty is encountered in obese patients.[150] Prior to insertion, the pharyngeal cuff is fully deflated and folded back against the breathing tube. The back of the cobra head and cuff are lubricated, taking care that the lubricant does not obstruct the grille. The patient's head is placed in the sniffing position. A jaw lift is performed and the distal end of the CPLA is directed straight back through the mouth between the tongue and hard palate. Modest neck extension (without a jaw lift maneuver) may aid the passage of the device as it turns toward the glottis at the back of the mouth. Once the CPLA traverses the back of the mouth, it usually turns caudally toward the larynx with minimal resistance, as the flexible distal tip guides the device downwards. The CPLA is properly seated above the glottis when modest resistance to further distal passage is encountered. Once inserted, the flexible tip lies behind the arytenoids, the cuff lies in the hypopharynx at the base of the tongue, and the ramp lifts the epiglottis. Then the cuff is inflated until the leak with PPV disappears. Indicators of correct placement are absence of leak on auscultation of the neck, bilateral breath sounds, absence of gastric insufflation, easily produced chest movement, and positive carbon dioxide detection. Exceeding a peak airway pressure of 25 cm H_2O with PPV is not recommended, even when testing for ventilation and cuff seal, because of the risk of gastric insufflation.

If the CPLA is not inserted far enough, inflation of the cuff may cause the tongue to protrude from the mouth of the patient. In this situation, the cuff should be deflated and the device advanced further, or a smaller-sized CPLA selected. It is possible to advance the cobra head beyond the laryngeal inlet, in which case ventilation will not be possible. The CPLA should be removed awake, with the airway protective reflexes intact.

What Are the Advantages of the CPLA Compared to the LMA?

The tube of the CPLA has a larger lumen than most EGDs and may be particularly useful in directing flexible endoscopic-assisted tracheal intubation,[151,152] especially when larger ETTs are indicated. An ETT of 8.0-mm ID can be advanced through the sizes 4 to 6 CPLA.[148] In addition, it has been made short enough such that its removal after insertion of an ETT is greatly facilitated. Although less reliable, blind tracheal intubation through the CPLA using a tracheal introducer (e.g., the ETI) may be possible.

Like many other EGDs, the insertion technique is simple and has been accomplished by personnel with little or no experience. Several small clinical studies reported that the CPLA has better airway sealing characteristics compared to the LMA.[153,154] Compared to the LMA, the pressures required to generate a leak were statistically higher for the CPLA.[155] This allows for more effective use in overweight patients with BMI of 25 to 35.[155] During gynecological laparoscopy, the CPLA provided similar insertion characteristics, but higher airway sealing pressures than the LMA.[156] However, Park et al.[157] showed that gastric insufflation, or ventilatory difficulty, may occur following the change of the position of the head and neck when using the CobraPLA, as compared to PLMA.

Khan et al.[158] reported successful use of the CPLA for ventilation following failed attempts in placing an LMA in patients with face and neck contractures, and limited mouth opening.

What Are the Disadvantages of the CPLA?

In comparison trials with LMA and LMAU, the CPLA took slightly longer to insert, and macroscopic blood occurred more frequently on the CPLA (seen on up to 40% of the devices after removal).[151,153,156] Although blood staining has been detected more frequently with the CPLA compared with other EGDs, there were no differences in airway morbidity.[159] Therefore, the clinical significance of these findings is uncertain.

The CPLA is not appropriate for patients with low lung compliance or increased airway resistance. The major disadvantage of the device is that it does not protect against aspiration and does not secure the airway as effectively as an ETT.[160] The mask aperture bars probably have no anatomical utility, and predispose to herniation of the pharyngeal structures on insertion and while in situ.[159]

Although it is rare, aspiration associated with use of the CPLA has been reported.[160,161] In fact, Cook and Lowe[160] terminated the CPLA evaluation study after two cases of serious pulmonary aspiration with the use of the CPLA, suggesting that the CPLA should be avoided in patients at risk of aspiration.

THE AMBU®-AURAONCE™ DISPOSABLE LARYNGEAL MASK

What Is the Ambu-AuraOnce Disposable Laryngeal Mask (ALM) and How Does It Differ from the LMA?

Unlike the reusable LMA, the Ambu-AuraOnce Laryngeal Mask (Ambu, Ballerup, Denmark [Figure 13.11]) is a disposable EGD.[162] It is made of polyvinyl chloride with an extra soft 0.4-mm cuff, providing a better seal that conforms well to the shape of the airway.[163] Similar to the LMAS, it incorporates a 70-degree preformed curvature that replicates natural oropharyngeal anatomy to facilitate insertion.[164] Unlike the LMA and LMAU, the bowl of the ALM lacks the aperture bars and therefore it would be easier to perform tracheal intubation through the airway tube of the ALM. The two horizontal lines on the airway tube can be used as indicators of proper depth of insertion of the ALM. The ALM has eight different sizes (sizes 1 and 1½ for infants, sizes 2 and 2½ for children, and sizes 3-6 for adults).

Since the introduction of the ALM in 2004, three other versions have been introduced:

- Ambu® Aura-i™ disposable laryngeal mask has the intubating capability using standard ETTs (Figure 13.12).
- Ambu® AuraFlex™ disposable laryngeal mask incorporates a nonkinkable, wire-reinforced airway. It is similar in design to the reusable LMA-Flexible.
- AuraGain disposable laryngeal mask is Ambu's latest laryngeal mask that facilitates rapid establishment of a safe airway by integrating gastric access and intubation capability in an anatomically curved single-use device.

How Is the ALM Inserted?

The insertion technique is similar to other EGDs. The cuff should be fully deflated and lubricated. The head of the patient should be placed in the "sniffing position." While many insertion techniques have been described, the manufacturer recommends the

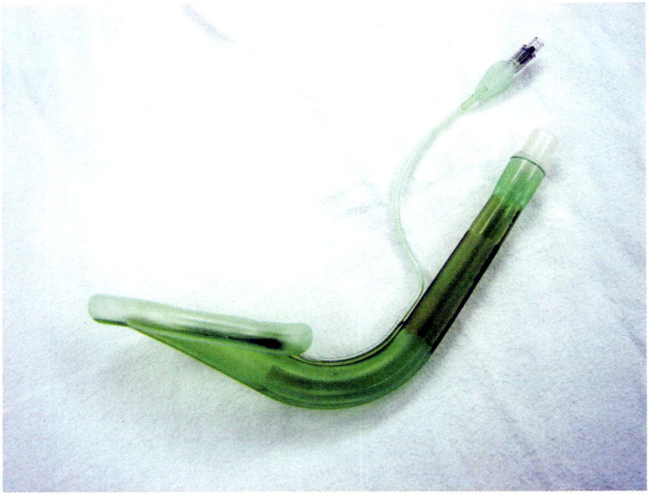

FIGURE 13.11. The Ambu-AuraOnce laryngeal mask.

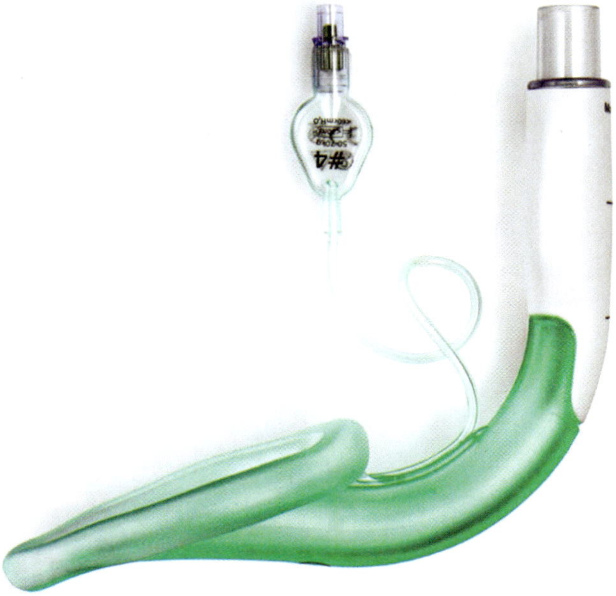

FIGURE 13.12. Ambu Aura-i disposable laryngeal mask has the intubating capability using standard ETTs.

"pencil insertion technique."[164] The airway tube is held by the dominant hand like a flute, with three fingers placed above the junction of the cuff and the tube and the thumb on the vertical line on the airway tube. As the tip of the cuff is placed inside the mouth, the ALM is inserted inward with a circular motion, pressing the contours of the hard and soft palate, and the ALM is then advanced into the hypopharynx until resistance is felt. The ALM is inserted correctly when the patient's incisors are between the two horizontal markings on the airway tube. The cuff is then inflated with sufficient air to obtain a seal, equivalent to intracuff pressures of approximately 60 cm H_2O. Like all EGDs, proper placement should be confirmed after insertion.

What Are the Advantages of the ALM Compared to the LMA?

According to the meta-analysis conducted by Baidya et al.,[165] device insertion is significantly faster with the ALM than with the LMAU, but similar to the LMA. The ALM also provides an oropharyngeal leak pressure higher than with the LMAU, and equivalent to that of the LMA.[165] Another advantage of the ALM over the LMA is the lack of aperture bars. In other words, tracheal intubation (either blindly or with the guidance of an FB) can be easily performed through the airway tube of the ALM following an airway rescue in a CICO situation.

What Are the Potential Clinical Uses of the ALM?

To investigate the clinical uses of ALM, a number of studies have been conducted during the last decade. In a meta-analysis conducted by Baidya et al.,[165] the investigators concluded that the ALM is similarly effective as the LMAU and LMA, and may be easier to insert than the other two devices. The incidence of complications associated with the use of the ALM is generally low.[162]

NONINFLATABLE CUFF EXTRAGLOTTIC DEVICE: STREAMLINED LINER OF THE PHARYNX AIRWAY (SLIPA)

What Is the SLIPA and How Does It Differ from the LMA?

The SLIPA (SLIPA Med, Cape Town, South Africa [Figure 13.13]) is a disposable EGD. It is designed for airway management during controlled ventilation.[166,167] The peculiar shape of the device provides a seal without the use of an inflatable cuff.

The body of the SLIPA is shaped like a hollow boot with "toe", "bridge," and "heel" prominences, designed to engage the mucosal lining of the patient's pharynx. Its hollow configuration and shape permit the entrapment of secretions, blood, or gastric contents in the device, theoretically reducing the risk of aspiration. The device is formed from soft plastic material, flexible enough to allow easy insertion. The hollow chamber flattens to facilitate insertion. After placement, the "toe" should sit in the hypopharynx. The "bridge," with its two lateral bulges, fits into the pyriform fossae, displacing tissue away from the posterior pharyngeal wall. The "heel" of the chamber anchors the SLIPA in position by sliding over the soft palate and into the nasopharyngeal opening. Toward the toe side of the bridge are smaller lateral bulges that coincide with the inferior cornus of the hyoid bone designed to relieve pressure on relevant nervous tissue, such as the superior laryngeal branch of the vagus.

How Is the SLIPA Inserted?

The SLIPA is inserted similarly to the LMA. The patient's head and neck should be placed in a sniffing position. Held in the dominant hand, the SLIPA is inserted in the midline of the mouth, pressed against the hard palate, and advanced until resistance is felt. A jaw lift may facilitate placement. The crescent shape of the toe minimizes the risk of downward folding of the epiglottis, which may lead to airway obstruction. The toe of the device slips easily into the esophagus, where it creates a seal. Kang et al.[168] reported that prewarming of the SLIPA appeared to improve the fitting of the laryngeal structure. After placement, the SLIPA returns to its preinsertion shape.

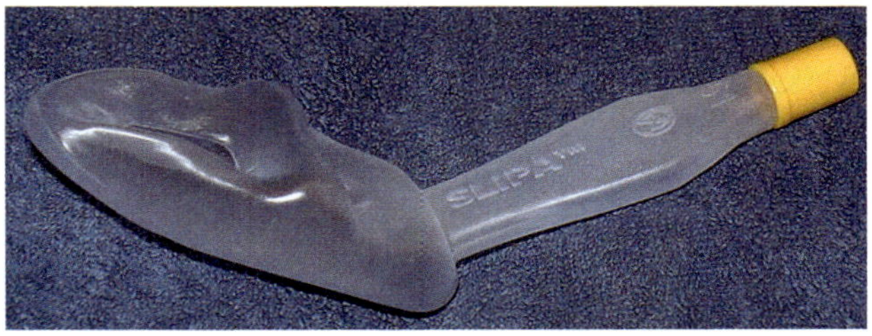

FIGURE 13.13. The SLIPA is shaped like a hollow boot with "toe," "bridge," and "heel" prominences, designed to engage the patient's pharynx. The hollow design feature permits the entrapment of liquids such as secretions, blood, and gastric fluids, thus preventing aspiration.

What Are the Advantages and Disadvantages of the SLIPA Compared to the LMA?

A systematic review and meta-analysis comparing SLIPA and LMA showed no difference between ease of insertion, oropharyngeal leak pressure, and quality of flexible bronchoscopic view of the larynx. The SLIPA compared to the PLMA had statistically lower rates of postoperative sore throat.[169] Additionally, insertion of the SLIPA device required 32% lower effector site concentration of remifentanil compared to LMA.[170] However, SLIPA insertion did have a higher incidence of bloodstaining after removal.[171]

What Are the Potential Clinical Uses of the SLIPA Device?

Based on the current available evidence, the SLIPA appears to have comparable efficacy and complications as the LMA, and may be used as a primary airway device for short surgical procedures.[148]

I-GEL

What Is the i-gel and How Does It Differ from the LMA?

The i-gel is a single-use EGD that is made of a thermoplastic elastomer gel. It has a noninflatable cuff, which can anatomically seal the pharyngeal, laryngeal, and perilaryngeal structures, with minimal risk of compression trauma. The device has an elliptical cross-sectional-shaped tube with a slight curve longitudinally to facilitate insertion and minimize axial rotation once it is placed (Figure 13.14). It also has an independent gastric drain tube and an integral bite block. It is available in sizes 3 to 5. A size 4 is recommended by the manufacturers for patients between 50 and 90 kg, making it the most common size for the normal adult population.

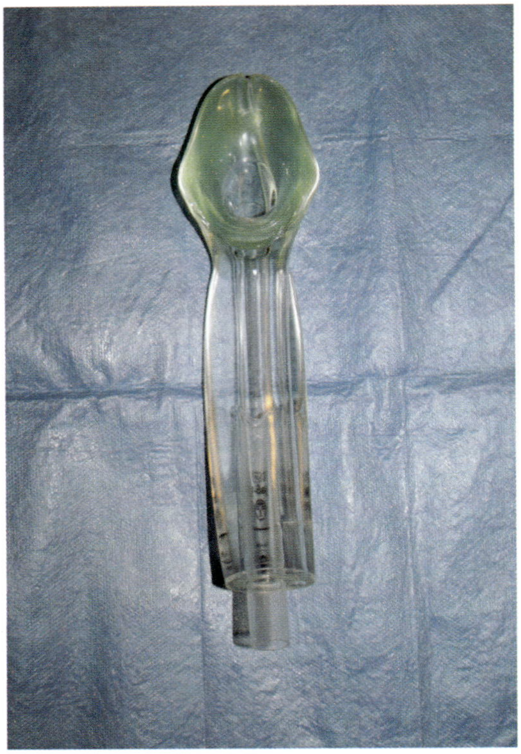

FIGURE 13.14. The i-gel device has a noninflatable cuff and an elliptical cross-sectional-shaped tube with a slight curve longitudinally to facilitate insertion. In addition, it also has an independent gastric drain tube and an integral bite block.

How Is the i-gel Inserted?

With the patient's head and neck placed in a "sniffing position," the well-lubricated i-gel is placed in the mouth and passed along the posterior pharynx until resistance is felt.[172] Insertion does not require an introducer or placement of the finger into the mouth, as the device is simply pushed into place. A 45-degree "twist" can be employed to facilitate insertion. The cuff does not require inflation of air following placement.

What Are the Advantages of the i-gel Compared to the LMA?

The insertion process requires one fewer step, as there is no air required for cuff inflation. The elastomer gel may provide a more efficient seal around the larynx after warming to body temperature.[173] In addition, the gel-filled cuff may potentially cause less direct trauma or pressure damage to the oropharyngeal mucosa. Unfortunately, at present, there are no clinical data to confirm this potential advantage. Compared to the LMA-Supreme, there is evidence that i-gel causes less postoperative laryngeal pain.[174]

The i-gel has a gastric drain tube which may offer added protection against the aspiration of regurgitated stomach contents. Two separate case reports have confirmed that this drainage tube provided protection against aspiration.[173,175] However, in a case series of 280 patients reported by Gibbison et al.,[176] three patients had regurgitation while using the i-gel. Although the i-gel completely protected the airway from aspiration of regurgitated stomach contents in two of these patients, it did not provide complete protection in the third patient. The investigators concluded that the efficacy of the drainage tube has not been confirmed, and further study is required to determine the safety profile of the device.

What Are the Disadvantages of the i-gel?

In a clinical evaluation study with 100 patients, Gatward et al.[177] found that the airway seal offered by the i-gel is inferior to other EGDs, such as the PLMA. In a cadaver study, Schmidbauer et al.[178] showed that both the PLMA and LMA provided a better seal of the esophagus than the i-gel airway. If there is a leak around the i-gel, it may have to be replaced with a different size, since there is no option of adding or withdrawing air from the cuff.

The drain tube of the i-gel is significantly smaller than the drainage tube of the PLMA. For instance, a French gauge 12 catheter can be inserted through the size 4 i-gel compared to a 16F catheter for a size 4 PLMA.[177] It is unknown if the smaller drain tube is adequate to provide equivalent protection of aspiration, compared with other EGDs with a larger drainage tube.

As many EGD devices are used in the prehospital setting, dislodgment during patient transportation is a very real concern. The i-gel required the least amount of force for dislodgment compared to LMA, LT, and ETT.[179] In addition, although i-gel has been found to be faster on insertion, it had less first insertion success rate compared to the LMAS.[180]

What Are the Clinical Uses of the i-gel?

Compared with seven other EADs (Airway Management Device, CobraPLA, Combitube, Laryngeal Tube, Laryngeal Tube Disposable [LT-D], Laryngeal Tube-Suction II® [LTS II], and the SLIPA), the i-gel has been shown to perform the best for ease of insertion into the airway during training on manikins by 10 anesthesiologists.[181]

In a clinical evaluation study involving 100 patients, Gatward et al.[177] reported that the i-gel was successfully inserted in all patients and allowed effective controlled ventilation in 98%. The investigators also commented that, while the airway seal offered by the i-gel may be inferior to other EGDs (such as the PLMA), it is still sufficient for controlled ventilation in most patients. Rates of failure, manipulations required, and complications were also very low for the i-gel in that study. In another prospective observational study with 71 patients, Richez et al.[182] confirmed the efficacy and safety of the i-gel airway device. A systematic review and meta-analysis did demonstrate that the i-gel was inserted in significantly shorter times than those of the LMA, ILMA, PLMA, LMAU, LT, CBT, and EasyTube; however, this was not associated with better overall first-attempt success rate.

The i-gel has been successfully used to provide ventilation in patients with a difficult airway in a number of case reports. Michalek et al.[183] reported successful placement of the i-gel under general anesthesia in two uncooperative patients with an anticipated difficult intubation (Hunter's and Waardenburg's syndromes). Oxygenation and ventilation were maintained using the i-gel, which was then used as a conduit for tracheal intubation using a pediatric FB.

Joshi et al.[184] reported the use of the i-gel as an airway rescue in a patient with scleroderma and predicted difficult intubation. Under general anesthesia, ventilation was difficult with a face mask, the LMA, and the PLMA, but ventilation was achieved easily with a size 4 i-gel. Others have also reported the use of the i-gel as a rescue airway device.[185]

In the Emergency Medical Service (EMS) systems in the United Kingdom, an EGD (the PLMA) was introduced into clinical practice as an alternative to emergency cricothyrotomy for the management of failed intubation in 2005.[186] The PLMA was initially chosen for the potential ability to ventilate and the presence of a gastric drainage channel to minimize aspiration. But, the i-gel has replaced the PLMA in 2010 for ease of insertion.[186]

BASKA MASK

What Is the Baska Mask?

The Baska Mask (BM; Logikal Health Products PTY Ltd, Morisset, NSW, Australia) is a relatively new EGD with a noninflatable cuff (self-energizing cuff), which can be molded to take up the shape of the airway around the glottis and provide a superior seal as compared to the LMA.[187] It also has some safety features (Figure 13.15): (1) a large sump cavity with two aspiratable gastric drain tubes; (2) a tab for manually flexing the mask to facilitate insertion; and (3) a suction elbow integral to one port with a second port acting as a free air flow access.[187]

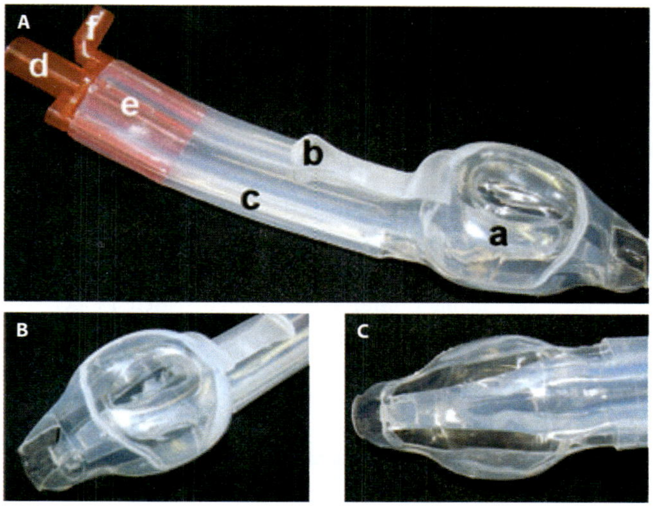

FIGURE 13.15. The Baska Mask. Panel (**A**): The Baska Mask has a noninflatable mask (a); a tab (b), which is used to flex the cuff during placement; a bite block (e) and a suction connector (f). It also has two channels, the side suction channel (c) and the central airway channel (d). Panel (**B**) shows a close-up view of the anterior (glottic) surface of the noninflatable cuff. Panel (**C**) shows the dorsal surface of the cuff with the pharyngeal drainage sump reservoir that drains into the bilateral suction channels. (Reproduced with permission from Alexiev V, Salim A, Kevin LG, et al. An observational study of the Baska® mask: a novel supraglottic airway. *Anaesthesia*. 2012;67(6):640-645.)

What Are the Advantages of the Baska Mask Compared to i-gel and LMA?

The BM is relatively easy to insert, with a first-time insertion success rate of >80% and nearly 100% successful on the second attempt. In comparison, the LMA has a higher first-time insertion success rate of >90%.[188] As this is a relatively new device, there is conflicting evidence on the insertion time of the BM compared to the i-gel. Multiple studies have noted that insertion of the BM can be completed in under 20 seconds, similar to the insertion time of the i-gel.[189–191]

A vital characteristic of the BM throughout the literature is its ability to obtain high airway seal pressure.[192,193] Compared to the i-gel and the LMAS, the BM has a superior airway seal pressure.[191,193,194] One unique aspect of the BM is that the airway seal pressure increases over time when compared to the insertion and 30 minutes after insertion.[195] This increased airway seal pressure has allowed it to be used in paralyzed patients using PPV and potentially less risky for gastric insufflation.[192,195,196] In a small study examining 90 patients undergoing laparoscopic cholecystectomy, the time for gastric tube insertion was significantly lower with the BM compared to the LMAS and i-gel.[191] Compared to endotracheal intubation, the BM has fewer pharyngolaryngeal complications such as cough, trauma, dysphonia, and sore throat.[197] There have been fewer complications compared to i-gel and LMAS.[190]

What Are the Disadvantages of the Baska Mask?

Statistically, studies have found that the time of insertion is slightly longer for the BM compared to i-gel and LMA; however, the question remains if the difference of seconds has any clinical significance.[198,199] The BM did require more attempts and optimization maneuvers than the first-generation LMA.[188] If the initial insertion attempts were unsuccessful, it has been described that upsizing the BM often resolved the issues.[188] Currently, the sizing of the BM is weight-based as per the manufacturer.

As with all EGDs, the BM is not a secure airway; however, with the ease of gastric suction and higher airway seal pressure, there is potential for lowering the risk of aspiration. At the present time, there are no reported cases of aspiration in the literature with the BM. The 4th National Audit Project of the Royal College of Anesthetists and the Difficult Airway Society (NAP4) has examined aspiration in the context of first-generation supraglottic devices and recommends second-generation devices to minimize the risk of aspiration.[43]

What Are the Clinical Uses of the Baska Mask?

As a newer generation EGD, the BM has been used in situations of failed airway similar to that of the i-gel and LMA. The increased airway seal pressure has demonstrated that it can be used to ventilate patients via positive pressure in paralyzed patients undergoing laparoscopic and gynecological procedures.[191–193]

SUMMARY

During the past two decades, EGDs, such as the LMA and the Combitube, have been shown to be effective and safe devices for delivering effective oxygenation and ventilation. In addition, many studies have shown that these devices can be used successfully to "rescue" patients with a failed airway. With the addition of newer second-generation EGDs on the market, many societies, such as the ASA Difficult Airway Management Algorithm, the Difficult Airway Society (UK), and the Canadian Airway Focus Group, recommend these devices as part of the failed airway algorithm. They ultimately leave the decision to the practitioner which device they choose.

The major disadvantage of all EGDs is their inability to completely seal the larynx and protect against aspiration. In addition, poor seal by any of these devices can lead to air leak on PPV and gastric insufflation. Newer designs of EGD, such as the Intubating LMA (or LMA-Fastrach), LMA-ProSeal, LMA-Supreme, LMA-Protector, King LTS-D®, Baska Mask, and i-gel have been developed to attempt to address these concerns.

As a result of the widespread acceptance and popularity of the original LMA, many newly designed reusable and disposable EGD devices have been introduced. There are no less than 25 EGDs currently available. Although many preliminary clinical studies have demonstrated the efficacy and safety of these devices, most of them involved only a small number of patients. More clinical studies with larger patient populations are needed to confirm these findings. Finally, these devices are not only effective airway management and airway rescue devices, but they can be used and learned easily, in contrast to face-mask ventilation (FMV) and endotracheal intubation. It is entirely reasonable to expect that these devices will supplant FMV as a rescue airway maneuver.

SELF-EVALUATION QUESTIONS

13.1. Which of the following is **NOT** true about the Laryngeal Tube (King LT)?

A. It cannot be used in patients with a history of latex allergy.

B. The Laryngeal Tube has two cuffs (pharyngeal and esophageal) but a single balloon for pressure control.

C. The Laryngeal Tube requires a mouth opening of at least 23 mm for its insertion.

D. The Laryngeal Tube cuffs should be inflated to a pressure of up to 60 cm H_2O using a manometer if possible.

E. A well-lubricated endotracheal tube can be passed blindly through the airway lumen of the LT.

13.2. Which of the following is **NOT** true with the use of the LMA?

A. In general, approximately 20 mL is required to inflate the cuff for a #3, 30 mL for a #4, and 40 mL for a #5 LMA.

B. The LMA should be inserted into the mouth with the index finger placed between the mask-tube junction.

C. The LMA cuff should be pressed against the hard palate during the insertion into the oropharynx.

D. Prior to insertion, the cuff should be completely deflated.

E. To facilitate placement, the LMA should be lubricated using lidocaine gel.

13.3. In comparison with tracheal intubation, which of the following is **NOT** an advantage of the LMA?

A. Improved hemodynamic stability on induction and during emergence

B. No risk of gastric aspiration

C. Reduced anesthetic requirements for airway tolerance

D. Lower frequency of coughing during emergence

E. A lower incidence of sore throat in adults

REFERENCES

1. Caplan RA, Posner KL, Ward RJ, Cheney FW. Adverse respiratory events in anesthesia: a closed claims analysis. *Anesthesiology.* 1990;72:828-833.
2. Kheterpal S, Martin L, Shanks AM, Tremper KK. Prediction and outcomes of impossible mask ventilation: a review of 50,000 anesthetics. *Anesthesiology.* 2009;110:891-897.
3. Langeron O, Masso E, Huraux C, et al. Prediction of difficult mask ventilation. *Anesthesiology.* 2000;92:1229-1236.

4. Mulcaster JT, Mills J, Hung OR, et al. Laryngoscopic intubation: learning and performance. *Anesthesiology*. 2003;98:23-27.
5. Miller DM. Third generation supraglottic airways: is a new classification needed? *Br J Anaesth*. 2015;115:634-635.
6. Apfelbaum JL, Hagberg CA, Connis RT, et al. 2022 American Society of Anesthesiologists practice guidelines for management of the difficult airway. *Anesthesiology*. 2022;136:31-81.
7. Agro FE, Pascarella G. Extraglottic airway devices: is the classification in generations really informative of properties and safety? *Minerva Anestesiol*. 2018;84:649-651.
8. Brimacombe J. A proposed classification system for extraglottic airway devices. *Anesthesiology*. 2004;101:559.
9. Law JA, Duggan LV, Asselin M, et al. Canadian Airway Focus Group updated consensus-based recommendations for management of the difficult airway: part 1. Difficult airway management encountered in an unconscious patient. *Can J Anaesth*. 2021;68:1373-1404.
10. Law JA, Duggan LV, Asselin M, et al. Canadian Airway Focus Group updated consensus-based recommendations for management of the difficult airway: part 2. Planning and implementing safe management of the patient with an anticipated difficult airway. *Can J Anaesth*. 2021;68:1405-1436.
11. Frerk C, Mitchell VS, McNarry AF, et al. Difficult Airway Society 2015 guidelines for management of unanticipated difficult intubation in adults. *Br J Anaesth*. 2015;115:827-848.
12. Ramaiah R, Das D, Bhananker SM, Joffe AM. Extraglottic airway devices: a review. *Int J Crit Illn Inj Sci*. 2014;4:77-87.
13. Bogetz MS. Using the laryngeal mask airway to manage the difficult airway. *Anesth Clin North Am*. 2002;20:863-870, vii.
14. Cook TM. The classic laryngeal mask airway: a tried and tested airway. What now? *Br J Anaesth*. 2006;96:149-152.
15. American Society of Anesthesiologists Task Force on Management of the Difficult Airway. Practice guidelines for the difficult airway. *Anesthesiology*. 1993;78.
16. Apfelbaum JL, Hagberg CA, Caplan RA, et al. Practice guidelines for management of the difficult airway: an updated report by the American Society of Anesthesiologists Task Force on Management of the Difficult Airway. *Anesthesiology*. 2013;118:251-270.
17. Kokkinis K. The use of the laryngeal mask airway in CPR. *Resuscitation*. 1994;27:9-12.
18. Stone BJ, Leach AB, et al. The use of the laryngeal mask airway by nurses during cardiopulmonary resuscitation. Results of a multicentre trial. *Anaesthesia*. 1994;49:3-7.
19. Law JA, Broemling N, Cooper RM, et al. The difficult airway with recommendations for management–part 2–the anticipated difficult airway. *Can J Anaesth*. 2013;60:1119-1138.
20. Law JA, Broemling N, Cooper RM, et al. The difficult airway with recommendations for management. Part 1: difficult tracheal intubation encountered in an unconscious/induced patient. *Can J Anaesth*. 2013;60:1089-1118.
21. Brimacombe JR. Placement phase. In: Brimacombe JR, ed. *Laryngeal Mask Anesthesia*. Philadelphia, PA: Saunders, Elsevier Ltd; 2005.
22. Garcia-Pedrajas F, Monedero P, Carrascosa F. Modification of Brain's technique for insertion of laryngeal mask airway. *Anesth Analg*. 1994;79:1024-1025.
23. Bignell S, Brimacombe J. LMA stability and fixation. *Anaesth Intensive Care*. 1994;22:746.
24. Kim GW, Kim JY, Kim SJ, Moon YR, Park EJ, Park SY. Conditions for laryngeal mask airway placement in terms of oropharyngeal leak pressure: a comparison between blind insertion and laryngoscope-guided insertion. *BMC Anesthesiology*. 2019;19:4.
25. Ozgul U, Erdil FA, Erdogan MA, et al. Comparison of videolaryngoscope-guided versus standard digital insertion techniques of the ProSeal laryngeal mask airway: a prospective randomized study. *BMC Anesthesiology*. 2019;19:244.
26. Brimacombe JR. Emergence phase. In: Brimacombe JR, ed. *Laryngeal Mask Anesthesia*. Philadelphia, PA: Saunders, Elsevier Ltd; 2005.
27. Deakin CD, Diprose P, Majumdar R, Pulletz M. An investigation into the quantity of secretions removed by inflated and deflated laryngeal mask airways. *Anaesthesia*. 2000;55:478-480.
28. Brimacombe J. The advantages of the LMA over the tracheal tube or facemask: a meta-analysis. *Can J Anaesth*. 1995;42:1017-1023.
29. Benumof JL. Laryngeal mask airway and the ASA difficult airway algorithm. *Anesthesiology*. 1996;84:686-699.
30. Keller C, Brimacombe J. Bronchial mucus transport velocity in paralyzed anesthetized patients: a comparison of the laryngeal mask airway and cuffed tracheal tube. *Anesth Analg*. 1998;86:1280-1282.
31. Verghese C, Brimacombe JR. Survey of laryngeal mask airway usage in 11,910 patients: safety and efficacy for conventional and nonconventional usage. *Anesth Analg*. 1996;82:129-133.
32. Keller C, Brimacombe J, Bittersohl J, Lirk P, von Goedecke A. Aspiration and the laryngeal mask airway: three cases and a review of the literature. *Br J Anaesth*. 2004;93:579-582.
33. Steuerwald MT, Braude DA, Petersen TR, Peterson K, Torres MA. Preliminary report: comparing aspiration rates between prehospital patients managed with extraglottic airway devices and endotracheal intubation. *Air Med J*. 2018;37:240-243.
34. Keller C, Sparr HJ, Brimacombe JR. Positive pressure ventilation with the laryngeal mask airway in non-paralysed patients: comparison of sevoflurane and propofol maintenance techniques. *Br J Anaesth*. 1998;80:332-336.
35. Keller C, Sparr HJ, Luger TJ, Brimacombe J. Patient outcomes with positive pressure versus spontaneous ventilation in non-paralysed adults with the laryngeal mask. *Can J Anaesth*. 1998;45:564-567.
36. Maltby JR, Beriault MT, Watson NC, Fick GH. Gastric distension and ventilation during laparoscopic cholecystectomy: LMA-Classic vs. tracheal intubation. *Can J Anaesth*. 2000;47:622-626.
37. Sidaras G, Hunter JM. Is it safe to artificially ventilate a paralysed patient through the laryngeal mask? The jury is still out. *Br J Anaesth*. 2001;86:749-753.
38. Bernardini A, Natalini G. Risk of pulmonary aspiration with laryngeal mask airway and tracheal tube: analysis on 65 712 procedures with positive pressure ventilation. *Anaesthesia*. 2009;64(12):1289-1294.
39. Devitt JH, Wenstone R, Noel AG, O'Donnell MP. The laryngeal mask airway and positive-pressure ventilation. *Anesthesiology*. 1994;80:550-555.
40. Johannigman JA, Branson RD, Davis K Jr, Hurst JM. Techniques of emergency ventilation: a model to evaluate tidal volume, airway pressure, and gastric insufflation. *J Trauma*. 1991;31:93-98.
41. Natalini G, Facchetti P, Dicembrini MA, Lanza G, Rosano A, Bernardini A. Pressure controlled versus volume controlled ventilation with laryngeal mask airway. *J Clin Anesth*. 2001;13:436-439.
42. Cook TM, Woodall N, Frerk C, Fourth National Audit Project. Major complications of airway management in the UK: results of the Fourth National Audit Project of the Royal College of Anaesthetists and the Difficult Airway Society. Part 1: anaesthesia. *Br J Anaesth*. 2011;106:617-631.
43. Cook TM, Woodall N, Harper J, Benger J, Fourth National Audit Project. Major complications of airway management in the UK: results of the Fourth National Audit Project of the Royal College of Anaesthetists and the Difficult Airway Society. Part 2: intensive care and emergency departments. *Br J Anaesth*. 2011;106:632-642.
44. Griffin RM, Hatcher IS. Aspiration pneumonia and the laryngeal mask airway. *Anaesthesia*. 1990;45:1039-1040.
45. Ismail-Zade IA, Vanner RG. Regurgitation and aspiration of gastric contents in a child during general anaesthesia using the laryngeal mask airway. *Paediatr Anaesth*. 1996;6:325-328.
46. Nanji GM, Maltby JR. Vomiting and aspiration pneumonitis with the laryngeal mask airway. *Can J Anaesth*. 1992;39:69-70.
47. Han TH, Brimacombe J, Lee EJ, Yang HS. The laryngeal mask airway is effective (and probably safe) in selected healthy parturients for elective Cesarean section: a prospective study of 1067 cases. *Can J Anaesth*. 2001;48:1117-1121.
48. Brimacombe JR. Pediatrics. In: Brimacombe JR, ed. *Laryngeal Mask Anesthesia*. Philadelphia, PA: Saunders, Elsevier Ltd; 2005.
49. Weiss M, Engelhardt T. Proposal for the management of the unexpected difficult pediatric airway. *Paediatr Anaesth*. 2010;20:454-464.
50. Guidelines for the basic management of the airway and ventilation during resuscitation. A statement by the Airway and Ventilation Management Working Group of the European Resuscitation Council. *Resuscitation*. 1996;31:187-200.
51. The American Heart Association. Guidelines 2000 for cardioplumonary resuscitation and emergency cardiovascular care. Part 11: neonatal resuscitation. *Circulation*. 2000;102:1343-1357.
52. Brimacombe JR. Difficult airway. In: Brimacombe JR, ed. *Laryngeal Mask Anesthesia*. Philadelphia, PA: Saunders, Elsevier Ltd; 2005:305-355.
53. Agro F, Brimacombe J, Carassiti M, Morelli A, Giampalmo M, Cataldo R. Use of a lighted stylet for intubation via the laryngeal mask airway. *Can J Anaesth*. 1998;45:556-560.
54. Hung OR. Light-guided tracheal intubation through the laryngeal mask airway. *Anesth Analg*. 1997;85:1415.
55. Berkow LC, Schwartz JM, Kan K, Corridore M, Heitmiller ES. Use of the Laryngeal Mask Airway-Aintree Intubating Catheter-fiberoptic bronchoscope technique for difficult intubation. *J Clin Anesth*. 2011;23:534-539.
56. Wong DT, Yang JJ, Mak HY, Jagannathan N. Use of intubation introducers through a supraglottic airway to facilitate tracheal intubation: a brief review. *Can J Anaesth*. 2012;59:704-715.
57. Langenstein H. The laryngeal mask airway in the difficult intubation. The results of a prospective study. *Anaesthesist*. 1995;44:712-718.

58. Williams PJ, Bailey PM. Comparison of the reinforced laryngeal mask airway and tracheal intubation for adenotonsillectomy. *Br J Anaesth.* 1993;70:30-33.
59. Sher M, Brimacombe J, Laing D. Anaesthesia for laser pharyngoplasty: a comparison of the tracheal tube with the reinforced laryngeal mask airway. *Anaesth Intensive Care.* 1995;23:149-153.
60. Quinn AC, Samaan A, McAteer EM, Moss E, Vucevic M. The reinforced laryngeal mask airway for dento-alveolar surgery. *Br J Anaesth.* 1996;77:185-188.
61. Brain AI, Verghese C, Addy EV, Kapila A, Brimacombe J. The intubating laryngeal mask. II: a preliminary clinical report of a new means of intubating the trachea. *Br J Anaesth.* 1997;79:704-709.
62. Wong JK, Tongier WK, Armbruster SC, White PF. Use of the intubating laryngeal mask airway to facilitate awake orotracheal intubation in patients with cervical spine disorders. *J Clin Anesth.* 1999;11:346-348.
63. Ferson DZ, Rosenblatt WH, Johansen MJ, Osborn I, Ovassapian A. Use of the intubating LMA-Fastrach in 254 patients with difficult-to-manage airways. *Anesthesiology.* 2001;95:1175-1181.
64. Brimacombe JR. Intubating LMA for airway intubation. In: Brimacombe JR, ed. *Laryngeal Mask Anesthesia.* Philadelphia, PA: Saunders, Elsevier Ltd; 2005:469-504.
65. Chan PL, Lee TW, Lam KK, Chan WS. Intubation through intubating laryngeal mask with and without a lightwand: a randomized comparison. *Anaesth Intensive Care.* 2001;29:255-259.
66. Dimitriou V, Voyagis GS, Grosomanidis V, Brimacombe J. Feasibility of flexible lightwand-guided tracheal intubation with the intubating laryngeal mask during out-of-hospital cardiopulmonary resuscitation by an emergency physician. *Eur J Anaesth.* 2006;23:76-79.
67. Wong DT, Woo JA, Arora G. Lighted stylet-guided intubation via the intubating laryngeal airway in a patient with Hallermann-Streiff syndrome. *Can J Anaesth.* 2009;56:147-150.
68. Pandit JJ, MacLachlan K, Dravid RM, Popat MT. Comparison of times to achieve tracheal intubation with three techniques using the laryngeal or intubating laryngeal mask airway. *Anaesthesia.* 2002;57:128-132.
69. Agro FE, Antonelli S, Cataldo R. Use of Shikani Flexible Seeing Stylet for intubation via the Intubating Laryngeal Mask Airway. *Can J Anaesth.* 2005;52:657-658.
70. Osborn IP. The intubating laryngeal mask airway (ILMA) is assisted by an old device. *Anesth Analg.* 2000;91:1561-1562.
71. Rich JM. Recognition and management of the difficult airway with special emphasis on the intubating LMA-Fastrach/whistle technique: a brief review with case reports. *Proc Bayl Univ Med Cent.* 2005;18:220-227.
72. Frappier J, Guenoun T, Journois D, et al. Airway management using the intubating laryngeal mask airway for the morbidly obese patient. *Anesth Analg.* 2003;96:1510-1515, table of contents.
73. Roblot C, Ferrandiere M, Bierlaire D, Fusciardi J, Mercier C, Laffon M. Impact of Cormack and Lehane's grade on Intubating Laryngeal Mask Airway Fastrach using: a study in gynaecological surgery. *Ann Fr Anesth Reanim.* 2005;24:487-491.
74. Asai T, Matsumoto H, Shingu K. Awake tracheal intubation through the intubating laryngeal mask. *Can J Anaesth.* 1999;46:182-184.
75. Mason AM. Use of the intubating laryngeal mask airway in pre-hospital care: a case report. *Resuscitation.* 2001;51:91-95.
76. Gercek E, Wahlen BM, Rommens PM. In vivo ultrasound real-time motion of the cervical spine during intubation under manual in-line stabilization: a comparison of intubation methods. *Eur J Anaesth.* 2008;25:29-36.
77. Henderson JJ, Popat MT, Latto IP, Pearce AC. Difficult Airway Society guidelines for management of the unanticipated difficult intubation. *Anaesthesia.* 2004;59:675-694.
78. Keller C, Brimacombe J, Kleinsasser A, Loeckinger A. Does the ProSeal laryngeal mask airway prevent aspiration of regurgitated fluid? *Anesth Analg.* 2000;91:1017-1120.
79. Handa-Tsutsui F, Kodaka M. Propofol concentration requirement for laryngeal mask airway insertion was highest with the ProSeal, next highest with the Fastrach, and lowest with the Classic type, with target-controlled infusion. *J Clin Anesth.* 2005;17:344-347.
80. Hwang JW, Park HP, Lim YJ, Do SH, Lee SC, Jeon YT. Comparison of two insertion techniques of ProSeal laryngeal mask airway: standard versus 90-degree rotation. *Anesthesiology.* 2009;110:905-907.
81. Howath A, Brimacombe J, Keller C. Gum-elastic bougie-guided insertion of the ProSeal laryngeal mask airway: a new technique. *Anaesth Intensive Care.* 2002;30:624-627.
82. Eschertzhuber S, Brimacombe J, Hohlrieder M, Stadlbauer KH, Keller C. Gum elastic bougie-guided insertion of the ProSeal laryngeal mask airway is superior to the digital and introducer tool techniques in patients with simulated difficult laryngoscopy using a rigid neck collar. *Anesth Analg.* 2008;107:1253-1256.
83. O'Connor CJ Jr, Borromeo CJ, Stix MS. Assessing ProSeal laryngeal mask positioning: the suprasternal notch test. *Anesth Analg.* 2002;94:1374-1375; author reply 5.
84. Cook TM, Brooks TS, Van der Westhuizen J, Clarke M. The Proseal LMA is a useful rescue device during failed rapid sequence intubation: two additional cases. *Can J Anaesth.* 2005;52:630-633.
85. Brimacombe J, Keller C. Aspiration of gastric contents during use of a ProSeal laryngeal mask airway secondary to unidentified foldover malposition. *Anesth Analg.* 2003;97:1192-1194, table of contents.
86. Keller C, Brimacombe J. Mucosal pressure and oropharyngeal leak pressure with the ProSeal versus laryngeal mask airway in anaesthetized paralysed patients. *Br J Anaesth.* 2000;85:262-266.
87. Qamarul Hoda M, Samad K, Ullah H. ProSeal versus Classic laryngeal mask airway (LMA) for positive pressure ventilation in adults undergoing elective surgery. *Cochrane Database Syst Rev.* 2017;7:CD009026.
88. Goldmann K, Jakob C. A randomized crossover comparison of the size 2 1/2 laryngeal mask airway ProSeal versus laryngeal mask airway-Classic in pediatric patients. *Anesth Analg.* 2005;100:1605-1610.
89. Goldmann K, Jakob C. Size 2 ProSeal laryngeal mask airway: a randomized, crossover investigation with the standard laryngeal mask airway in paediatric patients. *Br J Anaesth.* 2005;94:385-389.
90. Goldmann K, Roettger C, Wulf H. Use of the ProSeal laryngeal mask airway for pressure-controlled ventilation with and without positive end-expiratory pressure in paediatric patients: a randomized, controlled study. *Br J Anaesth.* 2005;95:831-834.
91. Lopez-Gil M, Brimacombe J. The ProSeal laryngeal mask airway in children. *Paediatr Anaesth.* 2005;15:229-234.
92. Lopez-Gil M, Brimacombe J, Barragan L, Keller C. Bougie-guided insertion of the ProSeal laryngeal mask airway has higher first attempt success rate than the digital technique in children. *Br J Anaesth.* 2006;96:238-241.
93. Lopez-Gil M, Brimacombe J, Garcia G. A randomized non-crossover study comparing the ProSeal and Classic laryngeal mask airway in anaesthetized children. *Br J Anaesth.* 2005;95:827-830.
94. Micaglio M, Bonato R, De Nardin M, et al. Prospective, randomized comparison of ProSeal and Classic laryngeal mask airways in anaesthetized neonates and infants. *Br J Anaesth.* 2009;103:263-267.
95. Cook TM, Lee G, Nolan JP. The ProSeal laryngeal mask airway: a review of the literature. *Can J Anaesth.* 2005;52:739-760.
96. Hohlrieder M, Brimacombe J, von Goedecke A, Keller C. Postoperative nausea, vomiting, airway morbidity, and analgesic requirements are lower for the ProSeal laryngeal mask airway than the tracheal tube in females undergoing breast and gynaecological surgery. *Br J Anaesth.* 2007;99:576-580.
97. Brown NI, Mack PF, Mitera DM, Dhar P. Use of the ProSeal laryngeal mask airway in a pregnant patient with a difficult airway during electroconvulsive therapy. *Br J Anaesth.* 2003;91:752-754.
98. Awan R, Nolan JP, Cook TM. Use of a ProSeal laryngeal mask airway for airway maintenance during emergency Caesarean section after failed tracheal intubation. *Br J Anaesth.* 2004;92:144-146.
99. Keller C, Brimacombe J, Lirk P, Puhringer F. Failed obstetric tracheal intubation and postoperative respiratory support with the ProSeal laryngeal mask airway. *Anesth Analg.* 2004;98:1467-1470, table of contents.
100. Vaida SJ, Gaitini LA. Another case of use of the ProSeal laryngeal mask airway in a difficult obstetric airway. *Br J Anaesth.* 2004;92:905; author reply.
101. Verghese C, Ramaswamy B. LMA-Supreme: a new single-use LMA with gastric access: a report on its clinical efficacy. *Br J Anaesth.* 2008;101:405-410.
102. Ali A, Canturk S, Turkmen A, Turgut N, Altan A. Comparison of the laryngeal mask airway Supreme and laryngeal mask airway Classic in adults. *Eur J Anaesth.* 2009;26:1010-1014.
103. Hosten T, Gurkan Y, Ozdamar D, Tekin M, Toker K, Solak M. A new supraglottic airway device: LMA-supreme, comparison with LMA-Proseal. *Acta Anaesthesiol Scand.* 2009;53:852-857.
104. Lee AK, Tey JB, Lim Y, Sia AT. Comparison of the single-use LMA supreme with the reusable ProSeal LMA for anaesthesia in gynaecological laparoscopic surgery. *Anaesth Intensive Care.* 2009;37:815-819.
105. LMA Protector™: Instructions for use. Product Monogram. In: Teleflex Medical M, NC, USA. Available at https://www.teleflexarcatalog.com/anesthesia-respiratory/airway/category/lma-sup-reg-sup-protector-sup-trade-sup-airway.
106. Tan LZ, Tan DJ, Seet E. Laryngeal mask airway protector: advanced uses for laparoscopic cholecystectomies. *Indian J Anaesth.* 2017;61:673-675.
107. Tan LZ, Tan DJA, Seet E. Use of the Laryngeal Mask Airway (LMA) Protector for shoulder surgeries in beach-chair position. *J Clin Anesth.* 2017;39:110-111.
108. Chang JE, Kim H, Lee JM, et al. A prospective, randomized comparison of the LMA-protector and i-gel in paralyzed, anesthetized patients. *BMC Anesthesiology.* 2019;19:118.

109. Tan LZ, An Tan DJ, Seet E. Laryngeal Mask Airway Protector for intubation and extubation in thyroid surgeries: a case report. *Indian J Anaesth.* 2018;62:545-548.
110. Practice guidelines for management of the difficult airway: an updated report by the American Society of Anesthesiologists Task Force on Management of the Difficult Airway. *Anesthesiology.* 2003;98:1269-1277.
111. Agro F, Frass M, Benumof JL, Krafft P. Current status of the Combitube: a review of the literature. *J Clin Anesth.* 2002;14:307-314.
112. Frass M, Frenzer R, Mayer G, Popovic R, Leithner C. Mechanical ventilation with the esophageal tracheal combitube (ETC) in the intensive care unit. *Arch Emerg Med.* 1987;4:219-225.
113. Frass M, Frenzer R, Rauscha F, Schuster E, Glogar D. Ventilation with the esophageal tracheal combitube in cardiopulmonary resuscitation. Promptness and effectiveness. *Chest.* 1988;93.
114. Frass M, Frenzer R, Zdrahal F, Hoflehner G, Porges P, Lackner F. The esophageal tracheal combitube: preliminary results with a new airway for CPR. *Ann Emerg Med.* 1987;16:768-772.
115. Frass M, Rodler S, Frenzer R, Ilias W, Leithner C, Lackner F. Esophageal tracheal combitube, endotracheal airway, and mask: comparison of ventilatory pressure curves. *J Trauma.* 1989;29:1476-1479.
116. Urtubia RM, Aguila CM, Cumsille MA. Combitube: a study for proper use. *Anesth Analg.* 2000;90:958-962.
117. Walz R, Davis S, Panning B. Is the Combitube a useful emergency airway device for anesthesiologists? *Anesth Analg.* 1999;88:233.
118. Butler BD, Little T, Drtil S. Combined use of the esophageal-tracheal Combitube with a colorimetric carbon dioxide detector for emergency intubation/ventilation. *J Clin Monit.* 1995;11:311-316.
119. Wafai Y, Salem MR, Baraka A, Joseph NJ, Czinn EA, Paulissian R. Effectiveness of the self-inflating bulb for verification of proper placement of the Esophageal Tracheal Combitube. *Anesth Analg.* 1995;80:122-126.
120. Bishop MJ, Kharasch ED. Is the Combitube a useful emergency airway device for anesthesiologists? *Anesth Analg.* 1998;86:1141-1142.
121. Brimacombe J, Berry A. The oesophageal tracheal combitube for difficult intubation. *Can J Anaesth.* 1994;41:656-657.
122. Mercer M. The role of the Combitube in airway management. *Anaesthesia.* 2000;55:394-395.
123. Staudinger T, Tesinsky P, Klappacher G, et al. Emergency intubation with the Combitube in two cases of difficult airway management. *Eur J Anaesth.* 1995;12:189-193.
124. Banyai M, Falger S, Roggla M, et al. Emergency intubation with the Combitube in a grossly obese patient with bull neck. *Resuscitation.* 1993;26:271-276.
125. Deroy R, Ghoris M. The Combitube elective anesthetic airway management in a patient with cervical spine fracture. *Anesth Analg.* 1998;87:1441-1442.
126. Klauser R, Roggla G, Pidlich J, Leithner C, Frass M. Massive upper airway bleeding after thrombolytic therapy: successful airway management with the Combitube. *Ann Emerg Med.* 1992;21:431-433.
127. Bercker S, Schmidbauer W, Volk T, et al. A comparison of seal in seven supraglottic airway devices using a cadaver model of elevated esophageal pressure. *Anesth Analg.* 2008;106:445-448, table of contents.
128. Krafft P, Roggla M, Fridrich P, Locker GJ, Frass M, Benumof JL. Bronchoscopy via a redesigned Combitube in the esophageal position. A clinical evaluation. *Anesthesiology.* 1997;86:1041-1045.
129. Calkins TR, Miller K, Langdorf MI. Success and complication rates with prehospital placement of an esophageal-tracheal combitube as a rescue airway. *Prehosp Disaster Med.* 2006;21:97-100.
130. Vezina D, Lessard MR, Bussieres J, Topping C, Trepanier CA. Complications associated with the use of the Esophageal-Tracheal Combitube. *Can J Anaesth.* 1998;45:76-80.
131. Zamora JE, Saha TK. Combitube rescue for Cesarean delivery followed by ninth and twelfth cranial nerve dysfunction. *Can J Anaesth.* 2008;55:779-784.
132. Bagheri SC, Stockmaster N, Delgado G, et al. Esophageal rupture with the use of the Combitube: report of a case and review of the literature. *J Oral Maxillofac Surg.* 2008;66:1041-1044.
133. McGlinch BP, Martin DP, Volcheck GW, Carmichael SW. Tongue engorgement with prolonged use of the esophageal-tracheal Combitube. *Ann Emerg Med.* 2004;44:320-322.
134. Agro F, Cataldo R, Alfano A, Galli B. A new prototype for airway management in an emergency: the Laryngeal Tube. *Resuscitation.* 1999;41:284-286.
135. Asai T, Shingu K. The laryngeal tube. *Br J Anaesth.* 2005;95:729-736.
136. Dumbarton TC, Hung OR, Kent B. Overinflation of a King LT Extraglottic Airway Device Mimicking Ludwig's Angina. *A & A Case Reports.* 2016;6:80-83.
137. Dorges V, Ocker H, Wenzel V, Schmucker P. The laryngeal tube: a new simple airway device. *Anesth Analg.* 2000;90:1220-1222.
138. Finteis T, Genzwuerker HV, Hinkelbein J, Roth H, Schmeck J. LMA-Unique, SoftSeal, LTD and LaryVent: bench model comparison of 4 single-use supraglottic airway devices to facemask ventilation. *Respiration.* 2004;21:65(A-262).
139. Wiese CH, Bahr J, Graf BM. "Laryngeal Tube-D" (LT-D) and "Laryngeal Mask" (LMA). *Dtsch Med Wochenschr.* 2009;134:69-74.
140. Genzwuerker HV, Fritz A, Hinkelbein J, et al. Prospective, randomized comparison of laryngeal tube and laryngeal mask airway in pediatric patients. *Paediatr Anaesth.* 2006;16:1251-1256.
141. Asai T, Murao K, Shingu K. Efficacy of the laryngeal tube during intermittent positive-pressure ventilation. *Anaesthesia.* 2000;55:1099-1102.
142. Marquez X, Marquez A. A new laryngeal tube. *Anesth Analg.* 2003;96:1842.
143. Asai T, Kawachi S. Pressure exerted by the cuff of the laryngeal tube on the oropharynx. *Anaesthesia.* 2001;56:911-912.
144. Agro FE, Galli B, Cataldo R, et al. Relationship between body mass index and ventilation with the Laryngeal Tube(R) in 228 anesthetized paralyzed patients: a pilot study. *Can J Anaesth.* 2002;49:641-642.
145. Bortone L, Ingelmo PM, De Ninno G, et al. Randomized controlled trial comparing the laryngeal tube and the laryngeal mask in pediatric patients. *Paediatr Anaesth.* 2006;16:251-257.
146. March JA, Tassey TE, Resurreccion NB, Portela RC, Taylor SE. Comparison of the I-Gel supraglottic and king laryngotracheal airways in a simulated tactical environment. *Prehosp Emerg Care.* 2018;22:385-389.
147. Genzwuerker HV, Vollmer T, Ellinger K. Fibreoptic tracheal intubation after placement of the laryngeal tube. *Br J Anaesth.* 2002;89:733-738.
148. Hooshangi H, Wong DT. Brief review: the Cobra Perilaryngeal Airway (CobraPLA and the Streamlined Liner of Pharyngeal Airway (SLIPA) supraglottic airways. *Can J Anaesth.* 2008;55:177-185.
149. Agro F, Barzoi G, Carassiti M, Galli B. Getting the tube in the oesophagus and oxygen in the trachea: preliminary results with the new supraglottic device (Cobra) in 28 anaesthetised patients. *Anaesthesia.* 2003;58:920-921.
150. Agro F, Carassiti M, Barzoi G, Millozzi F, Galli B. A first report on the diagnosis and treatment of acute postoperative airway obstruction with the CobraPLA. *Can J Anaesth.* 2004;51:640-641.
151. Gaitini L, Yanovski B, Somri M, Vaida S, Riad T, Alfery D. A comparison between the PLA Cobra and the Laryngeal Mask Airway Unique during spontaneous ventilation: a randomized prospective study. *Anesth Analg.* 2006;102:631-636.
152. Kusaka Y, Uda R, Son H, Akatsuka M. Successful fiberoptic tracheal intubation via Cobra PLA in a patient with an epiglottic tumor. *Masui.* 2009;58:474-476.
153. Andrews DT, Williams DL, Alexander KD, Lie Y. Randomised comparison of the Classic Laryngeal Mask Airway with the Cobra Perilaryngeal Airway during anaesthesia in spontaneously breathing adult patients. *Anaesth Intensive Care.* 2009;37:85-92.
154. Wronska-Sewruk A, Nestorowicz A, Kowalczyk M. Classic laryngeal mask airway vs COBRA-PLA device for airway maintenance during minor urological procedures. *Anestezjol Intens Ter.* 2009;41:73-77.
155. Yaghoobi S, Abootorabi SM, Kayalha H, Van Zundert TC, Pakpour AH. Efficacy of the New Perilaryngeal Airway (CobraPLA) Versus the Laryngeal Mask Airway (LMA) to improve oropharyngeal leak pressure in obese and overweight patients. *Tanaffos.* 2015;14:42-48.
156. Galvin EM, van Doorn M, Blazquez J, et al. A randomized prospective study comparing the Cobra Perilaryngeal Airway and Laryngeal Mask Airway-Classic during controlled ventilation for gynecological laparoscopy. *Anesth Analg.* 2007;104:102-105.
157. Park SH, Han SH, Do SH, Kim JW, Kim JH. The influence of head and neck position on the oropharyngeal leak pressure and cuff position of three supraglottic airway devices. *Anesth Analg.* 2009;108:112-117.
158. Khan RM, Maroof M, Johri A, Ashraf M, Jain D. Cobra PLA can overcome LMA failure in patients with face and neck contractures. *Can J Anaesth.* 2005;52:340.
159. van Zundert A, Brimacombe J, Kamphuis R, Haanschoten M. The anatomical position of three extraglottic airway devices in patients with clear airways. *Anaesthesia.* 2006;61:891-895.
160. Cook TM, Lowe JM. An evaluation of the Cobra perilaryngeal airway: study halted after two cases of pulmonary aspiration. *Anaesthesia.* 2005;60:791-796.
161. Farrow C, Cook T. Pulmonary aspiration through a Cobra PLA. *Anaesthesia.* 2004;59:1140-1141; discussion 1-2.
162. Hagberg CA, Jensen FS, Genzwuerker HV, et al. A multicenter study of the Ambu laryngeal mask in nonparalyzed, anesthetized patients. *Anesth Analg.* 2005;101:1862-1866.
163. Sudhir G, Redfern D, Hall JE, Wilkes AR, Cann C. A comparison of the disposable Ambu AuraOnce Laryngeal Mask with the reusable LMA Classic laryngeal mask airway. *Anaesthesia.* 2007;62:719-722.

164. The Ambu® AuraOnce™ Single Use Laryngeal Mask: Product Information.: ambu.
165. Baidya DK, Chandralekha, Darlong V, Pandey R, Maitra S, Khanna P. Comparative efficacy and safety of the Ambu((R)) AuraOnce() laryngeal mask airway during general anaesthesia in adults: a systematic review and meta-analysis. *Anaesthesia.* 2014;69:1023-1032.
166. Miller DM, Lavelle M. A streamlined pharynx airway liner: a pilot study in 22 patients in controlled and spontaneous ventilation. *Anesth Analg.* 2002;94:759-761; table of contents.
167. Miller DM, Light D. Laboratory and clinical comparisons of the Streamlined Liner of the Pharynx Airway (SLIPA) with the laryngeal mask airway. *Anaesthesia.* 2003;58:136-142.
168. Kang H, Kim DR, Jung YH, et al. Pre-warming the Streamlined Liner of the Pharynx Airway (SLIPA) improves fitting to the laryngeal structure: a randomized, double-blind study. *BMC Anesthesiology.* 2015;15:167.
169. Abdellatif AA, Ali MA. Comparison of streamlined liner of the pharynx airway (SLIPA) with the laryngeal mask airway Proseal for lower abdominal laparoscopic surgeries in paralyzed, anesthetized patients. *Saudi J Anaesth.* 2011;5:270-276.
170. Kim SH, Choi EM, Chang CH, Kim HK, Chung MH, Choi YR. Comparison of the effect-site concentrations of remifentanil for Streamlined Liner of the Pharynx Airway (SLIPA) versus laryngeal mask airway SoftSealTM insertion during target-controlled infusion of propofol. *Anaesth Intensive Care.* 2011;39:611-617.
171. Choi GJ, Kang H, Baek CW, et al. Comparison of streamlined liner of the pharynx airway (SLIPA) and laryngeal mask airway: a systematic review and meta-analysis. *Anaesthesia.* 2015;70:613-622.
172. i-gel User Guide. 2022. http://www.i-gel.com/lib/docs/instructions/i-gel%20user%20guide_UK.pdf. Accessed August 20, 2022.
173. Gabbott DA, Beringer R. The iGEL supraglottic airway: a potential role for resuscitation? *Resuscitation.* 2007;73:161-162.
174. Sharma R, MdA R. A comparative evaluation of LMA supreme and I-Gel in patients undergoing elective surgery with controlled ventilation. *Santosh Univ J Health Sci.* 2019;5:5-9.
175. Liew G, John B, Ahmed S. Aspiration recognition with an i-gel airway. *Anaesthesia.* 2008;63:786.
176. Gibbison B, Cook TM, Seller C. Case series: protection from aspiration and failure of protection from aspiration with the i-gel airway. *Br J Anaesth.* 2008;100:415-417.
177. Gatward JJ, Cook TM, Seller C, et al. Evaluation of the size 4 i-gel airway in one hundred non-paralysed patients. *Anaesthesia.* 2008;63:1124-1130.
178. Schmidbauer W, Bercker S, Volk T, Bogusch G, Mager G, Kerner T. Oesophageal seal of the novel supralaryngeal airway device I-Gel in comparison with the laryngeal mask airways Classic and ProSeal using a cadaver model. *Br J Anaesth.* 2009;102:135-139.
179. Davenport C, Martin-Gill C, Wang HE, Mayrose J, Carlson JN. Comparison of the force required for dislodgement between secured and unsecured airways. *Prehosp Emerg Care.* 2018;22:778-781.
180. An J, Nam SB, Lee JS, et al. Comparison of the i-gel and other supraglottic airways in adult manikin studies: systematic review and meta-analysis. *Medicine (Baltimore).* 2017;96:e5801.
181. Jackson KM, Cook TM. Evaluation of four airway training manikins as patient simulators for the insertion of eight types of supraglottic airway devices. *Anaesthesia.* 2007;62:388-393.
182. Richez B, Saltel L, Banchereau F, Torrielli R, Cros AM. A new single use supraglottic airway device with a noninflatable cuff and an esophageal vent: an observational study of the i-gel. *Anesth Analg.* 2008;106:1137-1139, table of contents.
183. Michalek P, Hodgkinson P, Donaldson W. Fiberoptic intubation through an I-gel supraglottic airway in two patients with predicted difficult airway and intellectual disability. *Anesth Analg.* 2008;106:1501-1504, table of contents.
184. Joshi NA, Baird M, Cook TM. Use of an i-gel for airway rescue. *Anaesthesia.* 2008;63:1020-1021.
185. Sharma S, Scott S, Rogers R, Popat M. The i-gel airway for ventilation and rescue intubation. *Anaesthesia.* 2007;62:419-420.
186. Lockey D, Crewdson K, Weaver A, Davies G. Observational study of the success rates of intubation and failed intubation airway rescue techniques in 7256 attempted intubations of trauma patients by pre-hospital physicians. *Br J Anaesth.* 2014;113:220-225.
187. Alexiev V, Salim A, Kevin LG, Laffey JG. An observational study of the Baska(R) mask: a novel supraglottic airway. *Anaesthesia.* 2012;67:640-645.
188. Alexiev V, Ochana A, Abdelrahman D, et al. Comparison of the Baska® mask with the single-use laryngeal mask airway in low-risk female patients undergoing ambulatory surgery. *Anaesthesia.* 2013;68:1026-1032.
189. Al-Rawahi SAS, Aziz H, Malik MA, Khan RM, Kaul N. A comparative analysis of the Baska mask vs proseal laryngeal mask for general anesthesia with IPPV. *Anaesth Pain & Intensive Care.* 2013;17:233-236.
190. Sachidananda R, Shaikh SI, Mitragotri MV, et al. Comparison between the Baska Mask® and I-Gel for minor surgical procedures under general anaesthesia. *Turk J Anaesthesiol Reanim.* 2019;47:24-30.
191. Sharma P, Rai S, Tripathi M, Malviya D, Kumari S, Mishra S. Comparison of LMA supreme, i-gel, and baska mask for airway management during laparoscopic cholecystectomy: a prospective randomized comparative study from North India. *Anesth: Essays Res.* 2022;16:42.
192. Garg A, Lamba NS, Ajai Chandra NS, Singhal RK, Chaudhary V. Supraglottic airway devices in short gynecological procedures: a randomized, clinical study comparing the Baska® mask and I-Gel® device. *J Family Med Prim Care.* 2019;8:1134-1137.
193. Tosh P, Kumar RB, Sahay N, Suman S, Bhadani UK. Efficacy of Baska mask as an alternative airway device to endotracheal tube in patients undergoing laparoscopic surgeries under controlled ventilation. *J Anaesthesiol Clin Pharmacol.* 2021;37:419-424.
194. Jadhav PA, Dalvi NP, Tendolkar BA. I-gel versus laryngeal mask airway-Proseal: comparison of two supraglottic airway devices in short surgical procedures. *J Anaesthesiol Clin Pharmacol.* 2015;31:221-225.
195. Mahajan SR, Mahajan M, Chaudhary U, Kumar S. Evaluation of Baska mask performance in laparoscopic cholecystectomy. *J Med Dent Sci.* 2018;17:74-78.
196. Verma N, Nigam A, Singam A. Comparative evaluation of Baska mask and LMA supreme in patients undergoing short surgical procedures under general anaesthesia. *J Evol Med Dent Sci.* 2020;9:2377-2381.
197. Ng CC, Sybil Shah MHB, Chaw SH, et al. Baska mask versus endotracheal tube in laparoscopic cholecystectomy surgery: a prospective randomized trial. *Expert Rev Med Devices.* 2021;18:203-210.
198. Foo LL, Shariffuddin II, Chaw SH, et al. Randomized comparison of the Baska FESS mask and the LMA Supreme in different head and neck positions. *Expert Rev Med Devices.* 2018;15:597-603.
199. Kara D, Sarikas CM. Comparison of the Baska and I-gel supraglottic airway devices: a randomized controlled study. *Ann Saudi Med.* 2019;39:302-308.

CHAPTER 14

Front-of-Neck Access

David T. Wong, Fabricio B. Zasso, and Kong Eric You-Ten

CASE PRESENTATION

The following clinical scenario highlights the importance of front-of-neck access (FONA) in perioperative anesthesia patient care:

A patient presented to the emergency department with significant stridor secondary to a neck mass extending just below his mandible. His past medical history included atrial fibrillation for which he was taking coumadin. Imaging demonstrated that the mass was a neck hematoma secondary to an overdose of coumadin with an INR >6. Due to a high risk of excessive bleeding that resulted in a difficult tracheotomy and severe hypoxemia, the patient underwent an awake flexible bronchoscopic intubation. A double set-up with a FONA was prepared and the neck landmarks for localization of the cricothyroid membrane (CTM) were identified using both palpation and ultrasonography. However, during the bronchoscopic intubation attempt, the patient experienced complete airway obstruction and oxygen desaturation. Without delay, the anesthesia practitioner performed an emergency FONA by accessing the trachea through the CTM using a size 10 scalpel blade, inserting a bougie, followed by a size 6.0 internal diameter endotracheal tube (ETT). Successful cricothyrotomy was confirmed with positive end-tidal CO_2, bilateral chest rises, and improved oxygen saturation to 96%. The patient was then transferred to the intensive care unit.

AIRWAY ANATOMY

What Anatomy Do I Have to Know to Perform a Front-of-Neck Access?

Access to the airway through the CTM requires a practical knowledge of the anatomy of the larynx, particularly the surface landmarks, and the important adjacent structures in the neck (also see Chapter 3).

In most adult males, the thyroid notch ("Adam's apple") is a prominent feature, which identifies the superior aspect of the thyroid cartilage. With the neck extended, palpation inferiorly from this point will often allow the practitioner to identify the inferior margin of the thyroid cartilage and the ringed-shaped cricoid cartilage below (Figure 14.1).

Between the inferior margin of the thyroid and cricoid cartilage is the CTM. The size of the membrane in adults is 22 to 33 mm wide and 9 to 10 mm high.[1] Should landmarks be difficult to palpate, the level of the CTM can be estimated by the finger stacking technique (or four-finger technique)[2]: with the head and neck in neutral position, the fifth finger is placed in the suprasternal notch; with all fingers in juxtaposition, the location of the index finger will approximate the level of the CTM. In addition, skin creases ("Launcelott Creases") in the anterior neck may also represent a useful visual landmark for estimating the level of the CTM. The study conducted at our institution demonstrated that with the head in the neutral position, in patients with two neck creases inferior to the mentum, the second skin crease was about 2.0 mm (median distance) above the cricoid cartilage[3] (Figure 14.2).

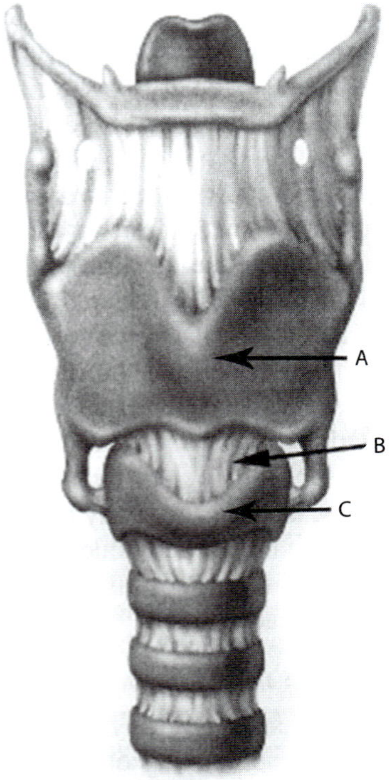

FIGURE 14.1. Anatomy of the larynx and trachea: **(A)** the thyroic cartilage; **(B)** the cricothyroid membrane; and **(C)** the cricoid cartilage.

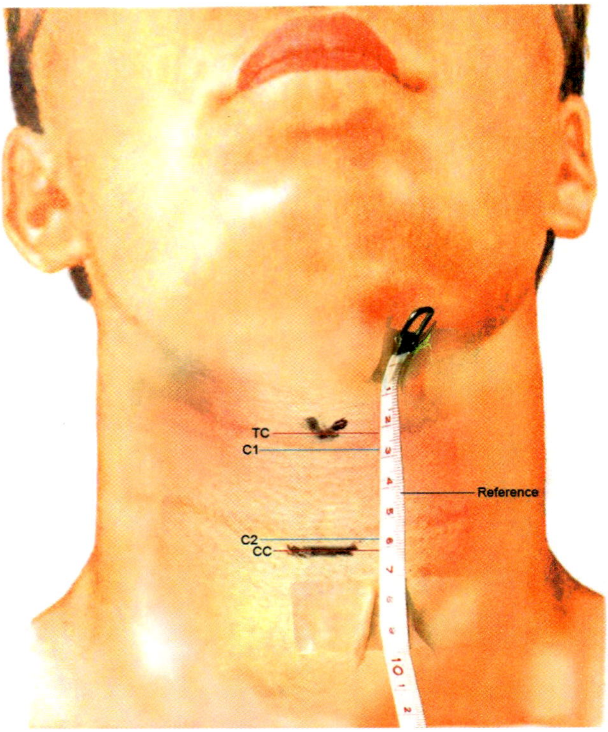

FIGURE 14.2. Surface landmarks of the anterior neck: thyroid cartilage (TC), first skin crease below mentum (C1), second skin crease below mentum (C2), and cricoid cartilage (CC).

The vocal cords are attached to the internal, anterior surface of the thyroid cartilage approximately 1 cm above its inferior border.[4] Care should be exercised in placing retraction instruments superior to the cricothyroid incision to minimize trauma to the vocal cords and body of the thyroid cartilage in the anterior midline. The only vascular structure of note in the vicinity of the CTM is the superior thyroid artery, which, in 54% of people, courses along its lateral border.[5] The left and right cricothyroid arteries, branches of their respective superior thyroid arteries, course medially and traverse the upper half of the CTM,[5] anastomosing in the midline. Injury to these vessels can be avoided by entering the CTM in its inferior half.

Other important anatomical structures include the hyoid bone and the thyroid gland with its central isthmus and possible presence of an attached pyramidal lobe. The airway itself is suspended by the hyoid bone lying superior to the thyroid cartilage. Identifying the hyoid bone is important to avoid mistaking the thyrohyoid space for the CTM. In patients with poorly palpable surface anatomy, the location of the hyoid bone can be estimated by extending a line from the mentum posteriorly, half the distance between the mentum and the angle of the mandible,[6] and distinguishing this underlying structure from the lower lying thyroid and cricoid cartilages. Identifying all the laryngeal structures, whether from top down or down up, is crucial prior to making a surgical incision.

The thyroid gland has a pyramidal lobe in up to 40% of patients.[7] The pyramidal lobe is highly vascular and has a propensity to come off the left side of the thyroid isthmus. Extension superiorly beyond the thyroid cartilage is often notable as a fibrous band, which is a remnant of the thyroglossal duct. Extension beyond the thyroid cartilage as high as the hyoid bone is very rare[8,9] and poses a small additional bleeding risk due to injury during cricothyrotomy.

What Approach Can Be Used to Identify the Neck Landmarks?

An approach advocated by the 2015 Difficult Airway Society Guidelines is the laryngeal handshake to identify the neck landmarks when performing an emergency FONA.[10] Using the non-dominant (ND) hand with the thumb on one side and four fingers on the other side placed just under the mandible, the tracheolaryngeal tract is grasped and stabilized. Starting at the hyoid cartilage, the thumb and fingers slide down over the thyroid laminae and the cricoid cartilage, while the index finger palpates the midline for the CTM located between the thyroid and cricoid cartilage. Anatomical advantages to perform a FONA via the CTM are that it is the most superficial structure of the airway tract in non-obese patients to access the trachea, is less vascularized to minimize bleeding, and the ring structure of the cricoid cartilage provides a relative protection of the posterior wall of the trachea during a cricothyrotomy.

Can the CTM Anatomical Landmark Be Better Defined?

Over the past decade, increasing evidence support the use of ultrasound-guided identification of the CTM puncture site prior

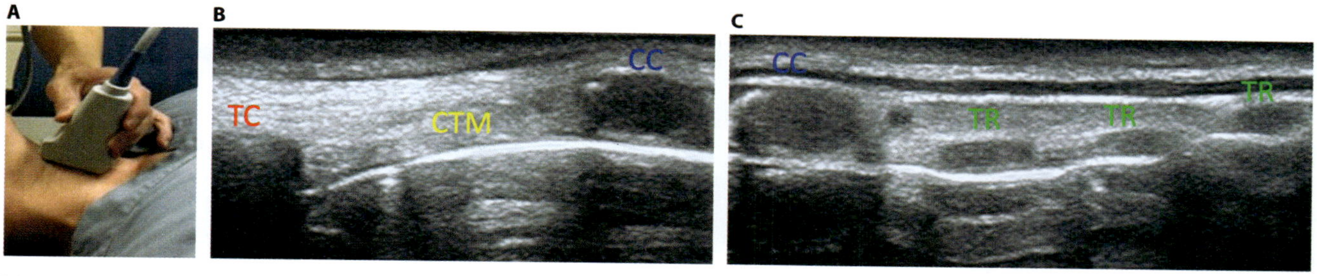

FIGURE 14.3. Ultrasound (US) identification of neck landmarks. **(A)** The US probe was placed on the longitudinal axis in the midline of a volunteer's neck with the probe indicator in the cephalad position. **(B)** The US images showing the cartilages as hypoechoic structures. The white hyperechoic lines are tissue-air artifacts with the lumen of the trachea below as reverberation artifacts. The US image shows the thyroid cartilage (TC—in red), cricothyroid membrane (CTM—in yellow), and cricoid cartilage (CC—in blue). **(C)** The cricoid cartilage (CC—in blue) is identified as an anterior and larger hypoechoic structure compared to the tracheal rings (TR—in green).

to induction of an elective or semi-elective patient suspected of having a difficult airway.[11,12] However, evidence is limited in the role of ultrasound of the airway in a "can't intubate, can't oxygenate" (CICO) emergency situation. Several studies showed that the CTM can be accurately, reliably, and expeditiously identified by bedside ultrasound (Figure 14.3). Studies have shown that practitioners accurately identified the CTM puncture site by palpation in only 10% to 30% of attempts.[13] The accuracy in CTM identification was even lower in individuals with high BMI, particularly in the non-pregnant[14] and pregnant[15] female population. Furthermore, there is a good correlation in identification of airway structures and dimension measurements between ultrasound and CT modalities in patients with normal[16] and abnormal[17] neck. Thus, in non-emergency cases with suspected or known difficult airway, especially in subjects with difficult CTM identification by palpation, a pre-procedure bedside ultrasound marking of CTM can be quite useful and potentially life-saving. In a study with cadavers, Siddiqui et al. demonstrated that ultrasound, compared to palpation, was more accurate in identifying the CTM and resulted in greater success and less complications of a cricothyrotomy.[18]

FRONT-OF-NECK AIRWAY

When Do You Perform a Cricothyrotomy? (Video 15)

An emergency cricothyrotomy is the last step in the CICO algorithm and is a potentially life-saving procedure where the benefit clearly outweighs the risk.[19] Studies reported that it is not the procedure itself, but the delay in performing the procedure that can lead to death and brain hypoxia in a CICO situation.[9,10] In the emergency situation when gas exchange cannot be established, a surgical airway is mandatory to prevent catastrophe. As such, there are no contraindications to a surgical airway. There are, however, certain issues that deserve consideration.

In acute or chronic inflammatory laryngeal pathology, and neoplastic disease, cricothyrotomy will likely be more difficult to perform and be subject to a greater incidence of subglottic stenosis (SGS). Obesity, injuries, and deformities of the neck may either distort the anatomy and/or render surface landmarks difficult to palpate; and uncontrolled hemorrhage may complicate the situation in the anticoagulated patient. Cricotracheal separation is an absolute contraindication to any procedures that utilize the CTM.

What Are the Most Common Techniques Used for FONA?

Five common methods of FONA through the CTM are outlined:

1. Open cricothyrotomy
2. Seldinger wire-guided cricothyrotomy
3. Scalpel bougie cricothyrotomy
4. Cannula over needle cricothyrotomy
5. Needle cricothyrotomy with narrow bore cannula

Can You Walk Me Through Each Method… Step by Step?

Preamble: Positioning of patient for cricothyrotomy for all techniques is critical. Sniffing position is not an optimal position for cricothyrotomy. Instead, the neck should be maximally extended by putting a row or towel between the shoulder blades, removing the pillow, and putting the head directly on the bed.

(1) Can You Describe the Open Cricothyrotomy Technique?[10,19] (Video 4)

Open cricothyrotomy is by far the simplest cricothyrotomy technique with the fewest equipment involved—a scalpel, tracheal hook (and Trousseau dilator) if available, and ETT.

Equipment

The instruments required are:

a) Scalpel with a #20 blade;
b) Tracheal hook (optional Trousseau dilator);
c) 6.0-mm ID cuffed ETT.

Technique: Scalpel, Retractor, ETT

1. Palpation of the CTM in a cadaver (Figure 14.4): The left (ND) hand is used to stabilize the larynx by grasping the body of the thyroid cartilage between the thumb and middle finger leaving the index finger free to palpate the cartilaginous structures;

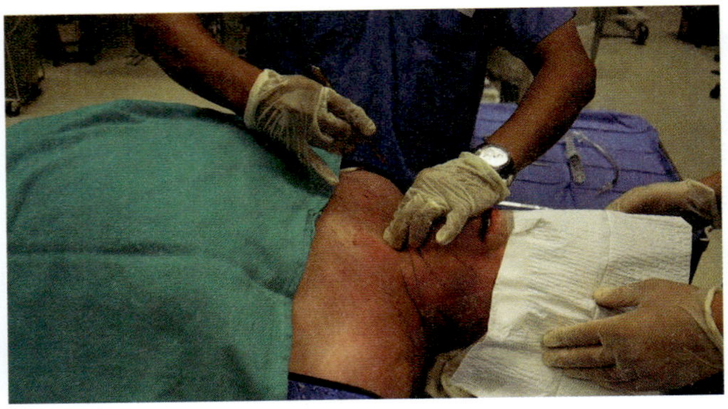

FIGURE 14.4. Open Cricothyrotomy Technique in a cadaver. Palpation of the cricothyrotomy membrane (CTM) in a cadaver: The left (non-dominant) hand is used to stabilize the larynx by grasping the body of the thyroid cartilage between the thumb and middle finger leaving the index finger free to palpate the cartilaginous structures.

2. A 4.0 cm *vertical, midline skin incision* (Figure 14.5);
3. A *transverse incision of the CTM* at the superior border of the cricoid cartilage;
4. *Retraction with a tracheal hook* (Figure 14.6); either superiorly, with potential trauma to the vocal cords or thyroid cartilage, or inferiorly, with less risk and perhaps better exposure due to a higher degree of mobility of the cricoid than the thyroid cartilage;

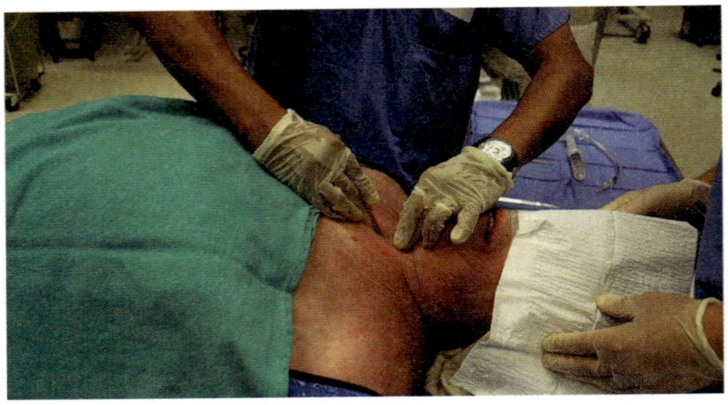

FIGURE 14.5. Open cricothyrotomy technique in a cadaver. A 4 cm vertical, midline skin incision is made followed by a transverse incision of the CTM at the superior border of the cricoid cartilage.

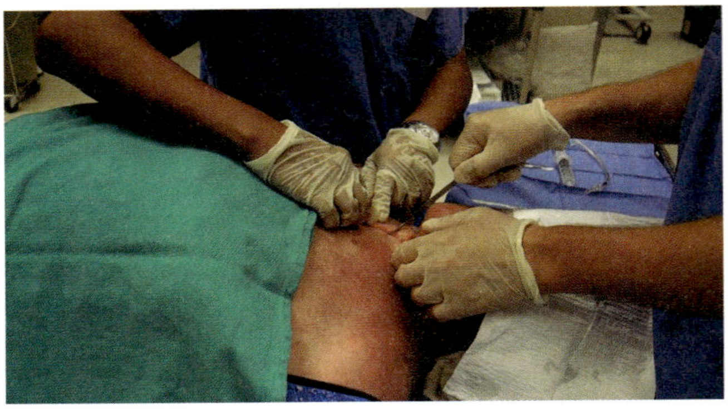

FIGURE 14.6. Open cricothyrotomy technique in a cadaver. Retraction with a tracheal hook superiorly.

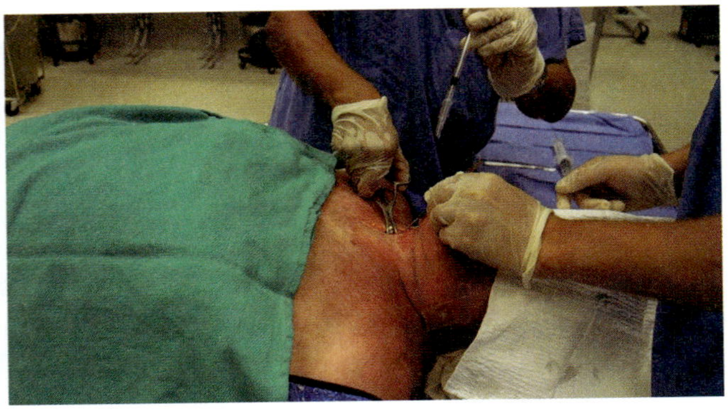

FIGURE 14.7. Open cricothyrotomy technique in a cadaver. Insertion of a Trousseau dilator (if available).

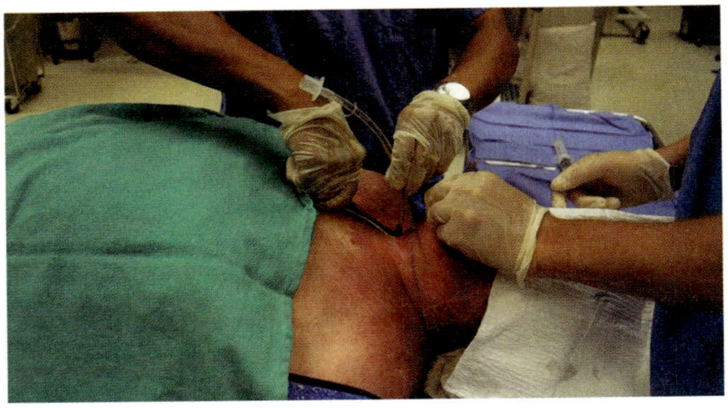

FIGURE 14.8. Open cricothyrotomy technique in a cadaver. A 6.0-mm ID ETT is inserted into the trachea through cricothyroid incision (or through the Trousseau dilator if used).

5. Optional step if available: Insertion of a *Trousseau dilator* to maintain the CTM opening. (Figure 14.7);
6. Insertion of a 6.0-mm ID cuffed ETT, through the CTM into the trachea (Figure 14.8);
7. Inflation of the cuff, ensuring the proper position, and removal of the tracheal hook or dilator;
8. Prior to securing the tube, it is important to confirm proper placement by $ETCO_2$, auscultation, or flexible endoscopy; a Chest X-ray should be obtained to determine proper tube position and to rule out any parenchymal lung injury or pneumothorax;
9. Current recommendations view a cricothyrotomy as a temporizing, life-saving measure. The cricothyrotomy tube may be removed later when the conditions leading to upper airway obstruction have resolved. Alternatively, the patient may undergo conversion to a traditional tracheotomy.

(2) What Is the Seldinger Wire-Guided Cricothyrotomy Technique and How Is It Done?[10,19–22]

Most practitioners are familiar with the wire-guided Seldinger technique from central venous cannula insertion, and surveys have shown that[20] airway practitioners were more comfortable with this approach than an open FONA approach. However, the NAP4[21] study revealed that the success rate of non-scalpel cricothyrotomy was less than 50%, while the success of open surgical cricothyrotomy was close to 100%. Furthermore, identifying accurately the CTM in an emergency "CICO" situation was in the realm of 30% and the technique was fraught with a multitude of issues, such as prolonged procedural time, kinking of the guidewire, creation of a false passage, and inability to adequately dilate and cannulate the airway.[22]

Equipment

There are several cricothyrotomy kits designed with this technique in mind and all with similar contents (Figure 14.9). They contain:

a) Scalpel with a #20 blade;
b) A 5- or 10-mL syringe;
c) 18-gauge cannula over needle (and/or a thin-walled introducer needle);
d) A guidewire;
e) A dilator;
f) Cuffed 5.0-mm ID or 6.0-mm ID airway tube.

Technique

1. A small vertical midline *scalpel stab incision* through the skin overlying the CTM;
2. Caudal insertion of an *18-gauge cannula* attached to a syringe (Figure 14.10);
3. Confirmation of cannula placement by *aspirating air*, advance cannula over needle, then removal of the needle and syringe; apply syringe to cannula to aspirate air confirming cannula location (Figure 14.11);
4. Insertion of a *guidewire* (Figure 14.12) and removal of the cannula, leaving the guidewire in the trachea;
5. After making a *small cut* of the CTM using the pointed scalpel along the guidewire, the cuffed airway *tube loaded onto the dilator* is advanced as a single unit, over the wire into the trachea (Figure 14.13);

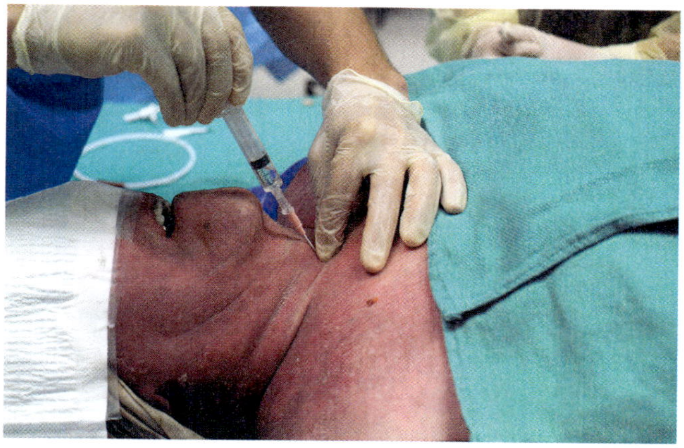

FIGURE 14.10. Seldinger wire-guided cricothyrotomy technique in a cadaver. Following a small vertical midline stab incision through the skin overlying the CTM, an 18-gauge cannula attached to a syringe is inserted through the CTM.

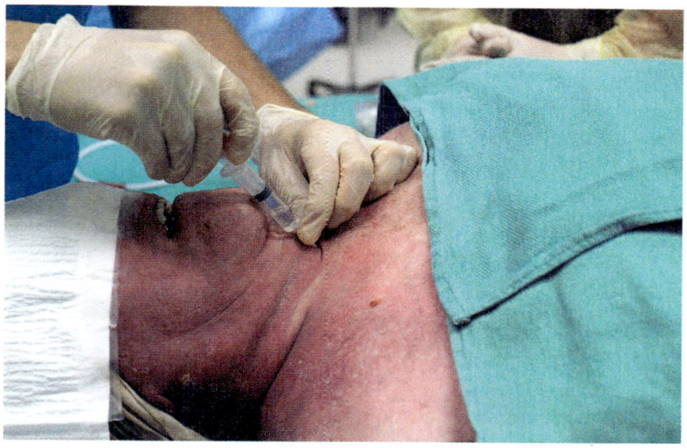

FIGURE 14.11. Seldinger wire-guided cricothyrotomy technique in a cadaver: Confirmation of cannula placement by *aspirating air*, advance cannula over needle, then removal of the needle and syringe. Apply syringe to cannula to aspirate air confirming cannula location.

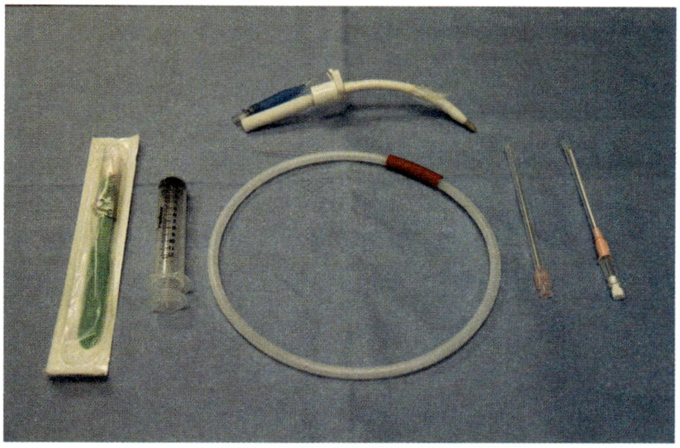

FIGURE 14.9. Equipment for Seldinger wire-guided cricothyrotomy technique: a scalpel blade, a syringe, an 18-gauge catheter over needle and/or a thin-walled introducer needle, a guidewire, a dilator, and a cuffed 5.0-mm ID airway tube.[23]

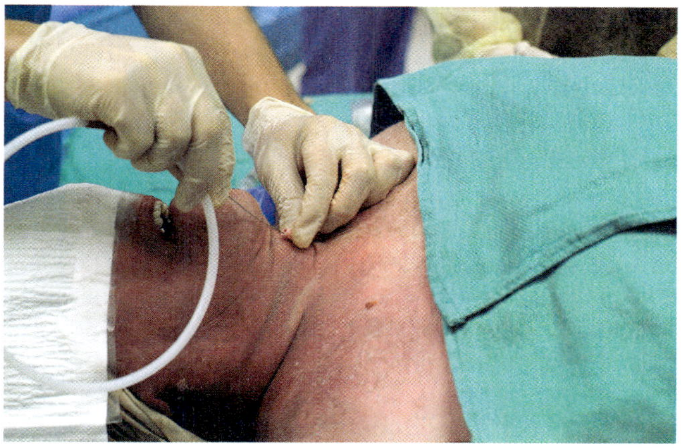

FIGURE 14.12. Seldinger wire-guided cricothyrotomy technique in a cadaver. A guidewire is inserted into the trachea through the cannula.

CHAPTER 14

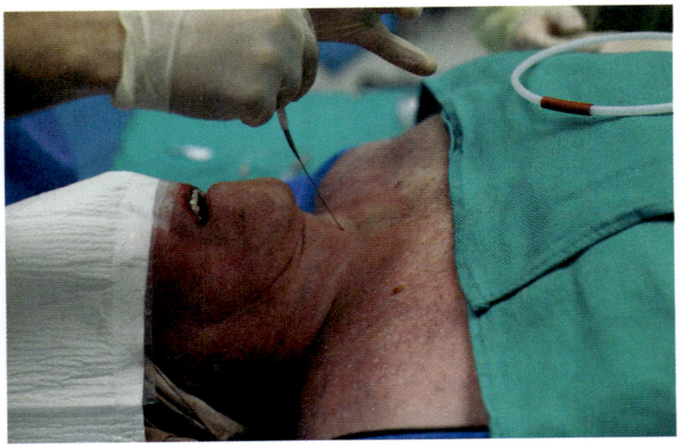

FIGURE 14.13. Seldinger wire-guided cricothyrotomy technique in a cadaver. After making a *small cut* of the CTM using the pointed scalpel along the guidewire, the cuffed airway *tube loaded onto the dilator* is advanced as a single unit, over the wire into the trachea.

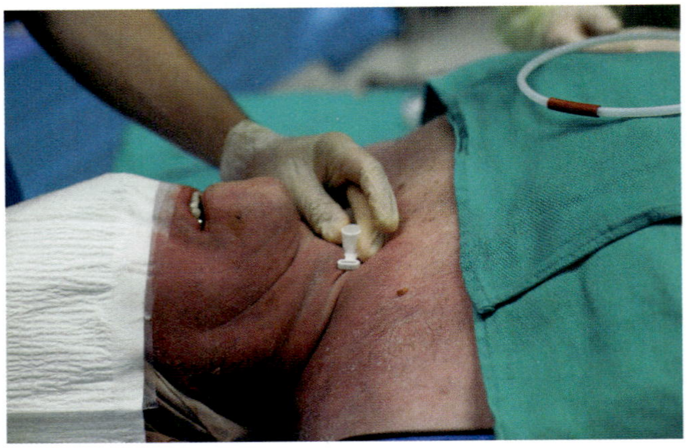

FIGURE 14.14. Seldinger wire-guided cricothyrotomy technique in a cadaver. Removal of dilator and guidewire leaving airway tube in trachea.

6. Removal of dilator and guidewire leaving airway tube in trachea (Figure 14.14);
7. Inflation of the airway tube cuff with air, ventilate;
8. Confirmation of proper tube placement by $ETCO_2$, auscultation, and if necessary flexible endoscopy.

Cook Medical (Bloomington, IN), the main North American supplier, provides three kinds of cricothyrotomy kits: (a) Seldinger wire-guided kit with a 6-mm ID uncuffed/5.0-mm ID cuffed tube, (b) Surgical kit with hook, Trousseau dilator 5-mm ID tube or (c) Universal kit with both the Seldinger and surgical components with a 5-mm ID tube.

(3) What Is a Scalpel Bougie Cricothyrotomy?[10,19] (Video 18)

This is a rapid technique requiring very little equipment—a scalpel, a tracheal tube introducer (bougie), and an airway tube. The main pitfall of the open surgical technique for an anesthesia practitioner is that most practitioners are unfamiliar with open scalpel cuts, which might lead to hesitation and delay in executing an emergency cricothyrotomy.[20] In contrast, the use of a bougie as an intermediary to insertion of an ETT is a familiar technique to most airway practitioners. With this technique, after a scalpel puncture of the CTM, a bougie is inserted, followed by advancing of an ETT over the bougie.

Equipment

a) Size 20 scalpel on a handle (size 10 scalpel may be used if size 20 is unavailable);
b) Tracheal tube introducer (bougie)—typically 4.7 to 5.0-mm OD, 60 to 70 cm in length;
c) 6.0-mm ID cuffed ETT.

Of note, as the typical bougie has an approximately 5.0-mm OD, the ETT chosen should be either 6.0-mm or 5.5-mm ID to minimize a size discrepancy between the bougie and ETT. A bigger ETT will result in a larger gap between the bougie and ETT and may make insertion of an ETT over a bougie more difficult.[24]

Technique: Scalpel Blade Size 20, Bougie 5.0-mm OD, Cuffed ETT 6.0-mm ID

1. Identify CTM with ND hand (Figure 14.15A);
2. *Make a stab incision* with *scalpel oriented horizontally* through CTM using dominant hand (Figure 14.15B). However, in a patient with difficult neck landmarks, make a vertical incision of 4 to 5 cm followed by a horizontal cut of the CTM.
3. *Rotate scalpel blade 90 degrees into a vertical* orientation (Figure 14.15C) and pull scalpel blade toward the practitioner, producing a triangular *wedged-shaped* hole (expansion in figure).
4. *Switch hands.* Grip the scalpel handle using the ND hand. Release dominant hand (Figure 14.15D).
5. With *bougie* aligned in a horizontal plane, oriented perpendicular to long axis of the patient, its tail pointing away from the practitioner, using the dominant hand, *insert the coude tip* of the bougie through the triangular wedged hole into the trachea (Figure 14.15E).
   (Alternatively, one can keep the scalpel handle in the dominant hand and use the ND hand to insert bougie. In the author's (DW) opinion, most practitioners are more familiar with bougie insertion using their dominant hand in the context of tracheal intubation, and will likely be more comfortable and effective with bougie insertion using the dominant hand in the context of cricothyrotomy).
6. Once the coude tip is in the trachea, rotate the bougie into the patient's sagittal plane and *advance caudally,* approximately 25 cm (Figure 14.15F).
7. *Advance the 6.0-mm ID ETT* over the bougie into trachea (Figure 14.15G) and then remove the bougie;
8. Verify correct ETT position with end-tidal capnography, auscultate, or flexible endoscope, if necessary.

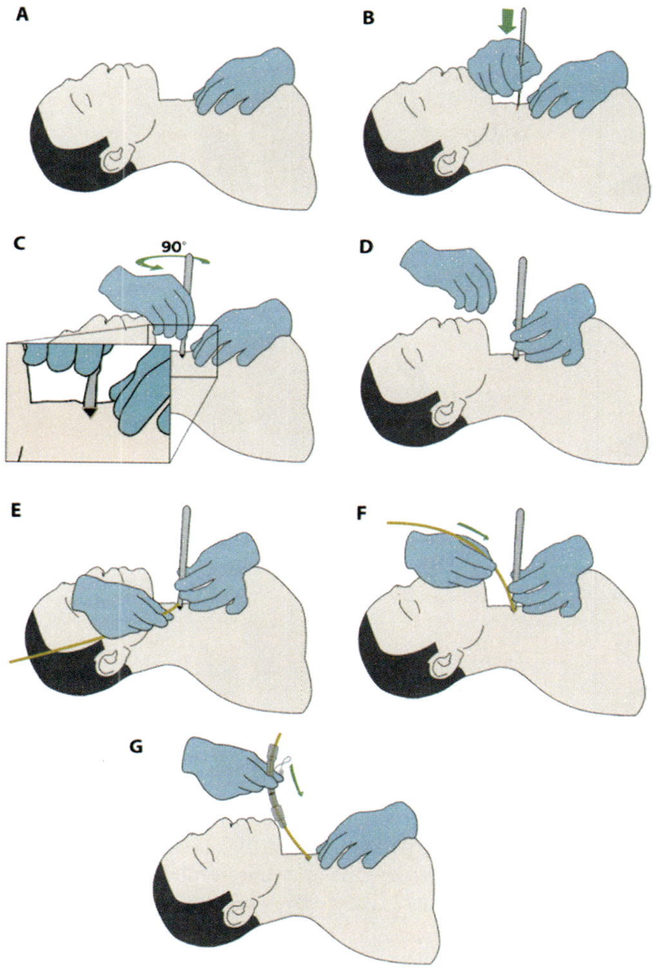

FIGURE 14.15. Scalpel bougie cricothyrotomy technique. (**A**) Identify CTM with the non-dominant (ND) hand. (**B**) *Make a stab incision* with *scalpel oriented horizontally* through CTM using dominant hand. (**C**) *Rotate scalpel blade 90 degrees into a vertical* orientation and pull scalpel blade toward the practitioner producing a triangular *wedged-shaped* hole (expansion in figure). (**D**) *Switch hands*. Grip the scalpel handle using the ND hand. Release dominant hand. (**E**) With *bougie* aligned in a horizontal plane, oriented perpendicular to long axis of the patient, its tail pointing away from the practitioner, using the dominant hand, *insert the coude tip* of the bougie through the triangular wedged hole into the trachea. (**F**) Once the coude tip is in the trachea, rotate the bougie into the patient's sagittal plane and *advance caudally*, approximately 15 cm. (**G**) *Advance the 6.0-mm ID ETT* over the bougie into trachea and then remove the bougie. (Reproduced with permission from Justin Wong, DDM.)

(4) What Is a Cannula over Needle Cricothyrotomy and How Is It Done?[25,26] (Video 5)

The cannula over needle cricothyrotomy technique consists of a pre-assembled cricothyrotomy tube snugly wrapped over either a large bore needle or a needle dilator. The cricothyrotomy device is inserted through the CTM into the airway using the exact same principle as an intravenous cannula over a needle. To illustrate the intravenous principle, once there is flashback of blood, the cannula is advanced over the needle into the vessel lumen. In the situation of the cricothyrotomy, once the needle is through the CTM into the airway, the cricothyrotomy cannula is advanced over the needle into the airway.

There are several commercialized cannula over needle cricothyrotomy kits; the most commonly used in North America are the Quicktrach I and II (VBM Medical Inc, Noblesville, IN)[25] and the PCK—Portex® Cricothyroidotomy Kit (Smiths Medical, Dublin, OH).[26] The Quicktrach does not require a skin incision. It is inserted directly through the skin and CTM, air aspiration, then advance cannula over needle. The PCK kit requires a skin incision, insertion of a Veress needle-dilator-tube assembly into the airway. Once airway entry is indicated by positive air aspiration and Veress needle indicator, the cricothyrotomy tube is advanced into the airway.

We will describe the cannula over needle technique using the Quicktrach II set.

Equipment

a) Pre-assembled Quicktrach cricothyrotomy: cricothyrotomy tube over needle as one piece;
b) Syringe.

Technique:

1. Locate the CTM;
2. Attach a syringe to the Quicktrach tube-needle set;
3. Puncture the skin and CTM with Quicktrach set at 90-degree angle of entry and confirm needle placement into the airway lumen with positive air aspiration (Figure 14.16A);
4. Change the angle of Quicktrach set to 45 degree with the needle tip pointing caudally (Figure 14.16B);
5. Remove red protector guard piece (upon puncture of the anterior airway lumen, the protector piece aims to prevent excessive depth of penetration of the needle, thereby reducing the risk of posterior airway wall damage or penetration) (Figure 14.16C);
6. Unclick and uncouple the airway tube from the needle (Figure 14.16D);
7. Advance cricothyrotomy tube over the needle to the limit until the airway tube hub abuts on patient's neck (Figure 14.16E);
8. Remove the syringe and needle together leaving airway tube in the trachea (Figure 14.16F);
9. Inflate tube pilot balloon;
10. Ventilate;
11. Confirm tube placement with end-tidal capnography, auscultation, or flexible endoscope, if necessary.

(5) Can You Describe the Needle Cricothyrotomy with Narrow Bore Cannula Technique?

The passage of a 12- to 14-gauge catheter through the CTM for the purposes of establishing an emergency airway is only a temporizing method at best. It provides short-term oxygenation until a definitive airway can be established, bearing in mind that the NAP4 study reported a high failure rate of 64% when needle cricothyrotomy was performed by anesthesiologists.[27] Many variations of this technique have been used in general relation to the availability of equipment. This technique should only be used with partial upper airway obstruction as a

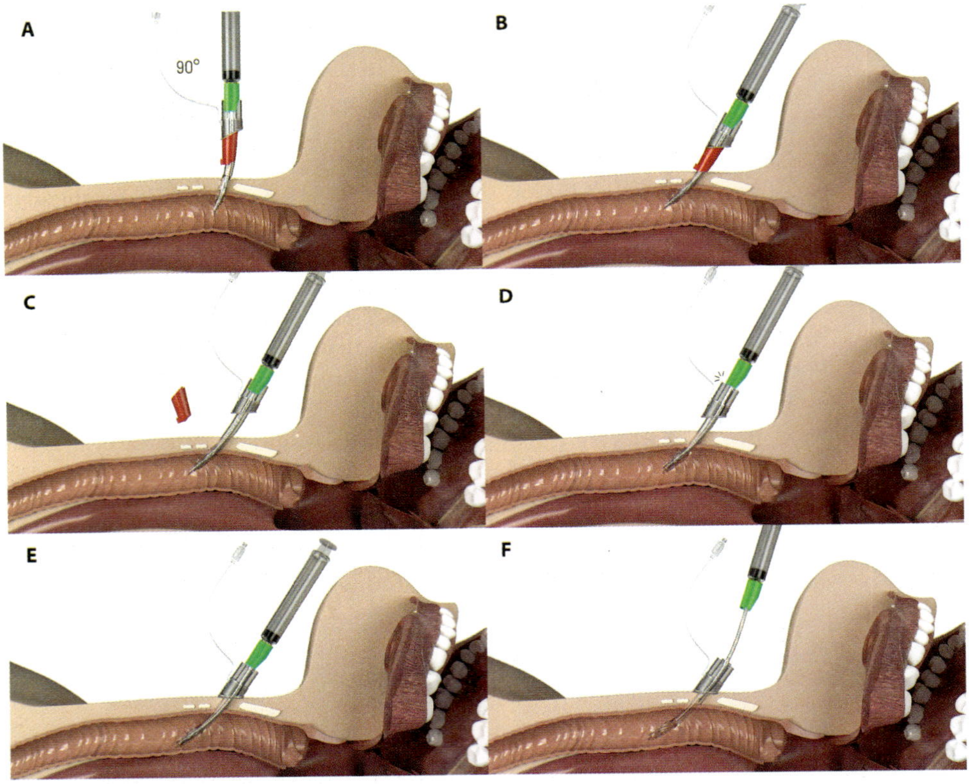

FIGURE 14.16. Cannula over needle cricothyrotomy technique using the Quicktrach II set. (**A**) Puncture CTM with Quicktrach at 90-degree angle of attack and confirm needle entry into the airway lumen with positive air aspiration. (**B**) Change the angle of Quicktrach tube needle set to 45 degree. (**C**) Remove the red protector guard piece. (**D**) Unclick and uncouple the airway tube from the needle. (**E**) Advance the cricothyrotomy tube over the needle to the limit. (**F**) Remove the syringe and needle together leaving airway tube in the trachea. (Reproduced with permission from VBM Medizintechnik GmbH.)

means of providing oxygenation until a definitive airway can be established in a "CICO" situation. One such technique is summarized as follows:

1. Caudal insertion of 14-g IV catheter, with a fluid-filled syringe attached, through the CTM;
2. Confirmation of position by aspiration air bubbles, and advancement of the catheter to its hub, while removing the needle and syringe;
3. Oxygenation utilizing one of several options;
4. To prevent air trapping, barotrauma, and pneumothorax/pneumomediastinum, it is critical that there is sufficient time for egress of gas following each ventilation.

Options that are available for the delivery of O_2 include jet ventilation, the O_2 flush valve on the anesthetic machine, and the anesthesia circuit itself. As mentioned above, it is essential that there is sufficient time and an available route for egress of gas. When using a high-pressure O_2 system to ventilate but without sufficient expiratory time for adequate gas exhaust can lead to serious barotrauma complications such as pneumothorax, pneumomediastinum, or subcutaneous emphysema.[27] An assistant should be instructed to manage the upper airway with all necessary maneuvers, including LMA, or other airway, and appropriate airway maneuvers. On a system of low-pressure oxygen delivery known as the Ventrain device, several case reports demonstrate adequate ventilation and active expiration via a narrow-bore catheter of mere 2- to 3-mm ID or long narrow transtracheal tube of 2.4 mm ID (https://www.ventinovamedical.com/wp-content/uploads/2021/04/MC031.00-Ventrain-Borchure-EN.pdf), even in fully obstructed airways, by using active expiration based on the Bernoulli Principle to avoid extreme intrapulmonary pressures and barotrauma-associated with high-pressure oxygen system.[28–31]

OTHER CONSIDERATIONS

What Are the Concerns in Establishing a Cricothyrotomy in Patients with a Deep Neck Infection?

Deep space neck infections are most common in the extremes of age. Underlying medical problems often accompany the afflicted elderly patient. Deep space infections can either variably occlude, or shift the airway, rendering what should be an easily managed airway into an emergency. Caution dictates that airway management should be performed in a controlled environment, preferably the operating room. A CT scan, if feasible, would greatly facilitate understanding of the altered anatomy but this may not be feasible in the severely compromised airway.

In the moderately affected airway, topical anesthesia and "awake" intubation using a flexible bronchoscope is the method of choice. If the airway is severely compromised, with total airway obstruction a possibility, an "awake" tracheotomy is the procedure of choice—to ensure a secure airway until the infection and its source can be treated.

Do You Have Any Concerns in Establishing a Cricothyrotomy in Children?

In children, as the laryngeal prominence does not develop until adolescence, surface landmarks are more difficult to palpate. The vertical dimension of the CTM is considerably smaller in children than in adults, with the result that an ETT may permanently damage the cartilaginous structures. There is an increased risk that the cricoid cartilage, the only completely circumferential supporting laryngeal structure, may be damaged. In addition, the airway of the child is more malleable, making posterior perforation a greater risk and the laryngeal mucosa more vulnerable to injury and SGS.[32] For all of these reasons, in an emergency situation, if transglottic tracheal tube placement cannot be accomplished, needle cricothyrotomy, or tracheotomy, is the method of choice in children 12 years of age or younger.[33]

What Are the Pros and Cons of Using Non-cuffed and Cuffed Tracheal Tubes for Cricothyrotomy?

The greatest risk of prolonged cricothyrotomy intubation is the development of SGS. Underlying medical illness and/or an element of gastroesophageal reflux, in conjunction with the mechanical disruption of intubation, may contribute to the development of SGS. Modern tracheostomy tubes are less likely to produce an inflammatory response in the mucosal airway, while low-pressure cuffs reduce mechanical trauma and its sequelae.

Cuffed tubes provide a seal in the airway to allow delivery of larger tidal volumes with lower airway pressures. However, cuffed tubes may be more difficult to insert in an emergency situation, due to their bulk and the risk of snagging the cuff on the edge of the surgical incision. This may tear the cuff and prevent an effective seal. It is critical that the simplest, safest, speediest, and most effective technique be used to re-establish a failed airway. Thus, a small, non-cuffed tube would be adequate for the primary goal of salvaging the airway and provision of oxygenation.

As patients requiring a surgical airway may have decreased lung compliance, positive pressure ventilation through a non-cuffed ETT can result in gas escaping from the proximal airway, resulting in inadequate ventilation. For this reason, either the Cook cuffed airway catheter or 5.0-mm ID cuffed ETT are the tracheal tubes of choice when establishing an emergency surgical airway.

What Immediate and Delayed Complications Should I Be Aware of?

In most studies, complication rates are higher for emergency than elective cricothyrotomy. In a series of 38 emergency cricothyrotomies, McGill et al[6] reported an overall complication rate of 40%. The most frequent complication identified by this group was misplacement of the ETT through the thyrohyoid membrane (i.e., above the larynx), instead of through the CTM. Other complications included execution time greater than three minutes, unsuccessful tube placement, and significant hemorrhage. One patient suffered a longitudinal fracture of the thyroid cartilage due to attempted placement of an 8.0-mm ID tube, resulting in significant long-term morbidity. In a similar series in 1989, Erlandson[34] reported a complication rate of 23%, related primarily to incorrect tube placement (10%) and hemorrhage (8%). Miklus et al.[35] reported on 20 patients requiring emergency cricothyrotomy in the field. In this study, there were no complications of tube misplacement, significant hemorrhage, or long-term morbidity in survivors. Gillespie et al.[36] reviewed 35 patients requiring emergency surgical airway over a six-year period and noted no differences in the overall complication rate between emergency tracheotomy and cricothyrotomy. Of particular note was that there were no long-term complications in the patients that received cricothyrotomy and were not subsequently converted to tracheotomy.[36]

Although rare, fatal hemorrhages have been reported as a result of laceration of the cricothyroid artery.[37] As this artery courses closer to the thyroid cartilage, there is a greater risk of hemorrhage if the incision is made in the upper half of the CTM.

Other complications include SGS, dysphonia due to laryngeal damage, tracheal cartilage fracture, endobronchial intubation, pulmonary aspiration, recurrent laryngeal nerve injury, esophageal perforation, and tracheo-esophageal fistula.[32]

Tissue emphysema (including subcutaneous and mediastinal emphysema) and barotrauma (including tension pneumothorax) have been reported as complications of jet ventilation and establishment of a surgical airway.[38] Weymuller[39] cautions that only practitioners experienced with transtracheal jet ventilation (TTJV) should attempt it in emergency airway management. He describes kinked or displaced transtracheal catheters, incoordination of respiratory effort, outlet obstruction, and distal airway secretions as the major problems encountered.

What Is the Historical Evolution of Surgical Tracheotomy?

Tracheostomy is one of the oldest surgical procedures in medical history.[40] Nevertheless, during the 19th and early 20th centuries, it was only performed in extreme circumstances (i.e., avoiding total upper airway obstruction from infectious processes in the larynx and trachea) due to high morbidity and mortality.[41] It was only in 1909 that Chevalier Jackson presented and described in detail the "modern" tracheotomy technique.[41,42]

In the last century, the introduction of endotracheal intubation, positive pressure ventilation, and advancements in intensive care led to increased requirements for long-term ventilation, which caused a significant modification in the indications for tracheotomy. Currently, the majority of tracheotomies are performed semi-electively for critically ill patients in the intensive care setting with mechanical ventilation.

What Are the Clinical Indications and Contraindications to Performing a Tracheotomy?

The indications for tracheotomy can be divided mainly into two categories: (1) to relieve upper airway obstruction from acute or chronic cases, such as extensive maxillofacial trauma, angioedema, obstructing upper airway tumors; (2) to facilitate ventilator support, including providing long-term ventilation, enable better pulmonary toilet, and easy weaning from mechanical ventilation. Absolute contraindications for tracheotomy are very rare (see Table 14.1).[43,44]

In Which Clinical Situations of Airway Obstruction Should a Tracheotomy Be Favored over a Cricothyrotomy?

The three principal aspects that should be considered for this decision are urgency of procedure, human resources, and cause of obstruction. Tracheotomy is a surgical procedure more complex than cricothyroidotomy, which requires some time to perform and surgeons with appropriate training and expertise. An acute loss of the airway with significant hypoxemia most likely would need a cricothyrotomy to provide oxygenation in an expedited time, which is usually done by airway practitioners including anesthesiologists (e.g., rapid progressing angioedema in the emergency department, CICO situation after anesthesia induction in an elective surgery).[45] However, these are less common events. In the majority of airway obstructions, there is time to have a trained surgeon performing a tracheotomy on an elective or semi-urgent basis. Additionally, the cause of obstruction should be contemplated. A peri-glottic tumor with unknown inferior extension increases the risk of damaging the tumor during the cricothyrotomy. When a deep neck infection with severe airway compromise is presented, a controlled open surgical technique should be the elected choice due to altered neck anatomy. Therefore, in these two situations, tracheotomy should be favored over cricothyrotomy.

TABLE 14.1. Indications and Contraindications for Tracheotomy

Indications	Contraindications
• Prolonged or expected prolonged intubation • Inability to manage secretions • Facilitation of ventilator support • Adjunct to major head and neck/oral maxillofacial surgery • Significant head and neck trauma	• Severe coagulopathy • Inadequate training in the procedure • Distal tracheal pathology

Is It Essential to Convert a Successful Cricothyrotomy to Tracheotomy?

The standard recommendation after a successful cricothyrotomy is conversion to tracheotomy within 72 hours due to the risk of SGS. This approach was advocated by Jackson a century ago,[46] and has been reinforced recently by other authors.[47,48] However, there is growing evidence in the literature that the risk of maintenance of cricothyrotomy for longer periods might not be as high as believed.[49,50] Additionally, the conversion per se might increase the risk of complications as shown by two case series.[51,52] In a failed intubation situation in an elective surgery resulting in an emergency cricothyrotomy, once the patient is awakened and stable, the airway may be safely decannulated in a short time with backup to reinsert an emergency airway. If the cricothyrotomy was done to deal with airway pathology such as tumor, it may be prudent to convert to a tracheotomy. More studies regarding the conversion from cricothyrotomy to tracheotomy are needed to establish a definitive answer for this question.

What Are the Potential Complications of Tracheotomy?

Creation of false passage, tube obstruction, and accidental decannulation are tracheostomy-related complications that are life-threatening. These complications demand prompt recognition and treatment to avoid patient hypoxia. Creation of false passage can either happen during primary placement or replacement of the tracheostomy tube. It should be suspected when, after the tracheostomy tube insertion, there is no end-tidal CO_2 detection and the patient cannot be manually ventilated. The possibility of a false passage can be ruled out under direct visualization using a flexible bronchoscope. When tracheostomy tube obstruction is suspected, it is essential to perform tracheal suction to remove blood or secretions that might be the source of obstruction. In the case of accidental decannulation, if the stoma is mature, a new tracheostomy tube needs to be inserted, or if the stoma is fresh, the patient is intubated orally and surgical service is consulted. In any of these scenarios, the patient's oxygenation has to be constantly assessed. Techniques to restore oxygenation that can be used include oral ventilation using either face mask or laryngeal mask (with stoma covered), stoma ventilation using a pediatric face mask, oral intubation or stoma intubation with a smaller ETT (6.0 cuffed).[53]

TABLE 14.2. Front-of-Neck Access Complications

Complications	Cricothyrotomy	Tracheotomy
Immediate	• Hemorrhage • False passage • Tracheal injury • Cricoid cartilage injury • Thyroid cartilage injury	• Hemorrhage • False passage • Pneumothora • xPneumomediastinum • Subcutaneous emphysema • Cricoid cartilage injury • Post-obstructive pulmonary edema
Early	• Accidental decannulation • Hemorrhage	• Accidental decannulation • Hemorrhage • Tube obstruction • Tube dislodgement
Late	• Tracheoesophageal fistula • Granuloma formation • Vocal cord paralysis • Scar formation • Subglottic stenosis • Infection/Neck abscess	• Tracheoesophageal fistula • Granuloma formation • Tracheocutaneous fistula • Tracheal injury • Scar formation • Subglottic stenosis • Tracheo-innominate artery fistula • Infection/Neck abscess

What Complications Are Associated with Front-of-Neck Access?

The complications of a FONA can be divided into three categories according to the timing: immediate (directly related to the surgical procedure), early postoperative (up to seven days of the surgical procedure), or late postoperative (beyond seven days of the surgical procedure) (see Table 14.2).[43,50,54]

SUMMARY

Front-of-neck access is a potentially life-saving procedure when airway practitioners encounter a "can't intubate, can't oxygenate" emergency situation. The options to oxygenate patients in this situation are cricothyrotomy and tracheotomy. There is a growing consensus amongst airway practitioners that anesthesiologists and emergency and critical care physicians should be able to perform an emergency cricothyrotomy. In this chapter, we describe the neck anatomy and how the landmarks should be recognized by palpation and ultrasonography. We also discussed the most common techniques, indications, and complications of cricothyrotomy.

Tracheotomy is a more complex procedure that should ideally be performed by surgical specialties including otolaryngologist, oral facial maxillary, and thoracic surgeons. Nevertheless, anesthesia practitioners may need to manage tracheotomy either during surgeries, in post-anesthetic setting, or the ward. Therefore, they should be knowledgeable about the indications, contraindications, and complications of this procedure, as discussed in this chapter.

SELF-EVALUATION QUESTIONS

14.1. Regarding the anatomy of the neck landmarks when performing a FONA, which of the following statements is NOT true?

A. The only vascular structure of note in the vicinity of the CTM is the superior thyroid arteries, which, in 54% of people, courses along its lateral border.

B. Identifying the hyoid bone is important to avoid mistaking the thyrohyoid space for the CTM.

C. Injury to cricothyroid arteries can be avoided by entering the CTM in its inferior half.

D. The hyoid cartilage is an important landmark, which in less than 10% of people, is inferior to the cricoid cartilage.

14.2. Regarding the scalpel-bougie-tube cricothyrotomy technique in adults, which of the following is NOT true?

A. The initial scalpel incision should be a horizontal midline incision.

B. The scalpel blade once inserted should be rotated 90 degrees to facilitate bougie insertion.

C. The bougie or tracheal tube introducer should be 19F in size.

D. The bougie should be 60 to 70 cm in length.

E. The ETT should be cuffed.

14.3. All of the following are complications of Front-of-Neck access EXCEPT:

A. Hemorrhage

B. Subglottic stenosis

C. False passage

D. Mediastinitis

E. Tracheal injury

REFERENCES

1. Kress TD, Balasubramaniam S. Cricothyroidotomy. *Ann Emerg Med.* Apr 1982;11(4):197-201.
2. Bair AE, Chima R. The inaccuracy of using landmark techniques for cricothyroid membrane identification: a comparison of three techniques. *Acad Emerg Med.* Aug 2015;22(8):908-914.
3. Kwofie K, Hung O, Hung C, Hung D, Hung H. The use of neck surface landmarks (Launcelott Creases) to locate the cricoid cartilage. *Anesthesiology.* 2008;109:176.
4. Bennett JD, Guha SC, Sankar AB. Cricothyrotomy: the anatomical basis. *J R Coll Surg Edinb.* 1996;41(1):57-60.
5. Dover K, Howdieshell TR, Colborn GL. The dimensions and vascular anatomy of the cricothyroid membrane: relevance to emergent surgical airway access. *Clin Anat.* 1996;9(5):291-295.
6. McGill J, Clinton JE, Ruiz E. Cricothyrotomy in the emergency department. *Ann Emerg Med.* Jul 1982;11(7):361-364.
7. Blumberg NA. Observations on the pyramidal lobe of the thyroid gland. *SAMJ.* 1981;59(26):949-950.
8. Kim DW, Jung SL, Baek JH, et al. The prevalence and features of thyroid pyramidal lobe, accessory thyroid, and ectopic thyroid as assessed by computed tomography: a multicenter study. *J Am Thyroid Assoc.* 2013;23(1):84-91.
9. Cook TM, Woodall N, Harper J, Benger J; Fourth National Audit Project. Major complications of airway management in the UK: results of the Fourth National Audit Project of the Royal College of Anaesthetists and the Difficult Airway Society. Part 2: intensive care and emergency departments. *Br J Anaesth.* 2011;106(5):632-642.
10. Frerk C, Mitchell VS, McNarry AF, et al. Difficult Airway Society 2015 guidelines for management of unanticipated difficult intubation in adults. *Br J Anaesth.* 2015;115(6):827-848.
11. You-Ten KE, Siddiqui N, Teoh WH, Kristensen MS. Point-of-care ultrasound (POCUS) of the upper airway. *Can J Anaesth.* 2018;65(4):473-484.
12. Kristensen MS. Ultrasonography in the management of the airway. *Acta Anaesthesiol Scand.* 2011;55(10):1155-1173.
13. Lamb A, Zhang J, Hung O, et al. Accuracy of identifying the cricothyroid membrane by anesthesia trainees and staff in a Canadian institution. *Can J Anaesth.* 2015;62(5):495-503.
14. Aslani A, Ng SC, Hurley M, McCarthy KF, McNicholas M, McCaul CL. Accuracy of identification of the cricothyroid membrane in female subjects using palpation: an observational study. *Anesth Analg.* 2012;114(5):987-992.
15. You-Ten KE, Desai D, Postonogova T, Siddiqui N. Accuracy of conventional digital palpation and ultrasound of the cricothyroid membrane in obese women in labour. *Anaesthesia.* 2015;70(11):1230-1234.
16. Prasad A, Yu E, Wong DT, Karkhanis R, Gullane P, Chan VW. Comparison of sonography and computed tomography as imaging tools for assessment of airway structures. *J Ultrasound Med.* 2011;30(7):965-972.
17. Siddiqui N, Yu E, Boulis S, You-Ten KE. Ultrasound is superior to palpation in identifying the cricothyroid membrane in subjects with poorly defined neck landmarks: a randomized clinical trial. *Anesthesiology.* 2018;129(6):1132-1139.
18. Siddiqui N, Arzola C, Friedman Z, Guerina L, You-Ten KE. Ultrasound improves cricothyrotomy success in cadavers with poorly defined neck anatomy: a randomized control trial. *Anesthesiology.* 2015;123(5):1033-1041
19. Law JA, Duggan LV, Asselin M, et al.; Canadian Airway Focus Group. Canadian Airway Focus Group updated consensus-based recommendations for management of the difficult airway: part 1. Difficult airway management encountered in an unconscious patient. *Can J Anaesth.* 2021;18:1-32.
20. Wong DT, Mehta A, Tam AD, Yau B, Wong J. A survey of Canadian anesthesiologists' preferences in difficult intubation and "cannot intubate, cannot ventilate" situations. *Can J Anaesth.* 2014;61(8):717-726.
21. Cook TM, Woodall N, Frerk C; Fourth National Audit Project. Major complications of airway management in the UK: results of the Fourth National Audit Project of the Royal College of Anaesthetists and the Difficult Airway Society. Part 1: anaesthesia. *Br J Anaesth.* 2011;106(5):617-631.
22. You-Ten KE, Wong DT, Ye XY, Arzola C, Zand A, Siddiqui N. Practice of ultrasound-guided palpation of neck landmarks improves accuracy of external palpation of the cricothyroid membrane. *Anesth Analg.* 2018;127(6):1377-1382.
23. Wong DT, Prabhu AJ, Coloma M, Imasogie N, Chung FF. What is the minimum training required for successful cricothyroidotomy?: a study in mannequins. *Anesthesiology.* 2003;98(2):349-353.
24. Asai T, Shingu K. Difficulty in advancing a tracheal tube over a fibreoptic bronchoscope: incidence, causes and solutions. *Br J Anaesth.* 2004;92(6):870-881.
25. Price TM, McCoy EP. Emergency front of neck access in airway management. *BJA Educ.* 2019;19(8):246-253.
26. Assmann NM, Wong DT, Morales E. A comparison of a new indicator-guided with a conventional wire-guided percutaneous cricothyroidotomy device in mannequins. *Anesth Analg.* 2007;105(1):148-154.
27. Duggan LV, Ballantyne SB, Law JA, Morris IR, Murphy MF, Griesdale DE. Transtracheal jet ventilation in the "can't intubate can't oxygenate" emergency: a systematic review. *Br J Anaesth.* 2016;117(suppl 1):i28-i38.
28. Willemsen MG, Noppens R, Mulder AL, Enk D. Ventilation with the Ventrain through a small lumen catheter in the failed paediatric airway: two case reports. *Br J Anaesth.* 2014;112(5):946-947.
29. Heuveling DA, Mahieu HF, Jongsma-van Netten HG, Gerling V.Transtracheal use of the Cricath cannula in combination with the Ventrain device for prevention of hypoxic arrest due to severe upper airway obstruction: a case report. *Anesth Analg Pract.* 2018;11(12):344-347.
30. Morrison S, Aerts S, Van Rompaey D, Vanderveken O. Failed awake intubation for critical airway obstruction rescued with the Ventrain device and an Arndt exchange catheter: a case report. *Anesth Analg Pract.* 2019;13(1):23-26.
31. Fearnley RA, Badiger S, Oakley R, Ahmad I. Elective use of the Ventrain for upper airway obstruction during high-frequency jet ventilation. *J Clin Anesth.* 2016;33:233-235.
32. Boon JM, Abrahams PH, Meiring JH, Welch T. Cricothyroidotomy: a clinical anatomy review. *Clin Anat.* 2004;17(6):478-486.
33. Elliott WG. Airway management in the injured child. *Intl Anesthesiol Clin.* 1994;32(1):27-46.
34. Erlandson MJ, Clinton JE, Ruiz E, Cohen J. Cricothyrotomy in the emergency department revisited. *J Emerg Med.* 1989;7(2):115-118.
35. Miklus RM, Elliott C, Snow N. Surgical cricothyrotomy in the field: experience of a helicopter transport team. *J Trauma.* 1989;29(4):506-508.
36. Gillespie MB, Eisele DW. Outcomes of emergency surgical airway procedure in a hospital-wide setting. *Laryngoscope.* 1999;109(11):1766-1769.
37. Schillaci CR, Iacovoni VF, Conte RS. Transtracheal aspiration complicated by fatal endotracheal hemorrhage. *N Engl J Med.* 1976;295(9):488-490.
38. Smith RB, Schaer WB, Pfaeffle H. Percutaneous transtracheal ventilation for anaesthesia and resuscitation: a review and report of complications. *Can Anaesth Soc J.* 1975;22(5):607-612.
39. Weymuller EAJr, Pavlin EG, Paugh D, Cummings CW. Management of difficult airway problems with percutaneous transtracheal ventilation. *Ann Rhinol Laryngol.* 1987;96(1 pt 1):34-37.
40. Karparvar Z, Goldenberg D. *Tracheotomy management: a multidisciplinary approach. Excerpt.* New York, NY: Cambridge University Press; 2011:2.
41. Kost K, Myers N. Tracheostomy; Operative Otolaryngology: Head and Neck Surgery. (Vol. 2, Ch. 68). Philadelphia, PA: Saunders; 2008: 577-594.
42. Jackson C. Tracheotomy. *Laryngoscope.* 1909;19:285-290.
43. American Academy of Otolaryngology Head & Neck Surgery (AAOHNS). 1999 Clinical Indicators Compendium. AAO-HNS Bull, 1999, October.
44. Freeman BD. Tracheostomy Update: When and How. *Crit Care Clin.* 2017;33(2):311-322.
45. Pracy JP, Brennan L, Cook TM, et al. Surgical intervention during a can't intubate can't oxygenate (CICO) event: emergency front-of-neck airway (FONA)? *Br J Anaesth.* 2016;117(4):426-428.
46. Jackson C. High tracheotomy and other errors: the chief causes of chronic laryngeal stenosis. *Surg Gynecol Obstet.* 1921;32:392-398.
47. Heffner JE. Tracheotomy application and timing. *Clin Chest Med.* 2003;24(3):389-398.

48. Thal ER, Weigelt JA, Carrico CJ. *Operative Trauma Management: An Atlas*. 2nd ed. New York, NY: McGraw-Hill Co, Inc; 2002:10.
49. Rehm CG, Wanek SM, Gagnon EB, Pearson SK, Mullins RJ. Cricothyroidotomy for elective airway management in critically ill trauma patients with technically challenging neck anatomy. *Crit Care*. 2002;6(6):531-535.
50. Francois B, Clavel M, Desachy A, Puyraud S, Roustan J, Vignon P. Complications of tracheostomy performed in the ICU: subthyroid tracheostomy vs surgical cricothyroidotomy. *Chest*. 2003;123(1):151-158.
51. Wright MJ, Greenberg DE, Hunt JP, Madan AK, McSwain NEJr. Surgical cricothyroidotomy in trauma patients. *South Med J*. 2003;96(5):465-467.
52. Altman KW, Waltonen JD, Kern RC. Urgent surgical airway intervention: a 3 year county hospital experience. *Laryngoscope*. 2005;115(12):2101-2104.
53. Emergency tracheostomy management. National Tracheostomy Safety Project. Accessed at https://www.tracheostomy.org.uk/storage/files/NTSP_GREEN_Tracheostomy_Algorithm.pdf on August 26, 2021.
54. Zasso FB, You-Ten KE, Ryu M, Losyeva K, Tanwani J, Siddiqui N. Complications of cricothyroidotomy versus tracheostomy in emergency surgical airway management: a systematic review. *BMC Anesthesiol*. 2020;20(1):216.

CHAPTER 15

Extracorporeal Membrane Oxygenation as a Support Strategy in the Management of the Difficult Airway

Rebecca Klinger, Michele Heath, Kimberly R Blasius, Sara Najmeh, and Mark Stafford-Smith

CASE PRESENTATION

The following two illustrative examples involving femoral VV-ECMO support for difficult airway management highlight its utility in the setting of (1) anticipated/elective and (2) unanticipated/emergency extremely difficult airway situations.

■ Case 1: Anticipated/Elective "Impossible" Airway

An otherwise healthy 28-year-old female with a friable inflammatory myofibroblastic tracheal malignancy complains of dyspnea and hemoptysis. The tumor mass is located mid-trachea on the left anterolateral wall causing significant tracheal obstruction (90%). Traditional difficult airway management strategies are anticipated to be successful in placing an endotracheal tube (ETT) in the trachea, but may fail to achieve ventilation and oxygenation because of the obstructing friable tracheal mass located distally. Additionally, the potential for major airway bleeding makes such a strategy likely to be unsafe, potentially compromising ventilation and any subsequent salvage efforts to re-secure the airway. A front-of-neck airway (FONA) in such circumstances (planned tracheotomy and emergency cricothyrotomy) would incur similar risks.

■ Case 2: Unanticipated/Urgent/Emergency "Impossible" Airway (i.e., Airway Crisis)

A 68-year-old male presents for urgent cardiac surgery (to address high-grade left main coronary artery disease and severe aortic stenosis). Beyond these cardiovascular conditions, pertinent history includes severe gastroesophageal reflux disease and limited head and neck mobility (due to radiation following excision of a squamous cell carcinoma from the base of the tongue). Preoperative airway exam reveals limited mouth opening and a Mallampati III score. Predicting a difficult airway, after thoughtful consideration and preparation, the anesthesiologist plans for flexible bronchoscopy-guided asleep tracheal intubation. Following denitrogenation, gentle initiation of anesthesia is achieved with intravenous propofol (without muscle relaxation), and face-mask ventilation (FMV) is possible. The anesthesiologist's attempts to pass a flexible bronchoscope, with video-laryngoscope assistance, into the airway through the mouth are unsuccessful. At this point, the patient develops trismus, which is additive to challenges presented by his preexisting limited mouth opening and prevents successful placement of an oral airway or laryngeal mask airway. The practitioner administers intravenous succinylcholine to achieve full muscle relaxation, but still cannot achieve transoral endotracheal intubation with either direct or video-assisted laryngoscopy. FMV becomes barely adequate and worsens and, presumably due to the effects of radiation and prior neck surgery, several attempts at needle cricothyrotomy also fail to access the airway.

INTRODUCTION

This text describes established difficult airway management strategies for the practitioner with a common theme involving simultaneously addressing the critical dual needs of the patient: (1) to preserve oxygenation and ventilation through the lung interface, while (2) safely securing the difficult airway. Yet what is the practitioner going to do in the rare, but terrifying, circumstance when such traditional techniques are considered unsafe, or worse fail? In this context, recent innovations now make available novel strategies that leverage support provided by extracorporeal membrane oxygenation (ECMO) to permit separation of these two tasks. By assuming control of respiratory functions without involving the lung interface, ECMO allows the practitioner to focus undistracted on securing the difficult airway. Published ECMO case reports and case series outlining successful management of challenging airways, often in extreme circumstances, have most commonly involved central airway obstruction and attest to the value of ECMO support as the newest fundamental addition to the armamentarium of the difficult airway practitioner.[1–5] A 2017 systematic review summarizes 36 publications on utilizing this approach to managing critical airway obstruction.[6] Furthermore, of the variety of options available, *femoral venovenous (VV)-ECMO* is typically the modality most suited for the management of difficult airway (in contrast to VV-ECMO using other venous locations, or venoarterial [VA] ECMO); rationales and other details are outlined below.

While conceptually, ECMO as a solution to airway management is deceptively appealing, as a strategy VV-ECMO is in fact complex to coordinate, expensive, and not without risk. Therefore, it generally remains reserved for occasional circumstances involving unique, highly complex difficult airway situations. Indeed, the challenge in accurately predicting the most eligible high-risk cases, such as total airway obstruction, means that a firm indication for VV-ECMO support in airway management is still controversial. While potentially suitable for both the anticipated and unanticipated difficult airway, VV-ECMO support is rarely used when other options would suffice, since its deployment requires the availability of a highly specialized team and extracorporeal circulation technology, sufficient time, and often at considerable expense. Furthermore, VV-ECMO support is not without its own set of potential complications, including bleeding, vascular injury, and thromboembolism. Outlined below, we describe clinical courses for the above-mentioned case examples involving anticipated and unanticipated difficult airway management with VV-ECMO support. We also summarize VV-ECMO technology and its use, and outline approaches—such as team training through simulation—to gain the most value from VV-ECMO support as a difficult airway adjunct (including, importantly, when such technology is not useful), whether introduction of such a service should be considered by an organization, and/or when elective referral to a center experienced in ECMO should be considered.

EXTRACORPOREAL MEMBRANE OXYGENATION

What Are the Different Types of Extracorporeal Membrane Oxygenation?

There are two main forms of ECMO differentiated by their access points to the circulation: venoarterial (VA) and venovenous (VV). VA-ECMO bypasses the heart and provides complete respiratory and circulatory support, akin to cardiopulmonary bypass as standardly used for heart surgery. VV-ECMO, on the other hand, is limited to replacement of respiratory function, returning blood to the venous system, and relying on the heart to otherwise support the circulation. In the context of difficult airway scenarios, VV-ECMO support is almost always sufficient. Only when hypoperfusion coexists (e.g., circulatory shock) is the added circulation support of VA-ECMO of value (e.g., compromised cardiac function or extracorporeal cardiac life support). Throughout the remainder of this chapter, we will primarily focus on the technology and considerations surrounding VV-ECMO (Video 31).

Discuss the ECMO Circuit Technology

VV-ECMO delivers oxygenation and removes carbon dioxide in venous blood which is then returned to the venous system. In other words, it functions *in series* with the lungs but without contributing to circulatory support. The path for blood flowing to the ECMO circuit starts with exiting the patient through a drainage cannula, which takes deoxygenated blood from the venous system through a specially coated (typically heparin) cannula. Venous blood subsequently transits through tubing to a pump, with sensors typically measuring oxygen saturation, hematocrit, and temperature. Centrifugal (nonpulsatile) pumps are standard, given their increased safety and reduced hemolysis relative to positive-displacement pulsatile pumps. Next in the circuit path is the device where gas exchange occurs: here a membrane interface between gas and blood facilitates oxygen enrichment (through oxygen gas administration) and removal of carbon dioxide (through alterations of the oxygen gas flow rate or "sweep"). The gas exchange device, commonly referred to as the "oxygenator," also permits rapid precise blood temperature control when a heater/cooler device is included. Due to the significant heat loss associated with extracorporeal circulation, a heater/cooler is commonly used to avoid hypothermia, unless the ECMO "run" is anticipated to be brief. After traversing the oxygenator, the oxygenated blood rejoins the patient through a return cannula (deliberately separated from the drainage cannula, in the originating vein, to avoid "recirculation"). Recirculation is a phenomenon unique to VV-ECMO that occurs when venous blood that has just completed passage through the ECMO circuit re-enters the ECMO circuit (usually due to inadvertent close proximity of the inflow and outflow cannulas), thus never re-entering the systemic circulation (Figure 15.1). Practically speaking, recirculation leads to insufficient return of oxygenated blood to the body, and implicitly permits more de-oxygenated blood to escape diversion to the

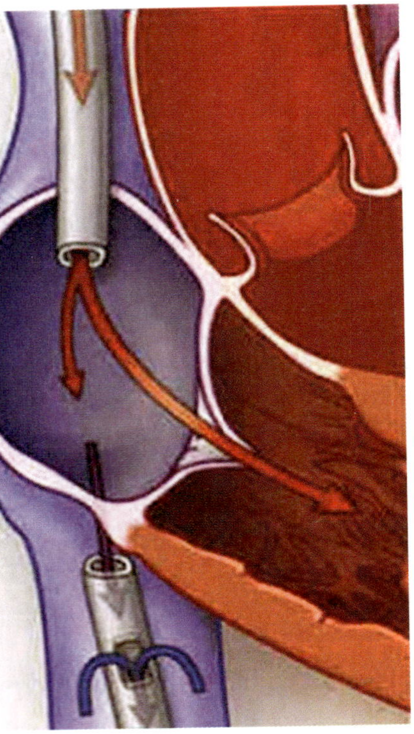

FIGURE 15.1. The image depicts recirculation, an effect that occurs when VV-ECMO inflow and outflow cannulas are too close to one another. In this example, the inflow cannula sits at the RA/IVC junction and drains deoxygssssenated venous blood (blue arrows) into the ECMO circuit. The outflow (i.e., return) cannula sits in the SVC and extends into the RA, returning oxygenated/decarboxylated blood from the ECMO machine to the RA (red arrows). Most of the returned blood passes across the tricuspid valve to eventually join the systemic circulation. However, if the inflow and outflow cannulas are too closely adjacent, some of the returning blood (smaller red arrow) can become re-entrained into the inflow cannula and returns to the ECMO machine without having contributed to the systemic circulation. (Reproduced with permission from Brodie D, Bacchetta M. Extracorporeal membrane oxygenation for ARDS in adults. *N Engl J Med.* 2011;365(20):1905-1914.)

ECMO circuit and passage directly on to the systemic circulation. Briefly, recirculation can seriously reduce the efficient/adequate delivery of oxygenated blood to the patient.

Ultimately, for patients undergoing VV-ECMO support, the net arterial blood oxygen content of blood (O_2 flux) exiting the left ventricle is composed of the admixture of (1) "ECMO-treated" systemic venous return and (2) "ECMO-untreated" systemic (shunt and coronary sinus) venous return, superimposed on (3) any gas exchange functions occurring in the native lung.[7]

Discuss the Cannulation Strategy

While the circuit technology for VV- and VA-ECMO are very similar, in terms of cannulation approach and management strategy, these two interventions are quite distinct. As highlighted above, when cardiac support is not required, VV-ECMO is employed to solely support the lungs.[8,9] During VV-ECMO, blood is both taken from and returned to a vein, with the blood being oxygenated extracorporeally in series with the lungs.[8] Typically two cannulas are required: (1) a venous drainage cannula, through which deoxygenated blood is removed from the body and pumped to the gas exchange device, and (2) a venous return cannula, often located in a separate vein, through which oxygenated blood is returned to the body (Figure 15.2).

When considering VV-ECMO generally, common peripheral venous cannulation site options include a femoral vein and an internal jugular (IJ) vein.[9] Alternately, a single specialized dual-lumen cannula (Avalon Elite® Bi-Caval Dual Lumen Catheter, Getinge AB, Göteborg, Sweden), designed specifically for use in the right IJ vein, can be used for both drainage and return flow[10] (Figure 15.3). Within the Avalon cannula, one multiorifice lumen drains deoxygenated venous blood from both the superior vena cava (SVC) and inferior vena cava (IVC) through a proximal and a distal port, respectively, while the second "return" lumen limits recirculation by directing oxygenated blood towards the right atrium (RA) and tricuspid valve.[7] The Protek Duo™ (Livanova, Boston, MA, USA) cannula employs similar dual-lumen principles and is also placed in the right IJ vein; however, the distal cannula tip is advanced into the main pulmonary artery. Notably, in addition to avoidance of recirculation, this cannula can also decompress the right ventricle, which is useful if isolated right ventricular (RV) failure is present.[7]

When considering VV-ECMO specific to the difficult airway, any neck-located cannulation approach has the serious potential to interfere with airway management. Hence, despite the convenience of such technology as a single dual-lumen right IJ vein cannula, typical cannulation in the setting of difficult airway involves bilateral single-lumen femoral vein access. Additionally, neck pathology as a source of the difficult airway (e.g., goiter) may make IJ vein access even more disadvantageous. To avoid recirculation with bilateral femoral vein cannulation, desired cannula placement is commonly verified using X-ray fluoroscopy. The tip of the inflow/drainage cannula is often advanced in the IVC, from 5 to 10 cm caudal to the IVC-RA junction, while the tip of the outflow/return cannula is usually advanced to rest within the RA itself.[7]

How Do You Manage the Physiological Changes of the VV-ECMO?

Careful monitoring and good communication among team members during ECMO implementation is key, particularly during the initiation phase when the significant physiologic consequences may involve hemodynamics and other effects that require clinical intervention. Baseline data is important to assess factors during ECMO initiation, such as arterial blood gas parameters, dilutional anemia (vs. transfusion), hypothermia, and hypotension. As outlined above, of the venous blood entering the heart, VV-ECMO-oxygenated blood contributes only a portion (which is oxygenated to a saturation of 100% and has CO_2 removed). Once initiated, VV-ECMO flow is gradually increased until a flow rate—desired, or maximum-achievable (determined by drainage cannula resistance)—is established.[11]

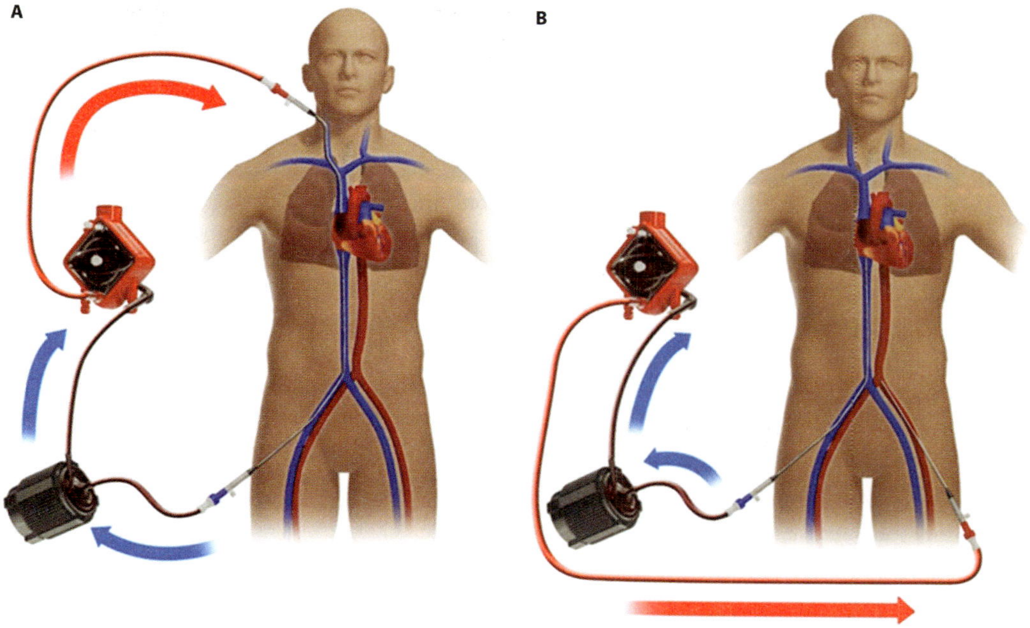

FIGURE 15.2. The two types of ECMO (V-V and V-A) are depicted. Typical VV-ECMO circuit configuration (**A**) involves an inflow cannula placed via a vein (e.g., femoral) that drains blood into the ECMO circuit, which is then pumped through an oxygenator where oxygenation/decarboxylation occurs, and then blood is returned to the patient via an outflow cannula placed in a distant vein (e.g., right IJ vein). In contrast, typical VA-ECMO circuitry (**B**) involves an inflow cannula placed in a vein (e.g., femoral), which drains blood into the ECMO circuit, which is then pumped through an oxygenator where oxygenation/decarboxylation occurs, and returned directly to the systemic circulation via an artery (e.g., femoral), providing both respiratory and circulatory support. (Reproduced with permission from Chang HH, Chen YC, Huang CJ, et al. Optimization of extracorporeal membrane oxygenation therapy using near-infrared spectroscopy to assess changes in peripheral circulation: A pilot study. *J Biophotonics*. 2020;13(10):e202000116.)

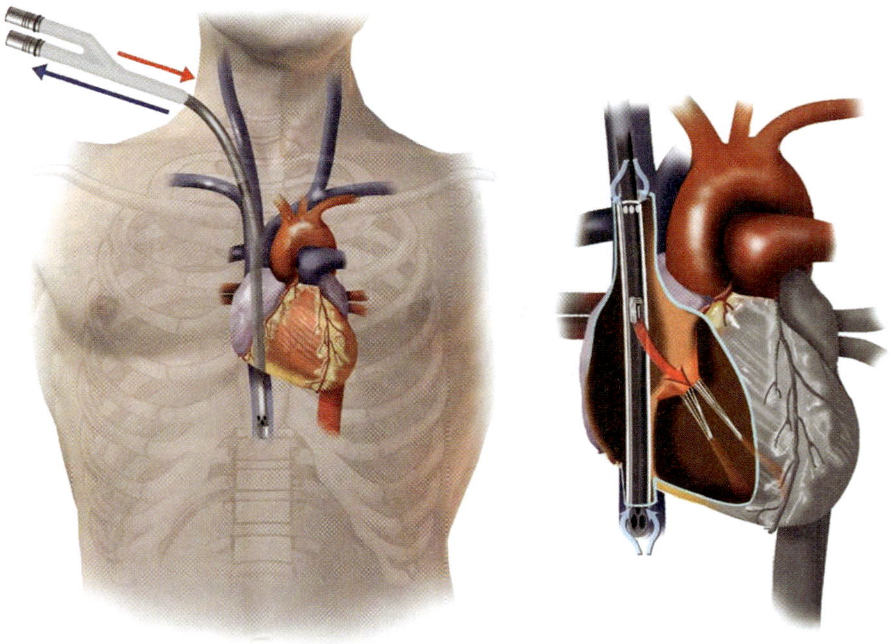

FIGURE 15.3. Depiction of dual-lumen cannula (Avalon) specifically designed for VV-ECMO support. Such single-lumen catheters simplify the setup of VV-ECMO while reducing the risk of recirculation. The cannula is placed via the right IJ vein and is guided by fluoroscopy or echocardiography so that the inflow side holes are positioned in the SVC and IVC to drain venous blood into the ECMO circuit, while the return side hole is positioned in the RA facing the tricuspid valve to direct return blood flow across the tricuspid valve. Although commonly utilized by VV-ECMO services, these cannulas are relatively unhelpful when VV-ECMO support is specifically for difficult airway management due to their requisite positing in the neck adjacent to the airway. (Reproduced with permission from Hirose H, Yamane K, Marhefka G, et al. Right ventricular rupture and tamponade caused by malposition of the Avalon cannula for venovenous extracorporeal membrane oxygenation. *J Cardiothorac Surg*. 2012;7:36.)

The desirable VV-ECMO flow rate for a specific patient is typically guided empirically by arterial oxygen saturation monitoring. At rest, adults consume 3 $mL \cdot kg^{-1} \cdot min^{-1}$ of oxygen (approximately 250 $mL \cdot min^{-1}$ for the average-sized individual). Assuming no contribution from lung function (e.g., the unventilated patient having a difficult airway managed), systemic arterial oxygen content becomes the simple combination of contents from the two blood sources entering the RA: (1) oxygenated "red" ECMO flow and (2) native "blue" venous flow (blood that avoids the ECMO circuit: total native venous flow = peripheral venous "escape" flow + coronary sinus flow). By extension, to conceptualize the effects of ECMO flow rates for a specific patient (e.g., to fully replace lung function), the following simplified equation can be used (applicable to the range of saturations functionally relevant to ECMO support): adapted from Bartlett[11]:

$$\frac{\text{Native } O_2 \text{ saturation} \times \text{native flow}}{\text{Cardiac output (total flow)}} + \frac{\text{ECMO } O_2 \text{ saturation} \times \text{ECMO flow}}{\text{Cardiac output (total flow)}} = \text{Desired (i.e., target) arterial } O_2 \text{ saturation}$$

Empirically, a target systemic arterial oxygen saturation of 80% to 90% is common. ECMO flow rate and oxygen saturation data are available from pump readings. Importantly, the above equation can be used to anticipate ECMO management challenges and options for intervention by predicting the effects on systemic oxygen saturation of changing physiologic conditions.[12]

- *Increased cardiac output.* If cardiac output (total flow) increases while ECMO flow (and thus delivered oxygen content) remains unchanged, one would expect the arterial oxygen saturation to decline. Notably, despite this decrease in the systemic arterial oxygen saturation, total oxygen supplementation to the body is unchanged and, therefore, should remain adequate in the setting of a rise in cardiac output.
- *Anemia.* A decrease in circulating hemoglobin concentration will reduce the total oxygen-carrying capacity and content of arterial blood and (for equivalent oxygen delivery to the body) result in lower oxygen saturation of returning native venous blood. When this desaturated venous blood mixes with ECMO blood the result is a further decrease in systemic arterial oxygen saturation.
- *Increased metabolism.* The hypermetabolic patient (e.g., due to sepsis, fever, agitation, shivering) increases total oxygen consumption such that, without adjusting ECMO flow, a resultant decrease in venous and arterial oxygen saturation occurs. Importantly, in the clinical setting, such physiologic demands can sometimes be so significant as to outstrip any available additional increase in oxygen delivery provided by ECMO.

What Are the Potential Problems Associated with Long-Term Use of ECMO?

Although ECMO episodes for difficult airway management can be relatively brief, in some cases, extended periods of support may be required even after the airway is secured, requiring practitioners to have an understanding of longer-term ECMO management strategies. Commonly, long-term ECMO patients receive mechanical lung ventilation, and the interplay of these interventions must be balanced. For example, ventilator tidal volume and VV-ECMO sweep gas flow rate both affect arterial CO_2 levels. Notably, combined titration to desired partial pressures for both CO_2 and O_2 levels is best achieved with guidance from arterial blood gas measurements. Generally, while maintaining lung protective ventilator settings, the ECMO sweep gas flow is adjusted to maintain a normal $PaCO_2$ of 40 mmHg while the ECMO flow rate is titrated to maintain the arterial O_2 saturation at 90%.[11] Typically, sweep gas is 100% oxygen, although occasional brief strategic lowering to 21% (room air) combined with lung ventilation can be used to assess functional lung recovery in some settings (see section *"How Do You Wean from VV-ECMO?"* later in the chapter). The ability to lower sweep gas oxygen levels while maintaining VV-ECMO flow to test for weaning readiness is a valuable feature of VV-ECMO.

When the VV-ECMO flow rate is at maximum and evidence suggests that oxygen delivery is still inadequate (e.g., worsening lactic acidosis), how can increased oxygen delivery be achieved? A first option is to raise the hemoglobin concentration (i.e., transfuse if anemia is present). A second more broadly applicable option is to increase the overall VV-ECMO flow by adding another venous drainage cannula. If a hypermetabolic state is suspected, specific concerns can be targeted to reduce oxygen consumption (e.g., cooling to address hyperthermia, muscle paralysis to address shivering). Sometimes recirculation produces inadequate oxygen delivery related to ECMO inefficiency (i.e., wasted ECMO oxygenation potential) amenable to improvement by re-positioning the ECMO cannulas.

As outlined above, recirculation is an important concern related to VV-ECMO management.[12] When ECMO-oxygenated "red" blood recirculates back to the VV-ECMO circuit due to inadequate separation of drainage and return cannulas, this blood does not participate in delivering oxygen to the patient, thus reducing the efficiency of ECMO. The effect is even more pronounced if cardiac output decreases, resulting in an increase in the proportion of recirculated ECMO blood relative to total cardiac output. Clues that recirculation is occurring include increasing ECMO circuit venous oxygen saturation and/or brightening of the color (i.e., oxygenation).[13]

Note that desired CO_2 clearance is always easier to achieve than desired oxygenation (due to the greater blood solubility of CO_2 vs. O_2). Hence, practically speaking, VV-ECMO management adjustments are almost always related to systemic oxygenation.[12] Restated, if CO_2 clearance is the primary goal of VV-ECMO, much lower ECMO flow rates can be used. An initial sweep gas flow rate of 2 liters per minute (lpm) is a good starting point, with titration based on arterial $PaCO_2$ blood gas determination. Importantly, decreasing $PaCO_2$ too rapidly may result in neurologic injury.[13]

Is Anticoagulant Necessary for ECMO?

Assuming sufficient flow rates to avoid stasis are maintained, the need for anticoagulation is a highly debated topic among ECMO practitioners. There is no consensus (even before any implications related to airway bleeding are considered) regarding the optimal level of anticoagulation required for VV-ECMO to balance the risks of thrombosis (under-anticoagulation) and hemorrhage (over-anticoagulation). Even the preferred method for anticoagulation monitoring is variable among institutions. A recent worldwide survey of ECMO centers yielded the following management trends for VV-ECMO[14]:

- Unfractionated heparin is the anticoagulant of choice in a majority of surveyed centers (96.7%).
- The preferred anticoagulation monitoring test varies considerably by center (activated partial thromboplastin time [APTT]: 41.8%; activated clotting time [ACT]: 30%; anti-factor Xa [anti-Xa] activity: 22.7%).
- Target anticoagulation goals (average lower-upper limits) considered therapeutic for VV-ECMO, by monitoring test, are as follows:
  - 50 to 60 seconds for APTT;
  - 170 to 200 seconds for ACT;
  - 0.3 to 0.5 IU/mL for anti-Xa.

Specific to difficult airway management, in the intraoperative setting where point-of-care ACT testing is likely to be available, we recommend the use of unfractionated heparin with ACT-based monitoring of the level of anticoagulation.

How Do You Wean from VV-ECMO?

When VV-ECMO is instituted, a plan for its intended weaning and discontinuation must also be in place. To emphasize this point, anticipated nonrecovery of lung function without a viable pathway towards ECMO decannulation (i.e., no "exit" plan) is the only *absolute contraindication* to initiating VV-ECMO.[13] In elective procedures where VV-ECMO support is used for difficult airway management, significant premorbid lung disease is rarely a major consideration. Rather, the goal of VV-ECMO is to temporarily replace lung function for the primary purpose of securing the airway in a safe, unrushed manner. In such difficult airway scenarios, native lung function is unlikely to be compromised. Nonetheless, ventilatory and oxygenation reserve are always assessed in preparation for ECMO discontinuation, to determine readiness. This can be achieved in one of two ways[13]: (1) reducing the VV-ECMO flow (generally to no less than 1-1.5 lpm to limit the risk of thrombosis), or (2) maintaining VV-ECMO flow but reducing the sweep gas oxygen level to 21%. In either scenario, the ability to maintain arterial oxygen saturation and CO_2 content with reasonable ventilator settings suggests eligibility for ending VV-ECMO support. The sweep gas flow rate can be reduced in a stepwise manner to OFF to determine the patient's unassisted ability to maintain $PaCO_2$ and an acceptable blood pH.

PATIENT MANAGEMENT

What Is the Role of VV-ECMO in Managing the Two Difficult Airway Cases Presented Above?

Hypothetical clinical courses for our two representative extreme difficult airway cases described earlier in the chapter, including the utility of VV-ECMO as an adjunct in their management, are outlined below.

Case 1. For the young female with a friable, airway-obstructing distal tracheal tumor at risk for irretrievable acute loss of the airway due to major bleeding, dual femoral venous cannulation permitted establishment of elective VV-ECMO as part of an airway management strategy. While still awake, the patient was positioned supine, and groins prepped and draped bilaterally. The surgeon administered copious local anesthesia infiltration (1% lidocaine) prior to achieving bilateral femoral venous access using Micropuncture® (Cook Medical, Bloomington, IN, USA) catheters. Through each catheter, guidewires were placed guided by fluoroscopy. Over these wires, the surgeon placed a 19 Fr *inflow* ECMO cannula and a 21 Fr *outflow* ECMO cannula. Unfractionated heparin was administered to achieve an ACT of greater than 200 seconds, and VV-ECMO flow was initiated at 2 lpm and titrated based on maintaining arterial blood gas oxygen saturation above 90%.

While still awake, full VV-ECMO support was initiated, and mask denitrogenation was followed by general anesthesia induction without any other airway interventions. The patient was moved to the right lateral decubitus position, and a right thoracotomy approach to the tumor permitted successful tumor resection and tracheal repair. After completion of the tracheal repair, with surgeon (intrathoracic) guidance, the anesthesiologist then secured the airway using a combination of careful direct oral laryngoscopy and bronchoscopic guidance of a 7.0-mm ID ETT such that the cuff was located just above the level of the tracheal repair. Following the successful initiation of positive pressure ventilation, prior to the end of surgery, VV-ECMO was cautiously weaned, guided by arterial oxygen saturation, and femoral venous cannulas were removed prior to awakening. Tracheal extubation of the patient occurred prior to departure from the OR. Recovery was otherwise uneventful.

Case 2. In this urgent cardiac surgical case, after anesthesia induction, an anticipated difficult airway evolved into an emergency with failure to secure tracheal intubation despite multiple attempts with advanced interventions. In this case, the ability to maintain marginal oxygenation and ventilation was achieved, but awakening was not considered a viable option due to difficulty in managing bleeding in the upper airway; hence, deployment of VV-ECMO immediately was identified as the best plan. An ECMO team was on call and immediately available in the cardiac surgery operating room. Once the ECMO team assembled, an intravenous bolus of unfractionated heparin was given, and the surgeon used ultrasound guidance to quickly place bilateral femoral venous cannulas over guidewires, and in a similar fashion to Case 1, VV-ECMO support was then instituted. Once VV-ECMO was established and ventilation and oxygenation stabilized through ECMO, the anesthesiologist made further attempts at securing the airway (in a considerably more controlled unhurried environment).

To highlight, even in the most resourced institutions, time from "go-call" to active deployment of ECMO support will not be sufficiently swift to make this intervention a good fit for management of the hypoxemic airway emergency. Based on local factors, emergency deployment may be as soon as 15 to 30 minutes but is highly variable among institutions, and often takes considerably longer to occur.

In the current case, a flexible bronchoscope was passed nasally without successful identification of the glottis. An otolaryngologist was consulted, and several further attempts were made with the flexible bronchoscope without success. Finally, together the otolaryngologist and anesthesiologist were able to access the airway percutaneously, achieving retrograde tracheal intubation with a 6.5-mm ETT passed over the retrograde guidewire. The intended cardiac surgical procedure was aborted due to the significant airway bleeding, and the patient was transferred under sedation with ECMO in place to the intensive care unit. Several days later, the patient underwent successful elective tracheotomy, and VV-ECMO was weaned and decannulated. Sometime later, the patient's medical condition was deemed not an emergency from a cardiac perspective that he was discharged to home and returned 3 weeks later with a functioning tracheotomy for the planned cardiac surgery. The cardiac surgery was uneventful and recovery smooth, including tracheotomy reversal several weeks following surgery.

Is There a Role for Simulation in ECMO Team Training?

The hypothetical cases presented summarize key features of real-life examples experienced by the authors where VV-ECMO support was successful, sometimes as a "last resort" strategy for management of the difficult/impossible airway. While in some ways the cases are similar, they also highlight the varied urgency and breadth of settings in which VV-ECMO may be employed as an adjunct rather than solution to facilitate the unrushed thoughtful use of other management strategies to safely secure the difficult airway. Most pertinent is that Case 2 involved *no opportunity* to anticipate the need for emergency VV-ECMO support, whereas Case 1 allowed for the controlled deployment of elective VV-ECMO. It is Case 2 that most exemplifies the value of a skilled team to promptly deploy VV-ECMO even when little or no warning is available. Detailed approaches to the financing, specific materials, and potential personnel that can create such a VV-ECMO team is beyond the scope of current chapter but suffice to say that successful models are emerging across many countries; these typically include the extremely difficult airway as one among many deserving indications for VV-ECMO (e.g., COVID-related respiratory failure). Nonetheless, it is key that such teams become proficient, not only in the deployment of VV-ECMO, but also the priorities that surround management of a difficult airway. Simulation can be a key part of rehearsing such activities.

Simulation is well-established as a training method for developing technical skills, improving teamwork, and enhancing patient safety and quality. The VV-ECMO for airway management is a rare and critical situation that is also complex in nature, requiring coordinated technical and team skills. Given these complexities, simulation can be a valuable tool to enhance team preparedness for cases where VV-ECMO will be used for difficult airway management. Simulation can offer many benefits, including but not limited to the ability to troubleshoot and optimize the process and the team dynamics, and developing a local protocol for VV-ECMO support for the difficult airway.

Deployment of VV-ECMO for managing the anticipated difficult airway calls for a multidisciplinary approach due to complex equipment needs coupled with a second team experienced in dealing with the difficult airway. Members of the difficult airway care team, while critical to the ultimate management of the airway, may not have experience initiating VV-ECMO. Clearly, simulation is an ideal modality for VV-ECMO initiation.

The simulation experiences must incorporate time for both a prebrief and a debrief. The simulation prebrief permits the team to be gathered to anticipate and plan for concerns, and allows the creation of a shared mental model for both VV-ECMO and airway management, including contingency plans, resources, and roles. Guidelines for the simulation experience should be presented to the team within the prebrief. During the simulation event, role clarity, care coordination, communication, and other team dynamics can actively be worked through and optimized. For example, the space available for the team to perform the task is crowded, and space logistics impact team effectiveness.

After simulation exercises, the debrief should allow team members to discuss the case and/or further develop a protocol and revise plans accordingly. The simulation may be repeated, paused, or fast forwarded, depending on the needs of the team, to optimize the process and team dynamics, and allow for an iterative approach.

Simulation logistics can be tailored to the circumstances and needs of any given institution. Ideally, the simulation scenario development involves faculty experienced in simulation methodology and content experts. See Chapter 67 for a detailed discussion of Simulation.

SUMMARY

Femoral VV-ECMO support may be useful to augment or replace lung function and facilitate unhurried management of the anticipated or unanticipated difficult airway. VA-ECMO is only required when left ventricular function is also compromised.

Establishing femoral VV-ECMO support requires not only specialized equipment but also specialized practitioners (e.g., surgeons, perfusionists, anesthesiologists) who are facile in this technology. Heparin anticoagulation requirements for VV-ECMO support are debated in the literature but are generally much lower than those for VA-ECMO or cardiopulmonary bypass. Oxygenation and carbon dioxide removal is easily achieved by adjusting of VV-ECMO flow rates and sweep gas rates. Failure to achieve these goals at appropriate settings should raise the concern of recirculation due to cannula malposition. Given the technical complexity and expertise required for successful implementation of VV-ECMO, simulation to define and rehearse team roles and practice technical skills should be undertaken. If VV-ECMO support is anticipated to be required for difficult airway management and the necessary technology and skilled practitioners are not available, patients should be referred to centers with established ECMO programs.

SELF-EVALUATION QUESTIONS

15.1. Which of the following *does not* reflect the role of ECMO in management of the difficult airway?

A. Separates gas exchange from securing the airway

B. An elective or emergency intervention

C. A lasting solution

D. Facilitates unhurried airway procedures

E. A temporary adjunct

15.2. Of the various types of ECMO, which is the preferred strategy for most difficult or impossible airway scenarios?

A. VA-ECMO: left femoral vein, right femoral artery

B. VV-ECMO: right internal jugular vein (Avalon Elite dual-lumen cannula)

C. AA-ECMO: left femoral artery, right femoral artery

D. VV-ECMO: left femoral vein, right femoral vein

E. VV-ECMO: right internal jugular vein (Protek Duo dual-lumen cannula)

15.3. What are the challenges for an institution previously without such a service, related to the introduction of ECMO (specifically as a difficult airway intervention)?

A. Financial support

B. Personnel expertise

C. Education of expert teams (airway and ECMO) on value/appropriate usage/complications

D. Role coordination (between expert teams, and among individuals)

E. All of the above

REFERENCES

1. Dunkman WJ, Nicoara A, Schroder J, et al. Elective venovenous extracorporeal membrane oxygenation for resection of endotracheal tumor: a case report. *A A Case Rep*. 2017; 9:97-100.
2. Kim JJ, Moon SW, Kim YH, Choi SY, Jeong SC. Flexible bronchoscopic excision of a tracheal mass under extracorporeal membrane oxygenation. *J Thorac Dis*. 2015;7:E54-E57.
3. Hong Y, Jo KW, Lyu J, et al. Use of venovenous extracorporeal membrane oxygenation in central airway obstruction to facilitate interventions leading to definitive airway security. *J Crit Care*. 2013;28:669-674.
4. Gourdin M, Dransart C, Delaunois L, Louagie YA, Gruslin A, Dubois P. Use of venovenous extracorporeal membrane oxygenation under regional anesthesia for a high-risk rigid bronchoscopy. *J Cardiothorac Vasc Anesth*. 2012;26:465-467.
5. Yunoki K, Miyawaki I, Yamazaki K, Mima H. Extracorporeal membrane oxygenation-assisted airway management for difficult airways. *J Cardiothorac Vasc Anesth*. 2018;32:2721-2725.
6. Malpas G, Hung O, Gilchrist A, et al. The use of extracorporeal membrane oxygenation in the anticipated difficult airway: a case report and systematic review. *Can J Anesth*. 2018;65:685-697.
7. Jayaraman AL, Cormican D, Shah P, Ramakrishna H. Cannulation strategies in adult veno-arterial and veno-venous extracorporeal membrane oxygenation: techniques, limitations, and special considerations. *Ann Card Anaesth*. 2017;20:S11-S18.
8. Lequier L, Horton SB, Mcmullan DM, Bartlett RH. Extracorporeal membrane oxygenation circuitry. *Pediat Crit Care Med*. 2013;14:S7-S12.
9. Squiers JJ, Lima B, Dimaio JM. Contemporary extracorporeal membrane oxygenation therapy in adults: fundamental principles and systematic review of the evidence. *J Thorac Cardiovasc Surg*. 2016;152:20-32.
10. Bermudez CA, Rocha RV, Sappington PL, Toyoda Y, Murray HN, Boujoukos AJ. Initial experience with single cannulation for venovenous extracorporeal oxygenation in adults. *Ann Thorac Surg*. 2010;90:991-995.
11. Bartlett RH. Physiology of extracorporeal gas exchange. *Compr Physiol*. 2020:879-891.
12. Bartlett RH, Conrad SA. The physiology of extracorporeal life support. In: Brogan TV, Lequier L, Lorusso R, MacLaren G, Peek G, eds. *Extracorporeal Life Support: The ELSO Red Book*, 5th ed. Ann Arbor, MI: Extracorporeal Life Support Organization; 2017.
13. Tonna JE, Abrams D, Brodie D, et al. Management of adult patients supported with venovenous extracorporeal membrane oxygenation (VV ECMO): guideline from the Extracorporeal Life Support Organization (ELSO). *ASAIO J*. 2021;67:601-610.
14. Protti A, Iapichino GE, Di Nardo M, Panigada M, Gattinoni L. Anticoagulation management and antithrombin supplementation practice during veno-venous extracorporeal membrane oxygenation. *Anesthesiology*. 2020;132:562-570.

SECTION 3

PREHOSPITAL AIRWAY MANAGEMENT

CHAPTER 16

What Is Unique About Airway Management in the Prehospital Setting?

Mark P. Vu, Michael F. Murphy, and Erik N. Vu

CASE PRESENTATION

On a stormy night in the countryside, a 72-year-old male driver falls asleep at the wheel and strays into oncoming traffic. A transport truck trying to avoid him strikes his small car. The car is crushed and the driver is trapped inside. Emergency medical services (EMS) are activated. Basic life support (BLS) medics and fire fighters arrive on the scene within 10 minutes. The patient is conscious with a Glasgow Coma Score of 13, BP 80/40 mmHg, HR 100 bpm, RR 26 breaths per minute, and O2 saturations of 82% prior to oxygen therapy.

UNIQUE PREHOSPITAL ISSUES

■ What Level of Airway Management Can We Expect from Prehospital Care Providers?

"A" is the cornerstone in the traditional ABCs, which form the foundation of BLS training for most prehospital providers. However, current tactical and military prehospital care prioritizes massive hemorrhage control over the airway. Military priority action sequence is MARCHE = Massive Hemorrhage/Airway/Respiratory/Circulatory/Headinjury/Everything Else. The type of training and skill sets varies significantly from country to country and the provider mix may be different from one jurisdiction to another within a country. For clarity, we will define four discrete levels of airway management provided in an EMS system. Each level assumes proficiency in the skills of the previous:

- First aid providers or "First Responders"—trained to apply supplemental O_2 by face-mask and perform artificial ventilation, typically face-mask ventilation (FMV), although in some jurisdictions extraglottic devices (EGDs) may be preferred at this level as first-line devices in place of FMV. Airway adjuncts at this level may include oral- and naso-pharyngeal airways.
- BLS providers—more experienced with FMV and these providers use EGDs, particularly Combitube™, King LT™, and laryngeal mask airways (LMAs) in some systems.
- Advanced life support (ALS) providers—typically perform laryngoscopy (direct or indirect) and endotracheal intubation, with or without the use of facilitating drugs, such as sedative-hypnotics and neuromuscular blocking agents. Emergency cricothyrotomy training is often included at this level.
- Critical care providers (e.g., typically Air Medical Transport or Critical Care Transport team members)—are permitted to perform rapid sequence intubation (RSI) using direct laryngoscope and usually other advanced airway techniques such as indirect laryngoscopy (e.g., video laryngoscopy) and cricothyrotomy. In some jurisdictions (most notably Europe and Australia), teams include other health care professionals, including registered nurses and physicians, as members of these multidisciplinary teams.

■ How Are Airway Management Protocols and Equipment Determined in Prehospital Care Systems?

In most North American systems, prehospital care providers perform delegated medical acts based on standardized medical protocols. In many European systems, physicians may be the usual prehospital care providers and, therefore, are less likely dependent on protocols. While protocols ought to reflect best clinical evidence, from a practical perspective, they are often limited by cost, training, competency maintenance, and space constraints. Over the past several years, there has been a movement in some jurisdictions away from protocols, and more toward treatment guidelines, allowing advanced prehospital care providers to exercise clinical judgment when managing airways. These guidelines allow for more flexibility to achieve predefined physiologic goals pertaining to airway management, with less emphasis on technical imperatives formerly used as markers of successful (or unsuccessful) airway management. For example, modern guidelines define successful airway management as the maintenance of oxygenation and ventilation by various means, other than simply placing an endotracheal tube (ETT).

Protocols or guidelines approved by the medical director of the EMS system determine the equipment necessary for prehospital care practice. The type and range of equipment available for managing the difficult airway in the prehospital setting are usually limited when compared to in-hospital settings. Even basic equipment, such as the endotracheal tube introducer (ETI; e.g., the Eschmann tracheal introducer, also known as the "gum-elastic bougie"),[1] laryngoscope blades, and ETT in an array of types and sizes, may be limited. Alternate intubating devices, such as the intubating LMA (ILMA or LMA®-Fastrach™) or lightwands (e.g., Trachlight™), often are not available due to limitations in space, training opportunities, cost, resterilization, and issues of skills maintenance. Rescue devices, such as the esophageal–tracheal Combitube, LMA, and the LMA-Unique™ (the disposable LMA), the King LT, and i-gel® are becoming more popular because they are relatively inexpensive, disposable, and are considered easier to use by prehospital care providers at varied levels of training.[2] However, ventilation using an EGD may not be appropriate in some clinical situations, particularly if adequate ventilation calls for an increase in peak airway pressure beyond the capabilities of a device to achieve an adequate seal, if the patient is sufficiently responsive to reject the device, or if protection against aspiration is preferred.[3] Surgical airway management devices[4] must be available in any system providing RSI. Critical Care EMS systems often differ from many ground systems because they carry more advanced equipment, such as the GlideScope™ video laryngoscope, or other devices.

What Unique Environmental Considerations Do Prehospital Care Providers Face When Managing the Airway?

The practitioner managing the airway is often confronted with an array of circumstances unique to the out-of-hospital environment, including:

- A chaotic scene;
- A dangerous scene (e.g., flood, fire, radiation, electrical wires down, toxic environment, assailant on the loose);
- Access to the patient and the airway which may be challenging due to a variety of factors:
  - an ongoing extrication;
  - position of the patient (e.g., seated, upside down). In non-trauma airway management, positioning may also present a problem (e.g., intubation performed lying prone and leaning on the elbows). Even with the patient on a stretcher in an ambulance or helicopter, an optimal position for airway management may be difficult to achieve.
- Other uncontrollable environmental conditions:
  - darkness inhibits full airway assessment and obscures subtle nonverbal communication cues among providers;
  - Bright sunlight may present similar problems, especially when tracheal intubation (TI) is performed using a laryngoscope or a lightwand;
  - Extremes of weather may present problems for patients, practitioners, and equipment (e.g., freezing temperature effects on plastic and metal objects);
  - An uncontrolled tactical environment, in which EMS may be deployed with police and be required to limit access to patients, or limit interventions performed in the various phases of tactical emergency casualty care;[5]
  - spectators, family, or friends of patients may require skilled handling.
- Lack of other essential equipment for airway management, e.g., suction;
- Uncontrolled human behavior in the prehospital setting may further interfere with airway management decisions and procedures:
  - distraught relatives challenging the focus of prehospital care providers;
  - knowledgeable and skilled assistants may be unavailable;
  - well-meaning first-aiders or bystander physicians may hamper efforts with inappropriately timed or out-of-context comments or actions.

Finally, management of an airway in the prehospital environment may have to be carried out amid the most adverse of surroundings and circumstances, e.g., a crime scene, on a dance floor, in a stadium.

Back to our case: ALS responders arrive on the scene 15 minutes later. The patient's level of consciousness is decreasing and he remains hypotensive. BLS providers have skillfully assisted ventilations with the FMV while other skilled rescuers attempt to extricate the patient from the wreckage. The Glasgow Coma Scale (GCS) is now 9, BP 80/40 mmHg, HR 120 bpm, and O_2 saturation 88%.

AIRWAY CONSIDERATIONS

What Are the Patient Factors that Influence Airway Management Decisions of a Prehospital Care Provider?

There are three related elements governing airway management in the field environment: time, anatomy, and (patho-) physiology (i.e., the clinical state of the patient).

Time Factors: When Is It Better to Wait?

All emergency airway management situations share this feature. In other words, they are "context sensitive" (see Chapter 7). It is well appreciated that geographic proximity to a hospital or trauma center does not correlate with out-of-hospital time (e.g., extrication delays), and as such, the prehospital care provider must often differentiate between an "indication" for a given airway management technique and the "need" to actually perform that intervention. Consider, for example, the following three cases:

- A 40-year-old male with sudden collapse of two blocks away from a hospital, GCS 6, with no cough or swallowing reflex, O2 saturations of 99%, and normal airway anatomy;
- The same 40-year-old male with sudden collapse, on a mountain side, two hours away from the nearest hospital, GCS 6, with no cough or swallowing reflex, O2 saturations of 99%, normal airway anatomy, and the only means to extricate the patient is via Helicopter Emergency Medical Services (HEMS) response; or
- The same 40-year-old man in a house fire who has stridor, O2 saturations of 70%, and evidence of upper airway burns.

In the first patient discussed above, the decision to intubate immediately will depend upon the anatomical assessment and time considerations. For example, if the transport time to a hospital is very short, it might be reasonable to wait (i.e., oxygenate and ventilate with FMV, protect with suction) until arrival at the ED where more resources are available. Training must emphasize that airway management means gas exchange and it does not always require intubation. We must avoid the trap of the "technical imperative"—just because it can be done, it should be done. In fact, there is growing evidence that in certain situations prehospital intubation may not necessarily improve outcomes and may be detrimental.[6,7]

On the other hand, in the second patient, despite stable physiology and no predictors of difficult anatomy, due to prolonged out-of-hospital time and the anticipation of aeromedical evacuation with limited access to the patient, it would be reasonable to take the time on the scene to place an advanced airway for oxygenation and ventilation as well as protection during flight and until arrival at a receiving hospital.

Likewise, in the third patient, with predicted difficult laryngoscopy and anticipated progression of airway edema, time is critical. A quick decision must be made and the provider must confidently follow the Emergency Difficult Airway Algorithm (Figures 2.11-2.14 in Chapter 2).

Anatomic Factors: How to Predict Difficulties in Different Airway Management Techniques?

The airway assessment is essentially an attempt to predict difficult direct and indirect laryngoscopy and intubation, difficult FMV, difficult EGD placement, and difficult cricothyrotomy based on an examination of external anatomic features (see Chapter 1). While recognizing that it may not be possible to assess the airway of some patients (e.g., unresponsive patients), this evaluation is a crucial component of prehospital airway management as it is in the hospital. It permits the airway practitioner to make appropriate airway management plans (Plans A, B, and C) that are most likely to be successful.

Patients with acceptable oxygen saturations and a short transport time, with or without predictors of difficult laryngoscopy and intubation, might be better served by a rapid transport to the nearest ED with more resources. This reflects context-specific decision balancing technical abilities (i.e., I can intubate) with physiologic goals (i.e., the patient is oxygenating and ventilating adequately), but also takes into consideration the poor predictive value of some of our airway assessment tools. In other words, though one may have predictors of easy direct laryngoscopy, once C-spine precautions are put in place, the patient's trachea may be difficult to intubate through standard means. Should clinical or time considerations preclude rapid transport for in-hospital airway management, the Emergency Difficult Airway Algorithm directs one to weigh carefully whether RSI, sedation, or awake intubation would be most appropriate. If any of these is unsuccessful, one should move promptly to the Failed Airway Algorithm (Chapter 2, Figure 2.14). Situations in which difficulty is predicted and airway management is urgently indicated may be better handled by an early call through dispatch for scene backup.

Most prehospital ALS and critical care providers are familiar with the necessity for an airway evaluation prior to each intubation, particularly if medications are to be administered to facilitate the procedure. However, this may be limited to predictors of difficult laryngoscopy and intubation rather than difficulty in other airway techniques (see Chapter 1), such as video laryngoscopy, EGDs, difficult FMV, and difficult surgical airway.

Clinical Factors: How Do the Clinical Condition and Presumed Diagnosis Affect Airway Management Decisions?

There are two clinical considerations in managing a difficult airway in the field setting: the indication for intubation and the underlying pathophysiology.

Indications for endotracheal intubation in the prehospital environment are similar to those in any other emergency.[8]

1. Failure to maintain adequate oxygenation;
2. Failure to maintain adequate ventilation (CO2 removal);
3. Failure to protect the airway;
4. The need for neuromuscular blockade;
5. The anticipated clinical course;
6. Uncompensated shock.

In practice, many patients may have more than one indication for endotracheal intubation.

Underlying Pathophysiology: The indications for intubation among various EMS systems may differ. The most common indication (up to two-thirds of all intubations) in a typical ground EMS system is cardiac arrest.[9] The remainder tend to be split evenly among respiratory failure (asthma, chronic obstructive lung disease, congestive heart failure, pulmonary embolism, pneumonia, anaphylaxis), nontrauma central nervous system conditions (coma, intracranial bleed/stroke, seizure, overdose), trauma (head injury, chest injury, neck injury, blood loss causing shock), and shock states (sepsis, cardiogenic, hypovolemic).

HEMS (also called rotorcraft Air Medical Transport [AMT]) rarely responds to primary cardiac arrest calls. These critical care teams are trained to manage patients who may require more advanced airway procedures, or those with a more complex pathophysiology.

In certain circumstances, a patient may have an indication for intubation but circumstances, such as predicted difficult airway and a short transport time to the ED, may sanction FMV and suction until intubation is possible. The weighing of "risk versus benefit" is illustrated in the example above (40-year-old man with a collapse and a short transport time vs. long transport time, vs. burn with time-sensitive pressures). Even in the face of an accepted indication for intubation, the potential benefits of prehospital intubation must be weighed within the context of the environment, time, anatomy, and pathophysiology.

What Alternatives Do Prehospital Providers Have in Managing a Difficult Airway?

Effective FMV technique (including two-handed mask hold requiring two providers if available or necessary) is essential to the prehospital care provider, particularly when the airway could be difficult and the transport time relatively brief.

Despite considerable controversy in the literature, the gold standard for definitive airway control remains the correct intratracheal placement of a cuffed ETT. According to the "Recommended Guidelines for Uniform Reporting of Data from Out-Of-Hospital Airway Management,"[10] there are four methods by which this can be achieved: direct oral laryngoscopy and intubation, nasotracheal intubation, tracheal intubation (TI) via oral rescue techniques (e.g., intubating LMA), and surgical rescue techniques (transtracheal jet ventilation and cricothyrotomy). These four methods may each be modified by five variables:

- oral approach—no facilitating sedative drugs or paralytics;
- nasal approach—no facilitating sedative drugs or paralytics;
- sedation-facilitated intubation—without the use of paralytics;
- RSI—with the use of paralytics and induction agents;
- other intubation techniques (e.g., digital, lightwand).

The actual number of options available to a given EMS system is driven by evidence-guided, rationale-based medical oversight, and limited by local culture, protocols, training, and equipment.

There is ample evidence that endotracheal intubation is not a benign intervention in the hands of inexperienced personnel.[11–13] Newer airway devices such as the LMA, King LT, i-gel, and the Combitube have been introduced and validated in the prehospital care setting.[3,14–19] These devices may be employed in two ways: as an alternative to endotracheal intubation in the cardiac arrest (or deeply comatose) patient by all levels of providers[3,15,18,20] or as a rescue device in the setting of failed intubation by ALS or critical care providers.[14,16]

An emerging alternative to endotracheal intubation in the respiratory failure patient is prehospital noninvasive positive pressure ventilation (NIPPV). Several case series have shown continuous positive airway pressure (CPAP) or bi-level ventilation (BiPAP) to be feasible and potentially beneficial in the prehospital setting.[21–23] Current evidence supports the use of CPAP in the prehospital setting for high-pressure pulmonary edema (i.e., CHF).[24] Prehospital critical care teams will often also use BiPAP in hypercapnic respiratory failure (e.g. secondary to chronic obstructive pulmonary disease).[25] Furthermore, based on case series and physiological principles, BIPAP can be used as a denitrogenation technique by critical care paramedics prior to transitioning to endotracheal intubation and formal mechanical ventilation.[26,27]

What Are the Challenges in Terminology Associated with Prehospital Airway Management?

Increasing attention is being paid to the many aspects of prehospital airway management. Research, discussion, education, and innovation in both devices and approaches have expanded. It is quite apparent that one approach does not fit all clinical situations in the ideal in-hospital environment, so it is folly to assume that it is any less complex in the prehospital setting in which there are more variables to consider. The clinical choices involved in airway management in the field setting may well be limited by personnel training, the realities of maintaining competence, and the devices and drugs available to field personnel. Using "patient outcome," rather than procedural outcome as the measure of success of airway management, one can begin to construct some useful definitions.

Inaccurate use of terms in three different risk/benefit clinical issues often makes the selection of the best airway management method to proceed within any clinical situation difficult. The three spectrums of risk/benefit are:

1. Pharmacology: which drug or combination of drugs should be administered;
2. Procedure/equipment: what procedure/equipment to use to facilitate the placement of a device;
3. Device: what device is most appropriate to oxygenate/ventilate the patient?

These confusions often lead to incorrect comparisons in research studies. If these three components are carefully separated from each other, it becomes apparent that interpretation of the results of a study comparing RSI versus EGDs is difficult rapid sequence airway (RSA).[28] The exact terminology eventually used is less important than the need to achieve consensus and consistency. However, separating these three decision points will be imperative, recognizing that the initial decision or plan may change with evolving clinical situations.

The most obvious use of vague terminology is in the area of the pharmacology of airway management. Many drugs and combinations of drugs can be used in facilitating prehospital airway procedures, particularly in what has been called "Rapid Sequence Intubation,"[29] "Rapid Sequence Airway,"[28] "Drug-Facilitated Intubation,"[30] "Drug-Assisted Intubation,"[31] "Delayed-sequence intubation,"[32] "Deep Sedation versus Awake Intubation,"[33] and others. For simplicity, these variations can be grouped into three categories:

1. Rapid Sequence, in which paralysis is preceded by an induction agent appropriate to the clinical state of the patient and the situation;
2. Sedation, in which the intent is to provide sedation, analgesia, or both;
3. Awake, in which topical anesthesia of the upper airway allows for lower sedative dose.

It might be said that clinically the difference between 2 and 3 above is "qualitative"; but the intent, and therefore the use of drugs, is clearly different. A lack of understanding of these differences can be both educationally confusing and clinically catastrophic. The use of deep sedation in a patient with a difficult airway without backup plans and essential equipment can lead to apnea, aspiration, profound physiologic disturbances, a failed airway, and ultimately, poor patient outcomes.

Should Tracheal Intubation Even Be Performed in the Field?

Both in and out of the hospital, inappropriate ventilation and inadequate oxygenation have been identified as primary contributors to preventable morbidity and mortality. It would seem reasonable, then, to assume that endotracheal intubation should be the gold standard in prehospital airway management. However, there has been considerable controversy as to whether patients requiring endotracheal intubation should have TI performed in the field or deferred until arrival at hospital. Several issues arise from this controversy:

- Trauma victims—There continues to be skepticism as to whether the intubation of trauma victims in the field improves survival. During the 1980s, it was generally felt that invasive airway management was ineffective in improving survival in urban environments but might be effective in longer transport environments.[34] Studies published during the 1990s gave conflicting results.[35–40] It might, at the very least, be anticipated that endotracheal intubation would be advantageous in patients with severe head injury. Early studies provided no clear direction[7,41–46] and a large trauma registry study found that prehospital intubation was associated with adverse outcomes after severe traumatic brain injury (TBI).[7] However, covariate adjustment in the same study suggests that management of the airway by an air medical team may improve outcomes. Unfortunately, as Zink and Maio[47] pointed out in an accompanying editorial, this is a retrospective association rather than a causation study. Importantly, these TBI studies raise questions about the downstream effects of drug choices, drug dosages, the physiology of transitioning from negative pressure-spontaneous ventilation to positive pressure ventilation, the type of positive pressure ventilation employed, and positive end-expiratory pressure (PEEP) among other things.
- Cardiac Arrest—In cardiac arrest patients, the issue of the efficacy of ETT remains unresolved.[48–52] To further add to the controversy, a study involving out-of-hospital cardiac arrest victims showed that patients who received cardiopulmonary resuscitation with only chest compressions had comparable survival outcomes compared to those who received chest compression and mouth-to-mouth ventilation.[53] A large prospective study to determine the incremented benefit of introducing ALS (including intubation) to a previously optimized system did not show a mortality benefit in cardiac arrest patients.[54] Furthermore, other observational studies have reported signals that advanced airway management is an independent predictor of worse neurological recovery after out-of-hospital cardiac arrest.[55]
- Children—Early studies in children showed that tracheal intubation by paramedics was associated with higher failure and complication rates than that in adults.[56] Results of subsequent studies have confirmed these early findings.[6,36,57–60] The only prospective trial to investigate the effectiveness of ground paramedics in performing TI in children showed that there was no increase in survival following TI as compared to that in the group treated with FMV.[6] This same study revealed concerns about TI displacement and the inability to recognize this catastrophic complication.[6] Many authorities maintain that these latter studies reflect inadequate training of paramedical personnel in TI of children. Furthermore, the literature does not resolve whether the field intubation of children with head injuries improves their outcomes.[61,62] In the final analysis, the emergency intubation of children is an uncommon and anxiety-provoking event for most paramedics. Both of these factors are likely to increase performance stress and failure rates, compared to the intubation of adults.

Recent studies have presented data and formed conclusions that challenge the basic, time-honored dogma of EMS airway management and question the best approach to the compromised airway in the prehospital environment. Furthermore, the development of other airway adjuncts (e.g., Combitube, King LT, LMA, i-gel, and CPAP) coupled with a reemphasis on standard FMV has changed the priority for prehospital endotracheal intubation and is a clear sign of maturity and success of the EMS.

It is becoming clear that airway management training and maintenance-of-competency programs are vital, as they will affect both psychomotor skill development and psychomotor skill decay, as well as context-specific decision-making that reflects current best-practice. Other issues such as equipment availability, the air versus ground environment, and the logistics associated with rural as opposed to urban critical care transport/ EMS suggest that a single, rigid approach to EMS airway management is inappropriate and cannot be supported.

Now to our case: ALS medics are unsuccessful in obtaining a definitive airway. Two IVs have been placed and a normal saline (NS) bolus administered. The patient has just been extricated (30 minutes later), boarded, and collared. The critical care crew has just landed at the scene. The patient now has a GCS of 7, a clenched jaw, BP 90/60 mmHg, HR 120 bpm, and an O2 saturation of 90% with assisted FMV with oxygen supplement.

MANAGEMENT OF THE AIRWAY IN THIS CASE

Prehospital RSI—What Does the Evidence Show?

The HEMS crew on the scene has the training and capability to perform an RSI on appropriate patients as part of their clinical mandate. This includes the use of an induction agent, followed in rapid sequence by a neuromuscular blocking agent and vasoactive agents (e.g., phenylephrine), in order to optimize intubating conditions and peri-intubation physiology, in order to increase the chances of successful endotracheal intubation and smooth transition to positive pressure ventilation.[29]

Until recently, the evidence in the EMS literature has not supported the use of RSI. Several recent, well-designed studies of ground systems have consistently shown suboptimal outcomes, or no difference in outcome, in patients suffering acute severe TBI in whom RSI is used to facilitate endotracheal intubation.[6,7,12,41,63] Head injury was deliberately chosen in these studies because prior reports have suggested that optimal oxygenation and ventilation of these patients improve outcomes. Therefore, it was assumed that successful endotracheal intubation would demonstrate a benefit.[64] A case-control study of prehospital RSI of severely head injured patients in 2003 identified increased mortality and morbidity in the RSI group when compared to patients who had TI performed in the ED following transport without RSI.[63] Though this study had methodological limitations that preclude generalizing their findings to all EMS systems that use RSI, an important message was the re-emphasis on protecting physiologic goals during airway management (i.e., SpO2, ETCO2, by any means), and de-emphasizing technical goals (i.e., achieving TI).

There have been attempts to determine the reasons for the poor outcomes associated with RSI in ground EMS services.

These explanations have included:

- increased on-scene time (average 15 minutes in one study);[65]
- lack of adequate training of the paramedics;[6,45,63]
- inappropriate hyperventilation and unrecognized hypoxemia during induction; and
- paralysis and attempts at intubation.[12]

Despite recent studies showing the lack of efficacy of RSI in the ground EMS systems, a distinct pattern of improved outcomes has emerged in the subpopulation of those patients in whom air medical transport (HEMS) had been utilized.[7,66–69] It would appear that the key to improved outcomes lies in the initial training and maintenance of competence (cognitive and psychomotor skills) for the prehospital providers.

Video Laryngoscopy in Prehospital Care

Video larygoscopy (VL) is becoming more common in routine emergency airway management practice as this technology becomes more affordable, more user friendly, and as practitioners become more familiar with its strengths and limitations. Hospital based consensus guidelines have embraced VL as a "first line" tool for tracheal intubation, but there is limited data in prehospital environments currently. Over time, as prehospital systems develop more experience with VL, and as VL technology evolves to meet the unique challenges of prehospital airway management, VL will find its place in the hierarchy of advanced tracheal intubation tools.

How Should a Critical Care Transport Team Proceed with the Management of the Airway in This Patient?

The HEMS crew elects to perform RSI using rocuronium (1.5 mg·kg^{-1})[70] *and ketamine (1.5 mg·kg^{-1}). A Grade 3 view of the laryngeal structures is obtained with no improvement of the view with the use of laryngeal manipulation. An Eschmann Tracheal Introducer is placed into the trachea and a 7.5-mm ID ETT is passed over it. A qualitative, colorimetric end-tidal CO2 (ETCO2) detector confirms tracheal tube placement. Adequate oxygen saturation is maintained during the procedure, and postintubation systolic blood pressure is 90 mmHg. To prevent hyperventilation, quantitative in-line ETCO2 monitoring is instituted postintubation and during transport.*

Other options for the pharmacologic approach to RSI in this patient could include succinylcholine as the paralytic (1.5 mg·kg^{-1}); etomidate and propofol (relatively contraindicated in hypovolemia) as the induction agents.

Because of its slow onset and associated hypotensive side effects at standard induction doses, midazolam may not be an ideal induction agent in EMS. Although the concept of "non-paralytic RSI" has been enshrined in some EMS systems, TI after the administration of an induction agent alone (without paralytic agent) is not supported by the literature and is not generally recommended.[71] In fact, success rates in intubation are generally lower and complications are higher with deep sedation when compared with RSI.[72–74]

It should be emphasized that full C-spine immobilization ought to be maintained during the intubation procedure. In the event TI failed, most EMS providers in this setting would use an EGD (e.g., King LT, LMA, i-gel, or Combitube). Cricothyrotomy (or an alternative percutaneous technique in young children) is a technique used by most advanced EMS providers. Continuous monitoring of oxygen saturation and ETCO2 should be maintained during transport in order to prevent hypoxemia, inadvertent hyper or hypoventilation, or extubation.

How Do Prehospital Providers Confirm and Maintain Intratracheal Placement of the ETT?

The consequences of an unrecognized, misplaced ETT may be devastating. Given the chaotic environment, the difficulty in employing the usual clinical verification signs and the increased movement and transfer of the patient, it is more difficult to recognize an esophageal intubation or dislodged endotracheal intubation in the prehospital setting than elsewhere. The exact number of unrecognized esophageal intubations is uncertain since many EMS systems do not gather these data. Inadvertent esophageal intubation rates in EMS have ranged from 1%[75] to 25%[76] based on verification of tube positioning by emergency physicians on arrival at the hospital. Very low rates are found in systems with specific tube verification protocols, ETCO2 monitoring, and ongoing performance improvement to ensure compliance. Unacceptably high rates are found when such protocols are not in place or tube placement verification devices are not available.

Prehospital care providers can confirm correct placement of the ETT in three ways: clinically, with mechanical esophageal detector devices (EDDs) or with a qualitative or quantitative ETCO2 detector. Clinical signs include visualization of the tube going through the vocal cords, mist condensation on the ETT, and auscultation of lungs and stomach. EDDs may take the form of a bulb or syringe aspiration device (Figures 16.1A and B). Carbon dioxide detectors may be colorimetric (Figure 16.2), digital capnometers, or continuous graphic display capnographs. End-tidal CO2 verification of correct ETT placement is the standard of care in EMS.[77]

The limitations of each of these techniques must be recognized. Carbon dioxide detection techniques tend to be less accurate in identifying correct placement of the ETT in patients with circulatory arrest, with reported false negative rates (carbon dioxide not detected, tube in the trachea) as high as 30% to 35%.[78] In patients with some circulation, carbon dioxide detection is reliable in confirming correct placement at 99% to 100% of the time.[78–82] Finally, one should also be aware that ETCO2 does not always correlate with PaCO2. As such, one should use caution employing ETCO2 alone during

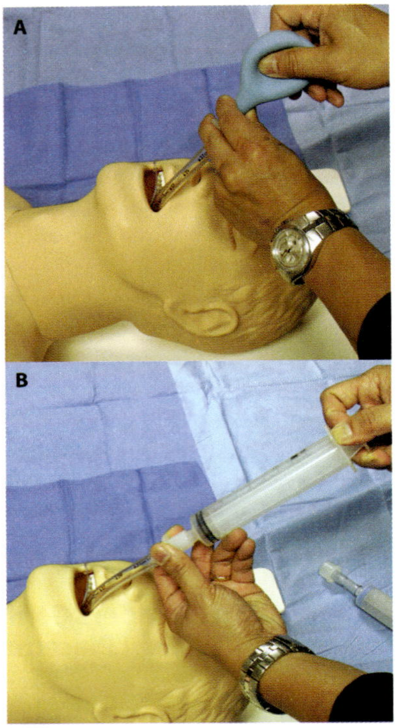

FIGURE 16.1. Esophageal detection devices (EDD): **(A)** The bulb type of EDD and **(B)** The syringe type of EDD.

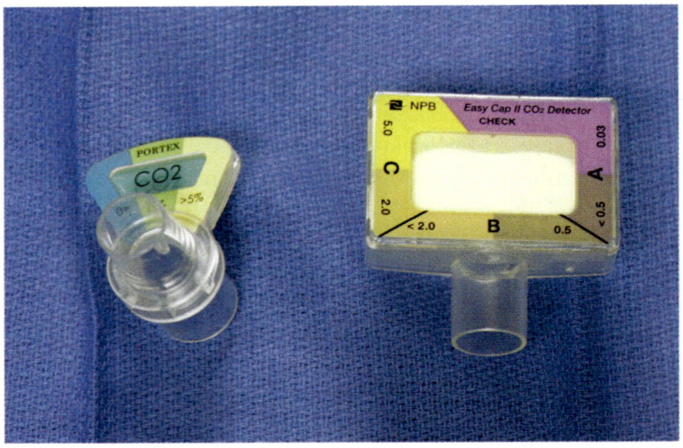

FIGURE 16.2. This figure depicts a typical qualitative end tidal carbon dioxide detection device.

"hyperventilation trials" in severe TBI patients with evidence of increased ICP, as ETCO2 may not accurately reflect PaCO2, pH, and the impact on cerebral blood flow.

Unlike carbon dioxide detection techniques, the EDD is not dependent on the presence of pulmonary blood flow. While some prehospital care systems use this device instead of carbon dioxide detection, the failure to detect esophageal intubation can be as high as 20%, suggesting that it should not be the only verification method used.[83] Physical examination techniques to verify placement of an ETT in the trachea, while neither sensitive nor specific, remain important adjuncts to carbon dioxide detection and EDD, particularly in patients in cardiac arrest.

Finally, the migration of an ETT from the trachea to the esophagus during transport is an ever-present hazard. It has been demonstrated that the continuous monitoring of exhaled carbon dioxide during the prehospital phase of care minimizes the risk of unrecognized displacement.[84]

In summary, while carbon dioxide detection remains the most reliable method of verifying tracheal placement of the ETT in prehospital care, the use of several methods of confirmation is superior to using just one method.

What Is the Postintubation Care of This Patient?

After successful endotracheal intubation, the ETT should be secured properly. It is also important to monitor oxygenation, ventilation, and hemodynamics continuously. Hyperventilation and the associated drop in $PaCO_2$ may adversely impact cerebral blood flow and perfusion in patients with closed-head injuries and hypotension in head-injured patients has a significant negative impact on survival.[64] It is also critical to consider the additive impacts of positive pressure ventilation and sedative/hypnotic medications on hemodynamic stability. Transition from negative-pressure, spontaneous ventilation to positive-pressure, assisted ventilation increases intrathoracic pressure and decreases venous return to the heart. In the context of prehospital patients with hypovolemia, this change in respiratory physiology can have a significant negative effect on blood pressure and end-organ perfusion. Moreover, loss of sympathetic tone after induction of anesthesia with hypnotic agents commonly results in a drop in blood pressure. The change in hemodynamics following intubation should be carefully anticipated and monitored, in order to prevent secondary end-organ injury and maintain organ perfusion. Strategies to mitigate hemodynamic variability include close attention to delivered tidal volume, minimizing external PEEP when appropriate, rapid volume administration (used by BLS and ALS providers) and the use of vaso-active agents, such as phenylephrine (used by clinicians).

SUMMARY

Airway management in the prehospital arena is difficult and fraught with realities that are unique to the environment. Individuals who provide prehospital airway management may vary widely in their training and experience. Although FMV is difficult to perform and may be replaced by EGDs which are easier to perform and equally as effective, FMV will continue to play a crucial role in prehospital airway management.

Induction and neuromuscular blocking agents are widely used in prehospital care. It would appear that health care providers (and systems) who have extensive training in airway management, intubate frequently, and participate in intensive skills maintenance and quality programs have improved intubation success rates and patient outcomes compared to those who do not. As with any airway practitioner employing these procedures, it is crucial that the medications are used correctly in appropriate patients (i.e., not in patients predicted to have a difficult airway) and the airway practitioner is capable of rescuing the airway (Plan B and Plan C) should Plan A fail (the Failed Airway).

Initial and continuous confirmation of ETT placement by capnometry, the use of EDDs, and clinical methods represent the current standard of care in the prehospital arena.

Finally, it is imperative that EMS training, protocols/guidelines, and maintenance of competencies for airway management emphasize the importance of peri-intubation physiology and the impact of any airway intervention on oxygenation, ventilation, and hemodynamic stability. These guiding principles should reflect the delicate balance and relationship between technical imperatives with physiology-guided goal-directed resuscitation endpoints.

SELF-EVALUATION QUESTIONS

16.1. Rapid sequence intubation by nonphysician prehospital care providers:

A. Is regulated by federal statute

B. Is safe in adults but not children

C. Is well established for paramedics

D. Is supported by the available evidence for critical care prehospital providers

E. Will replace EGDs in the foreseeable future

16.2. All of the following statements about "non-paralytic RSI" are correct **EXCEPT**:

A. Some jurisdictions permit paramedics to employ this technique.

B. It has been proven to be safer than "paralytic RSI."

C. It employs an induction agent at full dose but no neuromuscular blocking agent.

D. It provides an inferior view of the glottis.

E. It is felt to be more humane than intubating patients awake.

16.3. All of the following statements regarding qualitative, colorimetric end-tidal carbon dioxide determination in EMS are correct **EXCEPT**:

A. Continuous monitoring is indicated to identify inadvertent extubation during transport.

B. These devices enable one to adhere to the standard of care for confirmation of endotracheal intubation.

C. These devices are almost totally unreliable in patients having suffered a cardiac arrest.

D. They are more effective than esophageal detector devices in confirming endotracheal placement.

E. They are neither better nor worse than capnograpy in confirming correct endotracheal tube placement.

REFERENCES

1. Phelan MP, Moscati R, D'Aprix T, Miller G. Paramedic use of the endotracheal tube introducer in a difficult airway model. *Prehosp Emerg Care.* 2003;7:244-246.
2. Swanson ER, Fosnocht DE, Matthews K, Barton ED. Comparison of the intubating laryngeal mask airway versus laryngoscopy in the Bell 206-L3 EMS helicopter. *Air Med J.* 2004;23:36-39.
3. Rumball CJ, MacDonald D. The PTL, Combitube, laryngeal mask, and oral airway: a randomized prehospital comparative study of ventilatory device effectiveness and cost-effectiveness in 470 cases of cardiorespiratory arrest. *Prehosp Emerg Care.* 1997;1:1-10.
4. Marcolini EG, Burton JH, Bradshaw JR, Baumann MR. A standing-order protocol for cricothyrotomy in prehospital emergency patients. *Prehosp Emerg Care.* 2004;8:23-28.
5. Otten EJ, Montgomery HR, Butler FKJr. Extraglottic airways in tactical combat casualty care: TCCC Guidelines Change 17-01 28 August 2017. *J Spec Oper Med.* 2017;17:19-28.
6. Gausche M, Lewis RJ, Stratton SJ, et al. Effect of out-of-hospital pediatric endotracheal intubation on survival and neurological outcome: a controlled clinical trial. *JAMA.* 2000;283:783-790.
7. Wang HE, Peitzman AB, Cassidy LD, Adelson PD, Yealy DM. Out-of-hospital endotracheal intubation and outcome after traumatic brain injury. *Ann Emerg Med.* 2004;44:439-450.
8. Walls RM. The decision to intubate. In: Walls RM, Murphy MF, eds. *Manual of Emergency Airway Management.* Philadelphia, PA: Lippincott Williams and Wilkins; 2008:1-7.
9. Wang HE, Kupas DF, Paris PM, Bates RR, Yealy DM. Preliminary experience with a prospective, multi-centered evaluation of out-of-hospital endotracheal intubation. *Resuscitation.* 2003;58:49-58.
10. Wang HE, Domeier RM, Kupas DF, Greenwood MJ, O'Connor RE. Recommended guidelines for uniform reporting of data from out-of-hospital airway management: position statement of the National Association of EMS Physicians. *Prehosp Emerg Care.* 2004;8:58-72.
11. Deakin CD. Prehospital management of the traumatized airway. *Eur J Emerg Med.* 1996;3:233-243.
12. Dunford JV, Davis DP, Ochs M, Doney M, Hoyt DB. Incidence of transient hypoxia and pulse rate reactivity during paramedic rapid sequence intubation. *Ann Emerg Med.* 2003;42:721-728.
13. Nolan JD. Prehospital and resuscitative airway care: should the gold standard be reassessed? *Curr Opin Crit Care.* 2001;7:413-421.
14. Blostein PA, Koestner AJ, Hoak S. Failed rapid sequence intubation in trauma patients: esophageal tracheal combitube is a useful adjunct. *J Trauma.* 1998;44:534-547.
15. Calkins MD, Robinson TD. Combat trauma airway management: endotracheal intubation versus laryngeal mask airway versus combitube use by Navy SEAL and Reconnaissance combat corpsmen. *J Trauma.* 1999;46:927-932.
16. Della Puppa A, Pittoni G, Frass M. Tracheal esophageal combitube: a useful airway for morbidly obese patients who cannot intubate or ventilate. *Acta Anaesthesiol Scand.* 2002;46:911-913.
17. Doerges V, Sauer C, Ocker H, Wenzel V, Schmucker P. Airway management during cardiopulmonary resuscitation–a comparative study of bag-valve-mask, laryngeal mask airway and combitube in a bench model. *Resuscitation.* 1999;41:63-69.
18. Genzwuerker HV, Dhonau S, Ellinger K. Use of the laryngeal tube for out-of-hospital resuscitation. *Resuscitation.* 2002;52:221-224.
19. Tanigawa K, Shigematsu A. Choice of airway devices for 12,020 cases of nontraumatic cardiac arrest in Japan. *Prehosp Emerg Care.* 1998;2:96-100.
20. Tanigawa K, Takeda T, Goto E, Tanaka K. Accuracy and reliability of the self-inflating bulb to verify tracheal intubation in out-of-hospital cardiac arrest patients. *Anesthesiology.* 2000;93:1432-1436.
21. Craven RA, Singletary N, Bosken L, Sewell E, Payne M, Lipsey R. Use of bilevel positive airway pressure in out-of-hospital patients. *Acad Emerg Med.* 2000;7:1065-1068.
22. Kallio T, Kuisma M, Alaspaa A, Rosenberg PH. The use of prehospital continuous positive airway pressure treatment in presumed acute severe pulmonary edema. *Prehosp Emerg Care.* 2003;7:209-213.
23. Mosesso VNJr., Dunford J, Blackwell T, Griswell JK. Prehospital therapy for acute congestive heart failure: state of the art. *Prehosp Emerg Care.* 2003;7:13-23.
24. Thompson J, Petrie DA, Ackroyd-Stolarz S, Bardua DJ. Out-of-hospital continuous positive airway pressure ventilation versus usual care in acute respiratory failure: a randomized controlled trial. *Ann Emerg Med.* 2008;52:232-241, 241.e1.
25. Keenan SP, Sinuff T, Burns KE, et al. Clinical practice guidelines for the use of noninvasive positive-pressure ventilation and noninvasive continuous positive airway pressure in the acute care setting. *CMAJ.* 2011;183:E195-E214.
26. El-Khatib MF, Kanazi G, Baraka AS. Noninvasive bilevel positive airway pressure for preoxygenation of the critically ill morbidly obese patient. *Can J Anaesth.* 2007;54:744-747.
27. Hanouz JL, Lammens S, Tasle M, Lesage A, Gerard JL, Plaud B. Preoxygenation by spontaneous breathing or noninvasive positive pressure ventilation with and without positive end-expiratory pressure: a randomised controlled trial. *Eur J Anaesthesiol.* 2015;32:881-887.
28. Braude D, Richards M. Rapid Sequence Airway (RSA)—a novel approach to prehospital airway management. *Prehosp Emerg Care.* 2007;11:250-252.
29. Walls RM. Rapid sequence intubation. In: Walls RM, Murphy MF, eds. *Manual of Emergency Airway Management.* Philadelphia, PA: Lippincott Williams and Wilkins; 2008:23-35.

30. Wang HE, Kupas DF, Paris PM, Yealy DM. Factors associated with the use of pharmacologic agents to facilitate out-of-hospital endotracheal intubation. *Prehosp Emerg Care.* 2004;8:1-9.
31. Frascone RJ, Pippert G, Heegaard W, Molinari P, Dries D. Successful training of HEMS personnel in laryngeal mask airway and intubating laryngeal mask airway placement. *Air Med J.* 2008;27:185-187.
32. Weingart SD, Trueger NS, Wong N, Scofi J, Singh N, Rudolph SS. Delayed sequence intubation: a prospective observational study. *Ann Emerg Med.* 2015;65:349-355.
33. Kovacs G, Law JA. How to do awake intubations – oral and nasal. In: Kovacs G, Law JA, eds. *Airway Management in Emergencies.* New York, NY: McGraw-Hill; 2008:151-167.
34. Pepe PE, Stewart RD, Copass MK. Prehospital management of trauma: a tale of three cities. *Ann Emerg Med.* 1986;15:1484-1490.
35. Adnet F, Lapostolle F, Ricard-Hibon A, Carli P, Goldstein P. Intubating trauma patients before reaching hospital – revisited. *Crit Care.* 2001;5: 290-291.
36. Eckstein M, Chan L, Schneir A, Palmer R. Effect of prehospital advanced life support on outcomes of major trauma patients. *J Trauma.* 2000;48:643-648.
37. Frankel H, Rozycki G, Champion H, Harviel JD, Bass R. The use of TRISS methodology to validate prehospital intubation by urban EMS providers. *Am J Emerg Med.* 1997;15:630-632.
38. Karch SB, Lewis T, Young S, Hales D, Ho CH. Field intubation of trauma patients: complications, indications, and outcomes. *Am J Emerg Med.* 1996;14:617-619.
39. Liberman M, Mulder D, Sampalis J. Advanced or basic life support for trauma: meta-analysis and critical review of the literature. *J Trauma.* 2000;49:584-599.
40. Ruchholtz S, Waydhas C, Ose C, Lewan U, Nast-Kolb D. Prehospital intubation in severe thoracic trauma without respiratory insufficiency: a matched-pair analysis based on the Trauma Registry of the German Trauma Society. *J Trauma.* 2002;52:879-886.
41. Bochicchio GV, Ilahi O, Joshi M, Bochicchio K, Scalea TM. Endotracheal intubation in the field does not improve outcome in trauma patients who present without an acutely lethal traumatic brain injury. *J Trauma.* 2003;54:307-311.
42. Garner A, Crooks J, Lee A, Bishop R. Efficacy of prehospital critical care teams for severe blunt head injury in the Australian setting. *Injury.* 2001;32:455-460.
43. Garner A, Rashford S, Lee A, Bartolacci R. Addition of physicians to paramedic helicopter services decreases blunt trauma mortality. *Aust N Z J Surg.* 1999;69:697-701.
44. Murray JA, Demetriades D, Berne TV, et al. Prehospital intubation in patients with severe head injury. *J Trauma.* 2000;49:1065-1070.
45. Ochs M, Davis DP, Hoyt DB. Lessons learned during the San Diego paramedic RSI Trial. *J Emerg Med.* 2003;24:343-344.
46. Winchell RJ, Hoyt DB. Endotracheal intubation in the field improves survival in patients with severe head injury. Trauma Research and Education Foundation of San Diego. *Arch Surg.* 1997;132:592-597.
47. Zink BJ, Maio RF. Out-of-hospital endotracheal intubation in traumatic brain injury: outcomes research provides us with an unexpected outcome. *Ann Emerg Med.* 2004;44:451-453.
48. Adnet F, Jouriles NJ, Le Toumelin P, et al. Survey of out-of-hospital emergency intubations in the French prehospital medical system: a multicenter study. *Ann Emerg Med.* 1998;32:454-460.
49. Bissell RA, Eslinger DG, Zimmerman L. The efficacy of advanced life support: a review of the literature. *Prehosp Disaster Med.* 1998;13:77-87.
50. Eisen JS, Dubinsky I. Advanced life support vs basic life support field care: an outcome study. *Acad Emerg Med.* 1998;5:592-598.
51. Mitchell RG, Guly UM, Rainer TH, Robertson CE. Can the full range of paramedic skills improve survival from out of hospital cardiac arrests? *J Accid Emerg Med.* 1997;14:274-277.
52. Rainer TH, Marshall R, Cusack S. Paramedics, technicians, and survival from out of hospital cardiac arrest. *J Accid Emerg Med.* 1997;14:278-282.
53. Hallstrom A, Cobb L, Johnson E, Copass M. Cardiopulmonary resuscitation by chest compression alone or with mouth-to-mouth ventilation. *N Engl J Med.* 2000;342:1546-1553.
54. Stiell IG, Wells GA, Field B, et al. Advanced cardiac life support in out-of-hospital cardiac arrest. *N Engl J Med.* 2004;351:647-656.
55. Hasegawa K, Hiraide A, Chang Y, Brown DF. Association of prehospital advanced airway management with neurologic outcome and survival in patients with out-of-hospital cardiac arrest. *JAMA.* 2013;309:257-266.
56. Aijian P, Tsai A, Knopp R, Kallsen GW. Endotracheal intubation of pediatric patients by paramedics. *Ann Emerg Med.* 1989;18:489-494.
57. Boswell WC, McElveen N, Sharp M, Boyd CR, Frantz EI. Analysis of prehospital pediatric and adult intubation. *Air Med J.* 1995;14:125-127.
58. Brownstein D, Shugerman R, Cummings P, Rivara F, Copass M. Prehospital endotracheal intubation of children by paramedics. *Ann Emerg Med.* 1996;28:34-39.
59. Su E, Mann NC, McCall M, Hedges JR. Use of resuscitation skills by paramedics caring for critically injured children in Oregon. *Prehosp Emerg Care.* 1997;1:123-127.
60. Vilke GM, Steen PJ, Smith AM, Chan TC. Out-of-hospital pediatric intubation by paramedics: the San Diego experience. *J Emerg Med.* 2002;22:71-74.
61. Cooper A, DiScala C, Foltin G, Tunik M, Markenson D, Welborn C. Prehospital endotracheal intubation for severe head injury in children: a reappraisal. *Semin Pediatr Surg.* 2001;10:3-106.
62. Suominen P, Baillie C, Kivioja A, Ohman J, Olkkola KT. Intubation and survival in severe paediatric blunt head injury. *Eur J Emerg Med.* 2000;7:3-7.
63. Davis DP, Hoyt DB, Ochs M, et al. The effect of paramedic rapid sequence intubation on outcome in patients with severe traumatic brain injury. *J Trauma.* 2003;54:444-453.
64. Chesnut RM, Marshall LF, Klauber MR, et al. The role of secondary brain injury in determining outcome from severe head injury. *J Trauma.* 1993;34:216-222.
65. Ochs M, Davis D, Hoyt D, Bailey D, Marshall L, Rosen P. Paramedic-performed rapid sequence intubation of patients with severe head injuries. *Ann Emerg Med.* 2002;40:159-167.
66. Ma OJ, Atchley RB, Hatley T, Green M, Young J, Brady W. Intubation success rates improve for an air medical program after implementing the use of neuromuscular blocking agents. *Am J Emerg Med.* 1998;16:125-127.
67. Murphy-Macabobby M, Marshall WJ, Schneider C, Dries D. Neuromuscular blockade in aeromedical airway management. *Ann Emerg Med.* 1992;21:664-668.
68. Sing RF, Rotondo MF, Zonies DH, et al. Rapid sequence induction for intubation by an aeromedical transport team: a critical analysis. *Am J Emerg Med.* 1998;16:598-602.
69. Slater EA, Weiss SJ, Ernst AA, Haynes M. Preflight versus en route success and complications of rapid sequence intubation in an air medical service. *J Trauma.* 1998;45:588-592.
70. Levin NM, Fix ML, April MD, Arana AA, Brown CA3rd, Investigators N. The association of rocuronium dosing and first-attempt intubation success in adult emergency department patients. *CJEM.* 2021;23:518-527.
71. Werman HA, Schwegman D, Gerard JP. The effect of etomidate on airway management practices of an air medical transport service. *Prehosp Emerg Care.* 2004;8:185-190.
72. Lieutaud T, Billard V, Khalaf H, Debaene B. Muscle relaxation and increasing doses of propofol improve intubating conditions. *Can J Anaesth.* 2003;50:121-126.
73. McKeating K, Bali IM, Dundee JW. The effects of thiopentone and propofol on upper airway integrity. *Anaesthesia.* 1988;43:638-640.
74. McNeil IA, Culbert B, Russell I. Comparison of intubating conditions following propofol and succinylcholine with propofol and remifentanil 2 micrograms kg^{-1} or 4 micrograms kg^{-1}. *Br J Anaesth.* 2000;85:623-625.
75. Bozeman WP, Hexter D, Liang HK, Kelen GD. Esophageal detector device versus detection of end-tidal carbon dioxide level in emergency intubation. *Ann Emerg Med.* 1996;27:595-599.
76. Katz SH, Falk JL. Misplaced endotracheal tubes by paramedics in an urban emergency medical services system. *Ann Emerg Med.* 2001;37:32-37.
77. O'Connor RE, Swor RA. Verification of endotracheal tube placement following intubation. National Association of EMS Physicians Standards and Clinical Practice Committee. *Prehosp Emerg Care.* 1999;3:248-250.
78. MacLeod BA, Heller MB, Gerard J, Yealy DM, Menegazzi JJ. Verification of endotracheal tube placement with colorimetric end-tidal CO2 detection. *Ann Emerg Med.* 1991;20:267-270.
79. Grmec S. Comparison of three different methods to confirm tracheal tube placement in emergency intubation. *Intensive Care Med.* 2002;28:701-704.
80. Li J. Capnography alone is imperfect for endotracheal tube placement confirmation during emergency intubation. *J Emerg Med.* 2001;20:223-229.
81. Ornato JP, Shipley JB, Racht EM, et al. Multicenter study of a portable, hand-size, colorimetric end-tidal carbon dioxide detection device. *Ann Emerg Med.* 1992;21:518-523.
82. Takeda T, Tanigawa K, Tanaka H, Hayashi Y, Goto E, Tanaka K. The assessment of three methods to verify tracheal tube placement in the emergency setting. *Resuscitation.* 2003;56:153-157.
83. Hendey GW, Shubert GS, Shalit M, Hogue B. The esophageal detector bulb in the aeromedical setting. *J Emerg Med.* 2002;23:51-55.
84. Silvestri S, Ralls GA, Krauss B, et al. The effectiveness of out-of-hospital use of continuous end-tidal carbon dioxide monitoring on the rate of unrecognized misplaced intubation within a regional emergency medical services system. *Ann Emerg Med.* 2005;45:497-503.

CHAPTER 17

Airway Management of a Patient with Traumatic Brain Injury (TBI)

Edward T. Crosby

CASE PRESENTATION

An Advanced Life-Support Emergency Services unit brought a 35-year-old male into the emergency department on a backboard with a cervical collar in place. The patient was the driver of an all-terrain vehicle that rolled off the road and ejected him into a ditch. When a paramedic team arrived at the scene, the patient had a blood pressure of 90/50 mmHg, a heart rate of 120 bpm, a respiratory rate of 24 breaths per minute, and an oxygen saturation of 95% without supplemental oxygen. His Glasgow Coma Scale score was 7 (opened eyes to pain-2, moaned-2, abnormal flexion-3). The patient was given oxygen via nasal prongs and a non-rebreathing face mask, intravenous access was obtained, and an infusion of crystalloid was begun.

PREHOSPITAL CARE

The immediate management of the patient with traumatic brain injury (TBI) in a field setting should focus on stabilizing his condition while maintaining oxygenation and blood pressure. All patients with TBI have the potential for a cervical injury and should be immobilized at the scene and on transport to hospital.

■ Should Field Tracheal Intubation Be Performed in This Patient?

In this patient, ensuring oxygenation via a patent airway is of paramount importance, as hypoxia has a profound influence on neurological outcome. Indications for a field tracheal intubation include inadequate ventilation or oxygenation despite supplemental oxygen administration or the inability of the patient to protect the airway. A relative indication for intubation is the risk of losing the airway during transport and transport time must be considered. Studies of the outcome of prehospital airway management have yielded conflicting results, leaving little consistent evidence supporting field tracheal intubation in most patients with head injury who are oxygenated and ventilating at the time of transport.[1–6] The success rate of field intubation is correlated with the experience of the providers, and patient mortality may be increased when providers of limited experience perform prehospital intubation.[6–8] In the case presented, the patient was maintaining oxygenation and ventilation. His clinical course could not be certain, and it was reasonable for the field team to consider tracheal intubation. However, the patient had clenched teeth and was predicted to also pose difficult direct laryngoscopy (DL) intubation based on his short neck and cervical spine (C-spine) immobilization. A short transport time was anticipated, so field rapid sequence intubation (RSI) was not indicated.

■ What Additional Considerations Are Imposed by Field Conditions?

Several other priorities in clinical care must be addressed by the field team after initial patient stabilization.

Circulation

Hypotension is a critical factor associated with an increased morbidity and mortality in patients with TBI.[9–11] Blood pressure in the field should be monitored closely to avoid or correct hypotension. This patient presented with tachycardia and a field BP of 90/60 mmHg. With the poor outcome associated with hypotension in TBI patients, fluid resuscitation and perhaps the use of a vasopressor becomes a priority. However, the field team must weigh the benefit of securing IV access in the field with the risk of delayed transport to a trauma center. Ideally, IV access and fluid administration should occur during expeditious transport to the trauma center. It should be emphasized that isolated TBI rarely accounts for hypotension in trauma patients, and it is more likely to occur with multisystem injury[12]; if present, as with this patient, hemorrhage elsewhere must be suspected.

Neurologic Disability: Intracranial Pressure (ICP) and C-Spine (Best Motor Response)

ICP: The patient did not have unequivocal evidence of increased ICP, as his pupils were equal and reactive and the motor response was decorticating; there was no indication for paramedics to provide any field intervention for managing elevated ICP.[10] A potential pitfall in the management of the TBI patient is to assume that head trauma is entirely responsible for altered mental status. Consideration must also be given to other reversible causes of altered mental status, for example, hypoglycemia or intoxication, in addition to hypoxemia and hypotension.

C-spine immobilization: All patients with blunt trauma to the upper torso or neurological findings should be suspected of having spinal cord injury until proven otherwise. Although neurologic impairment is usually fully manifest at the time of injury in most patients with cervical spine injury (CSI), the implications of an unidentified spine injury are such that the routine use of immobilization devices is indicated.[13,14] Secondary neurological injuries are reported to occur in 4% to 30% of patients with delayed diagnosis of CSI who are not immobilized at the time of entry into care,[15,16] and in 2% to 10% of those who are immobilized.[17] Inadequate or misread imaging studies and clinically important distracting injuries have also been linked to missed CSI with secondary injury.[18,19] The probability of associated CSI is at least tripled with a Glasgow Coma Scale (GCS) score of 8 or less.[20–22] Despite concerns about the paucity of evidence supporting its benefit, cervical immobilization continues to be recommended and widely deployed in patients who either demonstrate neurological findings or cannot be adequately assessed at the time of field presentation following trauma.[23,24] The American Association of Neurological Surgeons and the National Association of EMS Physicians and the American College of Surgeons Committee on Trauma continue to recommend the prehospital use of a rigid cervical collar and supportive blocks on a backboard with straps.[25] Spinal immobilization is not without consequence, in that patients are at risk of aspirating if they seize, vomit, or lose protective airway mechanisms. In addition, collars may increase ICP and worsen ICP dynamics in patients with TBI,[26–29] probably by interference with cerebral venous drainage.[30] Finally, spinal immobilization has the potential to complicate airway management by worsening the laryngeal view obtained at DL.[31] With a history of TBI and GCS of 7, the presented patient was at significant risk of CSI, and spinal immobilization should be instituted before transport to hospital and maintained until the spine is cleared.

Analgesia/Sedation

Patients with moderate to severe TBI can experience episodes of agitation and combativeness, both of which tend to increase ICP and can pose safety risks to both the patient and the paramedic crew. Sedatives, such as benzodiazepines and opioid analgesics, are typically employed but, if given, the GCS score should first be determined, and the status of oxygenation and ventilation closely monitored after administration.

Transport Decisions

An early priority in the management of patients with moderate or severe brain injuries is transportation to the closest facility providing immediate access to neuroimaging and neurosurgical services. There is an improvement in outcomes for patients with acute subdural hematoma (SDH) who are managed expertly in the field, and expediently once they arrive in hospital.[32–34] Although many patients with TBI succumb within several hours of their injury, neurological damage may evolve and early and effective treatment may reduce the sequelae of TBI.[35] Reducing the length of time from the onset of clinical deterioration to operative treatment of an SDH is also significantly related to an improved outcome.[36]

EMERGENCY DEPARTMENT MANAGEMENT

The ambulance arrived at the emergency department (ED) after a 15-minute transport. While the patient was being transferred onto the gurney in the trauma bay, it was noted that he was obese (5′ 8″ [172 cm], 275 lb [125 kg], BMI 42.3 kg·m^{-2}). He had a hard cervical collar in place and was strapped to a short transport board. His BP was now 130/80 mmHg, HR 124 bpm, RR 24 breaths per minute with snoring respirations, and his SpO_2 was 90% on a non-rebreathing face mask. His GCS score had decreased to 6 (opened eyes to pain-2, moans-2, and intermittent decerebrate posturing-2) and it was noted that his right pupil was now 8 mm and unreactive; his left pupil was 4 mm and reacting sluggishly. A quick airway evaluation revealed that his teeth were still clenched; he had a 6-cm thyromental span and 4-cm hyothyroid distance. There was no evidence of blunt trauma to the neck, and the cricothyroid membrane was identifiable and palpable in the midline. Two large-bore IVs were secured, blood was drawn and sent for chemistries and type and cross match. The hematocrit on the venous blood gas was 45. Portable chest and pelvis radiographs in the trauma bay were normal. A cross-table lateral X-ray of the C-spine showed good alignment from C1–C7 and no prevertebral soft tissue swelling. A focused ultrasound examination of the abdomen was performed, which showed no free fluid in the abdomen; an attempt was made to perform a gastric scan, but reliable images could not be obtained. A stat neurosurgery consult was ordered.

Personnel from the CT imaging unit called, saying that they were ready to image the patient once he was stabilized. While the trauma team was deciding the best approach to protecting and securing the airway and managing the suspected increased ICP, the patient had a tonic–clonic seizure and was desaturated to a SpO_2 of 80%.

What Elements of Airway Management Must Be Considered in This Patient?

Patient outcomes after TBI are worse when hypoxemia occurs following injury; the immediate priority in this patient is restoring oxygenation.[10] The patient should receive supplemental oxygen and, if necessary, assisted face-mask ventilation (FMV) with 100% O_2 to restore SpO_2 to >90%. Once oxygen saturation has improved, attention can be turned to formulating a plan for tracheal intubation. Unless the seizure spontaneously terminates within 1 to 2 minutes, pharmacologic intervention with lorazepam would be indicated.

From the perspective of airway management, trauma patients secured on a backboard with cervical immobilization can appear intimidating. Notwithstanding, formal airway assessment may point to little anticipated difficulty (see sections "Difficult BMV: MOANS"; "Difficult DL Intubation: LEMON"; "Difficult VL Intubation: CRANE"; "Difficult Use of an EGA: RODS"; and "Difficult Cricothyrotomy: SHORT"; in Chapter 1). In this case, the patient's obesity predicts an increased likelihood of difficult FMV.[37,38] DL may also be difficult due to the patient's short neck and the C-spine immobilization. Manual in-line stabilization (MILS) applied during airway management increases the likelihood of obtaining a poor view during DL.[39] MILS also increases the magnitude of the forces which must be applied during DL to obtain a satisfactory view, which may increase the resultant neck movement.[40] Any trismus will likely resolve with muscle relaxant administration if used. Extraglottic airway (EGA) insertion may also be made more difficult but should succeed once pharmacologic paralysis is achieved. Finally, although obesity can make front-of-neck access more difficult, the cricothyroid membrane was felt to be easily palpable.

What Are the Goals During Intubation in the TBI Patient with C-Spine Precautions?

Our goals are to achieve first-pass success (FPS) with tracheal intubation while avoiding secondary neurologic injury by: (1) maintaining oxygenation; (2) avoiding decreases in cerebral perfusion pressure (CPP); and (3) minimizing movement of the head and neck. Attention must also be directed toward the prevention of gastric aspiration during the process.

How Should Tracheal Intubation Proceed?

Assessment of the patient reveals an uncooperative patient with features predicting an increased risk of both difficult mask ventilation and laryngoscopy (e.g., obesity, short neck, anticipated use of MILS). The importance of FPS is increasingly recognized and emphasized to minimize morbidity in emergency airway care; how best to achieve that outcome in each clinical scenario should be considered. A number of authors have reported an association between multiple intubation attempts, and complications in emergency airway management.[41–43] Rognås reported similar findings after analyzing prehospital endotracheal intubation in 636 patients.[44] Twenty-two percent of intubations required more than one attempt, and multiple attempts were associated with an increased overall incidence of complications. Brown et al. compared FPS using DL augmented by any of laryngeal manipulation, ramped patient positioning, or the use of a bougie (A-DL), with unaided video laryngoscopy (VL) in adult ED intubations in 11,714 patients (2016-2017).[45] FPS was significantly higher with all VL versus all A-DL, despite the VL group having more patients with predicted difficult airway. In addition, fewer esophageal intubations occurred with VL. Finally, Cabrini et al. performed a systematic review and meta-analysis of randomized controlled trials assessing outcomes of tracheal intubation in patients at risk for CSI undergoing surgery.[46] Eighteen trials enrolling 1972 patients were reviewed and a higher FPS was found with both VL and when pooling all flexible bronchoscopic techniques together. Postoperative neurological complications were 0.34% and there were no differences in complications among techniques deployed. To optimize the likelihood of FPS in this uncooperative patient, consideration should be given to deploying a VL during the performance of RSI. This plan confers the advantages of a high likelihood of FPS with VL under optimal intubating conditions with skeletal muscle relaxation. The use of opioid and sedative–hypnotic induction medications will help mitigate any laryngoscopy and intubation-induced increases in ICP.

How Can We Modify the Changing Cerebral Dynamics in TBI?

Elevated ICP is associated with worse outcomes in TBI, and high ICP refractory to treatment with worse outcomes still.[47] While its early measurement and management have not been conclusively linked to improved outcomes,[48] it is prudent to avoid any further increases in ICP in the brain-injured patient. ICP is determined by the contents of intracranial vault; the three normal contents are brain tissue, cerebrospinal fluid (CSF), and blood. Intracranial blood volume is influenced by CBF and is kept relatively constant by cerebral autoregulation; as blood pressure varies, cerebral vasoconstriction or vasodilatation occurs to maintain constant blood flow, volume, and pressure. The brain's ability to autoregulate blood flow is impaired or lost in TBI. Laryngoscopy and intubation may cause an increase in ICP through an increase in blood pressure (with disrupted autoregulation), increased venous pressures in a straining unparalyzed patient, or through a direct effect on ICP.

A second mediator of CBF is blood carbon dioxide (CO_2) tension. As blood CO_2 tension rises, so will CBF, leading to both increased intracranial blood volume and ICP. While aggressive hyperventilation in the patient with TBI is no longer recommended in the absence of signs of brain herniation, attention should be paid throughout the airway management process to maintaining normocarbia.[10,49] Cerebral perfusion pressure (CPP) is the driving force for blood flow to the brain and is measured by the difference between the mean arterial blood pressure (MAP) and the ICP, such that CPP = MAP – ICP. In the patient with disrupted autoregulation, decreases in MAP will decrease CPP while increases in MAP, if not accompanied by equivalent increases in ICP, may increase blood flow to, and oxygenation of, brain tissue. Current guidance recommends that the ICP be maintained below 20 mmHg, MAP between 100 and 110 mmHg, and CPP at or above 60 to 70 mmHg, in order to optimize brain perfusion.[10,49] Hypotension leading to a decrease in CPP, even for a very brief period, is especially harmful, and (as already mentioned) has been shown to be an independent predictor of increased mortality and morbidity in patients with a TBI.[9,50,51]

C-SPINE CONSIDERATIONS

Victims of major trauma often require several interventions, including definitive airway control, before a full assessment of the C-spine is possible. Without clinical clearance or radiographic evidence of an intact C-spine, an unstable injury should be assumed, and airway management is undertaken accordingly.

What Are the Causes of Neurologic Deterioration After Acute Cervical Cord Injury?

There are two principal categories of causes for neurological deterioration after acute CSI which may affect 5% to 6% of injured patients; they are either iatrogenic in nature or reflect natural progression of the injury process.[17] Most patients who experience deterioration present initially with obvious neurological findings, often complete cord (American Spinal Cord Injury Association Grade A [ASIA A]), and then get worse. Early progression is often associated with interventions such as traction and immobilization, and later deterioration is usually caused by progression of the injury secondary to inflammation and ischemia. Belanger et al. described subacute posttraumatic ascending myelopathy (SPAM) in patients with established cord injury occurring several days to a week postinjury, resulting in further neurological deterioration.[52] The condition occurs during a period when patients are otherwise stable and seems unrelated to interventions, mechanical compression, or instability; the precise cause or causes of the disorder remain unknown. It is important to remember when assessing for causes of the progression of neurological injury while providing care to these patients, that such syndromes are considered in the evaluation of worsening injury; there is a natural temptation to attribute the deterioration to temporally related clinical interventions when, in fact, these interventions may have had no impact on the progression of injury.[31]

What Is the Role of Emergency Airway Management in Causing Neurological Injury?

Several authors have described cases wherein catastrophic injuries in patients with injured, unstable, or otherwise vulnerable spines, were associated with (and attributed to) emergency airway management.[53–57] In all these instances, patient assessments for injury were deficient or absent, airway management was difficult and prolonged, and no efforts were made to limit the forces applied during laryngoscopy nor to constrain spinal movements. Farmer et al. linked intubation to neurological deterioration in a population of 1031 spine-injured patients admitted to a single spine center; 19 (1.84%) experienced worsening of their neurological condition while in care.[58] In four cases, deterioration was associated with intubation, one of which was emergency. Emanating out of these experiences, a more thoughtful approach evolved to identify patients at risk for spinal injury, instability, or vulnerability, to constrain spinal movements until injuries are ruled out, and to limit the number of efforts made and forces generated if airway interventions were required. More recently, considerable effort has been expended to assess whether approaches to the airway with alternatives to DL might result in improved patient outcomes following airway management in patients with vulnerable spines. Many of these elements will be addressed subsequently in this chapter.

Despite the anxiety among care providers regarding the potential for causing secondary neurological injury in an injured patient during a therapeutic intervention, the evidence suggests that the likelihood of that outcome is extremely low. Secondary injury or progression of neurological findings does not seem to be a common occurrence in patients who are presenting for care after trauma. Oto et al. reviewed published reports of secondary neurologic deterioration in the early stages of care after blunt CSI to describe its nature, context, and associated risk factors.[14] They identified 41 qualifying cases; in 30 cases, the new deficits were apparently spontaneous, and the original authors did not relate them to interventions. In the remainder, there was an attribution to a temporally associated precipitant, seven of which were possibly iatrogenic and included attempts at immobilization and performance of flexion/extension films. Oto et al. concluded that early neurological deterioration (secondary injury) is uncommon and often reflected a gradual worsening of condition without obvious precipitant. It was often consistent with inflammatory tissue response to injury, or with related sequelae such as thrombosis, hypotension, and hypoxia. Most reported events were not directly associated with mechanical movement and those that were associated with attempts to immobilize to constrain movements in injured and abnormal spines and not airway management.

Oto et al. noted that neurologic deterioration after the initiation of medical care may automatically and incorrectly be presumed to be a consequence of that care.[14] While they acknowledged that there might be a subset of secondary injury that is caused or exacerbated by movement and amenable to prevention via immobilization, in many incidents it was just as likely that the events were coincidental rather than causal; of note, five reported deteriorations occurred with full spinal precautions already in place. The authors concluded that clinicians and researchers should not assume that any deterioration occurring during medical interventions was avoidable, and to do so brings with it profound potential for misplaced liability. They echo Crosby who stated that neurologic deterioration in CSI patients is uncommon after airway management, even in high-risk patients undergoing urgent tracheal intubation, and that the deterioration may often reflect the progression of the injury state rather than an iatrogenic complication.[31]

What Are the Criteria Used for Cervical Spine Clearance?

The aim of cervical clearance is to quickly and accurately identify the patients who are unlikely to have sustained a spinal injury and to remove immobilizing devices once that has been done. That process is carried out by a combination of clinical clearance in alert patients (GCS ≥ 14), and radiographic clearance in patients who have lower GCS scores, or who fail clinical clearance strategies. Two clinical strategies have been promoted that focus on defining the population of injured patients that are deemed low-risk and who do not require further evaluations for spine injury. The National Emergency X-Radiography Utilization Study (NEXUS) defined a set of clinical criteria that patients need to meet to have them declared low risk for injury.[59] The Canadian C-Spine Rule (CCR) expands the list of criteria used in the evaluation to include the mechanism of injury and some physical additional physical examination information and has been found to be more sensitive and specific in defining the population at risk.[60] The use of such, or similar, strategies are core to the assessment of patients presenting with trauma. Unfortunately, in patients presenting with TBI with GCS < 14, assessment strategies relying on patient feedback no longer are clinically applicable.

What Range of C-Spine Movement Is Considered Within Physiologic Limits?

To allow for interpretation of the data on the impacts of airway manipulations on the movement of the C-spine, and the level of threat that may be imposed on the cord, the amount of motion that would indicate spinal instability and pathological movement should be defined. Panjabi et al. suggested that horizontal motion or displacement of one vertebral body on another exceeding 20% of vertebral body width (~3.5 mm in an adult), more than 11 degrees of relative angulation of adjacent cervical vertebrae, or greater than 1.4 mm of distraction between vertebrae is abnormal and would indicate instability.[61–63] These estimates provide the benchmark against which the results of many models of spinal injury are compared. Preexisting cervical abnormalities which result in canal stenosis increase the risk of neurologic consequences even inside these defined upper limits of normal movement.[64] In fact, there is evidence that these latter anomalies may be as important or more important in predisposing patients to peri-procedural spinal cord injury than is spinal instability.[65]

Does the Administration of Induction Agents and/or Muscle Relaxants Impact the C-Spine?

Historically, a view was advanced that CSI would be maintained stable by muscle spasms in the conscious patient, and that administration of an induction agent and muscle relaxant to the patient could release any "splinting" of an unstable segment by adjacent muscle spasm.[66] There is no published evidence that indicates that there is a clinically important increase in cervical spinal movement due solely to induction agent and muscle relaxant administration.

How Do Airway Opening Maneuvers and Mask Ventilation Impact the Movement of a Normal C-Spine?

Several radiographic studies have looked at the effects of airway opening maneuvers and FMV on C-spine movement. One cadaver study performed with no applied MILS found that chin lift and jaw thrust caused as much extension at C1–C2 as oral DL intubation.[67] A second cadaver study, using backboard, cervical collar, and tape found that more C-spine displacement occurred with FMV than with either oral or nasal tracheal intubation.[68] However, a subsequent study using elective surgical subjects with their heads taped in a neutral position found FMV to cause less movement than DL at multiple cervical motion segments.[69] Although conflicting in their results, these studies can at least be taken to indicate that cervical spinal movement may occur with basic airway interventions and appropriate C-spine precautions should be applied during all phases of airway management in patients at risk of CSI.

What Are the Impacts of Airway Maneuvers and Mask Ventilation in Cadaver Models of CSI?

Donaldson et al. studied the motion occurring during various airway maneuvers in a series of six cadavers with a surgically created unstable C1–C2 segment.[67] With the head stabilized, preintubation maneuvers (chin lift and jaw thrust) caused more narrowing of the space available for the spinal cord than DL or blind nasal intubation. In a subsequent cadaver series, this time with an unstable C5–C6 motion segment, the same investigators demonstrated similar movements caused by chin lift/jaw thrust and laryngoscopy.[70] Aprahamian et al. also studied a cadaveric specimen with a posteriorly destabilized C5–C6 segment and similarly reported that chin lift/jaw thrust caused as much or more movement at the site of injury as oral or nasal intubation.[71] Brimacombe et al. measured C-spine motion for six airway management techniques in cadavers with a posteriorly destabilized C3 vertebra.[72] Once again, chin lift/jaw thrust and oral intubation with DL caused significant antero-posterior (A-P) displacement of the unstable segment. Finally, Prasarn et al. measuring movement in nine human cadavers with a surgically created unstable C1–C2 injury, found that head tilt/chin lift caused significantly more angular motion in all planes, and more axial displacement and A-P translation, than the jaw thrust maneuver.[73] Although the measured movements in all reports typically were not excessive and were within previously described physiologic limits, the studies indicate that spinal movements do occur in injured spines with basic airway interventions. Caution should be exercised against applying excess forces to support the airway in at-risk patients.

How Does Laryngoscopy and Intubation Impact the Movement of the Normal C-Spine?

Radiographic studies on live and cadaveric subjects with intact C-spines demonstrate that DL causes considerable extension between the occiput and C2. Most movement occurs between the occiput and C1, with about half as much occurring between C1 and C2.[69,74–84] Lesser amounts of extension are seen in the subaxial spine (C2–C5).[69,75–77,83,84] From C5 to the cervicothoracic junction, a small amount of flexion occurs during laryngoscopy.[69,76,77] Actual tube passage causes slight additional superior rotation between the occiput and Cl, but little other movements.[74,85] There is evidence that exposing only a "minimum acceptable view" during laryngoscopy will reduce occiput to C2 extension.[74,85–87]

Does the Laryngoscope Blade Used Impact C-Spine Movement?

Several investigators have studied C-spine movement caused by different DL blades. Two studies in elective surgical patients found less head extension with Miller, as compared with Macintosh blade laryngoscopy.[88,89] However, other studies have failed to demonstrate a difference in motion between these two blade types.[90–92] Studies with the levering tip McCoy/CLM-type blades have also generated conflicting results: some reports indicate less movement with the use of the activated blade when compared to a Macintosh;[86,93] while others have not.[94,95] In cadaver injury models, one study showed that Miller DL resulted in significantly less axial distraction (1-2 mm) at the level of a surgically created C5–C6 transection than a DL with a Macintosh blade, whereas another with a similar model showed no difference.[71,94] At present, there is no evidence that a particular blade is preferred for DL when attempting to minimize movement of the C-spine,[96] nor that there are large differences in the cervical movements that would result with different blade types.

Is Any Laryngoscope Blade Superior for Exposing the Glottis with MILS Applied?

To date, there is no convincing evidence that any blade type is superior for exposing the laryngeal inlet during DL with applied MILS. However, several studies suggest that laryngoscopy using the levering tip McCoy/CLM blade with the tip activated may be helpful when a poor view is obtained in the setting of MILS. Three studies of the McCoy blade report improvement of a C-L Grade 3 view to 2 or better in 83% (MILNS alone),[97] to 86% (MILS with cricoid pressure),[98] and 92% (rigid cervical collar)[99] of cases, respectively compared with Macintosh blade DL. Santoni et al. reported that experienced anesthesiologists do apply greater force with the DL to obtain the best glottic view with MILS applied, than when MILS is not applied.[40] In that study, anterior laryngeal pressure to enhance the glottic view was not permitted, and so greater forces might have been transmitted through the DL than might have been necessary had anterior pressure been applied.

How Do Alternatives to DL Impact C-Spine Movement During Tracheal Intubation?

Many of the alternatives to DL, such as indirect optical or video laryngoscopes, appear to cause less movement of the C-spine during glottic visualization and tracheal intubation. Intubation with the Pentax Airway Scope (AWS) results in significantly less upper C-spine movement than DL, with both attempted full[100,101] and minimal acceptable[101] exposure of the cords. C-spine movement during AWS use is further reduced with passage of a tracheal tube introducer via the blade's delivery channel prior to endotracheal tube (ETT) advancement.[102] Compared with the Macintosh blade, Airtraq-facilitated intubation appears to cause less movement at some but not all of the studied C-spine motion segments.[77,103] However, a more recent cadaver study, using a surgically created unstable odontoid fracture, failed to demonstrate a significant difference in space available for the spinal cord at the C1–C2 segment between Airtraq, Macintosh, and McCoy DL exposure and intubation.[104] In this latter study, the DL blades were used to only expose a minimum (arytenoids) view, MILNS was applied, and a trans tracheal introducer (TTI) was passed prior to the ETT. The use of a GlideScope video laryngoscope (GVL) during MILS resulted in some reduction in midcervical (C2–C5) spine movement compared with DL in one study;[69] another failed to show a difference in spine movement at any level compared to that occurring during DL.[84] Studies with the Bonfils and Shikani optical stylets have also concluded that less C-spine movement occurred with the optical stylets compared to DL with a Macintosh blade.[69,105,106] Results with the intubating Laryngeal Mask Airway (ILMA or LMA-Fastrach) vary, with some studies showing small amounts of flexion of the upper C-spine during ILMA insertion and subsequent intubation with MILS,[107] while others have demonstrated extension, although not significantly different from that encountered during DL.[108] Use of the C-MAC D-blade resulted in less movement at the occiput-C1 motion segment in an immobilized spine compared to that measured with a DL with a Macintosh blade, but not in the lower motion segments.[109] Use of the Optiscope also resulted in less movement at the occiput to C1, C1–C2, and C2–C5 motion segments than with McGrath VL, during visualization and intubation in patients with MILS applied.[110] Tracheal intubation using a flexible bronchoscope (FB) results in less movement of the head and neck compared to DL,[108] GVL,[111] and LMA-Fastrach-facilitated[112] intubation in anesthetized patients. There is also less combined craniocervical movement from the occiput to C5 when the FB is combined with an intubating LMA, and compared to that seen with the C-MAC D-blade VL.[113] There is also less upper cervical movement when the FB is used compared to the McGrath VL for awake orotracheal intubation.[114]

The evidence supports the conclusion that many alternative devices result in less spinal movement at some C-spine motion segments compared with DL, and typically result in less extension of the head on the neck; the FB likely has the least impact of all. However, the movements created in all cases tend to be small, and the differences are smaller still. There is no evidence that a better neurological outcome results from the use of the alternative devices in patients at risk with CSI. Indeed, as discussed in the next section, the benefit of such alternatives is probably to optimize laryngeal visualization and FPS with MILS application during tracheal intubation.

Does MILS Prevent C-Spine Motion in Normal Patients and Injury Models?

MILS appears to restrain overall spinal movements occurring during DL in patients and cadaveric specimens with normal spines to within physiological levels and has less impact on airway interventions than do other forms of immobilization.[75,87,91] In injury models, Lennarson et al. reported that MILS did not eliminate movement at the injury level during intubation of a cadaver model with ligamentous C4–C5 disruption; however, the movements recorded during interventions were constrained to within physiological limits.[83,116] Gerling evaluated MILS as well as cervical collar immobilization on spinal movement during DL in a cadaver model with a C5–C6 transection injury.[117] There was less A-P displacement with application of MILS compared with the collar but the magnitudes of movements were small and within the physiological range. Turner studied 10 cadavers surgically destabilized at C4–C5 and reported that MILS did not significantly change the median motion seen during DL in any of angulation, distraction, or A-P displacement at the unstable level.[118]

Two comprehensive reviews on the topic support the notion that, while there may be some reduction in overall C-spine motion with MILS, movement at individual motion segments does still occur.[31,120] It may be that MILS represents one step in a process that emphasizes gentle and precise airway maneuvers to minimize C-spine movement when managing patients at risk for spinal injury.[31,71,119] Traction forces applied during MILS may endanger the spinal cord if there is a serious ligamentous injury; distraction may result at the site of a complete ligamentous injury when traction forces are applied.[116,120,121] Current recommendations which promote the use of MILS do not support the use of traction during airway interventions requiring C-spine precautions.

How Does Applied MILS Impact Airway Interventions?

Many trauma patients presenting to the ED arrive on a backboard immobilized with rigid cervical collar, sandbags, and tape. Unfortunately, any immobilization technique that restricts mouth opening will make laryngoscopy more difficult. In one study, 64% of patients immobilized with a collar, tape, and sandbags presented a Grade 3 or 4 view with DL, compared to only 22% of patients undergoing MILNS, with cervical collar removed.[120] Other studies concur that DL in patients stabilized with cervical collars will result in a greater than 50% incidence of C-L Grade 3 or 4 views.[94,121] Goutcher and Lochhead studied the effect of semirigid cervical collars on mouth opening in awake volunteers.[122] Mean mouth opening of 40 mm without a collar decreased to 26 to 29 mm with, and in a quarter of the subjects, mouth opening was reduced to 20 mm or less. A common pattern of practice is to remove the anterior element of the collar during laryngoscopy after the application of MILS. In general, when MILS is substituted for a rigid cervical collar, the glottic view obtained with DL improves and the incidence of C-L Grade 3 or 4 is reduced.[40,84,123–127] However, the application of MILS does increase the expected rate of both poor view with DL and failed first pass intubation when compared to the standard "sniffing" position.[126]

How Do Adjuncts and Alternatives Compare to DL for Intubation During Applied MILS?

The Eschmann Tracheal Introducer (gum elastic bougie) is a valuable adjunct to DL in the patient undergoing MILS, increasing both first pass and overall success rates compared to tube alone.[124] Studies of the GVL,[125,128,129] CMAC, VL with use of the Mac-style blade,[127] McGrath Series 5 video laryngoscope,[130] Pentax AWS,[85,125,131,132] Airtraq,[115,133–135] or optical stylets,[107,136] have documented one or more of: significantly improved laryngeal visualization;[125,126,134,135] improved success;[40,132,135] and lower intubation difficulty scores (IDS);[126,134–137] when compared to DL with a Macintosh blade in patient or cadaver studies with either applied MILS or cervical collar. Several series have evaluated the use of the LMA-Fastrach in patients with applied rigid collars: two have reported intubation success rates comparable to those obtained in unrestrained elective surgical patients;[138,139] and one that reported a poor success rate under these conditions had also included the application of cricoid pressure in the study protocol.[140] Suppan et al performed a systematic review and meta-analysis comparing any alternate intubation device with the DL with a Macintosh blade in human subjects with (C-spine) immobilization applied.[115] Twenty-four trials involving 1866 patients met the inclusion criteria for the analysis. With the use of alternative intubation devices, glottic visualization was improved and the risk of intubation failure was lower compared with the DL with a Macintosh blade. Many of the alternatives to DL applied in the patient undergoing tracheal intubation with MILS in place cause less neck movement, improved visualization, and higher rates of successful tracheal intubation.

Do EGAs Cause C-Spine Movement on Insertion?

In a cadaver study, both the LMA-Classic and LMA-Fastrach were found to transiently exert pressure on the upper cervical vertebrae during insertion, suggesting the potential to cause some degree of flexion in that location.[141] This was confirmed in a later in vivo study in which the LMA-Fastrach was seen to cause a small amount of flexion in the upper C-spine during insertion and a lesser amount upon removal.[142] C-spine movement was less during intubation with an LMA-Fastrach compared to C-MAC D-blade in 52 patients presenting for elective cervical discectomy, although FPS was 100% with the D-blade compared with 80% with the LMA.[143] In a cadaver model of a destabilized C3 segment, both the LMA-Fastrach and LMA-Classic caused posterior displacement of the unstable segment, yet significantly less than that caused by Combitube™ insertion and well within physiologic ranges.[72] There is a single case report associating posterior spinal ligament rupture, epidural hematoma formation, and cord compression, with persistent tetraplegia after elective LMA insertion in a patient presenting for laparoscopic cholecystectomy.[144] Although the authors attribute the injury to an unstable C-spine, there is no information in the case report as to the nature of the instability or how they made that determination. A ruptured and edematous posterior ligament was found during urgent surgical exploration and there was historical data that suggested that this was an evolving process in the days before surgery. Calder and McLeod take issue with the attribution of this injury to laryngeal mask insertion, noting that there was evidence of an evolving myelopathy in the days before injury.[145] Even if this injury were to be attributable to LMA insertion, it would have to be considered an extraordinarily rare event; in fact, it is likely not linked to airway management. Further, it does not diminish the role of EGA's as vital rescue oxygenation tools in difficult airway situations; their ability to facilitate reoxygenating a hypoxemic patient in a difficult/failed ventilation scenario would outweigh the potential risk posed by small movements of the C-spine, particularly if care is taken to minimize such movement.

How Does MILS Impact Insertion and Function of EGAs?

The presence of a cervical collar, or application of MILS without a collar, adversely impacts both first pass and overall success insertion rates with the LMA-Classic,[146] the LMA-Fastrach;[147] the Laryngeal Tube,[148] and the Combitube.[149] Comparative studies have indicated a slight advantage to the LMA-Proseal[150] and the LMA-Fastrach[151] when compared with the LMA-Classic under these conditions, and substantially better performance of the LMA-Fastrach when compared to the Laryngeal Tube.[152] Interestingly, in a study of the LMA-Supreme, once inserted, the application of a cervical collar increased the effectiveness of seal pressure from a median of 22 to 27 cm H_2O.[153] A small case series suggested a poor success rate with blind intubation through the LMA-Fastrach while wearing a neck collar with applied cricoid pressure.[154] However, larger series published subsequently, studying patients with immobilized spines without applied cricoid pressure, have reported that intubation success rates with blind[155–157] or FB-facilitated[158] intubation through the LMA-Fastrach appear to be similar to standard conditions.

How Does Front of Neck Access (FONA) Impact C-Spine Movement?

Although long considered a safe alternative in the presence of a CSI, the effect on C-spine movement of surgical cricothyrotomy has not been extensively studied. Gerling et al. studied C-spine movement during open surgical cricothyrotomy in a series of 13 cadavers with a complete C5–C6 transection.[159] A-P displacement was limited to 6.3% of C5 body width (i.e., 1-2 mm of subluxation), and axial distraction to <1 mm across the C5–C6 injury during the procedure. Using a similar injury model in a single cadaver, Donaldson et al. reported that A-P displacement was limited to 0.9 mm during tracheotomy.[70] As these movements are well within physiological levels, values from both studies would likely indicate that a FONA technique deployed to establish an airway should be safe in patients at risk for C-spine injury; efforts should be made to limit spinal movement during the intervention.

How Is Aspiration Risk Mitigated During Airway Management in Patients with Potential CSI?

Aspiration is common in emergency airway management and although death is relatively rare in absolute terms, morbidity is common and significant.[160] The Royal College of Anaesthetists 4th National Audit Project (NAP4), assessing the incidence and cause of airway-related deaths in anesthesia, reported that over 50% of airway-related deaths in anesthesia were a consequence of aspiration. Clinical assessment of the risk of aspiration historically has been based on the presence of patient risk factors; there is a high level of clinical uncertainty regarding risk associated with that assessment. One solution for reducing that uncertainty would be to deploy an objective method to determine the volume and nature of a patient's gastric content more accurately. Both experimental and clinical data demonstrate that ultrasound can do so.[161] Point-of-care gastric ultrasound (POCUS) is likely most useful when there is a high likelihood that the patient has a full stomach and, in this scenario, may help categorize the patient as either low or high risk of having a full stomach (e.g., "likely full stomach" or "likely empty stomach'").[162] Both the volume and nature of the gastric content may be estimated with POCUS. Unfortunately, the optimum position for accurate gastric scanning is the right lateral decubitus position, with a semi-recumbent (head elevated 45 degree) position being an alternative but less desirable position; the supine position is the least sensitive and least accurate patient position.[163] Although POCUS may help stratify injured patients as being at higher or lower risk for aspiration, based on assessment of the volume and nature of gastric contents, it may be difficult to safely position many patients at risk for C-spine injury for optimal imaging, with the result that scanning is not done in the best position for accuracy.

It is likely that, in a small cohort of patients, gastric POCUS will be adequate to reassure care providers that there is low risk of gastric regurgitation and aspiration during airway management. For many other patients in trauma scenarios, it is likely that the scans will either provide evidence of gastric content sufficient to represent an aspiration risk; or generate uncertain results, especially if performed in sub-optimal positions. In this setting, consideration needs to be given to strategies that may prevent regurgitation in at-risk patients; the most widely reviewed of these strategies is the application of cricoid pressure. The reader is referred to Chapter 5 for a more detailed discussion on the risks and benefits of cricoid pressure in emergency airway management. There has been considerable debate about the utility and efficacy of cricoid pressure, as well as its benefits and risks; no consensus has been reached.[164–166] There is no conclusive proof of its benefit, although many experienced anesthesiologists indicate that they would use it during induction in high-risk patients.[167] Although most anesthesiologists believe that a minimal risk of harm is associated with the application of cricoid pressure, a cohort is of the opinion that severe injury may result from its use, even though evidence in support of that view is rare and anecdotal.[168] The authors' opinion is that cricoid pressure reliably occludes the esophageal entrance[169] and may prevent aspiration in some patients, has low potential to meaningfully interfere with FPS or time to intubation,[170,171] and even lower to cause harm. It should be applied when there is a concern that the risk of regurgitation and aspiration is increased, and can be reduced or removed readily if its application results in difficulty in airway management.

With specific reference to the use of cricoid pressure in the patient with potential C-spine injury, a sizeable cohort of anesthesiologists express concern about the potential for exacerbating spinal injury with its application.[168] Although it could not be stated with certainty that it has never happened, given the paucity of reports alleging its occurrence, it must be an extraordinarily rare event. Radiographic studies (albeit in cadaveric specimens) have generally found that C-spine movements with the application of cricoid pressure are well within physiologic limits. In one study of six cadavers with intact C-spines, with 40N of applied cricoid pressure and using radiographs for assessment, Helliwell and Gabbott found a median A-P displacement of <1 mm.[172] In an earlier study of cadavers with a surgically created unstable C-spine at the C5–C6 level, Donaldson et al. reported a mean of 0.64 mm of A-P translation, 3.6 degrees of angulation, and 1 mm of spinous process distraction with cricoid pressure application.[70]

The decision to apply cricoid pressure in a patient with TBI must be considered in the context of the perceived risk of regurgitation and aspiration, as well as its potential for detrimental effects. Cricoid pressure may impact FMV, efforts to place or ventilate through an EGA, and laryngoscopy and intubation, although most of these effects can be readily managed.[166] Although cricoid pressure appears to result in radiographic movement that is within physiologic limits,[61] it may be prudent to reconsider its use in patients with known unstable lesions at or near the level of the cricoid cartilage (C5–C6). An alternative to cricoid pressure in this setting would be the application of left paratracheal pressure below the level of the identified lesion.[173] This would permit pressure to be placed to occlude the esophagus below the level of the identified injury, reducing the potential for aspiration, while also having relatively little impact on airway management.

How Safe Is It to Intubate the Trachea of the Patient with a Possible CSI?

There is no evidence that careful tracheal intubation with MILS applied results in secondary neurologic injury in patients with unstable CSI irrespective of the method used to intubate the trachea.[65,174–177] Oral intubation using DL was once deemed dangerous because it was thought to cause excessive spinal movement with the potential to cause neurological injury.[178] Many studies, both clinical and experimental, have also emphasized the role of movement during airway interventions as having the potential to precipitate secondary neurological injury in unstable spines. However, there seems to be little correlation between these studies and what is reported as the experience of many clinical centers; that carefully executed airway interventions are safe. It may be that the role of movement, especially those that are small in absolute terms, has been overemphasized in the literature in this regard. Rather than movement alone being responsible for injury, it is likely that the combination of preexisting pathologies that limit the spinal canal lumen and the space available for the cord (e.g., spondylolysis), or make the spine more brittle and vulnerable to injury with lesser forces (e.g., ankylosing spondylitis), may, in some patients, enhance the likelihood of injury with movement. Similar magnitudes of movements during airway management in acutely injured but otherwise normal spines may have little consequence compared to the latter group with preexisting conditions. McLeod and Calder reviewed case reports attributing the use of the DL in patients with spinal injury or pathology to subsequent injury.[179] They concluded that it was unlikely that the use of the DL was the cause of many of the myelopathies reported in most of the reports cited. As well, a report analyzing cases in the American Society of Anesthesiologists' Closed Claim database echoed the view that most case reports ascribing cord injury to intubation in patients with unstable injury failed to provide sufficient data to support conclusions regarding causation.[65] That same report noted that preexisting anomalies, such as spondylolysis and ankylosis, were common in patients who experienced perioperative cord injury, despite no evidence of spinal instability, difficult intubation, or excessive movement during airway management in these same patients.

As previously noted, multiple attempts at intubation with unrestricted spinal movement can lead to neurological injury in spine-injured patients.[53–57] However, the message that these reports emphasize is the need for prudently limiting both spinal movement and the number of attempts at intubation in patients at risk of a C-spine injury, and not that orotracheal intubation is contraindicated.

Which Is the Best Option for Intubation of the TBI Patient with Possible CSI?

Many authors have reported on the safe and successful use of DL in the management of patients with CSI for both elective and emergency intubations.[175,177,180–186] These studies are typically limited both by their small sample size and their retrospective nature, but they reveal that neurological deterioration in spine-injured patients is uncommon after airway management when appropriate care is provided, even in high-risk patients undergoing urgent tracheal intubation. Reassuring as they are, these studies are not sufficient to rule out the possibility that, on rare occasions, airway management undertaken in insolation or as part of a more complex clinical intervention, may result in neurological injury, even when provided with the utmost care. In addition, injured patients with preexisting spinal pathologies may be particularly susceptible to injury, even with carefully executed intubation. The use of a DL to facilitate intubation following induction of anesthesia in the patient with TBI (and at risk for CSI) is deemed an appropriate practice option by the American College of Surgeons, as outlined in the manual of Advanced Trauma Life Support Program® for doctors, and by experts in trauma, anesthesia, and neurosurgery.[31,176,179,181,187–189] Recognized advantages of the DL in this setting include its established effectiveness and clinician familiarity.

As noted in the previous discussions, the application of MILS during conventional laryngoscopy increases the forces applied with the DL to achieve an acceptable laryngeal view. Despite the increased force applied, the result is a lower grade view compared to no immobilization forces being applied. In scenarios where it is felt to be important to minimize forces transmitted to the spine, alternatives such as VL and FB may be deployed and are associated with high first pass and overall success.[115] In fact, a recent study reported that VL had largely supplanted not only DL but all other airway techniques in the emergency management of patients with CSI in a major trauma center.[190] VL was used alone (49.6%) or in conjunction with a FB (13.5%) in the majority of patients with most of the rest of the cases being managed with asleep FB-facilitated intubation (30.6%); the DL was rarely used. All tracheal intubations were performed in the presence of an immobilization technique and no cases of secondary neurological injury were attributed to airway management in this series of 252 patients. VL has also been demonstrated to be a more effective strategy in achieving salvage if DL has failed and should be deployed in preference to additional passes with DL if initial attempts are not successful. Finally, a range of VL types can achieve improved laryngeal views in this setting and are associated with higher first pass and overall success rates compared with the DL. VL is an acceptable alternative to the DL for intubation in the setting of both TBI and CSI and is likely to be increasingly deployed as the first-line technique in airway management in this setting in the future.

POSTINTUBATION CONSIDERATIONS

What Are the Postintubation Considerations in the Head-Injured Patient?

Objective confirmation (e.g., with an end-tidal CO_2 monitor) of correct tracheal placement of the ETT is essential. Recognizing the importance of maintaining CPP, blood pressure should be reassessed after airway interventions, and any unacceptable drop corrected with fluid and/or vasopressors. Pupils should be reassessed. After checking for optimal depth, the ETT should be well fixed, as many transfers will occur (e.g., to the diagnostic imaging department and thereafter to the ICU or operating room). If the patient's blood pressure permits, a slight head-up position can be achieved by placing the stretcher in the reverse Trendelenburg position. This will promote venous drainage and may help reduce elevated ICP if suspected.

The radiological investigation of choice in patients with suspected CSI is CT scanning; there is consistent evidence to demonstrate the diagnostic superiority of CT imaging compared with plain X-ray.[191–193] CT imaging of the (C-spine) should be performed at the same time as the cranial assessment for TBI. The 4th edition of the Brain Trauma Foundation TBI Guidelines (BTFG4) advises monitoring ICP in severe TBI and treating ICP > 22 mmHg.[194] While there is evidence that ICP management reduces in-hospital mortality, the long-term functional outcome may not be improved. Cerebral autoregulation is also impaired in TBI and cerebral blood flow is dependent on systemic blood pressure. For severe TBI, the BTFG4 advocates maintaining systolic blood pressure (SBP) at ≥ 100 mmHg for patients 50 to 69 years of age and ≥ 110 mmHg for patients 15 to 49 or > 70 years of age. Similarly, the BTFG4 set a cerebral perfusion pressure (CPP) goal of 60 to 70 mmHg. Maintaining a head position at 30 degrees, modest hyperventilation, and mannitol diuresis as temporizing measures to treat elevated ICP are recommended by the BTFG4.

Coagulopathies are common in severe TBI and are due to the release of tissue factor, which is in high concentrations in the brain; this leads to a consumptive coagulopathy.[195] This coagulopathy is associated with an almost 10-fold increase in death and worse cognitive outcomes in TBI survivors. Consequently, coagulopathies, including thrombocytopenia, should be promptly corrected in TBI patients. Although patients with isolated TBI typically do not require blood transfusion to treat anemia, they are routinely transfused with blood components to reverse the effects of anticoagulant and antiplatelet medications, and to correct comorbidities.[194] The risk of head injury-related death is reduced with tranexamic acid in patients with a mild-to-moderate head injury, but not in patients with severe head injury.[196] Treatment within 3 hours of injury is more effective than later treatment in patients with mild and moderate TBI, but time to treatment may not improve outcome in patients with severe head injury.

What Happened to this Patient?

As outlined in the section "Emergency Department Management" in this chapter, the patient's airway was fully assessed. The decision was made to perform RSI. Preparations included ensuring qualified help, and requisite airway equipment was at hand, together with a briefing of the team about the "Plan B" approach should difficulty be encountered. An assistant was delegated to provide in-line immobilization of the C-spine, following which the front of the patient's rigid collar was removed. Denitrogenation was provided with a tightly fitting face mask, and nasal prongs were applied with 10 L·min^{-1} of oxygen flow. RSI proceeded using fentanyl 100 µg, propofol 100 mg, and rocuronium 70 mg, and right paratracheal pressure was applied concurrent with induction. For tracheal intubation, laryngoscopy was performed with a Glidescope VL, using a #4 blade, and a styleted ETT. The ETT was passed and tracheal placement of the ETT was confirmed with visualization and a disposable end-tidal CO_2 detector, whereupon tracheal pressure was released. The anterior aspect of the rigid cervical collar was reapplied, and MILS was released. Continuous waveform capnography monitoring was instituted to confirm normocarbia. Vital signs were reassessed, with reference to the blood pressure. Decisions were then made about ongoing sedation and skeletal muscle relaxation, and arrangements were made for patient transfer to the diagnostic imaging department.

SUMMARY

Airway management of the patient with a head injury must be undertaken with an appreciation of the importance of avoiding secondary injury to both the brain and C-spine. Hypoxemia and hypotension must be avoided, and formal C-spine precautions must be observed. However, apart from these directives, the practitioner should take comfort in the knowledge that as long as reasonable precautions are undertaken, familiar airway interventions can be safely carried out for the patient with potential C-spine injury, including bag-mask ventilation, RSI, and tracheal intubation using carefully performed direct or video laryngoscopy. To the practitioner experienced in their use, alternative intubation techniques may be of value and may enhance the glottic view and increase the likelihood of FPS compared to DL when MILS is in place. Awake intubation of the patient with a known C-spine injury confers the opportunity to re-evaluate the patient's neurologic status postintubation, if they remain cognitively capable of cooperating in the process, before the induction of general anesthesia. Irrespective of the technique chosen, airway management in this setting should not proceed before a formal airway evaluation has been performed, needed personnel have been assembled and briefed, and the airway equipment necessary for the planned intervention readied.

SELF-EVALUATION QUESTIONS

17.1. Which of the following is contraindicated during intubation of the trauma patient with C-spine precautions and manual in-line stabilization (MILS) applied?

A. Removal of the front of the cervical collar

B. Oral intubation using direct laryngoscopy

C. Cricoid pressure

D. External laryngeal manipulation

E. None of the above

17.2. Which of the following interventions has been shown to improve neurologic outcome in the TBI patient?

A. Performing an awake fiberoptic intubation

B. Performing manual in-line stabilization during intubation attempts

C. Use of an alternative to direct laryngoscopy, such as a GlideScope

D. Avoiding oxygen desaturation

E. Aggressive hyperventilation to induce hypocapnia

17.3. Which of the following statements concerning patients with TBI is **TRUE**?

A. Improved neurological outcome is associated with the avoidance of direct laryngoscopy for intubation.

B. The unconscious TBI patient (GCS < 8) has a threefold chance of cervical spine injury.

C. Avoiding cervical spine movement during airway management is more important than avoiding transient hypoxia and hypotension.

D. The safest way of performing tracheal intubation is with the fiberoptic bronchoscope.

E. The use of muscle relaxants for intubation is contraindicated because they will interfere with subsequent neurological evaluation.

REFERENCES

1. Rajani RR, Ball CG, Montgomery SP, Wyrzykowski AD, Feliciano DV. Airway management for victims of penetrating trauma: analysis of 50,000 cases. *Am J Surg.* 2009;198:863-867.
2. Cobas MA, De la Pena MA, Manning R, Candiotti K, Varon AJ. Prehospital intubations and mortality: a level 1 trauma center perspective. *Anesth Analg.* 2009;109:489-493.
3. von Elm E, Schoettker P, Henzi I, Osterwalder J, Walder B. Pre-hospital tracheal intubation in patients with traumatic brain injury: systematic review of current evidence. *Br J Anaesth.* 2009;103:371-386.
4. Bernard SA, Nguyen V, Cameron P, et al. Prehospital rapid sequence intubation improves functional outcome for patients with severe traumatic brain injury: a randomized controlled trial. *Ann Surg.* 2010; 252:959-965.
5. Gravesteijn BY, Sewalt CA, Nieboer D, et al. Tracheal intubation in traumatic brain injury: a multicentre prospective observational study. *Br J Anaesth.* 2020;125:505-517.
6. Bossers SM, Schwarte LA, Loer SA, Twisk JWR, Boer C, Schober P. Experience in prehospital endotracheal intubation significantly influences mortality of patients with severe traumatic brain injury: a systematic review and meta-analysis. *PLoS ONE.* 2015;10(10):e0141034. doi:10.1371/journal. pone.0141034.
7. Lockey D, Crewdson K, Weaver A, Davies G. Observational study of the success rates of intubation and failed intubation airway rescue techniques in 7256 attempted intubations of trauma patients by pre-hospital physicians. *Br J Anaesth.* 2014;113:220-225.
8. Gellerfors M, Fevang E, Bäckman A, et al. Pre-hospital advanced airway management by anaesthetist and nurse anaesthetist critical care teams: a prospective observational study of 2028 pre-hospital tracheal intubations. *Br J Anaesth.* 2018;120:1103-1109.
9. Spaite DW, Hu C, Bobrow BJ, et al. The effect of combined out-of-hospital hypotension and hypoxia on mortality in major traumatic brain injury. *Ann Emer Med.* 2017;69:62-72.
10. Carney N, Totten AM, O'Reilly C, et al. *Guidelines for the Management of Severe Traumatic Brain Injury.* 4th ed. Brain Trauma Foundation; 2016.
11. Gravesteijn BY, Sewalt CA, Stocchetti N, et al. Prehospital management of traumatic brain injury across Europe: a CENTER-TBI study. *Prehosp Emerg Care* 2020: doi:10.1080/10903127.2020.1817210.
12. Mahoney EJ, Biffl WL, Harrington DT, Cioffi WG. Isolated brain injury as a cause of hypotension in the blunt trauma patient. *J Trauma.* 2003;55:1065-1069.
13. Colterjohn NR, Bednar DA. Identifiable risk factors for secondary neurologic deterioration in the CSI patient. *Spine.* 1995;20:2293-2297.
14. Oto B, Corey DJ, Oswald J, Sifford D, Walsh B. Early secondary neurologic deterioration after blunt spinal trauma: a review of the literature. *Acad Emerg Med.* 2015;22:1200-1212.
15. Reid DC, Henderson R, Saboe L, Miller JD. Etiology and clinical course of missed spine fractures. *J Trauma.* 1987;27:980-986.
16. Davis JW, Phreaner DL, Hoyt DB, Mackersie RC. The etiology of missed cervical spine injuries. *J Trauma.* 1993;34:342-346.
17. Harrop JS, Sharan AD, Vaccaro AR, Przybylski GJ. The cause of neurologic deterioration after acute cervical spinal cord injury. *Spine.* 2001;26:340-346.
18. Levi AD, Hurlbert RJ, Anderson P, et al. Neurologic deterioration secondary to unrecognized spinal instability following trauma – a multicenter study. *Spine.* 2006;31:451-458.
19. Lam C, Chen P-L, Kang J-H, Cheng K-F, Chen R-J, Hung K-S. Risk factors for 14-day rehospitalization following trauma with new traumatic spinal cord injury diagnosis: a 10-year nationwide study in Taiwan. *PLoS ONE.* 2017;12(9):e0184253. https://doi.org/10.1371/journal. pone.0184253.
20. Holly LT, Kelly DF, Counelis GJ, Blinman T, McArthur DL, Cryer HG. Cervical spine trauma associated with moderate and severe head injury: incidence, risk factors, and injury characteristics. *J Neurosurg.* 2002;96: 285-291.
21. Demetriades D, Charalambides K, Chahwan S, et al. Nonskeletal cervical spine injuries: epidemiology and diagnostic pitfalls. *J Trauma.* 2000;48:724-727.
22. Tian HL, Guo Y, Hu J, et al. Clinical characterization of comatose patients with cervical spine injury and traumatic brain injury. *J Trauma.* 2009;67:1305-1310.
23. Sundstrøm T, Asbjørnsen H, Habiba S, Sunde GA, Wester K. Preshospital use of cervical collars in trauma patients: a critical review. *J Neurotraum.* 2104;31:531-540.
24. Maschmann C, Jeppesen E, Rubin MA, Barfod C. New clinical guidelines on the spinal stabilization of adult trauma patients – consensus and evidence based. *Scand J Traum Resus Emerg Med.* 2019;27:77. https://doi. org/10.1186/s13049-019-0655-x.
25. White CC, Domeier RM, Millin MG, et al. Spinal precautions and the use of the long backboard—resource document to the position statement of the National Association of EMS Physicians and the American College of Surgeons Committee on Trauma. *Prehosp Emerg Care.* 2014;18(2):306-314.
26. Kolb JC, Summers RL, Galli RL. Cervical collar-induced changes in intracranial pressure. *Am J Emerg Med.* 1999;17:135-137.
27. Davies G, Deakin C, Wilson A. The effect of a rigid collar on intracranial pressure. *Injury.* 1996;27:647-649.
28. Mobbs RJ, Stoodley MA, Fuller J. Effect of cervical hard collar on intracranial pressure after head injury. *ANZ J Surg.* 2002;72:389-391.

CHAPTER 17

29. Hunt K, Hallworth S, Smith M. The effects of rigid collar placement on intracranial and cerebral perfusion pressures. *Anaesthesia*. 2001;56:511-513.
30. Stone MB, Tubridy CM, Curran R. The effect of rigid cervical collars on internal jugular vein dimensions. *Acad Emerg Med*. 2010;17:100-102.
31. Crosby ET. Airway management in adults after cervical spine trauma. *Anesthesiology*. 2006;104:1293-1318.
32. Zafrullah Arifin M, Gunawan W. Analysis of presurgery time as a prognostic factor in traumatic acute subdural hematoma. *J Neurosurg Sci*. 2013;57:277-280.
33. Tien HCN, Jung V, Pinto R, et al. Reducing time-to-treatment decreases mortality of trauma patients with acute subdural hematoma. *Ann Surg*. 2011;253:1178-1183.
34. Fountain DM, Kolias AG, Lecky FE, et al. Survival trends after surgery for acute subdural hematoma in adults over a 20-year period. *Ann Surg*. 2017;265:590-596.
35. Badjatia N, Carney N, Crocco TJ, et al. Guidelines for prehospital management of traumatic brain injury 2nd ed. *Prehosp Emerg Care*. 2008;12(suppl 1): S1-S52.
36. Bullock MR, Chesnut R, Ghajar J, et al. Surgical management of acute subdural hematomas. *Neurosurgery*. 2006;58:16-24.
37. Langeron O, Masso E, Huraux C, et al. Prediction of difficult mask ventilation. *Anesthesiology*. 2000;92:1229-1236.
38. Kheterpal S, Han R, Tremper KK, et al. Incidence and predictors of difficult and impossible mask ventilation. *Anesthesiology*. 2006;105:885-891.
39. Heath KJ. The effect of laryngoscopy of different cervical spine immobilisation techniques. *Anaesthesia*. 1994;49:843-845.
40. Santoni BG, Hindman BJ, Puttlitz CM. Manual in-line stabilization increases pressures applied by the laryngoscope blade during direct laryngoscopy and orotracheal intubation. *Anesthesiology*. 2009;110:24-31.
41. Bernhard M, Becker TK, Gries A, Knapp, K, Wenzel V. The first shot is often the best shot: first-pass intubation success in emergency airway management. *Anesth Analg*. 2015;121:1389-1393.
42. Mort TC. Emergency tracheal intubation: complications associated with repeated laryngoscopic attempts. *Anesth Analg*. 2004;99:607-613.
43. Duggan LV, Minhas KS, Griesdale DE, et al. Complications increase with greater than one endotracheal intubation attempt: experience in a Canadian adult tertiary-care teaching center. *J Clin Anesth*. 2014;26:167.
44. Rognås L, Hansen TM, Kirkegaard H, Tønnesen E. Pre-hospital advanced airway management by experienced anaesthesiologists: a prospective descriptive study. *Scand J Trauma Resusc Emerg Med*. 2013;21:58.
45. Brown CA III, Kaji AH, Fantegrossi A, Carlson JN, et al. Video laryngoscopy compared to augmented direct laryngoscopy in adult emergency department tracheal intubations: a National Emergency Airway Registry (NEAR) Study. *Acad Emerg Med*. 2020;27:100-108.
46. Cabrini L, Redaelli MB, Filippini M, et al. Tracheal intubation in patients at risk for cervical spinal cord injury: a systematic review. *Acta Anaesthesiol Scand*. 2020;64:443-454.
47. Miller JD, Butterworth JF, Gudeman SK, et al. Further experience in the management of severe head injury. *J Neurosurg*. 1981;54:289-299.
48. Chesnut RM, Temkin N, Carney N, et al for the Global Neurotrauma Research Group. A trial of intracranial-pressure monitoring in traumatic brain injury. *N Eng J Med*. 2012;367:2471-2481.
49. Hawryluk GWJ, Aguilera S, Buki A, et al. A management algorithm for patients with intracranial pressure monitoring; the Seattle International Severe Traumatic Brain Injury Consensus Conference (SIBICC). *Intens Care Med*. 2019;45:1783-1794.
50. Chesnut RM, Marshall LF, Klauber MR, et al. The role of secondary brain injury in determining outcome from severe head injury. *J Trauma*. 1993;34:216-222.
51. Volpi PC, Robba C, Rota M, Vargiolu A, Citerio G. Trajectories of early secondary insults correlate outcomes of traumatic brain injury: results from a large, single center, observational study. *BMC Emerg Med*. 2018;18:52. https://doi.org/10.1186/s.
52. Belanger E, Picard C, Lacerte D, Lavallee P, Levi ADO. Subacute posttraumatic ascending myelopathy after spinal cord injury. *J Neuro surg*. 2000;93:294-299.
53. Hastings RH, Kelley SD. Neurologic deterioration associated with airway management in a cervical spine-injured patient. *Anesthesiology*.1993;78:580-583.
54. Muckart DJ, Bhagwanjee S, van der Merwe R. Spinal cord injury as a result of endotracheal intubation in patients with undiagnosed cervical spine fractures. *Anesthesiology*. 1997;87:418-420.
55. Liang BA, Cheng MA. Efforts at intubation: cervical injury in an emergency circumstance? *J Clin Anesth*. 1999;11:349-352.
56. Oppenlander ME, Hsu FD, Bolton P, Theodore N. Catastrophic neurological complications of emergent endotracheal intubation: report of 2 cases. *J Neurosurg Spine*. 2015;22:454-458.
57. Powell RM, Heath KJ. Quadraplegia in a patient with an undiagnosed odontoid peg fracture. *J R Army Med Corps*. 1996;142:79-81.
58. Farmer J, Vaccaro A, Albert TJ, Malone S, Balderston RA, Cotler JM. Neurologic deterioration after cervical spinal cord injury. *J Spinal Disord*. 1998;11:192-196.
59. Hoffman JR, Wolfson AB, Todd K, Mower WR. Selective cervical spine radiography in blunt trauma: methodology of the National Emergency X-radiography Utilization Study (NEXUS). *Ann Emerg Med*. 1998;32:461-469.
60. Stiell IG, Wells GA, Vandemheen KL, et al. The Canadian C-spine rule for radiography in alert and stable trauma patients. *J Am Med Assoc*. 2001;286:1841-1848.
61. White AI, Panjabi M. *Clinical Biomechanics of the Spine*. 2nd ed. Philadelphia, PA: JB Lippincott; 1990.
62. Panjabi MM, Chen NC, Shin EK, Wang JL. The cortical shell architecture of human cervical vertebral bodies. *Spine*. 2001;26:2478-2484.
63. Panjabi MM, Thibodeau LL, Crisco JJ 3rd, White AA III. What constitutes spinal instability? *Clin Neurosurg*. 1988;34:313-339.
64. Turner CR, Block J, Shanks A, Morris M, Lodhia KR, Gujar SK. Motion of a cadaver model of cervical injury during endotracheal intubation with a Bullard laryngoscope or a Macintosh blade with and without in-line stabilization. *J Trauma*. 2009;67:61-66.
65. Hindman BJ, Palecek JP, Posner KL, et al. Cervical spinal cord, root, and bony spine injuries: a closed claims analysis. *Anesthesiology*. 2011;114: 782-795.
66. Walters FJM, Nott MR. The hazards of anaesthesia in the injured patient. *Br J Anaesth* 1977;49:707-720.
67. Donaldson WF 3rd, Heil BV, Donaldson VP, Silvaggio VJ. The effect of airway maneuvers on the unstable C1-C2 segment. A cadaver study. *Spine*. 1997;22:1215-1218.
68. Hauswald M, Sklar DP, Tandberg D, Garcia JF. Cervical spine movement during airway management: cinefluoroscopic appraisal in human cadavers. *Am J Emerg Med*. 1991;9:535-538.
69. Turkstra TP, Craen RA, Pelz DM, Gelb AW. Cervical spine motion: a fluoroscopic comparison during intubation with lighted stylet, GlideScope, and Macintosh laryngoscope. *Anesth Analg*. 2005;101:910-915.
70. Donaldson WF 3rd, Towers JD, Doctor A, Brand A, Donaldson VP. A methodology to evaluate motion of the unstable spine during intubation techniques. *Spine*. 1993;18:2020-2023.
71. Aprahamian C, Thompson BM, Finger WA, Darin JC. Experimental cervical spine injury model: evaluation of airway management and splinting techniques. *Ann Emerg Med*. 1984;13:584-587.
72. Brimacombe J, Keller C, Kunzel KH, Gaber O, Boehler M, Puhringer F. Cervical spine motion during airway management: a cinefluoroscopic study of the posteriorly destabilized third cervical vertebrae in human cadavers. *Anesth Analg*. 2000;91:1274-1278.
73. Prasarn ML, Horodyski M, Scott NE, Konopka G, Conrad B, Rechtine GR. Motion generated in the unstable upper cervical spine during head tilt-chin lift and jaw thrust maneuvers. *Spine J*. 2014;14: 609-614.
74. Sawin PD, Todd MM, Traynelis VC, et al. Cervical spine motion with direct laryngoscopy and orotracheal intubation. An in vivo cinefluoroscopic study of subjects without cervical abnormality. *Anesthesiology*. 1996;85: 26-36.
75. Watts AD, Gelb AW, Bach DB, Pelz DM. Comparison of the Bullard and Macintosh laryngoscopes for endotracheal intubation of patients with a potential cervical spine injury. *Anesthesiology*. 1997;87:1335-1342.
76. Turkstra TP, Pelz DM, Shaikh AA, Craen RA. Cervical spine motion: a fluoroscopic comparison of Shikani Optical Stylet vs Macintosh laryngoscope. *Can J Anaesth*. 2007;54:441-447.
77. Turkstra TP, Pelz DM, Jones PM. Cervical spine motion: a fluoroscopic comparison of the AirTraq Laryngoscope versus the Macintosh laryngoscope. *Anesthesiology*. 2009;111:97-101.
78. Hirabayashi Y, Fujita A, Seo N, Sugimoto H. A comparison of cervical spine movement during laryngoscopy using the Airtraq or Macintosh laryngoscopes. *Anaesthesia*. 2008;63:635-640.
79. LeGrand SA, Hindman BJ, Dexter F, Weeks JB, Todd MM. Craniocervical motion during direct laryngoscopy and orotracheal intubation with the Macintosh and Miller blades: an in vivo cinefluoroscopic study. *Anesthesiology*. 2007;107:884-891.
80. Mentzelopoulos SD, Tzoufi MJ, Papageorgiou EP. The disposition of the cervical spine and deformation of available cord space with conventional and balloon laryngoscopy-guided laryngeal intubation: a comparative study. *Anesth Analg*. 2001;92:1331-1336.
81. Hirabayashi Y, Fujita A, Seo N, Sugimoto H. Cervical spine movement during laryngoscopy using the Airway Scope compared with the Macintosh laryngoscope. *Anaesthesia*. 2007;62:1050-1055.

82. Houde BJ, Williams SR, Cadrin-Chenevert A, Guilbert F, Drolet P. A comparison of cervical spine motion during orotracheal intubation with the Trachlight® or the flexible fiberoptic bronchoscope. *Anesth Analg*. 2009;108:1638-1643.
83. Lennarson PJ, Smith D, Todd MM, et al. Segmental cervical spine motion during orotracheal intubation of the intact and injured spine with and without external stabilization. *J Neurosurg*. 2000;92:201-206.
84. Robitaille A, Williams SR, Tremblay MH, Guilbert F, Theriault M, Drolet P. Cervical spine motion during tracheal intubation with manual in-line stabilization: direct laryngoscopy versus GlideScope videolaryngoscopy. *Anesth Analg*. 2008;106:935-941.
85. Malik MA, Subramaniam R, Churasia S, Maharaj CH, Harte BH, Laffey JG. Tracheal intubation in patients with cervical spine immobilization: a comparison of the Airwayscope, LMA CTrach, and the Macintosh laryngoscopes. *Br J Anaesth*. 2009;102:654-661.
86. Sugiyama K, Yokoyama K. Head extension angle required for direct laryngoscopy with the McCoy laryngoscope blade. *Anesthesiology*. 2001;94:939.
87. Hastings RH, Wood PR. Head extension and laryngeal view during laryngoscopy with cervical spine stabilization maneuvers. *Anesthesiology*. 1994;80:825-831.
88. LeGrand SA, Hindman BJ, Dexter F, Weeks JB, Todd MM. Craniocervical motion during direct laryngoscopy and orotracheal intubation with the Macintosh and Miller blades: an in vivo cinefluoroscopic study. *Anesthesiology*. 2007;107:884-891.
89. Hastings RH, Hon ED, Nghiem C, Wahrenbrock EA. Force and torque vary between laryngoscopists and laryngoscope blades. *Anesth Analg*. 1996;82:462-468.
90. Hauswald M, Sklar DP, Tandberg D, Garcia JF. Cervical spine movement during airway management: cinefluoroscopic appraisal in human cadavers. *Am J Emerg Med*. 1991;9:535-538.
91. Majernick TG, Bieniek R, Houston JB, Hughes HG. Cervical spine movement during orotracheal intubation. *Ann Emerg Med*. 1986;15:417-420.
92. Hastings RH, Vigil AC, Hanna R, Yang BY, Sartoris DJ. Cervical spine movement during laryngoscopy with the Bullard, Macintosh, and Miller laryngoscopes. *Anesthesiology*. 1995;82:859-869.
93. Konishi A, Sakai T, Nishiyama T, Higashizawa T, Bito H. Cervical spine movement during orotracheal intubation using the McCoy laryngoscope compared with the Macintosh and the Miller laryngoscopes. *Masui*. 1997;46:124-127.
94. Gerling MC, Davis DP, Hamilton RS, et al. Effects of cervical spine immobilization technique and laryngoscope blade selection on an unstable cervical spine in a cadaver model of intubation. *Ann Emerg Med*. 2000;36:293-300.
95. MacIntyre PA, McLeod AD, Hurley R, Peacock C. Cervical spine movements during laryngoscopy. Comparison of the Macintosh and McCoy laryngoscope blades. *Anaesthesia*. 1999;54:413-418.
96. Grossman D, Schriger DL. Immobilization technique and blade choice in the endotracheal intubation of trauma patients: Miller time or much ado about nothing? *Ann Emerg Med*. 2000;36:351-353.
97. Uchida T, Hikawa Y, Saito Y, Yasuda K. The McCoy levering laryngoscope in patients with limited neck extension. *Can J Anaesth*. 1997;44:674-676.
98. Laurent SC, de Melo AE, Alexander-Williams JM. The use of the McCoy laryngoscope in patients with simulated cervical spine injuries. *Anaesthesia*. 1996;51:74-75.
99. Gabbott DA, Sasada MP. Tracheal intubation through the laryngeal mask using a gum elastic bougie in the presence of cricoid pressure and manual in line stabilisation of the neck. *Anaesthesia*. 1996;51:389-390.
100. Hirabayashi Y, Fujita A, Seo N, Sugimoto H. Cervical spine movement during laryngoscopy using the Airway Scope compared with the Macintosh laryngoscope. *Anaesthesia*. 2007;62:1050-1055.
101. Maruyama K, Yamada T, Kawakami R, Kamata T, Yokochi M, Hara K. Upper cervical spine movement during intubation: fluoroscopic comparison of the AirWay Scope, McCoy laryngoscope, and Macintosh laryngoscope. *Br J Anaesth*. 2008;100:120-124.
102. Takenaka I, Aoyama K, Iwagaki T, Ishimura H, Takenaka Y, Kadoya T. Approach combining the airway scope and the bougie for minimizing movement of the cervical spine during endotracheal intubation. *Anesthesiology*. 2009;110:1335-1340.
103. Hirabayashi Y, Fujita A, Seo N, Sugimoto H. A comparison of cervical spine movement during laryngoscopy using the Airtraq or Macintosh laryngoscopes. *Anaesthesia*. 2008; 63:635-640.
104. McCahon RA, Evans DA, Kerslake RW, McClelland SH, Hardman JG, Norris AM. Cadaveric study of movement of an unstable atlanto-axial (C1/C2) cervical segment during laryngoscopy and intubation using the Airtraq®, Macintosh and McCoy laryngoscopes. *Anaesthesia*. 2015;70:452-461.
105. Wahlen BM, Gercek E. Three-dimensional cervical spine movement during intubation using the Macintosh and Bullard laryngoscopes, the Bonfils fibrescope and the intubating laryngeal mask airway. *Eur J Anaesthesiol*. 2004;21:907-913.
106. Rudolph C, Schneider JP, Wallenborn J, Schaffranietz L. Movement of the upper cervical spine during laryngoscopy: a comparison of the Bonfils intubation fibrescope and the Macintosh laryngoscope. *Anaesthesia*. 2005;60:668-672.
107. Kihara S, Watanabe S, Brimacombe J, Taguchi N, Yaguchi Y, Yamasaki Y. Segmental cervical spine movement with the intubating laryngeal mask during manual in-line stabilization in patients with cervical pathology undergoing cervical spine surgery. *Anesth Analg*. 2000;91:195-200.
108. Sahin A, Salman MA, Erden IA, Aypar U. Upper cervical vertebrae movement during intubating laryngeal mask, fibreoptic and direct laryngoscopy: a video-fluoroscopic study. *Eur J Anaesthesiol*. 2004;21:819-823.
109. Paik H, Park H. Randomized crossover trial comparing cervical spine motion during tracheal intubation with a Macintosh laryngoscope versus a C-MAC D-blade videolaryngoscope in a simulated immobilized cervical spine. *BMC Anesthesiology*. 2020;20:201.
110. Nam K, Lee Y, Park H, Chung J, Yoon H, Kim TK. Cervical spine motion during tracheal intubation using an Optiscope versus the McGrath videolaryngoscope in patients with simulated cervical immobilization: a prospective randomized crossover study. *Anesth Analg*. 2019;129:1666-1672.
111. Wong DM, Prabhu A, Chakraborty S, Tan G, Massicotte EM, Cooper R. Cervical spine motion during flexible bronchoscopy compared with the Lo-Pro GlideScope. *Br J Anaesth*. 2009;102:424-430.
112. Brimacombe J, Keller C, Kunzel KH, Gaber O, Boehler M, Puhringer F. Cervical spine motion during airway management: a cinefluoroscopic study of the posteriorly destabilized third cervical vertebrae in human cadavers. *Anesth Analg*. 2000;91:1274-1278.
113. Swain A, Bhagat H, Gupta V, Salunke P, Panda NB, Sahu S. Intubating laryngeal mask airway-assisted flexible bronchoscopic intubation is associated with reduced cervical spine motion when compared with C-MAC video laryngoscopy-guided intubation: a prospective randomized cross over trial. *J Neurosurg Anesthesiol*. 2020;32:242-248.
114. Dutta K, Sriganesh K, Chakrabarti D, Pruthi N, Reddy M. Cervical spine movement during awake orotracheal intubation with fiberoptic scope and McGrath videolaryngoscope in patients undergoing surgery for cervical spine instability: a randomized control trial. *J Neurosurg Anesthesiol*. 2020;32:249-255.
115. Suppan L, Tramèr MR, Niquille M, Grosgurin O, Marti C. Alternative intubation techniques vs Macintosh laryngoscopy in patients with cervical spine immobilization: systematic review and meta-analysis of randomized controlled trials. *Br J Anaesth*. 2016;116:27-36.
116. Lennarson PJ, Smith DW, Sawin PD, Todd MM, Sato Y, Traynelis VC. Cervical spinal motion during intubation: efficacy of stabilization maneuvers in the setting of complete segmental instability. *J Neurosurg*. 2001;94:265-270.
117. Gerling MC, Davis DP, Hamilton RS, et al. Effects of cervical spine immobilization technique and laryngoscope blade selection on an unstable cervical spine in a cadaver model of intubation. *Ann Emerg Med*. 2000;36:293-300.
118. Turner CR, Block J, Shanks A, Morris M, Lodhia KR, Gujar SK. Motion of a cadaver model of cervical injury during endotracheal intubation with a Bullard laryngoscope or a Macintosh blade with and without in-line stabilization. *J Trauma*. 2009;67:61-66.
119. Manoach S, Paladino L. Manual in-line stabilization for acute airway management of suspected cervical spine injury: historical review and current questions. *Ann Emerg Med*. 2007;50:236-245.
120. Heath KJ. The effect of laryngoscopy of different cervical spine immobilisation techniques. *Anaesthesia*. 1994;49:843-845.
121. MacQuarrie K, Hung OR, Law JA. Tracheal intubation using Bullard laryngoscope for patients with a simulated difficult airway. *Can J Anaesth*. 1999;46:760-765.
122. Goutcher CM, Lochhead V. Reduction in mouth opening with semi-rigid cervical collars. *Br J Anaesth*. 2005;95:344-348.
123. Walls RM. Orotracheal intubation and potential cervical spine injury. *Ann Emerg Med*. 1987;16:373-374.
124. Nolan JP, Wilson ME. Orotracheal intubation in patients with potential cervical spine injuries. An indication for the gum elastic bougie. *Anaesthesia*. 1993;48:630-633.
125. Malik MA, Maharaj CH, Harte BH, Laffey JG. Comparison of Macintosh, Truview EVO2, Glidescope, and Airwayscope laryngoscope use in patients with cervical spine immobilization. *Br J Anaesth*. 2008;101:723-730.
126. Thiboutot F, Nicole PC, Trepanier CA, Turgeon AF, Lessard MR. Effect of manual in-line stabilization of the cervical spine in adults on the rate

of difficult orotracheal intubation by direct laryngoscopy: a randomized controlled trial. *Can J Anaesth*. 2009;56:412-418.
127. Byhahn C, Nemetz S, Breitkreutz R, Zwissler B, Kaufmann M, Meininger D. Brief report: tracheal intubation using the Bonfils intubation fibrescope or direct laryngoscopy for patients with a simulated difficult airway. *Can J Anaesth*. 2008;55:232-237.
128. Zamora JE, Nolan RL, Sharan S, Day AG. Evaluation of the Bullard, GlideScope, Viewmax, and Macintosh laryngoscopes using a cadaver model to simulate the difficult airway. *J Clin Anesth*. 2011;23:27-34.
129. Bathory I, Frascarolo P, Kern C, Schoettker P. Evaluation of the GlideScope for tracheal intubation in patients with cervical spine immobilisation by a semi-rigid collar. *Anaesthesia*. 2009:64:1337-1341.
130. Ilyas S, Symons J, Bradley WP, et al. A prospective randomised controlled trial comparing tracheal intubation plus manual in-line stabilisation of the cervical spine using the Macintosh laryngoscope vs the McGrath® Series 5 videolaryngoscope. *Anaesthesia*. 2014;69:1345-1350.
131. Enomoto Y, Asai T, Arai T, Kamishima K, Okuda Y. Pentax-AWS, a new videolaryngoscope, is more effective than the Macintosh laryngoscope for tracheal intubation in patients with restricted neck movements: a randomized comparative study. *Br J Anaesth*. 2008;100:544-548.
132. Komatsu R, Kamata K, Hoshi I, Sessler DI, Ozaki M. Airway scope and gum elastic bougie with Macintosh laryngoscope for tracheal intubation in patients with simulated restricted neck mobility. *Br J Anaesth*. 2008;101:863-869.
133. Maharaj CH, Buckley E, Harte BH, Laffey JG. Endotracheal intubation in patients with cervical spine immobilization: a comparison of Macintosh and Airtraq laryngoscopes. *Anesthesiology*. 2007;107:53-59.
134. Amor M, Nabil S, Bensghir M, et al. A comparison of Airtraq laryngoscope and standard direct laryngoscopy in adult patients with immobilized cervical spine. *Ann Fr Anesth Reanim*. 2013;32:296-301.
135. Koh JC, Lee JS, Lee YW, Chang CH. Comparison of the laryngeal view during intubation using Airtraq and Macintosh laryngoscopes in patients with cervical spine immobilization and mouth opening limitation. *Korean J Anesthesiol*. 2010;59:314-318.
136. Kihara S, Yaguchi Y, Taguchi N, Brimacombe JR, Watanabe S. The StyletScope is a better intubation tool than a conventional stylet during simulated cervical spine immobilization. *Can J Anaesth*. 2005;52:105-110.
137. Adnet F, Borron SW, Racine SX, et al. The intubation difficulty scale (IDS): proposal and evaluation of a new score characterizing the complexity of endotracheal intubation. *Anesthesiology*. 1997;87:1290-1297.
138. Moller F, Andres AH, Langenstein H. Intubating laryngeal mask airway (ILMA) seems to be an ideal device for blind intubation in case of immobile spine. *Br J Anaesth*. 2000;85:493-495.
139. Ferson DZ, Rosenblatt WH, Johansen MJ, Osborn I, Ovassapian A. Use of the intubating LMA-Fastrach in 254 patients with difficult-to-manage airways. *Anesthesiology*. 2001;95:1175-1181.
140. Wakeling HG, Nightingale J. The intubating laryngeal mask airway does not facilitate tracheal intubation in the presence of a neck collar in simulated trauma. *Br J Anaesth*. 2000;84:254-256.
141. Keller C, Brimacombe J, Keller K. Pressures exerted against the cervical vertebrae by the standard and intubating laryngeal mask airways: a randomized, controlled, cross-over study in fresh cadavers. *Anesth Analg*. 1999;89:1296-1300.
142. Kihara S, Watanabe S, Brimacombe J, Taguchi N, Yaguchi Y, Yamasaki Y. Segmental cervical spine movement with the intubating laryngeal mask during manual in-line stabilization in patients with cervical pathology undergoing cervical spine surgery. *Anesth Analg*. 2000;91:195-200.
143. Özkan D, Altinsoy S, Dolgun H, Ergil J, Dönmez A. Comparison of cervical spine motion during intubation with a C-MAC D-blade® and an LMA Fastrach®. *Der Anaesthesist*. 2019;68:90-96.
144. Edge CJ, Hyman N, Addy V, et al. Posterior spinal ligament rupture associated with laryngeal mask insertion in a patient with undisclosed unstable cervical spine. *Br J Anaesth*. 2002;89:514-517.
145. Calder I, McLeod AM. Neurological deterioration after laryngeal mask insertion. *Br J Anaesth*. 2003;90:702-703.
146. Gabbott DA, Sasada MP. Laryngeal mask airway insertion using cricoid pressure and manual in-line neck stabilisation. *Anaesthesia*. 1995;50: 674-676.
147. Komatsu R, Nagata O, Kamata K, Yamagata K, Sessler DI, Ozaki M. Intubating laryngeal mask airway allows tracheal intubation when the cervical spine is immobilized by a rigid collar. *Br J Anaesth*. 2004;93:655-659.
148. Asai T, Marfin AG, Thompson J, Popat M, Shingu K. Ease of insertion of the laryngeal tube during manual-in-line neck stabilisation. *Anaesthesia*. 2004;59:1163-1166.
149. Mercer MH, Gabbott DA. Insertion of the Combitube airway with the cervical spine immobilised in a rigid cervical collar. *Anaesthesia*. 1998;53:971-974.
150. Asai T, Murao K, Shingu K. Efficacy of the ProSeal laryngeal mask airway during manual in-line stabilisation of the neck. *Anaesthesia*. 2002;57:918-920.
151. Asai T, Wagle AU, Stacey M. Placement of the intubating laryngeal mask is easier than the laryngeal mask during manual in-line neck stabilization. *Br J Anaesth*. 1999;82:712-714.
152. Komatsu R, Nagata O, Kamata K, Yamagata K, Sessler DI, Ozaki M. Comparison of the intubating laryngeal mask airway and laryngeal tube placement during manual in-line stabilisation of the neck. *Anaesthesia*. 2005;60:113-117.
153. Mann V, Spitzner T, Schwandner T, et al. The effect of a cervical collar on the seal pressure of the LMA Supreme: a prospective, crossover trial. *Anaesthesia*. 2012;67:1260-1265.
154. Wakeling HG, Nightingale J. The intubating laryngeal mask airway does not facilitate tracheal intubation in the presence of a neck collar in simulated trauma. *Br J Anaesth*. 2000;84:254-256.
155. Komatsu R, Nagata O, Kamata K, Yamagata K, Sessler DI, Ozaki M. Intubating laryngeal mask airway allows tracheal intubation when the cervical spine is immobilized by a rigid collar. *Br J Anaesth*. 2004;93:655-659.
156. Nileshwar A, Thudamaladinne A. Comparison of intubating laryngeal mask airway and Bullard laryngoscope for oro-tracheal intubation in adult patients with simulated limitation of cervical movements. *Br J Anaesth*. 2007; 99:292-296.
157. Saini S, Bala R, Singh R. Evaluation of the Intubating Laryngeal Mask Airway (ILMA) as an intubation conduit in patients with a cervical collar simulating fixed cervical spine. *South Afr J Anaesth Analg*. 2017;23:40-44.
158. Mathew DG, Ramachandran R, Rewari V, Trikha A. Chandralekha. Endotracheal intubation with intubating laryngeal mask airway (ILMA), C-Trach, and Cobra PLA in simulated cervical spine injury patients: a comparative study. *J Anesth*. 2014;28:655-661.
159. Gerling MC, Davis DP, Hamilton RS, et al. Effect of surgical cricothyrotomy on the unstable cervical spine in a cadaver model of intubation. *J Emerg Med*. 2001;20:1-5.
160. Cook T, Frerk C. Fourth National Audit Project (NAP 4): Major complications of airway management in the United Kingdom Report and Findings. Chapter 19. Aspiration of gastric contents and of blood. The Royal College of Anaesthetists and the Difficult Airway Society; March 2011.
161. Perlas A, Mitsakakis N, Liu L, Cino M, Haldipur N, Davis L. Validation of a mathematical model for ultrasound assessment of gastric volume by gastroscopic examination. *Anesth Analg*. 2013;116:357-363.
162. Perlas A, Arzola C, Van de Putte P. Point-of-care gastric ultrasound and aspiration risk assessment" a narrative review. *Can J Anesth*. 2018;65: 437-448.
163. Koenig SJ, Lakticova V, Mayo PH. Utility of ultrasonography for detection of gastric fluid during urgent endotracheal intubation. *Intens Care Med*. 2011;37:627-631.
164. Salem NR, Khorasani A, Zeidan A, Crystal G. Crocoid pressure controversies: narrative review. *Anesthesiology*. 2017;126:738-752.
165. Zdravkovic M, Rice MJ, Brull SJ. The clinical use of cricoid pressure: first, do no harm. *Anesth Analg*. 2021;132:261-267.
166. Neilipovitz DT, Crosby ET. No evidence for decreased incidence of aspiration after rapid sequence induction. *Can J Anaesth*. 2007;54: 748-764.
167. Zdravkovic M, Berger-Estilita J, Sorbello M, Hagberg CA. An international survey about rapid sequence intubation of 10,003 anaesthetists and 16 airway experts. *Anaesthesia*. 2020;75:313-322.
168. Mistry R, Frei DR, Badenhorst C, Broadbent J. A survey of self-reported use of cricoid pressure among Australian and New Zealand anaesthetists: attitudes and practice. *Anaesth Int Care*. 2021;49:62-69.
169. Zeidan AM, Ramez Salem M, Mazoit JX, Abdullah MA, Ghattas T, Crystal GJ. The effectiveness of cricoid pressure for occluding the esophageal entrance in anesthetized and paralyzed patients: an experimental and observational Glidescope study. *Anesth Analg*. 2014;118:580-586.
170. Hung KC, Hung CT, Poon YY, et al. The effect of cricoid pressure on tracheal intubation in adult patients; a systematic review and meta-analysis. *Can J Anesth*. 2021;68:137-147.
171. White L, Dip G, Thang C, Hodson A, Melhuish T, Vlok R. Crocoid pressure during intubation; a systematic review and meta-analysis of randomized controlled trials. *Heart Lung*. 2020;49:175-180.
172. Helliwell V, Gabbott DA. The effect of single-handed cricoid pressure on cervical spine movement after applying manual in-line stabilisation—a cadaver study. *Resuscitation*. 2001;49:53-57.
173. Gautier N, Danklou J, Brichant JF, et al. The effect of force applied to the left paratracheal oesophagus on air entry into the gastric antrum during positive-pressure ventilation using a facemask. *Anaesthesia*. 2019;74: 22-28.

174. Talucci RC, Shaikh KA, Schwab CW. Rapid sequence induction with oral endotracheal intubation in the multiply injured patient. *Am Surg.* 1988;54:185-187.
175. Shatney CH, Brunner RD, Nguyen TQ. The safety of orotracheal intubation in patients with unstable cervical spine fracture or high spinal cord injury. *Am J Surg.* 1995;170:676-679.
176. Suderman VS, Crosby ET, Lui A. Elective oral tracheal intubation in cervical spine-injured adults. *Can J Anaesth.* 1991;38:785-789.
177. Meschino A, Devitt JH, Koch JP, Szalai JP, Schwartz ML. The safety of awake tracheal intubation in cervical spine injury. *Can J Anaesth.* 1992;39:114-117.
178. Walls RM. Orotracheal intubation and potential cervical spine injury. *Ann Emerg Med.* 1987;16:373-374.
179. McLeod AD, Calder I. Spinal cord injury and direct laryngoscopy—the legend lives on. *Br J Anaesth.* 2000;84:705-709.
180. Talucci RC, Shaikh KA, Schwab CW. Rapid sequence induction with oral endotracheal intubation in the multiply injured patient. *Am Surg.* 1988;54:185-187.
181. Shatney CH, Brunner RD, Nguyen TQ. The safety of orotracheal intubation in patients with unstable cervical spine fracture or high spinal cord injury. *Am J Surg.* 1995;170:676-679.
182. Holley J, Jorden R. Airway management in patients with unstable cervical spine fractures. *Ann Emerg Med.* 1989;18:1237-1239.
183. Rhee KJ, Green W, Holcroft JW, Mangili JA. Oral intubation in the multiply injured patient: the risk of exacerbating spinal cord damage. *Ann Emerg Med.* 1990;19:511-514.
184. Scannell G, Waxman K, Tominaga G, Barker S, Annas C. Orotracheal intubation in trauma patients with cervical fractures. *Arch Surg.* 1993;128: 903-905.
185. Wright SW, Robinson GG 2nd, Wright MB. Cervical spine injuries in blunt trauma patients requiring emergent endotracheal intubation. *Am J Emerg Med.* 1992;10:104-109.
186. Norwood S, Myers MB, Butler TJ. The safety of emergency neuromuscular blockade and orotracheal intubation in the acutely injured trauma patient. *J Am Coll Surg.* 1994;179:646-652.
187. Ball PA. Critical care of spinal cord injury. *Spine.* 2001;26:S27-S30.
188. Dunham CM, Barraco RD, Clark DE, et al. Guidelines for emergency tracheal intubation immediately after traumatic injury. *J Trauma.* 2003;55:162-179.
189. Mayglothling J, Duane TM, Gibbs M, et al. Emergency tracheal intubation immediately following traumatic injury: an Eastern Association for the Surgery of Trauma practice management guideline. *J Trauma Acute Care Surg.* 2012;73:S333-S340.
190. Holmes MG, Dagal A, Feinstein BA, Joffe AM. Airway management practice in adults with an unstable cervica spine: The Harborview Medical Center Experience. *Anesth Analg.* 2018;127:450-454.
191. Panczykowski DM, Tomycz ND, Okonkwo DO. Comparative effectiveness of using computed tomography alone to exclude cervical spine injuries in obtunded or intubated patients: meta-analysis of 14,327 patients with blunt trauma. *J Neurosurg.* 2011;115:541-549.
192. Como JJ, Diaz JJ, Dunham CM, et al. Practice management guidelines for identification of cervical spine injuries following trauma: update from the Eastern Association for the Surgery of Trauma Practice Management Guidelines Committee. *J Trauma.* 2009; 67: 651-659.
193. Ryken TC, Hadley MN, Walters BC, et al. Radiographic assessment. *Neurosurg.* 2013;72(Suppl 3):54-72.
194. Carney N, Totten AM, O'Reilly C, et al. Guidelines for the management of severe traumatic brain injury, 4th Edition. *Neurosurg.* 2017;80:6-15.
195. Stolla M, Zhang F, Meyer MR, Zhang J, Dong JF. Current state of transfusion in traumatic brain injury and associated coagulopathy. *Transfusion.* 2019;59;1522-1528.
196. The CRASH-3 trial collaborators. Effects of tranexamic acid on death, disability, vascular occlusive events and other morbidities in patiensts with acute traumatic brain injury (CRASH-3): a randomised, placebo-controlled trial. *Lancet.* 2019;394:1713-1723.

CHAPTER 18

Airway Management of an Unconscious Patient Entrapped After a Motor Vehicle Crash

Arnim Vlatten and Bjoern Hossfeld

CASE PRESENTATION

You are the emergency physician on duty for aeromedical transport calls. You are called to the scene of a motor vehicle collision in a remote area. Seventeen minutes into the flight, you hear from the on-scene paramedics that a young man hit a tree and flipped his car. He is the only occupant and is still trapped in the car. The rescuers have difficulty extricating him from the vehicle. On landing, you see firefighters preparing to use a heavy-extrication tool ("Jaws of Life"). As you exit the helicopter, the ground paramedic informs you that the accident scene is secure and that the patient is a 25-year-old obese man, unconscious, with stable vital signs. As you approach the vehicle, you note major front-end damage to the car, encroaching on the vehicle's interior, the airbag deployed, and the patient apparently unresponsive behind the steering column. The A- and B-column on the driver's side of the car appeared to have struck the left side of the patient's head, and both lower extremities are trapped under the dashboard. Vital signs are stable and he is unresponsive to pain. He is breathing spontaneously with high-flow oxygen delivered via a non-rebreather face mask; a cervical spine collar has been applied and two large-bore intravenous cannulas placed in the antecubital fossae.

PATIENT CONSIDERATIONS

■ What Are the Considerations in Extricating the Patient from the Vehicle?

Given that organized traffic control and firefighters ensure scene safety, the urgency of extrication must now be considered. A rapid extrication may be necessary in cases of impending arrest or uncontrollable bleeding. Priority is governed by "life before limb" and accepts the risk of further injuries to extremities and spine. A planned and deliberate rescue approach might be appropriate if there are no immediate life-threatening situations, such as a burning vehicle or markedly unstable vital signs. In the case of this patient, access had already been provided by the rescuers, permitting clinical assessment by emergency medical services (EMS) personnel and application of basic airway maneuvers and insertion of intravenous lines. Following initial medical interventions, the rescuers can then use a heavy-extrication tool to remove the roof of the vehicle and a hydraulic spreader to create space under the dashboard. The patient can then be extricated with full spine precautions.

■ What Are the Major Considerations According to the Trauma Guidelines?

According to the Prehospital Trauma Life Support (PHTLS) and Advanced Trauma Life Support (ATLS) guidelines, the primary assessment of a patient addresses the airway, breathing, circulation, and disability (ABCD).[1,2] After ensuring rescuer and patient safety and a short check for critical bleeding, airway management has the highest priority. In this unconscious patient, the airway is in jeopardy and needs to be secured early, and it must be assumed that the patient has suffered a severe traumatic brain injury. Oxygenation and ventilation are crucial steps in initial management to avoid hypoxemia and hypercarbia, both of which worsen any brain injury. With such extensive vehicle damage, injuries other than to the brain are very likely: cervical spine injury, pneumothorax or flail chest, and intraabdominal injuries–all must be considered once the airway is assured.

Because the patient's legs are impacted under the dashboard, early extrication is unlikely. Since the patient's vital signs are stable and a rapid extrication might increase the risk of cervical spine injury, a planned and careful extrication is preferable. Airway management remains a top priority even if the patient is still inside the vehicle.

Are There Any Special Considerations in This Case?

Special considerations in this case include urgent airway management in a difficult environment with limited patient access and resources. Access to a patient is usually gained by cutting the A- and B-column of the vehicle using the heavy-extrication tool and flipping the roof backward, a procedure that may be time-consuming. In this case, urgent airway management is necessary due to the traumatic brain injury with a resultant loss of airway reflexes. Tracheal intubation is the gold standard in securing a patient's airway. However, a possible cervical spine injury as well as limited neck movement, combined with reduced access to the patient's head will certainly make airway management using direct laryngoscopy (DL) extremely difficult if not impossible.

The benefit of endotracheal intubation in patients with severe traumatic brain injury in the prehospital setting is dependent on the experience of the provider[3] and its attempt may even worsen the outcome.[4] Mort found a positive correlation between complications and number of DL intubation attempts in the prehospital setting.[5] Data from these studies suggest that there should be a limit to the number of intubation attempts or that DL should be avoided in favor of alternative methods to secure the patient's airway.

AIRWAY MANAGEMENT

How Would You Assess the Patient's Airway?

Signs of an airway at risk and inadequate breathing, such as the sound of obstruction, gasping, indrawing, use of accessory muscles, and cyanosis can be evaluated within seconds at the scene and must not be missed. Airway evaluation should include a search for signs of airway trauma, neck trauma, and tracheal deviation. Several assessment tools can be used to evaluate a patient's airway and a search for (see Chapter 1). However, these assessment tools are of limited use in this prehospital setting due to limited patient access, unfavorable patient positioning, and the patient was unresponsive. Given the patient's unconscious state, position, and the difficulty of access, it must be assumed airway management would be challenging.

How Is the Airway Usually Managed in Trauma?

Beyond clinical signs of airway patency and adequacy of breathing, effective oxygenation and ventilation should be determined as quickly as practicable via pulse oximetry and end-tidal CO_2 measurement.[1,2] Oxygenation should be improved by high-flow oxygen via a non-rebreather face mask. All patients who are in acute respiratory distress or who are not breathing need immediate airway intervention. A rapid assessment of airway anatomy, appropriate to field conditions, must be done in case ventilatory assistance is required. While the mnemonic MOANS (see section "Difficult BMV: MOANS" in Chapter 1) may predict a difficult bag-mask ventilation (BMV), this assessment tool is not useful for an unresponsive patient. If BMV is difficult in this unresponsive patient due to airway obstruction (e.g., a large tongue), the obstruction can be relieved simply by lifting the chin or by the jaw-thrust maneuver, even though there may be a chance of aggravating C-spine injury. Similarly, the use of an oropharyngeal airway in an unconscious patient with no gag reflex or a nasopharyngeal airway in a patient with no facial or head trauma can be helpful in achieving a patent airway to facilitate BMV.

Patients with a Glasgow Coma Scale score of 8 or less require prompt tracheal intubation. Factors that may predict difficulties with advanced airway maneuvers have to be identified. The mnemonic LEMON (see section "Difficult DL Intubation: LEMON" in Chapter 1) helps predict a difficult DL. However, its use in an unresponsive patient is limited. If no difficulties are anticipated, tracheal intubation with or without drug assistance should follow. If unsuccessful, despite the use of adjuncts such as the Eschmann Tracheal Introducer (ETI, commonly known as "gum-elastic bougie"), extraglottic devices (EGDs) should be considered. In the case of inability to intubate the trachea and to ventilate the patient, a surgical airway should be established.[1,2]

What Are Your Airway Options in This Patient?

Due to the critical condition of this patient with suspected cervical spine injury and the difficult working environment, airway management would be challenging. The options will depend on the skills and level of training of the EMS practitioner. To avoid significant complications, advanced airway techniques should be attempted only by experienced EMS practitioners skilled in alternative methods of airway management. Practitioners with basic skills should rely on chin lift, jaw thrust, and tongue pull as basic airway maneuvers. However, the risk of hypoxemia and hypercarbia has to be balanced against the risk of further aggravating a spinal cord injury with jaw thrust maneuvers, in case a simple chin lift is not sufficient to clear the obstructed airway.

Basic airway maneuvers must be performed with caution and with regard to the cervical spine. In addition to the above-mentioned basic maneuvers, practitioners with advanced airway training should consider the placement of an EGD, such as a Laryngeal Mask Airway or Laryngeal Tube. The type of EGD used will be determined by the protocols of the EMS system. Experienced practitioners should at this point consider establishing a definitive airway using tracheal intubation. DL, video laryngoscopy (VL), intubating LMA, lightwand, or even cricothyrotomy may be used to provide oxygenation and ventilation. Each technique of airway management carries with it the risk of complications. These must be weighed against the risk of lethal hypoxemia coupled with the skills of the practitioner in the adverse environment of the field. Complications of placement of a definitive airway are esophageal intubation, aspiration, and hypoxemia as a result of prolonged intubation attempts. Regardless of the practitioner's experience and level of training, the number of intubation attempts should be limited, as repeated attempts increase the risk of morbidity and mortality.[5]

What Is the Role of the EGD in the Trauma Patient?

EGDs are the first alternative in the "cannot intubate, cannot oxygenate" situation. They have gained popularity as the primary prehospital airway management in a trauma patient.[6–9] Martin et al. reported a success rate of 94% in prehospital use of LMA in trauma patients with all insertions performed in 10 seconds or less. Adequate oxygenation and ventilation were provided with oxygen saturations ranging between 97% and 100% and end-tidal CO_2 between 24 and 35 mmHg.[6]

Multiple second-generation laryngeal masks have been introduced which incorporate an alternate channel for drainage of gastric contents and placement of a gastric tube. Second-generation laryngeal masks (see Chapter 13), for example, the LMA-Supreme, have even higher success rates in placement. Bosch et al. and Länkimäki et al. reported a successful placement of 100% by ground paramedics in prehospital airway management.[10,11] Laryngeal Tubes (see Chapter 13) have also gained some popularity in prehospital airway management. However, there are complications associated with the prehospital use of Laryngeal Tubes, such as significant tongue swelling, distention of the stomach, and significant bleeding due to malpositioning in the piriform sinus.[12]

In summary, EDG used in trauma patients have proven to be effective rescue devices with a very high success rate for proper placement; they reduce the need for DL as well as provide effective oxygenation and ventilation.

What Is Your Concern with Transporting This Patient with an EGD?

Placement of an EGD is an efficient technique for airway management in the prehospital setting. However, two considerations have to be kept in mind during the transport of a patient with an EGD in place. First, the EGD does not provide complete protection against aspiration. Case reports and studies have reported gastric distention and aspiration with the placement of an EGD similar to the LMA or the Laryngeal Tube.[6,12–14] Second-generation devices with a drainage tube at the distal end provide superior but not complete protection against aspiration.[14] The second concern in transporting a trauma patient with an EGD in place is potential malpositioning. Any change in the position of the EGD may impair or may seriously compromising oxygenation and ventilation. A cervical collar to maintain inline stabilization of the cervical spine may cause the EGD to shift or to partially obstruct the airway during transport.[7] Continuous monitoring of the positioning of the device and of effective ventilation must be provided.

What Are Your Options for a Definitive Airway?

The standard for a definitive airway still is endotracheal intubation with DL.[1,2] This requires the practitioner to be positioned above the head of the patient. In our case, the patient is sitting in the driver's seat, and it would be impossible for the clinician to attempt intubation above the patient's head until the roof of the vehicle is removed.

One alternative, the inverse intubation, is ventral approach for laryngoscopy directly facing the patient. This method is performed using the standard laryngoscope in the right hand.[15] The blade is used as a hook to allow a line-of-sight to the glottis. However, the significant anterior motion of the upper cervical spine may be necessary to achieve a line-of-sight to the glottic opening with the potential for complications.[16]

In recent years, multiple "look around the corner" devices as an alternative for DL have been introduced (see Chapter 11). The McGrath Series 5 video laryngoscope provides an indirect view of the glottic opening to allow the practitioner to face the patient from the front. Studies have shown that less movement of the cervical spine is produced during VL compared to standard DL.[17] The Airtraq, an optical laryngoscope using a series of lenses and mirrors, provides not only an indirect view of the glottic opening but also a guiding channel for the endotracheal tube. Both the Airtraq and McGrath Series 5 video laryngoscope were used in studies to compare their effectiveness in a trapped trauma patient simulation. Both devices had a 100% success rate compared to 88% with inverse DL. The intubation time was between 25 and 55 seconds for all three devices, and significantly longer compared to time for placement of EGDs.[17,18]

An alternative approach for endotracheal intubation is to use the Intubating LMA (LMA-Fastrach™) as an adjunct. This is a blind technique. The endotracheal tube is advanced blindly through the metal tube of the LMA-Fastrach into the trachea without visualization. In general, the position of the LMA-Fastrach needs to be adjusted by rotating or lifting the handle anteriorly to allow the endotracheal tube to pass easily through the vocal cords. This may increase the risk of cervical spine injury. In addition, this blind technique may also increase the risk of airway trauma. Overall, the success rate for correct tube placement is in the range of 75% to 90% (see Chapter 13). Another nonvisual technique for endotracheal intubation is the light-guided intubation using the lightwand (Trachlight™). The technique of intubation is well described in Chapter 12. However, since this device is not manufactured anymore since 2009, the experience with the use of this device may diminish over time.

Blind nasotracheal intubation is another approach in the prehospital field in spontaneously breathing patients.[19,20] Even with a low frequency of performance, the success rate is between 70% and 90%. However, the complication rate is reported as 13%.[19] Traumatic brain injuries with potential basal skull fractures and lack of respiratory efforts are contraindications for this technique.

Blind digital intubation (see Chapter 12) is a relatively simple and effective technique that is particularly useful in the emergency setting or under circumstances with limited resources and in which the practitioner cannot be positioned at the head of the patient, rendering direct laryngoscopic intubation impossible. Unfortunately, digital intubation is now often forgotten as a useful alternative technique in the case of an emergency[21] despite a cadaver study establishing that the overall success after 3 attempts may be as high as 90% when performed by emergency medicine residents and staff.[22]

However, the nonvisual techniques, the lightwand-guided, digital, and blind nasal intubation, require a certain skill set and should be restricted to practitioners with experience in those.

If ventilation and oxygenation cannot be provided by either bag-valve-mask, an EGD, or endotracheal intubation, a surgical cricothyrotomy is indicated.[1,2] Surgical cricothyrotomy can be performed quickly and safely in the field by appropriately trained practitioners using the ETI-assisted three-step technique (see Chapter 14).

How Was the Airway Managed in This Patient?

While you are assessing the overweight young patient trapped in the driver seat for any abdominal or thoracic injuries, you recognize sounds of airway obstruction. Going back to your "A" for airway in-patient assessment, you perform a gentle jaw thrust. While doing so, the patient is starting to clench his teeth. The oxygen saturation probe is showing 90% on 100% O_2 through a non-rebreather face mask. Since you plan for a careful extrication with the rescuers, you decide to sedate the patient to allow for airway control. After intravenous administration of 5 mg midazolam and 100 mg ketamine, you can open the mouth of the patient easily and insert a #4 LMA-Supreme™. With assisted spontaneous respiration, the oxygen saturation is increasing to 94% (Figure 18.1). After 10 minutes of technical rescue and extrication, the patient is placed on a spine board and transferred into the helicopter.

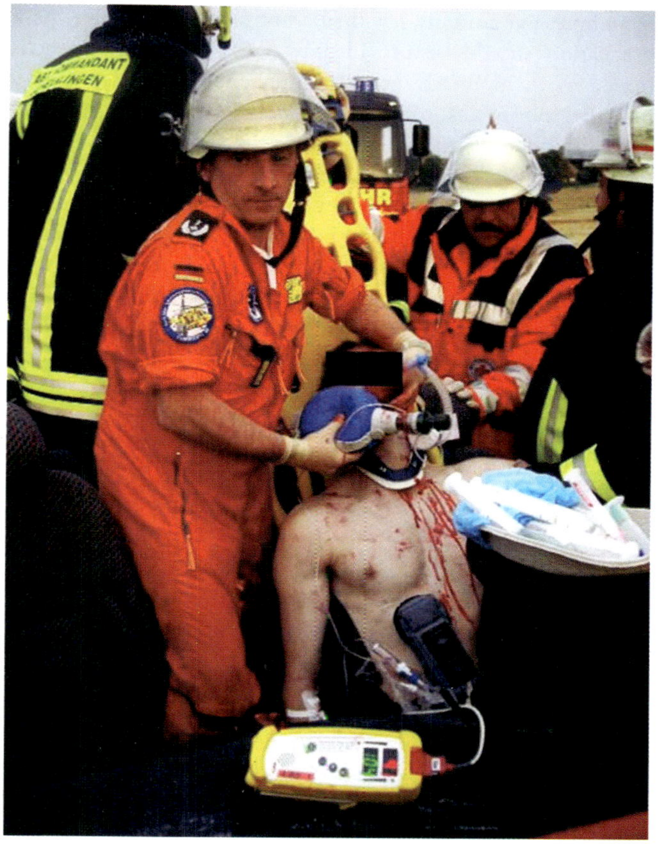

FIGURE 18.1. An unconscious patient still trapped in the vehicle. The roof of the vehicle is already removed by the surrounding firefighters. The airway is secured via a laryngeal mask airway. A spine board is placed once the driver seat is lowered, and the patient will be extricated from the vehicle with spine precautions.

Inside the helicopter, following the ABC protocol you reassess the patient. Due to the patient's obesity (an estimated weight of 95 kg) and his position on the spine board, the abdominal girth impairs ventilation; the oxygen saturation drops to 90%. You decide to secure the airway with an endotracheal tube. However, this patient presents several features of a difficult laryngoscopy. In addition to his obesity, he has a small chin with a reduced thyromental distance, a large overbite, and a potential cervical spine injury. You prepare for a DL with an ETI ready. After administering 140 mg succinylcholine intravenously, you perform a DL with a Mac#3 blade. You see nothing other than the tip of the epiglottis. One attempt with a blind insertion of the bougie fails. Your "plan B" was to reinsert the LMA-Supreme. Quickly, the LMA-Supreme is placed and the patient is ventilated, and the oxygen saturation rises to 92%. Considering a suboptimal oxygenation of an overweight patient with a nondefinitive airway on a long 35-minute flight to the nearest Level 1 trauma center, you decide to perform a surgical (open) cricothyrotomy. After removal of the anterior part of the cervical collar, while still maintaining controlled ventilation via LMA-Supreme, you prepare the neck with an antiseptic solution and make a vertical incision of the skin above the cricothyroid cartilage. You can easily palpate the cricothyroid membrane through the wound; you make a horizontal incision through the membrane and insert an ETI. Immediately you recognize correct placement by feeling the clicks of the tracheal rings. Guided by the ETI, you can advance a 6.0-mm ID endotracheal tube. Correct tube placement is confirmed by end-tidal CO_2 measurement. The oxygen saturation quickly improves to 96% on 100% FiO_2.

SUMMARY

Airway management of an unconscious and apneic patient trapped in a vehicle is one of the most challenging situations for prehospital practitioners. Due to limited access above the head inside the vehicle, standard airway techniques are impossible and the patient's airway needs to be managed face-to-face. The technique employed will depend on the field environment, the patient's condition, available airway resources, and the technical skill of the practitioner.

Following the ATLS guidelines, the focus should be on maintaining oxygenation and ventilation until there is access to the head or the patient is extricated from the vehicle. Basic airway techniques like chin lift, jaw thrust, and assisted bag-valve-mask ventilation should be provided by every prehospital practitioner. With more advanced training, more advanced airway measures can be instituted. These include the use of an EGD and endotracheal intubation. However, endotracheal intubation cannot be performed in the usual fashion and alternative techniques, such as inverse intubation or digital intubation, should be considered. Alternative devices, such as video laryngoscopes, can make face-to-face intubation easier. EGDs such as the Laryngeal Mask Airway or the Laryngeal Tube can easily be placed while facing the patient and can act as a bridge until greater access to the patient is possible and a more advanced airway can be secured. The technique used will depend mostly on the skill of the practitioner. As in all failed-airway scenarios, surgical cricothyrotomy may be necessary in order to oxygenate and ventilate the patient in the vehicle.

SELF-EVALUATION QUESTIONS

18.1. You are called to a motor vehicle collision, where the driver is trapped inside the car. The patient is unconscious and making ineffective respiratory efforts. How do you manage this patient?

A. Extricate the patient as soon as possible.

B. Insert a nasal airway to relieve airway obstruction.

C. Intubate the patient using a rapid sequence induction to avoid aspiration.

D. Following basic airway maneuvers to relieve obstruction, you attempt bag-mask-ventilation.

E. Since you are facing an impending loss of airway, you attempt a surgical cricothyrotomy.

18.2. Which of the following statements is INCORRECT?

A. The risk of aspiration during ventilation with an EGD is low.

B. EGDs are effective alternatives if endotracheal intubation should fail.

C. EGDs can be placed easily facing the patient from the front.

D. EGDs can be used successfully with a steep learning curve in practitioners unfamiliar with advanced airway techniques.

E. All EGDs are equally effective in the trauma population.

18.3. Which of the following may make airway management difficult in the trapped patient?

A. No access from above

B. Intraoral blood from head and neck injury

C. Suspected cervical spine injury

D. Acuity of the scene

E. All of the above

REFERENCES

1. National Association of Emergency Medical Technicians (NAEMT). *Prehospital Trauma Life Support*. 9th ed. Burlington, MA: Jones and Bartlett Publishers; 2018.
2. American College of Surgeons. *Advanced Trauma Life Support Student Course Manual*. 10th ed. Chicago, IL: American College of Surgeons; 2018.
3. Bossers SM, Schwarte LA, Loer SA, Twisk JW, Boer C, Schober P. Experience in prehospital endotracheal intubation significantly influences mortality of patients with severe traumatic brain injury: a systematic review and meta-analysis. *PLoS One*. 2015;10:e0141034.
4. Davis DP, Peay J, Sise MJ, et al. The impact of prehospital endotracheal intubation on outcome in moderate to severe traumatic brain injury. *J Trauma*. 2005;58:933-939.
5. Mort TC. Emergency tracheal intubation: complications associated with repeated laryngoscopy attempts. *Anesth Analg*. 2004;99:607-613.
6. Martin SE, Ochsner MG, Jarman RH, Agudelo WE, Davis FE. Use of the laryngeal mask airway in air transport when intubation fails. *J Trauma*. 1999;47:352-357.
7. Matioc AA, Wells JA. The LMA-unique in a prehospital trauma patient: interaction with semirigid cervical collar: a case report. *J Trauma*. 2002; 52:162-164.
8. Mason AM. Prehospital use of the intubating laryngeal mask airway in patients with severe polytrauma: a case series. *Case Rep Med*. 2009;2009:938531.
9. Shavit I, Aviram E, Hoffmann Y, Biton O, Glassberg E. Laryngeal mask airway as a rescue device for failed endotracheal intubation during scene-to-hospital air transport of combat casualties. *Eur J Emerg Med*. 2018;25:368-371.
10. Bosch J, de Nooji J, de Visser M, et al. Prehospital use in emergency patients of a laryngeal mask airway by ambulance paramedics is a safe and effective alternative for endotracheal intubation. *Emerg Med J*. 2014;31:750-753.
11. Länkimäki S, Alahuhta S, Silfvast T, Kurola J. Feasibility of LMA supreme for airway management in unconscious patients by ALS paramedics. *Scand J Trauma Resusc Emerg Med*. 2015;23:24.
12. Schalk R, Seeger FH, Mutlak H, et al. Complications associated with the prehospital use of laryngeal tubes—a systematic analysis of risk factors and strategies for prevention. *Resuscitation*. 2014;85:1629-1632.
13. Bernardini A, Natalini G. Risk of pulmonary aspiration with laryngeal mask airway and tracheal tube: analysis on 65 712 procedures with positive pressure ventilation. *Anaesthesia*. 2009;64:1289-1294.
14. Brimacomb J, Keller C. Aspiration of gastric contents during use of a ProSeal laryngeal mask airway secondary to unidentified foldover malposition. *Anesth Analg*. 2009;97:1192-1194.
15. Hilker T, Genzwuerker HV. Inverse intubation: an important alternative for intubation in the streets. *Prehosp Emerg Care*. 1999;3:74-76.
16. Smally AJ, Dufel S, Beckham J. Inverse intubation: potential for complications. *J Trauma*. 2002;52:1005-1007.
17. Schober P, Krage R, Van Groeningen D, Loer SA, Schwarte LA. Inverse intubation in entrapped trauma casualties: a simulator based randomized cross-over comparison of direct, indirect and video laryngoscopy. *Emerg Med J*. 2014;31:959-963.
18. Pap R, van Loggerenberg C. A comparison of airway management devices in simulated entrapment-trauma: a prospective manikin study. *Int J Emerg Med*. 2019;12:15.
19. O'Brien GJ, Danzl DF, Hooker EA, Daniel LM, Dolan MC. Prehospital blind nasotracheal intubation by paramedics. *Ann Emerg Med*. 1989; 18:612-617.
20. Zhang J, Lamb A, Hung O, Hung C, Hung D. Blind nasal intubation: teaching a dying art. *Can J Anaesth*. 2014;61:1055-1056.
21. Gordon G. Remember the simple digital alternative. *Anesth Analg*. 2004;98:1194.
22. Young SE, Miller MA, Crystal CS, Skinner C, Coon TP. Is digital intubation an option for emergency physicians in definitive airway management? *Am J Emerg Med*. 2006;24:729-732.

CHAPTER 19

Airway Management of a Motorcycle with a Full-Face Helmet Following an Accident

Mark P. Vu and Orlando R. Hung

CASE PRESENTATION

A 29-year-old male motorcyclist presents to the emergency department (ED) accompanied by a paramedic rescue team after being involved in a high-speed motor vehicle crash (MVC). The motorcyclist was traveling at approximately 65 km per hour (40 miles per hour) when he drove through an intersection and collided with a car. Although damage to the car was minimal, the motorcycle was severely damaged and the patient was found approximately 50 m (160 ft) from the point of impact. The patient's vital signs at the scene were: HR 110 beats per minute (bpm), BP 120/70 mmHg, RR 24 breaths per minute, and SpO_2 93% on room air. Paramedics placed the patient on a spine board and transferred him to the ED. In the ED, he complains of pain in his chest, difficulty breathing, and pain in his legs. He is wearing a nonmodular full-face helmet. His vital signs are found to be HR 120 bpm, BP 110/50 mmHg, RR 32 breaths per min, SpO_2 89%, and he is becoming confused. There is clinical evidence of a compound fracture of his right femur.

PATIENT CONSIDERATIONS

■ What Are the Initial Steps in the Management of This Patient?

The general principles of trauma care and resuscitation apply to this patient. An initial, rapid survey of the patient's vital functions is undertake, including immediately identification of sites of major hemorrhage, followed by assessment of airway, breathing and circulation.[1] Large bore intravenous access, oxygen and basic monitoring (pulse oximetry, ECG, and serial blood pressure readings) are instituted quickly. Supplemental oxygen had been provided in the field by placing an inverted simple face mask through the opening of the helmet, an acceptable maneuver if the helmet cannot be easily or safely removed for a primary survey. He is nonobese. His airway assessment shows that he is wearing a full-face, nonmodular type motorcycle helmet, obscuring his mouth from view. His nose and nares are visible above the line of the face shield portion of the helmet, and his anterior neck is visible and displays normal anatomy. Rapid examination of his chest demonstrates equal air entry bilaterally and his pulses are equal. Although the patient is protecting his airway, he is breathing and has an adequate blood pressure, after completion of the primary survey he may require intervention to control his airway and breathing.

■ Are There Recommendations in the Advanced Trauma Life Support® (ATLS®) Guidelines for the Removal of Helmets Prior to Transport?

There is currently no consensus regarding whether prehospital personnel should routinely remove a patient's helmet prior to transport to hospital. Individual patient factors and coexisting injuries will guide this decision. If possible, the helmet should remain in place unless emergency airway intervention or respiratory support is needed, in which case the helmet should be carefully removed in a manner that minimizes cervical spine motion. Most helmet removal techniques endorse a two-person approach; one person stabilizes the patient's head from below while another person carefully removes the helmet from above.[2] New safety innovations in motor sports helmets include specialized helmet removal systems that facilitate the safe, careful removal of a helmet from a patient (e.g., EQRS™, Shock Doctor Eject Helmet Removal System™). Prehospital personnel should be encouraged to consult with a hospital-based EMS physician if questions regarding patient care exist. Airway practitioners who provide first responder care to motor sports athletes wearing helmets should familiarize themselves with these specialized helmet release systems.

Are There Recommendations in the ATLS Guidelines for the Removal of Helmets Once the Patient Has Arrived in Hospital?

There is also no consensus on when or how a patient's helmet should be removed once the patient arrives in hospital. If the patient's condition is stable, the helmet can remain in place during the trauma assessment to minimize the potential for cervical spine movement. After a careful neurological assessment, and if the patient is in stable condition, removal of the helmet under fluoroscopy may be considered. If the patient's condition necessitates emergency airway or breathing support, the risks of providing airway management with the helmet in place should be carefully weighed against the risks of emergency removal of the helmet. These issues will be discussed later in this chapter.

Following a High-Speed Motorcycle Crash, What Other Injuries Might You Anticipate for This Patient?

Anticipating and identifying coexisting medical conditions in patients is important for practitioners. Alcohol is often a factor in motorcycle crashes and should be suspected in all cases.[3] A prospective study in 1996 involving 150 patients admitted to the emergency surgical service following an MVC showed that 37% were intoxicated with blood alcohol concentration[4] (BAC) greater than or equal to 100 $mg{\cdot}dL^{-1}$ or 0.1% (1% BAC by volume = 10 $mg{\cdot}mL^{-1}$, and the BAC legal limit is between 0.08% and 0.1% depending on the Province or State). Other causes for the crash should also be considered, including cerebrovascular accident, cardiac event, seizure, or intoxication from substances other than alcohol. A focused survey of the patient as suggested by the ATLS guidelines[1] will help to identify injuries that will significantly affect airway management decisions. Airway practitioners should presume that this group of patients will have a full stomach and are at high risk for a cervical spine injury. In addition, patients with open-face helmets are at higher risk of sustaining facial injuries, but these injuries are still possible in patients wearing full-face helmets. A rigorous assessment of the oropharynx, nasal passages, and ears is often difficult in patients wearing helmets and the benefits of a nasotracheal approach to endotracheal intubation should be weighed against the risks of this procedure in this patient population.

AIRWAY CONSIDERATIONS

What Types of Helmets Worn by Motorcyclists Can Pose Problems for Airway Management?

Motorcycle helmets can be grouped into two categories in the context of airway management: open-face and full-face. Open-face helmets cover the cranium, and sometimes cover the ears, but do not cover the neck, chin, mouth, or nose. These features make them less protective to the patient in the event of a crash. There is an increase in the likelihood of serious anterior neck and facial injuries affecting airway anatomy, but concurrently renders airway assessment and intervention more straightforward. Full-face helmets are more protective to patient's face in the event of a crash, but are a major hindrance to airway assessment and intervention since access to the mouth is practically impossible (Figure 19.1). Moreover, the removal of full-face helmets can be difficult, resulting in potentially significant cervical spine motion.[5,6] Laun et al.[7] conducted a study to evaluate the cervical spinal movement during the removal of a full-face helmet in 10 fresh cadavers with an experimental unstable fractured odontoid. Under fluoroscopy, there was significant movement of C1–C2 during helmet removal and dislocation of C1–C2 in two cases. Although the clinical significance of these findings in live patients is unknown, this study suggests that there is a potential risk of spinal cord injury during the removal of a full-face helmet.

An important variation of the full-face helmet is the "modular" full-face helmet (Figure 19.2). The design of this helmet allows the movement of the face shield portion of the helmet away from the face. This helmet design allows the effective conversion of a full-face helmet into an open-face configuration, making airway management with the helmet in place more feasible.

Should Helmets Always Be Removed in Order to Provide Airway Management?

Removal of helmets for airway management is case-dependent. There is currently no consensus on whether helmets should

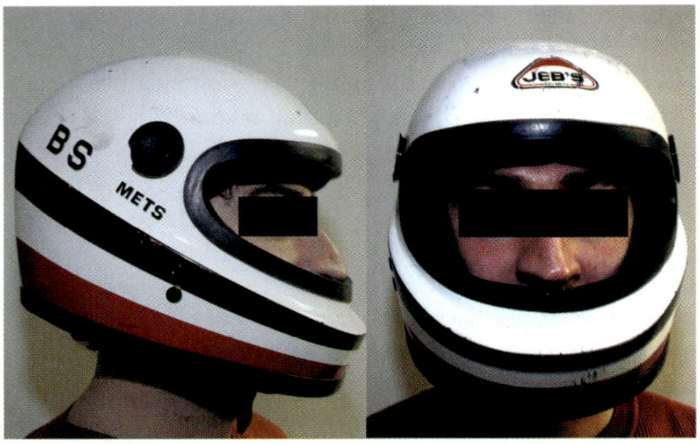

FIGURE 19.1. Full-face-type helmets present a challenge to airway practitioners. The patient's mouth is completely obscured by the face shield portion of the helmet (Left). In general, the nose and neck are readily accessible (Right). However, in some types of full-face helmets, access to the nose may be limited.

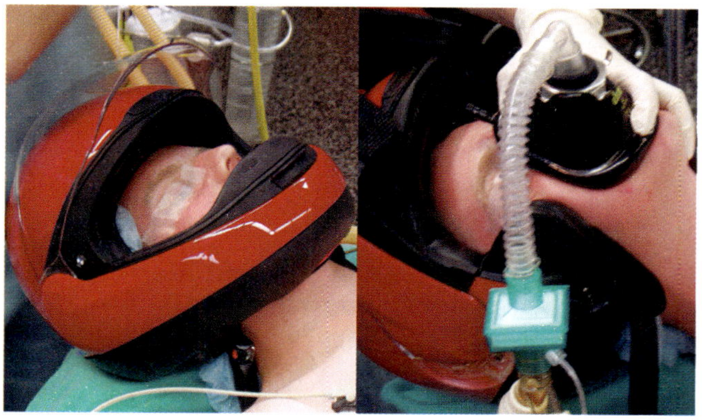

FIGURE 19.2. Modular-type helmets allow more options for airway interventions (Left). Displacement of the face shield cephalad (Right) allows full access to the patient's nose, mouth, and neck as well as ventilation using a face mask.

be routinely removed prior to airway management in trauma patients. There are concerns that cervical spine movement during helmet removal may be significant. Although the evidence of cervical spine movement during helmet removal has been supported by radiographic studies in cadavers, its clinical importance remains unknown. In prehospital care, the removal of helmets by paramedics is standard prior to airway management. However, in sports medicine it is sometimes recommended that emergency medical personnel have the tools to remove face shields in order to provide airway management with the helmet in place.[8] Some sports helmets brands now have "quick release" features that allow medical personnel to quickly and easily remove face masks to allow access to the airway without removing the helmet (e.g., Riddell Speedflex Helmet, Riddell™). Hospital-based airway practitioners should expect situations in which prehospital personnel have deferred definitive airway management until arrival at the hospital and therefore should be prepared for any scenario.

Describe a Systematic Approach to Manage the Airway of a Patient Wearing a Motorcycle Helmet

Assessment of any patient wearing a motorcycle helmet should be completed in the standard fashion aiming to assess the feasibility of providing oxygenation and ventilation by: (1) face mask; (2) extraglottic device (EGD); (3) tracheal intubation by direct and indirect laryngoscopy; or (4) a front-of-neck airway (FONA). The first part of the assessment of a patient wearing a motorcycle helmet is identifying whether the helmet is open-face or full-face configuration.

In a patient wearing an open-face helmet, airway management can be performed with the helmet in place and the patient's head can be manually stabilized by an assistant to minimize movement of the head and neck. Face-mask ventilation (FMV), EGD insertion, tracheal intubation, and FONA are commonly straightforward in this scenario. If the open-face helmet has a visor, it can be removed to optimize line-of-sight during direct laryngoscopy.

In a patient wearing a full-face helmet, the practitioner must now determine whether or not the helmet is a modular type. If it is a modular-type full-face helmet, the helmet may be left in place and the face shield portion can be carefully retracted superiorly to expose the face and neck. Once this is done, the airway can be managed with considerations similar to an open-face style helmet. It should be noted that a retracted face shield might obscure the line-of-sight during direct laryngoscopy. Alternative orotracheal intubating devices such as a lightwand, a video laryngoscope, or a rigid/flexible fiberoptic intubation device could be useful.

In a patient wearing a full-face helmet that is not modular, several important issues must be carefully considered. FMV and EGD insertion are practically impossible because access to the mouth and face is extremely limited by the face shield. Direct laryngoscopy is also impossible for the same reason. Access to the neck for a FONA is often possible and the anatomical landmarks for cricothyrotomy should be carefully assessed. At this juncture, the practitioner should decide: (1) Can the helmet be removed prior to airway management? (2) Should the helmet be removed prior to airway management? In many cases, it may be most appropriate to remove the helmet prior to airway interventions since this provides practitioners with the opportunity to properly assess the patient and optimally expose all relevant anatomy. Although there is no consensus on the proper technique for helmet removal, most authors advocate a two-person technique as described above. Helmets with specialized release mechanisms should be removed according to the manufacturer's instructions. These instructions can sometimes be found written on the sides of the helmet. Once the helmet is removed, oxygenation and ventilation can be provided in the standard fashion.

Should the Endotracheal Intubation Be Performed Awake?

In any patient wearing a motorcycle helmet, particularly a full-face helmet, difficulties in airway management can be expected. FMV is impossible in patients wearing a full-face helmet. Laryngoscopy is difficult or impossible with full-face helmets, as is EGD insertion. In light of this, an awake intubation approach should be considered and is a reasonable option in cooperative patients. Unfortunately, awake intubation in this group of patients is challenging because they are often uncooperative and have significant secretions or blood in their airway, limiting the efficacy of topical anesthesia and visualization. Practitioners must consider the challenges of an awake technique and be prepared to proceed to an alternative plan.

DIFFICULT SITUATIONS: WHEN THE HELMET CANNOT BE REMOVED

Describe How You Would Provide Oxygenation and Ventilation in a Situation Where You Cannot Remove a Nonmodular, Full-Face Helmet

Arguably the most challenging situation for a practitioner is when a patient wearing a full-face helmet needs oxygenation and ventilation but the helmet cannot be easily removed.

Many circumstances can make helmet removal difficult or impossible. Examples of such situations include patients with foreign objects penetrating the helmet and embedded in the skull and patients in whom removal of the helmet causes them extreme pain or distress, or individuals trapped in confined spaces where the helmet cannot be removed (e.g., inside a race car). A systematic assessment of the airway management options for this patient will show that FMV is impossible because the helmet's face shield obscures the mouth and chin. Similarly, insertion of an EGD is practically impossible because access to the mouth is also limited. The two remaining options are: (1) nasotracheal intubation or (2) FONA using a cricothyrotomy. Rapid assessment of the surgical landmarks relevant to an open cricothyrotomy is essential since this part of the patient's airway is usually unobstructed by the helmet or face shield. Securing the airway by a nasotracheal route is relatively simple and potentially useful and lifesaving. Airway practitioners familiar with nasotracheal intubation techniques should review the contraindications to this approach, such as evidence of basal skull fracture, prior to proceeding. Blind nasal intubation in a spontaneously breathing patient has a reasonable success rate among experienced practitioners. Two reports showed that the blind nasal intubating technique has a 90% success rate for prehospital trauma patients requiring an endotracheal tube (ETT).[9,10] However, the success of blind nasotracheal intubation is limited by practitioner skill. A flexible lightwand, such as the Trachlight™, loaded on a nasotracheal tube can be effectively used to achieve endotracheal intubation in a patient wearing a full-face helmet.[11] In this technique, transtracheal illumination using the lightwand indirectly confirms the proper placement of the nasotracheal tube.[12] If blood is present in the airway, the potential for a false passage in the airway makes a blind technique relatively contraindicated. Moreover, light-guided techniques may be difficult in prehospital environments where bright ambient light may make identification of transtracheal illuminated landmarks difficult. Using a flexible bronchoscope can be a helpful guide, especially in situations where blind techniques are contraindicated, but its efficacy may be limited by the presence of blood or secretions in the airway. Flexible endoscopic intubation can be performed with the patient awake and the nasopharyngeal mucosa topically anesthetized or with the patient under general anesthesia with muscle relaxation. The risks of each approach should be considered in the context of the patient's co-morbidities and the practitioner's familiarity with the techniques.

Airway practitioners are strongly advised to consider a "double set-up" plan that includes both a primary intubation approach (e.g., a light-guided nasotracheal intubation, flexible bronchoscope, etc.) and a secondary backup FONA approach for the patient wearing a full-face helmet that cannot be removed. Since the patient's neck is almost always accessible regardless of the type of helmet worn, a "double set-up" facilitates prompt airway control via a surgical access in case the primary plan is unsuccessful. Two separate equipment trays should be prepared: the first contains all the equipment needed for oral or nasotracheal access; the second tray contains all the instruments needed for a FONA (surgical airway). Having a second skilled practitioner available who is familiar with surgical airway access is ideal. Prior to initiating the airway intervention, the patient should be optimally positioned, the neck should be prepped and the airway management team should agree on clear "trigger points" that identify when the primary approach has failed and the secondary approach is to be undertaken (i.e., surgical airway).

How Do You Perform a Light-Guided Nasotracheal Intubation for This Patient If It Becomes Necessary?

An appropriately sized uncut ETT should be used. While it is not possible to warm and soften the ETT in this emergency situation, generous lubrication of the ETT will facilitate nasal intubation and minimize injury. The Trachlight (or a flexible lightwand) is prepared as previously described (see Chapter 12) with the stiff internal wire stylet removed so that the ETT/Trachlight (ETT/TL) unit is pliable and suitable for nasal intubation. Ideally, a vasoconstrictor, e.g., xylometazoline hydrochloride (Otrivin™) nasal spray (if available and time permits), should be administered prior to the insertion of the ETT/TL through the nostril. Following the placement of the ETT/TL tip into the nasopharynx, it is advanced gently into the glottic opening using the transillumination of the soft tissues of the anterior neck. As it is not possible to perform a jaw lift with the full-face helmet in place, a gentle jaw thrust with minimal neck movement can be performed by an assistant to elevate the tongue and epiglottis. Using the light glow, the tip of the ETT/TL is then guided to the glottic opening. When the tip of the ETT enters the glottic opening, a bright circumscribed glow can be seen readily just below the thyroid prominence and the ETT/TL unit is then advanced into the trachea.

The efficacy of Trachlight-facilitated nasotracheal intubation in patients wearing motor cycle helmets was demonstrated in a study in patients under general anesthesia.[11] A BMW System IV motorcycle helmet was used to demonstrate the feasibility of nasotracheal intubation with the face mask in the "down" position, and the modular design of the helmet also secondarily demonstrated that face-mask oxygenation and ventilation was easy to perform with the face mask in the "up" position (Figure 19.2). Transtracheal illumination was easily identified in the operating room setting and mean intubation times were relatively rapid with no complications (Figure 19.3).

How Do You Perform an Emergency Front-of-Neck Airway (Surgical Airway) for This Patient If It Becomes Necessary?

In a scenario where the patient's helmet cannot be physically removed and emergency airway management is necessary, a surgical airway should be considered. There are multiple approaches to surgical airway access (see Chapter 14). For non-surgeons or airway practitioners not familiar with emergency open tracheotomy techniques, a recommended approach is the tracheal introducer ("bougie")-facilitated open cricothyrotomy. This approach combines the speed of the open cricothyrotomy with the familiarity of the "bougie" (see Chapter 14). The "bougie"-facilitated cricothyrotomy requires the practitioner to

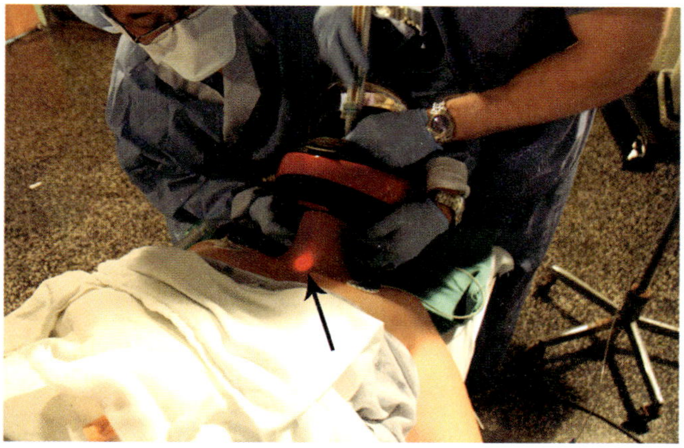

FIGURE 19.3. Light-guided nasotracheal intubation using a Trachlight through a full-face modular type helmet (BMW System IV helmet). With a gentle jaw thrust, the ETT/TL was inserted through the nostril and into the nasopharynx. When the tip entered the glottic opening, a bright circumscribed glow (*arrow*) was seen below the thyroid prominence.

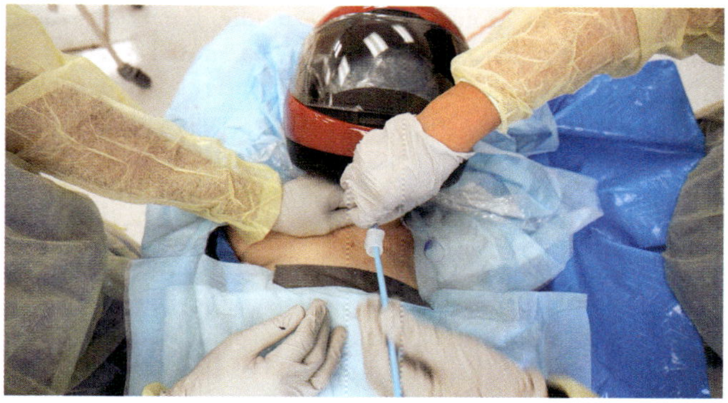

FIGURE 19.5. A "bougie"-facilitated open cricothyrotomy technique in a fresh-grade cadaver with a full-face helmet. Following the correct endotracheal placement of the "bougie," the ETT is then advanced over the "bougie" into the trachea.

use a scalpel to incise the skin of the anterior neck in a vertical midline incision, palpate the cricoid cartilage with a gloved finger, make a horizontal incision of the cricothyroid membrane with the scalpel, and pass a "bougie" into the trachea. It is the preference of the authors to perform the open "bougie"-facilitated cricothyrotomy in a patient with a full-face helmet standing (or kneeling if the patient is on the ground) on the left side of the patient with the nondominant hand (left hand of most practitioners) immobilize the trachea and the dominant hand to make the vertical midline incision (Figure 19.4), followed by the horizontal incision of the cricothyroid membrane and the insertion of the "bougie." The correct endotracheal position of the "bougie" is confirmed by the familiar "clicks" of the coude tip of the "bougie" passing over the anterior tracheal cartilages. The ETT is then advanced over the "bougie" into the trachea (Figure 19.5). Emergency "bougie"-facilitated cricothyrotomy has gained the endorsement of many advanced airway management experts as well as Emergency Medicine organizations due to the simplicity of the procedure, the availability of the equipment used, and its effectiveness.[13]

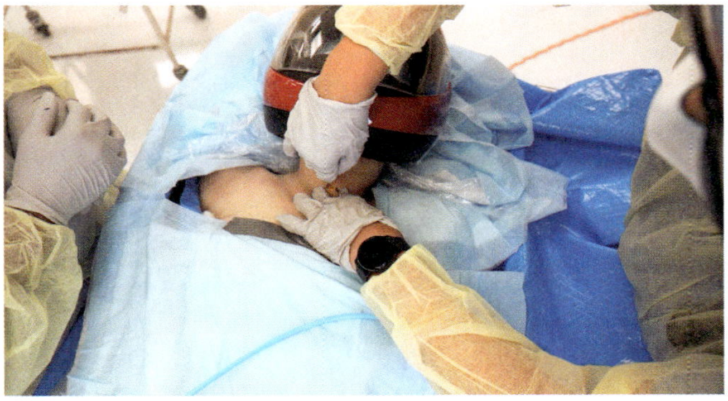

FIGURE 19.4. A "bougie"-facilitated open cricothyrotomy technique in a fresh-grade cadaver with a full-face helmet. The practitioner stands on the left side of the cadaver with the nondominant hand immobilizing the trachea and the dominant hand making the vertical midline incision.

Would Your Approach to Airway Management Change for a Patient Who Is Wearing a Sports Helmet?

The approach to a patient who is wearing a different type of protective helmet is similar.[14] Sports helmets can be open-face or full-face and can have various styles of face shields. Many of these face shields can be easily removed with simple tools, such as a screwdriver. For example, the cage of a football helmet can be easily removed using a cage removal tool that can instantly convert a caged and inaccessible airway into a manageable airway. Current recommendations suggest that injured athletes requiring emergency medical care should have their face shields removed and their helmets left in place for airway management.[15,16] This highlights the fact that sports helmets have face shields or cages that are easily removed and recognizes research suggesting that cervical spine motion is lessened when the helmet is left in place. Further consideration should be given to neutralizing c-spine movement by removing shoulder pads and other protective equipment if the helmet is removed for airway management.

SUMMARY

Airway management in patients wearing a helmet can present a major challenge to airway practitioners. The principles of airway management remain the same regardless of whether or not the patient is wearing a helmet; however, the type of helmet can significantly impact the options available to practitioners. It is worth remembering that almost all patients wearing a helmet are trauma patients, and so the usual considerations of full stomach, head injury, and cervical spine precautions are applicable. If a patient's airway can be managed with the helmet in place, this is often a safer option if an unstable cervical spine injury is suspected. Removing a helmet prior to airway management is often appropriate to optimize conditions for airway intervention, but should be done carefully. Rarely, situations occur where a patient's helmet cannot be removed but oxygenation and ventilation must be provided, and practitioners must have a plan and the skills to deal with this challenging situation.

SELF-EVALUATION QUESTIONS

19.1. You are about to perform a tracheal intubation in an unconscious, 29-year-old male motorcycle driver who was involved in a high-speed motor vehicle crash (MVC). His open-face helmet is in place. His airway examination is favorable, and he has no predictors of difficult facemask ventilation, extraglottic device insertion, or laryngoscopy. Regarding his helmet, which of the following statements is true?

A. A skilled assistant should maintain inline stabilization of the patient's head and neck during the airway intervention.

B. If the open-face style helmet is not obstructing the line-of-sight for laryngoscopy, it may remain in place during the airway intervention.

C. A rapid sequence induction (RSI) technique with a muscle relaxant is a reasonable choice to facilitate endotracheal intubation.

D. All of the above are true.

19.2. A 20-year-old motorcycle driver is involved in a high-speed MVC. He is brought to your hospital on a spine board still wearing his full-face-style helmet. His vital signs are stable and he is cooperative. He complains of pain in his left leg and his neck. You should:

A. Remove his helmet immediately and provide supplemental oxygen.

B. Carefully remove the helmet by yourself and ask the patient to inform you of any discomfort.

C. Ask the patient to carefully remove the helmet himself while you assist him.

D. Complete your primary survey assessment, provide oxygen through his helmet if necessary, and complete lateral C-spine X-rays with the helmet in place prior to removing the helmet with the assistance of a skilled colleague.

19.3. You assess a 50-year-old male motorcyclist who was involved in a high-speed MVC. He is wearing a modular full-face helmet with the face shield retracted. He is unconscious, breathing spontaneously, and is receiving oxygenation and ventilation via a i-gel placed in the field by paramedics after multiple failed attempts at laryngoscopy. He is obese and has a full beard. His SpO_2 on FiO_2 1.00 is 87%, BP 110/70, HR 100, RR 24 assisted. You quickly review this case with a colleague and decide that your safest plan to establish a definitive airway is:

A. Leave the Combitube in place indefinitely.

B. Replace the Combitube with an LMA.

C. Give succinylcholine, remove the Combitube and replace it with an orotracheal tube under direct laryngoscopy.

D. Perform a cricothyrotomy with the Combitube in place and the patient breathing spontaneously.

REFERENCES

1. American College of Surgeons: Committee on Trauma. *Advanced Trauma Life Support (ATLS STudent Course Manual)*. 10th ed. Chicago, IL: American College of Surgeons; 2018.
2. Tintinalli JE. *Emergency Medicine: A Comprehensive Study Guide*. New York, NY: McGraw Hill Professional Publishing; 2003.
3. Hurt H, Ouellet J, Thom D. *Motorcycle Accident Cause Factors and Identification of Countermeasures. Technical Report*. Traffic Safety Center, Los Angeles, CA: University of Southern California; 1981.
4. Mancino M, Cunningham MR, Davidson P, Fulton RL. Identification of the motor vehicle accident victim who abuses alcohol: an opportunity to reduce trauma. *J Stud Alcohol*. 1996;57:652-628.
5. Brimacombe J, Keller C, Kunzel KH, Gaber O, Boehler M, Puhringer F. Cervical spine motion during airway management: a cinefluoroscopic study of the posteriorly destabilized third cervical vertebrae in human cadavers. *Anesth Analg*. 2000;91:1274-1248.
6. Kolman JM, Hung OR, Beauprie IG. Evaluation of cervical spine movement during helmet removal. *Can J Anesth*. 2003;50:A18.
7. Laun RA, Lignitz E, Haase N, Latta LL, Ekkernkamp A, Richter D. Mobility of unstable fractures of the odontoid during helmet removal. A biomechanical study. *Unfallchirurg*. 2002;105:1092-1096.
8. Waninger KN. On-field management of potential cervical spine injury in helmeted football players: leave the helmet on! *Clin J Sport Med*. 1998;8:124-129.
9. Dauphinee K. Nasotracheal intubation. *Emerg Med Clin North Am*. 1988;6:715-723.
10. Weitzel N, Kendall J, Pons P. Blind nasotracheal intubation for patients with penetrating neck trauma. *J Trauma*. 2004;56:1097-1101.
11. Vu M, Guzzo A, Hung OR, et al. A novel method for endotracheal intubation in patients wearing full-face helmets. *World Congr Anesthesiol*. 2004;CD014.
12. Hung OR, Pytka S, Morris I, et al. Clinical trial of a new lightwand device (Trachlight) to intubate the trachea. *Anesthesiology*. 1995;83:509-514.
13. Frerk C, Mitchell VS, McNarry AF, et al. Difficult Airway Society 2015 guidelines for management of unanticipated difficult intubation in adults-dagger. *Br J Anaesth*. 2015;115:827-848.
14. Bowman TG, Boergers RJ, Lininger MR. Airway management in athletes wearing Lacrosse equipment. *J Athl Train*. 2018;53:240-248.
15. Laprade RF, Schnetzler KA, Broxterman RJ, Wentorf F, Gilbert TJ. Cervical spine alignment in the immobilized ice hockey player. a computed tomographic analysis of the effects of helmet removal. *Am J Sports Med*. 2000;28:800-803.
16. Swenson TM, Lauerman WC, Blanc RO, Donaldson WF3rd, Fu FH. Cervical spine alignment in the immobilized football player. Radiographic analysis before and after helmet removal. *Am J Sports Med*. 1997;25:226-230.

CHAPTER 20

Management of Opioid-Induced Respiratory Depression

David Hung, Ronald D. Stewart, and Orlando R. Hung

CASE PRESENTATION

A 34-year-old male was found unconscious and with abnormal breathing by his roommate. The patient has a known history of chronic pain as well as opioid use disorder who was recently started on daily sublingual Suboxone (a combination medication containing buprenorphine and naloxone). 911 was called and the roommate was instructed to check for a pulse which was present. He was instructed to administer the take-home naloxone kit provided by their pharmacy, for which 0.4 mg was given intramuscularly in the lateral thigh. Within 3 minutes the patient's eyes opened and he appeared to be breathing spontaneously. Paramedics arrived on scene 10 minutes later to find the male with a respiratory rate of 8 bpm, SpO_2 81%, a Glasgow Coma Scale (GCS) of 7 (E2V1M4), pupils 1 mm bilaterally, but with a strong carotid pulse. Blood pressures, heart rate, temperature, and blood glucose were within normal limits. Airway management was provided including face-mask ventilation (FMV) with an oropharyngeal airway (OPA) while an intravenous (IV) was established. A second dose of naloxone was administered intravenously at 0.4 mg. One minute later, the respiratory rate improved as well as GCS, from 7 to 14. The OPA was removed, and the patient was transported to the emergency department (ED) for ongoing assessment and management.

INTRODUCTION

How Common Is the Opioid-Related Overdose?

The opioid epidemic has been a global health crisis with a significant mortality and disease burden. In Canada, nearly 25,000 deaths were attributed to opioid toxicity deaths between 2016 and 2021. Increasing mortality has been attributed to two overarching themes: historical overprescription of opioids for pain and the contamination of illicit drugs with fentanyl, fentanyl analogues, and other opioids. Given this alarming number of opioid-related deaths, our strategic priority must be to reduce the risk of death of the opioid user.

Despite increasing mortality rates, there have been significant developments aimed at reducing opioid-related overdoses and death. These initiatives cross multiple domains, including patients, families, health care providers, the general public, and policymakers, and are described under three general pillars: primary prevention, access to treatment, and harm reduction. Primary prevention includes education to high-risk population groups, prescription monitoring programs, and increasing access to chronic pain specialists. Treatment access refers to expanding the availability of opioid agonist therapy (OAT) programs for medications such as methadone and buprenorphine, and ensuring that formularies cover costs. Lastly, the philosophy of "harm reduction" accepts the behavior as reality and shifts the focus from prosecution and focuses on reducing its harmful consequences such as infectious disease, incarceration, and death. Harm reduction strategies include safe injection sites, widely distributed naloxone kits, and Good Samaritan laws protecting individuals who seek to provide or receive medical assistance during illicit overdose who would otherwise fear criminal prosecution.[1]

Although it is abundantly clear that reducing opioid-related deaths is a multifaceted issue, the focus of this discussion will be on priorities for managing the airway in a patient who is unconscious from a suspected opioid overdose.

Discuss Briefly the Pharmacology of Opioids

Although numerous opioid receptor (OR) subtypes have been identified, only four have been established unequivocally: μ (MOR), κ (KOR), δ (DOR), and the nociception/orphanin FQ peptide receptor (NOP).[2] Each receptor elicits a different effect implying that knowing which opioids preferentially bind to which receptor allows one to predict the clinical effect. However, binding is usually not limited to a single receptor type accounting for the substantial crossover that is witnessed. Regardless, a basic understanding of the effects of each receptor remains important.

MOR can be subcategorized into two subtypes: MOR1 and MOR2. MOR1 is largely responsible for supraspinal analgesia and euphoria while MOR2 produces spinal-level analgesia and is implicated in respiratory depression. All MOR-agonists produce some degree of MOR2 activity. MORs can be found in the brain, medullary cough center, gastrointestinal (GI) tract, and peripheral nerves. KOR stimulation is responsible for spinal analgesia, diuresis and, most notably, miosis. Neither respiratory depression nor constipation has been associated with KOR activation. Although little is known about DOR, it has been implicated in supraspinal and spinal analgesia, modulation of MOR function, and inhibition of dopamine release.[3] Many different opioid agonists and antagonists bind to NOP, but its insensitivity to antagonism with Naloxone historically has contributed to its delayed acceptance as an OR subtype. Despite a lack of consensus, clinically it has been associated with anxiolysis and analgesia.[4]

What Is the Mechanism of Opioid-Induced Respiratory Depression (OIRD)?

OIRD is mediated through several mechanisms including respiratory rhythm generation by the central nervous system (CNS) via disruptions of the pre-Bötzinger complex of the medulla, and similarly diminishes the sensitivity of medullary chemoreceptors to hypercapnia.[2] Additionally, opioids depress the ventilatory response to hypoxemia. The combined loss of hypoxemic and hypercarbic drive eliminates the stimulus to breathe resulting in apnea.[5] Opioids exhibit approximately the same degree of respiratory depression across equianalgesic doses; however with agonist-antagonists or partial agonists such as buprenorphine, a relative ceiling of respiratory depression has been described.[6] This can be explained by the receptor subtypes on which they act; agonist-antagonist are either predominantly KOR or partial MOR-agonists.

What Are the Risk Factors for OIRD?

There are numerous risk factors that can predispose patients to OIRD which can be broadly categorized into prescription-specifics, patient factors, and polypharmacy. High opioid doses, prolonged duration of action, and extended-release formulations predispose patients to both dependence and OIRD. Patient factors include age (65 and over and 18-25), respiratory pathology including obstructive sleep apnea (OSA), asthma and chronic obstructive pulmonary disease (COPD), ischemic cardiac disease, cachexia, mobility restrictions, mental health disorders, or concomitant substance and/or alcohol use disorder. Polypharmacy is another contributing risk factor, especially for those who are prescribed benzodiazepines, sedatives/hypnotics, muscle relaxants, antipsychotics, or CNS depressants.

A recent case-controlled study in an adult hospitalized patient population by Boitor et al.[7] identified the risk factors for opioid-induced respiratory depression. These include renal and liver failure, concomitant administration of CNS depressants such as benzodiazepines, the first 24 hours of opioid administration, cardiac and respiratory disease, and advanced age.[7] In a surgical population, Gupta et al.[8] reported that elderly, female sex, presence of OSA, COPD, cardiac disease, diabetes mellitus, hypertension, neurologic disease, renal disease, obesity, two or more comorbidities, opioid dependence, use of patient-controlled analgesia, different routes of administration of opioids, and concomitant administration of sedatives are significant risk factors for postoperative OIRD.[8]

Discuss the Pharmacology of the Current Opioid Antagonists Available

Naloxone, naltrexone, nalmefene, and methylnaltrexone are competitive opioid antagonists at MOR, KOR, and DOR. They reverse the actions of opioid-agonists and cause withdrawal in opioid-dependent patients. Although all opioid antagonists have been shown to be safe to administer during overdose, naloxone's fast-onset and short-acting properties render an advantage over its long-acting counterpart nalmefene which can take 1 to 2 hours for peak effect.[9]

Naloxone can rapidly reverse opioid-induced respiratory depression (OIRD). While naloxone has a poor oral bioavailability (1-2%) due to its extensive hepatic first-pass metabolism, it is well absorbed through all parental routes including intravenous (IV), intramuscular (IM), subcutaneous (SC), sublingual (SL), inhalational (IN) or upper airway routes (e.g., endotracheal, nebulized, and intranasal), each with slightly-differing onsets of action. Traditional dosing is 0.4 mg IV/IM/SC/IN. However, in an opioid-dependent patient, such a dose may precipitate withdrawal symptoms. In an opioid-naive patient, withdrawal symptoms are not of concern. The main goal of opioid-receptor antagonism should be to restore respiratory effort, not CNS arousal. Therefore, depending on the clinical setting, naloxone can be administered initially IV at 0.04 mg to a maximum of 10 mg. The dose of administration is dependent on the properties of the opioid that induced overdose, where short-acting medications like fentanyl may be completely reversed with a small single dose of naloxone, while longer-acting agonists such as methadone or buprenorphine may require a continuous naloxone infusion.[10]

PATIENT MANAGEMENT

What Are the Appropriate Initial Responses When an Unresponsive Patient Is Found?

The approach to an undifferentiated, unresponsive patient in the prehospital setting is standardized based on the level of training of the bystander or health care provider as outlined in BLS/ACLS guidelines published by the American Heart Association.[11]

Using healthy apneic volunteers, Elam et al.[12] and then Safar et al.[13] demonstrated conclusively that sufficient ventilation could be achieved by laypersons, using the mouth-to-mouth technique. Citing these findings, they were instrumental in developing cardiopulmonary resuscitation (CPR) which was quickly validated and implemented worldwide. The widespread public adoption has been fundamental to improving the outcomes of out-of-hospital CPR and has saved countless lives.[14]

Despite this life-saving procedure, recent studies have reported reluctance of bystanders and health care providers to perform mouth-to-mouth ventilation (MTMV)[15] even though the number of infections related to resuscitation is estimated to be less than 1 in 200,000.[16] An alternative option to conventional CPR training is now recommended by the American Heart Association (AHA) for untrained rescuers, changing the sequence from the traditional ABCs to Chest compressions, then Airway, then Breathing (CAB).[17] This change is designed to encourage more rescuers to begin CPR with a compression-only technique, particularly when only one rescuer is available. Data from Japan's nationwide dissemination of recommendations for continuous chest compression CPR for lay rescuers showed that the implementation of compression-only CPR improved bystander CPR rates and increased survival.[18]

Regardless of a rescuer's level of training, chest compressions should be urgently applied to any unresponsive and pulseless patient, after confirming the rescuer's personal safety and calling for help. If ventilation and circulation are present in the unresponsive patient, the rescuer should next ensure that the airway is patent using a chin lift, jaw thrust, and then simply turning the patient on the side.

After ensuring adequate ventilation and circulation, the rescuer can then begin to determine the probable cause of unconsciousness and administer naloxone, if indicated. If there is strong clinical suspicion of an opioid-induced life-threatening emergency, such as known opioid use disorder, presence of OAT, prior history of OIRD, or risk factors as listed below, the approach to OR-agonist toxicity is dependent on the clinical setting. The mainstay in the initial management of a critically ill or unconscious patient should always start with the same standard; airway, breathing and circulation, recognizing the difference in approach for respiratory arrest with a pulse, and the presence of cardiac arrest. To note, Naloxone has no proven role in cardiac arrest. It is incorporated in both advance cardiac life support (ACLS) and basic life support (BLS) algorithms as it is generally accepted that some respiratory arrests are likely misclassified as cardiac arrest.[19]

In respiratory arrest secondary to opioid overdose, oxygenation and ventilation are typically sufficient to prevent death. Effective FMV with or without oral or nasal adjuncts is lifesaving. Administration of naloxone will decrease the duration of ventilatory support required and avoid invasive airway interventions such as tracheal intubation. As mentioned previously, initiating IV access and administering initial dose of naloxone at 0.04 mg is to re-establish respiratory drive while taking care to avoid precipitating withdrawal—not to restore arousal.

OR-agonist toxicity in the prehospital setting is managed following the same principles, depending on the level of resuscitative training of the provider. If a bystander comes across an unconscious person, immediately calling for help is priority. The American Heart Association updated BLS guidelines in 2015 to also include the administration of IM or IN naloxone in cases of opioid overdose integrated into the BLS algorithm for an unconscious patient.[20] Subsequently, in 2016 the Government of Canada updated the prescription drug list so that Naloxone, previously a prescription-only medication, can now be purchased or distributed without a prescription, increasing its access.[21]

It is important to emphasize that unless it is specifically known that the only offending agent is an OR-agonist, a broad differential diagnosis is required. If the ingestion is unknown, the classic toxidrome suspicious for OR-agonist toxicity is hypoventilation, miosis, altered mental status, and hypoperistalsis.

What Are the Potential Complications Associated with the Administration of Naloxone to Patients with a Presumed Opioid Overdose?

Naloxone administration in an opioid-naïve patient has not been reported to produce adverse effects. The most intense effects of opioid antagonist administration in the opioid-dependent patient mimic the symptoms of acute withdrawal with diaphoresis, rhinorrhea, mydriasis, vomiting, diarrhea, myalgias, insomnia, tachycardia, and hypertension. Precipitating withdrawal employing opioid antagonists in this population group usually causes a surge of catecholamines which can explain the increase in heart rate and blood pressure. More concerningly, in rare and severe cases, this surge can cause myocardial ischemia, heart failure, and CNS damage.[22] While violent reactions and behaviors are uncommon during acute withdrawal, Belz et al.[23] reported agitation or combativeness in 15% of the 164 patients treated with naloxone by emergency medical services responders. Noncardiogenic pulmonary edema has also been described in numerous case reports following naloxone administration. Lastly, as with any patient, if vomiting occurs there is a risk of aspiration pneumonitis which may complicate recovery. The risk of these complications may be reduced by using lower initial doses of naloxone, slowly titrating to effect.[24]

Discuss the Disposition of the Patient After Management

Careful attention is required in the administration of naloxone for OIRD so as not to precipitate withdrawal in opioid-dependent patients. If withdrawal occurs, supportive care and monitoring may be required. Careful observation of the patient after naloxone administration is crucial, but generally 2 hours should be sufficient if the patient is alert, oriented, and with stable vital signs. Special consideration must be given to those who required resuscitation or those who are on long-acting OAT such as methadone or buprenorphine.

SUMMARY

The opioid crisis is a global epidemic that has caused significant death and disability. It is prudent that practitioners advocate for reducing opioid-related deaths, focusing on primary prevention, access to treatment, and harm reduction. Empathy, while difficult to muster is an advisable course of action. If faced with OIRD, oxygenation and ventilation are typically sufficient to prevent death. Naloxone administration can reduce the duration of active airway management required and avoid unnecessary invasive airway interventions such as tracheal intubation.

CASE CONCLUSION

The patient was transported to the ED uneventfully; however, while waiting in the ED his level of consciousness declined, as did his respiratory rate and oxygen saturations. He was given another bolus dose of naloxone at 0.2 mg IV and started on an infusion of 0.3 $mg{\cdot}hr^{-1}$. Although he initially became tachycardic and restless with signs of acute withdrawal, this settled after 30 to 40 minutes. He was observed over the next 6 hours and did not require any subsequent airway intervention or OR antagonism. Prior to discharge, he admitted to purchasing illicit buprenorphine which he took in addition to his daily-dispensed dose of opioid. He agreed to follow up with his primary care provider and was given a new take-home naloxone kit.

SELF-EVALUATION QUESTIONS

20.1. Which of the following is **NOT** a potential side effect of naloxone when administered to a patient with opioid overdose?

A. Diaphoresis
B. Insomnia
C. Myocardial ischemia
D. Noncardiogenic pulmonary edema
E. Bradycardia

20.2. Which of the following is an example of harm reduction?

A. Education for health care providers on opioid agonist therapy
B. Increasing access to chronic pain specialists
C. Needle exchange program
D. Ensuring safe disposal of unused narcotics

20.3. Opioid Syndrome includes all of the following symptoms **EXCEPT:**

A. Mydriasis
B. Hypoventilation
C. Hypoperistalsis
D. Altered mental status

REFERENCES

1. Good Samaritan Drug Overdose Act. Ottawa: Canadian Department of Justice; 2017.
2. Pattinson KT. Opioids and the control of respiration. *Br J Anaesth.* 2008;100:747-758.
3. Henriksen G, Willoch F. Imaging of opioid receptors in the central nervous system. *Brain.* 2008;131:1171-1196.
4. Courteix C, Coudore-Civiale MA, Privat AM, Pelissier T, Eschalier A, Fialip J. Evidence for an exclusive antinociceptive effect of nociceptin/orphanin FQ, an endogenous ligand for the ORL1 receptor, in two animal models of neuropathic pain. *Pain.* 2004;110:236-245.
5. Lalley PM. Opioidergic and dopaminergic modulation of respiration. *Respir Physiol Neurobiol.* 2008;164:160-167.
6. Shook JE, Watkins WD, Camporesi EM. Differential roles of opioid receptors in respiration, respiratory disease, and opiate-induced respiratory depression. *Am Rev Respir Dis.* 1990;142:895-909.
7. Boitor M, Ballard A, Emed J, Le May S, Gelinas C. Risk factors for severe opioid-induced respiratory depression in hospitalized adults: a case-control study. *Can J Pain.* 2020;4:103-110.
8. Gupta K, Prasad A, Nagappa M, Wong J, Abrahamyan L, Chung FF. Risk factors for opioid-induced respiratory depression and failure to rescue: a review. *Curr Opin Anaesthesiol.* 2018;31:110-119.
9. Dixon R, Gentile J, Hsu HB, et al. Nalmefene: safety and kinetics after single and multiple oral doses of a new opioid antagonist. *J Clin Pharmacol.* 1987;27:233-239.
10. van Dorp E, Yassen A, Dahan A. Naloxone treatment in opioid addiction: the risks and benefits. *Expert Opin Drug Saf.* 2007;6:125-132.
11. American Heart Association. *Advance Cardiac Life Support and Basic Life Support Guidelines.* AHA;2020.
12. Elam JO, Brown ES, Elder JDJr. Artificial respiration by mouth-to-mask method; a study of the respiratory gas exchange of paralyzed patients ventilated by operator's expired air. *N Engl J Med.* 1954;250:749-754.
13. Safar P, Mc MM. Mouth-to-airway emergency artificial respiration. *JAMA.* 1958;166:1459-1460.
14. Gu XM, Li ZH, He ZJ, Zhao ZW, Liu SQ. A meta-analysis of the success rates of heartbeat restoration within the platinum 10 min among outpatients suffering from sudden cardiac arrest in China. *Mil Med Res.* 2016;3:6.
15. Wenzel V, Lindner KH, Prengel AW. Ventilation during cardiopulmonary resuscitation (CPR). A literature study and analysis of ventilation strategies. *Der Anaesthesist.* 1997;46:133-141.
16. Mejicano GC, Maki DG. Infections acquired during cardiopulmonary resuscitation: estimating the risk and defining strategies for prevention. *Ann Intern Med.* 1998;129:813-828.
17. American Heart Association. *American Heart Association Focused Updates on Adult and Pediatric Basic Life Support and Cardiopulmonary Resuscitation Quality.* AHA; 2017.
18. Iwami T, Kitamura T, Kiyohara K, Kawamura T. Dissemination of chest compression-only cardiopulmonary resuscitation and survival after out-of-hospital cardiac arrest. *Circulation.* 2015;132:415-422.
19. American Heart Association. *Highlights of the 2020 American Heart Association Guidelines for CPR and ECG.* AHA;2020.
20. American Heart Association. *Advance Cardiac Life Support & Basic Life Support Guidelines.* AHA; 2015.
21. Health Canada. Access to naloxone in Canada (including NARCAN™ Nasal Spray). In: Products DaH, ed. Ottawa: Health Canada; 2016.
22. Lassen CL, Zink W, Wiese CH, Graf BM, Wiesenack C. Naloxone-induced pulmonary edema. Case report with review of the literature and critical evaluation. *Der Anaesthesist.* 2012;61:129-136.
23. Belz D, Lieb J, Rea T, Eisenberg MS. Naloxone use in a tiered-response emergency medical services system. *Prehosp Emerg Care.* 2006;10:468-471.
24. Buajordet I, Naess AC, Jacobsen D, Brors O. Adverse events after naloxone treatment of episodes of suspected acute opioid overdose. *Eur J Emerg Med.* 2004;11:19-23.

CHAPTER 21

Extracorporeal Membrane Oxygenation (ECMO) in Airway Management in the Emergency Department

James Gould and David Hung

CASE PRESENTATION

Case 1

You are the attending Emergency Physician at a tertiary care facility, covering the Emergency Department (ED). A 55-year-old male patient presents to the ED with progressive dyspnea and weight loss over a 3-month period. He is otherwise known to have hypertension and diabetes and takes hydrochlorothiazide and metformin as his only medications. On arrival, he has significant stridor at rest, despite this his oxygen saturations are 98% on room air, he is afebrile, blood pressure 155/80. A computed tomography (CT) scan is performed which reveals a large compressive mass in his neck, arising from the thyroid, thought to represent a thyroid carcinoma. This mass is causing compression at the level of the glottis resulting in a 1 mm opening. Anesthesia and otolaryngology are consulted by the ED for assistance in planning surgical management. It is decided that the patient should undergo thyroidectomy, laryngectomy, and lymph node dissection. Given this anatomy, it is likely that face-mask ventilation (FMV), the use of extraglottic device (EGD), and tracheal intubation, including awake approach, will all be difficult. Furthermore, given the location of the tumor, front-of-neck airway (FONA) access under local anesthesia is excluded as an option. You consult your local cardiac surgeon about the possibility of initiating extracorporeal membrane oxygenation (ECMO) in the awake state, as a primary means of airway management.

Case 2

A 34-year-old female who is 3 weeks postpartum presents to the ED with progressive shortness of breath and weakness and chest pain. She appears unwell, with slight reduction in mentation, HR 115, BP 70/50, O_2 saturations 93% on 4 L·min^{-1} oxygen through nasal prongs (NP), with mild increase in work of breathing. Her skin is cold to touch, and she is making scant urine output. Laboratory results reveal an acute kidney injury, elevated troponin, and a lactate of 5.0 mmol·L^{-1}. ECG reveals a sinus rhythm tachycardia. Bedside ultrasound shows biventricular failure with presence of b-lines suggestive of pulmonary edema. She is diagnosed with cardiogenic shock on the presumed basis of postpartum cardiomyopathy. Resuscitation is initiated with high-flow nasal oxygenation, vasopressors, and inotropes. Unfortunately, there is no improvement in end-organ perfusion. You identify some decline in her oxygenation but that is currently being adequately managed noninvasively. You wonder if this young patient would be a candidate for venoarterial ECMO (VA-ECMO) for cardiac support. However, you are unsure if the patient requires intubation for such an intervention. Your concerns about tracheal intubation of this patient include the potential for decompensation during induction and complications of mechanical ventilation.

Case 3

A 64-year-old male collapses at a local museum shortly after complaining to his partner about chest pain. Emergency Medical Services (EMS) called and bystander cardiopulmonary resuscitation (CPR) is initiated. An automated external defibrillator (AED) is available immediately, and on initial analysis recommends and delivers a shock. EMS arrives within 6 minutes to find him in ventricular fibrillation (VF) and delivers two additional shocks without return of spontaneous circulation (ROSC). The patient has a history of hypertension, type-2 diabetes, and a strong family history of coronary artery disease. Standard advanced cardiac life support (ACLS) is initiated, and he receives multiple doses of IV epinephrine and amiodarone. Given the immediate proximity to local tertiary trauma center, the patient is transported and the ED team is alerted. You are the charge ED physician who receives the patch. Given the patient is in refractory VF, witnessed, with immediate CPR initiated by bystanders, and was within a short transport distance to the hospital, you wonder if this patient would be an appropriate candidate to initiate VA-ECMO for resuscitation.

INTRODUCTION

What Is ECMO?

ECMO refers to a method whereby a patient's blood is oxygenated outside of the body using a mechanical pump and oxygenator. This is done either by venovenous (VV) method where blood is extracted from the venous system, through a large peripherally placed cannula, oxygenated, and pumped back to the venous circulation, or by venoarterial (VA) method, whereby blood is extracted from the venous system and pumped back to the arterial circulation (Figure 21.1). In general, VV-ECMO is used to augment respiratory function, and VA-ECMO for cardiac function. The technique has a long-standing presence in the operating room dating back to the 1950s for use in cardiovascular surgery.[1] More recently, with the development of portable systems and percutaneous techniques, the concept of VV-ECMO and VA-ECMO has been used as a resuscitation tool outside of the operating room (OR). The term Extracorporeal life support (ECLS) refers to this use of ECMO in an emergency setting and extracorporeal cardiopulmonary resuscitation (ECPR) has been used to define the use of VA-ECMO in the setting of cardiac arrest. The utility of ECMO in the clinical setting is a relatively new modality, its use as a tool for primary "airway management" is largely theoretical and anecdotal, with little to no evidence published on the topic. In this chapter, we will review the theoretical concept of ECMO use in airway management and review some of the existing evidence to shed light on this rather novel concept.

What Constitutes a Difficult Airway?

The Canadian Airway Focus Group constitutes a difficult airway when an experienced practitioner anticipates or encounters difficulty in any or all of the following: face-mask ventilation (FMV), the use of an EGD, tracheal intubation, or emergency FONA.[2,3] Patient physiological factors can compound this difficulty. The difficulty one might face in airway management can be divided into anatomical difficulty and physiologic difficulty. Both difficulties carry the potential for adverse patient outcomes if not managed appropriately, and specific management strategies must be employed depending on either circumstance.

Anatomic Difficulty

Although many of the published predictors of difficulty of the classic four pillars of airway management are discussed in Chapter 1, a novel concept has recently emerged to address what is referred to as the "impossible" airway.[3] This refers to when an experienced practitioner anticipates difficulty with all four pillars of airway management. The scenario where FONA is anticipated to be difficult would include obstructions distal to the cricothyroid membrane or tracheotomy site, such as in tracheal tumors, mediastinal mass, head and neck tumors, and tracheal stenosis.[4] In these impossible scenarios, establishing

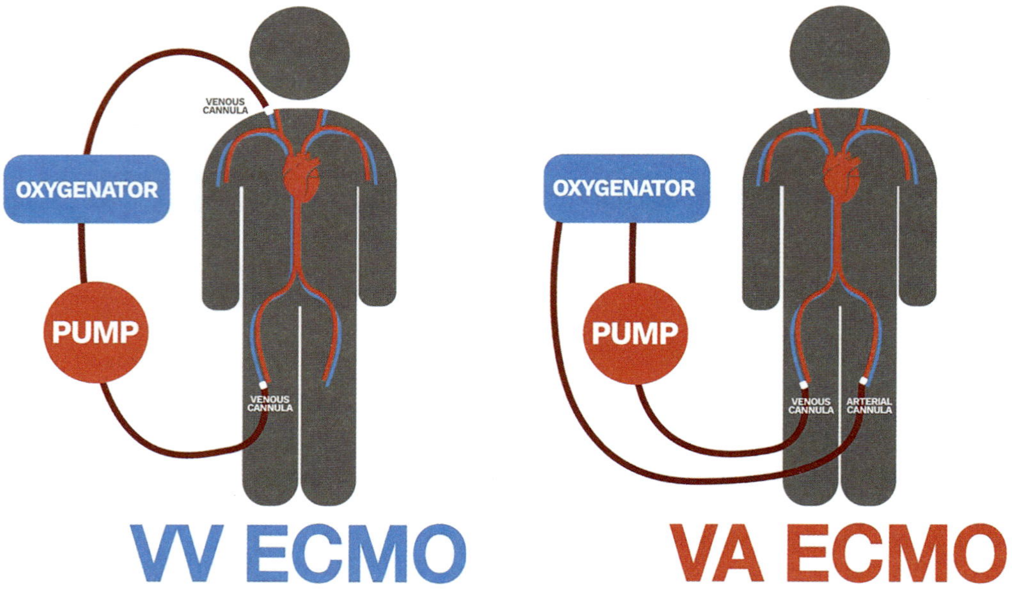

FIGURE 21.1. Schematic diagrams showing both the VV-ECMO and the VA-ECMO.

VV- or VA-ECMO prior to or as an alternative for airway management may be the safest option.[3] As such, expert opinion has considered implementing ECMO into airway management guidelines.

Physiologic Difficulty

Physiologic difficulty is an inherent feature of many emergency endotracheal intubations. These critically ill patients who require airway management are typically physiologically deranged. The process of intubation and transition to mechanical ventilation carries with it the potential for significant complications if these derangements are not recognized and adequately managed prior to and during airway management.[5] The physiologic impact of airway management includes the intubation phase and the postintubation mechanical ventilation stage. In general, emergency tracheal intubation includes provision of an induction agent and paralytic. All induction agents, even those thought to be hemodynamically favorable, have the potential to induce hypotension, either by their intrinsic properties, or by reduction in the patient's awareness and subsequent sympathetic response, i.e., vasomotor tone. Patients who are hemodynamically deranged to begin with, are likely at higher risk of this iatrogenic effect. Furthermore, the act of intubation induces a state of apnea, critically ill patients may be intolerant of that apneic period for a variety of reasons, mainly severe hypoxemia and metabolic acidosis. Loss of respiratory effort may result in a rapid decline in oxygenation in the setting of hypoxemia, or rapid worsening of acidosis in a patient who has lost their compensatory mechanisms.

The postintubation period carries its own set of physiologic effects on critically ill patients. Transition to positive pressure ventilation reduces preload and increases right ventricular afterload, two principles that may contribute to hemodynamic collapse in select patient populations.[6] Furthermore, mechanical ventilation may contribute to respiratory complications such as ventilator-associated pneumonia, need for tracheotomy, barotrauma, and acute respiratory distress syndrome (ARDS).

There are many strategies and technologies that can be employed to manage anatomically difficult airways, namely, awake intubation, and/or utilization of video laryngoscopy and flexible bronchoscopy to facilitate tracheal intubation. Furthermore, there are suggested strategies to manage the physiologically difficult airway, thus avoiding the negative physiologic effects of intubation and mechanical ventilation, namely, resuscitating a patient prior to intubation or employing lung protective ventilation strategies. However, there are cases where these strategies and technologies will be insufficient and an alternative approach using ECMO could be considered as a primary management strategy for these airways.

ECMO IN AIRWAY MANAGEMENT

How Can ECMO Be Used in Managing a Patient with an Anatomically Difficult Airway?

Where airway anatomy is incompatible with the principles of airway management, in situations described as the "impossible airway," ECMO may be the only option to provide oxygenation and ventilation.[3,7] This typically involves a significant obstruction distal to planned FONA or tracheotomy landmarks. Fundamentally, when pathology distorts anatomy such that the airway diameter is smaller than the external diameter of the endotracheal tube or tracheostomy tube (i.e., size 6-mm internal diameter [ID] ETT has an external diameter of 8.2 mm), ECMO should be considered.[8] One study suggests considering awake ECMO if advanced imaging shows an airway diameter of 5 mm or less.[9]

To date, the literature on ECMO for this purpose predominantly exists as case reports. The described pathology for severe airway obstructions includes tracheal tumor, tracheal stenosis, head and neck cancer, large mediastinal mass, primary lung cancer, benign thyroid goiter, esophageal cancer, malignant melanoma, and tracheal granulomas.[4,7]

One important acknowledgment in the existing evidence is that outcomes for ECMO in the anatomically difficult airway are likely better when used as a primary or prophylactic plan rather than as a rescue option, in the context of a failed alternative approach. In other words, if there is time and objective evidence of an anatomically impossible airway, ECMO should be considered as a primary approach. Unfortunately, some impossible airways will only be identified as such in hindsight, when in the absence of objective evidence of such an airway and once all other modalities have failed.

How Can ECMO Be Used in Physiologically Difficult Airway Management?

As stated previously, the physiologic consequences of airway management involve the effects of intubation and mechanical ventilation. The use of ECMO can be considered to avoid both of these effects. Specifically, employing ECMO as your primary strategy, or in other terms, performing "awake" ECMO without invasive mechanical ventilation, can avoid both these concerns. Both VV- and VA-ECMO can be performed peripherally under local anesthetic without any intubation or sedation. If initiated, these interventions could theoretically optimally manage oxygenation and ventilation in the setting of VV-ECMO and additionally hemodynamics, in the setting of VA-ECMO.

Two very important points should be noted. First, although implementation of an "awake" ECMO avoids the complications associated with intubation and mechanical ventilation, it carries with it a unique set of complications associated with the use of ECMO such as thromboembolism, bleeding, and infection. A risk-benefit analysis of such an approach must be considered. Formal scoring systems or guideline recommendations to help with that decision are nonexistent. Second, not all patients will be adequately oxygenated and ventilated with ECMO alone, requiring mechanical ventilation and or their mental status may require intubation. The hope with such patients would be that ECMO would allow for a shorter course of mechanical ventilation.

A recent propensity-score matched analysis[10] compared the use of peripheral VA-ECMO support in cardiogenic shock. A 7-year database was used to compare patients who received "awake" ECMO versus those who received traditional "non-awake" VA-ECMO, or in other words, initiation of ECMO while intubated and mechanically ventilated. Among 231 patients, 39% were "awake," and experienced significantly lower rates of pneumonia, tracheotomy, and renal replacement therapy. Moreover, the "awake" strategy was associated with a reduced 60-day (20% vs. 41%) and 1-year mortality (31% vs. 54%). Finally, mechanical ventilation at the time of ECMO cannulation was independently associated with 60-day mortality.

The use of awake VV-ECMO to reduce the complications of mechanical ventilation has been described in case reports and case series. The largest population of patients described are those awaiting lung transplant where ECMO is used as a bridge to their operation. A report of 26 patients receiving such a strategy showed shorter hospital and ICU stay.[11] An example of such a strategy involves use of ECMO in severely bronchospastic patients with obstructive lung disease to facilitate refractory CO_2 clearance. Since 2012, four case series have been published showing the successful use of ECMO without requiring invasive mechanical ventilation.[12] Finally, a case series of six patients with acute respiratory distress syndrome showed 3/6 successfully treated with VV-ECMO without any invasive mechanical ventilation.[13]

ECMO IN THE EMERGENCY DEPARTMENT

What Is ECPR?

Conventional cardiopulmonary resuscitation (CCPR) is performed to generate coronary perfusion pressure (CPP) and cardiac output (CO) during cardiac arrest. CPP dictates myocardial reperfusion which is vital to achieving the return of spontaneous circulation (ROSC) and CO dictates organ and cerebral perfusion to prevent ischemic damage.[14] CCPR in optimal circumstances produces a fraction of normal CO and CPP, with prolonged resuscitation increasing the risk of organ failure and hypoxic injury after ROSC.

ECPR is the implementation of VA-ECMO during the ongoing resuscitation of select patients in cardiac arrest due to reversible etiologies. ECPR increases blood flow and oxygen delivery as compared with CCPR and is considered an adjunct to conventional resuscitation. It is an invasive technique that requires an expert team, but it has been shown to improve survival outcomes in certain populations such as refractory ventricular fibrillation (VF).[15]

The main determinant of successful ECPR is the interval between patient collapse and initiation of ECPR. This period is further divided into two categories: "no-flow" state is the period after collapsing until the initiation of chest compressions and the "low-flow" state is the period after initiation of chest compressions to the initiation of ECPR. Studies to date examine predictors of survivability in both in-hospital cardiac arrest and out-of-hospital cardiac arrest as being correlated with minimizing low-flow times.

What Is the Evidence for ECPR?

The literature to support ECPR predominantly existed as observational cohort studies until 2020 when Yannopoulos et al.[16] published the first single-center, randomized control trial (RCT). It studied adult patients who met inclusion criteria of out-of-hospital cardiac arrest (OHCA) with rhythm of VF or pulseless VT, no ROSC after three defibrillation attempts, a body habitus that would accommodate the Lund University Cardiac Arrest System (LUCAS) device, and who had a transport time to the ED of less than 30 minutes. Patients were randomized into two groups: standard ACLS followed by coronary catheterization and ECPR followed by coronary catheterization. The results showed survival to hospital discharge with standard ACLS of 7%, congruent with global survival rates, but the ECPR group showed a 43% survival rate to hospital discharge.

What Is the Role of ECPR in the Prehospital Setting?

In OHCA, the historical emphasis for prehospital emergency care practitioners has been to stay on scene to provide CCPR, as opposed to rapid transport to the nearest facility. This is based on philosophy that the best patient outcome results from early ROSC which is associated with the treatment of reversible pathology and optimizing the quality of CPR, recognizing that during transport this is significantly reduced.[17]

In certain resource-rich, urban settings across the world, ECPR has been implemented in the prehospital setting. This has been described with numerous case studies and a small case series, with a prospective control trial comparing OCHA with prehospital ECPR recruiting in France.[18] Favorable outcomes have been reported, with the principle behind it being reducing low-flow state. However, it is a technique that has numerous logistical challenges. In the United Kingdom, this would be deployed by two consultant physicians and a clinical perfusionist. To operate 9 hours a day, 7 days a week that company estimates an annual cost of approximately 1 million US dollars.[14]

PATIENT MANAGEMENT

What Is the Patient Selection for ECPR in the ED or Prehospital Setting?

Indications and contraindications for ECPR vary across hospitals and experience levels of the emergency care teams. Due to the lack of RCTs for ECPR, there are no validated criteria for indications or patient selection. There are favorable outcomes associated with ECPR during certain conditions, and these are as follows: age <75, witnessed collapse and initiation of bystander CPR <5 minutes, initially shockable rhythm, no sustained ROSC within 15 minutes of CCPR, presumed reversible cause of cardiac arrest, and ensuring high-quality CPR.[19]

Similarly, unfavorable outcomes have been associated with the following: age >75, prolonged CCPR, cardiac arrest due to unsurvivable injury, low-quality CPR, clinical signs of irreversible brain damage or poor neurological prognosis, history of terminal illness, patient refusal or lack of informed consent with family, and low pH (<6.8).

What Are the Potential Complications Associated with ECPR in the Prehospital Setting?

Complications associated with ECPR in the prehospital setting are similar to those with initiating ECMO in-hospital; however, the resources to mitigate these are not as readily available. These complications include vascular injury or bleeding, failure to cannulate, limb ischemia, and infection.[14]

How Would You Manage the Presented Cases?

ECMO Case #1 (See Chapter 45 for a Detailed Management of a Patient with a Similar Obstruction)

The patient is brought to the operating room. Heliox™ is administered through a non-rebreathing mask. Under local anesthesia, ECMO cannulation is performed on the right femoral and internal jugular vein. Following that, VV-ECMO was initiated. Once oxygenation is ensured, anesthesia is induced and maintained throughout the case. Prior to incision, one attempt at tracheal intubation is attempted from above. Visualization of the glottis is difficult due to distorted anatomy; moreover, endotracheal tube advancement is not possible, reinforcing the appropriateness of ECMO use in this case. VV-ECMO is utilized as the prior means of oxygenation through the initial stages of the operation—tracheotomy. After tracheotomy, typical inhaled anesthetics are utilized, and the tumor is successfully resected.

ECMO Case #2

Cardiac surgery is consulted. It is decided to proceed with an "awake VA-ECMO" to avoid intubation and mechanical ventilation. Under local anesthesia, the patient is placed on peripheral VA-ECMO through the right femoral vessels. Her hemodynamics normalize and her clinical status improves with improved mentation and urine output. Her biochemical and end-organ state improve on laboratory work. During her stay in the intensive care unit, she develops left ventricular distension requiring decompression. Eventually, as her respiratory status improves, she is converted to a temporary biventricular assist device (BiVAD). Over the course of her ICU stay, her cardiac function improves and she is weaned from mechanical support, never having required mechanical ventilation outside of the operative period.

ECMO Case #3

Cardiac surgery is consulted prior to patient arrival and the attending agrees the patient is suitable for ECPR. The hospital ECPR team is activated, assembling cardiac surgery, anesthesia, and a perfusionist to the resuscitation area. Vascular access is obtained in the right femoral artery and vein under ultrasound guidance. The patient is successfully cannulated after confirmation of wire placement by transthoracic echocardiogram (TTE), and they are placed on ECMO pump flow. The patient is then stabilized and brought to the coronary catheterization lab where they are found to have a proximal left anterior descending artery occlusion with one drug-eluting stent deployed. They remain in cardiovascular ICU for 2 days, after which the ECMO pump is discontinued due to stable cardiac function. The patient has a prolonged recovery due to groin-site infection requiring IV antibiotics, but he survives hospital discharge with good neurological function.

SUMMARY

The utility of ECMO in clinical practice is rapidly expanding. As this expansion happens, we must consider the utility of ECMO as the primary modality for airway management. Keeping in mind that evidence is lacking, this should be a multidisciplinary process that uses sound clinical judgment, what little evidence does exist, and physiologic reasoning to determine the appropriateness of its use. In the interim, we should seek further investigations of this approach through clinical trials. In summary, as outlined in this chapter, we provide a conceptual framework for the potential use of ECMO in airway management in the ED including its use as primary oxygenation and ventilation in anatomically difficult or rather impossible airways, and in physiologically difficult airways, both in terms of avoiding physiologic consequences of intubation and subsequent physiologic consequences of mechanical ventilation. Additionally, ECPR has shown promising results in the ED for improving survival to hospital discharge, with ongoing research to evaluate its role in the prehospital setting.

SELF-EVALUATION QUESTIONS

21.1. Which of the following is an ***INCORRECT*** statement regarding ECMO?

A. VV-ECMO is generally used to augment respiratory function.

B. VA-ECMO can be used to augment both respiratory and cardiac failure.

C. ECMO has been proven to be an effective tool for primary airway management.

D. Portable unit of ECMO is available for prehospital use.

E. ECMO can be used in anatomically difficult airway management.

21.2. Which of the following is ***NOT*** a known complication of ECMO?

A. Vascular injury

B. Fluid volume depletion

C. Limb ischemia

D. Coagulopathy

E. Infection

21.3. ECPR should be avoided in which of the following situations?

A. Young patient

B. Healthy patient

C. CPR for <60 minutes

D. Irreversible cause of cardiac arrest

E. Experienced team

REFERENCES

1. Mosier JM, Kelsey M, Raz Y, et al. Extracorporeal membrane oxygenation (ECMO) for critically ill adults in the emergency department: history, current applications, and future directions. *Crit Care*. 2015;19:431. doi:10.1186/s13054-015-1155-7.
2. Law JA, Duggan LV, Asselin M, et al. Canadian Airway Focus Group updated consensus-based recommendations for management of the difficult airway: part 1. Difficult airway management encountered in an unconscious patient. *Can J Anaesth*. 2021;68(9):1373-1404. doi:10.1007/s12630-021-02007-0.
3. Law JA, Duggan LV, Asselin M, et al. Canadian Airway Focus Group updated consensus-based recommendations for management of the difficult airway: part 2. Planning and implementing safe management of the patient with an anticipated difficult airway. *Can J Anaesth*. 2021;68(9):1405-1436. doi:10.1007/s12630-021-02008-z.
4. Malpas G, Hung O, Gilchrist A, et al. The use of extracorporeal membrane oxygenation in the anticipated difficult airway: a case report and systematic review. *Can J Anaesth*. 2018;65(6):685-697. doi:10.1007/s12630-018-1099-x.
5. Kornas RL, Owyang CG, Sakles JC, Foley LJ, Mosier JM, Society for Airway Management's Special Projects Committee. Evaluation and management of the physiologically difficult airway: consensus recommendations from Society for Airway Management. *Anesth Analg*. 2021;132(2):395-405. doi:10.1213/ANE.0000000000005233.
6. Alviar CL, Miller PE, McAreavey D, et al. Positive pressure ventilation in the cardiac intensive care unit. *J Am Coll Cardiol*. 2018;72(13):1532-1553. doi:10.1016/j.jacc.2018.06.074.
7. Hung O, McAlpine J, Murphy M. Averting catastrophic outcomes: the fundamentals of "impossible" airways. *Can J Anaesth*. 2022;69(2):192-195. doi:10.1007/s12630-021-02117-9.
8. Gupta B, Gupta L. Significance of the outer diameter of an endotracheal tube: a lesser-known parameter. *Korean J Anesthesiol*. 2019;72(1):72-73. doi:10.4097/kja.d.18.00056.
9. Kim CW, Kim DH, Son BS, et al. The feasibility of extracorporeal membrane oxygenation in the variant airway problems. *Ann Thorac Cardiovasc Surg*. 2015;21(6):517-522. doi:10.5761/atcs.oa.15-00073.
10. Montero S, Huang F, Rivas-Lasarte M, et al. Awake venoarterial extracorporeal membrane oxygenation for refractory cardiogenic shock. *Eur Heart J Acute Cardiovasc Care*. 2021;10(6):585-594. doi:10.1093/ehjacc/zuab018.
11. Fuehner T, Kuehn C, Hadem J, et al. Extracorporeal membrane oxygenation in awake patients as bridge to lung transplantation. *Am J Respir Crit Care Med*. 2012;185(7):763-768. doi:10.1164/rccm.201109-1599OC.
12. Collaud S, Benden C, Ganter C, et al. Extracorporeal life support as bridge to lung retransplantation: a multicenter pooled data analysis. *Ann Thorac Surg*. 2016;102(5):1680-1686. doi:10.1016/j.athoracsur.2016.05.014.
13. Yeo HJ, Cho WH, Kim D. Awake extracorporeal membrane oxygenation in patients with severe postoperative acute respiratory distress syndrome. *J Thorac Dis*. 2016;8(1):37-42. doi:10.3978/j.issn.2072-1439.2016.01.32.
14. Singer B, Reynolds JC, Lockey DJ, O'Brien B. Pre-hospital extra-corporeal cardiopulmonary resuscitation. *Scand J Trauma Resusc Emerg Med*. 2018;26(1):21. doi:10.1186/s13049-018-0489-y.
15. Ahn C, Kim W, Cho Y, Choi KS, Jang BH, Lim TH. Efficacy of extracorporeal cardiopulmonary resuscitation compared to conventional cardiopulmonary resuscitation for adult cardiac arrest patients: a systematic review and meta-analysis. *Sci Rep*. 2016;6:34208. doi:10.1038/srep34208.
16. Yannopoulos D, Bartos J, Raveendran G, et al. Advanced reperfusion strategies for patients with out-of-hospital cardiac arrest and refractory ventricular fibrillation (ARREST): a phase 2, single centre, open-label, randomised controlled trial. *Lancet*. 2020;396(10265):1807-1816. doi:10.1016/S0140-6736(20)32338-2.
17. Olasveengen TM, Wik L, Steen PA. Quality of cardiopulmonary resuscitation before and during transport in out-of-hospital cardiac arrest. *Resuscitation*. 2008;76(2):185-190. doi:10.1016/j.resuscitation.2007.07.001.
18. Lamhaut L, Hutin A, Puymirat E, et al. A pre-hospital extracorporeal cardio pulmonary resuscitation (ECPR) strategy for treatment of refractory out hospital cardiac arrest: an observational study and propensity analysis. *Resuscitation*. 2017;117:109-117. doi:10.1016/j.resuscitation.2017.04.014.
19. Kim H, Cho YH. Role of extracorporeal cardiopulmonary resuscitation in adults. *Acute Crit Care*. 2020;35(1):1-9. doi:10.4266/acc.2020.00080.

SECTION 4

AIRWAY MANAGEMENT IN THE EMERGENCY DEPARTMENT

CHAPTER 22

Airway Management in the Emergency Department

John C. Sakles and Michael F. Murphy

CASE PRESENTATION

A 55-year-old man with a history of diabetes and hypertension presents to the emergency department (ED) with several days of worsening shortness of breath. He saw his primary care provider a week ago and tested positive for SARS-CoV-2. Upon arrival in the ED, he has a blood pressure of 94/52, a heart rate of 136, a respiratory rate of 34, a temperature of 100.9°F and a room air oxygen saturation of 66%. An intravenous (IV) is established and he is given a 1000 mL bolus of crystalloid and a norepinephrine infusion was started. He was placed on high-flow nasal oxygen (HFNO) with an FiO_2 of 100% and a flow of 40 $L{\cdot}min^{-1}$. A portable chest X-ray was performed which revealed diffuse patchy alveolar airspace disease.

INTRODUCTION

What Is It About Managing the Airway in the ED That Makes It "Different"?

Making critical, lifesaving decisions in the face of incomplete information is fundamental to the practice of emergency medicine. Expert management of the emergency airway is a defining skill of emergency medicine. Emergency physicians must be skilled in all aspects of airway management and must have immediate access to all necessary equipment and medications, including video laryngoscopes, extraglottic devices (EGDs), surgical airway equipment, induction agents, and neuromuscular blocking agents. Patients requiring emergency airway management typically present unexpectedly to the ED leaving little time for preparation and planning. Many of these patients have characteristics associated with difficult intubation and have significant physiologic derangements, but the urgency of the airway problem frequently prevents deferral or even consultation. Accordingly, the emergency physician must be both capable and constantly prepared to undertake skilled and timely intervention in patients in the ED and to plan an approach that takes into account all potential difficulties and incorporates within it backup plans (Plan B, Plan C, etc.).

Who Is Primarily Responsible for Managing the Airway in the ED?

Airway evaluation and management is a critically important aspect of resuscitation and establishing a patent airway to maintain oxygenation often takes precedence over all other activities. Identifying that the patient requires airway management does not necessarily mandate that the management be undertaken immediately; it simply establishes that early, deliberate airway management is indicated. In some cases, the patient will be apneic with an unprotected airway, and airway management will supersede virtually all other evaluation and management. In other cases, the practitioner will identify that early airway intervention is required, and plan to provide it early during the course of comprehensive and coordinated care.

The emergency physician has final responsibility for ensuring definitive management of the airway for patients presenting to the ED, which might, at times, require the assistance of other specialists such as anesthesiologists, otolaryngologists, or intensivists.

What Are the Indications for Tracheal Intubation in the ED?

The indications for tracheal intubation in the ED are straightforward:

- Inability of the patient to **maintain** or **protect** the airway
- Inability to maintain **adequate gas exchange**
- A **predictable** clinical deterioration in maintaining the airway or adequate gas exchange

Early establishment of a patent airway and provision of adequate oxygenation are critical to patient survival. Equally important is the ability to *predict* an impending loss of airway patency or gas exchange capability, particularly if the patient will be subjected to diagnostic studies in areas outside the ED or transported to another facility.

Subsequent decisions as to *how and when* the airway should be managed will depend on numerous factors, including the skills and experience of the practitioner, the equipment available, the anatomy of the airway, and the physiology of the patient.

Is There a Conceptual Framework Which the Emergency Physician Employs in Approaching the Airway in the ED?

It is widely recognized that a conceptual framework focusing on rapid airway evaluation, critical action analysis and performance, and facility with an array of airway management techniques minimizes the risk of failure and improves outcome.[1] To be precise, in an emergency, the airway practitioner must be capable of the following:

- Rapidly assessing the urgency of the situation and the patient's need for intervention
- Determining the best method of airway management for the particular circumstances at hand and having a backup plan in the event of failure
- Understanding the risks and benefits of each possible approach
- Optimizing the patient's cardiopulmonary status before intubation
- Deciding which pharmacologic agents to use and in what doses
- Managing the airway in the context of the patient's overall condition
- Using any of a number of airway devices to achieve a definitive airway while minimizing the likelihood, severity, and duration of hypoxemia or hypercarbia
- Recognizing when the planned airway intervention has failed and an alternative (rescue) technique is required
- Being able to rapidly identify when to call for assistance and what type of assistance might be required

HISTORY

How Did Airway Management in the ED Evolve to Where It Is Today?

Emergency airway management for much of history consisted of various forms of back-pressure/arm-lift "artificial respiration," or mouth-to-mouth, mouth-to-nose, and face-mask ventilation (FMV) by minimally trained practitioners until the 1960s when resuscitation research identified airway management failure as a crucial issue affecting the outcome.[2–5] By the early 1970s, tracheal intubation was recognized as an essential part of the skill set for physicians providing emergency care, but most physicians staffing emergency departments were trainees or practicing physicians with little or no formal training in emergency medicine. Intubation was generally accomplished without neuromuscular blocking agents, using either the oral or the nasal routes, sometimes requiring heavy sedation before airway management could be attempted. Intubation using a sedative, such as a benzodiazepine, often accompanied by an opioid, became a common practice despite its frequent failures and complications.

The advent of emergency medicine residency training programs in 1970 and the rapid growth of the specialty through the ensuing decades established a large cadre of trained emergency medicine specialists and led to the rapid deployment of neuromuscular blockade to facilitate tracheal intubation. By the late 1980s, the use of neuromuscular blockade for this purpose was well established in emergency medicine residency training programs, and had been dubbed "rapid sequence intubation" (RSI) in distinction to the anesthesia term "rapid sequence induction."[6] By the mid-to-late 1990s, neuromuscular blockade was widely used and it became evident that neuromuscular blockade not only made the technical task of intubation easier and faster but also resulted in greater success with lower complication rates.

However, a need clearly emerged for a consistent framework to identify patients at risk for difficult laryngoscopy and intubation, to develop a reliable approach to such patients, and to expand the rescue options beyond the single choice of cricothyrotomy.

The challenges facing emergency airway practitioners today include:

1. Restricting the use of neuromuscular blockade only to patients in whom there is a strong likelihood that tracheal intubation will be successful and that gas exchange can be maintained by some other technique in the event of failure
2. Selecting an alternative approach for those patients in whom a difficult or impossible intubation may be anticipated
3. Ensuring the success for alternative rescue devices or techniques in the event of intubation failure.

UNIQUE FEATURES

How Common Is the Difficult and Failed Airway in the ED?

Difficult direct laryngoscopic intubations are common in emergency practice, the incidence being as high as 20% of all emergency intubations. However, the incidence of intubation failure is quite uncommon, being in the 0.5% to 1.0% range. Moreover, the disaster of being unable to intubate or ventilate rarely occurs (0.1-0.5%).[6]

It is crucial to realize that in the case of a difficult intubation, the same standard applies as for a routine intubation; the practitioner must secure the trachea with a cuffed tracheal tube.

In the case of a failed airway (i.e., "can't intubate and can't oxygenate"), the approach is focused on rescue and keeping the patient alive and well-oxygenated.

Thus, the devices, techniques, and even the approach differ in these two situations. A difficult airway is managed in an "anticipatory" way; a failed airway is managed in a "reactive" way. In 2002, Walls coined the phrase "The 'Difficult Airway' is something you anticipate; the 'Failed Airway' is something you experience."[7]

What Is Unique About Airway Management in an ED?

Emergency airway management may be in an ED or extend beyond the ED for those locations where emergency practitioners are called to manage airways or to be directly responsible for their management by surrogate providers such as paramedics. These locations include the out-of-hospital setting, in-patient wards, intensive care units, diagnostic units such as the radiology department, and other sites.

Emergency airway management situations are characterized by several unique features:

- Clinical evaluation, not blood gases, is used to assess the adequacy of ventilation and judge the need for intubation in the acutely ill patient.
- The patient has a full stomach and is at high risk for aspiration.
- The airway must be secured with a cuffed tracheal tube. "Canceling the case," "awakening the patient," or significantly delaying airway management is not an option, nor in most cases, is any other form of airway management that does not protect the airway (beyond the temporary use of an EGD).
- Critical decisions must be made with less information than in almost any other setting. This, in fact, is the essence of emergency medicine and highlights the importance of expeditious and planned strategies for airway evaluation and management (see Chapters 1 and 2 for details).
- The need for intubation is ordinarily obvious, but in an emergency, the decision to intubate is often dependent on having knowledge of the natural course of the disorder or injury rather than on the patient's precise clinical status at the time of the evaluation. There are a few other situations in medicine in which judgment and knowledge of the *anticipated clinical course* of a disorder are so crucial.
- Erring on the side of caution:
    - Intubate earlier rather than later. Be especially cautious of penetrating neck wounds with evidence of injury to the airway itself (subcutaneous air) or the vascular system (hematoma—it does not have to appear to be "expanding"). Both the presence of such injuries and their apparent time course are important. The patient who presents 12 hours after sustaining a penetrating neck injury has withstood the test of time. A similarly appearing injury 10 minutes after injury is an unknown and must be assumed to present an imminent risk. Do not paralyze a patient (ordinarily RSI) if you are not confident that you can oxygenate the patient successfully with an FMV unit or an EGD. If these fail, a front-of-neck airway (surgical airway) is required, and this procedure must be planned for and cannot be considered a failure in airway management. Anticipating this procedure requires assessing the difficulty of each approach to managing the airway prior to embarking on Plan A (see Chapter 2).
    - Do not "sit on" patients with upper airway obstruction or insist on taking the patient out of the ED (e.g., to the computed tomography [CT] scan or to the operating room [OR]) unless it is absolutely clear that the patient's condition is stable enough and you are confident you can successfully secure the airway if needed. Observing the patient presents the risk that anatomy will worsen and obstruction will ensue, at which time the patient's trachea will be much more difficult to intubate and the need for doing so will be much greater. In addition, call for help early. Asking for help is not a failure.

How Should One Proceed in Managing the Airway in an Emergency?

Once it has been decided that intubation is indicated, the focus must be on what kind of airway problem is present, and what is the correct course of action (see Chapter 2).

- Is this a "Crash Airway" situation in which the patient is unconscious, unresponsive, and near death?
- Is this a "Difficult Airway" in which one anticipates difficulty with FMV, EGD use, laryngoscopy and intubation, or cricothyrotomy?
- If neither of these two situations exists, then RSI is the method of choice.
- Has a "Failed Airway" supervened?

This systematic approach to airway management in the ED takes into account all possible presentations, and properly identifying the type of airway situation permits the practitioner to select an appropriate course of action. Algorithms that address these situations are "expeditious management strategies" often used in crisis and are described in Chapter 2.

SUMMARY

RSI is the most common method of airway control in the ED. It is associated with a high rate of success; however, the complication rate in the critically ill is not insignificant. Some patients should not be paralyzed and successfully managing their airways will require alternative procedures, such as an awake tracheal intubation (ATI). The current challenge then is *how* to identify these patients in whom intubation or ventilation with face mask or EGDs would not suffice.

In the case presented here, the emergency physician recognized that the patient was in need of expeditious airway control. It was recognized that there were multiple factors that would complicate and make the management of the airway very difficult. Although laryngoscopy and intubation were not anticipated to be particularly difficult, this was considered a very high-risk airway due to significant physiologic derangements, including both severe hypoxemia and hypotension. The patient was unable to be adequately denitrogenated due to their underlying respiratory pathophysiology, making for a very short safe apnea time. Additionally, rescue oxygenation would likely be very difficult in the event of a failed intubation attempt due to the derecruitment of alveoli associated with RSI. Thus, it was felt by the practitioner that the patient was not a safe candidate for RSI. The decision was made to perform an awake intubation using a rigid video laryngoscope. Before this was attempted, the patient was set up for a potential surgical airway and had his cricothyroid membrane identified and marked. A surgical airway kit was readied and placed at the bedside. Five percent lidocaine ointment was applied topically to the oropharynx and the glottic inlet was anesthetized with 4% lidocaine solution using an atomizer. Using a C-MAC standard geometry video laryngoscope, the airway was easily visualized and the patient was quickly intubated on the first attempt. Once tracheal intubation was confirmed with capnography the patient was sedated to minimize the risk of accidental extubation.

SELF-EVALUATION QUESTIONS

22.1. All of the following are indications for emergency tracheal intubation **EXCEPT:**

A. Upper airway obstruction

B. Failure to protect the airway

C. Failure to maintain adequate oxygen saturations

D. The need for hyperventilation

E. Cardiac arrest

22.2. The emergency physician should be able to perform the following methods of airway management **EXCEPT:**

A. Cricothyrotomy

B. Rapid sequence intubation

C. Awake tracheal intubation

D. Tracheotomy

E. Extraglottic airway placement

22.3. Which of the following devices can be used for awake tracheal intubation?

A. Scalpel

B. Direct laryngoscope

C. Flexible endoscope

D. Hyperangulated video laryngoscope

E. All of the above

REFERENCES

1. Benumof J. The ASA difficult airway algorithm: new thoughts and considerations. 51st Annual Refresher Course Lectures and Clinical Update Program, #235. *American Society of Anesthesiologists*; 2000.
2. Daya M, Mariani R, Fernandes C. Basic life support. In: Dailey R, Simon B, Young G, Stewart R, eds. *The Airway: Emergency Management*. Philadelphia, PA: Mosby; 1992:39-61.
3. Safar P. Ventilatory efficacy of mouth-to-mouth artificial respiration; airway obstruction during manual and mouth-to-mouth artificial respiration. *J Am Med Assoc*. 1958;167:335-341.
4. Safar P, McMahon M. Mouth-to-airway emergency artificial respiration. *J Am Med Assoc*. 1958;166:1459-1460.
5. Safar P. History of cardiopulmonary resuscitation. *Acute Care*. 1986;12:61-62.
6. Walls R. Airway. In: Marx J, Hockberger R, Walls R, eds. *Rosen's Emergency Medicine: Concepts and Clinical Practice*. Philadelphia, PA: Mosby; 2009:2-20.
7. Murphy M, Walls RM. Identification of the difficult and failed airway. In: Walls RM, Murphy MF, eds. *Manual of Emergency Airway Management*. 3rd ed. Philadelphia, PA: Lippincott, Williams, Wilkins; 2008:81-93.

FURTHER READING

Ahmad I, El-Boghdadly K, Bhagrath R, et al. Difficult Airway Society guidelines for awake tracheal intubation (ATI) in adults. *Anaesthesia*. 2020;75(4):509-528.

April MD, Arana A, Reynolds JC, et al. Peri-intubation cardiac arrest in the emergency department: A National Emergency Airway Registry (NEAR) study. *Resuscitation*. 2021;162:403-411.

Cook TM, El-Boghdadly K, McGuire B, McNarry AF, Patel A, Higgs A. Consensus guidelines for managing the airway in patients with COVID-19: guidelines from the Difficult Airway Society, the Association of Anaesthetists the Intensive Care Society, the Faculty of Intensive Care Medicine and the Royal College of Anaesthetists. *Anaesthesia*. 2020;75(6):785-799.

Higgs A, McGrath BA, Goddard C, et al. Guidelines for the management of tracheal intubation in critically ill adults. *Br J Anaesth*. 2018;120(2):323-352.

Kornas RL, Owyang CG, Sakles JC, Foley LJ, Mosier JM. Evaluation and management of the physiologically difficult airway: consensus recommendations from Society for Airway Management. *Anesth Analg*. 2021;132(2):395-405.

Lentz S, Grossman A, Koyfman A, Long B. High-risk airway management in the emergency department. part I: diseases and approaches. *J Emerg Med*. 2020;59(1):84-95.

Lentz S, Grossman A, Koyfman A, Long B. High-risk airway management in the emergency department: diseases and approaches, part II. *J Emerg Med*. 2020;59(4):573-585.

Mosier JM, Hypes CD, Sakles JC. Understanding preoxygenation and apneic oxygenation during intubation in the critically ill. *Intensive Care Med*. 2017;43(2):226-228.

Mosier JM, Joshi R, Hypes C, Pacheco G, Valenzuela T, Sakles JC. The physiologically difficult airway. *West J Emerg Med*. 2015;16(7):1109-1117.

Myatra SN, Divatia JV, Brewster DJ. The physiologically difficult airway: an emerging concept. *Curr Opin Anaesthesiol*. 2022;35(2):115-121.

Natt BS, Malo J, Hypes CD, Sakles JC, Mosier JM. Strategies to improve first attempt success at intubation in critically ill patients. *Br J Anaesth*. 2016;117(suppl 1):i60-i68.

Russotto V, Myatra SN, Laffey JG, et al. Intubation practices and adverse peri-intubation events in critically Ill patients from 29 countries. *JAMA*. 2021;325(12):1164-1172.

Sakles JC, Pacheco GS, Kovacs G, Mosier JM. The difficult airway refocused. *Br J Anaesth*. 2020;125(1):e18-e21.

CHAPTER 23

Airway Management with Blunt Anterior Neck Trauma

David A. Caro, Ashley B. Norse, and Ryan S. Brandt

CASE PRESENTATION

A 25-year-old male drives into an unseen wire while he is snowmobiling. The wire strikes his anterior neck and throws him from his snowmobile. Paramedics are unsuccessful in placing an endotracheal tube (ETT) in the field. He arrives in the emergency department (ED) immobilized on a long spine board and with a cervical collar in place. He is unconscious, unresponsive to painful stimuli, and stridulous. Initial vital signs include a heart rate of 120 beats per minute, a blood pressure of 160/90 mmHg, a respiratory rate of 24 breaths per minute, and an oxygen saturation of 93% on room air. A non-rebreather oxygen mask is applied at a flush-flow rate, and his oxygen saturation increases to 97%.

Palpation demonstrates no obvious subcutaneous air, but there is a large abrasion across the anterior and lateral areas of the neck (Figure 23.1). Palpation of the larynx demonstrates crepitus and slight anatomic distortion. Plans begin immediately to further protect and secure the airway.

INITIAL PATIENT ASSESSMENT AND MANAGEMENT

■ What Are the Important Considerations in Evaluating This Patient?

Upon arrival at the ED, the team should follow a protocol that is consistent with the guidelines of the Subcommittee of Advanced Trauma Life Support® of the American College of Surgeons Committee on Trauma.[1–3] Careful but rapid airway assessment coupled with a high index of suspicion for associated injuries is a necessary step in the successful management of patients with this type of injury. The primary survey identifies an immediate airway concern, so airway management plans should immediately commence.

A young patient with no significant medical history should have adequate cardiorespiratory reserve if there are no concurrent traumatic injuries. His initial oxygen saturation is concerning, which prompts the addition of supplemental oxygen. His depressed level of consciousness could be due to a number of factors, including brain injury, and he might also have sustained a spinal cord injury. Head-injured patients have approximately 7% risk of an associated cervical spine fracture; the incidence of cervical spine fracture related to isolated blunt anterior neck trauma is difficult to adequately characterize, as it is such an infrequent event.[4–9] The airway practitioner must assume that this patient has a cervical spine fracture until proven otherwise.[2,10]

Other associated injuries can occur with this type of "clothesline injury." These include facial lacerations, vascular injuries, laceration of the trachea and/or esophagus,[11] and injury to the recurrent laryngeal nerve.[12] These injuries can present significant hazards to intubation. Vascular injuries and lacerations can result in hematoma formation that can impair visualization of the airway. Subcutaneous and submucosal emphysema can also impair visualization of the glottis. Incomplete tracheal

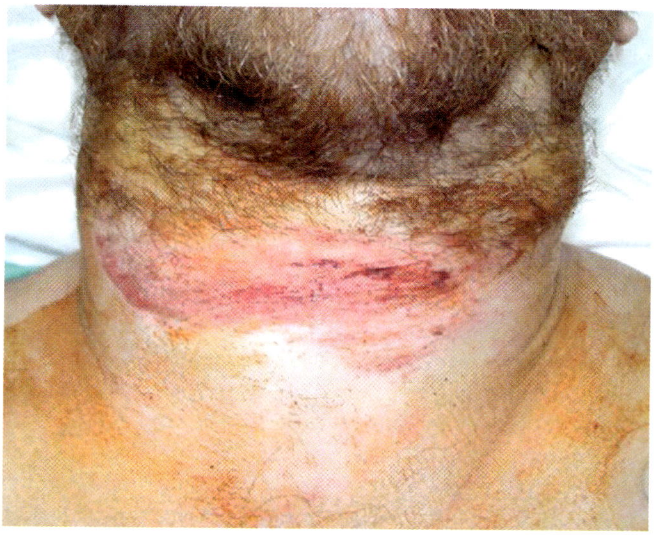

FIGURE 23.1. This "clothesline injury" patient has a large abrasion across the anterior and lateral areas of the neck.

disruption can result in the placement of an ETT in a false passage, with subsequent inability to ventilate. Complete tracheal disruption could result in retraction of the distal trachea into the thorax and complete inability to obtain a traditional or surgical airway.

What Are the Airway Priorities in This Patient?

The urgency of the presentation places the airway practitioner in a difficult situation. Unfortunately, a comprehensive evaluation of the airway will not be feasible, and computed tomography (CT) scanning of this tenuous patient could cause a delay that results in patient compromise.[13] It is possible to anticipate where difficulties will arise; however, rapid anatomic and physiologic evaluation of the patient is essential.

Anatomic considerations in this patient include the potential for laryngeal fracture, tracheal disruption, and an expanding hematoma that could impinge on the airway; all of these may be difficult to detect and could compromise airway patency.[14,15] Blunt anterior neck trauma can negatively influence all four components of initial airway management in this patient: facemask ventilation (FMV), use of extraglottic devices (EGDs), laryngoscopy/intubation, and cricothyrotomy.[16–18] FMV requires an open airway in addition to an adequate mask seal. Airway impingement or disruption might render FMV impossible. The airway distortion that can occur with a blunt neck injury could make EGD placement impossible. Hematoma formation could inhibit a laryngoscopic view and/or intubation. Tracheal disruption might make passage of an ETT difficult or impossible. Finally, depending on the location of the injury and the degree of tracheal injury, a front-of-neck airway (FONA) could be very difficult to secure.

The airway practitioner should anticipate difficult laryngoscopy, as well as the need to confirm continuity of the trachea as clear priorities in this patient. A clear view of the vocal cords is the first step, but supraglottic or glottic distortion may hinder visualization. Direct laryngoscopy (DL) may provide better control of the epiglottis and a more direct line of sight.[18] Video laryngoscopy (VL) can provide superior views of the glottis[19–21] with potentially less mobilization of the cervical spine[22–31] and may be preferable unless airway bleeding obscures the camera view. However, it must be understood that a clear view of the cords does not guarantee successful endotracheal intubation in this case. One must recognize that blunt anterior airway trauma may result in disruption or transection of the trachea distal to the glottis.[2] Tracheal transection may result in obstruction to tube passage or placement of the tube in a false passage through the tracheal disruption.[13,32] Orotracheal laryngoscopy cannot detect this injury and may lead to a false sense of security relative to the "ease" of intubation. One case series demonstrated six of seven tracheal disruptions to be at the cricothyroid/tracheal junction; four of these seven were successfully intubated while the others required emergency tracheotomy.[33]

Cricothyrotomy may also be very difficult in laryngeal trauma, as normal anatomic landmarks may be distorted, making it difficult to identify the larynx, the cricothyroid membrane, and the cricoid ring.[32,34] An open surgical technique is the preferred emergency FONA (see Chapter 14 for details). If the patient is awake, an initial midline skin incision under local anesthetic could help identify landmarks in this patient. Additionally, there is the possibility that the injury may be located distal to standard surgical airway landmarks leading to unsuccessful passage of the ETT.

AIRWAY MANAGEMENT

What Should We Consider in Managing This Patient's Airway?

This airway is not a "crash" airway, but it is a "difficult" one and needs to be secured urgently. Difficulty should be expected with FMV and laryngoscopy; the airway is possibly disrupted and neck mobility is limited. Difficulty can also be anticipated with EGD utilization and with cricothyrotomy (due to the potential for hematoma and laryngeal/tracheal distortion). The first step in the management of this patient is to summon help immediately, especially surgical assistance as an emergency tracheotomy might become necessary. Additionally, if extracorporeal membrane oxygenation (ECMO) is available at the institution, alert this team as well, as ECMO has been used in some instances of laryngeal trauma to allow time to safely perform a definitive airway.[35,36]

There is some time to formulate a plan. The identification of significant airway difficulty and the potential for irreversible airway compromise during the intubation attempt should stimulate the practitioner to utilize a difficult airway algorithm.[34,37] A facilitated look with a dissociative agent such as ketamine and topical anesthesia would be ideal in this circumstance. Careful sedation and topical anesthesia are appropriate in this patient, and in-line stabilization of the cervical spine is an absolute requirement. Coughing during the attempt could worsen the injury, or could further compromise a traumatized spinal cord. Be prepared with additional sedation and a paralytic agent for use either during intubation or once it is successfully achieved.

A difficult intubation should be performed by the most experienced laryngoscopist immediately available.[37–39] In-line stabilization of the cervical spine should be employed to prevent exacerbation of an unstable cervical injury. The laryngoscopy procedure of choice in this circumstance is intubation using a flexible bronchoscope (FB) in conjunction with VL.[39–42] VL is utilized to maintain an opening to the glottis. The FB can then be advanced into the airway to confirm airway patency, identify any tracheal injury, and serve as a stylet for the ETT to follow.[32,34,35] This technique permits visualization as one advances into the trachea and ensures that the ETT is not advanced into a blind passage. Traditional intubation with orotracheal, direct, or video laryngoscopy can result in the creation of false passages or pseudo-lumens which could compromise the patient's airway. Even the gentle placement of an Eschmann Introducer (EI; also known as "gum-elastic bougie") may create an airway obstruction in these patients,[1,2,39,43] although case reports exist of successful "bougie"-guided tracheal intubation in patients with tracheal-injury-producing, penetrating neck-wounds.[44] Confirmation of correct placement with an FB is important in these instances. A failed airway with inability to oxygenate via a face mask mandates an attempt at cricothyrotomy.[38,39]

■ Step by Step, What Is the Best Way to Intubate the Trachea of This Patient?

Timing is key. Rapidly assemble equipment, including FB if available, VL and/or DL equipment, while providing high-flow oxygen via non-rebreather face mask to denitrogenate. Additionally, a face-mask device should be opened and ready to use in the event of oxygen desaturation, and cricothyrotomy/tracheotomy equipment should be opened at the bedside and the patient's neck should be prepped and anesthetized for a potential attempt at a surgical airway in the event of decompensation due to inability to secure the airway. A suction catheter and additional airway adjuncts (such as oral and nasal airway devices) should be prepared. Additionally, an oral endoscopic intubation aid (e.g., the Berman break-away airway, the Williams oral intubating guide, the Ovassapian oral guide, or the Rapid Oral Tracheal Intubation Guidance System) or a track-intubation device would be helpful to allow a rapid, oral, flexible-bronchoscopic intubation attempt.[21,42]

The primary plan would be to perform VL-assisted, flexible-bronchoscopic intubation through an oral intubating guide or through an ETT placed at the cords.[2,32,34,35,39,42] In a pediatric patient, DL or VL oral intubation with a smaller-sized ETT might be preferable.[2] If the operator is "forced to act" and make a change in plans, change to an attempt at an oral DL or VL gently assisted with a bougie or a primary cricothyrotomy dependent on the airway practitioner's experience and capabilities, followed immediately by flexible-endoscopic confirmation.[2,38,39]

Adequate time for denitrogenation with a non-rebreather mask is essential to the success of this procedure. A well-oxygenated patient gives the airway practitioner a cushion of time in the event tracheal intubation is difficult and requires more time.[45] Steadily declining oxygen saturations may mandate assisted ventilation by a face mask. It is important to reiterate that EGDs are contraindicated in this patient as they may actually worsen the existing airway distortion. An immediate tracheotomy is indicated if oxygen desaturation occurs and the airway practitioner is unable to oxygenate with a face mask.[32,34,38]

Atomized 4% lidocaine or other agents used to provide topical anesthesia typically require 15 minutes to take effect, so the timing urgency must guide whether to use them or not.[46,47] Antisialogogues might be considered if time permits, although should not delay attempts at sedation and laryngobronchoscopy. Numerous sedating agents may be considered, including ketamine, propofol, midazolam, or etomidate. Ketamine (with or without propofol) is a good choice for this patient as it carries the benefit of analgesia, sedation, and maintenance of protective airway reflexes before the rare complication of associated laryngospasm, or emergence reaction.[48,49] Propofol and midazolam may have the advantage of practitioner's familiarity and ease of titration, although both drugs can potentially precipitate complete obstruction through a loss of muscle tone.[50,51] Dexmedetomidine might be a consideration if it is immediately available and extra help is present to allow the team to titrate the drip to effect.[52,53] The advantage of etomidate is its relative cardiovascular stability. However, the potential myoclonus associated with etomidate may place the potential unstable cervical spine and patency of a possible tenuous airway at risk.[54] While the use of neuromuscular blocking agents prior to intubation in difficult airways is debatable, the patient's obtundation complicates this scenario and might be necessary to facilitate actual ETT placement.[2,38] The amount of time the practitioner has to perform bronchoscopy and intubation will depend on the ability to maintain oxygen saturation. High-flow nasal oxygen during the bronchoscopic attempt might assist to provide prolonged maintenance of oxygenation.[55] A change of plan is indicated if glottic structures cannot be seen during the initial laryngoscopic look.

In the "can't intubate, can't oxygenate" (CICO) scenario, an immediate FONA is in order.[2,39] Open cricothyrotomy, or immediate bedside tracheotomy if surgery support is available, is preferable to percutaneous cricothyrotomy in this instance for the reasons stated above, including the creation of a false passage.[13,32,35] The open method allows the practitioner to identify the trachea and intubate under direct visualization if the distal end has not retracted into the thorax.[32,35] Blind attempts at finding a retracted, distal airway are rarely successful.[3,56]

OTHER CONSIDERATIONS

■ What Are the Concerns with Ventilation and Postintubation Care?

Once the trachea is intubated, ventilation takes priority. The use of end-tidal capnometry will ensure that the ETT is in the trachea and that the lower respiratory tree is being ventilated.[57]

Care must be taken to secure the ETT in place, as dislodgement could be disastrous. Immediate sedation is in order, as is continued protection of the cervical spine until fracture, dislocation, and ligamentous disruption of the cervical spine have been ruled out. Neuromuscular blockade at this point may also be in order if this patient is endangering his spine by excessive movement.

What Are Potential Postsurgical Complications Associated with "Clothesline Injuries"?

Following the repair of the laryngotracheal and cervical spine injuries, several serious postoperative complications may occur. These include voice compromise, recurrent laryngeal nerve damage, esophageal disruption, mediastinal infection, tracheoesophageal fistula, subglottic stenosis, neurologic injury, and carotid artery injury.[2,12,58,59] In a retrospective review of clothesline injury in children and adolescents (on all-terrain vehicles), between 1998 and 2003, Graham et al.[60] reported that all patients ($n = 7$) had significant neck and/or facial lacerations, with long-lasting disfigurement. One of the patients also had a functional impairment. Another retrospective review from 1995 to 2008 identified 35 pediatric patients with blunt laryngotracheal injuries; of the 11 "major" injuries, all required tracheotomy. Ultimately, all but one of these underwent decannulation.[61]

What Other Alternative Should Be Considered if Securing the Airway Is Not Possible for a Patient with a "Clothesline Injury"?

Extracorporeal circulation via a femoral–femoral cardiopulmonary bypass (CPB) or ECMO, placed with the use of local anesthesia and a portable unit, can be a lifesaving method of oxygenation and could have an important role in managing patients with a severely disrupted trachea. This can provide a safe solution for oxygenation when tracheal intubation or a surgical airway is either unsuccessful or too hazardous. However, establishment of a femoral–femoral bypass requires at least 15 to 20 minutes, even in experienced hands making it impractical and difficult to apply in emergency situations.[62]

SUMMARY

Blunt anterior neck injury poses a unique challenge to airway management and should be considered a difficult scenario. The airway practitioner must recognize the many barriers to airway management that can prevent intubation, including an obstructing hematoma or a transected trachea, and needs to quickly assemble an experienced team including surgical support, if available. Intubation using VL to provide the best views of the larynx, along with consistent oropharyngeal mouth opening, in conjunction with an FB to provide both indirect visualizations of an intact trachea and a stylet for ETT passage, is the ideal method of intubation in these patients. The intubation team should be prepared to obtain a surgical airway through the neck if the situation turns into a "CICO" scenario.

SELF-EVALUATION QUESTIONS

23.1. A patient presents with stridor and an oxygen saturation that is currently 85% and falling. What is the ventilation device of choice to attempt to provide oxygenation after passive means have failed?

A. Laryngeal Mask Airway
B. Intubating Laryngeal Mask Airway
C. Bag-valve-mask device
D. King LT™ Airway
E. Combitube™

23.2. What method of oxygenation can be used during bronchoscopic intubation in an attempt to maintain oxygen saturation?

A. Bilevel positive airway pressure
B. Non-rebreather mask
C. Nasal cannula or high-flow nasal oxygen
D. Continuous positive airway pressure
E. Venturi mask

23.3. What are the limitations of percutaneous cricothyrotomy in the setting of blunt anterior neck trauma with a concomitant laryngeal fracture?

A. Subcutaneous air may mimic intratracheal air, providing false localization.
B. Airway distortion may not allow readily identifiable, percutaneous airway structures.
C. Distal tracheal disruption may not be identified.
D. Advancement of the guidewire through the needle may be difficult.
E. All of the above.

REFERENCES

1. Butler AP, Wood BP, O'Rourke AK, Porubsky ES. Acute external laryngeal trauma: experience with 112 patients. *Ann Otol Rhinol Laryngol.* 2005;114(5):361-368.
2. Chatterjee D, Agarwal R, Bajaj L, Teng SN, Prager JD. Airway management in laryngotracheal injuries from blunt neck trauma in children. *Paediatr Anaesth.* 2016;26(2):132-138.
3. Edwards WH, Morris JA, DeLozier JB, Adkins RB. Airway injuries. The first priority in trauma. *Am Surg.* 1987;53(4):192-197.
4. Duggan LV, Griesdale DEG. Secondary cervical spine injury during airway management: beyond a "one-size-fits-all" approach. *Anaesthesia.* 2015;70(7):769-773.
5. Thompson WL, Stiell IG, Clement CM, Brison RJ, Canadian C-Spine Rule Study Group. Association of injury mechanism with the risk of cervical spine fractures. *CJEM.* 2009;11(1):14-22.
6. Mulligan RP, Friedman JA, Mahabir RC. A nationwide review of the associations among cervical spine injuries, head injuries, and facial fractures. *J Trauma.* 2010;68(3):587-592.
7. Verdonck P, de Schoutheete JC, Monsieurs KG, Van Laer C, Vander Poorten V, Vanderveken O. Penetrating and blunt trauma to the neck: clinical presentation, assessment and emergency management. *B-ENT.* 2016;Suppl 26(2):69-85.

8. Aufderheide TP, Aprahamian C, Mateer JR, et al. Emergency airway management in hanging victims. *Ann Emerg Med.* 1994;24(5):879-884.
9. Penney DJ, Stewart AHL, Parr MJA. Prognostic outcome indicators following hanging injuries. *Resuscitation.* 2002;54(1):27-29.
10. Nikolic S, Micic J, Atanasijevic T, Djokic V, Djonic D. Analysis of neck injuries in hanging. *Am J Forensic Med Pathol.* 2003;24(2):179-182.
11. Hamid UI, Jones JM. Combined tracheoesophageal transection after blunt neck trauma. *J Emerg Trauma Shock.* 2013;6(2):117-122.
12. LeJeune FE. Laryngotracheal separation. *Laryngoscope.* 1978;88(12):1956-1962.
13. Cheng J, Cooper M, Tracy E. Clinical considerations for blunt laryngotracheal trauma in children. *J Pediatr Surg.* 2017;52(5):874-880.
14. Stassen NA, Hoth JJ, Scott MJ, et al. Laryngotracheal injuries: does injury mechanism matter? *Am Surg.* 2004;70(6):522-525.
15. Sidell D, Mendelsohn AH, Shapiro NL, John MS. Management and outcomes of laryngeal injuries in the pediatric population. *Ann Otol Rhinol Laryngol.* 2011;120(12):787-795.
16. Pollack CV. The laryngeal mask airway: a comprehensive review for the Emergency Physician. *J Emerg Med.* 2001;20(1):53-66.
17. Donatelli J, Gupta A, Santhosh R, et al. To breathe or not to breathe: a review of artificial airway placement and related complications. *Emerg Radiol.* 2015;22(2):171-179.
18. Arino JJ, Velasco JM, Gasco C, Lopez-Timoneda F. Straight blades improve visualization of the larynx while curved blades increase ease of intubation: a comparison of the Macintosh, Miller, McCoy, Belscope and Lee-Fiberview blades. *Can J Anaesth.* 2003;50(5):501-506.
19. Lim HC, Goh SH. Utilization of a Glidescope videolaryngoscope for orotracheal intubations in different emergency airway management settings. *Eur J Emerg Med.* 2009;16(2):68-73.
20. Brown CA 3rd, Bair AE, Pallin DJ, Laurin EG, Walls RM, Investigators NEAR (near). Improved glottic exposure with the Video Macintosh Laryngoscope in adult emergency department tracheal intubations. *Ann Emerg Med.* 2010;56(2):83-88.
21. Li T, Jafari D, Meyer C, et al. Video laryngoscopy is associated with improved first-pass intubation success compared with direct laryngoscopy in emergency department trauma patients. *J Am Coll Emerg Physicians Open.* 2021;2(1):e12373.
22. Paik H, Park HP. Randomized crossover trial comparing cervical spine motion during tracheal intubation with a Macintosh laryngoscope versus a C-MAC D-blade videolaryngoscope in a simulated immobilized cervical spine. *BMC Anesthesiol.* 2020;20(1):201.
23. Dutta K, Sriganesh K, Chakrabarti D, Pruthi N, Reddy M. Cervical spine movement during awake orotracheal intubation with fiberoptic scope and McGrath videolaryngoscope in patients undergoing surgery for cervical spine instability: a randomized control trial. *J Neurosurg Anesthesiol.* 2020;32(3):249-255.
24. El-Tahan MR, El Kenany S, Khidr AM, Al Ghamdi AA, Tawfik AM, Al Mulhim AS. Cervical spine motion during tracheal intubation with King Vision™ video laryngoscopy and conventional laryngoscopy: a crossover randomized study. *Minerva Anestesiol.* 2017;83(11):1152-1160.
25. Kill C, Risse J, Wallot P, Seidl P, Steinfeldt T, Wulf H. Videolaryngoscopy with glidescope reduces cervical spine movement in patients with unsecured cervical spine. *J Emerg Med.* 2013;44(4):750-756.
26. Wong DM, Prabhu A, Chakraborty S, Tan G, Massicotte EM, Cooper R. Cervical spine motion during flexible bronchoscopy compared with the Lo-Pro GlideScope. *Br J Anaesth.* 2009;102(3):424-430.
27. Robitaille A, Williams SR, Tremblay MH, Guilbert F, Thériault M, Drolet P. Cervical spine motion during tracheal intubation with manual in-line stabilization: direct laryngoscopy versus GlideScope videolaryngoscopy. *Anesth Analg.* 2008;106(3):935-941.
28. Liu EHC, Goy RWL, Tan BH, Asai T. Tracheal intubation with videolaryngoscopes in patients with cervical spine immobilization: a randomized trial of the Airway Scope and the GlideScope. *Br J Anaesth.* 2009;103(3):446-451.
29. Kuo YM, Lai HY, Tan ECH, et al. Cervical spine immobilization does not interfere with nasotracheal intubation performed using GlideScope videolaryngoscopy: a randomized equivalence trial. *Sci Rep.* 2022;12(1):4041.
30. Gupta N, Rath GP, Prabhakar H. Clinical evaluation of C-MAC videolaryngoscope with or without use of stylet for endotracheal intubation in patients with cervical spine immobilization. *J Anesth.* 2013;27(5):663-670.
31. Yoon HK, Lee HC, Park JB, Oh H, Park HP. McGrath MAC videolaryngoscope versus optiscope video stylet for tracheal intubation in patients with manual inline cervical stabilization: a randomized trial. *Anesth Analg.* 2020;130(4):870-878.
32. Humenansky KM, Harris TM, Hoffman DM. Laryngotracheal separation following blunt neck trauma. *Am J Emerg Med.* 2017;35(4):669.e5-e669.e7.
33. Wu MH, Tsai YF, Lin MY, Hsu IL, Fong Y. Complete laryngotracheal disruption caused by blunt injury. *Ann Thorac Surg.* 2004;77(4):1211-1215.
34. Mercer SJ, Jones CP, Bridge M, Clitheroe E, Morton B, Groom P. Systematic review of the anaesthetic management of non-iatrogenic acute adult airway trauma. *Br J Anaesth.* 2016;117 Suppl 1:i49-i59.
35. Grewal HS, Dangayach NS, Ahmad U, Ghosh S, Gildea T, Mehta AC. Treatment of tracheobronchial injuries: a contemporary review. *Chest.* 2019;155(3):595-604.
36. Hamilton EC, Lazar D, Tsao K, Cox C, Austin MT. Pediatric tracheobronchial injury after blunt trauma. *J Trauma Acute Care Surg.* 2017;83(3):554-556.
37. Law JA, Duggan LV, Asselin M, et al. Canadian Airway Focus Group updated consensus-based recommendations for management of the difficult airway: part 2. Planning and implementing safe management of the patient with an anticipated difficult airway. *Can J Anaesth.* 2021;68(9):1405-1436.
38. Brown CA, Walls RM. Identification of the difficult and failed airway. In: Brown CA, Sakles JC, Mock NW, eds. *The Walls Manual of Emergency Airway Management.* 5th ed. Philadelphia, PA: Lippincott Williams & Wilkins; 2016:32-53.
39. Schaefer SD. Management of acute blunt and penetrating external laryngeal trauma. *Laryngoscope.* 2014;124(1):233-244.
40. O'Mara W, Hebert AF. External laryngeal trauma. *J La State Med Soc.* 2000;152(5):218-222.
41. Heidegger T, Starzyk L, Villiger CR, et al. Fiberoptic Intubation and Laryngeal Morbidity. *Anesthesiology.* 2007;107(4):585-590.
42. Sowers N, Kovacs G. Use of a flexible intubating scope in combination with a channeled video laryngoscope for managing a difficult airway in the emergency department. *J Emerg Med.* 2016;50(2):315-319.
43. Arndt GA, Cambray AJ, Tomasson J. Intubation bougie dissection of tracheal mucosa and intratracheal airway obstruction. *Anesth Analg.* 2008;107(2):603-604.
44. Steinfeldt J, Bey TA, Rich JM. Use of a gum elastic bougie (GEB) in a zone II penetrating neck trauma: a case report. *J Emerg Med.* 2003;24(3):267-270.
45. Mort TC. Preoxygenation in critically ill patients requiring emergency tracheal intubation. *Crit Care Med.* 2005;33(11):2672-2675.
46. Sun HL, Wu TJ, Ng CC, Chien CC, Huang CC, Chie WC. Efficacy of oropharyngeal lidocaine instillation on hemodynamic responses to orotracheal intubation. *J Clin Anesth.* 2009;21(2):103-107.
47. Xue FS, Liu HP, He N, et al. Spray-as-you-go airway topical anesthesia in patients with a difficult airway: a randomized, double-blind comparison of 2% and 4% lidocaine. *Anesth Analg.* 2009;108(2):536-543.
48. Gallo de Moraes A, Racedo Africano CJ, Hoskote SS, et al. Ketamine and propofol combination ("ketofol") for endotracheal intubations in critically ill patients: a case series. *Am J Case Rep.* 2015;16:81-86.
49. Jabre P, Avenel A, Combes X, et al. Morbidity related to emergency endotracheal intubation—a substudy of the KETAmine SEDation trial. *Resuscitation.* 2011;82(5):517-522.
50. Choi YF, Wong TW, Lau CC. Midazolam is more likely to cause hypotension than etomidate in emergency department rapid sequence intubation. *Emerg Med J.* 2004;21(6):700-702.
51. Win NN, Fukayama H, Kohase H, Umino M. The different effects of intravenous propofol and midazolam sedation on hemodynamic and heart rate variability. *Anesth Analg.* 2005;101(1):97-102.
52. Kunisawa T, Nagata O, Nagashima M, et al. Dexmedetomidine suppresses the decrease in blood pressure during anesthetic induction and blunts the cardiovascular response to tracheal intubation. *J Clin Anesth.* 2009;21(3):194-199.
53. Chu KS, Wang FY, Hsu HT, Lu IC, Wang HM, Tsai CJ. The effectiveness of dexmedetomidine infusion for sedating oral cancer patients undergoing awake fibreoptic nasal intubation. *Eur J Anaesthesiol.* 2010;27(1):36-40.
54. Guler A, Satilmis T, Akinci SB, Celebioglu B, Kanbak M. Magnesium sulfate pretreatment reduces myoclonus after etomidate. *Anesth Analg.* 2005;101(3):705-709.
55. Badiger S, John M, Fearnley RA, Ahmad I. Optimizing oxygenation and intubation conditions during awake fibre-optic intubation using a high-flow nasal oxygen-delivery system. *Br J Anaesth.* 2015;115(4):629-632.
56. Shweikh AM, Nadkarni AB. Laryngotracheal separation with pneumopericardium after a blunt trauma to the neck. *Emerg Med J.* 2001;18(5):410-411.
57. Hogg K, Teece S. Towards evidence based emergency medicine: best BETs from the Manchester Royal Infirmary. Colourimetric CO(2) detector compared with capnography for confirming ET tube placement. *Emerg Med J.* 2003;20(3):265-266.

58. Aouad R, Moutran H, Rassi S. Laryngotracheal disruption after blunt neck trauma. *Am J Emerg Med.* 2007;25(9):1084.e1-e2.
59. Smith DF, Rasmussen S, Peng A, Bagwell C, Johnson C. Complete traumatic laryngotracheal disruption–a case report and review. *Int J Pediatr Otorhinolaryngol.* 2009;73(12):1817-1820.
60. Graham J, Dick R, Parnell D, Aitken ME. Clothesline injury mechanism associated with all-terrain vehicle use by children. *Pediatr Emerg Care.* 2006;22(1):45-47.
61. Wootten CT, Bromwich MA, Myer CM. Trends in blunt laryngotracheal trauma in children. *Int J Pediatr Otorhinolaryngol.* 2009;73(8):1071-1075.
62. Belmont MJ, Wax MK, DeSouza FN. The difficult airway: cardiopulmonary bypass–the ultimate solution. *Head Neck.* 1998;20(3):266-269.

CHAPTER 24

Patient with Deadly Asthma Requires Tracheal Intubation

Lauren F. Becker and Anna Engeln

CASE PRESENTATION

Emergency Medical Services (EMS) presents with a 26-year-old female who is agitated and combative, in severe respiratory distress. Per EMS report, they have previously transported her for asthma "attacks" in the setting of polysubstance abuse. On chart review, you find that she has been intubated in the past, most recently 2 months ago during which she spent a week in the intensive care unit (ICU). During EMS transport, she received continuous aerosolized albuterol via nebulizer with minimal improvement and required restraints for agitation. On arrival at the Emergency Department (ED), she is speaking in one- to two-word sentences. She is more confused and is thrashing on the stretcher.

The patient is 5'2" (157 cm) tall and weighs 165 lb (74.8 kg), with a BMI of 30.5 kg·m^{-2}. Her vital signs are: heart rate of 134 beats per minute (bpm), respiratory rate of 30 breaths per minute, blood pressure of 130/80 mmHg, and oxygen saturation is 89% on 15 L·min^{-1} non-rebreather mask. She is using accessory muscles and is diaphoretic. She becomes more fatigued during your initial evaluation. You notice she has a short neck with a scar from prior cricothyrotomy, an obese habitus, and a recessed chin.

PATIENT EVALUATION

What Are the Patient's Vital Organ System Reserves?

CNS reserve: There is nothing to suggest that this patient will respond abnormally to standard weight-based doses of induction agents. Factors contributing to the patient's agitation may include stimulant intoxication, hypercarbia, and hypoxemia; none of these should significantly alter the patient's response to sedative-hypnotic induction agents.

Cardiovascular reserve: This young patient should theoretically have adequate cardiac reserve and normal systolic and diastolic function. Severe respiratory acidosis can potentiate myocardial depression associated with anesthesia induction agents, and chronic stimulant abuse may lead to abnormal baseline cardiac function due to cardiomyopathy. Many patients presenting with severe asthma exacerbation are hypovolemic due to a viral illness, dehydration, or inhaled stimulant abuse. When combined with the decrease in venous return due to air trapping and auto-PEEP seen with acute asthma, significant hypotension can result with induction for intubation.[1] This patient has been receiving high doses of albuterol, a β_2-agonist, which causes intracellular shifting of potassium. This shift may lead to serum hypokalemia and subsequent arrhythmias.[2]

Respiratory reserve: Patients with severe asthma have prolonged expiratory phases and air trapping.[3] As such, tidal volume (the amount of air that moves with each breath) is limited and respiratory reserve is minimal or nonexistent. Substantial ventilation-perfusion mismatch is present even before hypoxemia develops, which limits the ability to oxygenate and denitrogenate the lungs prior to induction.[4,5] Ventilatory support with noninvasive positive pressure ventilation (NIPPV) or intubation may be required in severe asthma as the patient becomes fatigued and unable to maintain gas exchange on their own. All these factors place the severe asthmatic at risk of rapid oxygen desaturation and worsening hypercapnia during rapid sequence intubation as they cannot tolerate apnea. Despite the risk of tracheal intubation of this patient, the real challenge lies in managing the patient in the postintubation phase of care.

AIRWAY EVALUATION AND MANAGEMENT OPTIONS

Employing the Mnemonics Suggested in Chapter 1, Does This Patient Have a Difficult Airway?

Yes! An obese face can make obtaining an appropriate seal for face-mask ventilation (FMV) difficult. In addition, both status asthmaticus and reduced chest wall mobility due to obesity create high airway pressures that are difficult to overcome with positive pressure FMV. Other than these factors, there appear to be no other predictors of difficulty in FMV when applying the mnemonic MOANS (see section "Difficult FMV: MOANS" in Chapter 1).

While the LEMON mnemonic (see section "Difficult DL Intubation: LEMON" in Chapter 1) suggests that an obese neck and recessed chin may make direct laryngoscopy difficult, there are predictors of difficult use of video laryngoscopy (VL) using the CRANE mnemonic (see section "Difficult VL intubation: CRANE" in Chapter 1). Subglottic stenosis is important to consider in this patient as she has experienced many tracheal intubations and a cricothyrotomy in the past, which may suggest an increased risk of scar tissue in the trachea. However, the geometry of her upper airway appears normal, and she has a Mallampati Class II airway. Her neck appears to be freely mobile.

In order to assess the feasibility of using an extraglottic airway device (EGD), the RODS mnemonic can be helpful (see section "Difficulty with an EGD: RODS" in Chapter 1). Restricted mouth opening is not an issue in this patient, and upper airway obstruction, while always a possibility, is not a major concern. However, her severe obstructive lung disease and compromised pulmonary compliance will limit the utility of a EGD and make the use of FMV difficult.

What Other Airway Concerns Do You Have for This Patient?

This patient in status asthmaticus has no respiratory reserve, has possible subglottic stenosis, and is at risk for rapid oxygen desaturation and hypotension during induction. Furthermore, the insertion of an endotracheal tube (ETT) in a person who is already in bronchospasm may worsen the bronchospasm.

Have We Medically Optimized Her Treatment Prior to Endotracheal Intubation?

Patients with severe asthma should undergo several medical interventions prior to performing tracheal intubation. The process of medical optimization may even allow the avoidance of intubation.

1. Oxygenation: Oxygen should be delivered to maintain saturations between 92% and 95% and begin denitrogenation in anticipation of intubation. Methods of oxygen delivery include nasal cannula at full flush combined with 15 $L \cdot min^{-1}$ through a non-rebreather oxygen mask, heated high-flow nasal cannula, or NIPPV. If intubation appears unavoidable, aim for an oxygen saturation of 100%, though this should not be maintained throughout as hyperoxia can worsen V/Q mismatch. Increasing the oxygen saturation in the blood leads to pulmonary vasodilation and increases perfusion areas of the lung with poor aeration, resulting in dead-space ventilation.
2. β_2-agonists: Short-acting β_2-agonists are the mainstay of treatment in asthma, typically via metered dose inhaler or nebulizer.[6] If patients are unable to cooperate with aerosolized β_2-agonists due to agitation or shallow respirations, terbutaline (a subcutaneous β_2-agonist) has been shown to be equally effective as albuterol in the treatment of acute asthma exacerbation.[7] This patient has been on a continuous nebulizer during transport but may still benefit from a trial of terbutaline if her agitation is interfering with her ability to cooperate with the nebulizer.
3. Anticholinergics: Anticholinergics are a mainstay of treatment in chronic obstructive lung disease and have been shown in meta-analysis to add a modest benefit to β_2-agonists in asthma as well.[8] Blocking cholinergic effects at muscarinic receptors can reduce smooth muscle contraction and minimize the release of secretions in large airways. The use of ipratropium bromide may reduce hospital admission rates.[9]
4. Magnesium: The effect of IV magnesium in acute asthma has been evaluated in two meta-analyses.[10,11] Seven trials were identified, and the investigators concluded there is evidence that magnesium improves pulmonary function and decreases hospitalization rates in severe asthma, although it has not been shown to reduce rates of intubation. As it is unlikely to cause harm, a trial of magnesium is reasonable in the severe asthmatic but should not delay intubation or other emergency interventions.
5. Steroids: Corticosteroids are recommended for all patients with acute moderate-to-severe asthma exacerbations, although administration will not affect immediate clinical status because time to onset takes a few hours and peak effect occurs around 24 hours.[12] Oral steroids are as good as IV steroids, and oral administration is generally preferred, but in this agitated and altered patient, a dose of IV corticosteroid is appropriate.

What Are the Possible Alternatives for Airway Management in Order to Avoid Intubation in This Patient?

NIPPV should be considered in patients with severe asthma; however, its use is dependent on mental status and the patient's ability to tolerate the device. This patient's mental status is altered, and she is uncooperative and is unlikely to tolerate NIPPV without sedation.

The use of NIPPV as a means of avoiding intubation in status asthmaticus has increased in popularity and is a valid option for initial airway management.[13,14] A 2012 Cochrane Review including six small heterogenous studies concluded that NIPPV might decrease rates of hospital admission and reduced respiratory rate (as a surrogate for decreased respiratory distress).[15] A multicenter retrospective cohort review published in 2016 suggested that patients who received NIPPV had better outcomes, but also found that failed NIPPV carried a higher mortality, though other studies have found failed NIPPV to carry no increased risk of mortality.[16,17] More recent studies have further supported that the use of NIPPV is safe and that it might reduce the need for invasive ventilation. In a study of 131 patients with worsening asthma and placed on NIPPV for ventilatory support, only four patients ultimately required intubation.[18]

To facilitate tolerance of NIPPV in an agitated patient, a trial of ketamine at lower doses (0.1-0.3 mg·kg^{-1}) may be carefully considered. In one study, this regimen was used to denitrogenate patients in preparation for intubation, but it was found that following the low-dose ketamine, several patients were able to tolerate the NIPPV, making intubation unnecessary.[19] In recent years, use of ketamine has become the mainstay in a trial of NIPPV, provided these patients are watched very carefully. The concept of delayed-sequence intubation, in which ketamine is given as an induction agent to facilitate denitrogenation and oxygenation prior to a paralytic, is an extension of the use of ketamine as a sedative during NIPPV.[20,21]

For multiple reasons, ketamine is the preferred induction agent or sedative for asthma. It increases circulating catecholamines and inhibits vagal outflow, while also dilating smooth muscle in both the vasculature and bronchioles.[22] These qualities make it more hemodynamically neutral than other induction agents and directly reverses the bronchospasm of acute asthma. Although case reports of dramatic improvement in pulmonary function with ketamine have driven its popularity,[23,24] no randomized studies have yet been performed to demonstrate ketamine's superiority over other induction agents. Small studies have shown improvement in oxygenation with patients treated with ketamine but have not shown changes in the overall outcome.[25] Although evidence remains limited, the mechanism of action and safety profile of ketamine suggest that it is the best agent for sedation and induction in acute asthma.

How Would You Proceed with Tracheal Intubation of This Patient?

If, after a trial of NIPPV with ketamine, the patient either continues to not tolerate NIPPV or their respiratory and/or mental status remain unstable, tracheal intubation should be considered. If the patient is unable to tolerate NIPPV, apneic oxygenation during intubation will be of paramount importance; both nasal cannula and non-rebreather should be placed on the patient prior to intubation.[26] If available, a heated high-flow nasal cannula is preferred to a low-flow nasal cannula for apneic oxygenation, although NIPPV is still superior for denitrogenation.[27]

1. **Equipment**
    - Person: The most experienced airway practitioner should attempt this airway, as the patient is unlikely to tolerate multiple or prolonged attempts.
    - Tube: Start with a 7.5-mm ID ETT (an 8.0-mm ID ETT for a male patient), but have a backup of smaller ETT prepared, especially in this patient who is at risk for subglottic stenosis with her history of prior cricothyrotomy.
    - Laryngoscope: Practitioners performing the intubation should use whatever laryngoscope they are most familiar with, although a video laryngoscope with a standard geometry blade is recommended.
    - Tracheal introducer (also known as a Bougie or Eschmann tracheal introducer): In airways with a risk for subglottic stenosis, having a bougie as an airway adjunct is important should there be difficulty in passing the ETT below the cords.
    - Surgical airway supplies: Although prior cricothyrotomy poses a risk for a difficult front-of-neck airway due to scar tissue and distorted anatomy, it may also indicate a previous difficult or failed tracheal intubation from above.
    - EGD: if this initial attempt fails, an EGD is a helpful rescue device, although poor lung compliance will make ventilation via an EGD challenging.
2. **Drugs**
    - Induction agent:
        1. Ketamine: 1-2 mg·kg^{-1}
        2. Etomidate: 0.3 mg·kg^{-1}
    - Paralytic:
        1. Succinylcholine: 1.5 mg·kg^{-1}
        2. Rocuronium: 1.2 mg·kg^{-1}
3. **Positioning**
    - During induction: Position the patient upright until paralytic is given, and continue to denitrogenate with NIPPV or heated high-flow nasal cannula.
4. **Laryngoscopy**
    - VL with a hyperangulated blade.
5. **Capnography**
    - In-line end-tidal CO_2 monitoring should be available as a quick and reliable way of confirming ETT placement.

POSTINTUBATION MANAGEMENT

What Is the Appropriate Postintubation Sedation Plan?

In order to maintain synchrony with the ventilator, prevent breath stacking and reduce auto-PEEP; deep sedation with medications to reduce respiratory drive are necessary. Propofol, ketamine, or fentanyl are all reasonable options.

Propofol is a GABA agonist with deep sedative effects, associated with significant respiratory depression at higher doses, and has some mild bronchodilatory effects.[28,29] Starting doses of 50 to 60 µg·kg^{-1}·min^{-1} are appropriate; note that this is a higher starting dose than used in traditional postintubation sedation as immediate deep sedation is desired. Beware of hypotension, which is a known complication of propofol.

Continue volume resuscitation as indicated, but a different sedative is preferred if hypotension is refractory to intravascular volume expansion.

Ketamine, with its previously discussed bronchodilatory effects via smooth muscle relaxation, is a good choice for sedation, but will not suppress respiratory drive. Its dissociative effects can achieve deep sedation and allow synchrony with the ventilator, but propofol is recommended as a first-line agent if the blood pressure can be maintained. Ketamine is associated with increased secretions, and coadministration with glycopyrrolate is recommended.[30]

Fentanyl and other opiates are respiratory depressants, but carry no physiologic benefit in the specific management of asthma. If the patient can hemodynamically tolerate a fentanyl infusion and has either not tolerated or not achieved adequate sedation with propofol or ketamine, fentanyl as an adjunct can be considered. The starting dose is usually 1 to 2 $\mu g \cdot kg^{-1}$ bolus, followed by an infusion of 1 to 7 $\mu g \cdot kg^{-1} \cdot hr^{-1}$, and keeping the dose low is recommended to reduce the long-term effects of opioid infusion. Morphine should be avoided due to histamine release and resultant worsening of bronchospasm.

What Are the Appropriate Ventilator Settings for This Patient?

All asthmatic patients have obstructed small airways and varying levels of alveolar hyperinflation. This hyperinflation leads to higher amounts of end-expiratory residual intra-alveolar gas and pressure, resulting in high levels of intrinsic PEEP or auto-PEEP. Elevations in auto-PEEP increase the risk for barotrauma. The primary goal of mechanical ventilation in the asthmatic is to allow for decompression of end-expiratory air-filled alveoli, while providing continuous in-line β_2-agonists to reduce airway obstruction. This goal is achieved by manipulating and assessing multiple ventilator parameters.

1. Inspiratory to expiratory ratio (I:E ratio): During normal exhalation, the airways collapse minutely due to changes in pressure; in the asthmatic, that collapse is exacerbated by an already decreased lumen. As such, exhalation takes significantly more time than inhalation in the setting of severe obstruction. A normal resting I:E ratio in a healthy individual is 1:2. In this patient, allowing a prolonged expiratory time, up to 1:5, is appropriate. A high inspiratory flow rate permits a longer expiratory phase.[31,32]
2. Minute ventilation (MV): Comprised of respiratory rate and tidal volume, MV represents the amount of air moved through the lungs in one minute. In order to prevent air trapping by allowing for alveolar decompression and facilitate prolonged exhalation, a lower respiratory rate and tidal volume are required. A respiratory rate of 10 and a tidal volume of 6 to 8 $mL \cdot kg^{-1}$ (based on ideal body weight) are appropriate starting parameters. The resultant lower MV leads to permissive hypercapnia, in which pCO_2 levels are allowed to rise to prevent barotrauma and the hemodynamic compromise, which can result from air trapping, wherein the high intrathoracic pressures impede cardiac preload and produce hypotension. The goal pH of permissive hypercapnia is 7.2, in which there is an isolated respiratory acidosis without metabolic component.[33–35]
3. Ventilator mode: There is no preferred mode for status asthmaticus; the goal is to maintain appropriate oxygenation and permissive hypercapnia without causing high plateau pressures. While pressure control mode allows for controlled peak pressures, the peak pressure in severe asthma will be high without fail, and volume control mode may be preferable. If using pressure control, the I:E ratio is adjusted directly by adjusting the inspiratory time parameter. If using volume control, the I:E ratio can be adjusted by increasing the peak flow rate. If using this mode, the "ramp" inspiratory waveform should be selected.
4. Plateau and peak pressure: The peak inspiratory pressure (PIP) factors in the resistance and compliance of the entire circuit. This measurement includes lungs, chest wall, airways, ETT, tubing, and the ventilator. In the recently intubated severe asthmatic, the peak pressure is expected to be high as severe airway obstruction contributed to the need for intubation. The plateau pressure is a much more important number to control. The plateau pressure is a measure of alveolar pressure; it removes the airways from the equation. An inspiratory hold can be performed on the ventilator which will yield the plateau pressure. Increasing plateau pressures are a sign of air-trapping; aim for a P-plat <25 to 30 cm H_2O. An expiratory hold maneuver is also possible and reveals the auto-PEEP present in the patient at a given time.
5. PEEP: As there is no parenchymal process driving alveolar collapse, high PEEP is not required. Keep the PEEP low, starting at 5 cm H_2O, ideally never going above 10 cm H_2O.[36]
6. FiO_2: Titrate FiO_2 to maintain O_2 saturation >90%. Decrease FiO_2 to below 60% as soon as possible, but do not make this a priority in the initial management of the ventilated asthmatic.[37]

In summary, after tracheal intubation of this patient, calculate her ideal body weight (50 kg). In pressure control mode, set the I:E ratio at 1:3-5. The respiratory rate is set at 8 to 10. The tidal volume is set at 6 $mL \cdot kg^{-1}$ (300 mL). Set the PEEP at 5 cm H_2O. After maintaining these settings for 5 minutes, do an inspiratory hold and measure the plateau pressure. If it is >30 cm H_2O, adjust the rate or expiratory time as needed. Do not be alarmed by high peak pressures; tolerate pressures ranging as high as 55 cm H_2O during initial management.

How Can Patient Synchrony with Ventilator Be Improved?

In certain cases, if plateau pressures are rising and air trapping is present, it is necessary to disconnect the patient from the ventilator and manually decompress the chest. After disconnection, place both hands on the patient's thorax at the anterior axillary line and firmly press inward and downward. You will hear a rush of air out of the ETT. Then, reconnect the patient to the ventilator and continue with the management strategy outlined above.

Deep sedation, with a goal Richmond Agitation-Sedation Scale (RASS) of −4 to −5, must be achieved.[38] Attempting different agents to identify the most effective sedation for the patient is often necessary. If synchrony persists despite appropriate sedation, a paralytic can be carefully considered.[39,40] Cisatracurium is the best choice as it is hemodynamically neutral, does not release histamine (which can be seen with succinylcholine), and does not require hepatic or renal clearance. Rocuronium can be considered; however, it has a shorter clinical duration than Cisatracurium. Paralysis should not be maintained longer than 24 hours, as it is associated with severe side effects including myopathy and delirium. However, as it provides time for the patient to rest their respiratory muscles and maintain ventilator synchrony, it is a useful option early in the course of the ventilated asthmatic.

ADDITIONAL CONSIDERATIONS

What Is the Clinical Utility of the Capnography Waveform?

The characteristic waveform of end-tidal CO_2 in severe asthma is a "shark fin" shape, in which the flow of air in the expiratory phase slows, and the slope of the end-tidal curve decreases. Applying end-tidal CO_2 and assessing the waveform in the prehospital setting and the ED has been studied in relation to improvements in spirometry. Hisamuddin et al. performed a prospective study that monitored 120 patients presenting with asthma exacerbation with both peak flow and end-tidal CO_2. While no statistically significant relationship between the two variables was found, they trended together.[41] In the severe intubated asthmatic who cannot participate in spirometry measurements, end-tidal CO_2 monitoring is another option, along with pressure measurements on the ventilator, to assess improvement with applied medical therapies.

What Is the Utility of Ultrasound in Managing the Airway of This Patient?

Use of ultrasound to identify pneumothorax is well established in studies looking at the Extended Focused Assessment with Sonography in Trauma (E-FAST) in identifying traumatic pneumothorax.[42] The sensitivity, while still low at approximately 60%, is higher than chest X-ray, which is approximately 50%.[43] While CT scan is the gold standard, with near 100% sensitivity, in the setting of the severe asthmatic in impending respiratory collapse, bedside studies are imperative and can rapidly guide the direction of care.

Identification of pneumothorax prior to intubation allows for placement of a chest tube and prevention of development of tension physiology with the increased thoracic pressure after intubation. Similarly, if the patient is decompensating after intubation, checking for a pneumothorax rapidly with bedside ultrasound is important. As it takes a large pneumothorax to cause significant respiratory and circulatory compromise, lung ultrasound in at least three views per lung is likely to detect it.[44]

In the Era of COVID-19, What Must the Emergency Department Practitioner Take into Account?

During initial management of the undifferentiated patient with severe respiratory failure, consideration must be given to COVID-19 infection. Even in a patient with a history of asthma and an examination consistent with asthma, the inciting factor for the exacerbation may be viral. Avoidance of aerosolizing procedures prior to negative COVID-19 result is recommended or even required by many ED protocols.

Nebulizer therapy is considered an aerosolizing procedure. Options to avoid open nebulization include: metered dose albuterol inhalers, subcutaneous terbutaline, and in-line nebulization during NIPPV if a viral filter is employed. Without a viral filter, NIPPV remains at risk for aerosolizing viral particles.

In managing any patient with respiratory failure in the ED, appropriate personal protective equipment (PPE), including an N-95 or approved respirator is paramount for protection of health care workers and patients.

SUMMARY

The patient with severe asthma constitutes a difficult airway even without anatomical features that might predict difficult laryngoscopy or intubation due to the fact that FVM and EGD rescue may be difficult or impossible because of limited respiratory reserve. Skilled medical management of a patient with status asthmaticus is essential and may even allow the avoidance of intubation. Initial medical management options include β_2-agonists, anticholinergics, corticosteroids, magnesium, and NIPPV. If tracheal intubation is deemed necessary, ketamine should be considered as the induction agent as it directly reverses the bronchospasm of acute asthma and is most hemodynamically neutral. A continuous infusion of ketamine may be of use for sedation following intubation. Careful postintubation management is essential. Ventilation strategies ought to include low tidal volumes (6 $mL \cdot kg^{-1}$) and respiratory rates (8-10 breaths per min) with long inspiratory to expiratory ratio (I:E 1:3-5) and a plateau pressure <25 to 30 cm H_2O. Deep sedation is necessary, and if patient's synchrony with the ventilator cannot be maintained, consider muscle paralysis. If plateau pressures are rising, consider air-trapping and treat with manual chest decompression. While tracheal intubation and management of the asthmatic patient is challenging, prudent use of these tools will help achieve the best patient outcome.

SELF-EVALUATION QUESTIONS

24.1. What is the preferred induction agent when intubating a patient with status asthmatics?

A. Etomidate

B. Ketamine

C. Propofol

D. Midazolam

24.2. You have successfully intubated your patient requiring intubation for status asthmatics. What is the most appropriate initial ventilator setting?

A. Elevated tidal volume of 10-12 $mL \cdot kg^{-1}$

B. Elevated PEEP at 10 cm H_2O

C. Elevated I:E ratio at 1:5

D. Elevated respiratory rate at 16 breaths per minute

24.3. In a patient with severe status asthmaticus, which of the following interventions is most effective at avoiding intubation?

A. Noninvasive positive pressure ventilation

B. IV magnesium

C. IV corticosteroids

D. Inhaled anticholinergic

REFERENCES

1. Horak J, Weiss S. Emergent management of the airway. New pharmacology and the control of comorbidities in cardiac disease, ischemia, and valvular heart disease. *Crit Care Clin.* 2000;16:411-427.
2. Bodenhamer J, Bergstrom R, Brown D, et al. Frequently nebulized beta-agonists for asthma: effects on serum electrolytes. *Ann Emerg Med.* 1992;21:1337-1342.
3. Hall J, Schmidt G, Wood L. *Principles of Critical Care.* 2nd ed. New York, NY: McGraw-Hill; 1998.
4. Sarkar M, Niranjan N, Banyal PK. Mechanisms of hypoxemia [published correction appears in Lung India. 2017;34(2):220]. *Lung India.* 2017;34(1):47-60. doi:10.4103/0970-2113.197116.
5. Rodriguez-Roisin R, Ballester E, Roca JR, Torres A, Wagner PD. Mechanisms of hypoxemia in patients with status asthmaticus requiring mechanical ventilation. The *American Review of Respiratory Disease.* 1989;139(3):732-739.
6. National Heart, Lung, and Blood Institute. National Asthma Education and Prevention Program (NAEPP), Expert Panel Report 2: Practical Guide for the Diagnosis and Management of Asthma. In: U.S. Department of Health and Human Services, Public Health Services, ed. National Institutes of Health Publication No. 97-4053; 1997.
7. Stauss R, Jawhari N. The treatment of asthma exacerbations with subcutaneous terbutaline. *J Allerg Clin Immun.* 2020;142(2):AB218.
8. Stoodley RG, Aaron SD, Dales RE. The role of ipratropium bromide in the emergency management of acute asthma exacerbation: a metaanalysis of randomized clinical trials. *Ann Emerg Med.* 1999;34:8-18.
9. Rodrigo GJ, Rodrigo C. The role of anticholinergics in acute asthma treatment: an evidence-based evaluation. *Chest.* 2002;121:1977-1987.
10. Alter HJ, Koepsell TD, Hilty WM. Intravenous magnesium as an adjuvant in acute bronchospasm: a meta-analysis. *Ann Emerg Med.* 2000;36:191-197.
11. Rowe BH, Bretzlaff JA, Bourdon C, Bota GW, Camargo CA Jr. Intravenous magnesium sulfate treatment for acute asthma in the emergency department: a systematic review of the literature. *Ann Emerg Med.* 2000;36:181-190.
12. Levy BD, Kitch B, Fanta CH. Medical and ventilatory management of status asthmaticus. *Intensive Care Med.* 1998;24:105-117.
13. Ganesh A, Shenoy S, Doshi V, Rishi M, Molnar J. Use of noninvasive ventilation in adult patients with acute asthma exacerbation. *Am J Ther.* 2015;22:431-434.
14. Garpestad E, Brennan J, Hill NS. Noninvasive ventilation for critical care. *Chest.* 2007;132:711-720.
15. Lim WJ, Mohammed Akram R, Carson KV, et al. Non-invasive positive pressure ventilation for treatment of respiratory failure due to severe acute exacerbations of asthma. Cochrane Database of Systematic Reviews 2012, Issue 12. Art. No.: CD004360.
16. Stefan MS, Nathanson BH, Lagu T, et al. Outcomes of noninvasive and invasive ventilation in patients hospitalized with asthma exacerbation. *Ann Am Thorac Soc.* 2016;13(7):1096-104.
17. Pallin M, Hew M, Naughton MT. Is non-invasive ventilation safe in acute severe asthma? *Respirology.* 2015;20:251-257.
18. Rasheed A, Latypov L, Gerolemou L, Vasudevan V. Utility of bilevel non-invasive positive-pressure ventilation (NIPPV) in patients with acute exacerbation of asthma. *Obstruct Lung Dis.* 2018;154(4):Suppl 786A.
19. Weingart SD, Trueger NS, Wong N, et al. Delayed sequence intubation: a prospective observational study. *Ann Emerg Med.* 2015;65:349-355.
20. Lentz S, Grossman A, Koyfman A, Long B. High-risk airway management in the emergency department. Part I: diseases and approaches. *J Emerg Med.* 2020;59(1):84-95.
21. Merelman AH, Perlmutter MC, Strayer RJ. Alternatives to rapid sequence intubation: contemporary airway management with ketamine. *West J Emerg Med.* 2019;20(3):466-471.
22. Huber FC Jr, Gutierrez J, Corssen G. Ketamine: its effect on airway resistance in man. *South Med J.* 1972;65:1176-1180.
23. L'Hommedieu CS, Arens JJ. The use of ketamine for the emergency intubation of patients with status asthmaticus. *Ann Emerg Med.* 1987;16:568-571.
24. Rock MJ, Reyes de la Rocha S, L'Hommedieu CS, Truemper E. Use of ketamine in asthmatic children to treat respiratory failure refractory to conventional therapy. *Crit Care Med.* 1986;14:514-516.
25. Hemmingsen C, Nielsen PK, Odorico J. Ketamine in the treatment of bronchospasm during mechanical ventilation. *Am J Emerg Med.* 1994;12:417-420.
26. Gleason JM, Christian BR, Barton ED. Nasal cannula apneic oxygenation prevents desaturation during endotracheal intubation: an integrative literature review. *West J Emerg Med.* 2018;19(2):403-411.
27. Ricard JD, Gaborieau B, Bernier J, Le Breton C, Messika J. Use of high flow nasal cannula for preoxygenation and apneic oxygenation during intubation. *Ann Transl Med.* 2019;7(Suppl 8):S380.
28. Schivo M, Phan C, Louie S, et al. Critical asthma syndrome in the ICU. *Clinic Rev Allerg Immunol.* 2015;48:31-44.
29. Pizov R, Brown RH, Weiss YS, et al. Wheezing during induction of general anesthesia in patients with and without asthma. A randomized, blinded trial. *Anesthesiology.* 1995;82(5):1111-1116.
30. Burburan SM, Xisto DG, Rocco PR. Anaesthetic management in asthma. *Minerva Anesthesiol.* 2007;73(6):357-365.
31. Corbridge TC, Hall JB. Techniques for ventilating patients with obstructive pulmonary disease. *J Crit Illn.* 1994;9:1027-1036.
32. Leatherman J. Mechanical ventilation for severe asthma. *Chest.* 2015;147:1671-1680.
33. Tuxen DV. Permissive hypercapnic ventilation. *Am J Respir Crit Care Med.* 1994;150:870-874.
34. Wiener C. Ventilatory management of respiratory failure in asthma. *JAMA.* 1993;269:2128-2131.
35. Bidani A, Tzouanakis AE, Cardenas VJ Jr, Zwischenberger JB. Permissive hypercapnia in acute respiratory failure. *JAMA.* 1994;272:957-962.
36. Tuxen D. Detrimental effects of positive end-expiratory pressure during controlled mechanical ventilation of patients with severe airflow obstruction. *Am Rev Respir Dis.* 1988;140(1).
37. Mosier JM, Hypes C, Joshi R, et al. Ventilator strategies and rescue therapies for management of acute respiratory failure in the emergency department. *Ann Emerg Med.* 2015;66:529-541.
38. Sessler CN, Gosnell MS, Grap MJ, et al. The Richmond Agitation-Sedation Scale validity and reliability in adult intensive care unit patients. *Am J Resp Crit Care Med.* 2002;166(10).
39. Brenner B, Corbridge T, Kazzi A. Intubation and mechanical ventilation of the asthmatic patient in respiratory failure. *Proc Am Thorac Soc.* 2009;6(4).
40. Papiris S, Kotanidou A, Malagari K, Roussos C. Clinical review: severe asthma. *Crit Care.* 2002;6(1):30-44.
41. Nik Hisamuddin NA, Rashidi A, Chew KS, Kamaruddin J, Idzwan Z, Teo AH. Correlations between capnographic waveforms and peak flow meter measurement in emergency department management of asthma. *Int J Emerg Med.* 2009;2(2):83-89.
42. Wilkerson RG, Stone MB. Sensitivity of bedside ultrasound and supine anteroposterior chest radiographs for the identification of pneumothorax after blunt trauma. *Acad Emerg Med.* 2010;17(1):11-17.
43. Husain LF, Hagopian L, Wayman D, Baker WE, Carmody KA. Sonographic diagnosis of pneumothorax. *J Emerg Trauma Shock.* 2012;5(1):76-81.
44. Kendall JL, Hoffenberg SR, Smith RS. History of emergency and critical care ultrasound: the evolution of a new imaging paradigm. *Crit Care Med.* 2007;35:S126-S130.

CHAPTER 25

An Uncooperative Patient with a History of a Difficult Intubation Requiring Tracheal Intubation in the Emergency Department

Katherine Mayer and Jarrod Mosier

CASE PRESENTATION

Police and paramedics are called to a busy intersection where a 28-year-old male was seen running through traffic and was presumeed to have been hit by a car. He was tackled by police and physically restrained until Emergency Medical Services (EMS) arrived and injected his thigh with 5 mg of intramuscular midazolam. Police left the scene, and the patient arrives at the emergency department by EMS 10 minutes after the midazolam injection. He is still agitated and uncooperative. The security staff place him in four-point restraints, and he is still combative. EMS has no identification on the patient, and he is not able to provide you with his past medical history. His heart rate is in the 140s and regular. He will not lie still enough to get a blood pressure measurement. The patient is screaming incomprehensible words mixed with profanities, with a faint inspiratory stridor as he gasps between fits. Peripheral pulses are strong and regular, skin is diaphoretic but warm, and you notice what appears to be a well-healed tracheostomy scar. You also notice a small laceration with underlying hematoma on the forehead.

PATIENT ASSESSMENT

How Should We Categorize This Extremely Agitated Patient, and What Physiologic Considerations Should We Be Aware of During Airway Management?

The differential for this patient's agitated delirium is broad and includes toxic ingestion and head injury—or both. Immediate rapid sequence intubation (RSI) without considering the underlying physiologic changes in severely agitated patients may result in rapid decompensation during intubation. In 2009, the American College of Emergency Physicians recognized the "excited delirium syndrome" into which this patient falls, though universal consensus on the definition is lacking.[1] Nonetheless, excited delirium is characterized by "incoercible psychomotor agitation and aggressiveness."[2] The pathophysiology of excited delirium is hypothesized to be related to high levels of endogenous catecholamines with concomitant use of stimulant drugs, most often cocaine.[2,3] Mortality from excited delirium is reported between 8.3% and 16.5%, and deaths are attributable to acute myocardial dysfunction.[2] There is a theorized connection between the hyperdopaminergic environment in the brain of patients with excited delirium and abnormal autonomic signaling. This is one explanation for sudden cardiovascular collapse seen in some patients with this syndrome.[4]

Pharmacologic treatment is often necessary to control the excited delirium and facilitate adequate assessment and preparation for intubation. Mild sedation allows for better anatomic assessment prior to intubation, and it is often vital for adequate denitrogenation. While medications to control agitation may be helpful in this way, emergency practitioners must also remember that these medications can also exert influence over the hemodynamic milieu, which can include autonomic dysregulation.

Many pharmacologic options exist for sedating severely agitated patients, including benzodiazepines, neuroleptics, ketamine, and dexmedetomidine. High doses of benzodiazepines require careful consideration, as high doses may be less hemodynamically neutral and are more likely to lead to respiratory depression. Neuroleptic agents can be effective as well, particularly in patients with known psychiatric disease. However, these agents can prolong the QT interval, increasing the risk of polymorphic ventricular tachycardia and cardiac arrest. Ketamine is often used in emergency settings for agitated delirium to dissociate patients and achieve behavioral control with low risk of respiratory depression.[5] Protocolized ketamine has been safely and effectively used for severely agitated patients in some prehospital settings.[5] However, in a patient experiencing maximal catecholamine surge, ketamine has two theoretical, if not hypothetical, potential downsides. The effects of ketamine administration in this patient may vary. The indirect sympathomimetic effect of ketamine may worsen the catecholamine surge. In addition, it is also possible that in this patient, the reserves of endogenous catecholamines may already be exhausted. Ketamine can also cause direct myocardial depression that may predominate in this patient.

The goal of controlling agitation with ketamine may come at the cost of either of these hemodynamic effects. Dexmedetomidine may control behavior and improve the underlying hemodynamics through its α_2-agonist effects.[6,7] Remifentanil as well may be an option in these patients, though it is a potent respiratory depressant.[8] Whichever medication is used, preintubation agitation should be treated to allow for adequate airway evaluation and preparation. Ongoing hemodynamic and respiratory monitoring is essential as any of these medications can precipitate respiratory arrest despite a favorable safety profile.

What Are the Anatomic Considerations When Intubating a Patient with a Prior Tracheotomy?

The most serious concern when intubating a patient with a prior tracheotomy is unrecognized tracheal or subglottic stenosis. While this is a concern for any patient with a previous intubation, particular risk develops in patients who have experienced longer durations of mechanical ventilation. The incidence of postintubation and post tracheotomy tracheal stenosis ranges from 10% to 22%, but only about 1% to 2% have severe symptomatic stenosis.[9] The most common location of tracheal stenosis in patients with a history of prolonged intubation is at the prior endotracheal balloon/cuff site, and at the stoma site in patients with a history of prior tracheotomy.[9] The fundamental risk with subglottic or tracheal stenosis, as it relates to airway management, is the potential inability to pass an endotracheal tube (ETT) past the stenosis, or inability to ventilate due to resistance across the stenotic region. Even emergency cricothyrotomy may not lead to effective ventilation in a patient with severe tracheal stenosis that is distal to the cricothyrotomy location.

AIRWAY MANAGEMENT

What Are the Airway Management Options for This Patient?

One must assess the patient for potential anatomically difficult laryngoscopy and ETT placement, face-mask ventilation (FMA), or extraglottic device (EGD) rescue oxygenation. Additionally, one must consider the patient's underlying pathophysiology (oxygenation/ventilation and hemodynamics) when proceeding with denitrogenation, apnea, induction medications, and transition to positive pressure ventilation. If not done thoughtfully, the risk of peri-intubation cardiac arrest, or other complications, increases. This patient's agitation poses problems with any assessment, either anatomic or physiological. In general, there are three potential options:

1. *Rapid sequence induction.* In this case, the patient is induced with the sedative and paralytic prior to denitrogenation and without assessment for difficulty. While not a *forced-to-act* scenario in the traditional sense of an impending complete airway obstruction, one is *forced to induce* the patient in order to prepare for intubation. The risks of this approach include all of those found with an unidentified, unprepared for difficult airway, lack of denitrogenation, and unmitigated underlying physiological disturbances.
2. *Spontaneously breathing intubation.* The benefit of maintaining spontaneous breathing during intubation in this patient is the restored ability to denitrogenate, and more options for ventilation and oxygenation available in the face of unrecognized difficulty, such as the discovery of a stenotic trachea. Spontaneously breathing intubations require a fine balance between safety and success. The worst-case scenario when maintaining spontaneous breathing during intubation is a hypopneic or apneic patient from sedation but yet is not optimized for laryngoscopy without a paralytic in the face of recognized or anticipated difficulty. Thus, traditionally, spontaneously breathing intubations are performed with topicalization of the airway to facilitate airway manipulation and have an awake, cooperative patient. Sometimes, low-dose sedatives are required for anxiolysis but still facilitate a cooperative patient with spontaneous respiration. Unfortunately, neither is an option with this patient, which leaves dissociation or deeper sedation the only option to facilitate laryngoscopy while maintaining spontaneous respiration. The risks of this deeper sedation or dissociation without muscle paralysis include the risk of a suboptimal glottic view, airway trauma, and aspiration from a patient not completely passive during laryngoscopy.
3. *Delayed sequence intubation (DSI).* Delayed sequence intubation was described to address the risks associated with deeper sedation or dissociation without paralysis in a spontaneously breathing intubation outlined above. With this technique, behavioral control is achieved with a dissociative dose of ketamine to facilitate denitrogenation. The neuromuscular blocking agent is then given after denitrogenation to optimize intubating conditions. The difference between

dissociated intubation and DSI is the addition of a paralytic in the delayed sequence approach, once denitrogenation has been achieved. The concept of achieving behavioral control to facilitate airway evaluation and denitrogenation, however, is theoretically agnostic to the medication given. The risks of DSI include: apnea with the ketamine dose; undesirable side effects of ketamine or an evaluation after dissociation that warrants a more awake and cooperative patient in a now dissociated and uncooperative patient; and the aspiration of gastric content.

The best option will depend on the complex relationship between anatomic, physiological, and situational factors. For each option to be viable, there must be adequate staff, experience, and equipment to perform any of the three. In this patient, there is anticipated potential difficulty given the tracheotomy history within the context of a physiologically fragile milieu presenting an unpredictable response to ketamine or any other sedative. Of the options, RSI would result in an apneic patient without denitrogenation and potential difficulty. Spontaneously breathing intubation is the safest approach but impractical given the excited delirium and likely high doses of sedatives required to obtain behavioral control. This option would result in an overly sedated but still not optimized patient. DSI in this patient has its risks—those outlined previously and also an unpredictable response to ketamine—yet provides the best option to allow for denitrogenation, time for physiologic optimization, and appropriate airway assessment, yet still provides the optimized intubation conditions with the paralytic.

How Do You Denitrogenate an Uncooperative Patient?

Denitrogenation requires three things to be successful at providing an adequate apnea time to perform laryngoscopy and intubation. In the agitated delirium patient, this will likely require added time in order to properly position the patient after induction. The three necessary variables are: (1) adequate functional residual capacity (FRC), (2) complete removal of the nitrogen within the FRC, and (3) availability of that oxygen reservoir to resaturate hemoglobin as it passes through the pulmonary circulation. To most effectively resaturate hemoglobin, the oxygen reservoir should be deep and not rapidly consumed, and the alveolar-capillary interface in the lungs would be without inflammation or congestion, in order to minimize "shunting." Shunting results when blood flows to areas in the lungs that are not able to participate in gas exchange (such as in pulmonary edema, atelectasis, or pneumonia). Hyperactive or delirious/agitated patients have several potential barriers to denitrogenation. First, they may be uncooperative to any face mask or high-flow oxygen source on the face, which dramatically diminishes the ability to denitrogenate. Second, the catecholamine surge, if present, comes with increased cardiac output and peripheral oxygen consumption. Third, if the agitated delirium is the result of intoxication or head injury, there may be cardiogenic, inflammatory, or neurologically driven pulmonary edema or aspiration pneumonitis present. These factors combine to create a patient who may have an inadequately denitrogenated FRC, which may be further impacted by pulmonary edema, shunt physiology, and increased peripheral oxygen consumption. In addition, if the patient is hyperthermic from sympathomimetic overdose, the oxyhemoglobin dissociation curve is shifted rightward, all of which can increase the likelihood of rapid desaturation of these patients upon induction.

Consequently, as described above, you are left with a decision to either induce the patient with RSI, which implies trying to denitrogenate after induction, or make the patient pharmacologically compliant with denitrogenation or a DSI. With RSI, induction would be followed immediately with denitrogenation using FMA (or an EGD) and a PEEP valve. Pharmacological compliance options for sedatives include: midazolam or propofol (with the risk of depressed respiratory drive); dexmedetomidine or remifentanil (which are short-acting and may not be potent enough to control the agitation); and dissociation with ketamine. Regardless, once sedatives are given in any form, the practitioner must be prepared for rapid decompensation and should be ready for tracheal intubation, rescue oxygenation, and emergency front-of-neck access (FONA).

How Do You Secure the Airway of This Patient?

Preintubation assessment in this patient is difficult because of the agitated delirium; thus, the practitioner must be broadly prepared for any outcome. This includes medication selection for induction and the potential hemodynamic decompensation; thus, vasopressors should be prepared even if the patient is hypertensive and hyperdynamic prior to induction. The difficult airway cart should be on hand with proper equipment to execute Plan B, C, etc., and for rescue oxygenation/ventilation. Since this patient has a history of a tracheotomy and stridor on exam, one must expect potential tracheal stenosis, and preparations should be made accordingly in case the laryngoscopy or ETT advancement fails. This includes a second-generation EGD, a flexible bronchoscope, and progressively smaller ETTs. A strategy should be developed and communicated to the team so that the team can move as one in the event of a crisis.

The ideal induction medication will preserve hemodynamic stability and result in rapid sedation. To that end, etomidate, ketamine, and propofol are all excellent options but doses should be considered carefully as all induction agents have some dose-response effect on hemodynamics. If RSI is the plan, we recommend paralysis in typical RSI fashion to optimize first-pass success. It is likely that this agitated patient has experienced significant muscular activation, and the risk of rhabdomyolysis is high.[10] As such, a nondepolarizing paralytic such as rocuronium (1.2 $mg{\cdot}kg^{-1}$) should be used over succinylcholine due to the possibility of hyperkalemia from acute renal failure.

The technical approach to intubating this patient hinges upon the recognition that this patient's oxygen saturation may drop quickly and there may be tracheal stenosis, making it difficult to pass the ETT. While it is vital to be broadly prepared, it is also important to consider practitioner's familiarity and muscle memory. It would be unwise to try an unfamiliar technique for the first time. Laryngoscopy should occur as it normally would, and the adaptation to tracheal intubation with possible tracheal stenosis lies in having smaller than typical ETTs. We would recommend placing a tracheal introducer (commonly known as "bougie") through the vocal cords as a Plan A approach so that smaller ETTs can be exchanged over the "bougie" if needed. The smallest ETT that can fit over an adult "bougie" is a 6.0-mm ID. If a "bougie" is unable to be passed easily, or the patient's oxygen saturation decreases quickly, the next step is placement of a second-generation EGD to maintain gas exchange. A flexible bronchoscope can be passed through the EGD while maintaining oxygenation and ventilation, and if a pediatric bronchoscope is used, a 5.0-mm ID ETT can be passed over the scope. If there is still difficulty, and gas exchange can be maintained with the EGD, it is important not to make repeated intubation attempts to avoid trauma and swelling at the site of stenosis and convert a "can't intubate, can oxygenate" into a "can't intubate, can't oxygenate" scenario.

In most patients that have an immediate need for RSI, the best approach is laryngoscopy with a backup plan of rescue oxygenation, including potential emergency FONA. In patients with tracheal stenosis, however, the backup options are more nuanced and challenging. In severe tracheal stenosis, a cricothyrotomy will likely not bypass the area of stenosis, so maintaining gas exchange with an EGD becomes the rescue airway while arranging for rigid bronchoscopy or emergency open tracheotomy.

What Is the Postintubation Management Plan for the Patient?

Once the airway is secure, ongoing sedation and ventilator management will become the focus. Importantly, higher doses of sedating agents may be needed in this phase of treatment, both due to the preexisting agitation and due to the possibility of a smaller than typical ETT, which can lead to patient discomfort and ventilator dyssynchrony once the paralytic has worn off. Endotracheal tube diameter maintains an inverse relationship to flow and work of breathing.[11] High inspiratory flow rates lead to more turbulent flow and increased work of breathing. As such, if a 6.5-mm ID ETT is placed, one can expect high peak pressures to be delivered by the ventilator in order to provide adequate flow through a smaller diameter ETT.[12] The acceptable ventilator pressure thresholds may need to be set higher to allow adequate flows and tidal volumes to be delivered to the patient. Due to flow limitations of a smaller ETT, increased time may be required to deliver (and subsequently remove) a typical 6 $mL \cdot kg^{-1}$ tidal volume breath. A slower inspiratory and expiratory time is often not tolerated by patients unless deeply sedated and sometimes even paralyzed. For all these reasons, deep sedation in patients with small ETTs will likely be required for both gas exchange and ventilator synchrony. It is prudent to obtain an ABG just after intubation, during the early stabilization period following intubation, and whenever ventilator adjustments are made. The excited delirium patient has several reasons to have a metabolic acidosis (AKI, hyperthermia, lactic acidosis), and adequate ventilation as assessed by blood gas measurements is critical to ensure appropriate respiratory compensation and a pH >7.20.

Lastly, in patients with tenuous airways, physical restraints are especially indicated as a final means to prevent accidental self-extubation.

SUMMARY

Agitated delirium presents multiple challenges with airway management. First, uncooperative and combative patients make airway assessment difficult or impossible. Second, denitrogenation is challenging and often not possible until patients are either pharmacologically compliant or after induction of anesthesia. Third, the precipitating factor for agitated delirium presents physiological challenges that may increase the risk of morbidity and mortality associated with intubation—whether from neurological decompensation or cardiovascular collapse. These challenges are exacerbated in patients with a history of, or risk factors for, an anatomically difficult intubation. To successfully manage these patients' airways, careful consideration must be given to developing a strategy for hemodynamically stable induction of anesthesia, denitrogenation, and rapid progression through plans to place an ETT or rescue oxygenate. Overpreparation can be understated and will often be the difference between a successful safe intubation and a tragic catastrophe.

SELF-EVALUATION QUESTIONS

25.1. What is the primary pharmacological principle when performing a spontaneously breathing intubation?

A. Induction dose sedative without a neuromuscular blocking agent

B. Dissociative dose ketamine

C. Topical anesthesia of the upper airway

D. Low-dose sedatives

25.2. You plan for RSI in a patient without any apparent difficult airway predictors. Your first attempt fails because of an inability to pass an endotracheal tube past a stenotic lesion. The patient starts to desaturate. What is the next best step?

A. Continue to attempt with smaller tube sizes until something fits across the lesion.

B. Insert a rigid stylet and force the tube across the stenosis.

C. Insert a second-generation EGD.

D. Perform a cricothyrotomy.

E. Insert a tracheal introducer and then mask ventilate.

25.3. You have a combative, uncooperative patient that requires intubation to facilitate workup for a head injury. The patient is a normal appearing 70 kg male, and vital signs include tachycardia (124), hypertension (188/110), afebrile (37.9), and saturation 95% on room air. Chest radiograph shows no pneumothorax or infiltrates. You are unable to obtain any laboratory studies or imaging until the patient is intubated and restrained. So, you decide to perform RSI. What is the biggest threat to preoxygenation in this patient?

A. Shunt physiology

B. Decreased functional residual capacity

C. Oxygen consumption

D. Denitrogenation

REFERENCES

1. DeBard M, Adler J, Bozeman W, et al. *White Paper Report on Excited Delirium Syndrome*. American College of Emergency Physicians, 2009.
2. Gonin P, Beysard N, Yersin B, et al. Excited delirium: a systematic review. *J Soc Acad Emerg Med*. 2018;25:552-565.
3. Otahbachi M, Cevik C, Bagdure S, et al. Excited delirium, restraints, and unexpected death: a review of pathogenesis. *Am J Forensic Med Pathol*. 2010;31:107-112.
4. Mash DC. Excited Delirium and Sudden Death: A syndromal disorder at the extreme end of the neuropsychiatric continuum. *Front Physiol*. 2016;7:435.
5. Mo H, Campbell MJ, Fertel BS, et al. Ketamine safety and use in the emergency department for pain and agitation/delirium: a health system experience. *West J Emerg Med*. 2020;21:272-281.
6. Tobias JD. Dexmedetomidine to control agitation and delirium from toxic ingestions in adolescents. *J Pediatr Pharmacol Ther*. 2010;15:43-48.
7. Carrasco G, Baeza N, Cabre L, et al. Dexmedetomidine for the treatment of hyperactive delirium refractory to haloperidol in nonintubated icu patients: a nonrandomized controlled trial. *Crit Care Med*. 2016;44:1295-1306.
8. Barbic D, Andolfatto G, Grunau B, et al. Rapid agitation control with ketamine in the emergency department (RACKED): a randomized controlled trial protocol. *Trials*. 2018;19:651.
9. Zias N, Chroneou A, Tabba MK, et al. Post tracheostomy and post intubation tracheal stenosis: report of 31 cases and review of the literature. *BMC Pulm Med*. 2008;8:18.
10. Takeuchi A, Ahern TL, Henderson SO. Excited delirium. *West J Emerg Med*. 2011;12:77-83.
11. Pfitzner J. Poiseuille and his law. *Anaesthesia*. 1976;31:273-275.
12. Shapiro M, Wilson RK, Casar G, et al. Work of breathing through different sized endotracheal tubes. *Crit Care Med*. 1986;14:1028-1031.

CHAPTER 26

Airway Management for the Burn Patient

Laeben Lester and Darren Braude

CASE PRESENTATION

A 57-year-old man was brought to the Emergency Department (ED) by Emergency Medical Services (EMS) with burns to the head, face, and chest secondary to smoking while on 2 L·min^{-1} of oxygen via nasal cannula for COPD. There was no reported loss of consciousness. Albuterol was nebulized, an 18-gauge IV was placed, and IV fluids and fentanyl administered. Upon arrival to the ED, the patient is awake and alert but in obvious pain with mild respiratory distress. He speaks in full sentences with a hoarse voice. His blood pressure is 152/91, with a heart rate of 112 beats per min, breathing 26 times per min, with an oxygen saturation of 97% while receiving oxygen through a non-rebreathing mask, and his temperature is 36.8°C. Lungs' sounds are remarkable for diffuse wheezing with fair air movement.

The patient is noted to be 6′3″ and 110 kg (30.2 kg·m^{-2}). Further rapid evaluation reveals deep partial- to full-thickness burns to the perioral region, anterior neck, and upper chest wall. Despite these burns, the patient still has full mouth opening greater than three finger breaths (approximately 5 cm), with a thyromental distance of three finger breaths (approximately 5 cm) and the larynx is more than two finger breaths (approximately 3 cm) below the hyoid. The Mallampati class is I. The nasal hairs are singed, and there is mild erythema to the tongue and posterior pharynx with a small intact blisters noted. He has full range of motion of the neck but laryngeal landmarks are difficult to appreciate due to a combination of obesity and burns.

PATIENT ASSESSMENT

What Are the Airway Evaluation Considerations in This Patient?

Airway evaluation and management for the acute burn patient builds on standard airway evaluation and management with the added complexities associated with both inhalational and external burns, and the potential for coexisting toxicological injuries from carbon monoxide and cyanide. In addition, it is critical to consider the potential for the dynamic evolution of inhalational and topical burn injury; an airway initially at low risk for difficulty can progress and become very difficult if edema ensues and leads to obstruction.

This patient currently has predictors of moderate difficulty in all four dimensions of airway management: face-mask ventilation (FMV), laryngoscopic intubation, front-of-neck airway (FONA), and extraglottic device (EGD) rescue. The likelihood of toxicological issues is low in this case, given there was no prolonged smoke exposure, no loss of consciousness, and mental status is currently normal with relatively reassuring vital signs.

What Are Signs and Symptoms of Inhalational Injury?

Inhalational injury is a major contributor to the morbidity and mortality associated with burns and is a critical component to the evaluation and management of the airway. Inhalational injury is primarily associated with fires in enclosed space, especially when there is loss of consciousness. Signs and symptoms of inhalational injury may include dyspnea, hoarseness, hot potato voice, stridor, respiratory distress, use of accessory muscles, cough, deep burns to the face or neck, singed nares, carbonaceous sputum, and blistering or edema of the oropharynx. Initial and serial nasopharyngoscopic evaluation of the upper and/or lower airway is increasingly performed in many centers to help with the diagnosis of inhalational injury and to monitor progression and may represent the most important advancement in airway management of burn patients.[1–4] Recently, ultrasonic evidence of tracheal thickening has been used as a marker of inhalational injury.[5]

What Is the Time Course for Airway Injury to Manifest and Worsen and How Does This Impact Decisions?

Airway edema can progress early and rapidly or at any time during the first 12 to 24 hours, or longer, making airway management significantly harder.[6–8] Likewise, burned skin to the face, neck, and torso can become less elastic, and significant swelling can occur from inflammation and third spacing during fluid resuscitation (often hugely iatrogenic), compounding airway and ventilation issues. Thus, early intubation has traditionally been emphasized in patients with inhalational injury and may be supported by an increased risk of difficult airway in burned patients intubated in a delayed fashion at burn centers compared to earlier in their course at the initial receiving hospital.[8] That said, some have suggested that burn patients are intubated at too high a rate, suggesting more sensitive and specific objective methods of evaluation of the likelihood of progression are needed, such as serial nasopharyngoscopic evaluation.[9,10] One study based on retrospective data of patients, extubated within 2 days of intubation, suggests lower risk of the need for intubation prior to transfer to a burn center when the burns are nonflame injury (such as scald injury), are not in an enclosed space, are less than 20% total body surface area, not third-degree burns to the face, and the distance to the burn center requires less than 3 hours of transfer time.[10]

Recently, Moshrefi and colleagues reported on a case series of 51 burn patients with external signs of burn injury who would meet standard criteria for intubation but were evaluated with serial endoscopic nasolaryngoscopy—in this series, only one patient required intubation after serial nasolarynoscopy.[4] Freno and colleagues reported on a case series of 210 patients undergoing nasolaryngoscopy for evaluation of inhalational injury.[2] Of the 22 symptomatic patients, 14 had laryngoscopic findings of inhalation injury, of which 7 were felt to be severe enough to require intubation. Of the remaining 188 asymptomatic patients, 53 had positive nasolaryngoscopic findings but only 2 required intubations; none of the patients without nasolaryngoscopic findings of inhalation injury required intubation.

We believe that because of this evidence and the increased availability of small bronchoscopes and nasolaryngoscopes, fewer burn patients will require intubation. However, when there is concern for inhalational injury and progression of disease, early intubation remains the pragmatic and recommended approach, especially when patients present to nonburn centers without nasopharyngoscopic capability and/or long transfer times.

What Additional Features of Burns Can Affect the Airway?

Burns to lips, cheeks, and neck can affect access to the larynx, making FMV, EGD placement, and laryngoscopy more difficult. Burns to the neck can impact head positioning, affecting EGD placement, laryngoscopy, and cricothyroidotomy. Likewise, injury and edema to the oropharynx can make FMV, intubation, and EGD challenging. Injury to the trachea, bronchial tree, and lungs can make oxygenation and ventilation difficult, and are particularly worrisome in injuries with steam or other super-heated gases. Importantly, chest wall burns can lead to restricted ventilation and may require escharotomy.

What Toxicities Should Be Considered?

Common inhalation and fire-related toxicities include carbon monoxide and cyanide. Screening for carbon monoxide can be performed quickly in the ED. In general, burn victims should be treated with 100% oxygen as a presumptive treatment for carbon monoxide poisoning, while simultaneously allowing for denitrogenation in anticipation of airway management. Cyanide toxicity should be considered in any unconscious patients, or patients with cardiac arrest or prearrest, profound hemodynamic instability, and markedly elevated lactates found in a smoke-filled environment. Empiric therapy with cyanocobalamin should be considered along with toxicology consultation. Additional products of combustion may contribute to airway injury but most do not have specific diagnostic tests or antidotes. Intoxication with alcohol and drugs are potential comorbid conditions in burn patients and should be considered along with vigilance for other ingestions associated with a suicide attempt.

What Other Concerns Do You Have for This Patient?

In this case, there is no suggestion of traumatic injury. However, burns associated with blast injuries, vehicle collisions, or other situations involving blunt trauma with the subsequent potential for spinal injury should be considered early as it may affect airway management.

Ongoing or impending hypovolemic shock is an important consideration in the treatment of burn victims and must be considered in choosing induction agents and in preparation for pre- and postintubation management.

AIRWAY MANAGEMENT

What Are the Prehospital Airway Management Considerations?

In EMS systems that do not include medication-facilitated airway management in their scope of practice, the decision process for spontaneously breathing patients is quite simple and focuses on basic airway management and rapid transport, or summoning critical care transport teams when the risk for airway deterioration is considered high and transport times long. Blind nasotracheal intubation may be considered, though has generally fallen out of favor. For EMS teams with the option for medication-facilitated airway management, the thought process and considerations discussed here are relevant. Patients with a strong possibility of inhalation injury or serious facial burns and/or long transport times should undergo early intubation prior to transfer when possible, unless an endoscopic examination can be performed with reassuring findings. Deferring intubation to the receiving hospital may be preferable in borderline cases to ensure all the necessary resources for a difficult airway are available.

What Are the Airway Management Considerations in This Case?

In this patient, anticipation of the potential for increased difficulty associated with FMV, laryngoscopic intubation, extraglottic airways, and FONA should be considered, given the burns to the face, neck, and oropharynx and the potential for inhalational injury, and the mechanical effects of burns to the chest wall on ventilation. It is likely that this patient will worsen before they get better and early intubation is advised, though endoscopic nasopharyngeal examination could be considered to exclude serious inhalation if it could be performed expeditiously. This is not a crash airway and there is time for optimal denitrogenation and preparation.

What Procedures Should Be Used to Intubate the Trachea of This Patient?

The best choices for airway management in this patient are rapid sequence intubation (RSI) with video-laryngoscopic (VL) intubation if it can be performed before there is further progression of injury, or awake intubation. Awake intubation is always a safe choice in such cases and could include endoscopic intubation via the mouth or nose, or direct laryngoscopy (DL) or VL following airway topicalization and with the patient in the seated position, using techniques described further in this book. Awake FONA such as cricothyrotomy or tracheotomy may also be considered when there is real concern about the likelihood of RSI/rescue success and the equipment or expertise for awake intubation is not available.

In this case, early RSI with VL was considered to have a high likelihood of success. Given the predicted difficulties, a self-inflating bag with PEEP valve connected and an appropriately sized EGD were prepared and ready and the neck prepared for a FONA (double setup). Denitrogenation with albuterol nebulizer was utilized throughout the preintubation phase as it was maintaining good saturations. In addition, a nasal cannula was placed to allow for passive oxygenation during the apneic phase of the RSI. RSI was performed with ketamine and rocuronium, and intubation was successful on the first attempt with VL with a hyperangulated blade (C-MAC® Dblade) with no change in the oxygen saturation. Tracheal tube placement was confirmed using end-tidal CO_2.

Are There Unique Pharmacologic Considerations for the Burn Victim?

It is important to provide adequate analgesia from the outset. Ketamine and etomidate should be considered in the patient with potential or real hypovolemia and hypotension; otherwise, any induction agent would be appropriate. In this case, ketamine may have additional benefits in treating the bronchospasm and pain. In burn victims, more than 24 to 48 hours after injury, succinylcholine has been associated with life-threatening hyperkalemia and should be avoided. However, in acute burns, succinylcholine is a safe choice for RSI. Lidocaine could be considered in this patient due to the bronchospasm but is unlikely to add much benefit.

POSTINTUBATION MANAGEMENT

What Other Issues Should Be Considered Following Tracheal Intubation?

Immediately after tracheal intubation is confirmed and the tube secured, attention must be given to breathing, circulation, and maintenance of analgesia and sedation. The patient with inhalational injury is at risk for serious oxygenation and ventilation issues, even without comorbid pulmonary conditions. Bronchospasm may be more common and usually responds to β_2-agonists. Pulmonary toilet may be necessary due to endobronchial sluffing and alveolar edema. Maintenance of a clear endotracheal tube (ETT) is essential as inspissation of mucous can cause complete obstruction of the ETT and require ETT exchange.[11]

Assurance of hemodynamic stability is critical and hypotension should be anticipated in the immediate postintubation phase as the triumvirate of hypovolemia, sedative drug administration, and positive pressure ventilation can lead to cardiovascular collapse. When hemodynamic stability is assured, postintubation analgesia and sedation should be administered per local guidelines, with consideration of minimizing the risk for ICU delirium.

In severe chest wall burns, especially those that are circumferential, escharotomy may be necessary to allow adequate ventilation with lower ventilatory pressures. Neck escharotomy may also need to be performed in very rare situations.

SUMMARY

Airway evaluation and management for the acutely burned patient builds on the standard airway approach, adding consideration of possible inhalational injury, external burns, and toxicological exposure to the process. Special consideration to the potential for progression of inhalational and topical burn injury is critical in deciding if and when intubation should occur and how to best manage the airway. Endoscopic nasopharyngeal examinations have a role in assessing for inhalation injury and the need for intubation.

CHAPTER 26

SELF-EVALUATION QUESTIONS

26.1. Factors associated with challenges in airway management in patients with acute burns include:

A. Hypovolemia

B. Inhalational Injury

C. Airway Edema

D. Mechanical effects of burns to the face, neck, and thorax

E. All of the above

26.2. The approach to airway evaluation and management in the burn patient should include:

A. The standard approach to airway evaluation and management

B. Intubation for all patients who present with burn injuries

C. Consideration for potential for co-existing toxicological injuries

D. A completely unique approach

E. A and C only

26.3. Burns to the face, neck, and torso can:

A. Make FVM more difficult

B. Make EGD placement more difficult

C. Make laryngoscopy and endotracheal tube placement more challenging

D. Make front-of-neck airway more challenging

E. All of the above

REFERENCES

1. Bai C, Huang H, Yao X, et al. Application of flexible bronchoscopy in inhalation lung injury. *Diagn Pathol.* 2013;8:174.
2. Freno D, Sahawneh J, Harrison S, Sahawneh T, et al. Determining the role of nasolaryngoscopy in the initial evaluation of upper airway injury in patients with facial burns. *Burns.* 2018;44:539-543.
3. Madnani DD, Steele NP, de Vries E. Factors that predict the need for intubation in patients with smoke inhalation injury. *Ear Nose Throat J.* 2006;85(4):278-280.
4. Moshrefi S, Skeckter CC, Shepard K, et al. Preventing unnecessary intubations: a 5-year regional burn center experience using flexible fiberoptic laryngoscopy for airway evaluation in patients with suspected inhalation or airway injury. *J Burn Care Res.* 2019;40(3):341-346.
5. Kameda T, Fujita M. Point-of-care ultrasound detection of tracheal wall thickening caused by smoke inhalation. *Crit Ultrasound J.* 2014;6(1):11.
6. Dries DJ, Endorf FW. Inhalation injury: epidemiology, pathology, treatment strategies. *Scand J Trauma Resusc Emerg Med.* 2013;21:31.
7. McCall JE, Cahill TJ. Respiratory care of the burn patient. *J Burn Care Rehabil.* 2005;26(3):200-206.
8. Esnault P, Prunet B, Cotte J, et al. Tracheal intubation difficulties in the setting of face and neck burns: myth or reality? *Am J Emerg Med.* 2014;32(10):1174-1178.
9. Mackie DP, van Dehn F, Knape P, et al. Increase in early mechanical ventilation of burn patients: an effect of current emergency trauma management? *J Trauma.* 2011;70(3):611-615.
10. Romanowski KS, Palmieri TL, Sen S, Greenhalgh DG. More than one third of intubations in patients transferred to burn centers are unnecessary: proposed guidelines for appropriate intubation of the burn patient. *J Burn Care Res.* 2016;37(5):e409-e414.
11. Cancio LC. Airway management and smoke inhalation injury in the burn patient. *Clin Plastic Surg.* 2009;36(4):555-567.

CHAPTER 27

Airway Management in a Patient with Angioedema

Genevieve McKinnon

CASE PRESENTATION

This 42-year-old black female presents to the emergency department (ED) 2 hours after the onset of facial swelling that has now progressed to difficulty in breathing.

She has no previous history of tissue swelling and there is no family history of disorders characterized by tissue swelling. Her past medical history is remarkable only for newly diagnosed hypertension. She is otherwise healthy, without any history of drug allergies. Last week, her primary care physician started her on lisinopril, an angiotensin-converting enzyme inhibitor (ACEI) antihypertensive.

Upon presentation to the ED, her vital signs are as follows: heart rate 100 bpm, respiratory rate 22 bpm, blood pressure 165/90 mmHg, oxygen saturation 96% on room air, and temperature 37°C.

The patient is seated upright (Figure 27.1) with markedly edematous lips and face. She has a muffled voice ("hot potato voice") and is having difficulty swallowing her own secretions. There is no audible stridor. The remainder of the physical examination is within normal limits.

DIAGNOSIS

What Is the Pathophysiology of Angioedema?

Angioedema is characterized by the abrupt onset of localized, transient, nonpitting swelling of the skin, deep subcutaneous tissues, and mucosal membranes of the upper respiratory and gastrointestinal tracts. Affected areas may be erythematous or skin-colored, and typically have ill-defined margins without urticaria. Angioedema develops due to a local increase in permeability of the submucosal or subcutaneous capillary vessels, causing local plasma extravasation into the interstitial space. This results in transient swelling of well-demarcated areas. This process is mediated by the localized or systemic release of vasoactive substances, most frequently histamine or bradykinin.[1–4]

Angioedema can progress rapidly, particularly with histamine-mediated reactions, and constitute a medical emergency when involving the oropharynx, pharynx, and larynx due to the imminent risk of airway obstruction. Importantly, this airway swelling may develop into a potentially difficult airway, making airway management such as intubation quite challenging. Although the presenting clinical signs and symptoms are similar, the biochemical cascade initiated by histamine is distinct from that mediated by bradykinin.[5] Therefore, it is imperative that practitioners have a comprehensive understanding of the underlying pathophysiologic processes in order to appropriately treat patients presenting with angioedema.

How Is Angioedema Classified?

There are various classification schemes that attempt to organize the different forms of angioedema into a comprehensive yet useful structure. A biochemical basis for classification with a focus on the pathophysiologic processes will be discussed. In general, this approach organizes angioedema into allergic (immune) or nonallergic (nonimmune) forms. Specifically, allergic angioedema

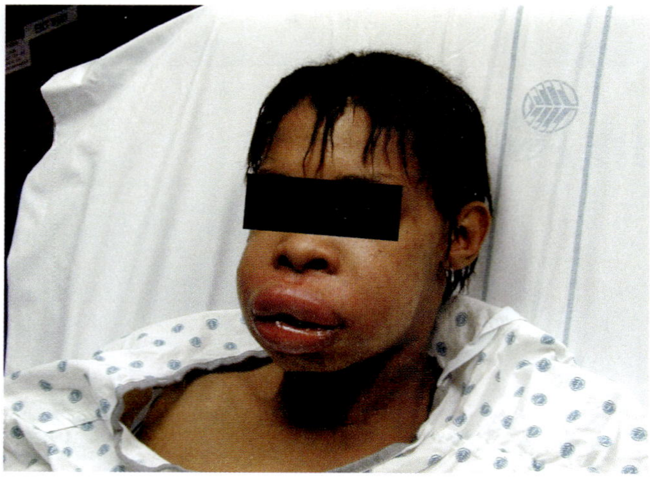

FIGURE 27.1. Patient with angioedema.

is mediated by histamine while the majority of nonallergic angioedema is mediated by increased plasma and tissue concentrations of bradykinin. Importantly, histaminergic reactions also include nonallergic hypersensitivity reactions, also known as anaphylactoid reactions or pseudoallergic angioedema.[6,7]

Nonallergic angioedema can be further organized into hereditary angioedema (HAE) and acquired angioedema (AAE) most commonly involving the renin-angiotensin system. This form is most commonly seen with ACEIs and referred to as AAE-ACEI. AAE can also be in the form of acquired C1-inhibitor deficiency that is distinct from HAE. The last category of nonallergic angioedema is idiopathic edema (IAE), which is a diagnosis of exclusion.[8–10] In this chapter, we will focus exclusively on ACEI-induced angioedema and will not explore the other forms of AAE.

Allergic Angioedema

Histamine-mediated (histaminergic) or allergic angioedema occurs through an immunoglobulin E (IgE), Type 1 hypersensitivity immune response and involves exposure to a previously sensitized allergen. Repeat exposure to that allergen causes cross-linking of IgE bound on mast cells, resulting in mast cell degranulation and release of preformed mediators, including histamine and tryptase. Excess histamine causes increased local vasodilation and vascular permeability, leading to plasma extravasation into the interstitial space resulting in angioedema.[1,8,11]

Allergic hypersensitivity reactions range from mild skin symptoms to life-threatening anaphylaxis. In its most extreme form, anaphylaxis is a systemic reaction of sudden onset that results in a spectrum of symptoms, including most frequently hypotension secondary to vasodilation and loss of intravascular volume, upper airway angioedema, and respiratory compromise. In highly sensitized individuals, systemic reactions can occur within minutes following intravenous injection resulting in profound cardiovascular collapse, severe laryngeal angioedema, and possibly death by asphyxia in a patient with an unsecured airway.[8,11–13]

Mast cell degranulation can also occur without previous sensitization and instead occurs upon first exposure to a trigger in a dose-dependent fashion. This reaction is nonallergic but clinically indistinguishable from true allergic (IgE)-mediated hypersensitivity. For this reason, the European Academy for Allergy and Clinical Immunology proposed that all reactions be described as anaphylaxis at the time of presentation and categorically divided into allergic or nonallergic hypersensitivity only after diagnostic investigation has been completed.[14] For the purpose of simplicity and consistency, we will adopt that nomenclature in this chapter as well.

Perioperative Anaphylaxis

Perioperative anaphylaxis is a serious complication of anesthesia and has been reported with variable frequency. In 2018, the 6th National Audit Project (NAP6) of the Royal College of Anaesthetists performed a prospective one year study of anaphylaxis related to anesthesia and surgery. All hospitals in the National Health Service (NHS) in the United Kingdom were surveyed and more than 3 million anesthetics were reviewed.[9] The audit found an incidence of anaphylaxis in every 1 per 10,000 anesthetics. It was determined that antibiotics accounted for 47% of reactions, neuromuscular blocking agents (NMBAs) were implicated 33% of the time, chlorhexidine skin preparation solution 9%, and intravenous blue dye 5% of the time.

Other reviews conducted have found an incidence of clinical anaphylaxis during anesthesia to be as high as 1 in 1250, which may suggest that anaphylaxis occurs more frequently than previously measured or reported. However, these findings must be interpreted with caution as it is possible that the rising incidence of anaphylaxis may also be attributable to improved identification and reporting of anaphylactic reactions.[7,15]

Regardless of reported incidence, these reviews suggest that antibiotics remain a major cause of anaphylaxis in other countries as do NMBAs, chlorhexidine, and dyes. Latex-induced allergies appear to be stable or declining and local anesthetic reactions are uncommon. Newer agents such as sugammadex are emerging as potent allergens causing IgE-mediated anaphylaxis, while older drugs such as aprotinin continue to be a major cause of allergic reactions in cardiovascular surgery.[11,13,16,17]

Perioperative anaphylaxis has several unique features, which influence the identification of the reaction and management of patients under anesthesia at the time of the event. First, most drugs are administered intravenously (IV), thereby causing the most rapid and severe reactions. Second, particularly around the time of anesthesia induction and emergence, there are several IV drugs given concurrently, which routinely disrupt normal physiology and may result in hypotension, bronchospasm/high airway pressures, and possibly even elicit a rash. Commonly, these physiological derangements are attributed to the effects of anesthetic agents and not to an anaphylactic reaction, possibly resulting in a lag time for specific management. Lastly, these reactions occur in the presence of an anesthesia practitioner trained in managing anaphylaxis and therefore timely management prevents the vast majority of deaths in the operating room.[9]

Although perioperative anaphylaxis occurs in a monitored setting whilst under the care of an attending anesthesia practitioner, deaths may occur even with immediate identification and appropriate treatment. The reporting rate of perioperative mortality varies by country and ranges from less than

2% in Western Australia to ~4% in the Unites States, United Kingdom, France, and Japan.[9,17]

Nonallergic Angioedema

Hereditary Angioedema HAE is a rare, potentially life-threatening condition characterized by recurrent, self-limiting episodes of facial, laryngeal, genital or extremity swelling, and abdominal pain. The reported prevalence ranges between 1 in 10,000 and 1 in 150,000 people but is generally quoted as 1 in 50,000 individuals. No ethnicity or gender predominance has been found.[18,19]

There are several different forms of HAE genetically identifiable. Type 1 HAE (HAE-1), which is the most common form, is characterized by decreased levels of functional C1INH in the plasma, while Type 2 (HAE-2) is characterized by expression of a dysfunctional C1INH protein resulting in low functional levels of C1INH. Type 3 HAE, although clinically indistinguishable from Types 1 and 2, is characterized by normal production and function of complement C4 and C1INH. Most but not all patients are women, and there is a close association with estrogen as a precipitant of attacks of angioedema.[20–22]

The primary role of C1INH is to regulate activation of the complement system, the contact system, and the coagulation cascade. Decreased activity, either by deficient levels or dysfunctional activity of C1INH, results in an abnormal increase in the activation of C1 and subsequent excessive formation of the enzyme kallikrein. The excess kallikrein transforms kininogen into kinins, including bradykinin. Bradykinin, the primary biologic mediator responsible for nonallergic angioedema, binds to receptors on endothelial cells causing increased vascular permeability (edema, swelling, and ascites), vasodilation (congestion, erythema, and hypotension), and contraction of nonvascular smooth muscle (cramps, spasms, and pain).[21]

HAE attacks can be unpredictable in frequency and severity and may be triggered without warning, causing significant anxiety for patients and caregivers. HAE attacks are often spontaneous without a clear trigger, although local tissue trauma and emotional stress have been identified as precipitants. Frequently, the trauma is considered to be minor and can be as innocuous as prolonged sitting on a hard surface or clapping of the hands. Dental and surgical trauma are well-recognized precipitators of an acute attack.[18]

Patients with known HAE should have a predetermined comprehensive management plan that includes access to treatment in acute attacks and a prophylactic strategy, when indicated, such as prior to elective surgery. Bradykinin-mediated angioedema is not responsive to standard angioedema treatment modalities used for mast cell-mediated anaphylactic angioedema, such as corticosteroids, antihistamines, and epinephrine.[18,19,21,23]

Fortunately, there are effective targeted therapies available for the treatment of acute HAE attacks. C1INH concentrates, which can be plasma-derived (e.g., Berinert or Cinryze) or recombinant (e.g., Ruconest), replace the deficient (HAE-1) or dysfunctional (HAE-2) endogenous proteins. Treatment increases the plasma levels of C1INH and helps to regulate all systems involved in the production of bradykinin, thereby interrupting the pathways responsible for systemic effects.[21] The other therapies are bradykinin-pathway antagonists aimed at reducing the production of bradykinin (Ecallantide) or acting as a competitive antagonist to the B2 bradykinin receptor (Icatibant).[2,20,21]

Acquired Angioedema

Angiotensin-Converting Enzyme Inhibitor-Induced Angioedema ACEIs are a first-line agent for hypertension, heart failure, and diabetic nephropathy and one of the most commonly prescribed medications in the general population. In addition to beneficial therapeutic effects of inhibiting the conversion of angiotensin I to angiotensin II, the suppression of ACE also results in reduced degradation of bradykinin leading to increased levels of bradykinin and subsequent vasodilation and tissue swelling.[24] Angioedema has also been demonstrated to occur with the angiotensin II receptor blockers (ARBs) although at a much lower incidence. There is a modest increase in risk for ARB-induced angioedema in patients who have previously experienced ACEI-induced angioedema, so caution must be exercised when discontinuing an ACEI in favor of an ARB.[25]

According to the literature, the incidence of ACEI-induced angioedema ranges from 0.1% to 0.7% of all patients using ACEIs[2,26–28] and accounts for approximately one-third of all patients presenting to the ED with angioedema.[29] In the omapatrilat versus enalapril (OCTAVE) antihypertensive trial, the investigators identified independent risk factors including increased incidence in black patients, age greater than 65, history of drug rash, and history of seasonal allergies.[28] Additional risk factors identified in other research include Hispanic patients, female gender, history of smoking, increasing age, transplant recipients, and patients on immunosuppressive therapy. Approximately 55% of all ACEI-induced angioedema cases occur within 3 months of starting the medication, with the remainder occurring anywhere from weeks to years after starting the drug.[26,28] Discontinuation of the ACEI will resolve the angioedema, though the risk of recurrent angioedema attacks may persist for weeks. Patients who have experienced an angioedema attack and who continue with ACEI therapy are at significant risk of recurrence within 5 years.[2]

Unfortunately, there is no known effective pharmacologic intervention for ACEI-induced angioedema. Unlike allergic/histamine-mediated angioedema, nonallergic/bradykinin-mediated angioedema does not respond to conventional therapies such as antihistamines and corticosteroids and are poorly responsive to epinephrine.[30] Although there have been studies investigating the possible application of bradykinin pathway antagonist such as those used in HAE, results have been mixed and further research is required in this field.[31–33] The emergency care of ACEI-induced angioedema continues to be acute airway management and discontinuation of the medication.

EVALUATION

What Is the General Clinical Course of Angioedema?

The onset of allergic/histamine-mediated anaphylaxis is rapid and often life-threatening if not treated appropriately. The clinical course of nonallergic/bradykinin-mediated ACEI-induced angioedema is often subacute but extremely unpredictable. Life-threatening presentations requiring airway interventions do occur and are reported in up to 20% of these patients.[2] This variability may reflect a spectrum of patients from those with acute severe disease to those with a less acute presentation who were intubated for concerns of disease progression. It is extremely difficult to predict which patients who present with a stable airway will progress to a requirement for airway intervention. Since the clinical course of angioedema, especially ACEI-induced, is very unpredictable, and potentially life-threatening, it is recommended that these patients be admitted to an environment where they can be properly evaluated and closely monitored.[30,34]

What Investigations Can Be Done to Assess the Severity of Angioedema?

The unpredictable clinical course of angioedema demands that each of these patients be triaged as "emergencies" to a resuscitation area of the ED and attended to immediately by nursing and physician staff. Evaluation and management are carried out concurrently, as are appropriate in patients with life-threatening conditions. It is often obvious that the airway is in immediate jeopardy, and this should trigger calling for assistance and implementing a strategy to safely secure the airway. Airway management in these patients requires time to execute safely; therefore, calling early for expert assistance should be a priority.

Nasopharyngoscopy

If one has the luxury of time and possesses the skill, the severity of airway compromise may be assessed by flexible nasopharyngoscopy. It is prudent to prepare for this procedure as though one were intending to perform an awake endoscopic-guided nasal intubation. This assumes that one has judiciously anesthetized/topicalized the nasopharyngeal passage and prepared a nasotracheal tube through which the endoscope is passed in case the findings mandate intubation. It is preferable that the scope used for this procedure be of sufficient length and stiffness to guide an endotracheal tube into the trachea. When available, and clinically appropriate, a flexible bronchoscope (FB) may be preferred over a nasopharyngoscope as it is of larger caliber and may facilitate easier passage of the endotracheal tube. This must be weighed against the size of the airway and the potential to cause complete obstruction with the scope in the presence of severe tissue swelling.

Repeated nasopharyngoscopic evaluation at regular intervals may be indicated in the event where immediate tracheal intubation is NOT necessary; however, caution must be exercised. Any manipulation of the upper airway carries a risk of triggering a complete airway obstruction and therefore, prior to undertaking nasopharyngoscopy, there should be a plan in place to proceed with intubation via the nasopharyngoscope should the patient become hypoxemic with evidence of obstruction. In addition, it would be prudent that the backup plan includes the immediate ability to perform a front-of-neck airway (FONA)/cricothyrotomy in the event that intubation through the nasopharyngoscope is not possible.

Care must be taken with topicalization as it may precipitate loss of airway tone and cause airway obstruction in a tenuous airway. However, a practitioner may have no choice but to employ topicalization in an attempt to secure the airway. Nonvisual/manual techniques such as blind nasal intubation and light-guided techniques are relatively contraindicated due to the potential for airway distortion and the risk of producing further trauma and bleeding.

Point-of-Care Ultrasound (POCUS)

During routine and emergency intubation and endoscopy, it is possible to generate aerosols, as many patients will cough or sneeze during upper airway topicalization and introduction of the FB. Therefore, these procedures have been determined to be aerosol-generating procedures (AGPs) that have the potential to place the airway management team at risk of exposure to SARS-CoV-2 and other respiratory viruses. In addition, most current recommendations require the use of personal protective equipment (PPE) during airway management of known, suspected, or untested patients with COVID-19.[35–37]

In an effort to reduce the exposure of airway teams during these procedures, and the subsequent required use of PPE, airway POCUS has been suggested as a noninvasive, non-AGP alternative to nasopharyngoscopy to evaluate the severity of laryngeal and upper airway angioedema.[38,39] In addition, it has been used to confirm endotracheal intubation, assess depth of endotracheal tube (ETT) placement, and to reconfirm ETT position after transportation.[40–42]

Portable ultrasound machines are readily available in most EDs and operating rooms (ORs), however, they do require a more thorough and time-consuming decontamination process after use. Handheld POCUS platforms on tablets or smartphones may simplify these challenges. They are easily decontaminated or protected with an ultrasound probe sleeve, require a single skilled practitioner, and can be utilized at the bedside without transportation of critically unstable patients.[42] In addition, a growing number of handheld POCUS products offer an expanding number of features, including artificial intelligence (AI)-assisted diagnosis, wireless connectivity, and rechargeable batteries, making purchasing and use a more accessible option for out-of-hospital or remote community airway management.[43]

AIRWAY MANAGEMENT

How Should This Patient's Airway Be Managed?

Some patients with angioedema have had prior episodes and may be able to provide some reassurance that this episode will resolve under close observation. This may be true in the small percentage of patients with known HAE 1-2 or recurrent allergic angioedema with known triggers and exposure. It is much more likely that the clinical course will be unpredictable and warrants careful evaluation and monitoring with preparation for airway intervention in the event that the angioedema worsens and warrants tracheal intubation.

The decision for airway intervention will be based largely on the clinical signs of respiratory distress: difficulty in swallowing saliva, muffled voice, stridor, accessory respiratory muscle use, dyspnea, agitation, and hypoxemia. Objective information obtained from nasopharyngoscopy and airway POCUS will help inform this decision, but will largely support the clinical gestalt.[30]

Laryngeal involvement, characterized by stridor, hoarseness, and voice change indicates impending complete airway obstruction and mandates an aggressive approach. This would include preparations for a "double setup" that includes a plan for airway management above the larynx (intubation) and surgical airway management below the larynx (FONA/surgical airway). Although early airway management is indicated for patients with rapidly progressive and severe upper and/or lower airway compromise, a trial of epinephrine is nearly always indicated, particularly when the etiology is unknown.[30,34,44,45]

Airway planning and management is driven by the guidelines for management of the difficult airway.[46] Rapid sequence induction (RSI) is rarely an option in these patients, however, in patients without features of a difficult airway, but in whom there is concern for worsening angioedema leading to obstruction, an RSI with an induction agent and paralytic may be used to facilitate intubation. This can be accomplished with either direct laryngoscopy or flexible bronchoscopic intubation; however, video laryngoscopy may result in a faster time to intubation and improved first-pass success.[30]

If there is evidence of airway obstruction or the airway is determined to be difficult, the next step will depend on the practitioner's access to, and ability to use a FB. If an experienced practitioner is available, then intubation using FB ought to be performed with immediate FONA/cricothyrotomy as backup. The nasal route for the FB-guided intubation is ordinarily much easier for those who infrequently perform endoscopic intubations. In the event one does not have, or cannot use, an FB, then an "awake look" using either a direct or video laryngoscope may help create a more informed decision to intubate the trachea awake or to move to an awake FONA. Again, it is important to employ judicious topicalization to avoid worsening an already tenuous airway.[30,46]

It is often a difficult decision to use sedative-hypnotic agents to facilitate airway evaluation and management in patients with upper airway obstruction as even small doses of these sedative agents may precipitate a complete upper airway obstruction. Titrated small doses of ketamine, remifentanil, and dexmedetomidine may be used to achieve cooperation, and sedation but must be used judiciously.

There may be instances when a patient presents in extremis with evidence of obstruction causing ventilatory compromise and resulting in hypoxia. These patients will likely not tolerate any form of topicalization or nasopharyngoscopy due to distress and the inability to cooperate fully with the procedure. In these cases, there should be a discussion regarding an awake FONA as a primary airway technique. However, this is an advanced procedure and will require the coordination of multiple services including anesthesia, emergency medicine, and ideally, otorhinolaryngology. If a formal tracheotomy is to be the first choice, and it is safe to transport the patient, then ideally, arrangements should be made to perform the tracheotomy in the formal operating room rather than a procedure or trauma room in the ED. This is to ensure that all skilled personnel, equipment, and medication are readily available in the event of difficulty. In addition, the operating rooms will likely be larger, able to accommodate the multiple services required, fully equipped with an anesthesia machine and drug cart, and in closer proximity to perfusion services.

In rare cases, with patients presenting with severe obstruction requiring an awake tracheotomy approach, there may be significant concern regarding worsening hypoxemia during the procedure or loss of the airway entirely. In these cases, it may be advisable to consider planned extracorporeal membrane oxygenation (ECMO) prior to beginning the FONA attempt.[46] However, it must be stated that the practicality and logistics of organizing ECMO, transporting an unstable airway to the OR, successfully cannulating vessels with a patient in extremis, and then proceeding with the FONA attempt present such a challenge without guarantee of success that it may not be possible to entertain.

SUMMARY

The incidence of angioedema has increased dramatically over the past two decades with the introduction of ACEIs for the treatment of hypertension. The clinical course of any angioedema episode is unpredictable regardless of underlying etiology. For this reason, securing the airway early is a safer course than "watching and waiting." Commonly administered medications including intravenous steroids, antihistamine, and epinephrine are of marginal value in bradykinin-mediated angioedema, and utilization of these agents ought not delay airway intervention. Intubation over an FB may be the preferred technique; the nasal route being recommended for those who perform flexible intubation infrequently. Employing judicious topical anesthesia may enable one to intubate using direct or indirect laryngoscopy; however, there must be an appreciation of the risk of converting a marginally patent airway into complete airway obstruction and a "can't intubate, can't oxygenate" (CICO) situation. The Plan B option of surgical airway performed under local anesthesia with the patient awake must be considered as a backup, or in some cases, even a primary method of securing the airway.

As with all cases of upper airway obstruction, one must appreciate that while the patient may have "stable" vital signs, the airway is exceedingly "unstable"!

SELF-EVALUATION QUESTIONS

27.1. ACE-inhibitor-induced angioedema patients:

A. Usually respond to subcutaneous and aerosolized epinephrine
B. Have an unpredictable clinical course with respect to the airway
C. Can usually be safely observed as long as they do not have stridor
D. Usually respond to high-dose intravenous steroids
E. Can be managed with fresh frozen plasma

27.2. All of the strategies for definitive airway management are acceptable in patients with angioedema EXCEPT:

A. Awake intubation using a flexible bronchoscope
B. Awake intubation under direct laryngoscopy

C. Rapid sequence intubation

D. Cricothyrotomy

E. Tracheotomy

27.3. Which of the following symptoms would suggest a marginally patent airway that requires definitive airway management?

A. Stridor

B. Muffled voice

C. Oxygen desaturation

D. Difficulty managing secretions

E. Use of accessory muscles

REFERENCES

1. Grigoriadou S, Longhurst HJ. Clinical immunology review series: an approach to the patient with angio-oedema. *Clin Exp Immunol.* 2009;155(3):367-377.
2. Kaplan AP, Greaves MW. Angioedema. *J Am Acad Dermatol.* 2005;53(3):373-388.
3. Zuraw BL, Bernstein JA, Lang DM, et al. A focused parameter update: hereditary angioedema, acquired C1 inhibitor deficiency, and angiotensin-converting enzyme inhibitor-associated angioedema. *J Allergy Clin Immunol.* 2013;131(6):1491-1493.e25.
4. Zuraw BL, Christiansen SC. HAE pathophysiology and underlying mechanisms. *Clin Rev Allergy Immunol.* 2016;51(2):216-229.
5. Bernstein JA, Moellman J. Emerging concepts in the diagnosis and treatment of patients with undifferentiated angioedema. *Int J Emerg Med.* 2012;5(1):39.
6. Bas M, Adams V, Suvorava T, Niehues T, Hoffmann TK, Kojda G. Nonallergic angioedema: role of bradykinin. *Allergy.* 2007;62(8):842-856.
7. Volcheck GW, Mertes PM. Local and general anesthetics immediate hypersensitivity reactions. *Immunol Allergy Clin North Am.* 2014;34(3):525-546, viii.
8. Castells M, Bonamichi-Santos R. Drug hypersensitivity. In: *Clinical Immunology.* London: Elsevier; 2019:649-667.e1.
9. Harper NJN, Cook TM, Garcez T, et al. Anaesthesia, surgery, and life-threatening allergic reactions: epidemiology and clinical features of perioperative anaphylaxis in the 6th National Audit Project (NAP6). *Br J Anaesth.* 2018;121(1):159-171.
10. Marcelino-Rodriguez I, Callero A, Mendoza-Alvarez A, et al. Bradykinin-mediated angioedema: an update of the genetic causes and the impact of genomics. *Front Genet.* 2019;10:900.
11. Simons FER, Ebisawa M, Sanchez-Borges M, et al. 2015 update of the evidence base: World Allergy Organization anaphylaxis guidelines. *World Allergy Organ J.* 2015;8(1):32.
12. Winters M. Clinical practice guideline: initial evaluation and management of patients presenting with acute urticaria or angioedema. American Academy of Emergency Medicine (AAEM). Position Statement; 2021.
13. Simons FER, Ardusso LR, Bilò MB, et al. International consensus on (ICON) anaphylaxis. *World Allergy Organ J.* 2014;7(1):9.
14. Johansson SGO, Bieber T, Dahl R, et al. Revised nomenclature for allergy for global use: Report of the Nomenclature Review Committee of the World Allergy Organization, October 2003. *J Allergy Clin Immunol.* 2004;113(5):832-836.
15. Savic LC, Kaura V, Yusaf M, et al. Incidence of suspected perioperative anaphylaxis: a multicenter snapshot study. *J Allergy Clin Immunol Pract.* 2015;3(3):454-455.e1.
16. Grattan CEH, Borzova E. Urticaria, angioedema, and anaphylaxis. In: Rich RR, Fleisher TA, Shearer WT, et al., eds. *Clinical Immunology.* 5th ed. London: Elsevier; 2019:585-600.e1.
17. Mertes PM, Volcheck GW, Garvey LH, et al. Epidemiology of perioperative anaphylaxis. *Presse Médicale.* 2016;45(9):758-767.
18. Ghazi A, Grant JA. Hereditary angioedema: epidemiology, management, and role of icatibant. *Biol Targets Ther.* 2013;7:103-113.
19. Nzeako UC, Frigas E, Tremaine WJ. Hereditary angioedema: a broad review for clinicians. *Arch Intern Med.* 2001;161(20):2417-2429.
20. Bork K. A decade of change: recent developments in pharmacotherapy of hereditary angioedema (HAE). *Clin Rev Allergy Immunol.* 2016;51(2):183-192.
21. Maurer M, Magerl M, Ansotegui I, et al. The international WAO/EAACI guideline for the management of hereditary angioedema—The 2017 revision and update. *Allergy.* 2018;73(8):1575-1596.
22. Santacroce R, D'Andrea G, Maffione AB, Margaglione M, d'Apolito M. The genetics of hereditary angioedema: a review. *J Clin Med.* 2021;10(9):2023.
23. Patel G, Pongracic JA. Hereditary and acquired angioedema. *Allergy Asthma Proc.* 2019;40(6):441-445.
24. Burks AW, Holgate ST, O'Hehir RE, et al., eds. *Middleton's Allergy: Principles and Practice.* 9th ed. Amsterdam: Elsevier; 2020.
25. Haymore BR, Yoon J, Mikita CP, Klote MM, DeZee KJ. Risk of angioedema with angiotensin receptor blockers in patients with prior angioedema associated with angiotensin-converting enzyme inhibitors: a meta-analysis. *Ann Allergy Asthma Immunol.* 2008;101(5):495-499.
26. Miller DR, Oliveria SA, Berlowitz DR, Fincke BG, Stang P, Lillienfeld DE. Angioedema incidence in US veterans initiating angiotensin-converting enzyme inhibitors. *Hypertension.* 2008;51:1624-1630.
27. Banerji A, Blumenthal KG, Lai KH, Zhou L. Epidemiology of ACE inhibitor angioedema utilizing a large electronic health record. *J Allergy Clin Immunol Pract.* 2017;5(3):744-749.
28. Kostis JB, Kim HJ, Rusnak J, et al. Incidence and characteristics of angioedema associated with enalapril. *Arch Intern Med.* 2005;165(14):1637-1642.
29. Sandefur BJ, E Silva LOJ, Lohse CM, et al. Clinical features and outcomes associated with angioedema in the emergency department. *West J Emerg Med.* 2019;20(5):760-769.
30. Moellman JJ, Bernstein JA, Lindsell C, et al. A consensus parameter for the evaluation and management of angioedema in the emergency department. *Acad Emerg Med.* 2014;21(4):469-484.
31. Bernstein JA, Moellman JJ, Collins SP, Hart KW, Lindsell CJ. Effectiveness of ecallantide in treating angiotensin-converting enzyme inhibitor–induced angioedema in the emergency department. *Ann Allergy Asthma Immunol.* 2015;114(3):245-249.
32. Cai G, Barber C, Kalicinsky C. Review of icatibant use in the Winnipeg Regional Health Authority. *Allergy Asthma Clin Immunol.* 2020;16(1):96.
33. Sinert R, Levy P, Bernstein JA, et al. Randomized trial of icatibant for angiotensin-converting enzyme inhibitor–induced upper airway angioedema. *J Allergy Clin Immunol Pract.* 2017;5(5):1402-1409.e3.
34. Bernstein JA, Cremonesi P, Hoffmann TK, Hollingsworth J. Angioedema in the emergency department: a practical guide to differential diagnosis and management. *Int J Emerg Med.* 2017;10(1):15.
35. Brown J, Gregson FKA, Shrimpton A, et al. A quantitative evaluation of aerosol generation during tracheal intubation and extubation. *Anaesthesia.* 2021;76(2):174-181.
36. Dhillon RS, Rowin WA, Humphries RS, et al. Aerosolisation during tracheal intubation and extubation in an operating theatre setting. *Anaesthesia.* 2021;76(2):182-188.
37. Nestor CC, Wang S, Irwin MG. Are tracheal intubation and extubation aerosol-generating procedures? *Anaesthesia.* 2021;76(2):151-155.
38. Chao TN, Atkins JH, Qasim Z, Kearney JJ, Mirza N, Rassekh CH. Airway management of angioedema patients during the COVID-19 pandemic. *World J Otorhinolaryngol: Head Neck Surg.* 2020;6(Suppl 1):S36-S39.
39. Schick M, Grether-Jones K. Point-of-care sonographic findings in acute upper airway edema. *West J Emerg Med.* 2016;17(6):822-826.
40. Gottlieb M, Olszynski P, Atkinson P. Just the facts: point-of-care ultrasound for airway management. *Can J Emerg Med.* 2021;23(3):277-279.
41. Sun JT, Chu SE, Fan CM, Sim SS. Trans-tracheal ultrasound: a feasible method for endotracheal tube position reconfirmation during COVID-19 pandemic. *Hong Kong J Emerg Med.* 2021;28(6):383-384.
42. Yau O, Gin K, Luong C, et al. Point-of-care ultrasound in the COVID-19 era: a scoping review. *Echocardiography.* 2021;38(2):329-342.
43. Khanji MY, Ricci F, Patel RS, et al. Special article - the role of hand-held ultrasound for cardiopulmonary assessment during a pandemic. *Prog Cardiovasc Dis.* 2020;63(5):690-695.
44. Bentsianov BL, Parhiscar A, Azer M, Har-El G. The role of fiberoptic nasopharyngoscopy in the management of the acute airway in angioneurotic edema. *Laryngoscope.* 2000;110(12):2016-2019.
45. Mudd PA, Hooker EA, Stolz U, Hart KW, Bernstein JA, Moellman JJ. Emergency department evaluation of patients with angiotensin converting enzyme inhibitor associated angioedema. *Am J Emerg Med.* 2020;38(12):2596-2601.
46. Law JA, Duggan LV, Asselin M, et al. Canadian Airway Focus Group updated consensus-based recommendations for management of the difficult airway: part 2. Planning and implementing safe management of the patient with an anticipated difficult airway. *Can J Anesth Can Anesth.* 2021;68(9):1405-1436.

CHAPTER 28

Airway Management for Penetrating Facial Trauma

David A. Caro, Ashley B. Norse, and Jessica A. Ryder

CASE PRESENTATION

A 70-year-old depressed man presents after attempted suicide by shooting himself with a handgun held under his jaw. He is seated upright and leaning forward when paramedics arrive on the scene and refuses to lie supine due to facial bleeding. He is kept in position to optimize airway patency and is expeditiously transported to the nearest emergency department (ED). The patient presents to the ED in tripod position with obvious bleeding from his mouth. His anterior mandible is missing, and he is holding a non-rebreather oxygen mask in front of his face. His oxygen saturation is 95% and has been stable during transport. Vital signs include a pulse of 85 beats per minute, a blood pressure of 175/90 mmHg, a respiratory rate of 22 breaths per minute, and a temperature of 37°C. Upon initial examination (Figure 28.1), he has ongoing oral hemorrhage and is completely missing his anterior mandible. The patient is awake and has a GCS of 15. In light of his injuries, he is kept upright on the gurney in anticipation of tracheal intubation (for airway protection).

PATIENT ASSESSMENT

■ What Are the Airway Evaluation Considerations for This Patient?

This patient presents with multiple clinical issues that may influence his airway management.[1] The missing anterior mandible is a dramatic presentation, but standard trauma management principles apply.[2,3] His airway does require management for airway protection and the anticipated clinical course. However, this is not a "crash" intubation situation (because his oxygen saturation is >90% and he is stable). Therefore, a rapid evaluation of the airway for anticipated difficulty is possible.[4] If this were a "crash" scenario (e.g., vital signs become unstable or patient becomes hypoxemic), an emergency cricothyrotomy might be the most appropriate initial approach.[2,4]

The presence of orofacial disruption will likely hinder face-mask ventilation (FMV) due to a poor mask seal and attempts at FMV may create subcutaneous emphysema further distorting tissues. Similarly, with the associated hemorrhage, soft-tissue edema, and the presence of foreign bodies (teeth, clots, etc.), the use of an extraglottic device (EGD) may be difficult. Laryngoscopy will likely be complicated by the presence of blood, tissue edema, and possible airway disruption. However, the absence of mandibular resistance might actually make visualization easier. Additionally, it is always wise to consider cervical spine injury in the setting of head trauma, but this case is special. Maintenance of strict cervical spine precautions in this instance, such as lying the patient supine or placing the patient in a cervical collar, could result in aspiration and obstruction of the airway.[3] In this instance, maintaining the patient in a position of relative comfort in an upright, sitting position allows the patient to keep their airway open and clear of bleeding, and also provides the airway practitioner an opportunity for further assessment in planning the airway approach. This airway is classified as "difficult," specifically for potential anatomic

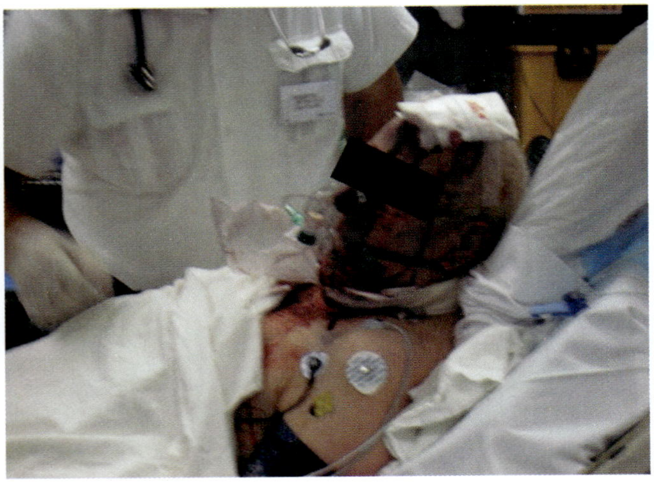

FIGURE 28.1. The patient in the emergency department sitting with a non-rebreather oxygen mask.

challenges that may be encountered during laryngoscopy or any attempt at mask ventilation.

How Does Airway Assessment Proceed in the Setting of Disrupted Anatomy?

Penetrating facial injuries can present significant difficulties in isolating landmarks. A "look, listen, feel" approach to airway evaluation is wise. Critical structures to initially identify include the tongue, the hypopharynx, and the larynx. The tongue frequently remains present in penetrating facial injuries but can also be disrupted by the trauma. Key to airway evaluation is identification of the glottis at the base of the tongue. Hence, sequential visualization of the anatomy from the base of the tongue can direct the airway practitioner to the glottis. Abnormal airway sounds, such as gurgling, stridor, or the inability to phonate may indicate impending airway compromise. Palpation of airway anatomy might allow for identification of otherwise unrecognizable structures, such as the grossly abnormal tongue, mandible, etc., and will also allow the practitioner to identify the position of the larynx in the neck to localize the target for cricothyrotomy, if it is necessary.

How Is Airway Hemorrhage Managed in This Circumstance?

Patient positioning is paramount.[3–5] Severe hemorrhage requires consideration of sitting the patient upright or rolling the patient into a lateral decubitus position to allow gravity to assist with moving blood out of the airway. It merits emphasizing that gravity can also work against the airway practitioner if the patient is forced to lie supine when hemorrhage is severe. Adequate suction is a necessity; plan to have at least two devices available to allow for adequate suction. Direct pressure with 4 × 4 gauze might be of use if the bleeding site is within reach. Topical vasoconstricting medications will most likely be unsuccessful. Injected lidocaine with epinephrine is an occasional consideration once airway stability is confirmed.

How Often Is a Penetrating Facial Injury Associated with Cervical Spine Injury?

The incidence of associated cervical spine fracture with severe *blunt* facial trauma ranges from 1% to 6% of patients.[3,6–9] While incidence of cervical spine fracture with penetrating facial wounds can be relatively high (8.1%-23%),[5,10,11] there are no case reports of penetrating facial/head injury in a *neurologically intact* patient that has resulted in an unstable cervical spine fracture. Immediately forcing a patient who has sustained a penetrating facial injury into a cervical collar or supine positioning might result in catastrophe. Caution and common sense should guide emergency medical service (EMS) personnel and the emergency airway practitioner. If no concomitant trauma issues exist (e.g., a fall from a height after the penetrating wound), allowing the patient to stay in a position of comfort can be lifesaving.

What Other Concerns Do You Have for This Patient?

Oxygenation will be difficult, as any mask device will not provide a good seal and will also serve to pool blood and further compromise the airway.[2,5] Alternatives to non-rebreather masks or face mask devices include blow-by oxygen with a non-rebreather mask held in front of the airway, and nasal oxygen by a high-flow nasal cannula. If nostrils are intact, both modes might be employed simultaneously.

If induction of anesthesia is deemed necessary, a cerebral protective sedative (e.g., propofol, benzodiazepines, or barbiturates) is warranted, but care must be taken not to induce or exacerbate hypotension. Based on patient assessment, a "facilitated," sedation-only approach might be the preferred method of managing this patient's airway. Etomidate is attractive because of its relative hemodynamic stability, and its neutral effects on intracranial pressure (ICP).[12–18] Ketamine may allow "facilitated cooperation," provide analgesia, and allow further assessment of the patient's airway.[19–22] Recent evidence supports the use of ketamine even in the instance of head trauma as the concern for ICP rises with the use of ketamine is offset by the increase in cerebral perfusion pressure.[21–27] The choice of agents is of particular importance when caring for patients with a diminished cardiac reserve, such as those with severe cardiac disease, those who are critically ill, or patients who are elderly. These patients are more prone to a hypotensive response than are healthier patients with similar injuries.

What Investigations Are Warranted for This Patient Before Proceeding to Airway Management?

Adequate oxygen delivery is a priority in managing patients with trauma. Airway intervention usually takes precedence over any further investigation or intervention. Some may argue that plain film imaging of the face and neck may give additional information related to the destructive path of the projectile, which may help plan the approach to the airway. However, the value of such imaging is questionable and is insufficient in its ability to exclude a potential spinal injury and should not delay airway management.[2,3] Concurrent resuscitation and evaluation is key to trauma care, meaning that relevant investigations are underway at the same time when airway intervention is undertaken and do not delay management.

AIRWAY MANAGEMENT

What Are the Airway Management Considerations One Needs to be Aware of?

Anticipate difficult laryngoscopy, difficult EGD placement, and difficult (actually, impossible) FMV. Focus on patient positioning for laryngoscopy, as the volume of bleeding and the mechanical stability of the airway might preclude supine positioning.[3,4,28] The preferred method in such a patient would be a "sedated" look, with the patient seated upright or in the lateral decubitus position.[28] An "awake" intubation will be challenging to execute, as topical anesthesia will be difficult or impossible in this bloody airway, and will also require significant time to take effect. Rapid sequence intubation (RSI) is an option, but the airway practitioner must realize that it will be impossible to rescue the patient if oxygen desaturation occurs during laryngoscopy, so they will be placed into a "forced to act" scenario.[4] Failure to visualize the glottis or successfully pass an oral endotracheal tube (ETT) is a significant possibility in this patient, as first-pass success rates diminish with "soiled" airways when using either direct laryngoscopy (DL) or video laryngoscopy (VL) in such circumstances.[4,29] Additionally, the efficacy of many of the common alternative devices would also be compromised. The EGDs, such as the intubating laryngeal mask or the King LT airway, require intact hypopharyngeal structures to seat correctly, and so might be difficult to place. Indirect vision with VL, such as the GlideScope®, C-MAC®, or flexible bronchoscopy, may be obscured in the presence of significant volumes of blood.[2,29,30] Regardless of approach, prepare for a surgical airway as part of a double setup if airway attempt failure occurs.[1,31]

What Procedure Should Be Used to Intubate the Trachea of This Patient?

Preparation for any emergent airway begins by assembling standard intubating equipment, alternative airway devices, and a surgical airway kit.[1] Oxygenation with a non-rebreather mask should be initiated as early as possible,[32] and strong consideration should be given for apneic oxygenation with a nasal cannula during the intubation attempt.[33–36] The non-rebreather will probably need to be held slightly away from the face to avoid pooling of blood due to significant bleeding. Continuous nasal oxygenation during laryngoscopy attempts might provide oxygenation support during this vulnerable period of time.[37,38] Uncontrolled epistaxis may impede this process, can lead to aspiration, and may require immediate packing or cauterization. Having two, functioning, rigid suction devices is essential.

Timing and positioning are also important considerations. The patient is able to maintain his airway while he is sitting up. This positioning allows blood, bone fragments, and macerated tissue to be displaced away from the airway. In contrast, immediately placing the patient supine strictly for concern of cervical spine injury or reflexively resorting to typical airway management positioning could place his already tenuous airway at undue risk.[28,39] Given the soft tissue disruption and continued hemorrhage, one would anticipate that he would quickly obstruct his airway in a supine position. Help should be summoned from other experienced airway practitioners and surgical colleagues to be immediately available to assist in managing this patient.[4] Once all preparations for the difficult airway have been made, the practitioner needs to determine what plan to employ for airway management.

The pharmacologic strategy, in this case, would include a "sedated" look with immediate intubation when the glottis is visualized. Ketamine is a potent analgesic, has favorable hemodynamic properties, and, most importantly, should allow the patient to maintain their airway reflexes while facilitating laryngoscopy and intubation.[4,40–44] RSI, and in particular, neuromuscular blockade, in this instance is an option; however, the airway practitioner must recognize that if oxygen desaturation occurs during the intubation attempt, there will not be rescue oxygenation techniques that can reverse hypoxemia. This would create a "forced to act" scenario and would require an immediate surgical airway. If a "forced to act" is present when the patient arrives, an RSI might be considered as part of a double setup with immediate concurrent initiation of a cricothyrotomy.[1,4,45,46]

The actual intubation plan will be dictated by the actual clinical scenario. Multiple paths could be envisioned. An upright but semirecumbent patient could be approached with oral laryngoscopy with the practitioner on a step stool and coming over the patient. For a patient who is leaning forward and unable to tolerate any supine position, an alternative would be reversed-blade laryngoscopy, also known as the "Tomahawk" technique, with either the DL or the VL.[47] This technique requires the airway practitioner to hold the laryngoscope upside down in the right hand while standing and facing the patient who is seated upright. The blade is then used to "walk" back along the top of the tongue while applying gentle pressure down-and-away from the airway to open the mouth for visualization. An assistant is required to hold the patient's head from coming forward once either of these approaches commence. Another alternative would be to lie the patient in a lateral decubitus position (see Figures 28.2 and 28.3) for an attempt with a facilitated look and oral laryngoscopy; this may provide a different view of the airway that might allow successful intubation. In severe cases where the maneuver is not immediately successful in obtaining a view of the glottis and any portion of the tongue remains intact, a zero-silk on a curved needle can be placed through the tongue and the airway pulled anteriorly under the blade to allow the glottis to be delivered up into visualization, but this technique might require further sedation or analgesia. Alternatively, a pair of Babcock forceps can be used to grasp the tongue and pull the airway anteriorly. Once airway structures are visualized, the airway can be immediately intubated. Plan not to use Sellick's maneuver (cricoid pressure), which has fallen out of favor, as no literature exists to support benefit and mounting evidence

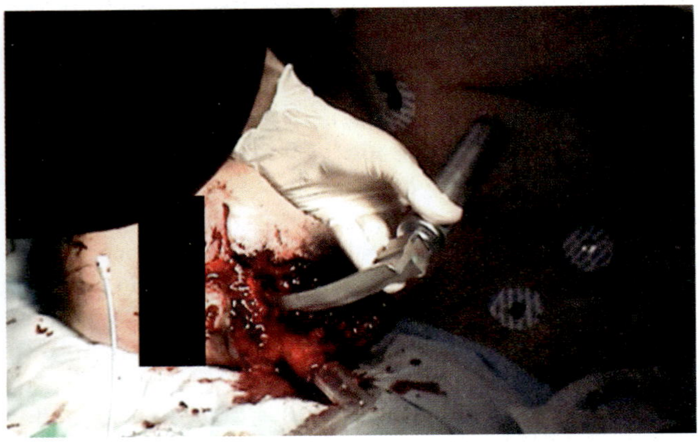

FIGURE 28.2. Direct laryngoscopy in lateral decubitus position in a patient with penetrating facial trauma.

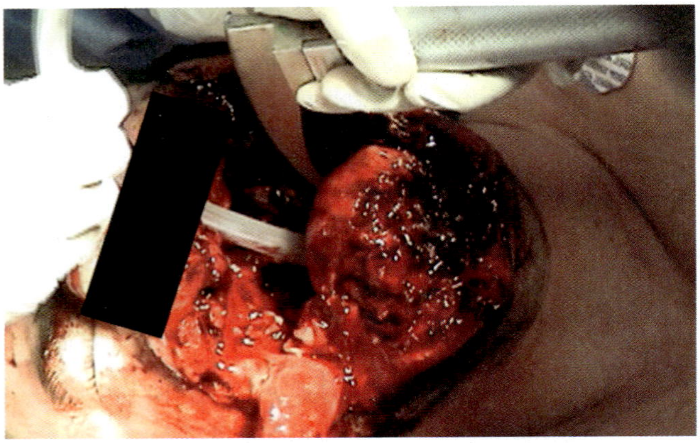

FIGURE 28.3. Laryngoscopic intubation in lateral decubitus position in a patient with penetrating facial trauma.

of it causing difficulty with intubation, mask ventilation, and EGD use.[28–31,34,48–52] Finally, an awake tracheotomy or cricothyrotomy could be considered as a primary approach if an oral and/or nasal route is predicted to be impossible.

A sequence of predetermined steps should be employed if primary laryngoscopy or oxygenation failure occurs. The patient's neck should be prepped for a surgical airway prior to the initial awake look approach, and cricothyrotomy equipment should be opened and ready for use. Traumatic airway management has a higher failure rate than other types of airway cases,[3] and cases such as this are prime examples of why that is the case. The emergency airway practitioner should be comfortable with performing a cricothyrotomy if the situation dictates.

POSTINTUBATION CONSIDERATION

■ What Other Issues Should Be Considered Following Tracheal Intubation?

Capnography, if available, or capnometry should be used to confirm ETT placement. Securing the ETT is critical and challenging in this case. Traditional tracheal taping may not be successful due to excessive bleeding or secretions. The practitioner might need to use a dedicated ETT holder that screws onto the ETT and is held in place by Velcro straps, or for short-term stabilization, a length of IV tubing can be used to wrap around the neck and then encircle the ETT, allowing the airway practitioner to wrap the ends around the ETT and tie off in a knot to keep the tube in place. Importantly, the patient should be adequately sedated to prevent accidental extubation, and pain control should be addressed.

SUMMARY

A penetrating maxillofacial injury can significantly impair both the ability to provide face-mask ventilation and perform laryngoscopy. Careful consideration must be given to approach this difficult airway. The lessons from this patient are that standard patient positioning may not be possible in such scenarios, alternative approaches must be considered, and backup plans must be ready in the event that the trachea cannot be intubated orally.

SELF-EVALUATION QUESTIONS

28.1. The patient presents in tripod position to maintain adequate breathing. Blow-by oxygen is provided by mask. Appropriate strategies to initially secure the airway would *NOT* include:

A. Keep the patient seated upright during awake look.
B. Attempt blind nasal intubation.
C. Assemble equipment for cricothyrotomy.
D. Call for immediate assistance from a surgical colleague.
E. Use personal protective equipment.

28.2. In the above scenario, when would a primary cricothyrotomy be appropriate?

A. On initial presentation
B. Once the surgical colleague arrives
C. After the initial attempt at awake look fails while oxygen saturation is 98%
D. Persistent oxygen desaturation
E. With nasal hemorrhage that prevents blind nasal intubation

28.3. The incidence of associated unstable cervical spine fracture in a neurologically intact patient with penetrating facial trauma:

A. Is negligible
B. Is not a concern provided a cervical collar that provides rigid immobilization is used
C. Ranges from 1% to 2.6% of patients
D. In some studies, approaches 20%
E. Has never been studied

REFERENCES

1. Law JA, Duggan LV, Asselin M, et al. Canadian Airway Focus Group updated consensus-based recommendations for management of the difficult airway: part 2. Planning and implementing safe management of the patient with an anticipated difficult airway. *Can J Anesth*. 2021;68(9):1405-1436.
2. Barak M, Bahouth H, Leiser Y, El-Naaj IA. Airway management of the patient with maxillofacial trauma: review of the literature and suggested clinical approach. *Biomed Res Int*. Published online 2015. doi:10.1155/2015/724032.
3. Perry M, Morris C. Advanced trauma life support (ATLS) and facial trauma: can one size fit all? Part 2: ATLS, maxillofacial injuries and airway management dilemmas. *Int J Oral Maxillofac Surg*. 2008;37(4):309-320.
4. Brown CA, Walls RM. Identification of the difficult and failed airway. In: Brown CA, Sakles JC, Mick NW, eds. *The Walls Manual of Emergency Airway Management*. 5th ed. Philadelphia, PA: Lippincott Williams & Wilkins; 2016.
5. Demetriades D, Chahwan S, Gomez H, Falabella A, Velmahos G, Yamashita D. Initial evaluation and management of gunshot wounds to the face. *J Trauma*. 1998;45(1):39-41.
6. Ardekian L, Gaspar R, Peled M, Manor R, Laufer D. Incidence and type of cervical spine injuries associated with mandibular fractures. *J Craniomaxillofac Trauma*. 1997;3(2):18-21.
7. Bayles SW, Abramson PJ, McMahon SJ, Reichman OS. Mandibular fracture and associated cervical spine fracture, a rare and predictable injury. Protocol for cervical spine evaluation and review of 1382 cases. *Arch Otolaryngol Head Neck Surg*. 1997;123(12):1304-1307.
8. Beirne JC, Butler PE, Brady FA. Cervical spine injuries in patients with facial fractures: a 1-year prospective study. *Int J Oral Maxillofac Surg*. 1995;24(1 Pt 1):26-29.
9. Haug RH, Wible RT, Likavec MJ, Conforti PJ. Cervical spine fractures and maxillofacial trauma. *J Oral Maxillofac Surg*. 1991;49(7):725-729.
10. Medzon R, Rothenhaus T, Bono CM, Grindlinger G, Rathlev NK. Stability of cervical spine fractures after gunshot wounds to the head and neck. *Spine*. 2005;30(20):2274-2279.
11. Liu FC, Halsey JN, Hoppe IC, Ciminello FS, Lee ES, Granick MS. A single-center review of facial fractures as the result of high-speed projectile injuries. *Eplasty*. 2018;18:e16.
12. Guldner G, Schultz J, Sexton P, Fortner C, Richmond M. Etomidate for rapid-sequence intubation in young children: hemodynamic effects and adverse events. *Acad Emerg Med*. 2003;10(2):134-139.
13. Gauss A, Heinrich H, Wilder-Smith OH. Echocardiographic assessment of the haemodynamic effects of propofol: a comparison with etomidate and thiopentone. *Anaesthesia*. 1991;46(2):99-105.
14. Jellish WS, Riche H, Salord F, Ravussin P, Tempelhoff R. Etomidate and thiopental-based anesthetic induction: comparisons between different titrated levels of electrophysiologic cortical depression and response to laryngoscopy. *J Clin Anesth*. 1997;9(1):36-41.
15. Bramwell KJ, Haizlip J, Pribble C, VanDerHeyden TC, Witte M. The effect of etomidate on intracranial pressure and systemic blood pressure in pediatric patients with severe traumatic brain injury. *Pediatr Emerg Care*. 2006;22(2):90-93.
16. Modica PA, Tempelhoff R. Intracranial pressure during induction of anaesthesia and tracheal intubation with etomidate-induced EEG burst suppression. *Can J Anaesth*. 1992;39(3):236-241.
17. Sharda SC, Bhatia MS. Etomidate compared to ketamine for induction during rapid sequence intubation: a systematic review and meta-analysis. *Indian J Crit Care Med*. 2022;26(1):108-113.
18. April MD, Arana A, Schauer SG, et al. Ketamine versus etomidate and peri-intubation hypotension: a national emergency airway registry study. *Acad Emerg Med*. 2020;27(11):1106-1115.
19. Green SM, Roback MG, Krauss BS, et al. Unscheduled procedural sedation: a multidisciplinary consensus practice guideline. *Ann Emerg Med*. 2019;73(5):e51-e65.
20. Green SM, Roback MG, Kennedy RM, Krauss B. Clinical practice guideline for emergency department ketamine dissociative sedation: 2011 update. *Ann Emerg Med*. 2011;57(5):449-461.
21. Leede E, Kempema J, Wilson C, et al. A multicenter investigation of the hemodynamic effects of induction agents for trauma rapid sequence intubation. *J Trauma Acute Care Surg*. 2021;90(6):1009-1013.
22. Baekgaard JS, Eskesen TG, Moo Lee J, et al. Ketamine for rapid sequence intubation in adult trauma patients: a retrospective observational study. *Acta Anaesthesiol Scand*. 2020;64(9):1234-1242.
23. Zanza C, Piccolella F, Racca F, et al. Ketamine in acute brain injury: current opinion following cerebral circulation and electrical activity. *Healthcare (Basel)*. 2022;10(3):566.
24. Kuza CM, To J, Chang A, et al. A retrospective data analysis on the induction medications used in trauma rapid sequence intubations and their effects on outcomes. *Eur J Trauma Emerg Surg*. 2022 Jun;48(3): 2275-2286. 2021.
25. Gregers MCT, Mikkelsen S, Lindvig KP, Brøchner AC. Ketamine as an anesthetic for patients with acute brain injury: a systematic review. *Neurocrit Care*. 2020;33(1):273-282.
26. Bhaire VS, Panda N, Luthra A, Chauhan R, Rajappa D, Bhagat H. Effect of combination of ketamine and propofol (ketofol) on cerebral oxygenation in neurosurgical patients: a randomized double-blinded controlled trial. *Anesth Essays Res*. 2019;13(4):643-648.
27. Kramer N, Lebowitz D, Walsh M, Ganti L. Rapid sequence intubation in traumatic brain-injured adults. *Cureus*. 2018;10(4):e2530.
28. Raja AS, Laurin EG. Distorted airways and acute upper airway obstruction. In: Brown CA, Sakles JC, Mick NW, eds. *The Walls Manual of Emergency Airway Management*. 5th ed. Philadelphia, PA: Lippincott Williams & Wilkins; 2016.
29. Sakles JC, Corn GJ, Hollinger P, Arcaris B, Patanwala AE, Mosier JM. The impact of a soiled airway on intubation success in the emergency department when using the GlideScope or the direct laryngoscope. *Acad Emerg Med*. 2017;24(5):628-636.
30. Brar MS. Airway management in a bleeding adult following tonsillectomy: a case report. *AANA J*. 2009;77(6):428-430.
31. Apfelbaum JL, Hagberg CA, Caplan RA, et al. Practice guidelines for management of the difficult airway: an updated report by the American Society of Anesthesiologists Task Force on Management of the Difficult Airway. *Anesthesiology*. 2013;118(2):251-270.
32. Mort TC. Preoxygenation in critically ill patients requiring emergency tracheal intubation. *Crit Care Med*. 2005;33(11):2672-2675.
33. Silva LOJE, Cabrera D, Barrionuevo P, et al. Effectiveness of apneic oxygenation during intubation: a systematic review and meta-analysis. *Ann Emerg Med*. 2017;70(4):483-494.e11.
34. Caputo N, Azan B, Domingues R, et al. Emergency department use of apneic oxygenation versus usual care during rapid sequence intubation: a randomized controlled trial (The ENDAO Trial). *Acad Emerg Med*. 2017;24(11):1387-1394.
35. Pavlov I, Medrano S, Weingart S. Apneic oxygenation reduces the incidence of hypoxemia during emergency intubation: a systematic review and meta-analysis. *Am J Emerg Med*. 2017;35(8):1184-1189.
36. Binks MJ, Holyoak RS, Melhuish TM, Vlok R, Bond E, White LD. Apneic oxygenation during intubation in the emergency department and during retrieval: a systematic review and meta-analysis. *Am J Emerg Med*. 2017;35(10):1542-1546.
37. Engström J, Hedenstierna G, Larsson A. Pharyngeal oxygen administration increases the time to serious desaturation at intubation in acute lung injury: an experimental study. *Crit Care*. 2010;14(3):R93.
38. Taha SK, Siddik-Sayyid SM, El-Khatib MF, Dagher CM, Hakki MA, Baraka AS. Nasopharyngeal oxygen insufflation following pre-oxygenation using the four deep breath technique. *Anaesthesia*. 2006;61(5):427-430.
39. Gibbs MA, Raja AS, Gonzalez MG. The Trauma Patient. In: Brown CA, Sakles JC, Mick NW, eds. *The Walls Manual of Emergency Airway Management*. 5th ed. Philadelphia, PA: Lippincott Williams & Wilkins; 2016.
40. Driver BE, Prekker ME, Reardon RF, et al. Success and complications of the ketamine-only intubation method in the emergency department. *J Emerg Med*. 2021;60(3):265-272.
41. Merelman AH, Perlmutter MC, Strayer RJ. Alternatives to rapid sequence intubation: contemporary airway management with ketamine. *West J Emerg Med*. 2019;20(3):466-471.
42. Sibley A, Mackenzie M, Bawden J, Anstett D, Villa-Roel C, Rowe BH. A prospective review of the use of ketamine to facilitate endotracheal intubation in the helicopter emergency medical services (HEMS) setting. *Emerg Med J*. 2011;28(6):521-525.
43. Begec Z, Demirbilek S, Onal D, Erdil F, Toprak HI, Ersoy MO. Ketamine or alfentanil administration prior to propofol anaesthesia: the effects on ProSeal laryngeal mask airway insertion conditions and haemodynamic changes in children. *Anaesthesia*. 2009;64(3):282-286.
44. Heffner AC, Deblieux PMC. Anesthesia and sedation for awake intubation. In: Brown CA, Sakles JC, Mick NW, eds. *The Walls Manual of Emergency Airway Management*. 5th ed. Philadelphia, PA: Lippincott Williams & Wilkins; 2016.
45. Patanwala AE, Stahle SA, Sakles JC, Erstad BL. Comparison of succinylcholine and rocuronium for first-attempt intubation success in the emergency department. *Acad Emerg Med*. 2011;18(1):10-14.
46. Law JA, Broemling N, Cooper RM, et al. The difficult airway with recommendations for management–part 2–the anticipated difficult airway. *Can J Anaesth*. 2013;60(11):1119-1138.

47. Silverton NA, Youngquist ST, Mallin MP, et al. GlideScope versus flexible fiber optic for awake upright laryngoscopy. *Ann Emerg Med.* 2012;59(3):159-164.
48. Levitan RM. Cricoid Pressure Impedes First Pass Intubation Success and Contributes to Difficult Laryngoscopy in Emergency Airway. In: *2006 Annual Meeting of the Society for Acadamic Emergency Medicine (SAEM 2006).* 2006. http://search.proquest.com/docview/39933623?accountid=10920. Accessed on July 16, 2022.
49. Harris T, Ellis DY, Foster L, Lockey D. Cricoid pressure and laryngeal manipulation in 402 pre-hospital emergency anaesthetics: essential safety measure or a hindrance to rapid safe intubation? *Resuscitation.* 2010;81(7):810-816.
50. Palmer J, Ball DR. The effect of cricoid pressure on the cricoid cartilage and vocal cords: an endoscopic study in anaesthetised patients. *Anaesthesia.* 2000;55(3):263-268.
51. Corda DM, Riutort KT, Leone AJ, Qureshi MK, Heckman MG, Brull SJ. Effect of jaw thrust and cricoid pressure maneuvers on glottic visualization during GlideScope videolaryngoscopy. *J Anesth.* 2012;26(3):362-368.
52. Salem MR, Khorasani A, Zeidan A, Crystal GJ. Cricoid pressure controversies: narrative review. *Anesthesiology.* 2017;126(4):738-752.

CHAPTER 29

Airway Management in a Patient with a Deep Neck Infection

Alexander Poulton

CASE PRESENTATION

A 32-year-old man (Figure 29.1) presented to the emergency department (ED) with dysphagia, dysphonia, and dyspnea. Further inquiry revealed a 1-week history of right-sided jaw pain. This was initially treated with oral antibiotics and analgesics by his family doctor while awaiting an appointment with his dentist. He saw his dentist the preceding day and had an abscessed second molar tooth extracted from his right mandible. Unfortunately, his pain continued and he developed swelling and fever, prompting him to present to the ED. His past medical history was unremarkable. Aside from his recent prescriptions for penicillin and hydromorphone, he was on no medications. He had no known allergies.

INTRODUCTION

Discuss the Incidence and Etiology of Deep Neck Infections in Adults

Deep neck infection (DNI) remains a frequently encountered condition in both children and adults.[1] Pediatric data from the United States estimates the incidence of DNI at 4.6 per 100,000.[2] The management of the patient whose airway is compromised due to a DNI is a challenge for even the most experienced practitioner. Fortunately for acute care practitioners, severe life-threatening presentations of DNI are relatively uncommon.[3] As in this case, adult DNI is often odontogenic in origin. Most patients are aged 40 to 60 and there is a predominance of males. Risk factors include diabetes mellitus,[4,5] hematological malignancies, and positive HIV status.[6,7] In pediatric patients, pharyngotonsillitis remains the most important cause of DNI.[1]

Discuss the Relevant Anatomic Relationships of the Deep Neck Spaces

A detailed description of the anatomy of the neck is beyond the scope of this chapter; however, a basic understanding is helpful to understand the potential consequences of DNIs. At least 11 deep neck spaces exist within a complex framework of cervical fascial planes. These fascial planes function to contain DNIs so long as their resistance is not overcome. However, once overcome, they serve to direct infectious spread.[8] The deep neck spaces are often classified relative to their relationship to the hyoid with those above (including peritonsillar and submandibular), below (including pretracheal), and those that involve the entire neck (including retropharyngeal and danger space) differentiated.

The retropharyngeal space is located posterior to the pharynx and esophagus, running from the skull base to the mediastinum. The alar fascia posterior to this space is the only barrier to infectious spread to the danger space (which allows spread to the superior mediastinum and severe infection in the form of mediastinitis).[9] Patients with retropharyngeal infection can present with severe neck pain and rigidity, often maintaining their neck in flexed position, greatly complicating surgical and nonsurgical airway management approaches.[10]

The submandibular space exists between the mylohyoid muscle and the skin. The apices of the second and third molar

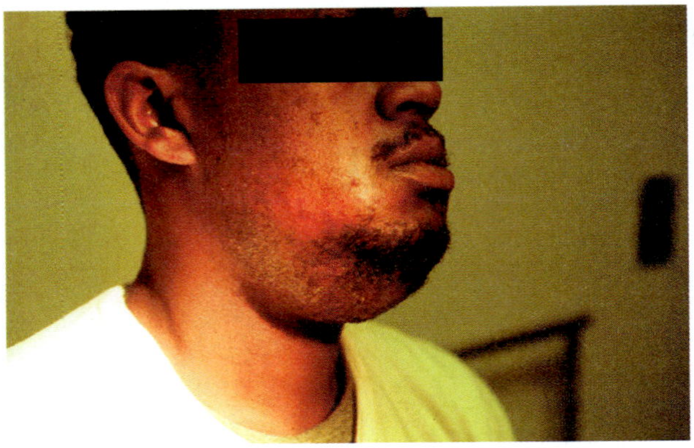

FIGURE 29.1. This 32-year-old man presented with dysphagia, dysphonia, and dyspnea. There was marked swelling on the right side of the neck. Due to marked discomfort, he was unable to protrude his tongue for proper pharyngeal evaluation.

teeth typically pierce below the mylohyoid and create a pathway for infection to spread to this space. Infection here leads to swelling that typically progresses from inferolateral mandible and spreads medially. This space has an open posterior boundary allowing spread to secondary spaces. Infection can lead to pronounced elevation and protrusion of the tongue. If infection spreads to include the submandibular along with submental and sublingual spaces bilaterally, the infection is known as Ludwig's angina.[1]

■ Do All Deep Neck Infections Require Airway Intervention?

Most patients with DNIs can be managed conservatively without surgical intervention and do not require intervention to maintain the patient's airway.[11,12] A conservative approach with antibiotics and potentially steroids may be all that is required, especially with small abscess pockets involving a single neck space.[1,13] Needle aspiration followed by antibiotics may suffice for abscesses unlikely to resolve with conservative management alone, such as peritonsillar abscesses. However, some patients will require transoral or transcervical incision and drainage. Although patients may present with altered phonation and upper airway dyspnea, severe airway compromise is uncommon. Despite this fact, careful repeated assessment of the patient's airway is important given the risk of deterioration and the fact that airway compromise is the leading cause of mortality in these patients.[3]

■ What Is Ludwig's Angina?

This potentially life-threatening infection of the floor of the mouth was first described in 1836 by Wilhelm Frederick von Ludwig. The condition has also been called morbus strangulatorius, angina maligna, and garotillo (Spanish for "hangman's loop"). These older terms reflect the high mortality rate, typically by total airway obstruction, in the days before antibiotics.

Ludwig's angina is defined as severe bilateral gangrenous cellulitis and edema of the submandibular, submental, and sublingual spaces. "Woody" swelling of the submandibular area in a febrile patient with a history of jaw pain is the classic presentation. The infection may cause swelling and displacement of the tongue and epiglottis that can impair the ability to swallow and clear secretions. Total airway obstruction may result from progressive swelling or from laryngospasm secondary to aspiration of purulent secretions, or both.[14] Ludwig's angina typically requires aggressive intervention, including surgical drainage and definitive airway management, in addition to antibiotic therapy, intravenous steroids, and nebulized epinephrine.[15,16]

ASSESSMENT OF THE PATIENT

■ Why Might Airway Management Be Difficult in Patients with Ludwig's Angina?

Patients with Ludwig's angina or a retropharyngeal abscess have the potential for difficulty with all aspects of standard airway management: face-mask ventilation (FMV), ventilation using extraglottic devices (EGDs, e.g., LMA), laryngoscopy and tracheal intubation, and surgical airway access. Extracorporeal membrane oxygenation (ECMO) has been advocated as a potential option for predicted severely difficult airways; however, the need for near supine positioning if femoral access is required and implementation time make this less than ideal in Ludwig's angina.[17] In addition, the potential for physiologic derangements including hypoxemia, acid-base disturbances, and sepsis can create a scenario known as a *physiologically difficult airway*.[18]

The oropharyngeal and sublingual swelling leads to significant displacement of the tongue. With progression, deep-space infection may track and involve the periglottic region. Stridor represents a late presentation with impending airway collapse. FMV if required would be a challenge and necessitate high airway pressures to produce adequate gas flow. High-flow nasal oxygenation would be better tolerated and may bypass the obstructive oropharyngeal pathology. These patients are often dependent on position for airway patency and so maintaining an upright posture and avoiding sedation when possible is prudent. It may prove difficult or impossible to open the airway of the sedated or unconscious patient due to loss of muscle tone and the resultant further narrowing of the airway. Copious secretions may increase the risk of laryngospasm, and tongue swelling may preclude use of an oral airway. A nasal airway is an option but bleeding could possibly trigger laryngospasm.

Upward displacement of the tongue by the infection can make insertion of any of the EGDs difficult or impossible. Additionally, EGDs that are able to navigate past the tongue may be ineffective due to glottic edema, and the patient remains susceptible to laryngospasm.

Secretions and edema, particularly tongue swelling, will make direct laryngoscopy more difficult regardless of the type of blade chosen. Nuchal rigidity, trismus, or both may preclude insertion of the laryngoscope blade. While nuchal rigidity and trismus may improve with sedation or muscle relaxants, there is no guarantee that these agents will be effective. Blind intubation techniques, such as the Intubating Laryngeal Mask Airway and lighted stylets (such as the Trachlight™) would not generally be considered for first-line use in these patients as these techniques run the risk of disrupting infected tissue and potentially soiling the airway. Furthermore, these nonvisual intubating techniques could result in laryngospasm during the intubation attempt. Typically, these patients have heavy secretions and may have bleeding, limiting the use of indirect visual techniques such as the flexible and rigid intubating scopes and video laryngoscopes (VLs). Similar to the direct laryngoscope (DL), even low-profile VL blades may not be able to reach the posterior oropharynx due to trismus. In advanced cases of Ludwig's angina, oral intubation with any instrument may not be possible due to limited oral access. Most experts would advocate either a nasal intubation or a surgical approach as a primary approach, particularly in the presence of trismus.

Unfortunately, performing a surgical airway in this patient population is difficult. The anatomy is often distorted due to swelling and hyperemic tissues may increase the likelihood of bleeding. In some patients, the abscess may involve the area surrounding the trachea. Supine positioning of the patient to perform a surgical airway may worsen dyspnea and reduce the patient's cooperation. Additionally, nuchal rigidity may limit the patient's ability to extend their neck to allow for surgical access to the trachea.

All possible options of ventilation and oxygenation in Ludwig's angina are fraught with danger. The ultimate airway management decision will be made based on the urgency of the clinical circumstance, the available resources, the careful setting of priorities, and the experience of the airway team (emergency and anesthesia practitioners and ENT surgeons).

Discuss the Role of Diagnostic Imaging in Assessing These Patients

A lateral neck X-ray is often performed in these situations. This imaging may demonstrate submandibular or retropharyngeal swelling and epiglottic thickening but seldom provides enough information to direct management independently.

The advent of the CT scan has revolutionized the ability to accurately assess the swollen, inflamed neck. CT scans with IV contrast provide excellent visualization of the severity and location of infection involving different neck spaces. The CT scan can also determine the presence or absence of infected jugular vein thrombosis (Lemierre syndrome). However, CT cannot always reliably differentiate the purulent collection of an abscess from generalized edema secondary to the infection, termed phlegmon. Unfortunately, in the presence of a rapidly deteriorating airway, it will usually be necessary to proceed with emergency airway management before a CT examination of the neck becomes available. Even in patients with "stable" airways, a CT scan may not be possible prior to definitive airway management because the patient may be unable to lie flat. In these cases, a CT scan to better determine the extent of the infection should be performed only after safely securing airway. Some CT scanners can accommodate patients with elevated head positioning but the risk-benefit ratio of transport to the CT area prior to airway control in patients with such advanced disease must be carefully weighed.[19]

While ultrasound is commonly employed to assess neck masses in general, the airways and the larynx are rarely included in these assessments. As technology and skills improve, some authors have suggested that point-of-care ultrasonography play more of a role in management of these patients.[20] This could potentially alleviate the problems of positioning and radiation associated with CT, and provide useful information quickly.

Discuss the Technique of Nasopharyngoscopy and Its Role in the Management of Patients with Deep Neck Infections

Nasopharyngoscopy is a safe and simple technique. Anesthesia practitioners, otolaryngologists, and emergency practitioners should become familiar to this technique. Following the application of topical vasoconstrictor and local anesthetic, the flexible nasopharyngoscope is passed into the nasopharynx. Care should be taken not to apply local anesthetic or vasoconstrictor to the glottis as this could trigger laryngospasm. With the flexible nasopharyngoscope, the glottis and periglottic anatomy can be viewed from above without the risk of provoking laryngospasm. The technique is usually first done in the ED as part of the initial evaluation, and repeated at the bedside or in the operating room (OR) as required to provide an ongoing evaluation of the airway. Serial nasopharyngoscopic assessments become particularly important if conservative airway management is decided upon. Documentation of nasopharyngoscopic assessment is also helpful in determining the safety of patient transport to the imaging suite.[1]

How Was This Patient Assessed?

On examination, he appeared anxious and in severe discomfort. He was febrile with a temperature of 38.7°C. His respiratory rate was 26 breaths per minute. His heart rate was 104 beats per minute and his blood pressure was 132/76 mmHg. His oxygen saturation was 91% on a non-rebreather face mask. He had a marked decrease in the range of motion of his neck. Significant swelling and erythema was observed extending from the right submandibular region, crossing the midline, and down the neck to include his left upper chest. Mouth opening was limited in this patient due to moderate trismus, and the patient's tongue appeared elevated.

A lateral X-ray of the neck was remarkable for submandibular and retropharyngeal swelling along with a diminished airway caliber (Figure 29.2).

Nasopharyngoscopy was performed in the ED by the ENT resident and revealed right lateral pharyngeal swelling and posterior displacement of the epiglottis obscuring the vocal cords.

How Do You Assess the Severity of Airway Obstruction?

Airway obstruction is assessed clinically by history and physical examination. Oxygen saturation, respiratory rate, stridor, tracheal tug, intercostal indrawing, and use of accessory muscles are assessed and changes are noted. Lateral X-ray (Figure 29.2) and CT scan of the head and neck can quantify the degree of obstruction. It is worth bearing in mind that these imaging

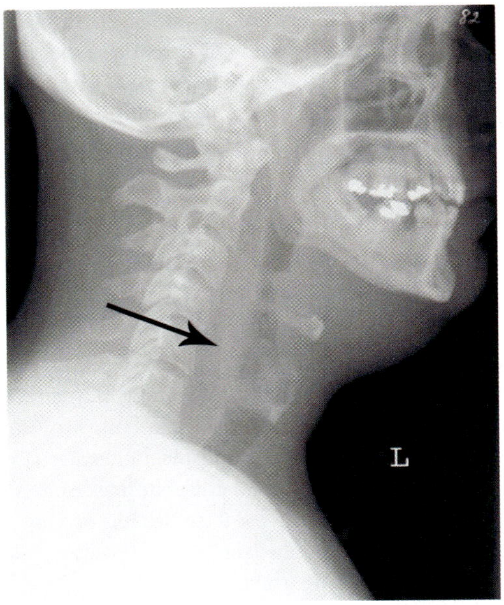

FIGURE 29.2. Although this lateral X-ray view of the head and neck did not show any obvious sign of airway obstruction, it showed an increase in prevertebral soft tissue (swelling of the posterior pharyngeal wall) (arrow), an important diagnostic sign of retropharyngeal abscess.[21] There was also a loss of normal lordotic curvature of the spine.

modalities typically provide static images and the obstruction may appear worse at varying stages of the respiratory cycling than others. Skilled practitioners may also be able to assess airway obstruction with ultrasound.[20] Nasopharyngoscopy is particularly useful, in that it allows for a dynamic assessment of the obstruction. However, due to the risk of sudden deterioration in this patient with severe stridor, a clear airway management plan should be articulated with the team prior to proceeding with nasopharyngoscopy in a monitored setting.

AIRWAY MANAGEMENT

What Are the Indications for Establishing a Definitive Airway in Patients with Deep Neck Infections?

Indications for definitive airway management in these patients include impending or anticipated progression to airway obstruction and the need for general anesthesia to be able to drain the abscess and gain control of infectious source. While some advocate for a decision based on percentage of airway obstruction, the ultimate decision to secure the airway should be made in collaboration with a team of care providers including the emergency and anesthesia practitioners and the ENT surgeon.[1] There is some evidence that it may be prudent to intervene at an earlier stage in at-risk patients, such as those with diabetes mellitus.[4] In some instances, the emergency practitioner may be forced into airway intervention if the patient is acutely decompensating. Once the decision to intervene is made, anesthesia practitioner and ENT surgeon, if not already involved, should be immediately consulted. These patients are ideally managed in the operating room with access to a full suite of operative equipment, provided that the transfer can be done safely and complete airway obstruction is not imminent.

What Was the Plan in This Case?

Given the severity of the obstruction and the patient's worsening symptoms, the decision was made to establish a definitive airway. Anesthesia was immediately consulted and the plan was made to proceed to the OR for definitive airway management, followed by surgical drainage of the abscess.

Do These Patients Require a Primary Surgical Airway or Can an Attempt Be Made to Intubate the Trachea from Above?

Once the need to secure the airway has been established, the next decision is whether to attempt tracheal intubation from above (either oral or nasal) or to go directly to a front-of-neck airway (FONA). In the "stable" patient, this generally refers to an awake tracheotomy done by an experienced ENT surgeon. Local anesthesia infiltration with minimal sedation (e.g., remifentanil 0.05-0.1 $\mu g \cdot kg^{-1} \cdot min^{-1}$) is usually all that is needed to ensure patient cooperation and provide an antitussive effect when the procedure is performed by a competent surgeon. In rare circumstances, an awake cricothyrotomy may be indicated if surgical expertise or time is not available. The choice of airway should be a joint decision of the anesthesia practitioner and surgeon based on the predicted difficulties of each of the following: FMV, EGD ventilation, laryngoscopic intubation, alternative intubation, and FONA. The skill and experience of the airway team will also affect this decision. In a review by Potter et al., the investigators found that primary surgical airways appeared to be favored by otolaryngologists, while oral and maxillofacial surgeons favored oral or nasal intubation.[22]

Discuss the "Double-Setup" and Plan C

In many cases, it will be reasonable to make a nonsurgical attempt to secure the airway. The specific route (awake, asleep, oral vs. nasal) will be discussed below. But it is critical to have a well-developed Plan B (and sometimes Plan C). The "Double Setup" is the recommended approach for most of these cases, meaning that the surgical team is ready to obtain FONA, should attempts to secure the airway from above by the anesthesia practitioner fail. This may involve having the surgical team gowned and gloved, equipment laid out, and the patient's neck marked and prepped. Many times, a formal tracheotomy can be performed; however, in the event of emergent airway compromise, a cricothyrotomy may be the better choice.

The FONA typically represents Plan B and this may solve the airway problem. Surgical access could, however, prove difficult for any of the reasons discussed above. Loss of the airway during tracheotomy has been reported and such an eventuality must be prepared for with "Plan C."[23] This will typically involve an awake patient breathing spontaneously with sedation (IV or inhalation) to facilitate patient cooperation, but in rare circumstances could require muscle relaxation and attempts to optimize airway management from above while efforts to obtain surgical access continue.

Discuss the Pros and Cons of Securing the Airway in the Awake or Anesthetized Patient

One must decide whether to perform tracheal intubation awake or asleep. As discussed above, these patients invariably have features that pose problems in airway management. The safest initial approach with these patients is to manage the airway while they are awake. Sedation may indeed be necessary in some cases, but it is preferred to keep the patient cooperative and spontaneously breathing. Ketamine (0.5-1 mg·kg^{-1}), low-dose remifentanil infusion (0.05-0.1 µg·kg^{-1}·min^{-1}), or dexmedetomidine (0.2-1 µg·kg^{-1} over 10 minutes) may prove useful. Sedative medications, including dexmedetomidine, may promote upper airway collapse and impair respiratory drive so the use should be selective and based on the patient's condition.[24] Whether medication is used or not, clear communication with the patient with repeated reassurance and a confident demeanor on the part of the practitioner is critical. The patient will typically need to be maintained in a sitting or semi-sitting position in order to help preserve the airway, which will increase comfort and help ensure the patient's cooperation.

Discuss Reasons Why an Awake Intubation May Be Unsuccessful

While awake intubation remains the safest initial approach to airway management, it is important to realize that sudden deterioration with a complete airway obstruction may occur even in a fully awake or minimally sedated patient.[21,25–27] Reports of complete airway obstruction and failed bronchoscopic intubation emphasize the importance of managing these patients under "double setup."[28] Inadequate airway anesthesia, airway practitioner inexperience, oversedation, copious secretions, and bleeding are all reasons an awake intubation could fail. It is also worth emphasizing that delay in definitive airway management and natural progression of disease could lead to complete obstruction while preparing to access the airway in severe cases.

What Is the Alternative Plan If Awake Intubation Fails or Is Not an Option?

If an awake intubation fails or is not possible, then a complete, but rapid, reassessment of the situation is in order. The next safest approach may be an awake FONA, provided that the patient still has a patent airway and is at least minimally cooperative. In the rapidly deteriorating or actively uncooperative patient, a primary FONA may not be a practical alternative. It may then become necessary to induce general anesthesia in a patient with multiple predictors of difficulty across all modalities of airway management, certainly a less-than-ideal circumstance.

Discuss Options If General Anesthesia Becomes Necessary to Secure the Airway

Should it be necessary to induce general anesthesia, the "ideal" approach is a matter of opinion. There are "pros and cons" with respect to all of the available choices. Induction of general anesthesia in this setting should always be done under "double setup" conditions, as discussed above.

Perhaps the classic approach is an inhalation induction, attempting to induce general anesthesia while preserving spontaneous respiration. Inhalation induction followed by laryngoscopy with an appropriate model of blade (Macintosh, Miller, or other) and intubation is a common practice in young children with airway obstruction since awake intubation is rarely a practical option.

Inhalation induction of adults with airway obstruction may be more difficult, in that the relatively longer excitement phase predisposes to aspiration, laryngospasm, or both. As anesthetic depth increases, complete airway obstruction can also occur due to the loss of muscle tone. Inhalation induction typically requires at least some degree of patient cooperation but can be accomplished without it.[29] As with awake intubation, it is critical to have a well-rehearsed backup plan (Plans B and C). Preservation of spontaneous ventilation under anesthesia may also be accomplished by utilizing IV agents. However, compared to inhalation agents, it may be more difficult to achieve the goal therapeutic window whereby spontaneous ventilation is preserved and the adequate depth of anesthesia reached.

Rapid sequence intubation (RSI) should not be a first-line management option in these patients. However, in the event that the airway is completely lost, consideration should be given to use of muscle relaxants to eliminate the possibility of complete laryngospasm and facilitate trial of intubation, FMV, or EGD ventilation while attempts to achieve FONA continue.

Discuss the Pros and Cons of "Nasal or Oral" Intubation

Following the decision to attempt intubation from above, the next decision is whether to use the nasal or oral route. Each has its advantages and drawbacks.

The nasal route bypasses the tongue (which may be swollen and elevated) and often provides a convenient passage to the glottic opening. At one time, blind nasal intubation was a common choice in these patients, but with the general availability of flexible bronchoscopes, this technique is now seldom indicated. Furthermore, blindly advancing the endotracheal tube (ETT) into the glottic opening may rupture the abscess with resultant soiling of the trachea and the potential for purulent secretions to trigger laryngospasm.[30] The risk of epistaxis is a potential concern with the nasal approach, as bleeding may hamper visualization and could also trigger laryngospasm.

The oral approach avoids the risks of nasal bleeding and also allows for application and administration of high-flow nasal oxygenation throughout the intubation process, which may prevent or delay the onset of hypoxemia.[31] Unfortunately, massive tongue swelling combined with trismus, often seen in patients with Ludwig's angina, can make an oral intubation impossible.

How Can One Minimize the Risk of Bleeding Associated with Nasal Intubation?

The risk of bleeding during nasal intubation is a risk to be aware of when using this approach (see section "Preparation for Awake Intubation" in Chapter 3 for more detail). Epistaxis may be minimized with the liberal use of topical vasoconstrictors (e.g., xylometazoline) and by using a small ETT (7.0-mm ID or smaller for adults). However, a larger ETT (7.0-mm ID or greater) is advantageous in that it allows for the use of the adult flexible bronchoscope with its superior optics and suction capabilities. ETTs (including nasal RAE ETTs) may be made less damaging to tissues by softening the tubes in warm saline prior to use and using a suitable lubricant when advancing the ETT.

The practice of "dilating up the nasal passage" using different sizes of nasopharyngeal airway may also decrease bleeding and allow for the passage of a larger tube (see section "Flexible Bronchoscopic Intubation" in Chapter 10 for more detail).[32] Following application of local anesthesia and vasoconstrictors, a small soft nasopharyngeal airway lubricated with 2% lidocaine jelly can be inserted into the nasal passage. The right nasal passage (larger in most people) is preferred unless there are anatomic reasons to preferentially use the left naris.[33] If resistance is encountered, the opposite naris can be tried. The process can then be repeated with the next larger size nasopharyngeal airway until finally the largest possible nasopharyngeal airway split longitudinally can be placed and used as a guide through which to pass the bronchoscope. The split nasopharyngeal airway can then be removed before subsequent passage of the ETT over the bronchoscope.

What Is the Best Tool to Facilitate Intubation?

For the most part, the tool that one chooses to facilitate intubation in these patients is less important than the approach discussed above. The technique chosen should reflect the practitioner's skill, experience, and comfort with the technique, the available resources, and the safety and practicality of the chosen technique. Blind techniques are discouraged due to risks of soiling the airway and of possible laryngospasm. For reasons discussed earlier, techniques that allow visualization of the airway are preferred, usually direct-visualization laryngoscopy, indirect-visualization laryngoscopy using a VL, indirect-visualization using a flexible bronchoscope, or a combination of these methods. Other methods may be acceptable provided the practitioner is skilled in their use.

Discuss the Advantages and Disadvantages of Flexible Bronchoscopic Intubation

Flexible bronchoscopic intubation (FBI) offers the advantage of being able to visualize and navigate "around the obstruction" and is usually well tolerated in the awake patient. Unfortunately, heavy secretions, bleeding, or both, may limit the usefulness of the FBI. Smaller flexible bronchoscopes, in particular, may struggle to manage secretions via their suction channel. Unfortunately, larger bronchoscopes necessitate larger ETTs, which may be more difficult to deliver past the area of obstruction. Additionally, as the ETT is advanced blindly over the bronchoscope during intubation, careful attention is required to avoid rupturing the abscess and soiling the airway with infective materials. FBI may be more difficult in the unconscious patient with decreased muscle tone, but if attempted, may be best done in combination with a VL.[34,35] The combined approach, where feasible, offers numerous advantages, including ability to increase space for the bronchoscope in the oropharynx, indirect visualization of the ETT as it passes along the bronchoscope, and the ability to shelter bronchoscope from active secretions. However, the technique is limited by equipment availability, required amount of mouth opening to position the VL, and the need for a second practitioner to hold the VL in place.[36]

Discuss the Advantages and Disadvantages of Direct Laryngoscopy

Direct laryngoscopy may be advantageous in the presence of heavy secretions or a soiled airway, although the degree of benefit is disputed.[37] It can be performed quickly, allows complete visualization of the ETT passing into the trachea, and is the historical technique of choice in the unconscious patient. However, direct laryngoscopy is highly stimulating and may not be tolerated in the awake patient, particularly if much force is needed to expose the glottis. The ability to use this technique will be severely limited if not made impossible by any degree of trismus.

Describe the Plan to Secure the Airway in This Patient

In the operating room, the airway was re-evaluated and, in consultation with the ENT surgeon, the decision was made to perform an awake nasotracheal intubation using a flexible bronchoscope under "double setup" conditions.

The patient was positioned semi-sitting and standard monitors were applied. Supplemental oxygen was delivered with nasal prongs featuring end-tidal CO_2 monitoring during preparation and airway anesthesia. A low-dose infusion of remifentanil (0.05 $\mu g \cdot kg^{-1} \cdot min^{-1}$) was administered intravenously to improve cooperation and provide an antitussive effect. The neck was prepped and the surgical team was gowned and gloved, ready to perform an emergency FONA (Plan B). A VL with a low-profile hyperangulated blade was made available at the patient's bedside to assist with the nasotracheal bronchoscopic intubation if needed.

Discuss Airway Anesthesia for Patients with Ludwig's Angina

There are multiple techniques to anesthetize the airway and these are discussed in detail in Chapter 3. The chosen technique depends largely on the preference of the practitioner. However, care must be taken to avoid early stimulation of the airway, which can result in fatal laryngospasm.[38]

Inflammation and infection can, in theory, decrease the efficacy of local anesthetics due to changes in local pH. However, this is generally not of any clinical significance. Heavy secretions, bleeding, or both, can decrease the amount of local anesthetic that actually reaches the mucosa and this should be taken into account, but there are many reports of successful airway anesthesia in the presence of significant infection.[39]

How Was Airway Anesthesia Achieved in This Case?

Airway anesthesia was achieved with a combination of lidocaine ointment, lidocaine cotton tip swabs, and atomized lidocaine. Xylometazoline (Otrivin nasal spray, Novartis Consumer Health Canada Inc, Mississauga, ON) was applied to both nasal passages in hopes of decreasing bleeding potential. Approximately 2.0 cm of 5% lidocaine ointment was applied to the back of the tongue with a tongue depressor, primarily to facilitate VL assistance if required. The EZ Spray 100 atomizer (Alcove Medical Corporation, Houston, TX) was then used to deliver 10 mL of 4% lidocaine to the patient's nasal passages. Atomized lidocaine spray during vigorous inhalation is very effective at topicalizing the glottis; however, in this case, care was taken to focus the anesthetizing effect on the nasal passages. Lidocaine-soaked long cotton-tipped applicators were then used to apply 4% lidocaine to posterior nasal cavity. Transmucosal superior laryngeal nerve block was not performed due to the possibility of disrupting the abscess and potentially soiling the airway.

How Was This Patient's Airway Secured?

The patient was asked to take a deep breath while occluding each naris independently. The right appeared more patent and was dilated as described above (see section "How Can One Minimize the Risk of Bleeding Associated with Nasal Intubation?" in this chapter for more detail) so that an 8.0-mm nasal airway was easily accepted. A 7.0-mm nasal ETT was softened in warm saline, cuff fully deflated, and appropriately lubricated. The ETT was then gently advanced into the nasopharynx. An adult 5.2-mm FB was then passed through the ETT. The anatomy was abnormal with an inflamed, posteriorly displaced, and leftward deviated epiglottis obscuring the view of the laryngeal inlet. Despite the patient's trismus, he was able to provide just enough mouth opening to attempt to advance a low-profile hyperangulated VL blade into the oropharynx. Thus, to assist with visualization, a GlideScope® hyperangulated Titanium blade (Verathon Medical, Bothwell, WA) was then advanced in the posterior oropharynx which improved the ability to view the laryngeal inlet with the bronchoscope and increased the space available to advance past the vocal cords. The bronchoscope was directed into the trachea until the carina was in view and the ETT was then gently advanced into the trachea over the bronchoscope under indirect visualization on the VL screen. Following the end-tidal CO_2 confirmation of successful tube placement, general anesthesia was induced with sevoflurane inhalation.

Surgical drainage of the abscess was then accomplished without incident. Following 36 hours of ventilation in the ICU, tracheal extubation took place uneventfully and the patient made a full recovery.

SUMMARY

It is clear that there is no single approach that will satisfy all potential circumstances when managing the airway for patients with a DNI. The ultimate decision must be based on the specific patient presentation, local resources, and the skillset of the airway management team.

In 2002, Jenkins et al.[40] surveyed Canadian anesthesia practitioners regarding their choice of airway management for specific patient presentations. For patients presenting with dysphagia due to retropharyngeal abscess, 70% chose an awake approach, 23% chose inhalation induction, and only 7% chose an IV induction of anesthesia. In terms of primary airway technique, 50% chose FBI, 37% chose direct laryngoscopy, and 8% chose primary surgical airway. McDonnough et al.[41] performed at retrospective review of adult patients admitted through the ED with a primary diagnosis of Ludwig's angina from 2006 to 2014 in the United States. Of 5855 patient requiring admission, 8% required airway intervention with 42% of those patients receiving a surgical airway. A 2004 study by Bross-Soriano et al. reported on 107 patients with Ludwig's angina over 18 years.[5] Surgical airway was required in 28%, when nasal intubation failed or was not possible, highlighting the concept of the "double setup."

DNIs resulting in airway compromise provide challenges for both the airway practitioner and the surgeon who are dependent on each other for a successful outcome. The likelihood of a satisfactory result is enhanced by early involvement of the entire airway management team and collaborative planning for the challenges predicted.

SELF-EVALUATION QUESTIONS

29.1. What is Ludwig's angina?

A. Epiglottitis
B. Unstable angina
C. Deep neck infection and edema involving the entire floor of the mouth
D. Lingual tonsillitis
E. Mediastinitis

29.2. Which of the following airway management strategies may be difficult in patients with Ludwig's angina?

A. Face-mask ventilation
B. Ventilation using extraglottic devices
C. Direct laryngoscopy
D. Surgical airway
E. All of the above

29.3. Which of the following is *NOT* an acceptable intubating technique in managing patients with Ludwig's angina?

A. Surgical airway
B. Flexible bronchoscopic intubation
C. Blind intubation using an Intubating LMA
D. Laryngoscopic intubation
E. Intubation using a GlideScope

REFERENCES

1. Christian J, Felts C, Beckmann N, Gillespie MB. Deep neck and odontogenic infections. In: *Cummings Otolaryngology: Head and Neck Surgery*. 7th ed. Elsevier; 2020:141-154.
2. Adil E, Tarshish Y, Roberson D, Jang J, Licameli G, Kenna M. The public health impact of pediatric deep neck space infections. *Otolaryngol Head Neck Surg*. 2015;153(6):1036-1041.
3. Karkos PD, Leong SC, Beer H, Apostolidou MT, Panarese A. Challenging airways in deep neck space infections. *Am J Otolaryngol*. 2007;28(6):415-418.
4. Boscolo-Rizzo P, da Mosto MC. Submandibular space infection: a potentially lethal infection. *Int J Infect Dis*. 2009;13(3):327-333.
5. Bross-Soriano D, Arrieta-Gómez JR, Prado-Calleros H, Schimelmitz-Idi J, Jorba-Basave S. Management of Ludwig's angina with small neck incisions: 18 years experience. *Otolaryngol Head Neck Surg*. 2004;130(6):712-717.
6. Parhiscar A, Har-El G. Deep neck abscess: a retrospective review of 210 cases. *Annals Otol Rhinol Laryngol*. 2001;110(11):1051-1054.
7. Mathew GC, Ranganathan LK, Gandhi S, et al. Odontogenic maxillofacial space infections at a tertiary care center in North India: a five-year retrospective study. *Int J Infect Dis*. 2012;16(4):e296-e302.
8. Vieira F, Allen SM, Stocks RMS, Thompson JW. Deep neck infection. *Otolaryngol Clin North Am*. 2008;41(3):459-483.
9. Ma C, Zhou L, Zhao JZ, et al. Multidisciplinary treatment of deep neck infection associated with descending necrotizing mediastinitis: a single-centre experience. *J Int Med Res*. 2019;47(12):6027-6040.
10. Grisaru-Soen G, Komisar O, Aizenstein O, Soudack M, Schwartz D, Paret G. Retropharyngeal and parapharyngeal abscess in children—epidemiology, clinical features and treatment. *Int J Pediatr Otorhinolaryngol*. 2010;74(9):1016-1020.
11. Sichel JY, Dano I, Hocwald E, Biron A, Eliashar R. Nonsurgical management of parapharyngeal space infections: a prospective study. *Laryngoscope*. 2002;112(5):906-910.
12. Mayor GP, Millán JMS, Martínez-Vidal A. Is conservative treatment of deep neck space infections appropriate? *Head and Neck*. 2001;23(2):126-133.
13. Lawrence R, Bateman N. Controversies in the management of deep neck space infection in children: an evidence-based review. *Clin Otolaryngol*. 2017;42(1):156-163.
14. Neff SPW, Merry AF, Anderson B. Airway management in Ludwig's angina. *Anaesth Intensive Care*. 1999;27(6):659-661.
15. Bridwell R, Gottlieb M, Koyfman A, Long B. Diagnosis and management of Ludwig's angina: an evidence-based review. *Am J Emerg Med*. 2021;41:1-5.
16. Macdonnell SPJ, Timmins AC, Watson JD. Adrenaline administered via a nebulizer in adult patients with upper airway obstruction. *Anaesthesia*. 1995;50(1):35-36.
17. Malpas G, Hung O, Gilchrist A, et al. The use of extracorporeal membrane oxygenation in the anticipated difficult airway: a case report and systematic review. *Can J Anesthesia*. 2018;65(6):685-697.
18. Mosier JM, Joshi R, Hypes C, Pacheco G, Valenzuela T, Sakles JC. The physiologically difficult airway. *Western J Emerg Med*. 2015;16(7):1109-1117.
19. Souza FJF de B, Evangelista AR, Silva JV, Périco GV, Madeira K. Cervical computed tomography in patients with obstructive sleep apnea: influence of head elevation on the assessment of upper airway volume. *J Brasil Pneumol*. 2016;42(1):55-60.
20. Narendra PL, Vishal NS, Jenkins B. Ludwig's angina: need for including airways and larynx in ultrasound evaluation. *BMJ Case Rep*. 2014;2014:bcr2014206506.
21. Ho AMH, Chung DC, To EWH, Karmakar MK. Total airway obstruction during local anesthesia in a non-sedated patient with a compromised airway. *Can J Anesth*. 2004;51(8):838-841.
22. Potter JK, Herford AS, Ellis E. Tracheotomy versus endotracheal intubation for airway management in deep neck space infections. *J Oral Maxillofacial Surg*. 2002;60(4):349-354; discussion 354-355.
23. McGuire G, El-Beheiry H, Brown D. Loss of the airway during tracheostomy: rescue oxygenation and re-establishment of the airway. *Can J Anesth*. 2001;48(7):697-700.
24. Lodenius Å, Maddison KJ, Lawther BK, et al. Upper airway collapsibility during dexmedetomidine and propofol sedation in healthy volunteers: a nonblinded randomized crossover study. *Anesthesiology*. 2019;131(5):962-973.
25. Shaw IC, Welchew EA, Harrison BJ, Michael S. Complete airway obstruction during awake fibreoptic intubation. *Anaesthesia*. 1997;52(6):582-585.
26. McGuire G, El-Beheiry H. Complete upper airway obstruction during awake fibreoptic intubation in patients with unstable cervical spine fractures. *Can J Anesth*. 1999;46(2):176-178.
27. Mason RA, Fielder CP. The obstructed airway in head and neck surgery. *Anaesthesia*. 1999;54(7):625-628.
28. Pahl C, Yarrow S, Steventon N, Saeed NR, Dyar O. Angina bullosa haemorrhagica presenting as acute upper airway obstruction. *Br J Anaesth*. 2004;92(2):283-286.
29. Smith Charles E, Fallon WF. Sevoflurane mask anesthesia for urgent tracheostomy in an uncooperative trauma patient with a difficult airway. *Can J Anaesth*. 2000;47(3):242-245.
30. Neff SPW, Merry AF, Anderson B. Airway management in Ludwig's angina. *Anaesth Intensive Care*. 1999;27(3):659-661.
31. Weingart SD, Levitan RM. Preoxygenation and prevention of desaturation during emergency airway management. *Ann Emerg Med*. 2012;59(3):165-175.
32. Hall CEJ, Shutt LE. Nasotracheal intubation for head and neck surgery. *Anaesthesia*. 2003;58(3):249-256.
33. Boku A, Hanamoto H, Hirose Y, et al. Which nostril should be used for nasotracheal intubation: the right or left? A randomized clinical trial. *J Clin Anesth*. 2014;26(5):390-394.
34. Lenhardt R, Burkhart MT, Brock GN, Kanchi-Kandadai S, Sharma R, Akça O. Is video laryngoscope-assisted flexible tracheoscope intubation feasible for patients with predicted difficult airway? A prospective, randomized clinical trial. *Anesth Analg*. 2014;118(6):1259-1265.
35. Sharma D, Kim LJ, Ghodke B. Successful airway management with combined use of GlideScope® videolaryngoscope and fiberoptic bronchoscope in a patient with Cowden syndrome. *Anesthesiology*. 2010;113(1):253-255.
36. Poulton A, Hung D, Hung O. Combined video-laryngoscope and flexible bronchoscope intubation technique: a case report and systematic review. *Trends Anaesth Crit Care*. 2020;30:e56.
37. Sakles JC, Corn GJ, Hollinger P, Arcaris B, Patanwala AE, Mosier JM. The impact of a soiled airway on intubation success in the emergency department when using the GlideScope or the direct laryngoscope. *Acad Emerg Med*. 2017;24(5). doi:10.1111/acem.13160.
38. Brimacombe J, Berry A, van Duren P. Use of a size 2 LMA to relieve life-threatening hypoxia in an adult with quinsy [4]. *Anaesth Intensive Care*. 1993;21(4):475-476.
39. Ovassapian A, Tuncbilek M, Weitzel EK, Joshi CW. Airway management in adult patients with deep neck infections: a case series and review of the literature. *Anesth Analg*. 2005;100(2):585-589.
40. Jenkins K, Wong DT, Correa R. Management choices for the difficult airway by anesthesiologists in Canada. *Can J Anesth*. 2002;49(8):850-856.
41. McDonnough JA, Ladzekpo DA, Yi I, Bond WR, Ortega G, Kalejaiye AO. Epidemiology and resource utilization of Ludwig's angina ED visits in the United States 2006–2014. *Laryngoscope*. 2019;129(9):2041-2044.

SECTION 5

AIRWAY MANAGEMENT IN THE INTENSIVE CARE UNIT (ICU)

CHAPTER 30

Unique Airway Management Issues in the Intensive Care Unit

Nicola Jarvis and Matteo Parotto

CASE PRESENTATION

A 56-year-old male was the driver of a motorcycle involved in a motor vehicle crash. The primary survey performed by the trauma team reveals the patient to have a patent airway, with spontaneous breathing and clear, bilateral breath sounds. His circulation is normal with strong pulses present in all limbs and no signs of external hemorrhage. His Glasgow Coma Scale is 14 of 15 due to slight confusion. Secondary survey reveals rib fractures on the left and several orthopedic injuries including a broken tibia and femur on the left and a pelvic fracture. Several hours after the injury, the patient is brought to the operating room (OR) for surgical repair of the long bone fractures and external fixation stabilization of the pelvic fracture under general anesthesia.

He is admitted to the ICU immediately after the surgery, and is extubated uneventfully shortly thereafter. For the first 2 days after the injury, the patient requires high doses of opioids to control his pain from the rib fractures. Late in the evening of the third postoperative day, he spikes a temperature of 38.9°C, and is having trouble clearing his secretions with coughing. His respiratory rate is 32 per minute; his oxygen saturation is 92% on a non-rebreather face mask (NRB); his heart rate is 120 beats per minute; and his blood pressure is 160/85 mmHg. He is complaining of dyspnea and severe pain. The patient looks tired and has obvious use of accessory muscles of respiration. A chest radiograph reveals volume loss and airspace disease with air bronchograms in the right lower lobe but no pneumothorax.

The house staff is alerted by the patient's nurse. A first-year resident is on call with a senior fellow in critical care medicine (CCM). After their assessment and discussion with the attending staff by telephone, the house staff team proceeds with tracheal intubation. Based on the examination of the airway, no difficulties are anticipated with the tracheal intubation itself. The respiratory therapist prepares the usual equipment while oxygen is administered by NRB. The resident physician administers 2 mg of midazolam intravenously, and with the patient placed in semi-Fowler position at 45 degrees makes an attempt at intubation using direct laryngoscopy (DL) under the supervision of the senior fellow. The first attempt results in esophageal intubation. Oxygen saturation dips into the high 80s. After repositioning the patient's head and neck, and recovery of the saturation into the low 90s, this time employing a bag-mask unit with oxygen flow at 15 $L \cdot min^{-1}$, a second attempt is performed by the resident. Despite using a tracheal introducer (also known as "gum elastic bougie") and the backward upward right pressure (BURP) laryngeal maneuver, the attempt is again unsuccessful.

A third attempt at tracheal intubation under DL is made by the CCM fellow following the administration of propofol 100 mg and succinylcholine 120 mg, but this also fails. After this intubation attempt, it becomes more difficult to manually ventilate the patient using bag mask. It is unclear if this is because neuromuscular function has returned or if it is related to deteriorating lung compliance. The patient needed several boluses of vasopressor to treat hypotension during this last intubation attempt, probably related to high bag-mask ventilation (BMV) pressures coupled with the circulatory effect of the propofol. Recognizing the seriousness of the situation, the CCM fellow requests that some more airway equipment be made available in the event that they cannot secure the airway. The respiratory therapist reports that some of the difficult airway equipment is down the hall in a locked room, and that he needs to leave to acquire the items requested. None of the staff involved in the resuscitation are aware of what exactly is available on this cart, but clearly, not having it in the room from the beginning was an error in judgment.

The fellow now requests that the anesthesia team be called to assist with securing the airway. A video laryngoscope (VL) is brought from the OR by a senior anesthesia resident and is used to successfully intubate the trachea of the patient. VL reveals significant swelling of the supraglottic structures and vocal cords.

Those involved in the care of this patient recognized that this situation could have had a more negative outcome. A multidisciplinary meeting was scheduled to debrief and review options for improving their approach to airway management in the ICU employing a Root Cause Analysis (RCA) methodology and intended to implement systematic changes that are preventative in nature.

INTRODUCTION

Is Airway Management in the ICU Associated with More Complications Compared to the OR?

One of several important messages from the UK's 4th National Audit Project (NAP4) was that airway complications occurred more commonly in the ICU than the OR.[1] When adverse airway events did occur, they were more likely to result in death or serious neurological injury (61%) compared to adverse airway events in the OR (14%). Chacko et al. reported on critical incidents in a closed 18-bed, multidisciplinary unit over a 33-month period.[2] Airway-related incidents accounted for 32.8% of all reported incidents, with the most common being accidental extubation. In this study, there were 32 incidents (11.4% of those reported) that led to adverse outcomes, including four deaths, all of which were due to airway-related events.

Not only are airway events more common, but emergency intubations are more likely to result in adverse cardiovascular and respiratory outcomes. A recent international prospective study of 2964 patients from 197 sites across five continents that looked at emergency intubations performed outside the OR (INTUBE study) found that major adverse events peri-intubation occurred in 45.2% of cases. Cardiovascular instability was observed in 42.6% of all patients undergoing emergency intubation, severe hypoxemia in 9.3%, and cardiac arrest in 3.1%.[3]

When comparing intubation outcomes of patients who had been intubated both in ICU and the OR, the ICU attempts had a higher rate of poor glottic visualization, lower first-pass intubation success, and were associated with more complications such as hypoxemia, hypotension, and esophageal intubation than those in the OR.[4] This would suggest that more is at play than simply the patient's airway anatomy.

Needham et al.[5] reported on factors that contributed to airway events that had been collected as part of the Intensive Care Unit Safety and Reporting System, a voluntary anonymous reporting system developed in conjunction with the Society of Critical Care Medicine and used in 18 ICUs across the United States over a 12-month period. There were 841 incidents reported with 78 airway events. More than half of the airway events were considered preventable and about 20% of the patients with airway reports sustained a physical injury and had an actual or anticipated prolonged hospital length of stay associated with the event. They noted that factors for improvement that might reduce adverse outcomes included adequate ICU staffing and the use of skilled assistants.

Equally, from the NAP4 data, there were strong signals that higher rates of out-of-hours intubations and less-experienced operators performing the intubations may have contributed to the worse outcomes.[1]

In reality, a multitude of factors are likely to contribute to the poorer outcomes in ICU patients, namely, factors related to the patient population, those related to the staff, and those related to the intensive care environment itself.[6]

Why Is the ICU Patient More Likely to Experience Adverse Events in the Peri-Intubation Period?

Patients requiring intubation in ICU are often severely compromised in more than one organ system and have limited physiological reserve. In some, the primary indication for intubation will be cardiac arrest or hemodynamic instability, and this is a particularly vulnerable group. Unsurprisingly, the incidence of cardiac arrest in the ICU setting is as high as 2% to 3%, much higher than the 0.068% rate in the operating room.[7] Cardiovascular instability will be worsened by the induction of anesthesia even with cautious use of induction drugs. It often requires the delegation of medication and hemodynamic management to an experienced physician while others attend to the airway.

In other patients, respiratory compromise may be the indication for intubation, and thus patients undergoing ICU intubation may already have been subjected to optimization attempts such as supplemental oxygen delivery, BiPAP (via mask or more recently, helmet), and position changes. Denitrogenation prior to induction therefore may not offer the usual "apneic buffer" present in the nonemergency setting.

Other patient complexities that contribute to difficult intubation include the need for *re*intubation, which inherently has greater risks associated, even in the absence of airway changes. Furthermore, the pathology that has led to the patient's ICU admission may also make airway visualization more challenging, such as massive transfusion, anaphylaxis, and associated airway swelling.

How Does Staffing in the ICU Add to the Difficulties in Airway Management?

Commonly, tracheal intubations in the ICU are performed outside of regular working hours when more experienced help may be harder to summon,[8] which is "context sensitive." This is often when more junior staff and fewer people are available. De Jong et al. developed and then validated the MACOCHA tool to assess risk of difficult intubation and serious adverse events for patients facing intubation in the ICU.[9] One of the risk factors for adverse events and difficult intubation was found to be the absence of an anesthesiologist, and so this has been incorporated into the risk score.

During the COVID-19 pandemic, an emphasis was placed on minimizing the number of intubation attempts in an effort to reduce risk to patients and health care workers. Subsequently, airway interest groups endorsed intubation being performed by experienced airway practitioners. In some observational trials, this care package (typically in conjunction with high use of VL) resulted in higher rates of first-pass intubation success,[10] than other recent studies of intubations performed outside the OR and where less experienced airway practitioners were more likely to perform the intubation, in association with lower rates of VL use.[3]

What Are the Environmental Factors Affecting Intubation Management in the ICU?

Even when the airway practitioner managing intubation has much experience and can manage straightforward airways, it is when difficulties are encountered, and intubation plan B (and C and D) need to come into effect, that the problems with the intubation environment become obvious. Equipment may differ, both in content and layout, from that available elsewhere in the hospital, or in other environments the team may have worked. The delay in accessing equipment can take up precious time as oxygen levels fall, pushing the patient further toward their physiological limits.

AIRWAY MANAGEMENT IN THE ICU

How Can We Address the Patient's Poor Physiologic Reserve to Reduce the Risk of Peri-Intubation Events?

Denitrogenation is more difficult in the critically ill patient population, making oxygen desaturation during airway management a common adverse event. Oxygen desaturation is associated with serious complications such as cardiovascular collapse, global hypoxia-related brady-asystolic arrest, dysrhythmias, neurologic injury, or death. There are important physiological reasons for such limited respiratory reserve:

- Increased oxygen consumption in the critically ill patient leads to reduced safe apnea time, and an increased alveolar-arterial gradient makes the saturation of hemoglobin less efficient with a given functional residual capacity.[11]
- This is compounded by an increased shunt fraction in some patients related to diffusion block (e.g., pulmonary edema) and reductions in FRC.
- Predictable reduction in FRC related to obesity, position (increased closing capacity), lung disease, etc., attenuates safe apnea time even further.

Several strategies may be employed in improving denitrogenation and prolonging the safe apnea period. These include[12]:

- Positioning the patient in a semirecumbent position
- Continuous nasal cannulae at 10 to 15 $L \cdot min^{-1}$
- Noninvasive ventilation if oxygen saturations are 90% or less, titrating peep to between 5 and 15 cm H_2O
- Use of a PEEP valve during BMV to augment the patient's tidal volume

Pre-emptive or continuing use of Transnasal Humidified Rapid-Insufflation Ventilatory Exchange (THRIVE)[13] (e.g., Optiflow®) should be considered. Simple high-flow nasal oxygenation does not assist with ventilation in apneic patients and therefore arterial carbon dioxide concentrations will rise at a predictable rate. However, the Optiflow system has been shown to provide some degree of ventilation, as measured by slower rise of carbon dioxide over time.

Denitrogenation should be provided for at least 3 minutes, situation acuity permitting. Delayed sequence intubation (DSI),[14] employing ketamine titration balancing continued patient ventilation with CNS obtundation, has been used successfully in critically ill patients to aid the denitrogenation process; however, recent data may suggest a higher risk of complications with this approach compared with either topical anesthesia without sedation or with RSI.[15]

Hypotension at the time of intubation is more common in critically ill patients and is associated with an increased mortality. Risk factors associated with an increase in postintubation hypotension are septic shock, renal failure, respiratory failure, and increased age.[16] Right ventricular failure is an especially difficult condition to manage should it pre-exist, or result from the acute respiratory event. Several strategies are useful in addressing this important complication; ensuring patent intravenous access, assessing the need for a fluid bolus prior to intubation (in the absence of pulmonary edema), having vasopressor therapy immediately available, and in some cases, pre-emptively administered as a bolus by continuous infusion prior to induction of anesthesia.

In addition to limited cardiopulmonary reserve, other important concerns, such as hepatic and renal dysfunction, a "full stomach" (e.g., patients on continuous tube feeding), and altered neurological function are also common in this patient population.

It is not uncommon in the ICU population for patients to be extubated and then need to be reintubated at a later time in their care. A prospective database of 1053 ICU intubations revealed that subsequent intubations have an even higher risk of complications compared to the first intubation.[17] This increase in complications occurred without there being a measurable increase in predicted technical difficulty. The main complications were hypotension and hypoxemia. This study highlights the importance of recognizing that these patients are at higher risk of these complications and the need to strive to avoid them with proper preparation.

Intensive care patients are as complex as the environment in which they are cared for. The airway practitioner tasked with airway management in this setting must be aware of these factors and make sound decisions, often very quickly, to improve patient outcomes.

What Are the Pharmacologic Considerations for Airway Management in the Critically Ill?

Several of the pharmacologic agents routinely used in an elective situation could be harmful to a critically ill patient with a limited reserve. A detailed discussion on the pharmacology of intubation can be found in Chapter 4. Much has been debated about the best pharmacologic approach to facilitate airway management in the critically ill. Some have endorsed the use of awake intubation in patients whose physiological derangements are so great that the use of usual anesthesia induction drugs, even in reduced doses, produces too great a risk.[18] However, skills to perform this and the standard of care are not necessarily held by all ICU practitioners, nor are trained staff available at the time of all emergency intubations. Subsequently, the more common question in the ICU will be: how can practitioners provide the best conditions for intubation with the least amount of risk?

The ideal induction agent should provide good conditions for tracheal intubation without adversely impacting the cardiac contractility or systemic vascular resistance. Historically, etomidate has been used as an induction agent in the hemodynamically fragile patient because it is thought to have a favorable hemodynamic response compared to propofol. The KEEP PACE trial examined the use of ketamine/propofol admixture versus etomidate in a heterogenous, critically ill population and found similar hemodynamic outcomes in both groups, and higher rates of adrenal insufficiency in the etomidate group in those patients tested for this complication.[19] This is consistent with the pre-existing concern that use of even a single bolus of etomidate is associated with adrenal insufficiency and increased mortality.[20] Although ketamine/propofol were not found to be superior to etomidate, the similar hemodynamic outcomes suggest it is a reasonable alternative to etomidate in the setting of an emergency intubation in the ICU.

Another pharmacological question that is raised is whether the use of neuromuscular blocking drugs (NMBDs) to facilitate endotracheal intubation improves success rates and reduces complication rates in the critically ill population, as has been demonstrated in Emergency Medicine.[21] One side of the debate argues that NMBD will improve first-attempt success, thus reducing complications associated with repeated attempts at intubation. The other side argues that proper personnel, training, and equipment may not be in place to handle an emergency complication if not able to ventilate and intubate. A Cochrane review examining the effects of avoidance or use of neuromuscular blocking agents found that avoidance was associated with greater difficulty with intubation, and risk of upper airway discomfort and trauma, though evidence quality in this review was considered only low to moderate.[23]

If NMBDs *are* used, the choice of a depolarizing option is associated with more rapid desaturation than nondepolarizing,[12] perhaps due to the increase in oxygen consumption secondary to muscle fasciculations. In addition, the potential risk of hyperkalemia with succinylcholine may indicate rocuronium as a preferable alternative.

Several factors other than pharmacologic agents may contribute to severe hemodynamic instability in the critically ill patient (e.g., institution of positive pressure ventilation [PPV], especially in the presence of hypovolemia). It is best to prepare for and expect hemodynamic instability associated with airway management in these patients regardless of the agents used by pre-emptively administering vasopressors by infusion or boluses depending on the situation. These recommendations were incorporated into guidelines for the emergency intubation of the critically ill patient.

What Can Be Done About the Staffing and Physical Environment in ICU to Affect Better Airway Outcomes?

Several approaches have been identified to improve the culture of safety and optimize the care of airway emergencies outside the operating room. Some institutions have organized a group of multidisciplinary experts to focus on improving safety and quality improvement with respect to airway management, such as one institution's so-called DART (Difficult Airway Response Team).[23] This approach focuses on safety monitoring, quality improvement, availability of equipment in key locations, an educational program, and a response team that is deployed in an anticipated or unanticipated difficult airway situation.

The COVID-19 pandemic saw a renewed focus on team-based intubation efforts. In an attempt to reduce adverse patient outcomes and minimize risk of aerosol-related transmission of disease to the practitioners involved, intubation teams were adopted internationally. Many teams instituted a protocolized approach to intubation management. Underlying themes in these protocols, endorsed by professional groups included: experienced airway practitioner to perform intubation, use of VL, use of drugs to facilitate rapid sequence induction or modified rapid sequence induction, preparation of vasopressors, use of a reproducible set of equipment, employing simulation opportunities to familiarize team members with protocols.[24,25]

Recommendations about the contents of a difficult airway trolley/cart for use outside of the OR are discussed in Chapter 63. Principles of organizing a difficult airway trolley/cart for ICU center on making available, in a structured way, advanced airway equipment that is familiar due to its use in other parts of the hospital. Equipment should include airway adjuncts to facilitate ventilation (e.g., extraglottic devices) and tracheal intubation (e.g., tracheal tube introducer [bougie]); alternatives to DL (VLs, intubating extraglottic devices); airway exchange catheters (AECs); and front-of-neck access (FONA) equipment to facilitate cricothyrotomy (the "scalpel and bougie" FONA is the technique of choice now endorsed by the Difficult Airway Society [DAS] and the Canadian Airway Focus Group [CAFG]).

Cook et al.[26] conducted a survey of practice in the United Kingdom to evaluate improvements since NAP4, and remaining gaps in practice in areas where recommendations had been made. Immediate access to a difficult airway trolley/cart was one of the areas of greatest compliance, and existed in 80% of respondents in the ICU. Just over 70% of difficult airway trolleys/carts matched those trolleys/carts present in other areas of the hospital. Lowest rates of departmental compliance surrounded the use of continuous capnography for all patients with tracheal tubes (68%) and all ICU staff trained to interpret capnography.[26] Ongoing audits regarding compliance to these recommendations is an important step in improving airway safety culture in the ICU.

Equipment for awake flexible bronchoscopic intubation should also be immediately available given its emergence as an alternative to asleep intubation in physiologically and anatomically challenging airways. See Chapter 3 for detailed discussion on how to perform an awake tracheal intubation.

Is There Any Advantage to the Use of Video Laryngoscopy in the Critical Care Unit?

Prior to the COVID-19 pandemic, there were strong arguments for the ready availability of VLs on all difficult intubation trolleys/carts, and accessibility to these VLs in all parts of the hospital where intubations occurred. The initial primary reason that VL was adopted for COVID-19 intubations was to increase the "mouth to mouth" distance between intubating practitioner and patient, and thus reducing risk of transmission of disease during the procedure of intubation. Other important benefits that the VL afforded were access to a laryngoscope that is often considered a "salvage" device, that is, it is normally used when intubation with a standard laryngoscope fails and thus using it as a first-line device may result in better first-pass intubation success.[27–30]

VL also affords the experienced airway practitioner a more effective means by which to supervise learning intubators, and allows for a "shared airway," where the whole team can visualize potential difficulties and more promptly assist. The use of hypercurved or hyperangulated VL blades (e.g., GlideScope AVL—Video-Laryngoscopy, Verathon Inc, Bothell, WA) can be reserved for the patient presenting with more difficult laryngoscopic anatomy to further aid in laryngeal visualization, recognizing that tube delivery can be slightly more challenging with their use.

OTHER CONSIDERATIONS

What Educational Techniques Could Be Employed to Facilitate Competency in the ICU Setting?

There are several components to learning how to manage an airway in a critically ill patient. Because these patients are at high risk of physiologic decompensation, it takes a skilled practitioner and team approach to immediately respond to a rapidly changing clinical situation. The trainee needs to become competent with technical skills and nontechnical skills. Some of the technical skills are denitrogenation, optimizing the patient's head and neck position, manual BMV, and endotracheal intubation. The nontechnical skills are related to situational awareness and crisis resource management. High-fidelity simulation may be an ideal environment for these skills to be taught in a nonthreatening environment for the learner without any risk to a real patient. Teaching and simulation training has been covered in Chapter 67 of this book.

Exposure to a cadaver training session has been shown to improve self-reported percent of glottis opening (POGO) scores by CCM fellows.[31] They were also able to report a 98% first-attempt success rate in the clinical setting following the session. In this report, the critical care training program used five surgical grade cadavers with a different clinical scenario at each station to demonstrate a variety of anatomical challenges (spontaneously breathing in need of BMV assistance, cervical spine collar in situ, beard, full teeth, emesis or blood obstructed view, etc.). Chapter 67 describes these models in detail.

Multidisciplinary in situ simulation could also be an important way to improve the quality and safety of airway management in the ICU. This exercise allows all team members, including nurses, respiratory therapists, and physician trainees to work together to improve their response to an airway management situation in the ICU. This type of simulation takes place in the actual clinical environment where team members use equipment and resources they have at hand in everyday practice. Wheeler et al.[32] described their experience with this type of simulation training and how it is useful in identifying gaps in knowledge, threats to patient safety, and improve teamwork behaviors.[33]

How Important is Troubleshooting the Complications of Tracheotomy to the ICU Physician?

NAP4 identified that 50% of the cases and 60% of the deaths in ICU involved complications of tracheotomy.[1] In ICU, planning should recognize that tracheostomy tube may inadvertently fall out. Tracheostomy tube displacement occurred most frequently in obese patients and during patient movement, during sedation holidays (e.g., sudden awakening and coughing or manually removing a tube), or during airway interventions (e.g., tracheal suction or nasogastric tube placement). Further, delayed diagnosis of displacement, in the absence of capnography was reported repeatedly in by NAP4, and it is not a new finding.[33]

What Is the Role for Waveform Capnography in the ICU?

It can be categorically recommended that *continuous* waveform capnography be employed in ICU for all intubated and ventilated patients. Further, capnography is now the standard of care for confirming correct tracheal placement of device, such as an endotracheal or tracheostomy tube, and emphasis is placed on the concept that a *flat trace* in the newly arrested patient means that the device is NOT in the trachea unless confirmed by flexible bronchoscopy.

NAP4 identified that the diagnosis of esophageal intubation was hampered by lack of capnography.[1] They further found that the misinterpretation of a flat capnograph when esophageal intubation occurred during cardiac arrest and attributed to circulatory arrest was incorrect. It has been recognized for many years that during cardiopulmonary resuscitation (CPR), capnography is not flat but indicates a low concentration of expired gas.[34,35]

How Should a Tracheal Tube Cuff Leak Be Approached in the Critically Ill Patient?

Endotracheal tube (ETT) cuff leaks can occur in the intubated patient. This can lead to problems with mechanical ventilation and loss of lower airway protection against aspiration of secretions or gastric contents. In the critically ill patient, ETT exchange can be risky because of apnea intolerance from high FiO_2, PEEP, or minute ventilation requirements, or in those with new or normally difficult airway anatomy. An important first step in troubleshooting a presumed cuff leak is to confirm that the cause of leak is indeed nonremediable: one critical care study documented that of 18 ETT exchanges for a putative cuff leak, in only seven cases was a defective tracheal tube cuff or pilot valve apparatus confirmed to be the source of the leak.[36] Other causes of apparent cuff leak include cephalad migration of the tube, cuff underinflation, inadvertent placement of an oro- or nasogastric tube through the glottis, or a mid-sized tracheal tube.[37] These findings suggest that before embarking on a potentially risky tube change, diagnostic maneuvers such as VL should be considered to confirm that the cuff of the ETT is appropriately located below the glottis. If indeed an ETT does need to be exchanged due to a leak or other reason, considerations must be given to where (e.g., in the ICU or OR), how (should an AEC be used for ETT exchange?), or will safety be maximized by conversion to tracheotomy (rather than risky ETT exchange?), and by whom this will most safely occur. In the high-risk patient, ETT exchange over an AEC is recommended. When used, a higher first-attempt success and lower complication rate has been shown when facilitated by VL rather than DL.[38]

How Should Tracheal Extubation Proceed in the Critically Ill Patient with a Difficult Airway?

Tracheal extubation should occur as soon as the patient is deemed ready with respect to gas exchange and has a level of consciousness sufficient to maintain upper airway patency, manage secretions, and protect the lower airway. Nonetheless, planned extubation is always elective and should occur only when conditions have been optimized and appropriate plans put in place.

If upper airway edema is suspected, additional evaluation of the larynx with nasopharyngoscopy, VL, or various cuff leak assessment maneuvers is recommended (see Chapter 31). Without a doubt, there is a significant incidence of failure of extubation in the critically ill population. Therefore, the extubation of the ICU patient must be accompanied by a viable plan for reintubation. The plan should include an assessment of the anticipated difficulty of tracheal re-intubation, together with an assurance that equipment and expertise for the reintubation is readily available. In addition, for the patient with suspected difficult airway anatomy (e.g., recently fused neck; suspected or known airway edema), consideration should be given to extubation over an 11- or 14-Fr Airway Exchange Catheter® (AEC, Cook Critical Care), to be used as a placeholder to facilitate re-intubation if needed. Thomas Mort studied 354 ICU and OR difficult airway patients who were extubated over an AEC.[38] Fifty-four patients who required reintubation over the AEC were compared with 36 patients in whom the AEC had already been removed. First-attempt success for reintubation over the AEC was 87%, in contrast to 14% without an AEC in-situ. Airway-related complications were also significantly less in the AEC group. For those reintubated over an AEC, in most cases, the failure of extubation occurred within 10 hours of the original extubation.[39]

SUMMARY

Critically ill patients needing airway interventions are at higher risk for life-threatening complications. They are more likely to experience hypoxemia and hypotension during the time of tracheal intubation. This is associated with an increased mortality and risk of serious anoxic injury. Specific clinical interventions can be used to minimize these complications. These include careful positioning, denitrogenation, preloading with an intravenous fluid bolus, and using vasopressor therapy when required.

With respect to the case presented at the beginning of the chapter, several measures at the institutional level could be implemented to improve the quality of care provided by their team. The organization could focus on improving the availability of equipment immediately available to the team in the ICU. Educational programs can be implemented to improve the basic skill level of the ICU staff and multidisciplinary team members, as were enacted in many centers at the start of the COVID-19 pandemic.

SELF-EVALUATION QUESTIONS

30.1. What are the two most common complications associated with intubation in the ICU patient?

A. Dental injury and mucosal laceration
B. Dysrhythmia and hypertension
C. Hypotension and hypoxemia
D. Cannot Ventilate, Cannot Intubate

30.2. All of the following are reasonable approaches to a quality improvement program that may improve outcomes associated with intubations in the ICU, EXCEPT:

A. Practicing in-situ multidisciplinary simulation
B. Difficult Airway Response Team (DART)
C. Reviewing what airway equipment is immediately available in the ICU
D. Limiting laryngoscopes models to direct laryngoscopes only

30.3. All of the following are reasons why hypoxemia/desaturation is more common during airway interventions in the critically ill patient, EXCEPT:

A. Increased oxygen may decrease their drive to breath
B. Decreased functional residual capacity (FRC)
C. Increased arterial—alveolar gradient
D. Increased oxygen consumption

REFERENCES

1. Cook TM, Woodall N, Harper J, Benger J, Fourth National Audit P. Major complications of airway management in the UK: results of the Fourth National Audit Project of the Royal College of Anaesthetists and the Difficult Airway Society. Part 2: Intensive care and emergency departments. *Br J Anaesth.* 2011;106(5):632-642.
2. Chacko J, Raju HR, Singh MK, Mishra RC. Critical incidents in a multidisciplinary intensive care unit. *Anaesth Intensive Care.* 2007;35(3):382-386.
3. Russotto V, Myatra SN, Laffey JG, et al. Intubation practices and adverse peri-intubation events in critically ill patients from 29 countries. *JAMA.* 2021;325(12):1164-1172.
4. Taboada M, Doldan P, Calvo A, et al. Comparison of tracheal intubation conditions in operating room and intensive care unit. *Anesthesiology.* 2018;129(2):321-328.
5. Needham DM, Thompson DA, Holzmueller CG, et al. A system factors analysis of airway events from the Intensive Care Unit Safety Reporting System (ICUSRS). *Crit Care Med.* 2004;32(11):2227-2233.
6. Mosier JM, Sakles JC, Law JA, Brown CA 3rd, Brindley PG. Tracheal intubation in the critically ill. where we came from and where we should go. *Am J Respir Crit Care Med.* 2020;201(7):775-788.
7. Olsson GL, Hallen B. Cardiac arrest during anaesthesia. A computer-aided study in 250,543 anaesthetics. *Acta Anaesth Scand.* 1988;32(8):653-664.
8. Boylan JF, Kavanagh BP. Emergency airway management: competence versus expertise? *Anesthesiology.* 2008;109(6):945-947.
9. De Jong A, Rolle A, Molinari N, et al. Cardiac arrest and mortality related to intubation procedure in critically ill adult patients: a multicenter cohort study. *Crit Care Med.* 2018;46(4):532-539.
10. Ahmad I, Jeyarajah J, Nair G, et al. A prospective, observational, cohort study of airway management of patients with COVID-19 by specialist tracheal intubation teams. *Can J Anaesth.* 2021;68(2):196-203.
11. Mosier JM, Hypes CD, Sakles JC. Understanding preoxygenation and apneic oxygenation during intubation in the critically ill. *Intensive Care Med.* 2017;43(2):226-228.
12. Weingart SD, Levitan RM. Preoxygenation and prevention of desaturation during emergency airway management. *Ann Emerg Med.* 2012;59(3):165-175.
13. Patel A, Nouraei SA. Transnasal Humidified Rapid-Insufflation Ventilatory Exchange (THRIVE): a physiological method of increasing apnoea time in patients with difficult airways. *Anaesthesia.* 2015;70(3):323-329.
14. Weingart SD. Preoxygenation, reoxygenation, and delayed sequence intubation in the emergency department. *J Emerg Med.* 2011;40(6):661-667.
15. Driver BE, Prekker ME, Reardon RF, et al. Success and complications of the ketamine-only intubation method in the emergency department. *J Emerg Med.* 2021;60(3):265-272.
16. Heffner AC, Swords DS, Nussbaum ML, Kline JA, Jones AE. Predictors of the complication of postintubation hypotension during emergency airway management. *J Crit Care.* 2012;27(6):587-593.
17. Elmer J, Lee S, Rittenberger JC, Dargin J, Winger D, Emlet L. Reintubation in critically ill patients: procedural complications and implications for care. *Crit Care.* 2015;19:12.
18. Lapinsky SE. Endotracheal intubation in the ICU. *Crit Care.* 2015;19:258.
19. Smischney NJ, Nicholson WT, Brown DR et al. Ketamine/propofol admixture vs etomidate for intubation in the critically ill: KEEP PACE Randomized clinical trial. *J Trauma Acute Care Surg.* 2019;87(4):883-891.
20. Albert SG, Ariyan S, Rather A. The effect of etomidate on adrenal function in critical illness: a systematic review. *Intensive Care Med.* 2011;37(6):901-910.
21. Walls RM, Brown CA 3rd, Bair AE, Pallin DJ, Investigators NI. Emergency airway management: a multi-center report of 8937 emergency department intubations. *J Emerg Med.* 2011;41(4):347-354.
22. Lundstrøm LH, Duez CHV, Nørskov AK, et al. Effects of avoidance or use of neuromuscular blocking agents on outcomes in tracheal intubation: a Cochrane systematic review. *Br J Anaesth.* 2018;120(6):1381-1393.
23. Mark LJ, Herzer KR, Cover R, et al. Difficult airway response team: a novel quality improvement program for managing hospital-wide airway emergencies. *Anesth Analg.* 2015;121(1):127-139.
24. Cook TM, El-Boghdadly K, McGuire B, McNarry AF, Patel A, Higgs A. Consensus guidelines for managing the airway in patients with COVID-19: guidelines from the Difficult Airway Society, the Association of Anaesthetists the Intensive Care Society, the Faculty of Intensive Care Medicine and the Royal College of Anaesthetists. *Anaesthesia.* 2020;75(6):785-799.
25. Brewster DJ, Chrimes N, Do TB, et al. Consensus statement: Safe Airway Society principles of airway management and tracheal intubation specific to the COVID-19 adult patient group. *Med J Aust.* 2020;212(10):472-481.
26. Cook TM, Woodall N, Frerk C. A national survey of the impact of NAP4 on airway management practice in United Kingdom hospitals: closing the safety gap in anaesthesia, intensive care and the emergency department. *Br J Anaesth.* 2016;117(2):182-190.
27. Hypes CD, Stolz U, Sakles JC, et al. Video laryngoscopy improves odds of first-attempt success at intubation in the intensive care unit. A propensity-matched analysis. *Ann Am Thorac Soc.* 2016;13(3):382-390.
28. Kory P, Guevarra K, Mathew JP, Hegde A, Mayo PH. The impact of video laryngoscopy use during urgent endotracheal intubation in the critically ill. *Anesth Analg.* 2013;117(1):144-149.
29. Noppens RR, Geimer S, Eisel N, David M, Piepho T. Endotracheal intubation using the C-MAC(R) video laryngoscope or the Macintosh laryngoscope: a prospective, comparative study in the ICU. *Crit Care.* 2012;16(3):R103.
30. Silverberg MJ, Li N, Acquah SO, Kory PD. Comparison of video laryngoscopy versus direct laryngoscopy during urgent endotracheal intubation: a randomized controlled trial. *Crit Care Med.* 2015;43(3):636-641.
31. Wise EM, Henao JP, Gomez H, Snyder J, Roolf P, Orebaugh SL. The impact of a cadaver-based airway lab on critical care fellows' direct laryngoscopy skills. *Anaesth Intensive Care.* 2015;43(2):224-229.
32. Wheeler DS, Geis G, Mack EH, LeMaster T, Patterson MD. High-reliability emergency response teams in the hospital: improving quality and safety using in situ simulation training. *BMJ Qual Saf.* 2013;22(6):507-514.
33. Thomas AN, McGrath BA. Patient safety incidents associated with airway devices in critical care: a review of reports to the UK National Patient Safety Agency. *Anaesthesia.* 2009;64(4):358-365.
34. Deakin CD, Morrison LJ, Morley PT, et al. Part 8: Advanced life support: 2010 International Consensus on Cardiopulmonary Resuscitation and Emergency Cardiovascular Care Science with Treatment Recommendations. *Resuscitation.* 2010;81(1):e93-e174.
35. Falk JL, Rackow EC, Weil MH. End-tidal carbon dioxide concentration during cardiopulmonary resuscitation. *New Engl J Med.* 1988;318(10):607-611.
36. Kearl RA, Hooper RG. Massive airway leaks: an analysis of the role of endotracheal tubes. *Crit Care Med.* 1993;21(4):518-521.
37. El-Orbany M, Salem MR. Endotracheal tube cuff leaks: causes, consequences, and management. *Anesth Analg.* 2013;117(2):428-434.
38. Mort TC, Braffett BH. Conventional versus video laryngoscopy for tracheal tube exchange: glottic visualization, success rates, complications, and rescue alternatives in the high-risk difficult airway patient. *Anesth Analg.* 2015;121(2):440-448.
39. Mort TC. Continuous airway access for the difficult extubation: the efficacy of the airway exchange catheter. *Anesth Analg.* 2007;105(5):1357-1362.

CHAPTER 31

Management of Extubation of a Patient with an "Impossible Airway" Following Cervical Spine Fusion

Jade Panzarasa and Michael J. Wong

CASE PRESENTATION

A 75-year-old man with ankylosing spondylitis and previous C2–T12 spinal fusion presented with a C4–C5 chance fracture after a fall (Figure 31.1). While neurologically intact, this unstable fracture required emergency fixation. He had a predicted difficult airway due to severe fixed kyphosis with his chin approximating his chest and was Mallampati IV on inspection. Awake orotracheal intubation using flexible bronchoscope was performed with difficulty due to marked cervical kyphosis but was successful after several attempts. Spinal stabilization surgery in prone position was uneventful. Postoperatively, he was transferred to the intensive care unit (ICU), intubated and sedated, to permit careful extubation planning.

EXTUBATION PLANNING

■ What Are the General Strategies for Optimizing Successful Extubation?

Because extubation failure is increasingly recognized as a cause of airway management-related morbidity and mortality, contemporary guidelines now address this critical component of airway management.[1–3] In general, tracheal extubation should be performed thoughtfully, intentionally, and electively, allowing for sufficient time to identify patients at risk of extubation failure and to make contingency plans accordingly. It is important to remember that the overarching goal during extubation is to ensure adequate oxygenation by any means necessary.

General strategies for approaching tracheal extubation are as follows:

1) Determining appropriateness for low-risk extubation. The degree of mechanical ventilatory support should be weaned as early as possible after the initial indication for intubation has resolved, when the patient is hemodynamically stable with metabolic derangements addressed. Oxygenation should be adequate with a minimized fraction of inspired oxygen. Additionally, the patient should be awake, cooperative, and have adequate return of strength with full reversal of neuromuscular blockade;
2) Denitrogenation for 3 to 5 minutes to optimize physiologic reserve and apnea tolerance;
3) Placements of a bite block to prevent occlusion of endotracheal tube (ETT) and possible resultant negative pressure pulmonary edema;
4) Suctioning of the oropharynx, ideally under direct visualization to minimize risk of trauma and exacerbation of airway edema; and,
5) Mitigating the risk of exaggerated laryngeal reflexes. Breath holding, coughing, bucking, and laryngospasm are all possible consequences of stimulating the airways during tracheal extubation. They all have the potential to exacerbate physiologic compromise from increased arterial blood pressure, bleeding from surgical sites, or obstruction of the airway. Strategies to minimize these reflexes should be considered, including the use of opioids, dexmedetomidine, and topical lidocaine via the ETT.[3,4]

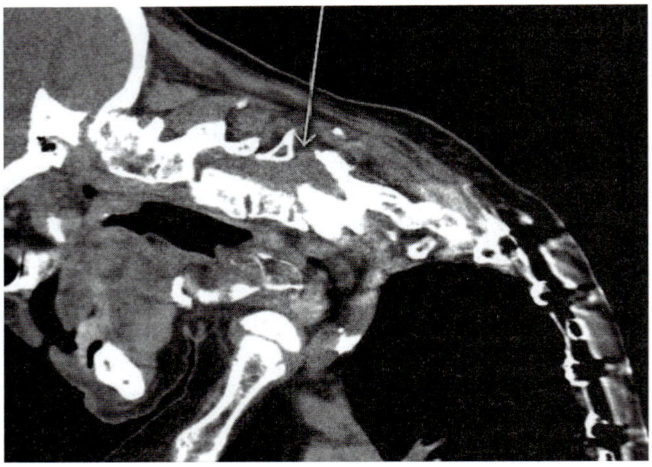

FIGURE 31.1. This computed tomography image of the patient shows a chance fracture at C4–C5 (arrow) and the anatomic distortion of the patient's spine due to ankylosing spondylitis and previous spinal fusion. The fixed position between the patient's jaw and chest can be seen here as a radiologic predictor of difficult airway.

What Is Failed Extubation?

Extubation failure occurs when the patient is unable to adequately maintain oxygenation, ventilation, airway patency, secretion clearance, or airway protection. Airway management after failed extubation poses a challenge that is fundamentally unique from the original intubation, resulting from multiple interacting factors that are both environmental in nature (e.g., unfamiliarity with the intubating setting, poor access to equipment and personnel, and underlying urgency) and changes in the patient's underlying physiology (e.g., hypoxemia, agitation, aspiration, airway edema, or hemodynamic instability).

Closed claims analysis has revealed significant morbidity associated with failed extubation, including hypoxic brain injury and death.[5] In the operating room and post-anesthesia care unit, extubation failure occurs in up to 0.45% of cases, while the rate of extubation failure is much higher (15%) in the critical care setting.[6–8] Critically ill patients are more likely to fail extubation compared to routine postoperative patients due to underlying pathology that may predispose them to impaired neurologic status, altered lung mechanics, and diminished strength.

What Is an At-Risk Extubation, and What Additional Strategies Are Considered?

The at-risk extubation refers to a situation where the ability to oxygenate or maintain a patent airway after the removal of the ETT is uncertain.[1] Such patients may be anticipated to either be physiologically intolerant to tracheal extubation or loss of mechanical ventilatory support, or they may have anatomical factors that make airway management difficult. Airway obstruction may contribute to extubation failure and has a myriad of contributing factors, such as tracheal or soft tissue collapse, airway edema, compressing neck hematoma, laryngospasm, or accumulation of respiratory secretions.[8]

In the at-risk extubation, additional measures should be undertaken prior to removal of the ETT. If there are reversible causes for anticipated difficult airway management (e.g., trauma, masses, bleeding, foreign body, or edema from anaphylaxis or thermal injury), then the cause must be eliminated, and the airway returned to its normal anatomic state before extubation. However, at times the underlying cause of airway difficulty may be irreversible (e.g., obesity, tracheomalacia, arthritis).

Further evaluation by flexible bronchoscopy through the in-situ ETT allows for assessment of blood or debris in the airway. Bronchoscopic visualization around the ETT can help identify upper airway edema, which has been implicated as the cause of extubation failure in approximately 15% of cases.[9,10]

The cuff-leak test is another method of assessing airway edema in high-risk patients and involves deflation of the ETT cuff while listening for an audible air leak or measuring the volume lost during each respiratory cycle (see Chapter 38 for more details about the cuff-leak test).[11] There is no established cut-off for quantitative cuff-leak testing, though a threshold of around 110 mL (in patients with mechanical ventilation) is often used in clinical practice.[12] Although the absence of a cuff leak (a failed cuff-leak test or a negative test) has a high specificity as a predictor for airway edema, both qualitative and quantitative approaches have low sensitivity for predicting postextubation airway obstruction, so close monitoring is still desirable after extubation. Additionally, a negative test (i.e., lack of cuff leak despite absence of laryngeal edema) carries the risk of prolonging extubation. In cases where an air leak is absent but the patient is otherwise ready for extubation, administration of systemic corticosteroids (i.e., methylprednisolone 20 mg) at least 4 hours prior to extubation attempt is a reasonable choice to potentially reduce airway edema and improve first-time extubation success.[13] Repeat cuff-leak testing after such administration of corticosteroids is not routinely required.

Additionally, consideration of extubation using an airway exchange catheter (AEC) may be advisible.[1–4] These devices are long hollow catheters with a distal side port that may permit some degree of emergency manual or jet ventilation, though this carries a high risk of barotrauma and is generally avoided.[1] AECs are placed through the ETT, which is then subsequently removed, creating a direct conduit to the trachea. An AEC can be temporarily left in place while assessing whether the patient can tolerate extubation, and it subsequently can facilitate reintubation by acting as a guide for ETT advancement.

What Is an Impossible Airway?

In recent years, there has been increasing awareness of a rare subset of patients for whom all four fundamental airway management techniques (i.e., face-mask ventilation [FMV], extraglottic airway placement, laryngoscopy, and front-of-neck access [FONA]) have a high risk of failure.[1,14,15] These patients may be considered as having a potentially "impossible airway."

Although by necessity, airway management in such cases was traditionally undertaken despite the high risk of failure, in recent decades, advancements in technology and availability of extracorporeal membrane oxygenation (ECMO) have begun to establish it as an additional contingency for maintaining oxygenation in such critical patients.

EXTRACORPOREAL MEMBRANE OXYGENATION (ECMO)

What Is ECMO?

ECMO is a form of life support used for decades in the setting of severe cardiac and/or respiratory dysfunction (Video 31).[16] In critical care, ECMO is traditionally employed as a bridge-to-recovery, or as a bridge-to-transplant when native heart or lung function is unlikely to improve. There are primarily two distinct configurations that may be chosen based on the underlying indication, namely venovenous (VV) or venoarterial (VA) ECMO. While the overarching goal for both modes is oxygen delivery and carbon dioxide elimination, VV-ECMO is principally used for severe respiratory failure, whereas VA-ECMO is used when hemodynamic support is required (e.g., cardiogenic shock).

The necessary components of an ECMO circuit include a drainage cannula to receive deoxygenated blood, a membrane lung (oxygenator), a blood pump, a blood warmer, and a return cannula to provide oxygenated and decarboxylated blood to the patient.[17,18] In VV-ECMO, the drainage cannula is usually placed in the right femoral vein, while the return cannula is usually inserted into the right internal jugular vein.[16–18] It is also possible to use one double-lumen (i.e., bicaval) cannula for VV-ECMO, rather than inserting two separate cannulas; placed into the right internal jugular vein, a bicaval cannula simultaneously drains both inferior and superior vena cavae via two separate ports while providing blood return through a middle port.

In VA-ECMO, venous drainage is again typically achieved through femoral vein cannulation.[17] The femoral artery is most commonly accessed for return cannula placement, with oxygenated blood directed retrogradely into the descending aorta. Alternatively, subclavian and axillary arteries may be suitable for a return cannula. It is worth noting that femoral artery cannulation may place patients at risk of ipsilateral limb ischemia, which may require surgical intervention.[19] To mitigate this risk, it is common practice to place a distal perfusion cannula at the time of primary cannulation.[20]

What Are the Contraindications to ECMO?

The contraindications to ECMO are generally relative in nature, balancing the risks of complications arising from ECMO support against the therapy's potential benefit.[16] Such relative contraindications include intolerance of systemic anticoagulation and poor vascular access. An important absolute contraindication is the presence of severe irreversible conditions incompatible with survival or quality of life (e.g., end-stage malignancy) (see Chapters 15 and 21). For VA-ECMO specifically, aortic dissection or severe aortic regurgitation are also absolute contraindications.

How Can ECMO Be Used to Support Management of the Difficult Airway?

Over the past decade, there has been increasing recognition of the "impossible airway,"[21] in which the four fundamental techniques of oxygenation (i.e., FMV, extraglottic airway device ventilation, tracheal intubation, or FONA) have a high risk of failure.[15] Some situations that might produce "impossible" airway include massive head and neck trauma, tracheal transection, upper airway anatomical obstruction, or massive hemoptysis.[14] While uncommon, the "impossible" airway presents a stressful clinical conundrum with potentially catastrophic patient outcomes. Thus, as ECMO therapy is increasingly employed worldwide over the past two decades,[22] so too has its use to aid in airway management.[23–25] As suggested by Malpas and colleagues in a systematic review of case reports, the planned use of ECMO as an adjunct for difficult airway management allows for indefinite maintenance of tissue oxygenation until a definitive airway may be secured in a controlled environment.[23]

More recently, there has been specific interest in the use of ECMO for certain patients deemed at risk during extubation.[15] Traditionally, practitioners have depended on a limited armamentarium to manage the at-risk extubation. For patients at risk of upper airway obstruction, established strategies include extubation to helium-oxygen (Heliox),[26] mask-delivered high-flow oxygen or continuous positive airway pressure, or extubation through an AEC.[27] Unfortunately, some series report a 13% failure rate of intubating over an AEC,[28] which is far from reassuring when other options are limited. While it is possible to provide rescue oxygenation via an AEC, this may be difficult to manage in practice, and there is risk of serious complications, including barotrauma and pneumothorax. The use of ECMO support provides predictable oxygenation and carbon dioxide elimination while contingency plans for extubation or definitive airway management may be put into place.

What Personnel and Resources Are Required for ECMO Cannulation?

ECMO is a resource-intensive form of life support, requiring not only specialized equipment but also an expert multidisciplinary team to manage the patient on ECMO.[21] These team members include cardiothoracic surgeons, perfusionists, intensivists, critical care nurses, and respiratory therapists. Additionally, the maintenance of ECMO relies on robust ancillary support, such as timely access to laboratory tests of coagulation, as well as blood products. Given these significant requirements, ECMO availability is limited to specialized centers, and early referral to such institutions is prudent if a patient is anticipated to have an "impossible" airway or if they are deemed likely to develop one.

What Are the Risks of ECMO?

The risk of airway loss in the at-risk extubation must be weighed against the potential of serious complications associated with ECMO therapy. As such, the choice to pursue ECMO as an aid to airway management must not be taken lightly.[16,29,30] Risks of ECMO include coagulopathy, hemorrhage, vascular injury, and air embolism.

Systemic anticoagulation is typically required during ECMO because the components of the ECMO circuit are foreign materials that readily activate the clotting cascade,[31] and thrombosis of the oxygenator or other circuit components may be catastrophic. Although there is increasing experience with the use of heparin-bonded circuits without systemic anticoagulation,[31,32] this practice is currently limited to patients unable to tolerate anticoagulation (e.g., refractory hemorrhage) and is not routinely recommended.[33] After decannulation, it is very common for patients on ECMO to have local thrombus formation at the sites of cannulation.[34]

Hemorrhage is a common complication of ECMO, owing to systemic anticoagulation and coagulopathy arising from ECMO therapy itself (e.g., acquired von Willebrand disorder, platelet consumption).[35] It is also possible for vascular injury to occur during cannulation itself, or with inadvertent ECMO cannula migration after placement. In VA-ECMO, cannulation of the femoral artery places patients at risk of critical limb ischemia, a risk that is at least partially mitigated with the use of a peripheral perfusion cannula.[20]

Other critical events may occur during ECMO, and the expertise of the ECMO team is essential to avoid morbidity and mortality.[36] Accidental decannulation is an ECMO emergency, which may lead to rapid exsanguination and massive air embolism. ECMO pump failure is another feared complication, requiring immediate repair or replacement while pump flow is maintained using a hand crank or backup pump. ECMO flow and/or oxygenation may also be impaired by suboptimal positioning of cannulas, kinking of cannulas or circuit tubing due to poor patient positioning, and elevated cardiac output greatly in excess of pump flows.

In long-term ECMO support, other common complications include renal failure requiring dialysis, nosocomial pneumonia, sepsis, hemolysis, hepatic dysfunction, and gastrointestinal bleeding.[29] However, some of these adverse outcomes are related to the underlying critical illness that necessitated ECMO therapy. It appears that brief ECMO cannulation to facilitate airway management has a relatively low risk of severe complications.[37]

What Cannula Configuration Is Appropriate to Support Airway Management?

Oxygenation may be maintained with VV-ECMO. As discussed above, the most common access sites for VV-ECMO are the femoral and internal jugular veins which, respectively, allow for drainage of deoxygenated blood from the inferior vena cava and for return of oxygenated blood to the superior vena cava. However, internal jugular vein cannulation may itself interfere with airway management, owing to the unwieldy nature of the circuit tubing at the patient's head. Additionally, some causes of difficult airway may inherently render internal jugular vein access technically challenging (e.g., large head and neck tumors, cervical spine fusion). In such instances, some authors advocate for bilateral femoral vein cannulation.[21]

How Is ECMO Cannulation Performed?

While some centers have sufficient resources and support to routinely allow for ECMO cannulation to occur routinely in the ICU,[38] in most instances, cannulation in the operating room is preferred for both the ECMO team and anesthesia practitioners. The operating room also tends to be a more conducive environment for establishment of a surgical airway when anatomical factors make this challenging. Discussions with all team members will be needed to determine which specific clinical area will be ideal for cannulation.

A Seldinger technique is usually sufficient for vascular access in both VV- and VA-ECMO, though cut-down is also an option depending on the surgical team's preference and patient anatomy.[16] A supine position is generally ideal for cannulation. Using real-time ultrasound visualization and sterile technique with full surgical drapes and gowns, guidewires are placed in the target vessels. Sequential dilatation is then performed along the guidewires to accommodate the desired cannula size, usually around 23 Fr. A bolus of intravenous heparin (50-100 $U{\cdot}kg^{-1}$) is given just prior to cannula placement. Cannula positioning is confirmed by transthoracic or transesophageal echocardiography or, less commonly, fluoroscopy prior to securely suturing the cannulas in place and initiating the ECMO pump. A minimal flow rate (e.g., 1 $L{\cdot}min^{-1}$) is required in order to prevent cannula and circuit thrombosis.

Due to recent postoperative status, some patients with "impossible" airway requiring extubation may be deeply sedated or under general anesthesia at the time of cannulation, while others may be already weaned to a minimal level of sedation after a longer period in the ICU. Using percutaneous techniques, ECMO cannulation may be performed with local anesthetic with or without sedation.[16] In some instances, sedation during cannulation may improve patient comfort and avoid forceful spontaneous respiration that might cause air embolism.

How Is Tracheal Extubation Performed After ECMO Cannulation Is Complete?

Safe and successful ECMO use in the setting of airway management depends on having adequate time for appropriate cannula placement. Cannulation often requires a half hour to accomplish, not including the time needed for the ECMO team to assemble and have equipment at hand, including a primed ECMO circuit. Although pre-emptive guidewire placement with "ECMO stand-by" for emergency cannulation is occasionally described,[39] this arrangement is not ideal. There may be unforeseen difficulties during vessel dilation or cannula advancement, and there can be little time to spare when faced with severe airway obstruction after failed extubation.

If ECMO is to be used seriously as part of the extubation strategy for the at-risk airway, cannulas should be inserted and secured prior to any airway manipulation, otherwise, there will not likely be enough time for ECMO initiation before risking permanent hypoxic neurologic injury. In existing guidelines, the operating room is suggested as the location for extubation of the at-risk airway[1] and this continues to be true when ECMO support is provided for backup. As with extubation of any at-risk airway, adjunctive strategies for extubation should be considered. This may include AECs, flexible bronchoscopes, extraglottic airway devices, Heliox, high-flow oxygen, and continuous positive airway pressure. Whereas cannulation is most effectively performed with the patient positioned supine, the semi-upright position is ideal for extubation, owing to improved diaphragmatic expansion and pulmonary toileting, increased functional residual capacity, and reduction of airway edema.[40]

How Can Oxygenation Be Maintained in the Event of Airway Loss?

With the ECMO cannulas in place and connected to the circuit, it is straightforward to continue oxygenation in the event of airway obstruction after extubation. The primary determinants of gas exchange on ECMO are the ECMO flow rate, the sweep gas flow, and the sweep gas FiO_2 (usually set to 100%). While the ECMO pump is operating, the team may proceed with the next steps for definitive airway management, which may include further medical optimization of reversible causes for airway obstruction, or FONA distal to the level of obstruction. Aside from the bulk of the circuit components, patients remain comfortable on ECMO support and have no specific sedation requirements.

When and How Should Decannulation Take Place?

If the patient is able to maintain airway patency with adequate oxygenation, the FiO_2 may be decreased and/or stopped. While there are few data to suggest an optimal time for decannulation, it is reasonable to discontinue the ECMO cannulas if there is no further concern for airway compromise after 24 hours. For VV-ECMO, decannulation by the cardiothoracic surgeon may be performed in the ICU at the bedside. While percutaneous closure devices are increasingly used in VA-ECMO decannulation, this procedure is generally still performed in the operating room. Because there is a high rate of cannula site thrombosis, it is recommended, regardless of ECMO duration or anticoagulation regimen, that patients undergo duplex ultrasonography after decannulation.[34] If there is evidence of cannula site thrombosis, patients usually require systemic anticoagulation until resolution of any such clots.

TRACHEAL EXTUBATION

The patient at the beginning of this chapter represented an at-risk extubation due to a combination of pre-existing and postoperative factors. Limited mouth opening and neck extension made FMV, extraglottic airway placement, DL, and VL challenging. Initial awake intubation with a flexible bronchoscope was difficult, in spite of good patient cooperation and prior to the development of potential airway edema postoperatively. Moreover, lack of access to the patient's anterior neck meant that emergency FONA was impossible to achieve; otolaryngology and cardiac surgery assessment concluded that positioning for tracheotomy was so limited that median sternotomy would be required to permit adequate surgical exposure. As such, in the event of failed extubation, there was potential that this patient's airway could render oxygenation and ventilation impossible.

Extubation, therefore, required careful planning to be carried out effectively and safely. Through a collaborative effort involving anesthesia practitioners, cardiac surgeons, perfusionists, intensivists, and otolaryngologists, it was decided that the tracheal extubation should take place in the operating room over an AEC with pre-emptive ECMO cannula placement to ensure ongoing oxygenation in case the airway became difficult to manage. Initiation of VV-ECMO via internal jugular and femoral vein cannulation would have been the preferred approach. However, cannulation would be technically challenging due to anatomical factors (i.e., limited access to neck vessels, bilateral femoral atherosclerotic plaques, presence of pacemaker leads in region of axillary vessels, and large body habitus. Due to these technical factors and equipment availability, the team opted to pursue VA-ECMO via unilateral femoral artery and vein, recognizing the higher risk of morbidity with VA-ECMO (e.g., limb ischemia, arterial injury) compared to VV-ECMO. Additionally, there was no specific need for hemodynamic support from VA-ECMO.

Optimal conditions for extubation were then established. The patient was brought to the operating room and placed in a semi-reclined position. The presence of a cuff leak was confirmed and nasopharyngoscopy was performed to exclude upper airway edema. Bronchoscopy then confirmed proper ETT tip positioning above the carina, allowing a lidocaine ointment-coated AEC to be subsequently placed through the ETT. Sedation was weaned. Spontaneous ventilation was confirmed, and oxygenation was adequate without requiring assistance from the ECMO circuit. The ETT was then carefully removed and the AEC left in place. This was well tolerated and the patient was able to breathe comfortably with satisfactory oxygen saturation. After 30 minutes of uneventful observation, the AEC was subsequently removed and the patient was brought back to the ICU. The patient underwent ECMO decannulation 24 hours later.

SUMMARY

Failed extubation is a dreaded complication associated with morbidity and mortality, so pre-emptive strategies are often undertaken to optimize the chance of successful tracheal extubation. Yet for certain patients, there remains an unacceptably high risk for subsequent failure of re-intubation, face-mask ventilation, extraglottic device placement, or front-of-neck access (i.e., the "impossible airway"). Because of anticipated difficulties when attempting these four fundamental methods of oxygenation, for such patients, it is prudent to consider pre-emptive extracorporeal membrane oxygenation (ECMO) cannulation to ensure adequate oxygen delivery in the event of extubation failure. ECMO support is resource-intensive and technically demanding, requiring an experienced specialist team and ancillary support; hence, this is undertaken in quaternary referral centers.

SELF-EVALUATION QUESTIONS

31.1. The "impossible airway" refers to a situation with anticipated difficulty in which methods of oxygenation?

A. Face-mask ventilation
B. Extraglottic device placement
C. Tracheal intubation
D. Front-of-neck access
E. All of the above

CHAPTER 31

31.2. Which of the following are possible complications of ECMO support?

A. Hemorrhage

B. Air embolism

C. Vascular injury

D. Thrombosis of cannula sites or circuit components

E. All of the above

31.3. Which of the following personnel or resources are usually required in order to use ECMO as an adjunct for oxygenation in the at-risk extubation?

A. Perfusionist to operate and troubleshoot ECMO pump

B. Cardiothoracic surgeon or other trained proceduralist to perform cannulation

C. Critical care nurse experienced in caring for patients on ECMO support

D. Point-of-care assays, or timely access to laboratory tests, for monitoring systemic anticoagulation

E. All of the above

REFERENCES

1. Law JA, Duggan LV, Asselin M, et al. Canadian Airway Focus Group updated consensus-based recommendations for management of the difficult airway: Part 2. Planning and implementing safe management of the patient with an anticipated difficult airway. *Can J Anesth*. 2021;68(9):1405-1436.
2. Apfelbaum JL, Hagberg CA, Connis RT, et al. 2022 American Society of Anesthesiologists practice guidelines for management of the difficult airway. *Anesthesiology*. 2021. doi:10.1097/aln.0000000000004002.
3. Difficult Airway Society Extubation Guidelines Group, Popat M, Mitchell V, et al. Difficult Airway Society guidelines for the management of tracheal extubation. *Anaesthesia*. 2012;67(3):318-340.
4. Parotto M, Cooper RM, Behringer EC. Extubation of the challenging or difficult airway. *Curr Anesthesiol Reports*. 2020;10(4):334-340.
5. Peterson GN, Domino KB, Caplan RA, Posner KL, Lee LA, Cheney FW. Management of the difficult airway: a closed claims analysis. *Anesthesiology*. 2005;103(1):33-39.
6. Frutos-Vivar F, Esteban A, Apezteguia C, et al. Outcome of reintubated patients after scheduled extubation. *J Crit Care*. 2011;26(5):502-509.
7. Thille AW, Harrois A, Schortgen F, Brun-Buisson C, Brochard L. Outcomes of extubation failure in medical intensive care unit patients. *Crit Care Med*. 2011;39(12):2612-2618.
8. Cavallone LF, Vannucci A. Extubation of the difficult airway and extubation failure. *Anesth Analg*. 2013;116(2):368-383.
9. Epstein SK, Ciubotaru RL. Independent effects of etiology of failure and time to reintubation on outcome for patients failing extubation. *Am J Resp Crit Care*. 1998;158(2):489-493.
10. Thille AW, Richard JCM, Brochard L. The decision to extubate in the intensive care unit. *Am J Resp Crit Care*. 2013;187(12):1294-1302.
11. Adderley RJ, Mullins GC. When to extubate the croup patient: the "leak" test. *Can J Anaesth*. 1987;34(3):304-306.
12. Kuriyama A, Jackson JL, Kamei J. Performance of the cuff leak test in adults in predicting post-extubation airway complications: a systematic review and meta-analysis. *Crit Care*. 2020;24(1):640.
13. Girard TD, Alhazzani W, Kress JP, et al. An Official American Thoracic Society/American College of Chest Physicians clinical practice guideline: liberation from mechanical ventilation in critically ill adults. Rehabilitation protocols, ventilator liberation protocols, and cuff leak tests. *Am J Resp Crit Care*. 2016;195(1):120-133.
14. Hung O, McAlpine J, Murphy M. Averting catastrophic outcomes: the fundamentals of "impossible" airways. *Can J Anaesth*. 2021:1-4.
15. Phipps SJ, Meisner JG, Watton DE, Malpas GA, Hung OR. The role of ECMO in the "at-risk" tracheal extubation. *A&A Pract*. 2018;12(2):41-43.
16. Extracorporeal Life Support Organization. ELSO guidelines for cardiopulmonary extracorporeal life support, version 1.4. 2017.
17. Kelly B, Carton E. Extended indications for extracorporeal membrane oxygenation in the operating room. *J Intensive Care Med*. 2020;35(1):24-33.
18. Quintel M, Bartlett RH, Grocott MPW, et al. Extracorporeal membrane oxygenation for respiratory failure. *Anesthesiology*. 2020;132(5):1257-1276.
19. Yau P, Xia Y, Shariff S, et al. Factors associated with ipsilateral limb ischemia in patients undergoing femoral cannulation extracorporeal membrane oxygenation. *Ann Vasc Surg*. 2019;54:60-65.
20. Ranney DN, Benrashid E, Meza JM, et al. Vascular complications and use of a distal perfusion cannula in femorally cannulated patients on extracorporeal membrane oxygenation. *ASAIO J*. 2018;64(3):328-333.
21. Yunoki K, Miyawaki I, Yamazaki K, Mima H. Extracorporeal membrane oxygenation-assisted airway management for difficult airways. *J Cardiothor Vasc An*. 2018;32(6):2721-2725.
22. Extracorporeal Life Support Organization. ECLS Registry Report. 2007.
23. Malpas G, Hung O, Gilchrist A, et al. The use of extracorporeal membrane oxygenation in the anticipated difficult airway: a case report and systematic review. *Can J Anesth*. 2018;65(6):685-697.
24. Karim AS, Son AY, Suen R, et al. Pre-intubation veno-venous extracorporeal oxygenation in patients at risk for respiratory decompensation. *J Extra Corpor Technol*. 2020;52(1):52-57.
25. Kim CW, Kim DH, Son BS, et al. The feasibility of extracorporeal membrane oxygenation in the variant airway problems. *Ann Thorac Cardiovas Surg*. 2015;21(6):517-522.
26. Ho AMH, Dion PW, Karmakar MK, Chung DC, Tay BA. Use of heliox in critical upper airway obstruction. Physical and physiologic considerations in choosing the optimal helium:oxygen mix. *Resuscitation*. 2002;52(3):297-300.
27. Duggan LV, Law JA, Murphy MF. Brief review: Supplementing oxygen through an airway exchange catheter: efficacy, complications, and recommendations. *Can J Anesth*. 2011;58(6):560.
28. McLean S, Lanam CR, Benedict W, Kirkpatrick N, Kheterpal S, Ramachandran SK. Airway exchange failure and complications with the use of the Cook Airway Exchange Catheter®. *Anesth Analg*. 2013;117(6):1325-1327.
29. Zangrillo A, Landoni G, Biondi-Zoccai G, et al. A meta-analysis of complications and mortality of extracorporeal membrane oxygenation. *Crit Care Resusc*. 2013;15(3):172-178.
30. Lafçı G, Budak AB, Yener AÜ, Cicek OF. Use of extracorporeal membrane oxygenation in adults. *Heart Lung Circ*. 2014;23(1):10-23.
31. Mazzeffi M. Patient blood management in adult extracorporeal membrane oxygenation patients. *Curr Anesthesiol Rep*. 2020;10(1):147-156.
32. Galvagno SM, Shah NG, Cornachione CR, Deatrick KB, Mazzeffi MA, Menaker J. Long term veno-venous extracorporeal life support without intravenous anticoagulation for diffuse alveolar hemorrhage. *Perfusion*. 2019;34(6):523-525.
33. Olson SR, Murphree CR, Zonies D, et al. Thrombosis and bleeding in extracorporeal membrane oxygenation (ECMO) without anticoagulation: a systematic review. *ASAIO J*. 2020;67(3):290-296.
34. Menaker J, Tabatabai A, Rector R, et al. Incidence of cannula-associated deep vein thrombosis after veno-venous extracorporeal membrane oxygenation. *ASAIO J*. 2017;63(5):588-591.
35. Sniderman J, Monagle P, Annich GM, MacLaren G. Hematologic concerns in extracorporeal membrane oxygenation. *Res Pract Thromb Haemost*. 2020;4(4):455-468.
36. Patel B, Arcaro M, Chatterjee S. Bedside troubleshooting during venovenous extracorporeal membrane oxygenation (ECMO). *J Thorac Dis*. 2019;11(Suppl 14):S1698-S1707.
37. Hong Y, Jo KW, Lyu J, et al. Use of venovenous extracorporeal membrane oxygenation in central airway obstruction to facilitate interventions leading to definitive airway security. *J Crit Care*. 2013;28(5):669-674.
38. Menaker J, Dolly K, Rector R, et al. The lung rescue unit—does a dedicated intensive care unit for venovenous extracorporeal membrane oxygenation improve survival to discharge? *J Trauma Acute Care*. 2017;83(3):438-442.
39. Padilla C, Conte AH, Ramzy D, et al. Utilization of "stand-by" extracorporeal membrane oxygenation in a high-risk parturient with methamphetamine-associated cardiomyopathy undergoing dilation and evacuation. *Case Reports*. 2017;8(5):105-108.
40. Karmarkar S, Varshney S. Tracheal extubation. *Continuing Educ Anaesth Critical Care Pain*. 2008;8(6):214-220.

CHAPTER 32

Airway Management of a Patient in a Halo Jacket with Acute Obstruction of a Reinforced Tracheal Tube

Dietrich Henzler

CASE PRESENTATION

A 52-year-old worker of normal body habitus was injured in a fall from approximately 15 feet (5 m) of height. He sustained fractures to the vertebral bodies of C3 and C4, and a C5 transverse process fracture. He was retrieved by an ambulance team and admitted to the hospital in a hemodynamically stable condition. His breathing on admission was noted to be "normal," albeit with decreased air entry to the right side. An infiltrate on chest X-ray was consistent with aspiration. Neurologically, the patient was awake and alert. He had evidence of a Brown-Sequard syndrome with an almost complete paralysis of his left limbs and a sensory deficit on his right.

The patient's neck had been placed in a rigid cervical collar at the scene and he was given oxygen via face mask. Tracheal intubation was performed uneventfully by awake flexible bronchoscopic intubation in the operating room (OR) for dorsal fixation of his C-spine. Completion of internal fixation by ventral stabilization was planned at a later date and in the interim, the patient was placed in a halo frame for external fixation (Figure 32.1). He was then transferred to the intensive care unit (ICU) intubated and ventilated, as his oxygen requirements had increased to 60%. An aspiration pneumonia was suspected and he was sedated and ventilated according to a lung-protective ventilation strategy.

Past medical history included hypertension, gastroesophageal reflux disorder (GERD), and a question of significant alcohol consumption.

By day 3 of his ICU admission, the pulmonary situation had improved marginally. He still required a FiO_2 of 0.45 and was breathing spontaneously with a pressure support of 12 cm H_2O and positive end-expiratory pressure (PEEP) of 10 cm H_2O. Attempts to wean the pressure support had failed at that point, resulting in tachypnea and oxygen desaturation. Thick purulent sputum was being suctioned from his endotracheal tube (ETT) twice per shift, and he was receiving empiric antibiotics to treat his presumed pneumonia.

Agitation had become a major issue, thought to be delirium tremens secondary to alcohol withdrawal. A cranial CT had ruled out posttraumatic intracerebral hemorrhage as underlying cause. The patient was difficult to manage, often requiring more than one nurse at the bedside, and he had tried to remove lines and ETT with his functioning hand. For this reason, he required passive restraints and sedation.

On day 4, the bedside nurse called urgently to report that the patient had bitten on the tube in severe agitation. To prevent kinking of the tube during surgery, the patient had been intubated with a wire-reinforced (armored) ETT, and had not undergone exchange to a regular ETT prior to transfer to the ICU. The reinforced ETT was now flattened at the level of the patient's teeth, causing acute obstruction by its significantly reduced inner diameter (Figure 32.2). The patient was being inadequately ventilated, with a drop of SpO_2 and minute ventilation, together with hemodynamic decompensation.

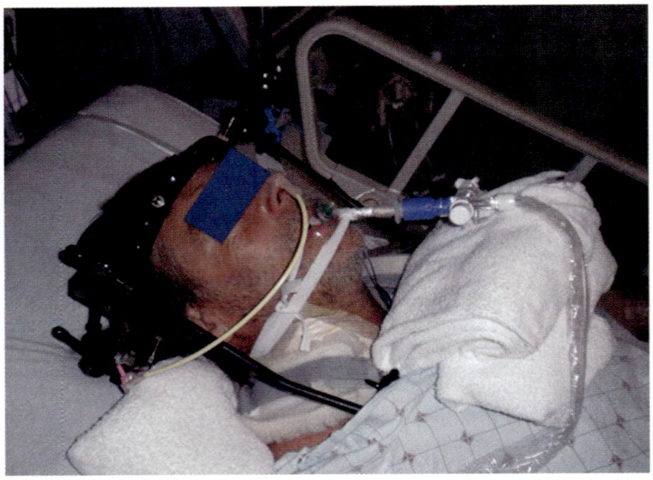

FIGURE 32.1. Patient with Halo frame for stabilization of cervical spine fractures.

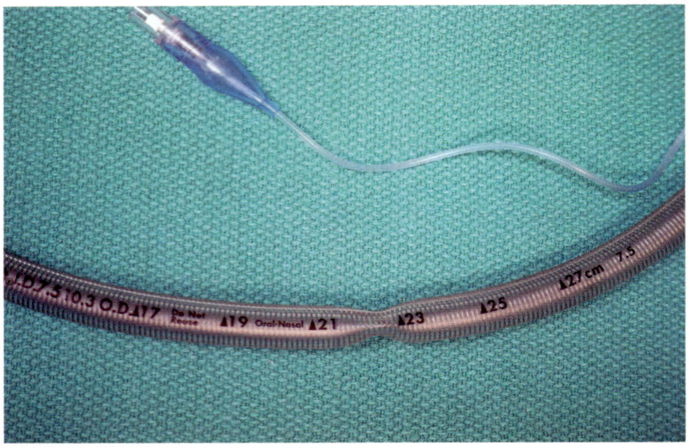

FIGURE 32.2. Reinforced tube with almost complete obstruction caused by biting on the metal armored part.

PATIENT CONSIDERATIONS

Medical Considerations

Is the Patient at Acute Risk of Suffering Harm?

Hemodynamics and gas exchange must be included in the assessment of the acute need for emergency treatment. While an SpO_2 of 87% is certainly abnormally low, it might not impose an acute danger to the patient in the short term. Two factors are important: whether the patient has organs at risk of hypoperfusion (and thus cellular hypoxia) and if sufficient oxygen-carrying capacity exists to compensate for a lower oxygen saturation.

Oxygen-carrying capacity (or oxygen delivery) depends on cardiac output, hemoglobin concentration, and hemoglobin oxygen saturation. The patient was slightly anemic (Hgb 110 $g{\cdot}dL^{-1}$), although with an increase in heart rate from 81 to 105 $beats{\cdot}min^{-1}$ following development of the tube obstruction, some compensation had occurred by increasing cardiac output to maintain oxygen delivery.

The patient was not known to have coronary artery or cerebrovascular disease; he had no specific risk factors and was thus unlikely to have hypoperfusion of vital organs. As such, a borderline SpO_2 could be tolerated for a short period of time.

On the other hand, acute obstruction of the artificial airway leads to severe dyspnea and increased respiratory effort. The patient is forced to increase respiratory drive thus generating more negative inspiratory pressure to maintain tidal volume. This can be quite dangerous for the risk of developing negative pressure pulmonary edema (NPPE). We can conclude that this patient needs urgent troubleshooting including an emergency ETT exchange to prevent further harm.

What Are the Management Options for This Situation?

In a prospective multi-center study involving 426 ICU patients, Boulain[1] reported that 57 episodes of self-extubation occurred in 46 patients (11%), and of the 46 patients, 18 did not require re-intubation after their first (or only) episode of self-extubation. Therefore, it is necessary to assess the patient's ability to breathe unassisted and determine the need for further ventilatory assistance. While it is possible that a subgroup of self-extubated patients not yet capable of completely breathing on their own may be amenable to noninvasive ventilation (NIV), this patient's halo frame precluded NIV due to technical constraints.

Indicators for the ability to ventilate include respiratory rate, the patient's work of breathing, and gas exchange. In this patient, an increase in heart and respiratory rate and the decrease in SpO_2, combined with clearly visible usage of accessory muscles of respiration indicated the need for further ventilatory support. His respiratory failure is likely multifactorial, including the aspiration pneumonia and compromised intercostal and diaphragmatic muscular function due to his high spinal cord injury. As the patient needs further ventilatory assistance, an ETT exchange is indicated.

Airway Considerations

What Should Be the Initial Management?

First, the patient should be placed on FiO_2 of 1.0 to improve oxygenation. This increased the SpO_2 to 91%, which helped to buy some time to adequately prepare for the procedure. Secondly, the respiratory drive has to be reduced to decrease the risk of NPPE. Therefore, sedation is increased and the patient received 10 mg of morphine IV. The inspiratory pressure from the ventilator has to be increased to overcome airway resistance. To help with expiration and prevent from dynamic hyperinflation, an artificial cuff leak was created by deflating the ETT cuff to the point of an audible leak during expiration. In this manner, some degree of minute ventilation was maintained, as not all of the delivered tidal volume escaped and the patient continued spontaneous breathing efforts.

Alternative approaches in the case of life-threatening hypoxemia should aim to temporarily restore oxygenation until a definitive airway can be placed. The existing ETT, if ineffective, can be removed and the patient's respiratory efforts assisted with face-mask ventilation (FMV). Ventilation can be improved by use of an oropharyngeal airway, if tolerated. However, in most cases, even with a leaky cuff, some ventilation can be maintained by hyperventilating with high flows and respiratory rate (>30 breaths per min), mimicking high-frequency ventilation.

The high-frequency oscillation (HFO) mode of ventilation can provide sufficient oxygenation even with a cuff leak. Indeed, during routine use of HFO, a cuff leak is sometimes purposefully used to improve ventilation. It is an ideal rescue maneuver in a situation where a patient's oxygen desaturates and cannot be ventilated by other means. This option could be considered before a leaky tube was removed. HFO would be the preferred technique in this situation if a patient had profound gas exchange impairment, such as ARDS, to be used until arrangements for safe ETT exchange were made.

There should always be alternatives at hand in case the first attempt to reintubate the patient fails following removal of the faulty ETT. These can follow the ASA algorithm for the difficult airway and might include, but are not confined to, smaller ETTs; alternatives to direct laryngoscopic (DL) intubation such as a video laryngoscope (VL) with a hyperangulated blade; an appropriately sized extraglottic device (EGD, ideally a second-generation EGD with a conduit for intubating); flexible bronchoscope and cricothyrotomy equipment. Additional expert help should be obtained: a difficult situation such as this can always be better managed with the support of further medical and nursing staff. Calling for additional expertise is not a sign of incompetence, but of professionalism!

How Might the Presence of a Halo Jacket Impact Airway Management?

The presence of a Halo Jacket can adversely impact all facets of airway management. In this case, the initial tracheal intubation was performed awake using a flexible bronchoscopic, and the DL view had not been assessed thereafter. The Halo Jacket fixes the head in a neutral position and prevents any flexion or extension of the neck (Figure 32.1). With attempted DL, it is likely that at best a Cormack/Lehane (C-L) grade 3 view will be achieved. Tracheal intubation is more likely to succeed with alternatives to DL, such as a flexible bronchoscope or a VL with a hyperangulated blade, although these can also fail in this scenario (see Chapters 10 and 11). Should intubation fail and the patient require oxygenation by positive pressure ventilation between attempts, FMV could also prove challenging due to limited motion of the cervical spine (see Chapter 8), and for the same reason, EGD insertion may be difficult. Finally, front-of-neck airway (FONA) is usually performed with the head extended, so this can also be expected to be somewhat more difficult in the patient with a Halo Jacket.

In this agitated and uncooperative patient, it is unlikely that application of topical airway anesthesia, light sedation, and "awake look" assessment (e.g., by VL) will be an option. However, deeper sedation carries the risk of respiratory depression and apnea. Alternative approaches must be considered.

What Other Risks Are Inherent in This Situation?

Enteral nutrition imposes an additional risk for aspiration while the airway is unprotected. Enteral feeds should be stopped immediately and the feeding tube suctioned to clear as much content as possible from the stomach.

An already agitated patient may well get more delirious if ventilatory support suddenly stops and hypoxemia develops. Sedation will also be needed to have the patient tolerate the tube exchange procedure. On the other hand, should reintubation fail during tube exchange, preservation of spontaneous ventilation will add a margin of safety. When practical, nonpharmacological ways of calming the patient ("talk-down" and reassurance with the help of additional staff) cannot be overestimated (although unlikely to help the patient described in this scenario). If needed, short-acting drugs, such as propofol, are preferred.

The stenosis of the armored tube poses a significant risk for inducing an NPPE by forced inhalation efforts against a closed airway. This risk is even more relevant in severe agitation where breathing efforts are massively increased.

The reasons for the patient's continuing need for mechanical ventilation are weakness and pneumonia. Weakness alone as a cause of respiratory failure could be treated by noninvasive ventilation (NIV). However, in this case, severe agitation is a contraindication to NIV and as previously suggested, the Halo Jacket will cause difficulty with its application. Pneumonia, on the other hand, causes edema, atelectasis, and ventilation-perfusion mismatch, resulting in hypoxemic respiratory failure. To aggravate the situation, the loss of PEEP due to the cuff leak will lead to even more atelectasis formation in unstable regions. Furthermore, functional residual capacity (FRC) will be reduced, increasing the patient's susceptibility to hypoxemia. As the combination of these factors increases, the risk of rapidly developing hypoxemia and tube exchange should not be deferred for long, and when done, should be performed with attention to maintaining patient oxygenation during the process.

Although a leak is clearly audible, other significant alterations of the airway should be anticipated. Mucosal swelling from inflammation and general edema, and displacement of tissue from the previous trauma may cause physical impediment to the placement of a new ETT or total obscuring of laryngeal inlet anatomy after the defective tube is removed.

AIRWAY MANAGEMENT PLAN

What Is the Best Strategy to Secure the Airway and Avoid Complications?

In evaluating the different options, one has to consider the following key points:

- How much time is there to act?
- What equipment is available?
- What technical skills are available?
- For the tube exchange, should spontaneous ventilation be maintained or ablated?

The first question has already been answered: even though the patient is temporarily stable, he will not tolerate the present situation for a prolonged period of time. The necessary equipment should be obtained immediately from a difficult airway cart and additional expertise. In an ICU airway emergency, the needed equipment is rarely available at the bedside.

Contents and location of the airway equipment cart within the ICU should be well known. If necessary, additional equipment should be obtained from the OR.

Which procedure to choose will depend partially on the skills and experience of the attending practitioner. While there is much to be said for using familiar techniques and equipment, if time permits, additional expertise can be obtained to perform a less familiar technique (e.g., tracheotomy), if indicated.

Preservation of spontaneous respiration during the tube exchange will provide the advantage of helping to maintain oxygenation for a short period of time should placement of the new ETT prove problematic after removal of the defective one. However, this patient is agitated, and will likely have to be deeply sedated for the procedure, putting him at risk of apnea. The downside of an unconscious, apneic patient (i.e., having to manage gas exchange, airway patency, and airway protection) would then occur without the upside of conditions optimized by a neuromuscular blocking agent. On the other hand, choosing to deliberately ablate spontaneous respirations with an induction dose of sedative/hypnotic and use of a neuromuscular blocking agent will provide optimal conditions for the tube exchange but should occur only with an appreciation of (and preparations for) the difficulty that may be encountered during the procedure.

What Options Exist for Exchanging the Endotracheal Tube?

As pointed out above, obstruction of the upper airway imposes a significant risk for the placement of a new endotracheal tube (ETT). With any procedure requiring complete removal of the ETT from the airway before placement of the new one, there is a chance that the new ETT might not pass into the trachea.[3] This could be caused by displacement, collapse, or swelling of tissue, which was previously held open by the ETT.

For the tube exchange, a few options exist. With appropriate preparation, the defective ETT can simply be removed and a new one placed. For this option, as discussed above, it must be appreciated that intubation by DL will most likely not succeed. Other options such as the lightwand or VL (e.g., GlideScope®) are more likely to succeed,[2] but (a) the equipment must be available and (b) the practitioner must be experienced in its use. Use of an airway exchange catheter would be judged preferably in many situations; however, in this case, the tube exchanger is likely not to pass through the stenotic ETT. Alternatively, if direct intubation of the trachea fails, a tracheal tube introducer (also known as "bougie") could be introduced first and the ETT be advanced over the introducer under indirect view using a VL.

If an experienced surgeon is immediately available, a surgical airway (FONA or tracheotomy) will result in an almost 100% success rate, although it is the most invasive option. The complication rate, including risk of significant bleeding, false cannula passage, pneumothorax, and infection, has been quoted to be as high as 12.5% in elective tracheotomy[5] and even higher in emergencies. However, surgical airway in this setting would help avoid the risks inherent in a difficult tube exchange, and might be considered if time permits and there is a high probability that the patient will go on to tracheotomy anyway in the coming days or weeks. Otherwise, it will be a fallback option should other techniques fail for technical or time-critical reasons.

Lastly, in a desperate situation, one could try to improve upper airway conditions by removing the Halo Jacket. The dorsal fixation has been done; thus, the risk of injuring the spinal cord by flexing of the neck is less than initially. However, it is unknown whether such maneuver would be safe, and, as explained before, there is no guarantee that intubating conditions will actually be improved. On the other hand, FMV with two hands technique would be easier without the Halo while the cervical spine could be stabilized manually by another person. Removal of the Halo would be appropriate only if all other options have failed and the patient is at risk of acute hypoxemic injury.[6]

To summarize the options:

- Plan A: Intubation with VL
- Plan B: Intubation of the trachea with a tracheal introducer and advance the ETT under VL view over the catheter
- Plan C: Use of an intubating laryngeal mask airway (LMA-Fastrach®)
- Rescue plan: Surgical airway, removal of halo frame.

What Medications Can Be Used to Facilitate the Procedure?

The use of sedation in the ICU has decreased to much lower levels in recent years. Very few patients will tolerate a tube exchange without increasing their sedation, unless awake, cooperative, and with well-topicalized upper airway. Compared to elective intubation in the OR, the emergency intubation of critically ill patients carries a much higher risk of complications, for example, postintubation hemodynamic instability, which is associated with a significant mortality.[4] Vasomotor insufficiency, impaired organ perfusion and microcirculation, an increased sympathetic tone, and lower oxygen delivery (a combination of anemia, hypoxemia, and low cardiac output) place these patients at high risk for profound hypotension, arrhythmia, and myocardial hypoperfusion, to name just the most vital consequences of short-term instability. Careful planning and the choice of drugs have a great impact on preventing hemodynamic instability. Although difficult to predict whether a patient will develop hemodynamic instability, it is important to have a plan in place to treat this early, before it becomes life-threatening. Generally, it is not the particular combination of drugs, but the way they are administered that has the greatest effect on preserving hemodynamic stability.

The choice of drugs should reflect the level of sedation desired, anticipated effects on hemodynamics, and their interactions with patient physiology. The ideal drug has a short duration of action, is metabolized independently from liver and kidney function, has minimal cardiodepressant or vasodilating effects, and can be easily titrated to the desired degree of sedation. Often, no single drug has all these attributes, so a combination of drugs may be necessary.

Propofol is a readily titratable agent, increasingly used for long-term sedation in the ICU. It has dose-dependent cardiodepressant and vasodilating effects.

Benzodiazepines have classically been used for sedation in the ICU but tend to have longer half-lives, a dependency on liver metabolism, and the risk of creating delirium. Short-acting benzodiazepines, such as midazolam, are preferred for procedural sedation.

Etomidate is an ultrashort-acting sedative with little effect on hemodynamics. Unfortunately, even a single dose can induce adrenocortical depression, although the clinical significance of this remains uncertain.

Ketamine has sedative and analgesic properties, while respiratory function and hemodynamic stability are preserved. In contrast to other hypnotic drugs, it causes a dissociative state in which patients tolerate uncomfortable or painful stimuli. Ketamine can cause hallucinations, which has led to substantially decreased use for many years. However, due to the increasingly recognized importance of hemodynamic stability, ketamine has experienced a revival in recent years.

Opioids are standard analgesics often used as adjuncts for procedures such as tracheal intubation. While potentially cardioprotective (by preventing tachycardia), in the context of a critically ill patient, they can cause hypotension by suppressing sympathetic drive.

Neuromuscular blocking agent may be used in conjunction with a sedative/hypnotic agent to optimize intubating conditions provided an airway assessment has been performed that suggests tracheal intubation will succeed, or that fallback options such as ventilation using a face mask or EGD will be possible should intubation attempts fail. With a hemiparesis of 72 hours' duration, succinylcholine should be avoided in this patient for the potential risk of life-threatening hyperkalemia.

PROCEDURE

What Preparations Were Made for the Tube Exchange?

Tube exchange using a VL with a hyperangulated blade was the chosen technique, as such an approach is the least invasive combined with a good success rate. A GlideScope was obtained within minutes from the OR for the purpose. The plan was determined as follows:

1. A second person skilled in airway management (e.g., anesthesia practitioner, respiratory therapist) was called to the bedside.
2. One additional nurse was called to assist with calming the patient, administering drugs, charting or calling for additional help if needed.
3. Tube feeds were confirmed off, and the stomach suctioned through the nasogastric tube. A rigid tonsil suction catheter connected by tubing to the wall suction outlet was placed close to the patient's head, who was placed in 30-degree head of bed elevation. The bed was moved away from the wall to increase working space.
4. A call was made to the OR to ensure that a surgeon would be immediately available if needed.
5. The following airway management supplies were gathered at the bedside: An adult-sized tracheal tube introducer; a complete conventional intubation kit with laryngoscopes and Macintosh 3 & 4 blades (lights checked), a GlideScope, a flexible bronchoscopy cart with monitors and optical stylet (e.g., C-MAC Video Stylet, KARL STORZ), ETTs sizes 7- to 9-mm ID; oropharyngeal and nasopharyngeal airways; Ambu® bag with oxygen reservoir and face masks of appropriate size; #4 and 5 LMA-Classic and intubating LMAs (LMA-Fastrach); xylocaine spray and gel; and an emergency cricothyrotomy kit. An 8.5-mm ID ETT was opened, styleted to an appropriate shape, and its outside lubricated with xylocaine gel.
6. The following drugs were prepared: propofol infusion, s-ketamine, midazolam, and rocuronium. An additional vasopressor was not deemed necessary as a norepinephrine infusion of 0.05 $\mu g{\cdot}kg^{-1}{\cdot}min^{-1}$ was already running to maintain an adequate mean arterial pressure.
7. It was confirmed that the patient's FiO_2 had already been increased to 1.0. Nasal prongs were applied to the patient, through which oxygen was administered at 15 $L{\cdot}min^{-1}$. The patient was informed about the upcoming procedure.

Airway Exchange Procedure

Before all equipment and additional staff could be present at the bedside, despite sedation, the patient deteriorated with severe agitation due to increased respiratory effort. The ETT had to be removed urgently. Assisted FMV was undertaken with a two-handed technique. Despite the use of an oropharyngeal airway, ventilation was not sufficient, caused by difficulties in handling of the face mask within the constraints of the halo frame.

A critical situation as this requires quick decisions. If spontaneous breathing is preserved, the patient might further agitate with the risk of gagging, regurgitation, aspiration, and laryngospasm. On the other hand, if going apneic with deep sedation and paralysis, there is a risk of severe hypoxemia if the airway is not established in time.

A decision was made to proceed with administration of induction doses of a hypnotic and neuromuscular blocking agent immediately, to optimize airway management conditions. Anesthesia and muscle relaxation were achieved with propofol 1.5 $mg{\cdot}kg^{-1}$ and 1.2 $mg{\cdot}kg^{-1}$ rocuronium (an increase in norepinephrine infusion was necessary to ensure hemodynamic stability). Because difficult FMV was encountered earlier, a #4 LMA-Classic was placed to provide acceptable ventilation and oxygenation. The LMA was then removed and the oropharynx was suctioned to remove secretions. Standing behind the patient's head, a second practitioner introduced the GlideScope into the oropharynx without resistance. However, the glottis could not be visualized easily since mouth opening was reduced due to the rigid fixation of the head. A new 8.5-mm ID ETT, loaded with an intubating stylet was then advanced under VL view. With a hyperangulated blade VL, it is important to preformat the ETT with the malleable intubation stylet with a similar curvature as the distal portion of laryngoscope blade (resembling the letter "J"), so the tip of the ETT can be adequately directed to glottic inlet. In this case, the styleted ETT was shaped to an excessive curvature and could not be advanced into the trachea without force. Because of the extreme angulation of the styleted ETT, the tip of the ETT was caught by the anterior aspect of the glottis and the ETT could not be brought in-line with the axis of the larynx. The procedure had to be aborted and a #4 LMA-Fastrach was inserted to facilitate ventilation.

After short consideration, the plan to use the LMA-Fastrach intubating tube was aborted for the need to change the tube to a high-volume low-pressure cuffed ETT with 8.5-mm ID afterward, which would be another airway exchange procedure in a risky situation.

Once the SpO_2 had reached 96% and would not increase further, the LMA-Fastrach was removed and secretions suctioned. The Storz C-MAC Video Stylet loaded with an 8.5-mm ID ETT connected to a monitor was used and precurved to follow the pharyngeal arch. Doing so, the special situation of decreased mouth opening and inability to flex the neck can be overcome without the disadvantages of a flexible bronchoscope that can easily be misguided by anatomical structures. One practitioner performed a jaw thrust while the second practitioner gently advanced the C-MAC Video Stylet from the retromolar space with guidance from the video display. The C-MAC Video Stylet has a deflectable tip, which is operated by a lever at the handle (see Chapter 11). The glottis was visualized without difficulty and the ETT passed through the glottis without impingement on soft tissue. One practitioner held the C-MAC Video Stylet in place, while the other advanced the ETT under videoscopic vision. The ETT cuff was inflated, and the C-MAC Video Stylet removed. The self-inflating resuscitator bag was connected and ventilation resumed. Correct ETT placement was confirmed by $ETCO_2$. The procedural time without ventilation was less than 20 seconds for each step, and the patient's oxygen saturation did not drop below 88% during the intubation. The patient was then reconnected to the mechanical ventilator and the SpO_2 increased to 98% soon after. A chest X-ray showed that the ETT tip was 4 cm above the carina, with no evidence of pneumothorax or atelectasis.

Considerations About the Use of Reinforced ETT in the ICU

Reinforced tubes are often used whenever kinking could be an issue, for example, this can occur during OR procedures when the head (and airway) is not accessible to the anesthesia practitioner, such as in neurosurgery or ENT surgery. Placing a patient in a prone or sitting position inherently poses a risk to the ETT, which can result in kinking and complete airway obstruction if the OR table or equipment is moved. In such cases, an armored tube would be an appropriate choice.

If extubation at the end of the procedure is not possible, and the patient has to be weaned off mechanical ventilation for a prolonged period of time, the reinforced tube is not the best choice, as demonstrated in this case. Formerly, reinforced tubes had been useful in nasal intubation, since it cannot be occluded by clenching of the teeth. However, the risk of bleeding from the septum and a higher incidence of sinusitis and pneumonia have led to completely discard nasal intubation in long-term ventilation. An alternative in patients ventilated only for a few hours may be the use of a bite block if orally intubated, such as an oropharyngeal airway. In any case, changing the ETT to a regular, nonarmored tube should be considered as soon as possible following surgery.

SUMMARY

An acutely obstructed ETT due to biting on the wire-reinforced component represents an indication for immediate tube exchange, since sufficient ventilation is often impossible and there is a great risk of developing NPPE. A careful, but timely plan is important to safely restore mechanical ventilation without causing additional harm to the patient.

In a difficult airway situation, such as fixation of the neck in a halo frame, an exit strategy (e.g., emergency surgical airway) should be in place. If time permits, additional staff and all equipment needed should be at the bedside before the procedure begins.

The procedure should not be completed without sedative/hypnotic and paralysis. If sedation alone is to be used, it should be titrated to achieve just the level needed to tolerate the procedure. Oversedation is associated with the risk of hemodynamic instability and complications.

When possible, ETT exchange in a patient with predictors of difficult airway management should be facilitated with an airway exchange catheter. Safety is further enhanced by indirect laryngoscopy using a VL during the exchange procedure, for example, to help avoid impingement of the tip of the ETT on laryngeal structures. After the exchange, correct tube placement should be confirmed by capnography, and intrathoracic complications excluded by chest X-ray.

SELF-EVALUATION QUESTIONS

32.1. Which of the following methods is NOT suitable for the exchange of an endotracheal tube in a patient with anticipated difficult airway, such as in a halo jacket?

A. Video laryngoscopy
B. Flexible bronchoscopic intubation
C. Direct laryngoscopy with a McCoy blade
D. Airway exchange catheter
E. Tracheotomy

32.2. A possible complication during an airway exchange is:

A. Massive bleeding
B. Increased abdominal pressure
C. Acute respiratory failure
D. Ventilator-associated pneumonia (VAP)
E. Acute airway obstruction

32.3. All of the following can be tried if the tracheal tube cannot be advanced over the tube exchanger through the glottis EXCEPT:

A. Counterclockwise rotation of the tube
B. Gentle pressure to force the tube through the glottis
C. Lubrication of the tip of the tube
D. Jaw thrust
E. Assist with video laryngoscopy

REFERENCES

1. Boulain T. Unplanned extubations in the adult intensive care unit: a prospective multicenter study. Association des Reanimateurs du Centre-Ouest. *Am J Respir Crit Care Med.* 1998;157(4 Pt 1):1131-1137.
2. Huang SJ, Lee CL, Wang PK, Lin PC, Lai HY. The use of the GlideScope® for tracheal intubation in patients with halo vest. *Acta Anaesthesiol Taiwan.* 2011;49(3):88-90.
3. McLean S, Lanam CR, Benedict W, Kirkpatrick N, Kheterpal S, Ramachandran SK. Airway exchange failure and complications with the use of the Cook Airway Exchange Catheter®: a single center cohort study of 1177 patients. *Anesth Analg.* 2013;117(6):1325-1327.
4. Mort TC. Tracheal tube exchange: feasibility of continuous glottic viewing with advanced laryngoscopy assistance. *Anesth Analg.* 2009;108:1228-1231.
5. Mort TC, Braffett BH. Conventional versus video laryngoscopy for tracheal tube exchange: glottic visualization, success rates, complications, and rescue alternatives in the high-risk difficult airway patient. *Anesth Analg.* 2015;121(2):440-448.
6. White AN, Wong DT, Goldstein CL, Wong J. Cervical spine overflexion in a halo orthosis contributes to complete upper airway obstruction during awake bronchoscopic intubation: a case report. *Can J Anaesth.* 2015;62(3):289-293.

CHAPTER 33

A Patient with Suspected or Known COVID-19: Oxygenation and Airway Management

Louise Ellard and David T. Wong

CASE PRESENTATION

Case 1: ICU Patient with Acute Respiratory Failure, Now Requiring Intubation

A previously well 55-year-old, 90 kg man presented to hospital 3 days earlier with fever, muscle aches, and mild respiratory symptoms. He spent the first 48 hours of his hospital stay in the ward before being admitted to intensive care with increasing oxygen requirements and progressive respiratory symptoms. Due to worsening oxygen saturation and fatigue, the intensive care team determined that he required intubation.

The intubation team was assembled, comprising a staff anesthesia practitioner, airway assistant, personal protective equipment (PPE) spotter, and the patient's bedside nurse in intensive care unit (ICU). The patient was moved to a negative pressure isolation room in the ICU for intubation.

The intubation team donned airborne level PPE, including a fit-tested respirator mask, goggles, face shield, full-length gown, and two pairs of gloves. An intubation pack for a male patient (including an 8.0-mm ID endotracheal tracheal [ETT], anesthesia mask, size 4 and 5 extraglottic airway devices [EGDs], Guedel and nasopharyngeal airways, and disposable hyperangulated blades for the video laryngoscope [VL]) was brought into the negative pressure room, which already had a prepared VL with a stand-alone monitor screen. Only the intubation team were present in the room, with the doors closed.

At the time of intubation, the patient had oxygen saturations of 92% on 10 L oxygen via a non-rebreathing mask. His BP was 150/75 and HR 110. An intravenous cannula and arterial line were both in-situ. Following adequate denitrogenation using a tight-fitting face mask and self-inflating bag, apneic oxygenation using humidified high-flow nasal oxygen (HFNO) was used due to the potential for severe hypoxemia. To reduce the risk of hypotension, intravenous fluids are administered at the time of induction and vasopressors are prepared. The chosen induction drugs were midazolam 2 mg, ketamine 150 mg, and rocuronium 100 mg. Cricoid pressure was applied, and the patient was intubated swiftly on the first attempt. The ETT cuff was inflated and the ICU ventilator connected, with in-line suction. Once the ETT position was confirmed with $ETCO_2$ and by observing equal chest movement, cricoid pressure was removed and lung protective ventilation commenced. The single-use airway equipment was immediately disposed of into a plastic bag along with the outer pair of gloves for the airway operator and assistant.

One at a time, the intubation team left the room, doffing their gown and gloves in the negative pressure room and entering the anteroom. Within the anteroom, after performing hand hygiene, the eye shield and goggles were removed. Hand hygiene was repeated and the respirator mask removed. Hand hygiene was performed again before leaving the room.

After completion of the room resting time, the patient was moved out of the negative pressure room and into a COVID-designated ICU bay. The negative pressure room was thoroughly cleaned and reset for the next intubation.

Case 2: Known/Suspected COVID Patient Coming to Operating Room (OR) for Emergency Surgery

A household contact of a patient with recently diagnosed COVID developed right iliac fossa pain and presented to the emergency department. A COVID swab was taken, the patient managed as suspected COVID, and admitted to the surgical ward for an appendectomy.

When the COVID-designated OR was available, the patient, who was wearing a surgical mask, was transported via a dedicated lift and pathway by staff wearing airborne level PPE, including a fit-tested respirator mask, face shield, full-length gown and gloves, directly into the operating theater. The COVID operating theater had been adjusted to be negative pressure relative to the set-up and ancillary rooms and contained minimal equipment. At the time of induction and intubation, only the anesthesia practitioner and anesthesia assistant were in the room—wearing airborne-level PPE. The theater was only accessible via the set-up and anesthesia rooms, with hoarding in place to prevent movement in or out of the theater via other doors.

The patient had a rapid sequence induction and the airway was secured with an ETT. Immediately after the ETT was secured, the airway equipment was safely disposed and the anesthesia practitioner and assistant removed their outer pair of contaminated gloves. After the aerosol settling time was complete, the remaining staff entered the room and surgical preparations were made.

After surgery, the surgical staff again left the OR and the doors were closed. When it was appropriate to do so, the patient was extubated. A surgical mask was placed under the oxygen mask and the patient recovered in the OR for approximately 30 minutes. Once the patient was clinically ready for discharge to the ward, ward staff retrieved the patient directly from the operating theater, again wearing appropriate PPE.

BACKGROUND INFORMATION ON CORONAVIRUS AND CORONAVIRUS DISEASE

What Causes Coronavirus Disease?

On December 31, 2019, the WHO China Country Office was informed of cases of pneumonia of unknown etiology (unknown cause) detected in Wuhan City, Hubei Province of China.[1] This enveloped RNA coronavirus was subsequently named by the World Health Organization (WHO) as Severe Acute Respiratory Syndrome Coronavirus 2 (SARS-CoV-2) with a resulting disease known as Coronavirus disease 2019 (COVID-19). A pandemic was declared on March 11, 2020 and has caused an enormous burden on worldwide health care systems. As of January 21, 2022, there have been over 340 million confirmed cases and 5.57 million deaths worldwide.[2]

How Is Coronavirus Disease Spread?

This highly contagious virus is spread via respiratory droplets (>5 μm in diameter)[3] and most likely through airborne transmission of smaller particles (<5 μm in diameter) which may remain airborne for prolonged periods of time.[4] Early in the pandemic, a high percentage of cases were seen in treating clinicians.[5,6]

What Clinical Features Are Typical?

The COVID-19 case fatality rate (global fatality rate approximately 1.6%)[2] is lower than for SARS[6] with clinical features lying on a spectrum from asymptomatic illness to acute hypoxic respiratory failure requiring admission to intensive care units. Fever, fatigue, muscle aches, and cough are common symptoms. Treatment is largely symptomatic, including oxygen therapy for hypoxemic patients with some specific pharmacological therapies introduced recently. Currently recommended pharmacological therapies include steroids such as dexamethasone, monoclonal antibodies including sotrovimab and tocilizumab, and antiviral agents such as remdesivir.[7] A worldwide vaccination program began in 2021, with over 9 billion doses administered as of early 2022.[2]

AIRWAY MANAGEMENT IN PATIENTS WITH COVID-19

What Methods Can Be Used to Avoid Intubation in Patients with COVID-19?

Some patients with COVID-19 will require intubation and mechanical ventilation due to acute hypoxic respiratory failure. However, methods to reduce the need for intubation including noninvasive ventilation and prone positioning can be considered, to reduce patient harm associated with prolonged intubation and potential harm to staff from the spread of the virus during the intubation itself.

HFNO can be considered in the management of acute hypoxic respiratory failure, although theoretical concerns exist surrounding the aerosolization of infectious particles[5,8] and the potential for harm due to delaying inevitable intubation.[9] Although some trials show an increase in droplet dispersion with increasing flow rates,[10] the extent to which HFNO is aerosol generating remains debated and uncertain. When used, the patient should be closely monitored for worsening respiratory status.[11,12] The addition of a standard surgical mask over a properly fitted HFNO device may reduce droplet dispersion from exhaled gas flow.[6,13,14] Use of HFNO in single airborne isolation rooms[12] with a preference for a negative pressure room is supported by the WHO Guidelines.[15]

The use of HFNO in hypoxic patients with COVID-19 needs to balance the benefits and risks to both patients and staff and airborne precaution PPE should be used.[14–17]

Personnel and PPE

What PPE Is Recommended When Caring for Patients with COVID-19?

PPE is the final barrier of a system to protect staff and other patients from COVID-19 transmission[4] alongside other important considerations including limiting visitors to hospitals, cohorting or isolation of patients with known or suspected COVID-19 and limiting personnel in the vicinity of patients with COVID-19. Cleaning regimes and appropriate disposal of equipment and waste management are also important.[4]

Droplet precautions aim to prevent droplet and contact transmission and airborne precautions prevent droplet, contact, and airborne transmission.[4] Airborne precautions should be used when any aerosol-generating procedure is performed in patients with COVID-19[3,9,12,18] or there is the potential for suspended aerosolized secretions.[4,19] In some countries, following outbreaks in health care workers, updated advice required the use of airborne PPE for all contact with COVID-19 patients[20,21] and aerosol-generating procedures in all patients, not just those who are COVID-positive, given the high asymptomatic carrier rate.[22]

Droplet and contact precautions include a surgical mask, face shield, gown, and gloves.[3] Airborne precautions include a fit-tested and fit-checked high-filtration mask, goggles or visor, long-sleeve fluid-repellent gown and gloves.[4] Hand hygiene must be meticulous before and after all procedures.[18] Eye protection using either a full-face shield or goggles is recommended, as inoculation of the conjunctival mucus membrane is a potential mode of transmission.[23] The use of double gloves[6,19,24,25] reduces wrist exposure and is associated with less contamination than single gloving.[26,27]

What Respiratory Protection Is Recommended?

Adequate airborne respiratory protection includes either a fit-tested respirator mask or a powered air-purifying respirator (PAPR). Respiratory protection masks include fit-tested N95, filtering facepiece (FFP) 2 or FFP 3 respirators. N95 masks can be worn for up to 4 hours if undamaged.[4]

The respirator mask should be individually fit tested,[3,4,14,23,28] and if achieving and maintaining a good fit cannot be guaranteed during the whole aerosol-generating procedure, PAPR is highly recommended.[23,29]

Powered air-purifying respirators have a hose attached to a high-efficiency particulate air (HEPA) filter. PAPRs provide eye, face, and neck protection and are generally more comfortable to wear and can be used if the user has facial hair.[20,25,30,31] Hooded models do not require fit testing and therefore eliminate poor respiratory fit concerns.[32] However, there are downsides, including expense, challenging communication, impossible auscultation,[32] and a higher risk of contamination during doffing.[20]

What Are the Recommendations for Donning and Doffing PPE?

Supervised donning and doffing[12,14,19] remains a critical step in avoiding cross-infection. This includes checking of proper PPE prior to entering the room and replacement of heavily soiled PPE components immediately following aerosol-generating procedures.

Doffing is the highest risk time for self-contamination[3,29,30] and should be considered a "critical moment" when nothing except communication relating to doffing itself should be discussed.[3] A buddy system and doffing checklist are useful[3,4,9,33] including the removal of respiratory protection last, in the anteroom or outside of the patient's room if an anteroom is not available. Complex PPE can result in contamination during doffing, which is a consideration when using items such as coveralls and PAPR.

How Can Staff Prepare?

Simulation-based training should be considered to evaluate OR set-ups and workflows, especially in-situ simulation in the actual clinical environment.[32] Simulation is also useful to allow staff to practice PPE donning and doffing.[12] It is also important to practice closed-loop communication and the use of simple instructions, as communication is hampered by all forms of respiratory protection.[9]

Airway Equipment

What Airway Equipment Is Recommended?

The suggested airway equipment is outlined in Table 33.1. Single-use airway equipment should be used wherever possible[6,9,12,25,32] and the use of a tracheal intubation pack,[9,12] or separate dedicated COVID airway cart can be considered[6] to ensure all necessary equipment is in the room at the time of the intubation attempt.

Immediate careful disposal of airway equipment including the face mask and laryngoscope into a plastic bag or dedicated tray is essential.[24,34,35] Pre-COVID practices including storage of used airway equipment on the anesthesia cart should be discouraged.[34] Following completion of the case/airway management, decontamination of surfaces and equipment and careful waste management is important.[9]

Equipment to help minimize aerosolization, including clamps and inline suction,[36] should be readily available and are discussed in further detail below. One recommended set-up for inline suction, viral filter and CO_2 detector is shown in Figure 33.1.

What Modifications Should Be Made to the Anesthesia Machine?

Anesthetic monitors/machines can be covered with plastic wrap to decrease the risk of contamination and facilitate decontamination.[23,32] A viral HEPA filter is placed between the face mask

TABLE 33.1. Suggested Specific Airway Equipment for COVID-19 Patients

- Single-use equipment wherever possible
- HFNO or low-flow nasal cannula for apneic oxygenation
- Anesthesia face mask
- Circle circuit, Mapleson circuit, or self-inflating bag
- In-line suction
- Clamp
- HEPA filters (between face mask and breathing circuit, and on the expiratory limb of the anesthesia machine)
- CO_2 detector
- Video laryngoscope with a stand-alone monitor screen
- Airway rescue equipment (Guedel airway, second-generation extraglottic airway, FONA kit)
- Induction drugs

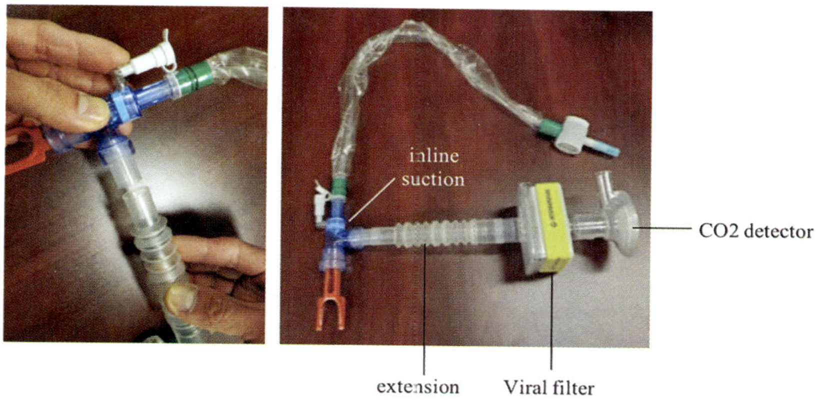

FIGURE 33.1. Suggested set-up of in-line suction, HEPA viral filter, and CO_2 detector. (Reproduced with permission from University of Toronto, Department of Anesthesiology and Pain Medicine. Protected Code Blue Guidelines.)

and breathing circuit[43] and on the expiratory limb of the circle circuit on the anesthesia machine.[30,32,33,35] Some organizations advise placing filters on both inspiratory and expiratory limbs to prevent the erroneous placement of a single filter.[12,14]

Are Barrier Enclosures Recommended?

Barrier enclosures systems such as "aerosol boxes" were largely motivated by a lack of available PPE[37] with the assumption that these systems would add to the protection for staff members. However, in a series of manikin/simulation studies, these enclosures have been shown to reduce the speed and ease of intubation,[38–41] provide a false sense of security,[35,37] and compromise PPE integrity.[35,37,40] The potential for secondary aerosolization also exists after barrier removal.[35,37] Although protective shields and barrier-enclosure systems were approved by the FDA under an emergency use authorization in May 2020, safety and performance concerns prompted revoking of this permit in August 2020.[25,42] Barrier enclosures are not recommended.

Location for Airway Management

What are the Room Requirements for Intubation of COVID Patients?

Aerosol-generating procedures in COVID-19 patients are ideally undertaken in a negative pressure room, to avoid the release of pathogens outside of the room, thus protecting other health care workers and patients.[4,9,11,32,43] A minimum of 12 air changes per hour is recommended.[6,9,11] An associated anteroom, with a separate entrance to don and doff PPE, is ideal.[6,20,43] If negative pressure rooms are not available, options include disabling positive pressure flow,[4,6] maximizing the number of air changes per hour to restrict aerosol dispersion outside the room[6,35] and use of a portable HEPA filter to remove small particulate matter from the air.[6,11]

What Operating Room Modifications Should Be Made?

Dedicated ORs for patients with COVID-19 should be used wherever possible, with restricted entry points.[23,24,32] Organizations can consider using dedicated hallways and patient transport routes for COVID-19 patients.[12] Recovery of patients following anesthesia could occur within the OR itself, to restrict contamination to a single location, rather than the use of a traditional postanesthetic care unit.[24,32]

Who Should Intubate and Be in the Room?

Intubation should be performed by the health care worker who is most experienced with airway management to minimize the duration and number of attempts and therefore the risk of transmission.[9,11,18,23,30,32,33] The number of health care workers participating in the intubation should be limited.[4,6,9,12,18] A team huddle prior to commencing airway management is useful to ensure all required equipment is in the room, avoiding the need for staff to leave and re-enter.[32] In some organizations, the establishment of a specific tracheal intubation team can be considered if the case load is sufficient.[9]

Risks to Personnel Associated with Airway Management

What Is an Aerosol Generating Procedure?

Many airway activities are considered to be aerosol-generating procedures including tracheal intubation, tracheotomy, extubation, face-mask ventilation, respiratory suctioning, and bronchoscopy.[9] Extraglottic airway placement and use is generally not included in lists of aerosol-generating procedures, however, it is logical to consider this as a potentially aerosol-generating procedure, and if the airway leak persists during ventilation, this risk may persist.[4]

Two recent studies aimed to address the evidence gap surrounding the generation of aerosols during airway management. Brown et al.[44] performed particle analysis in four ultraclean ventilation ORs and concluded that intubation was not an aerosol-generating procedure.[44] Dhillon et al.[45] also sought to answer this question and concluded that face-mask ventilation, tracheal tube insertion, and cuff inflation all generated small particles that remained suspended in airflows, with the largest particle count associated with positive pressure face-mask ventilation.[45] Given the absence of overwhelming evidence to the contrary, airway management should be considered to potentially generate aerosols and appropriate PPE should be used.

SECTION 5

What Risks Are Posed to Health Care Workers Involved in Airway Management?

Health care workers who contracted SARS in Toronto during the 2003 epidemic were more likely to have been involved in airway-related procedures such as tracheal intubation, noninvasive ventilation, tracheotomy, and manual ventilation before intubation.[18,46]

The voluntary self-reporting "intubate COVID" registry captured 1718 health care workers (HCW) performing 5148 intubation procedures on COVID-19 patients in 17 countries. The primary endpoint was found in 10.7% of reporters, including laboratory-confirmed COVID-19, admission to the hospital with COVID-19-related symptoms, or self-isolation due to COVID-19-related symptoms.[47] However, only 3.1% reported laboratory-confirmed COVID-19 infection. The majority (87.9%) of these intubators wore PPE conforming to WHO minimum standards for aerosol generating procedures.[47]

Names of all participating health care workers participating in airway management should be recorded to facilitate contact tracing if required.[30]

Preparation for Intubation

How Should Denitrogenation Be Performed?

In COVID-19 patients requiring intubation, hypoxemia is common prior to and during intubation.[19] Recommendations for oxygenation of COVID-19 patients are outlined in Table 33.2. HFNO for denitrogenation prior to intubation is generally discouraged[9,23,25,32,33,35,48] and instead a tight-sealing face mask, attached to a HEPA filter and a two-hand vice grip is suggested.[6,9,18,25,35] The rationale for this recommendation includes reduced effectiveness of HFNO when compared to traditional denitrogenation,[25,49,50] lack of an endpoint as ETO_2 cannot be measured with HFNO,[25,49] and the aforementioned concerns about viral dispersion and aerosolization with HFNO use.[25] When compared with the use of HFNO for the treatment of acute hypoxic respiratory failure, the use of HFNO for denitrogenation results in closer proximity of the treating clinician to the patient's airway.

Should Apneic Oxygenation Be Used?

When considering the best option for apneic oxygenation following the administration of muscle relaxants and prior to successful intubation, a variance of opinion appears in the literature. There is a preference for low-flow nasal oxygen[25,33,35] and if required due to hypoxemia, face-mask ventilation with a well-sealed face mask or placement of an extraglottic airway.[25]

TABLE 33.2. Recommendations for Peri-intubation Oxygenation of COVID-19 Patients

- Denitrogenation—preference for tight-sealing face mask, HEPA filter, with two-hand vice grip
- HFNO for denitrogenation prior to intubation is generally discouraged
- ETO_2 to confirm effectiveness (target > 90% if possible)

Apneic oxygenation

- Low-flow nasal oxygen
- Face-mask ventilation with a well-sealed face mask if necessary
- Placement of an extraglottic airway if necessary

Intubation

Which Induction Technique Is Recommended?

The use of checklists should be considered when performing tracheal intubation in COVID-19 patients to protocolize processes and aid preparedness.[9] Intubation steps and recommendations are outlined in Table 33.3.

A rapid sequence induction is recommended using rocuronium 1.2 $mg{\cdot}kg^{-1}$ or succinylcholine 1.5 $mg{\cdot}kg^{-1}$ to ensure full neuromuscular blockade before attempting tracheal

TABLE 33.3. Intubation of COVID-19 Patients

- Use of an intubation checklist
- Use disposable airway equipment
- Rapid sequence induction
- Rocuronium may be preferred to succinylcholine to avoid potential for paralysis to wear off
- Avoid face-mask ventilation of the patient where possible
- Consider avoidance of cricoid pressure in fasted/low-aspiration risk patients and remove if difficulty encountered with intubation
- Use a VL with a stand-alone monitor screen
- Inflate cuff prior to starting ventilation
- Confirm ETT position with $ETCO_2$ and bilateral chest movement (not auscultation)
- Monitor airway cuff pressure to avoid a leak
- Use an in-line suction system
- Minimize circuit disconnections
- Ensure HEPA filter attached to ETT

Suggested modification to awake intubation technique in patients with COVID-19

- Minimize the number of personnel in the room[59]
- Avoid HFNO[48]
- Use an antisialogogue[25]
- Use local anesthetic-impregnated swabs, cotton pledges, and nerve blocks instead of atomized local anesthetic or transtracheal local anesthesia infiltration[25,33,51]
- Consider an increased dose of remifentanil to obtund the coughing reflex[33,48,51]
- Use single-use bronchoscopes with a separate screen[6,25,33,35,51]
- Consider ATI with a VL[33,35]
- Use a smaller size ETT to reduce arytenoid impingement and subsequent coughing[6,33]
- Avoid the nasal route as it may have a particularly high viral particle load[25]
- Consider using an endoscopy mask to enclose the patient's mouth and nose during the procedure[25]

intubation.[9,32,33,35] Rocuronium may be preferred to succinylcholine to avoid the potential for paralysis to wear off and the patient to cough if intubation attempts are prolonged.[6,12,19] The use of ketamine as a sole induction agent may reduce the loss of sympathetic drive at induction.[30]

It is ideal to avoid face-mask ventilation of the patient[12,32] but if that is not possible, a tight mask seal and small tidal volumes (at low pressure) should be administered.[18,23,30,32] If the patient is adequately fasted and the risk of aspiration is deemed low, the use of cricoid pressure is discouraged, as it requires the assistant to lean closer to the patient's airway, increasing the chance of exposure to aerosols.[35] As always, cricoid pressure should be removed if it causes difficulty in ventilation or intubation.

Is Video Laryngoscopy Recommended?

The use of a video laryngoscope with a stand-alone monitor screen is strongly encouraged to increase the distance of the operator from the airway[9,12,19,30,32] and increase the chance of first-pass success.[9,11,19] Given that PPE can hamper vision during laryngoscopy,[19] the larger laryngeal view with VL could be beneficial to intubation success.[32] As for other airway equipment, a disposable device is preferred.[33] Removal of the tracheal introducer or stylet following intubation should be done with caution to avoid the spread of secretions.[6,9]

How Is ETT Position Confirmed?

Auscultation is difficult and not recommended whilst wearing PPE[12,35] as it can contaminate the stethoscope and operator.[6] Instead, continuous waveform capnography and observation of equal bilateral chest wall expansion is recommended to confirm ETT position.[9,20]

What Complications Are Commonly Seen Following Intubation of COVID-19 Patients?

Complications following intubation of COVID-19 patients may include hypoxemia, hypotension, pneumothorax, and even cardiac arrest.[19]

It should be noted that in addition to known anatomic predictors, physiological difficulty exists in many patients with COVID-19 as they may be hypoxemic, require urgent/emergency intubation and are at risk of hemodynamic instability during intubation.[25]

How Is Aerosolization Minimized in an Intubated Patient?

The cuff should be inflated to seal the airway prior to starting ventilation[9,12,32,35] and the airway cuff pressure should be monitored to avoid a leak.[9]

If tracheal suction is required, the use of an in-line suction system is recommended instead of open suction.[6,9,12,32,35] Although circuit disconnections should be minimized, if required ventilation should be paused, the ETT clamped, and the HME filter left in-situ.[9,32] Clamping the ETT can result in accidental damage to the tube and pilot balloon, therefore clamping close to the ETT connector over a gauze is suggested.[6]

Is Awake Intubation Discouraged?

The decision to proceed with an awake tracheal intubation (ATI) technique must be taken carefully, given the potential for significant aerosol generation.[19,23,32] Specific concerns with awake bronchoscopic intubation techniques include local anesthetic atomization that may aerosolize the virus[6,9,18,51] and patient coughing.

If an awake technique is used, the modifications in Table 33.3 are suggested. It is important to note that to date, cross infection of HCW has not been reported during ATI, therefore it should be utilized when a difficult airway is anticipated, especially when tracheal intubation after induction of anesthesia is considered unsafe.[14]

Relevance of Airway Algorithms/Guidelines in COVID-19 Patients

How Does the Management of COVID-19 Patients Differ from Published Airway Guidelines?

The principles of the various airway guidelines are applicable to a COVID-19 patient. The main difference is the added emphasis on the safety of health care workers and other patients. Strategies to minimize the risk of aerosolization and the spread of infection are paramount. Guidelines for airway management in COVID-19 patients[9] suggest the use of a standard failed tracheal intubation algorithm with a cognitive aid if difficulty arises, such as the Difficult Airway Society (DAS) guidelines,[52] the Canadian Airway Focus Group (CAFG) guidelines,[53,54] and the ASA guidelines.[55] If airway rescue is required after a failed intubation attempt, a 2nd generation extraglottic device (EGD) with an improved seal is recommended[9,35] and ideally one that also allows tracheal intubation.[6] Subsequent intubation attempts can be made through an intubating EGD using a flexible bronchoscope.[25]

What Technique Is Recommended If a "Can't Intubate Can't Oxygenate" (CICO) Is Encountered?

If front-of-neck access is required, most guidelines recommend a scalpel-bougie-tube technique or other surgical FONA to minimize aerosolization, rather than a cannula technique and transtracheal jet ventilation,[6,9,25,35] although the evidence surrounding this recommendation is not strong.

Tracheotomy Considerations

What Are the Specific Concerns with Performing Tracheostomy in COVID-19 Patients?

Using data from China during SARS, HCW who performed tracheotomies had 4.1 times greater odds of contracting the virus than controls who did not perform tracheotomy.[56] The national tracheotomy safety project outlines measures to reduce the risk associated with tracheotomies in patients with COVID-19.[57]

What Modifications Are Suggested for Tracheotomy Creation in Patients with COVID-19?

In addition to the general principles of aerosol reduction, specific modifications are suggested for the anesthesia practitioner assisting with tracheotomy in patients with COVID-19. It is ideal to have the most experienced operator perform the tracheotomy to minimize the total time that staff are exposed[58] and to delay tracheotomy until active COVID-19 disease is resolved if possible.[9,58] The patient should be adequately paralyzed[55] and ventilation ceased prior to tracheal incision.[48,56] The use of suction during the procedure[56] should be minimized.

Extubation Strategy

How Can the Risk of Aerosolization at the Time of Extubation Be Minimized?

Increasingly, it is considered that extubation results in more aerosols than intubation.[6,44] Some strategies to limit the risk at the time of extubation are outlined in Table 33.4.

Routine Management of Patients Presenting for Surgery During COVID

How Has Routine Anesthesia Management Been Affected by COVID?

During the course of the COVID-19 pandemic, in-person reviews have largely been replaced by telemedicine. This may lead to unanticipated airway difficulties that are not preempted prior to the day of surgery. Wherever possible, use of regional anesthesia over general anesthesia can avoid many of the concerns with airway management.[23,32] If general anesthesia is required, a lower threshold for intubation is suggested to allow controlled ventilation and avoid an airway leak.[9,30,32] Prophylactic antiemetics are recommended toward the end of the procedure to reduce the risk of vomiting and consequent viral spread.[6,32,35]

TABLE 33.4. Suggested Modification to Extubation Technique in Patients with COVID-19

- Remove unnecessary personnel from the room prior to extubation[6]
- Use airborne-level PPE for all personnel in the room[60]
- Extubate in a negative pressure room wherever possible[60]
- Use medications to minimize cough during emergence including dexmedetomidine, lidocaine (IV or intracuff) and opioids such as remifentanil[9,12,25,61–63] with dexmedetomidine having the highest cumulative likelihood to decrease cough.[63]
- Avoid use of airway exchange catheters[9,35]
- Consider changing an ETT to an extraglottic airway before emergence[9]
- Use low-flow oxygen in preference to high-flow nasal cannula[9]
- Place a standard surgical mask on the patient as soon as possible after extubation[9]
- Manage the patient in a head-up position, with the operator positioned behind the head of the patient[6]

SUMMARY

The COVID-19 pandemic has created an enormous burden on health systems around the world. There has been a large volume of literature describing safe airway management for patients to optimize outcomes and protect staff.

Many patients with COVID-19 will require intubation, either due to respiratory compromise or an intercurrent surgical problem requiring operative management. The established principles in existing airway algorithms and guidelines apply. Given the absence of evidence to the contrary, airway management should be considered as aerosol-generating, and therefore close attention to the safety of staff and other patients is paramount.

Airway practitioners should be using the highest available level of PPE. Denitrogenation is to be optimized using a tight-fitting face mask with FiO_2 of 1.0. Once denitrogenation is completed, induction drug and high-dose rocuronium should be given to ensure rapid paralysis for tracheal intubation. No face-mask ventilation should be performed unless oxygen saturation is prior to the establishment of muscle relaxation. A video laryngoscopy with hyperangulated blade should be used as the first-line instrument to optimize first-pass intubation success. For patients with a higher index of suspicion of a difficult airway, an awake intubation may be performed using airborne PPE precautions. Extubation is an aerosol-generating procedure and should be performed cautiously.

SELF-EVALUATION QUESTIONS

33.1. Which of the following is an important strategy to protect staff who are performing or assisting with airway management in patients with COVID-19?

A. Airway management should occur in a positive pressure room to remove aerosols from the room.

B. A minimal number of staff should be in the vicinity of the patient during airway management.

C. Droplet and contact precautions are advised for all aerosol-generating procedures.

D. All of the above.

33.2. Which precautions are suggested if an awake intubation is required in a patient with COVID-19?

A. Full PPE including airborne precautions should be used.

B. Atomization of local anesthetic is best avoided.

C. An antisialagogue is recommended.

D. All of the above.

33.3. Which of the following statements regarding peri-intubation oxygenation or ventilation of patients with COVID-19 is true?

A. High-flow nasal oxygen is the preferred strategy for denitrogenation of patients prior to intubation.

B. Apneic oxygenation is not recommended due to concerns about aerosolization and spread of infection.

C. Denitrogenation prior to intubation is ideally performed with a tight-fitting face mask and two-hand "vice" grip.

D. Face-mask ventilation following administration of muscle relaxants is recommended as many patients will experience hypoxemia.

REFERENCES

1. WHO. https://www.who.int/emergencies/disease-outbreak-news/item/2020-DON229. Accessed January 20, 2022.
2. WHO Coronavirus (COVID-19) dashboard. https://covid19.who.int. Accessed January 24, 2022.
3. Lockhart SL, Duggan LV, Wax RS, Saad S, Grocott HP. Personal protective equipment (PPE) for both anesthesiologists and other airway managers: principles and practice during the COVID-19 pandemic. *Can J Anaesth.* 2020;67(8):1005-1015.
4. Cook TM. Personal protective equipment during the coronavirus disease (COVID) 2019 pandemic – a narrative review. *Anaesthesia.* 2020;75(7):920-927.
5. Li J, Fink JB, Ehrmann S. High-flow nasal cannula for COVID-19 patients: low risk of bio-aerosol dispersion. *Eur Respir J.* 2020;55(5).
6. Thiruvenkatarajan V, Wong DT, Kothandan H, et al. Airway management in the operating room and interventional suites in known or suspected COVID-19 adult patients: a practical review. *Anesth Analg.* 2020;131(3):677-689.
7. Ontario COVID-19 Drugs and Biologics Clinical Practice Guidelines Working Group. Clinical practice guideline summary: recommended drugs and biologics in adult patients with COVID-19. Ontario COVID-19 Science Advisory Table. 2022; Version 9.0. https://covid19-sciencetable.ca/sciencebrief/clinical-practice-guideline-summary-recommended-drugs-and-biologics-in-adult-patients-with-covid-19-version-9-0/. Published Jan 21, 2022. Accessed January 24, 2022.
8. Agarwal A, Basmaji J, Muttalib F, et al. High-flow nasal cannula for acute hypoxemic respiratory failure in patients with COVID-19: systematic reviews of effectiveness and its risks of aerosolization, dispersion, and infection transmission. *Can J Anaesth.* 2020;67(9):1217-1248.
9. Cook TM, El-Boghdadly K, McGuire B, McNarry AF, Patel A, Higgs A. Consensus guidelines for managing the airway in patients with COVID-19: guidelines from the Difficult Airway Society, the Association of Anaesthetists the Intensive Care Society, the Faculty of Intensive Care Medicine and the Royal College of Anaesthetists. *Anaesthesia.* 2020;75(6):785-799.
10. Loh N, Tan Y, Taculod J, et al. The impact of high-flow nasal cannula (HFNC) on coughing distance: implications on its use during the novel coronavirus disease outbreak. *Can J Anaesth.* 2020;67(7):893-894.
11. Alhazzani W, Moller MH, et al. Surviving Sepsis Campaign: guidelines on the management of critically ill adults with Coronavirus Disease 2019 (COVID-19). *Intensive Care Med.* 2020;46(5):854-887.
12. Greenland JR, Michelow MD, Wang L, London MJ. COVID-19 Infection: implications for perioperative and critical care physicians. *Anesthesiology.* 2020;132(6):1346-1361.
13. Leonard S, Strasser W, Whittle JS, et al. Reducing aerosol dispersion by high flow therapy in COVID-19: high resolution computational fluid dynamics simulations of particle behavior during high velocity nasal insufflation with a simple surgical mask. *J Am Coll Emerg Physicians Open.* 2020;1(4):578-591.
14. Wei H, Jiang B, Behringer E, et al. Controversial topics regarding airway management in COVID-19 patients: updated information and international expert consensus recommendations. *Br J Anaesth.* 2020;126(2):361-366.
15. WHO. Clinical management of COVID-19. Interim guidance. https://www.who.int/publications/i/item/clinical-management-of-covid-19. World Health Organisation; 2020. Accessed on February 4, 2021.
16. Leung CCH, Joynt GM, Gomersall CD, et al. Comparison of high-flow nasal cannula versus oxygen face mask for environmental bacterial contamination in critically ill pneumonia patients: a randomized controlled crossover trial. *J Hosp Infect.* 2019;101(1):84-87.
17. Hui DS, Chow BK, Lo T, et al. Exhaled air dispersion during high-flow nasal cannula therapy versus CPAP via different masks. *Eur Respir J.* 2019;53(4).
18. Orser BA. Recommendations for endotracheal intubation of COVID-19 patients. *Anesth Analg.* 2020;130(5):1109-1110.
19. Yao W, Wang T, Jiang B, et al. Emergency tracheal intubation in 202 patients with COVID-19 in Wuhan, China: lessons learnt and international expert recommendations. *Br J Anaesth.* 2020;125(1):e28-e37.
20. Wax RS, Christian MD. Practical recommendations for critical care and anesthesiology teams caring for novel coronavirus (2019-nCoV) patients. *Can J Anaesth.* 2020;67(5):568-576.
21. Jin Y, Cai L, Cheng Z, et al. A rapid advice guideline for the diagnosis and treatment of 2019 novel coronavirus (2019-nCoV) infected pneumonia. *Mil Med Res.* 2020;7(4).
22. Jessop ZM, Dobbs TD, Ali SR, et al. Personal protective equipment for surgeons during COVID-19 pandemic: systematic review of availability, usage and rationing. *Br J Surg.* 2020;107(10):1262-1280.
23. Awad ME, Rumley JCL, Vazquez JA, Devine JG. Perioperative considerations in urgent surgical care of suspected and confirmed covid-19 orthopaedic patients: operating room protocols and recommendations in the current COVID-19 pandemic. *J Am Acad Orthop Surg.* 2020;28(11):451-463.
24. Dexter F, Parra MC, Brown JR, Loftus RW. Perioperative COVID-19 defense: an evidence-based approach for optimization of infection control and operating room management. *Anesth Analg.* 2020;131(1):37-42.
25. Foley L, Urdaneta F, Berkow L, et al. Difficult airway management in adult coronavirus disease 2019 patients: statement by the Society of Airway Management. *Anesth Analg.* 2021;133(4):876-890.
26. Verbeek JH, Rajamaki B, Ijaz S, et al. Personal protective equipment for preventing highly infectious diseases due to exposure to contaminated body fluids in healthcare staff. *Cochrane Database Syst Rev.* 2020;5:CD011621.
27. Nicolle L. SARS safety and science. *Can J Anaesth.* 2003;50:983-988.
28. ECDC. European Centre for Disease Prevention and Control. Personal protective equipment (PPE) needs in healthcare settings for the care of patients with suspected or confirmed 2019-nCoV. Stockholm; 2020.
29. Forrester JD, Nassar AK, Maggio PM, Hawn MT. Precautions for operating room team members during the covid-19 pandemic. *J Am Coll Surg.* 2020;230(6):1098-1101.
30. Lee D, Ma M, Parotto M, Wasowicz M. Intubtion outside of the operating room: new challenges and opportunities in the COVID-19 era. *Curr Opin Anaesthesiol.* 2020;33(4):608-611.
31. Mick P, Murphy R. Aerosol-generating otolaryngology procedures and the need for enhanced PPE during the COVID-19 pandemic: a literature review. *J Otolaryngol Head Neck Surg.* 2020;49(1):29.
32. Wong J, Goh QY, Tan Z, et al. Preparing for a COVID-19 pandemic: a review of operating room outbreak response measures in a large tertiary hospital in Singapore. *Can J Anaesth.* 2020;67(6):732-745.
33. Sorbello M, El-Boghdadly K, Di Giacinto I, et al. The Italian coronavirus disease 2019 outbreak: recommendations from clinical practice. *Anaesthesia.* 2020;75(6):724-732.
34. Fujishiro A, Saito T, Asai T. COVID-19: be aware of contaminated airway devices. *J Anesth.* 2020;34(6):960-961.
35. Patwa A, Shah A, Garg R, et al. All India difficult airway association (AIDAA) consensus guidelines for airway management in the operating room during the COVID-19 pandemic. *Indian J Anaesth.* 2020;64(Suppl 2):S107-S115.
36. University of Toronto, Department of Anesthesiology and Pain Medicine. Protected Code Blue Guidelines. https://anesthesia.utoronto.ca/code-blue-protected. Accessed February 1, 2021.
37. Sorbello M, Rosenblatt W, Hofmeyr R, Greif R, Urdaneta F. Aerosol boxes and barrier enclosures for airway management in COVID-19 patients: a scoping review and narrative synthesis. *Br J Anaesth.* 2020;125(6):880-894.
38. Laack TA, Pollok F, Sandefur BJ, Mullan AF, Russi CS, Yalamuri SM. Barrier enclosure for endotracheal intubation in a simulated covid-19 scenario: a crossover study. *West J Emerg Med.* 2020;21(5):1080-1083.
39. Clariot S, Dumain G, Gauci E, Langeron O, Levesque E. Minimising COVID-19 exposure during tracheal intubation by using a transparent plastic box: a randomised prospective simulation study. *Anaesth Crit Care Pain Med.* 2020;39(4):461-463.
40. Begley JL, Lavery KE, Nickson CP, Brewster DJ. The aerosol box for intubation in coronavirus disease 2019 patients: an in-situ simulation crossover study. *Anaesthesia.* 2020;75(8):1014-1021.
41. Noor Azhar M, Bustam A, Poh K, et al. COVID-19 aerosol box as protection from droplet and aerosol contaminations in healthcare workers performing airway intubation: a randomised cross-over simulation study. *Emerg Med J.* 2021;38(2):111-117.
42. FDA. Protective barrier enclosures during the COVID-19 pandemic may increase risk to patients and healtcare providers – letter to healthcare providers. https://www.fda.gov/medical-devices/letters-health-care-providers/protective-barrier-enclosures-without-negative-pressure-used-during-covid-19-pandemic-may-increase2020. Accessed on February 4, 2021.
43. Wexner SD, Cortes-Guiral D, Gilshtein H, Kent I, Reymond MA. COVID-19: impact on colorectal surgery. *Colorectal Dis.* 2020;22(6):635-640.

44. Brown J, Gregson FKA, Shrimpton A, et al. A quantitative evaluation of aerosol generation during tracheal intubation and extubation. *Anaesthesia.* 2021;76(2):174-181.
45. Dhillon RS, Rowin WA, Humphries RS, et al. Aerosolisation during tracheal intubation and extubation in an operating theatre setting. *Anaesthesia.* 2021;76(2):182-188.
46. Tran K, Cimon K, Severn M, Pessoa-Silva CL, Conly J. Aerosol generating procedures and risk of transmission of acute respiratory infections to healthcare workers: a systematic review. *PLoS One.* 2012;7(4):e35797.
47. El-Boghdadly K, Wong DJN, Owen R, et al. Risks to healthcare workers following tracheal intubation of patients with COVID-19: a prospective international multicentre cohort study. *Anaesthesia.* 2020;75(11):1437-1447.
48. Ahmad I, Wade S, Langdon A. Awake tracheal intubation in a suspected COVID-19 patient with critical airway obstruction. *Anaesth Rep.* 2020;8(1):28-31.
49. Hanouz JL, Lhermitte D, Gerard JL, Fischer MO. Comparison of pre-oxygenation using spontaneous breathing through face mask and high-flow nasal oxygen: A randomised controlled crossover study in healthy volunteers. *Eur J Anaesthesiol.* 2019;36(5):335-341.
50. Tan PCF, Millay OJ, Leeton L, Dennis AT. High-flow humidified nasal preoxygenation in pregnant women: a prospective observational study. *Br J Anaesth.* 2019;122(1):86-91.
51. Phipps SJ, Scott AC, Legge CE. Awake tracheal intubation during the COVID-19 pandemic – an aerosol-minimising approach. *Anaesth Rep.* 2020;8(2):101.
52. Frerk C, Mitchell VS, McNarry AF, et al. Difficult Airway Society 2015 guidelines for management of unanticipated difficult intubation in adults. *Br J Anaesth.* 2015;115(6):827-848.
53. Law JA, Duggan LV, Asselin M, et al. Canadian Airway Focus Group updated consensus-based recommendations for management of the difficult airway: part 1. Difficult airway management encountered in an unconscious patient. *Can J Anaesth.* 2021;68(9):1373-1404.
54. Law JA, Duggan LV, Asselin M, et al. Canadian Airway Focus Group updated consensus-based recommendations for management of the difficult airway: part 2. Planning and implementing safe management of the patient with an anticipated difficult airway. *Can J Anaesth.* 2021;68(9):1405-1436.
55. Apfelbaum J, Hagberg C, Caplan R, Blitt C, Connis R, Nickinovich D. Practice guidelines for management of the difficult airway. An updated report by the American Society of Anesthesiologists Task Force on Management of the difficult airway. *Anesthesiology.* 2013;118(2):251-270.
56. Tay J, Khoo M, Loh W. Surgical considerations for tracheostomy learned from the svere acute respiratory syndrome outbreak. *JAMA Otolaryngol Head Neck Surg.* 2020;146(6):517-518.
57. NTSP. National Tracheostomy Safe project. Multidisciplinary COVID-19 tracheostomy guidance. http://www.tracheostomy.org.uk/storage/files/Multidisciplinary%20COVID_19%20tracheostomy%20guidance%2030_4_20.pdf2020. updated April 30 2020. Accessed on February 4, 2021.
58. Gosling AF, Bose S, Gomez E, et al. Perioperative considerations for tracheostomies in the era of COVID-19. *Anesth Analg.* 2020;131(2):378-386.
59. Ip V, Tham C. COVID-19 Pandemic: Negative pressure tent during atomization of local anesthetic for awake fibreoptic intubation. *Anesth Analg.* 2020;131(3):e178-e189.
60. Kangas-Dick A, Swearingen B, Wan E, Chawla K, Wiesel O. Safe extubation during the COVID-19 pandemic. *Respiratory Medicine.* 2020;170:1-3.
61. D'Silva DF, McCulloch TJ, Lim JS, Smith SS, Carayannis D. Extubation of patients with COVID-19. *Br J Anaesth.* 2020;125(1):e192-e195.
62. Yang SS, Wang NN, Postonogova T, et al. Intravenous lidocaine to prevent postoperative airway complications in adults: a systematic review and meta-analysis. *Br J Anaesth.* 2020;124(3):314-323.
63. Tung A, Fergusson NA, Ng N, Hu V, Dormuth C, Griesdale DEG. Medications to reduce emergence coughing after general anaesthesia with tracheal intubation: a systematic review and network meta-analysis. *Br J Anaesth.* 2020;S0007-0912(20)30012-X. doi:10.1016/j.bja.2019.12.041.

CHAPTER 34

Airway Management of the ICU Patient with Both a Predicted Anatomically Difficult Airway and Physiologically Difficult Airway

Nicola Jarvis and Matteo Parotto

CASE PRESENTATION

Mr. R was a 68-year-old male presenting for coronary bypass graft surgery and aortic valve replacement for severe aortic stenosis, and triple vessel coronary artery disease.

His past medical history was significant for ankylosing spondylitis and kyphosis that had rendered him relatively immobile, except when walking slowly with the assistance of a four-wheel walker. Relating to his spinal disease he had a restrictive respiratory deficit on his lung function tests and baseline oxygen saturation on room air of 92%. His preoperative echo showed a reduced left ventricular ejection fraction of 30%.

His preoperative airway assessment revealed severe kyphosis, with a fixed cervical spine, unable to extend, flex, or rotate. He had full native dentition, mouth opening of 3 finger breadths, and a Mallampati score of 4.

The anesthesia practitioner decided to perform an awake flexible bronchoscopic intubation for his bypass surgery. This decision was based on the airway assessment outlined above informed by a history of awake flexible bronchoscopic intubations being performed for his previous surgeries. The intubation went smoothly, as did the operation. The patient was extubated in the intensive care unit on postoperative day 1. He was found to have suffered an acute kidney injury and had low urine output. His overall fluid balance was over 5 L positive for the preceding 24 hours. Over the course of the 2 hours postextubation, he exhibited increased work of breathing and escalating oxygen requirements. An arterial blood gas showed a mixed respiratory and metabolic acidosis, with a PaO_2 of 50 mmHg on a non-rebreathing face mask at 15 $L{\cdot}min^{-1}$ oxygen flow. His most recent postextubation chest X-ray was consistent with pulmonary edema. A decision was made by the intensive care unit (ICU) fellow to reintubate the patient emergently.

The ICU fellow felt that the intubation needed to be performed expeditiously and decided to perform the intubation employing a hyperangulated video laryngoscope with a styleted endotracheal tube (ETT).

Oxygen was administered via a non-rebreather face mask at 100% FiO_2. Two milligrams of midazolam and 100 mg of succinylcholine were administered. Oxygen saturation before the attempt at laryngoscopy was 88%. The first attempt at laryngoscopy revealed that it was difficult to insert the video laryngoscope blade into the patient's mouth due to the handle abutting the patient's chest. The fellow found that attempts to optimize the position in the ICU bed were difficult as they, and the other people in the room, were not familiar with this new type of bed and were unable to manipulate the bed precisely to the position they wanted.

They called for help from someone else in the ICU familiar with the new bed and asked for the on-call anesthesiologist to be paged overhead to assist. While this was happening the patient's oxygen saturation fell to 82%, and the systolic blood pressure decreased from 130 to 75 mmHg. The fellow performed bag-mask ventilation (BMV) on the patient effectively and asked for the bedside nurse to administer phenylephrine to treat the blood pressure. The oxygen saturation improved to 88% and systolic BP to 95 mmHg.

An attendant familiar with the bed arrived and was able to move the position enough that the laryngoscope blade could be inserted into the patient's mouth. And although an adequate view of the cords was obtained, the curve of the styleted-ETT could not deliver it to the larynx. Again, the oxygen saturations fell, this time to 75%. The on-call anesthesiologist arrived from the operating room (OR) and took over attempts at intubation and was also unable to pass the ETT with the stylet. He tried to pass a Frova Bougie and despite achieving a good view of the cords yet again, was unable to manipulate the bougie through the vocal cords. At this point, the anesthesiologist asked the nurses for a flexible bronchoscope to be brought into the room. Some confusion followed when a bronchoscopy tower with no bronchoscope arrived, but eventually, the nurses found the disposable flexible bronchoscope in one of the equipment rooms and brought this to the patient's bedside.

Meanwhile, the anesthesiologist and ICU fellow had reverted to BMV to improve the oxygen saturation further, though they struggled to achieve an adequate seal and the saturations only came up to 82%. Epinephrine IV infusion had been started, achieving a systolic blood pressure of 85 mmHg. The anesthesiologist then employed both a video laryngoscope and a flexible bronchoscope simultaneously as a flexible guide, with the ETT loaded on it. This allowed placement of the ETT between the cords. The patient's oxygen saturation returned to above 95% with positive pressure ventilation and the blood pressure normalized. After several days of optimal diuresis, the patient's oxygen requirements decreased and he was extubated uneventfully.

INTRODUCTION

What Is Unique About the Difficult Airway in the Intensive Care Unit Compared to One Encountered in the Operating Room?

More airway management related complications occur outside the OR than inside it, including the intensive care unit.[1] The reasons for this in the ICU are multifactorial and include the physiological state of the patient requiring emergent intubation, staffing and their airway skills, and the physical environment, including equipment available.[2] The critically ill patient with the predictably difficult airway presents even more challenges than might be present had that same patient presented electively for surgery in the OR.

The Physiologically Stressed Patient Has Less Reserve

Intubations occurring in the ICU are almost always emergency intubations due to deterioration of a patient's condition in one or more organ systems, or in the event of cardiac arrest. Irrespective of laryngeal view grade, ICU patients are more likely to require multiple attempts at laryngoscopy compared to those intubated in the OR,[3] resulting in a greater risk of hypoxemia, aspiration, and cardiac arrest.[4] The patient who is already physiologically compromised tolerates repeated intubation attempts poorly.

Time Pressures of Emergency Intubations

An airway practitioner faced with a deteriorating patient may feel pressured to secure the patient's airway quickly to facilitate rapid support of their respiration, circulation, or other failing organ. In most hands, the fastest technique is a rapid sequence induction/intubation (RSI). Most ICU patients will not tolerate the pharmacodynamic changes of typical RSI drugs in doses used for otherwise healthy individuals. Medication selection and dosing are crucial components in inducing these patients safely. This factor, particularly when coupled with a difficult airway, makes it prudent to briefly "apply the brakes," rather than rush into an RSI. Although actions need to occur quickly, the airway practitioner at the bedside should remember that the patient with an oxygen saturation of 90% and a respiratory rate of 35 per minute while breathing for themselves is better off than the patient who has been paralyzed for intubation but found, after multiple intubation attempts, to be impossible to oxygenate as their oxygen saturations fall relentlessly.

Environmental Factors Specific to the Intensive Care Unit

In addition to physiological challenges, there are distinct human and environmental factors that contribute to stressors in this already challenging clinical scenario.[2]

Human factors influence the actions and decisions of clinicians, nurses, respiratory therapists, and auxiliary ICU staff. Significant disparities in experience and skills among staff often exist in ICU over the course of a 24-hour period. Ordinarily, those with more experience are concentrated during the daytime, and those less experienced are present overnight. Compounding this factor, staffing numbers are generally higher during the day and lower at night in most units. Intubations in the ICU are performed by intensive care clinicians in most hospitals. Training and ongoing skills maintenance for advanced airway techniques vary among clinicians, as does any single clinician's ability to perform these tasks for patient who is physiologically compromised.

The COVID-19 pandemic prompted the creation of "intubation teams" in many hospitals. Groups of clinicians (doctors, nurses, anesthesia assistants, or respiratory therapists) practiced airway algorithms and Personal Protective Equipment (PPE) protocols, and then they were the team called upon to perform all of the emergency intubations in the hospital over a period of time. Protocolization of intubation attempts, with emphasis on video laryngoscopy for first intubation attempts, resulted in high first-pass success rates.[5] Prior to COVID, literature on intubation teams was relatively limited, though this concept had been explored.[6] Although the majority of intubations in COVID-19 are not anatomically difficult intubations, what this experience has taught us is that the protocolization of airway techniques, familiarity of teams with other team members, and the airway equipment being used, results in high first-pass success rates. Extrapolating this experience to the ICU, the infrequently-performed advanced airway techniques of awake intubation and emergency front-of-neck access (eFONA) would potentially be better performed by teams familiar with the performance of these tasks either in the OR, or, for eFONA, in a simulated environment.

What Needs to Be Considered When Choosing Your Approach to the Anatomically and Physiologically Difficult Intubation?

Assessment of the Patient's Airway

If afforded the luxury of taking a history from the patient (or their family) about previous intubation attempts, or having this information available in the patient's health record, this can very quickly alert the airway practitioner to potential difficulty. Regardless of this information, an airway examination is crucial in anticipating difficulty. Detsky et al. reviewed studies from 1946 to 2018 to determine which airway examination characteristics were the best predictors of difficult intubation.[7] Sixty-two studies including 33,559 patients found the best predictor was the inability of the lower incisors to touch the top lip, followed by shorter hyomental distance, retrognathia, and Wilson score. These all had a higher positive likelihood ratio than the commonly used Mallampati score equal to or greater than 3.

In some instances, intubation will need to be performed in the event of cardiac arrest, or when the patient can't participate in an airway exam for other reasons. When this situation arises, there is still crucial information an experienced clinician will absorb quickly upon entering the patient's room, the so-called end-of-the-bed-o-gram. Such things include obvious facial hairs, facial or neck deformities and immobility, head and neck radiation, obviously short thyromental distance, or extreme obesity. If faced with these features, an immediate request for difficult airway equipment and extra staff should be made.

Clinical State of the Patient

Advanced planning cannot take place for the patient that suffers a sudden need for airway management (e.g., cardiac arrest), and the airway management team is left with no option other than to progress down the standard algorithm of attempts to oxygenate the patient: best laryngoscopy, BMV, extraglottic devices (EGDs), or eFONA.

Alternatively, while the patient is deteriorating but has not yet arrested, airway practitioners should consider how rapidly the deterioration is taking place and if there are any temporizing measures that can be performed (e.g., fluid resuscitation, inotropes/vasopressors administration, or control of rapid arrhythmias) prior to intubation that could make induction and asleep intubation safer. The rapidity of their decline will also inform the decision to perform an awake intubation if this is the most appropriate option, given the patient's airway anatomy or physiologic state.

Skills of Staff and Equipment Available

An emergency intubation in a physiologically challenging patient is not the time to be performing an awake flexible bronchoscopic intubation for the first, second, or third time! Not all ICU practitioners are comfortable performing an awake intubation. In many cases, there may be practitioners in the facility who possess such skills that can be drawn on to assist in the ICU.

Since the National Audit Project 4 (NAP4) in the United Kingdom, the creation of a difficult intubation trolley/cart has been strongly endorsed. The cart and contents are the same throughout the hospital and reflect the structure of a difficult airway algorithm. The term "universality" indicates that wherever an intubation needs to occur in the hospital, the equipment is the same and in the same location from cart to cart. This familiarity has been shown to improve intubation performance.

When faced with a truly challenging airway, the most comfortable intubating environment for most anesthesia practitioners is the OR. With a deteriorating patient there may not necessarily be time to reach the OR, and moving the patient may cause more instability. For this reason, ICUs should have all the equipment needed for awake intubation including flexible bronchoscopes, video laryngoscopes, topicalization drugs, and the means to apply them. Critical care staff are gaining increasing exposure to advanced airway techniques and equipping the ICU to deal with such emergencies adequately should mean that the most comfortable place for the difficult intubation is in the ICU.

Incorporating Airway Examination, Patient Condition, and Staff Experience

The MACOCHA score uses examination and clinical information to predict the absence of a difficult airway and is specifically designed for and validated in ICU patients.[8] This study validated this score and also found that the presence of difficult intubation (three or more attempts at laryngoscopy) was associated with much higher complication rates of cardiovascular and respiratory complications.

The MACOCHA score incorporates:

- Patient airway factors:
  - Malampatti score 3 or 4 — 5 points
  - Obstructive sleep apnea (OSA) — 2 points
  - Reduce mobility of cervical spine — 1 point
  - Limited mouth opening <3 cm — 1 point
- Factors related to pathology
  - Coma (GCS <8 as the reason for intubation) — 1 point
  - Severe hypoxemia (SpO_2 <80%) — 1 point
- Factor related to operator
  - Nonanesthesiologist — 1 point

Score of 0 = easy intubation; Score of 12 = very difficult.

Use of this score is increasingly being incorporated into ICU intubation checklists as a reminder to assess for predicted difficult intubation.

TECHNIQUES TO SECURE THE DIFFICULT AIRWAY IN THE INTENSIVE CARE UNIT

Awake Flexible Bronchoscopic Intubation

Avoiding the apnea and hemodynamic compromise associated with induction and paralysis for endotracheal intubation is arguably the safest way to intubate those at the highest risk of respiratory and cardiovascular collapse.[2,9] Couple with this the fact that in the patient with a difficult airway, awake flexible bronchoscopic intubation is considered the gold standard,[10] there is a growing argument to support awake flexible bronchoscopic intubation as the safest option in the anatomically and physiologically challenging airway. There will be occasions when an airway practitioner will decide that the risk of delaying intubation to allow for airway topicalization and an awake approach, is greater than the risk of intubation failure, and so alternate options (see section "Optimized Intubation Plan After Induction of Anesthesia Including 'Double Set-Up'") would need to be employed. But in the physiologically challenged patient in whom the intubation is expected to be very challenging, and there is time to topicalize the airway, an awake flexible bronchoscopic intubation should be utilized. In light of their instability, however, a specific approach will be needed (summarized in Table 34.1). The approach described in the following text is based on the Difficult Airway Society's four-step structure when planning awake flexible bronchoscopic intubation.[11]

Oxygen Delivery

The ICU patient in extremis will have much greater oxygen requirements than the typical patient undergoing awake flexible bronchoscopic intubation in the OR, particularly if the indication for the intubation is respiratory failure. At a minimum, a high-flow nasal cannula (HFNC) is strongly recommended, at a rate of 30 to 70 L·min^{-1} (DAS, 2020). In patients with concurrent right heart failure and pulmonary hypertension, nasal noninvasive ventilation can be used for the administration of inhaled pulmonary vasodilators which has been described in case series.[12] Positioning the patient head up to optimize functional residual capacity and respiratory mechanics is also recommended in physiologically challenged patients.[13]

TABLE 34.1. Awake Tracheal Intubation (ATI) Current Guidelines and Alterations in the Physiologically Challenged ICU Patient

	Current Consensus Suggestions (DAS, CAFG)[10,11]	Alterations for the Physiologically Challenged Patient
Oxygenation	High-flow nasal prongs 30-70 L·min^{-1}	No alteration, could also consider nasal CPAP or administer inhaled pulmonary vasodilator.
Topicalization	(See also Chapter 3.) 5% lidocaine ointment via a tongue depressor to the base of tongue; followed by up to 15 mL of 3% or 4% atomized lidocaine to airway; followed by 3% or 4% lidocaine-soaked pledgets in the pyriform recesses via Jackson cross-over forceps. Max dose topical lidocaine should not exceed 9 mg·kg^{-1}	May have less cooperation from patient for inhalation during atomization, may have to rely on a "spray-as-you-go" through the endoscope technique. Avoid cocaine due to the risk of coronary vasospasm and tachycardia from systemic absorption.
Sedation and adjuncts	Remifentanil 0.05 µg·kg^{-1}·min^{-1} via IV infusion pump Other options: *Sedation* dexmedetomidine bolus 0.5-1 µg·kg^{-1} followed by infusion 0.3-0.7 µg·kg^{-1}·hr^{-1} *Analgesia:* Fentanyl bolus 0.5-1 mcg·kg^{-1}, subsequent doses of 0.5 mcg·kg^{-1} if required. Alfentanil bolus 5 µg·kg^{-1}, subsequent doses of 1-3 µg·kg^{-1} as required. Atropine or glycopyrrolate is commonly used for antisialogogue effects.	Sedation may not be required if the patient is obtunded from hypoxemia, hypercarbia, or another cause, (though altered sensorium may make things more difficult). If required, use small doses and titrate judiciously. Sedation should be managed by a separate clinician. If an antisialagogue is to be used, note the onset of antisialogogue effect of glycopyrrolate and atropine is 15-20 minutes, and in an emergency there may not be time to wait for this. The decision to use an antisialogogue should be weighed against the risk of extreme tachycardia in the already physiologically stressed patient.
Perform	Appropriate ETT choice may be nasal or oral depending on operation and pathology. Patient sitting up. Confirmation of ETT placement before induction of anesthesia.	Oral route is preferable due to the ability to use larger diameter ETT, and tolerated better than nasal ETT for longer periods of ventilation. If nasal ETT is the only way to establish an airway an early tracheostomy to be considered if a long period of ventilation required. Positioning the patient sitting up is better for respiratory mechanics but may necessitate vasopressors support for cardiovascular stability.

Abbreviations: ETT, endotracheal tube; LAST, local anesthetic toxicity.

Topicalization

Many topicalization techniques involve significant patient cooperation, such as having the patient inhale as the clinician administers lidocaine via an atomizer. Some patients are in a state of distress, or even periarrest, prior to ICU intubation, so any topicalization that occurs must take place quickly and be as nonstimulating as possible. If the patient is having difficulty coordinating their inhalation with the atomization of lidocaine or has only poor respiratory effort, then pretopicalization of the vocal cords and trachea may be suboptimal. In this case, more reliance on the "spray as you go" approach may be necessary. For this approach, once the vocal cords are visualized with the bronchoscope, lidocaine is sprayed directly on them via the working channel of the bronchoscope. The patient often coughs and it is necessary to wait further time for the coughing to settle and the local anesthesia to work. Spraying more lidocaine below the cords may also be necessary.

Sedation and Adjuncts

Most physiologically challenged ICU patients will tolerate sedation poorly, and over-sedation is a common complication of awake flexible bronchoscopic intubation, even in well patients.[14] In the unwell patient, concomitant hypoxemia or hypercarbia may render the patient sedated or obtunded, thus diminishing any sedation requirements. Regardless, sedation needs to be administered cautiously, in the lowest dose possible, if at all.

DAS guidelines for awake tracheal intubation (ATI) suggest remifentanil infusion as the first-line sedative agent. Alternatives to remifentanil suggested in this latest guideline include propofol infusion, midazolam, dexmedetomidine infusion, fentanyl, or alfentanil as small boluses.[11] The doses suggested are likely too great for the unwell ICU patient, causing deleterious effects like excessive sedation, further hypoxia, or cardiovascular collapse. Studies elucidating this further are relatively limited. Case reports of physiologically challenged patients undergoing awake flexible bronchoscopic intubations for respiratory failure describe the safe use of a variety of low-dose sedative techniques including 50 to 100 μg of fentanyl, 40 to 50 mg of ketamine, 1 to 8 mg of midazolam, or etomidate 10 mg.[12] Until more evidence becomes available regarding these dosages, the safest approach for an experienced airway practitioner will be to titrate sedation cautiously, and use only if strictly necessary.

Antisialagogues are often used in the OR to facilitate topicalization and improve visualization of the airway. Two problems arise in the emergency ICU intubation. First, the time of onset for the antisialagogue effect of both glycopyrrolate and atropine is approximately 15 to 20 minutes after intravenous administration. Generally, this is outside of the acceptable time frame for an emergency intubation. Second, both agents, but more so for atropine, will cause tachycardia long before the desired antisialogogue effect begins. This may be detrimental in the patient who already has precarious hemodynamics, so the risks and benefits need to be considered in the context of the patient's current physiological state. If an antisialogogue is not used a small suction catheter can be placed via the nose that sits in the posterior pharynx to provide continuous pharyngeal suction.[15]

Awake intubation for ICU patients has been described in case reports and series. Johannes et al. described 9 patients with right heart failure and pulmonary hypertension requiring intubation for respiratory failure.[12] All patients were successfully intubated with an awake flexible bronchoscopic technique while receiving minimal sedation and being concomitantly oxygenated via either nasal noninvasive ventilation (NIV) or oxygen via HFNC.

Proposed physiological benefits of this technique include:

- Systemic vascular tone is maintained by avoiding larger doses of systemic anesthesia.
- Upright positioning favors better ventilation/perfusion (V/Q) matching in most patients.
- Spontaneous ventilation avoids hypoventilation and hypoxemia, thus limiting these effects on pulmonary vascular resistance.
- Nasal delivery of oxygen (NIV or HFNC with some peak end expiratory pressure) can also occur with pulmonary vasodilator therapy, maintains alveolar recruitment, and can assist with splinting the upper airway to maintain patency.[12]

Performance of the Awake Flexible Bronchoscopic Intubation

ETT choice will depend on whether an oral approach to the airway is possible. The oral approach is generally considered to be preferable to a nasal intubation because a larger ETT can be used, and because nasal tubes are poorly tolerated for longer periods, with common complications being nasal pressure sores and sinusitis.

The sitting position strikes a good compromise between optimal respiratory mechanics (for most patients) and a workable practical position for the performance of awake flexible bronchoscopic intubation. Additionally, this position may be a more comfortable one for the patient with certain cardiovascular pathologies, e.g., mitral stenosis, and acute pulmonary edema. If the patient has cardiovascular instability this may necessitate additional vasopressors to maintain mean arterial pressure throughout the procedure.

Awake Video Laryngoscopy (VL) for Intubation

This technique has gained additional popularity over the last 5 to 10 years, particularly among younger anesthesia practitioners who have more familiarity with VL than they do with flexible bronchoscopes. Systematic review and meta-analysis found awake VL to be associated with a shorter intubation time and similar success rates and safety profiles compared to flexible bronchoscopic intubation.[16] Considerations concerning awake VL intubation are the same as for awake flexible bronchoscopic intubation.

Compared to the awake flexible bronchoscopic technique, the equipment (i.e., video laryngoscope) for this technique may be more readily available. The best-tolerated VL blade is likely to be a hyperangulated video laryngoscope, preferably a "low profile" blade that requires less mouth opening, so it should be available in all ICU difficult airway trolleys.

Positioning for awake VL may either be supine or sitting up at 45 degrees (semi-Fowler). The supine position may be poorly tolerated in patients with compromised respiratory status.

Optimized Intubation Plan After Induction of Anesthesia Including "Double Set-Up"

If there is no time to topicalize the airway and perform an awake intubation, or the patient is not cooperative enough for this to take place, intubation after induction of anesthesia should be attempted.

Airway practitioners dealing with this scenario are facing at least two distinct challenges: (1) maintaining or not worsening the physiological state of the patient while administering sedation and paralysis and (2) securing a difficult airway. For this reason, the airway team looking after the patient should be organized in a way that separates these two tasks, and delegates the responsibility of drug administration and hemodynamics to an experienced team member, and management of the intubation to a separate experienced team member (or two).

The approach to intubation, and plan must be explicitly stated by the team, should address each of the four fundamental methods of ensuring oxygenation of the patient, namely, (A) laryngoscopy, (B) EGDs, (C) –BMV, and (D) FONA or cricothyrotomy. The 2021 Canadian Airway Focus Group guidelines[10] recommend the use of a "double set-up" for anticipated very difficult intubation when there is not sufficient time to perform an awake flexible bronchoscopic intubation. In addition to the usual equipment required for plans A, B, and C, they also recommend preparing FONA by opening the necessary equipment, marking the cricothyroid membrane on the neck (with ultrasound assistance as needed), and allocating a separate airway team member to be at the bedside ready to perform this task if called upon. The team briefing should also discuss triggers to proceed to FONA. Having the set-up ready partly diminishes the mental hurdle of FONA as emblematic of failure; rather, it is part of the airway management plan.

Awake Tracheotomy

This technique is not uncommon as a means of establishing an airway in patients with upper airway obstruction presenting emergently to the OR. In this instance, the awake tracheotomy is performed by an experienced surgeon, and the patient is supported by anesthesia care. Sometimes these patients have other comorbidities that may render them physiologically challenged, however, the primary reason they are in the OR is for relief of upper airway obstruction, not any other indication for intubation. Surgeons and anesthesia practitioners alike would most likely prefer OR environment over the ICU.

Awake tracheotomy as a first-line technique to secure a difficult airway in the ICU (where there is a separate indication for intubation outside of the airway itself) is a rare occurrence with little reported literature, and if this were to be undertaken it would need to be with adequately skilled practitioners with the availability of all necessary equipment.

Role of Extracorporeal Membrane Oxygenation (ECMO) Devices

The use of ECMO has increased significantly over the last 10 years, both in the number of centers utilizing this technique and the number of patients receiving it.[17] Typically ECMO for respiratory failure is employed when a patient has ongoing respiratory failure despite mechanical ventilation and thus, they are already intubated. As such it is rarely instituted in patients who are not intubated.

However, at institutions familiar with the placement of ECMO cannula in spontaneously breathing patients, if a patient is expected to be impossible to intubate or the above-mentioned methods of establishing oxygenation are expected to be unsuccessful, this is a feasible option. ECMO or CPB (cardiopulmonary bypass) for patients with airway pathology that either makes intubation impossible or where intubation is not expected to improve oxygenation (e.g., distal tracheal pathology) has been described in numerous case reports and series and summarized in a systematic review by Malpas et al. looking specifically at a priori cannulation, not as a salvage technique in failed intubation.[18] Most of these cases involve short periods of ECMO/CPB, performed in the OR, until tracheal intubation was performed another way (e.g., surgical tracheotomy) or the airway obstruction/pathology was surgically resolved.

Use in patient whose respiratory failure for reasons other than what makes their intubation difficult are limited, but have been described, such as in the case of respiratory failure due to pneumonia in a patient with severe tracheal abnormality associated with TB-related spinal deformity.[19] In this particular patient, ECMO was instituted after attempts at flexible bronchoscopic intubation had failed.

The choice of whether to employ venovenous (VV)-ECMO versus venoarterial (VA)-ECMO depends on the presence of concurrent circulatory failure, with VV-ECMO being reserved for those with respiratory failure only. Choosing VA-ECMO for a patient without circulatory failure can result in relatively de-oxygenated blood being delivered to the cerebral and coronary circulation, and hyperoxygenated blood delivered to the abdomen and lower body. Despite this potential problem, VA-ECMO has been described in a patient with expected difficult intubation and expected difficult tracheotomy due to large thyroid cancer who had no subsequent neurological sequelae from this ECMO configuration.[18]

SUMMARY

Intubations in the ICU are almost always emergencies. Patients who possess both a physiologically and anatomically challenging airway require special consideration and may need to draw upon the resources and expertise of staff beyond the ICU. In the whirlwind of activity that occurs in emergency intubation, there may be undue pressure to perform endotracheal intubation without consideration for the potential for intubation failure, and the consequences that result. As with all patients, a history of previous intubations and examination of the airway play a critical role in determining the safest management option.

If there is time to tropicalize the airway, many would suggest an awake flexible bronchoscopic or awake video laryngoscopic intubation as the best option. If the intubation is an emergency, the next best option is the "double set-up" incorporating FONA cricothyrotomy in the plan. ECMO is another option for centers equipped and experienced in performing this on spontaneously ventilated patients, recognizing that the technical aspects of cannula insertion differ from performing it on intubated, mechanically ventilated patients.

SELF-EVALUATION QUESTIONS

34.1. The following are all potential predictors of difficult intubation EXCEPT:

A. Ability to bite top lip with bottom incisors

B. Cervical spine immobility

C. Short hyomental distance

D. Obstructive sleep apnea history

34.2. In a patient with respiratory failure in the intensive care unit and impending respiratory arrest, what factors inform the approach to intubation?

A. Previous successful intubation techniques

B. Current patient condition and how quickly they are deteriorating

C. Airway examination

D. Skills of the attending clinician

E. All of the above

34.3. Team members required for optimal care of patients with physiological and anatomically challenging airway might include all of the following EXCEPT:

A. Clinician dedicated to the administration of drugs and hemodynamic control

B. Clinician allocated to perform front-of-neck access

C. Clinician allocated to be primary airway operator

D. Clinician dedicated to perform insertion of nasogastric tube following induction of anesthesia but prior to endotracheal intubation

REFERENCES

1. Cook TM, Woodall N, Harper J, Benger J, Fourth National Audit P. Major complications of airway management in the UK: results of the Fourth National Audit Project of the Royal College of Anaesthetists and the Difficult Airway Society. Part 2: intensive care and emergency departments. *Br J Anaesth.* 2011;106(5):632-642.
2. Mosier JM, Sakles JC, Law JA, Brown CA 3rd, Brindley PG. Tracheal intubation in the critically ill. Where we came from and where we should go. *Am J Respir Crit Care Med.* 2020;201(7):775-788.
3. Taboada, M., Doldan, P., Calvo, A., et al. Comparison of tracheal intubation conditions in operating room and intensive care unit. *Anesthesiology.* 2018;129(2):321-328.
4. Mort TC. Emergency tracheal intubation: complications associated with repeated laryngoscopic attempts. *Anesth Analg.* 2004;99(2):607-613.
5. Ahmad I, Jeyarajah J, Nair G, et al. A prospective, observational, cohort study of airway management of patients with COVID-19 by specialist tracheal intubation teams. *Can J Anaesth.* 2021;68(2):196-203.
6. Mark LJ, Herzer KR, Cover R, et al. Difficult airway response team: a novel quality improvement program for managing hospital-wide airway emergencies. *Anesth Analg.* 2015;121(1):127-139.
7. Detsky ME, Jivraj N, Adhikari NK, et al. Will this patient be difficult to intubate? The rational clinical examination systematic review. *JAMA.* 2019;321(5):493-503.
8. De Jong A, Rolle A, Molinari N, et al. Cardiac arrest and mortality related to intubation procedure in critically ill adult patients: a multicenter cohort study. *Crit Care Med.* 2018;46(4);532-539.
9. Lapinsky SE. Endotracheal intubation in the ICU. *Crit Care.* 2015;19:258.
10. Law JA, Duggan LV, Asselin M, et al. Canadian Airway Focus Group updated consensus-based recommendations for management of the difficult airway: part 2. Planning and implementing safe management of the patient with an anticipated difficult airway. *Can J Anaesth.* 2021;68(9):1405-1436.
11. Ahmad I, El-Boghdadly K, Bhagrath R, et al. Difficult Airway Society guidelines for awake tracheal intubation (ATI) in adults. *Anaesthesia.* 2020;75(4):509-528.
12. Johannes J, Berlin DA, Patel P, et al. A technique of awake bronchoscopic endotracheal intubation for respiratory failure in patients with right heart failure and pulmonary hypertension. *Crit Care Med.* 2017;45(9): e980-e984.
13. Kornas R, Owyang C, Sakles J, Foley L, Mosier, J. On behalf of the Society for Airway Management's Special Projects Committee Evaluation and Management of the Physiologically Difficult Airway: Consensus recommendations from Society for Airway Management. *Anesth Analg.* 2021;132(2)-395-405.
14. El-Boghdadly K, Onwochei DN, Cuddihy J, Ahmad I. A prospective cohort study of awake fibreoptic intubation practice at a tertiary centre. *Anaesthesia.* 2017;72(6):694-703.
15. Hannig KE, Hauritz RW, Jessen C, Grejs AM. Acute awake fiberoptic intubation in the ICU in a patient with limited mouth opening and hypoxemic acute respiratory failure. *Case Rep Anesthesiol.* 2019:6421910. doi:10.1155/2019/6421910.
16. Alhomary M, Ramadan E, Curran E, Walsh SR. Videolaryngoscopy vs. fibreoptic bronchoscopy for awake tracheal intubation: a systematic review and meta-analysis. *Anaesthesia.* 2018;73(9):1151-1161.
17. Extracorporeal Life Support Organization (ELSO). ECLS registry report, International Summary. https://www.elso.org/registry/internationalsummaryandreports/internationalsummary.aspx. Accessed on April 19, 2023.
18. Malpas G, Hung O, Gilchrist A, et al. The use of extracorporeal membrane oxygenation in the anticipated difficult airway: a case report and systematic review. *Can J Anaesth.* 2018;65(6):685-697.
19. Kakizaki R, Bunya N, Uemura S, Narimatsu E. Successful difficult airway management with emergent venovenous extracorporeal membrane oxygenation in a patient with severe tracheal deformity: a case report. *Acute Med Surg.* 2020;7(1):e539.

CHAPTER 35

Management of the Difficult and Failed Airway in the ICU: Honing Our "Verbal Dexterity"

Peter G. Brindley and Jarrod M. Mosier

CASE PRESENTATION

A respiratory arrest occurs in the surgical ward. The patient is an elderly man in a cervical halo, 3 days after admission following a motor vehicle crash. Soon after a "code-blue" is called overhead to which both the intensive care unit (ICU) resident and the anesthesia/anesthesiology resident respond. Upon arrival, 15 other people are crowded into the room, including many students who were receiving a lecture nearby. The noise level is so high that it is impossible to hear anyone calling out instructions. It is also impossible to tell if someone is leading the resuscitation or preparing for intubation.

Two nurses are taking turns performing chest compressions and a respiratory therapist is performing appropriately slow bag-mask ventilation. The anesthesia resident goes to the head of the bed. He starts making suggestions: "perhaps we could intubate"; "maybe it's time for others to take over compressions" and, "I think someone needs to lead this resuscitation." Unfortunately, nobody picks up on his initial polite hints. As such, he believes he has tried but there is no point trying again if nobody will listen. Rather than escalating his concerns he becomes silent and stands at the head of the bed silently hoping somebody will hand him a laryngoscope and endotracheal tube. The ICU resident goes to the patient's right groin to insert a central line and shouts for "someone," or "anyone" to get him "the damn equipment." He is angry when nobody does and starts berating the others for being "lousy team mates."

A surgical resident arrives at this point and asks if the patient might have a postoperative pulmonary embolus and whether there are contraindications to thrombolysis. He announces that if the patient survives they ought to get "a 12-lead ECG and a bedside echo," and then he walks away. Meanwhile, the nurses performing chest compressions have become exhausted but do not know how to ask for replacements. As such they cease compressions and it is 30 seconds before another person takes over.

The anesthesia/anesthesiology resident uses this pause in chest compressions to attempt intubation, but fails. He does not know (or ask) if anyone has airway skills so tries four more times before causing an airway bleed and hence returning to bag-mask ventilation. The patient has been pulseless for 45 minutes. A nurse suggests calling the ICU attending physician. She arrives and finds a clear Do-Not-Resuscitate order on the chart. At this point, resuscitative efforts are ceased and the patient is declared dead. Several of the team members try to leave and one states dismissively: "well, he was a DNR so it doesn't matter." Instead, the attending/consultant insists they remain for an immediate debrief. She states that crisis management skills, and especially the communication skills, need to be improved. All nod their heads sagely, but when they try to be more specific the intensivist and other team members are unsure what to say.

INTRODUCTION

Why Dedicate a Chapter to Communication Skills in the Difficult and Failed Airway?

The above case includes clinical errors. However, as correctly pointed out by the Senior Intensivist, the crisis management skills and in particular, communication was especially poor. In another high-stakes industry, namely aviation, pilots can summarize their job as: "navigate, aviate, and communicate."[1] Pilots could also argue that they "fly by voice." All of this suggests that planes are flown as much by communication as by the plane's instruments.[1–4] Accordingly, those of us managing difficult and failed airways should learn to "oxygenate; ventilate; communicate" and to "resuscitate by voice."[2,3] This is because of all the human factor and crisis management skills the most important appears to be communication.[2–6]

This chapter supplements the discussion of Human Factors and Teamwork outlined in Chapter 6. Logically, if communication means to "share, join, unite, or make understanding common,"[2] then, much of what it means to create a good airway team, or to become a team member, means being a good team communicator.[2–4] However, just as teamwork—namely both leadership and followership—does not come naturally nor does crisis communication, these skills must be learned.[2–15] For these reasons, this chapter will focus on practical communication skills that can be applied to the difficult and failed airway, wherever they occur. Readers are strongly encouraged to read widely given the importance of this topic. They should also accept that being an expert airway practitioner includes being an expert airway communicator.[2–4]

Many of the ideas contained within this chapter are not native or unique to medicine (or to these authors). Instead, like the previous chapter these ideas have been translated from other high-consequence low-tolerance professions; most notably aviation. As previously stated, we should not overdo the comparison between aviation and acute care medicine. After all, planes do not take off during inclement weather, whereas the failed airway forces practitioners to routinely "fly into the storm." However, poor cockpit communication—especially between junior and senior crew—has long been understood to be one of the commonest reasons why mechanically-sound planes crash.[3–5] This is mirrored in acute medical crisis (such as the difficult and failed airway) where poor communication is recognized as a key component in preventable medical error and preventable death.[3–9] The difference is that medicine has only recently embraced deliberate communication instruction. We should accept that medicine has been a relative laggard, and that there is no more (justifiable) time to waste.

In short, this chapter on medical communication is part of medicine's long-overdue patient safety catch-up. It is also an effort to move beyond terror or hubris when it comes to the difficult and failed airway in ICU. Especially in "ectopic areas," such as the ICU, emergency room, or radiology suite (as compared to the comparatively controlled operating theatre), where a difficult airway can quickly deteriorate into a failed airway. With the risk of hyperbole, communication could be thought of as the resuscitation team's "oxygen." If so then "communication anoxia" is dangerous to the team's brain in the same way that airway anoxia is dangerous to the patient's brain. Bad communication impairs our ability to identify, predict, and coordinate. This is why we must not compound the dangers of "cannot intubate cannot oxygenate" airways by having "cannot intubate cannot communicate" teams. Fortunately, these practical skills can be taught, maintained, and mastered.

UNDERSTANDING COMMUNICATION

What Are the Basics of Communication and Communication Error?

Our communication shortfalls can be neatly summarized using a quote from Rall and Gaba: "Meant is not said; said is not heard; heard is not understood; understood is not done."[6] However, it is also important not to oversimplify something as complex as communication. The first insight is that communication is more than just talking. Good communication is a key skill that helps (or hinders) relationship building, bolsters (or stalls) information exchange and aids (or impairs) task execution.[2–4] Communication is also more than just what is said. It also includes how it is said and how it is understood.[2] As a result, nonverbal communication (which includes posture, facial expressions, gestures, and eye contact), as well as paraverbal communication (which includes pacing, tone, volume, and emphasis) are at least as important as the words that are used, or mumbled, or merely thought, but not adequately shared.[2,3] Moreover, these attributes have become more complicated now that masks and other isolation gear are muffling voices and hiding facial expressions.

Understanding communication as verbal, paraverbal, and nonverbal is especially important when there may be incongruence between the words used and the facial expression or the tone.[2–4] For example, if we say: "I don't need your help with this intubation" but in a tone that suggests otherwise then listeners are likely to downplay the verbal in favor of the nonverbal. Alternatively, they may base their response upon prior interactions (i.e., "he never wants help from anyone…no matter what he is now saying"). As such, we need to 'say what we mean and mean what we say,' and build a reputation as a straight but empathic talker. At best incongruence can increase misinterpretation, at worst it erodes teamwork (how members interact) and taskwork (how members get things done).[2–4] Congruence is even more important when those involved are unfamiliar to each other, or when the medical situation is novel.[2–4] In addition, practitioners should understand that we really cannot NOT communicate. Failing to say anything can also send its own unintended message: silence may be misinterpreted as a lack of concern or unwillingness to work with others.

Aviation made a priority of flattening the authority gradient.[5] A practical strategy is to teach, and model, "horizontal communication."[2,3] This means that all members of the team are authorized—in fact obligated—to speak up, and to do so clearly, regardless of rank.[5] Moreover, aviation has mandated "transmitter-orientated" communication (where it is the speaker's responsibility to be understood), rather than "receiver-orientated" communication (where it is the listeners responsibility to unravel what was meant).[5] However, making communication more deliberate means that we also promote active listening.[2] This requires that we confirm understanding and demand clarification, regardless of seniority, embarrassment or consequence. All team members take responsibility for how messages are delivered, received, understood, and carried out.[2–5,8]

If we compare communication to a drug, it would be one of our most potent 'therapies.' Similarly, like a drug, communication is not one-size-fits-all, nor a panacea. Like a drug, it should be used in the right dosage at the right time and tailored to the patient's needs. Like a drug, communication can also be either a "placebo" (i.e., good communication makes things better) or "nocebo" (i.e., bad communication makes things worse).[2,3] Rudeness can be profoundly detrimental (akin to a toxic drug); so can excessively passive language (akin to administering the wrong drug). Better communication should be expected to decrease litigation, maintain the hospital reputation, and bolster an individual's reputation. Regardless, all of this emphasizes why communication is everybody's business: it should be taught to trainees, expected from practitioners, supported by administration, and corrected when it errs.[2–4,11]

What Are Some Relevant Communication Models, and How Could They Be Adapted to the Difficult and Failed Airway?

Shannon and Weaver worked for Bell Laboratories approximately 50 years ago. They developed a model for verbal telephone communication that has been widely shared. It can still be applied to medicine decades later.[2] Simply put, transmitters (i.e., speakers) encode messages and receivers (i.e., listeners) decode them. However, both must be on the same channel (in medicine this equates with possessing similar situational awareness and emotional states), and there should be minimal interference (in the context of airway management means minimizing chaos, stress, and cognitive bias). They also identified the danger of "channel-overload" (translated to airway management means we must avoid communication that is unnecessarily complex). "Overload," which often results in indecision occurs unless the receiver can filter data into usable information. The practical point is that a skilled practitioner will receive data (i.e., "his oxygen saturation is dropping despite bag-mask ventilation"), but be able to turn this into actionable information (i.e., "we have a failed airway").[2]

Shannon's communication model has limitations. For example, complex communication also requires *meaning* (i.e., "we need to cric NOW"). *Meaning* is harder to encode, transmit, and decode. This is why we cannot assume that co-workers have reached the same conclusions about the patient's airway as we have. In airway management terms, this is why even the term "emergency surgical airway" may not be *fit-for-task* if the surgeon assumes tracheotomy when you meant cricothyrotomy.[2] Regardless, Shannon's model describes communication as unidirectional (transmitter to receiver), while medical decision-making is commonly multidirectional across disciplines and across hierarchies.[2–4,11]

Location (i.e., a noisy operating theatre or trauma bay) ought not to affect information transmission, but it does affect communication quality, impact, and efficiency. In other words, location can affect understanding and meaning. For example, when the transmitter and receiver are no longer face-to-face, communication loses important nonverbal cues.[2] This is why communication while wearing masks and the *medical telephone call* are important to practice. It is also why confirming understanding by routinely summarizing and "repeating back" offers an important fail-safe.[2–4,11] The more that communication is impaired (i.e., you are wearing a mask, background noise, an unfamiliar team) the more we need to speak clearly and confirm understanding. This is why norms such as demanding closed-loop communication or words to be repeated back should not be regarded as patronizing or superfluous, but rather potentially life-saving.

Modern communication models focus on relationships, not simple tasks. The "four mouths and four ears model"[2] has a sender and a listener separated by a message with four equal sides: (1) content; (2) relationship; (3) self-revelation; and (4) appeal. *Content* refers to facts and words. *Relationship* posits that senders reveal (consciously and unconsciously) how they regard receivers through specific words, intonations, and nonverbal signals. Senders indicate how they feel about themselves, namely a form of *self-revelation.* Finally, there is an *appeal* (or request) such that messages encourage the receiver to do (or not do) something. These four dimensions apply to both talker and listener: we "speak with four mouths" and "listen with four ears." This is often unconscious and depends upon the mental state, expectation, and previous interactions.[2] Notably, the sender cannot fully force the listener's mind (and vice-versa). Here is a practical airway management example: When one anesthesiologist says to another, "What do you want me to do?" they might presume that they asked an unambiguous question respecting the listener's knowledge and abilities. Though intended to be a neutral question, intonation might suggest otherwise. For example, the sender may have implied his inability to make a difficult decision or perhaps expressed frustration about the patient's condition ("he's too sick for me; I don't know what to do!"). The sender's self-revelation could be viewed to portray "appropriate concern for the patient" or "resignation" ("I don't have the time/training/authority for this airway…just tell me and I'll do it"). The request or appeal (albeit unstated) might be an attempt to subtly persuade the second anesthesiologist to assume control (i.e., "I'm outside of my comfort zone, what do you want me to do?"). In contrast, senior medical practitioners may be reluctant to seek help or surrender control. In this case, communication should unequivocally state what each person will do (i.e., "you will be intubator one; I will perform intubation attempt two while you prepare for an extraglottic device").

The listener listens with four ears, though either may be more or less open. For example, a content-based response should respond with objectivity (i.e., "because you could not intubate, I will insert an extraglottic device"). If the second medical practitioner hears the self-revelation he/she might reply: "I am comfortable taking over, but please stay as I will need your ongoing help." If the second medical practitioner is attuned to the relationship dimension, or they had previously had a fraught interpersonal relationship, then they may be more defensive (i.e., "why are you asking me; are you just trying to transfer the blame?"). Only rarely will the listener have the state of mind to decipher the appeal: "so what I think you're telling me is…" Regardless, this model shows how communication can create a virtuous cycle that builds cooperation, or a vicious cycle that destroys it.[2–4]

PRACTICAL COMMUNICATION STRATEGIES IN THE DIFFICULT AND FAILED AIRWAY

How Do We Speak Up in a Crisis?

Health care workers may not speak due to stress, overload, or uncertainty, or simply because they do not have readily available phrases.[12] Similarly, aviation talks about pilots suffering from "helmet fire" and about black box silence for minutes before a crash.[1–3] Instead of risking silence, we can teach standardized verbal responses. An example would be: "direct laryngoscopy has failed, what is our plan B and C?" Another would be: "I am unclear what has happened; please summarize?" Other team members need verbal strategies to rapidly become part of the team. A simple example could be "I am from Anesthesia; how can I help?" Over time, familiar lines also offer more than those few words suggest. For example, the explicit statement: "can't intubate, can't oxygenate" is more than just a slogan, it also implicitly communicates far more than those words alone. It should trigger the team of the need to "get help"; "get the difficult airway kit"; and also that "we have permission to perform a cricothyrotomy." It also means that team members understand the full consequences of "can't intubate, can't oxygenate." Regardless, it means that leaders need to be sufficiently verbally dexterous to communicate with both experienced and inexperienced teams (Table 35.1).

When team members are familiar with the situation or the situation is routine, implicit communication (i.e., using minimal words and assuming everyone knows their role) is perfectly acceptable. The best example perhaps is the Formula 1 pit crew whose only job is to change tires: a task that the team has practiced countless times. A corollary might be imagined: the more immature the team, the more unfamiliar the team members, the more the situation veers from an algorithm, the more we require explicit verbal coordination.

The danger of overreliance upon implicit communication in airway management is that it assumes that health care workers with varying experiences and disparate backgrounds will have a common understanding. For example, as the senior anesthesiologist you might assume that by placing a series of airway adjuncts on the patient's chest, you have adequately communicated to the entire team that you are more concerned about this airway than usual ("if Dr X is setting up all these equipment then he must be predicting difficulty, so I should too"). Unfortunately, however, implicit communication also fails to acknowledge the power of denial ("I don't believe that this airway will be difficult...therefore it won't be") or the heuristic bias (i.e., "anesthesia succeeded with direct laryngoscopy the last five times, so it will not be difficult this time").

TABLE 35.1. Practical Strategies to Improve Verbal Communication in the Difficult and Failed Airway

- Perform regular airway simulation exercises with all team members
- Practice active-listening
- Model "transmitter-oriented language"
- Ban "mitigating language"; ban rudeness
- Three **C**'s: cite names; be clear/concise; close the loop
- Structure communication using "**SBAR**" and "repeat-backs"
- "Call out" when significant changes occur
- Practice "escalating assertiveness"
- Avoid "somebody"/"anybody" comments
- Respect communication "sterility"; control interruptions

As stated above, we need tools to be sure that "we say what we mean and mean what we say." Therefore, we need to recognize the difficult airway AND declare it. Other high-task professions do not leave communication to chance. The military and aviation have used SBAR (**S**ituations, **B**ackground, **A**ssessment, **R**ecommendation) as a communication framework. While it can be overly formal—especially when team members are either familiar with each other or if the problem is routine—it offers a useful construct for junior staff, and for unfamiliar situations.[13] A simple example could be:

- Situation: "this is Dr X, I need your help now."
- Background: "I cannot oxygenate or ventilate this patient with facial trauma."
- Assessment: "We have a failed airway."
- Recommendation: "Bring me the surgical airway kit."[3,13]

The three "C's of communication" stipulate that:

- We must **cite** names (to avoid diffusion of responsibility).
- We must be **clear** and **concise** (to avoid confusion).
- Most importantly, we must **close-the-loop** (to confirm that it has been done).[2–4,8,12]

"Closing the loop" means that we reinforce (or amplify) our instructions by demanding feedback. For example, when we direct a specific person to intubate the trachea and to tell us when it is done (or tell us the end-tidal CO_2). This also means we do not just ask a colleague to increase oxygen percentage but rather: "John, increase to 100% oxygen...and call out the saturation every minute" or "Jane, immediately poke for an arterial blood gas...and bring the result back to me," or "set up a cricothyrotomy kit ...and tell me when ready." In other words, while there may be many ways to "close the loop," confirmation requires that the instruction was heard, understood, and done.

A potential additional "C" includes "crowd control." This directs that there are enough people present ("we do not have someone who can do a surgical airway, go and get me Dr X"), or that we have the right people present ("can you do a surgical airway: yes or no?"), and that too many people are present ("thank you for responding, but we need to clear out all but the following people...").

How Do We Make Ourselves Heard in a Crisis?

In addition to getting aviators to speak up, they are taught how to be acknowledged. Therefore, they learn how to use a variety of levels or grades of assertiveness.[2–5,12,14–16] For example, aviation's three-step model teaches C.U.S: I'm **C**oncerned; I'm **U**ncomfortable; this is a **S**afety issue. Aviation's four-step

P.A.C.E communication progresses from **P**robing to **A**lerting to **C**hallenging to **E**mergency language. Other aviation constructs include up to six steps. Regardless, the intention is to offer strategies from least to most direct. For example, the six-step approach includes the "hint" (e.g., "should things look like this?"); "preference" (e.g., "I would suggest..."); "query" (e.g., "what do you think?"); "shared suggestion" (e.g., "you and I could"); "statement" (e.g., "we need to") and "command" (e.g., "do this now!"). Of note, those actively listening should also pick up on the escalating urgency, and react accordingly. It is worth re-emphasizing that leaders understand that crisis communication is as much about listening as talking. As stated before (see Chapter 6) while leadership skills are very important, so are good followership skills.

Without instruction, junior team members may only hint (i.e., "perhaps you would like to try something other than repeated laryngoscopy?"), and, if ignored, fail to escalate their assertiveness.[5] On the other extreme, without instruction, senior team members may rely too heavily upon blunt commands (i.e., "give me that laryngoscope now").[5] This style is certainly unequivocal, and is needed when team members have repeatedly failed to appreciate the seriousness of a situation. However, it can destroy the team structure if routinely used as the initial, or the only, communication style.[7] With the same purpose in mind, aviation also teaches a five-step model of advocacy and confirmation.[12] The following includes aviation examples and airway corollaries: "Attention Getter" ("Captain/Doctor"). "State Your Concern" ("We're low on fuel/the patient is desaturating"). "State The Problem as You See It" ('I don't think we can land/I think we need to intubate now'). "State a solution" ("Let's re-route to a closer airport/ I'll get the difficult airway kit"). "Obtain Agreement" (e.g., "Okay, Captain/Doctor?").[12]

What Other Communication Strategies Can Be Applied to the Difficult and Failed Airway?

Another strategy is the "call out"[12] where we alert the team with important changes (i.e., "he's now desaturating").[15] Similarly, the "step back method" means we force a "time-out." This compels the team to reassess assumptions ("I know you think you saw the tube pass the cords, but what is the end-tidal CO_2"). The "repeat back method"[12] provides a safety check by repeating in order to confirm mutual understanding (i.e., "so is the next step extraglottic airway or cricothyroidotomy?"). The "read back method"[12] means we confirm a verbal order before processing it (i.e., "okay, so first you want the difficult airway kit in the room, then you want the videoscope in your left hand").

While team members are encouraged to speak up, contributions must be task-focused and appropriately timed. Aviation's "Sterile Cockpit Rule" means that no "non-operational talk" is permitted during critical phases such as taxi, take-off, or landing.[3,17,18] Of note, it applies to all those in the cockpit to enforce it, not just those currently talking.[3,17,18] This can be readily adapted to medical crises such as airway management.[2–4] For example, in less-critical situations we should confirm if others are able to focus their attention ("I want you present during this potentially difficult airway, do you have time?"). In more critical situations we can demand attention ("Stop that conversation and focus on this difficult airway"). The anesthesia practitioner (or intensivist) is in his or her critical phase during the induction of anesthesia and awakening. Therefore, others must avoid unnecessary noise or distraction. They should also learn not to take offense if asked to be quiet. Once the operation is underway, surgeons are in their critical phase and it is just as important for anesthesia practitioners to avoid unnecessary interruptions or disturbances. This includes loud music and phone conversations. In other words, all members are responsible for creating the right environment so that the right team communication can be leveraged to benefit the patient.[3,4]

Ambiguous or noncommittal speech (aka "mitigating speech") is common prior to airline crashes, as well as during medical crises.[5] This is why, during crises, we must replace comments like "perhaps we need to consider a surgical airway," or "we should think about an extraglottic device," with "get me the cric kit now" and "if this intubation fails then we are immediately moving to an attempt at extraglottic device, followed by cricothyrotomy." Junior medical practitioners (or those that feel "unsafe" in their role) may mitigate speech to show deference when embarrassed, or if unsure.[2–4] Interestingly, if time permits then "mitigating language" can be harmless, and can even aid team building (i.e., "no urgency, but if you get a moment could you give me some advice with this patient?"). However, if the wrong communication tool is used during a crisis it can be no less dangerous than the wrong airway technique. As stated, it is about being as dexterous with your voice as with your hands.

Overcautious language is inappropriate during crises, just as overly dogmatic language can be inappropriate at less critical times. Crisis communication should still be polite but must be unambiguous ("John, your next job is to intubate, do it now, please"). Communication must also be addressed to a specific person to avoid diffusion of responsibility.[2–4,8] This is why comments like "could someone?" and "does anybody?" can be as dangerous as using the wrong piece of airway equipment.[2] However, just as we need to control communication during a crisis we need to loosen the reigns once it has abated. As a result, at other times we also need to promote more free-flowing communication. This is essential for debriefing conflict management, and stress relief. In other words, communication is also essential to keep the team resilient for the next difficult or failed airway, and to build teams that the best wish to work on.[2]

SUMMARY

Communication is likely the most important nontechnical skill when it comes to the difficult and failed airway. This is especially true in the ICU where orders (such as "give this drug now," or "get me this piece of equipment") are frequently carried out by nurses while procedures (i.e., intubations, insertion of extraglottic devices) are usually performed by medical practitioners. In other words, teamwork is essential, and teamwork needs communication. Given its importance, "verbal dexterity" should not be assumed to be innate and nor should it be left to chance. First, we need to understand that communication is more than just words: it incorporates verbal, paraverbal, and nonverbal aspects. Moreover, incongruence between verbal, paraverbal, and nonverbal communication increases the likelihood of error. Fortunately, practical strategies do exist and can be readily translated from other high-stakes industries and applied to the difficult and failed airway.

Understanding the basics of communication may help those charged with managing the difficult and failed airway better manage the team and help mitigate an evolving crisis. Ultimately, though, practical strategies can be applied. These include learning and practicing standardized lines such as "can't intubate; can't oxygenate," announcing clearly when there is a difficult or failed airway and preannouncing a plan A, B, and C. Other strategies include S.B.A.R (**S**ituation, **B**ackground, **A**ssessment, and **R**ecommendation) and using the three **C**s (citing names, being **C**lear and **C**oncise, and most importantly using **C**losed-loop communication). However, in addition to speaking up, we need to ensure that our concerns are heard and acknowledged.

There are practical strategies to help health care workers become increasingly assertive. There is a three-step model using C.U.S: **C**oncerned; **U**ncomfortable; **S**afety issue, and a four-step P.A.C.E model: **P**robing; **A**lerting; **C**hallenging; **E**mergency language. A five-step model has health care workers use an "Attention Getter"; then "State Your Concern"; then "State The Problem As You See It"; then "State a solution" and finally "Obtain Agreement." A six-step model uses the "hint"; "preference"; "query"; "shared suggestion"; "statement," and "command" (e.g., "do this now!"). Regardless, all progress from least to most direct. Moreover, communication is not all about talking. Listeners should also recognize the escalating urgency, and react accordingly.

Those charged with managing the difficult and failed airway can also use a deliberate "call out" to obtain attention, and a "repeat back" whenever there is doubt. They should also avoid mitigating or overly cautious language and could manage interruptions by translating aviation's sterile cockpit rule. Finally, and so that there is no doubt, it is worth ending by reemphasizing that the best functioning airway team will understand crisis communication is as much about active listening as talking.

SELF-EVALUATION QUESTIONS

35.1. Regarding patient outcome, communication during acute medical crises:

A. Is certainly important but not as important as factual recall or manual skill

B. Is very important outside on the wards, but far less important in the operating theater

C. Appears to be the most important nontechnical skill and likely the greatest determinant of teamwork and crisis management

D. Cannot be taught, so we need to hire innate communicators

E. All of the above

35.2. The following is true about basic medical communication:

A. Verbal communication is more important than paraverbal or nonverbal communication.

B. Incongruent communication occurs when verbal, paraverbal, and nonverbal communication appear to be out-of-sync.

C. Communication can be understood using a three-voices and three-ears model: words; interpretation; meaning.

D. Shannon and Weaver, two physicians, developed a communication model initially intended for medical practitioners, but now relevant to all health care workers.

E. "Silence is golden": do not speak up unless asked to by the leader.

35.3. Which of the following is true?

A. Assertiveness can be taught using models that initially came from aviation and include three, four, five, or six steps.

B. The three Cs of communication stand for: Cite the priorities; Calm the team; Close the loop.

C. Mitigating language is helpful in a crisis so that people do not feel intimidated.

D. The "call out" and "repeat back methods" should be avoided in a medical crisis because they create too much noise.

E. Aviation's Sterile Cockpit Rule means everybody has to be quiet in case the captain needs to speak.

REFERENCES

1. Skygod quotes. http://www.skygod.com/quotes/cliches.html. Accessed July 2015.
2. St Pierre M, Hofinger G, Buerschaper C. *Crisis Management in Acute Care Settings: Human factors and team psychology in a high stakes environment.* New York: Springer; 2008.
3. Cyna AM, Andrew MI, Tan SGM, Smith AF, eds. *Handbook of Communication in Anaesthesia and Critical Care. A Practical Guide to Exploring the Art.* Oxford University Press; 2011.
4. Brindley PG, Reynolds SF. Improving verbal communication in critical care medicine. *J Crit Care.* 2011;26:155-159.
5. Gladwell M. The ethnic theory of plane crashes. In: Gladwell M, ed. *Outliers.* New York: Little, Brown & Co; 2008:177-223.
6. Rall M, Gaba D. Human performance and patient safety. In: Miller R, ed. *Miller's Anesthesia.* Philadelphia, PA: Elsevier Churchill Livingstone; 2005: 3021-3072.
7. Aron D, Headrick L. Educating physicians prepared to improve care and safety is no accident: it requires a systematic approach. *Qual Saf Health Care.* 2002;11:168-173.
8. Gaba DM, Fish KJ, Howard SK. *Crisis Management in Anesthesiology.* New York: Churchill Livingstone; 1994.
9. Gawande A. The checklist. In: Gawande A, ed. *The Checklist Manifesto.* New York: Henry Holt and Company; 2009:32-48.
10. Brindley PG. Patient safety and acute care medicine: lessons for the future, insights from the past. *Crit Care.* 2010;14(2):217-222.
11. Brindley PG, Smith KE, Cardinal P, Leblanc F. Improving medical communication: skills for a complex (and multilingual) world. *Can Respir J.* 2014;21:89-91.
12. Dunn EJ, Mills PD, Neily J, Crittenden MD, Carmack AL, Bagian JP. Medical team training: applying crew resource management in the Veterans Health Administration. *Jt Comm Qual Patient Saf.* 2007;33(6): 317-325.

13. SBAR Institute for Healthcare Improvement. SBAR Technique for Communication: a situational briefing model. http://www.ihi.org/IHI/Topics/PatientSafety/SafetyGeneral/Tools/SBARTechniqueforCommunicationASituationalBriefingModel.htm. Accessed August 2015.
14. Leonard M, Graham S, Bonacum D. The human factor: the critical importance of effective communication in providing safe care. *Qual Saf Health Care*. 2004;13(suppl):i85-90.
15. Fischer U, Orasanu J. Cultural diversity and Crew Communication 1999. http://www.lcc.gatech.edu/~fischer/AIAA99.pdf. Accessed July 2015.
16. Besco, RO. To intervene or not to intervene? The copilots 'catch 22': Developing flight crew survival skills through the use of 'P.A.C.E'. 1994. http://www.crm-devel.org/resources/paper/PACE.PDF. Accessed July 2015.
17. Airbus flight operations briefing notes. Human performance: managing interruptions and distractions. http://www.skybrary.aero/bookshelf/books/176.pdf. Accessed July 2015.
18. The Sterile Cockpit Rule Aviation Safety Reporting System (ASRS) 1993. http://asrs.arc.nasa.gov/publications/directline/dl4_sterile.htm. Accessed July 2015.

SECTION 6

AIRWAY MANAGEMENT IN THE OPERATING ROOM

CHAPTER 36

Airway Management Considerations for Robotic-Assisted Laparoscopic Prostatectomy

Susan Galgay

CASE PRESENTATION

A 65-year-old man presents for robotic-assisted laparoscopic prostatectomy (RALP). He is an ex-smoker with 50 pack-years of smoking and chronic obstructive pulmonary disorder (COPD). He is on salbutamol puffers as needed. He has no allergies. He weighs 90 kg (198 lb) and is 165 cm (5'4") tall (BMI 33.1 kg·m^{-2}). His oxygen saturation on room air was 95%.

Preoperative airway assessment reveals no predictors of difficult laryngoscopic intubation with Mallampati score of II, thyromental distance 3 finger breaths (5 cm), and normal range of cervical spinal motion and full dentition. Following induction with fentanyl, propofol, and rocuronium, a Cormack/Lehane Grade 2 view of the larynx is visualized via direct laryngoscopy using a # 3 Macintosh blade. The trachea is intubated using a 7.5 mm ID endotracheal tube (ETT) and secured at 24 cm at the lips. A 14 Fr orogastric (OG) tube is inserted and confirmed in the stomach via aspiration of a small amount of gastric contents. A gauze bite block is placed, and the eyes are protected with tape and hard goggles.

The patient is placed in steep Trendelenburg position with a tilt of 30 degree and secured using bean bag restraint. Pneumoperitoneum is achieved with a peak insufflation pressure of 12 mmHg and the robot docked in place.

INTRODUCTION

■ What Is the Robotic-Assisted Laparoscopic Prostatectomy (RALP)?

RALP, also known as robotic-assisted radical prostatectomy [RARP]) is a minimally invasive procedure utilizing pneumoperitoneum to visualize intra-abdominal contents.[1] The instruments are attached to an immobile robot via bulky arms that are remotely manipulated by the surgeon. The robot allows a higher degree of precision and better visualization of tissues than a standard laparoscopic technique. The goal of this technique is reduced surgical blood loss, decreased postoperative pain, and a shorter hospital stay than a traditional radical prostatectomy.[2] Limited access to the patient due to the bulky robot, unintended injury from the robot, ensuring a completely immobile patient, and steep Trendelenburg position plus pneumoperitoneum with subsequent potential difficult ventilation are but a few of the anesthetic concerns with robotic-assisted prostate/pelvic surgery.

■ What Are Your Concerns When a Patient Is Placed in the Steep Trendelenburg Position for a Prolonged Period of Time?

Intra-abdominal robotic-assisted surgery involves gaining access to the desired anatomy via a traditional laparoscopic approach. The ports and instruments are placed by the surgeon and pneumoperitoneum is attained. The patient is then positioned head down, the robot rolled into position, and the instruments attached, typically to 4 to 6 arms. The robot is then docked and at this point, the patient is essentially attached to the robotic instruments and immovable. The robot is bulky, limiting access to the patient for assessment, airway adjustment, vascular access, and emergency procedures. Additionally, unanticipated injury is possible from the arms and instruments touching the patient. The surgeons then control the robot remotely leaving one assistant to assist in the procedure directly manipulating laparoscopic instruments.

Robotic-assisted prostatectomy requires extreme head-down positioning, 30 to 40 degrees while in the lithotomy position combined with pneumoperitoneum with the arms tucked at the sides. Once the robot is docked, there is little access to the patient for any further monitors, line, or ETT adjustments.

This position is complicated by the risk of stretch, pressure, and ischemic injury to nerves. In the extreme head-down position there is potential for compression and stretch of the brachial plexus with the use of shoulder braces to prevent the patient from sliding cephalad. At our center, a specially formed compressive bean bag along with anti-slip cushions are used to prevent patient movement and avoid direct pressure on the shoulders and brachial plexus. In addition, the common peroneal nerve must be free from pressure in the lithotomy position. As the legs may be elevated for a prolonged time, care must be taken to avoid unduly low mean arterial pressure (MAP) as the elevated limbs may potentially be underperfused and prone to ischemic nerve injury and compartment syndrome.

Cardiovascular changes may include increased systemic vascular resistance, increased MAP, increased myocardial oxygen consumption, and decreased renal, portal, and splanchnic flow. Difficulty in performing cardiopulmonary resuscitation due to the presence of the docked robot and extreme positioning is ever-present.

The respiratory system is also severely impacted. Since gravitational forces push the abdominal contents and diaphragm cephalad, the functional residual capacity (FRC) is reduced with a resultant predisposition for atelectasis. Increased pulmonary blood flow and gravitational force on mediastinal structures further impede FRC and pulmonary compliance. Vital capacity is decreased, and peak airway pressures are elevated. Hypercarbia and respiratory acidosis may result.[3]

Cerebral blood flow and intracranial and intraocular pressures are all increased. Release of catecholamines and activation of the renin-angiotensin system occurs.

Airway considerations include difficult ventilation with high airway pressure, potential for upper airway edema, and impaired access due to the docked robot.

AIRWAY MANAGEMENT

In the Setting of RALP, What Is the Differential Diagnosis of High Airway Pressures and How Would You Address Them?

High airway pressure is not an uncommon occurrence during surgery and is often easily managed. Diagnosing and treating the source of high airway pressure must be promptly assessed and managed. In this situation, with limited patient access and a fixed surgical position due to a docked robot, examination of the patient may prove difficult. High on the differential is endobronchial intubation. Even though the ETT is still observed to be 24 cm at the lips as initially secured when supine, due to the combination of extreme head-down positioning and pneumoperitoneum, the trachea may move cephalad and thereby lead to a mainstem ETT placement.[4] Evidence shows the combination of a steep Trendelenburg position and the creation of pneumoperitoneum may decrease the distance from the carina to the vocal cords by up to 1 cm.[5] Other studies show that it is pneumoperitoneum alone that may be the cause of endobronchial intubation. Chang et al.[6] demonstrated that shortening of the "carina to tube tip difference" observed on pneumoperitoneum and not displacement of the ETT with position change was the culprit. The lungs may be easily compressed and shifted upward with the creation of pneumoperitoneum, thus pushing the mobile carina cephalad and decreasing the ETT tip-to-carina distance. However, the upper trachea is connected to the muscles and ligaments of the larynx and maintains a relatively fixed position. It is recommended that the ETT be positioned mid-trachea at the outset and its position checked after positioning and the creation of the pneumoperitoneum to avoid endobronchial intubation during the surgical procedure.

Mitigating and corrective actions such as switching to 100% oxygen and manual mode of ventilation to assess lung compliance while notifying the surgical team should be the initial steps, followed by auscultation of the lungs bilaterally to ensure correct ETT positioning and ensuring ventilator synchrony with additional muscle paralysis if necessary. In the event repositioning is indicated, the ETT cuff may be deflated, and the tube is carefully withdrawn while actively listening to the breath sounds. When bilateral breath sounds are confirmed the ETT may be resecured in place. Alternatively, and perhaps more safely, a flexible bronchoscope can be used to correctly position the ETT tip in the mid-trachea.

Light anesthesia (with a cough) is probably the most common cause of intra-operative high airway pressure, which can be easily treated (e.g., increase anesthesia depth and muscle paralysis). Other potential sources of high airway pressures must also be sought. These include obstructed ETT with secretions or aspirations, kinked circuit or tube, valve misfunction on the ventilator, bronchospasm (secondary to tracheal irritation or COPD), pulmonary edema, pneumothorax, and anaphylaxis.

One novel cause of difficult ventilation and high airway pressures noted by Pathan et al.[7] is complete ETT occlusion due to pneumoperitoneum while in a steep Trendelenburg position. Despite the withdrawal of the ETT, repeated airway obstruction occurred with abdominal insufflation. After assessment using a flexible bronchoscope, it was determined that during pneumoperitoneum insufflation, the trachea, diaphragm, and mediastinal structures shifted such that the ETT was occluded in the absence of a murphy eye in the tube. Once the ETT was switched to a conventional ETT with a murphy eye, the case proceeded uneventfully.

After Ruling Out Other Causes as Stated Earlier, High Airway Pressures Are Still Noted with a Peak Inspiratory Pressure (PIP) of 35 Cm H_2O. How Would You Address This Problem?

The initial steps should include ruling out catastrophic causes such as pneumothorax and tension pneumothorax secondary to barotrauma. Checking with the surgical team to ensure minimal pneumoperitoneum inflation pressures are used is an easy first intervention. Commonly, switching ventilation settings will be helpful. In the setting of RALP, Choi et al.[8] reported that the use of pressure-controlled ventilation (PCV) resulted in lower peak airway pressures and greater dynamic compliance compared to volume-controlled ventilation (VCV). In PCV, inspiratory flow is delivered by a decelerating flow pattern; thus, the flow rate naturally decays as the patient's lungs fill on inspiration. As such, adequate tidal volumes may be achieved at lower PIPs because laminar flow is promoted and a more even distribution of gasses is achieved. Decelerating flow wave pattern is associated with a significant reduction in total resistance, improved pulmonary compliance, decreased dead space ventilation, and improved oxygenation.[9]

How Common Are Pneumothorax, Pneumomediastinum, and Subcutaneous Emphysema (SCE) Associated with RALP and What Are the Appropriate Management Steps?

In the setting of high insufflation pressures, insufflated CO_2 may traverse the diaphragm via a natural hiatus and cause increased intrathoracic pressures and difficulty with ventilation. Cessation of insufflation should resolve these problems. Slow reinsufflation and maintenance of pressures less than 12 mmHg should limit the impact of this event.

The risk of SCE increases with maximal $ETCO_2$ greater than or equal to 50 mmHg, operative time greater than 200 minutes, six or more port sites and older patients.[10] Should SCE develop in prefascial planes and contribute in this way to pneumothorax, pneumomediastinum and pneumopericardium may result.

Diagnosis of pneumothorax is made clinically by absence of breath sounds and hyperresonance on percussion on the affected side. Upright chest X-ray (CXR) shows the absence of lung markings on the affected side, while ultrasound may show the absence of typical lung sliding with respiration. Due to the limited access to the patient and docked robot, CXR is not feasible. Diagnosis will be based on clinical assessment and possibly, ultrasound examination.

Prompt cessation of insufflation should resolve these issues. Overall, hypercarbia may persist with resultant acid-base disturbances. Maintenance of controlled ventilation is indicated until the resolution of acid-base derangements.

Tension pneumothorax may result from barotrauma secondary to high mechanical ventilation pressures. In this scenario, hemodynamic instability may ensue. Immediate recognition, communication, and treatment of this complication are imperative. Elevated jugular venous pressure (JVP), trachea deviation away from the affected side and absence of previously present breath sounds are hallmarks of this complication. Management includes placing the patient on 100% oxygen, communicating the suspicion to the surgical team, and rapidly decompressing the tension pneumothorax with a large bore IV cannula placed in the second intercostal space in the midclavicular line of the affected side. Improvement of both hemodynamics and ventilation should occur. Definitive treatment with a surgically placed chest tube in the fifth intercostal space just anterior to the midaxillary line should follow.

After 4 Hours of Surgical Time, the Pneumoperitoneum Is Released, the Robot Undocked, and the Patient Returned to The Supine Position. Upon Examination, Facial Edema and Chemosis Are Noted. What Are Your Immediate Concerns Regarding Emergence and Extubation?

Several hours of steep Trendelenburg positioning can lead to edema of the head and neck and a reduction in pulmonary compliance. Clinical swelling of the face and upper airway with venous stasis is common. Chemosis has been associated with decreased nasal airflow thus indicating upper airway edema and potential for postextubation stridor and need for reintubation.

Fluid restriction to a total volume of less than 2 L of crystalloid is recommended to reduce the risk of upper airway swelling and is restricted to no more than 800 mL given prior to completion of the vesicourethral anastomosis.[10]

The patients should be returned to the supine or slightly head-up positions as soon as possible after robot undocking to facilitate venous drainage and limit edema.

Other risk factors for laryngeal edema in addition to that from positioning and excessive fluid loading. These include high endotracheal cuff pressure, traumatic intubation, and hypoalbuminemia.

A high index of suspicion for laryngeal edema should be present. Prior to extubation, the patient should be otherwise optimized with a complete reversal of muscle paralysis and adequate spontaneous ventilation. A cuff-leak test or endoscopic examination of the laryngeal inlet may be warranted (see Chapter 38).

In Addition to Facial Swelling, There Is Also Substantial Facial SCE. Video Laryngoscopy Shows SCE in the Airway (see Figure 36.1). Discuss Your Management

SCE of the upper airway and hypopharynx may cause compression of tissues and acute complete airway obstruction upon extubation. Endoscopic airway examination may be useful to evaluate glottic edema due to fluid, ETT positioning, and SCE. The patient should remain intubated and transferred to the intensive care unit for observation until the SCE is resolved, pCO_2 normalized, and normal acid-base status returned. Extubation should require the patient be weaned from controlled ventilation, alert, and have a reassuring endoscopic examination of the glottis with resolution of the SCE and airway edema.

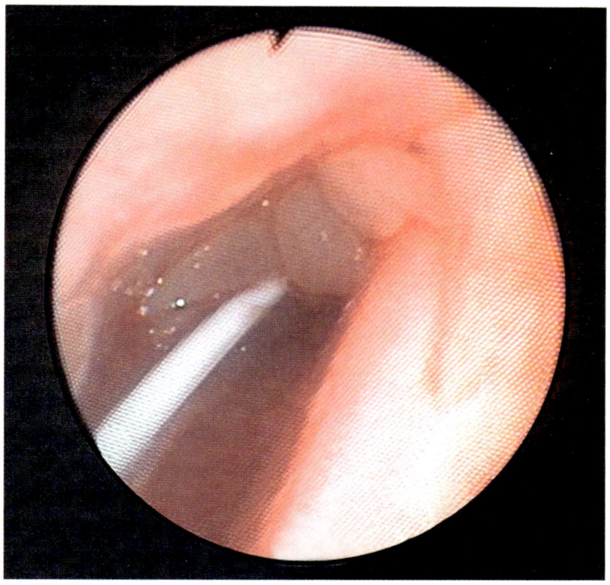

FIGURE 36.1. Subcutaneous emphysema of the airway of a patient following robotic-assisted laparoscopic prostatectomy (RALP).

SUMMARY

RALP has several anesthesia considerations for the airway practitioner. Steep Trendelenburg position combined with pneumoperitoneum may lead to unintentional mainstem intubation and high airway pressures.

Ventilation may also be challenging due to positioning and pneumoperitoneum leading to complications from barotrauma such as pneumothorax, tension pneumothorax, and SCE. Extreme positioning and limited access to the patient due to the robot may cause difficulty in assessing and diagnosing these complications. A high index of suspicion for airway obstruction postextubation should be maintained and potentially delayed extubation for the resolution of upper airway edema. A careful extubation plan should be in place and preparation made for immediate reintubation.

SELF-EVALUATION QUESTIONS

36.1. Which of the following is true for robotic-assisted laparoscopic prostatectomy (RALP)?

A. Allows a rapid return of urinary function

B. Reduces blood loss

C. Promotes a higher rate of potency recovery

D. Reduces length of hospital stay

E. All of the above

36.2. Physiologic changes associated with robotic-assisted laparoscopic prostatectomy (RALP) include all **EXCEPT:**

A. Decreased FRC

B. V/Q mismatch

C. Increased SVR

D. Increased CVP

E. Decreased ICP

36.3. Factors contributing to high airway pressures during robotic-assisted laparoscopic prostatectomy (RALP) include:

A. Steep Trendelenburg position

B. Pneumoperitoneum

C. Endobronchial intubation

D. Light anesthesia

E. All of the above

CHAPTER 36

REFERENCES

1. Yaxley JW, Coughlin GD, Chambers SK, et al. Robot-assisted laparoscopic prostatectomy versus open radical retropubic prostatectomy: early outcomes from a randomised controlled phase 3 study. *Lancet.* 2016;388:1057-1066.
2. Ilic D, Evans SM, Allan CA, Jung JH, Murphy D, Frydenberg M. Laparoscopic and robotic-assisted versus open radical prostatectomy for the treatment of localised prostate cancer. *Cochrane Database Syst Rev.* 2017; 9:CD009625.
3. Irvine M, Patil V. Anaesthesia for robot-assisted laparoscopic surgery. *Continuing Education in Anaesthesia Critical Care and Pain.* 2009; 9(4):125-129.
4. Iqbal H, Gray M, Gowrie-Mohan S. Anaesthesia for robot-assisted urological surgery. In: Holmes K, ed. *Anesthesiologists. Tutorial 408.* WFSA; 2019.
5. Lee JR. Anesthetic considerations for robotic surgery. *Korean J Anesthesiol.* 2014;66:3-11.
6. Chang CH, Lee HK, Nam SH. The displacement of the tracheal tube during robot-assisted radical prostatectomy. *Eur J Anaesthesiol.* 2010;27:478-480.
7. Pathan H, Gulati S. A case of airway occlusion in robotic surgery. *J Robot Surg.* 2007;1:169-170.
8. Choi EM, Na S, Choi SH, An J, Rha KH, Oh YJ. Comparison of volume-controlled and pressure-controlled ventilation in steep Trendelenburg position for robot-assisted laparoscopic radical prostatectomy. *J Clin Anesth.* 2011;23:183-188.
9. Pillai SA. *Mechanical Ventilation Made Easy.* Jaypee Brothers Medical Pub; 2009.
10. Gainsburg DM. Anesthetic concerns for robotic-assisted laparoscopic radical prostatectomy. *Minerva Anesthesiol.* 2012;78:596-604.

CHAPTER 37

Airway Management of a Patient with a History of Radiation Therapy

Carrie L. Goodine

CASE PRESENTATION

A 79-year-old male presents with an open right clavicle fracture secondary to osteoradionecrosis. He is scheduled for a right neck dissection, clavicle debridement, and potential left pectoralis major flap.

Three years back, he underwent a tonsillectomy and then a selective right neck dissection and brachial plexus exploration for squamous cell carcinoma. This was followed by a 5-week course of high-dose cisplatin chemotherapy and radiation. Progression of radiation damage resulted in eventual clavicle fracture and protrusion through the skin.

The remainder of his past medical history is significant for osteoarthritis, controlled hypothyroidism, and acid reflux. Other past surgical history includes hip and knee arthroplasties and inguinal hernia repair. He quit smoking 30 years back, consumes little alcohol, and exercises regularly. His medications include amoxicillin/clavulanate, acetaminophen, celecoxib, rabeprazole, and levothyroxine.

On examination, he is in no apparent distress. His vital signs are: blood pressure 130/80, heart rate 76 beats per minute, respiratory rate 18 breaths per minute, temperature 36.5°C, and oxygen saturation 98% on room air. He is 183 cm tall and weighs 84 kg (BMI 25.1 $kg{\cdot}m^{-2}$). Auscultation of his chest yields normal heart sounds with no extra heart sounds or murmurs, and clear breath sounds bilaterally.

Airway examination reveals a Mallampati III classification. Mouth opening, thyromental distance, and mandibular protrusion were within normal limits. Neck extension is severely limited (see Figure 37.1). He has full natural dentition. Examination and palpation of his neck reveal woody, indurated tissue extending from his right ear superiorly to larynx anteriorly, to the dressing that covers the open wound mid-clavicle (see Figures 37.1 and 37.2). His larynx is immobile.

INTRODUCTION

What Anatomic and Pathophysiologic Changes Occur Following Radiotherapy to the Structures of the Oral Cavity and Neck?

Radiotherapy inflicts a radiochemical injury to both normal and malignant cells.[1] The damage is related to the total radiation dose and the method of radiotherapy delivery. In order to achieve adequate tumor control, damage to normal tissues is inevitable.[1–3] Radiation also activates various cellular signaling pathways that lead to the release of proinflammatory and profibrotic cytokines and vascular injury.[4] Early (acute) tissue toxicities from radiotherapy are arbitrarily considered to occur within 90 days of the commencement of treatment, and late effects beyond 90 days of treatment.[2,5] Early side effects are observed during or shortly after a course of radiotherapy, whereas late effects manifest after a latent period and may not be evident until years following the radiotherapy.[2,6] In general, tissues with rapidly dividing cell populations such as mucous membranes and skin demonstrate acute effects of radiation (mucositis, desquamation), whereas those with slowly proliferating cells such

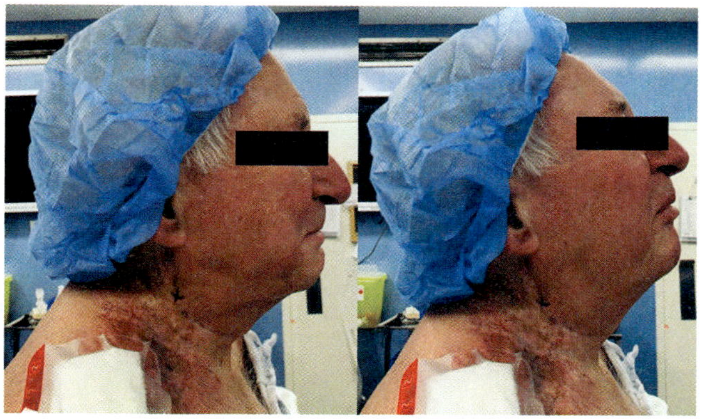

FIGURE 37.1. Limited cervical spine extension in a patient with history of right neck dissection and radiotherapy.

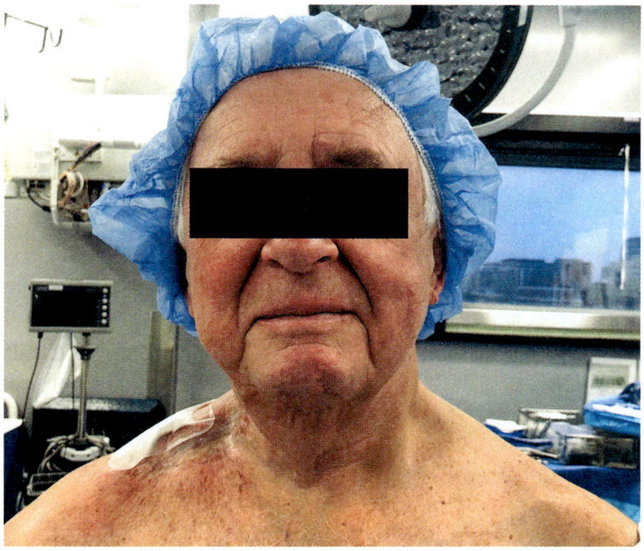

FIGURE 37.2. Appearance of the external neck following right neck dissection and radiotherapy. Note the telangiectasia, loss of normal skin creases, and thickened appearance of the anterior neck on the irradiated side.

as organ parenchyma, connective and vascular tissues demonstrate late effects (edema, fibrosis).[2,7] The severity of the late effects of radiation therapy in general cannot be predicted by the severity of the acute effects.[7] Late radiation sequelae are usually irreversible and progressive, with increasing severity over time.[2] Progression of late effects has been reported up to 34 years after therapy.[4]

Mucosal Damage

Following radiation therapy to the oral cavity, pharynx, or larynx, the mucous membranes can become erythematous within 1 week, and develop areas with white pseudomembranes (mucositis) at about 2 weeks.[7] The patches of mucositis may coalesce by the third week.[7] This acute mucosal reaction usually heals within 2 to 4 weeks following the completion of radiotherapy, although ulceration and necrosis can occur.[6] Late effects of radiation on the mucosa are characterized by thinning or atrophy of the epithelium, telangiectasia, dryness, a loss of mucosal mobility, submucosal induration, and occasionally chronic ulceration and necrosis.[8] The mucosa is fragile and more susceptible than normal to mechanical injury.[7]

Laryngeal Edema

Edema is seen in the subcutaneous or submucosal soft tissue in the early phase following radiotherapy, can persist for 6 to 12 months,[9] and can become chronic.[5,10] Edema occurs when vascular permeability is increased by inflammatory mediators or when venous or lymphatic passages are obstructed[11] and is associated with the duration of radiotherapy treatments, dose per fraction, total number of fractions, and the interval between fractions.[12]

Laryngeal cartilage covered by normal mucous membrane usually tolerates conventional fractionated high-dose radiation therapy.[6,7] However, arytenoid edema, chondritis, vocal cord palsy,[3,13] and rarely, chondronecrosis can occur (see Figures 37.3B, 37.4B, 37.5, 37.6, 37.7B, and 37.8).[1] Laryngeal edema can occur at any time following the completion of radiation therapy[14] and can produce airway compromise.[10]

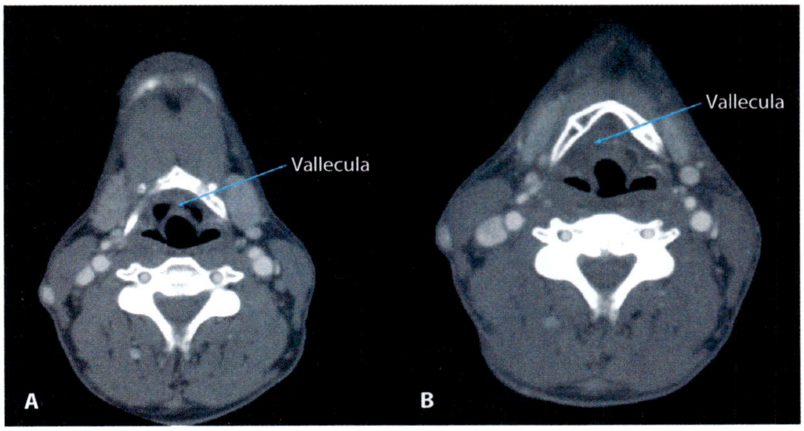

FIGURE 37.3. CT scans of the head and neck at the level of the vallecula. **(A)** Normal soft tissues of the upper airway with normal vallecula. **(B)** Postradiotherapy soft tissue swelling in the vallecula.

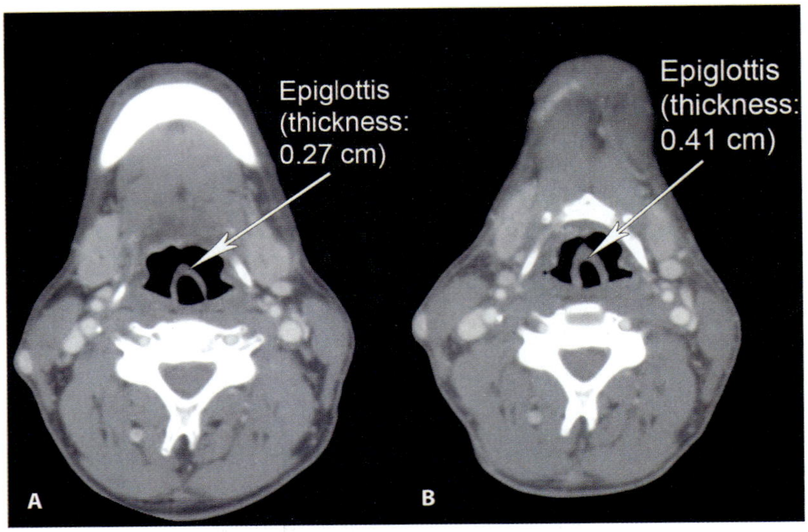

FIGURE 37.4. CT scans of the head and neck. **(A)** Normal epiglottis. **(B)** Postradiotherapy thickening of the epiglottis.

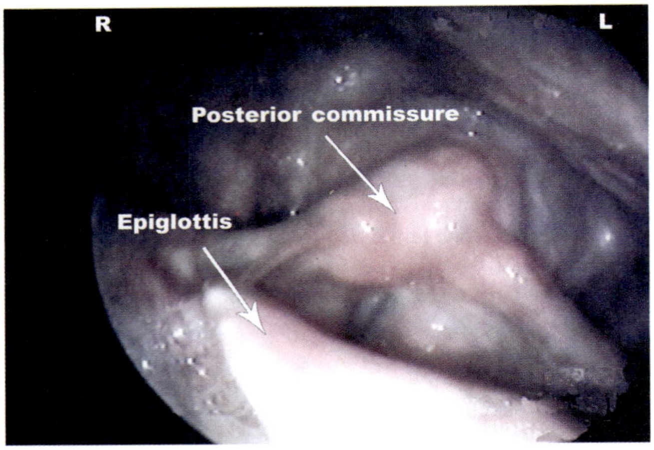

FIGURE 37.5. Laryngeal inlet view through a bronchoscope shows a normal epiglottis. Note the sharp leaf-like edge along the right lateral aspect.

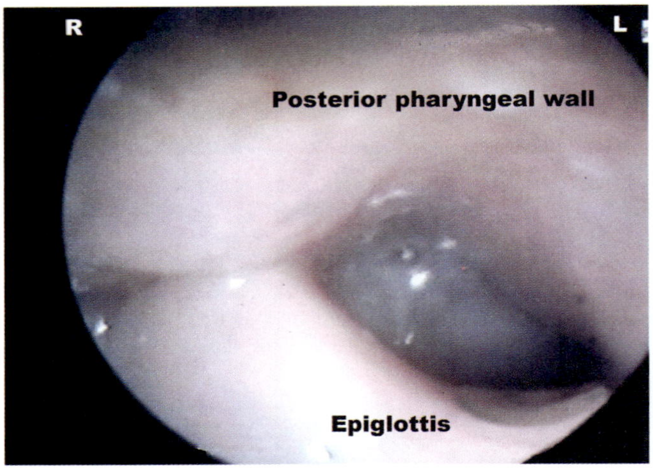

FIGURE 37.6. Laryngeal inlet view through a bronchoscope shows the appearance of the edematous epiglottis following radiotherapy.

Radiotherapy-induced laryngeal edema occurs on a continuum from mild to severe,[12] and can be graded from 0 (absent) to 4 (necrosis).[15] After radiotherapy for head and neck cancer, 15% to 59% of patients develop ≥ Grade 2 laryngeal edema within 2 years.[16] Grade 2 (moderate) edema is not associated with significant or symptomatic airway obstruction.[15] However, severe laryngeal edema (Grade 3) may cause airway obstruction and require an urgent tracheotomy.[16] Laryngeal chondronecrosis (Grade 4) has been reported to occur up to 22 years following radiotherapy.[10]

Laryngeal edema which persists for more than 3 months after radiotherapy may suggest the presence of residual or recurrent tumor[16] and local recurrence in about 50% of patients was noted to be associated with persistent laryngeal edema.[16]

Tissue Fibrosis

Fibrosis is one of the most common delayed radiation-associated manifestations.[7] Radiation of fibroblasts leads to induced differentiation and a significant increase in collagen deposition[17]; this upregulation may persist and be resistant to housekeeping processes that normally terminate fibrogenesis.[18]

Radiation fibrosis usually appears in subcutaneous tissues within 6 to 12 months of treatment,[7] although it can occur as early as 4 to 12 weeks.[8] The fibrosis tends to be slowly progressive,[7] nonhomogeneous, and variable in extent and severity from site to site.[19] The severity of the fibrosis increases when high total doses of radiation and large fraction sizes are used.[6] The risk of developing moderate to severe fibrosis has been reported to be about 40%.[5] The affected soft tissue loses elasticity and subcutaneous fat[8] and is indurated to palpation.[1,8] In the presence of moderate to severe fibrosis, contracture of the tissues also occurs.[1] In severe cases, the soft tissues develop a woody consistency and may form a hard mass fixed to the skin and underlying muscle or bone (see Figures 37.1 and 37.2).[7] Fibrotic contractures of neck tissue can produce a limitation of neck extension.[8,20]

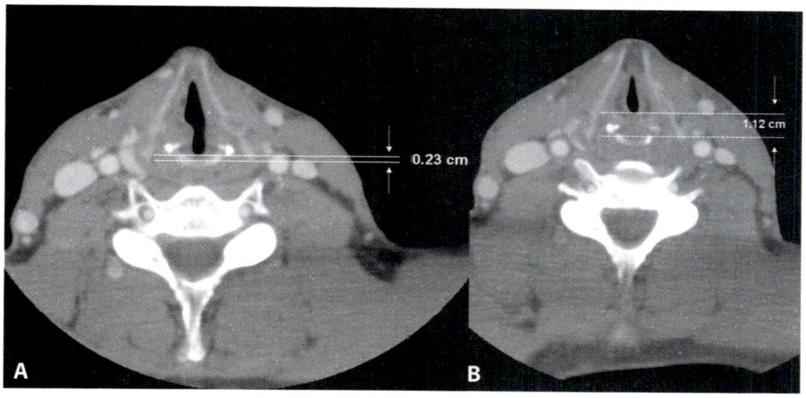

FIGURE 37.7. CT scans of the head and neck. **(A)** Normal soft tissue thickness at the posterior commissure (0.23 cm); and **(B)** Edema at the level of arytenoid cartilages and the posterior commissure (1.12 cm) following radiotherapy.

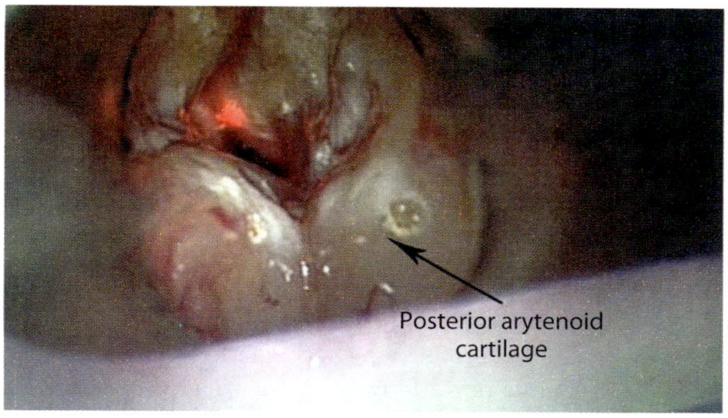

FIGURE 37.8. Laryngeal inlet view through a bronchoscope shows the appearance of the arytenoid cartilages and adjacent supraglottic area following radiotherapy. Note the extensive thickening and tissue distortion.

Voluntary and involuntary muscles exposed to high-dose irradiation can also develop fibrosis. Fibrotic changes in the muscles of mastication (the temporalis, masseter, and pterygoid muscles) may result in trismus.[7] The temporomandibular joint itself is however relatively resistant to ankylosis secondary to radiation injury.[7] Radiotherapy has been reported to reduce mouth opening by 18% (SD, 17%) within 12 months of follow-up.[21,22] Although trismus may be apparent during the course of radiation therapy, it may not become apparent until 3 to 6 months after radiotherapy.[21] The prevalence of trismus after radiotherapy for head and neck cancer has been reported to be between 5% and 38%.[22,23]

Radiation-induced fibrosis may affect airway patency and protection. Fibrosis of the pharyngeal musculature can produce swallowing dysfunction[24] and a predisposition to aspiration.[3] Stenosis of the pharynx or supraglottic larynx can occur and lead to airway compromise.[7,25–27] Stenosis of the larynx at the glottic level, associated with fixation of the vocal cords due to a scar at the posterior glottis, is not unusual after radiotherapy for carcinoma of the larynx.[27] Choanal stenosis thought to be associated with severe mucosal reaction followed by fibrosis has also been reported after radiotherapy for nasopharyngeal carcinoma.[28] Radiotherapy in head and neck cancer patients has also been associated with the development of obstructive sleep apnea.[29] The cause is likely multifactorial and may include persistent mucosal edema, decreased elasticity, increased fibrosis, and poor pharyngeal constriction.[29]

Radiation therapy can also produce vascular injury which includes intimal thickening, atheroma formation, and fibrosis of the media and adventitia.[7] The capillary network is particularly vulnerable to radiotherapy and obstruction can occur due to endothelial cell injury and thrombosis.[18] Telangiectasia and atrophy are common late effects[17,18] and a reduction in the microvascular network can ultimately lead to ischemia.[19] Tissue ischemia may be a consequence of or contribute to the radiation injury.[18] Narrowing or obstruction of larger arteries can also occur, as can occlusive thrombosis.[19] The changes in the vessel walls are similar to those associated with atherosclerosis due to aging.[8] Symptomatic carotid atherosclerosis can be a result of cervical irradiation and may require surgical intervention.[14]

Xerostomia and Dental Caries

Radiation injury to the salivary glands produces a decrease in saliva production and a change in the composition of saliva.[7] Typically, about 60% to 65% of the total salivary volume is produced by the parotid glands, 20% to 30% by the submandibular glands, and 2% to 5% by the sublingual glands.[7] The remainder of the salivary volume is produced by anonymous minor salivary glands distributed throughout the oral cavity and pharynx and which are variable from patient to patient.[7] The degree of salivary gland dysfunction depends on the volume of the glands included in the radiation field and the total dose administered.[7] It is usually not possible to irradiate the pharynx or the upper jugular nodes without irradiating the submandibular glands; however, the parotid and submandibular glands can be partially shielded during treatment.[6] Intensity-modulated radiotherapy can also be used to preserve salivary flow.[30,31] A significant reduction in salivary flow occurs within 1 week of fractionated radiotherapy to the head and neck.[7] Salivary flow may become barely measurable by the end of a 6- to 8-week course of treatment and the xerostomia may be permanent.[8] Xerostomia causes discomfort, alters taste acuity, and contributes to a deterioration in dental hygiene.[7]

The diminished salivary flow has an altered electrolyte content and reduced pH, and promotes dental decay as the normal oral microflora is altered to a highly cariogenic microbial population.[7] In the absence of stringent measures to protect the teeth, caries can develop within 3 to 6 months and lead to the complete destruction of dentition within 3 to 5 years.[7] Dental extractions from an irradiated mandible can precipitate osteoradionecrosis.[6]

What Other Systemic Effects Occur Following Radiotherapy?

Hypothyroidism occurs in 5% to 10% of patients who undergo irradiation of the lower neck,[6] and fibrosis of the apical segments of the lungs can also occur.[7]

Patients with collagen vascular diseases such as scleroderma, rheumatoid arthritis, and systemic lupus erythematosus appear to have an increased incidence and severity of late normal tissue radiation toxicity[18] and comorbidities with impaired vascularity such as diabetes and hypertension may have an adverse effect. Age may also be a factor.[4]

AIRWAY MANAGEMENT

What Airway Management Difficulties Can Be Anticipated Following Radiotherapy to the Oral Cavity, Pharynx, Larynx, or Neck?

Radiotherapy to the oral cavity, pharynx, larynx, or neck can result in limited mouth opening, limited cervical spine extension, the noncompliant immobile fibrotic soft tissue in the floor of the mouth and pharynx, edema and fibrosis of the laryngeal walls,[30] and vocal cord dysfunction.[13] Airway management can be difficult in the presence of these anatomic changes. The degree of difficulty for each management modality is dependent on the site and the extent of the altered anatomy.

Can Ventilation by Face Mask or Extraglottic Device Be Anticipated to Be More Difficult?

In a review of 53,041 general anesthetics in whom FMV had been attempted, Kheterpal et al. identified 77 cases of **impossible** FMV (0.15%).[32] Of the 77 patients who were impossible to ventilate using a face mask, 19 (25%) also demonstrated difficult intubation. However, the incidence of difficult intubation in the subgroup of patients with neck radiation was not provided.[32] Both univariate and multivariate analyses demonstrated neck radiation to be the most significant clinical predictor of impossible FMV. Of the subgroup of 310 patients with neck radiation, 3 could not be ventilated using a face mask. In a subsequent study, Kheterpal et al. reported an incidence of 0.4% for difficult FMV combined with difficult laryngoscopy in a series of 176,679 patients undergoing general anesthesia.[33] Neck mass or radiation was an independent predictor of difficult FMV combined with difficult laryngoscopy.[33] FMV and laryngoscopy serve as primary rescue techniques for each other and the inability to ventilate using a face mask in the setting of a difficult intubation has significant potential for morbidity and mortality.[33,34]

Giraud et al. assessed the ease of FMV and laryngeal mask airway (LMA®) placement in nine patients after oral or cervical radiation.[20] FMV was easy for all nine patients. All five of the oral radiotherapy patients had limited mouth opening, and LMA placement was difficult but successful. Two patients with severe limitation of mouth opening (0.7 and 0.5 cm) required retromolar passage of the LMA. Once successfully passed, ventilation was satisfactory in all five patients. LMA placement was easy in the 4 patients who had received *cervical* radiation, but positive-pressure ventilation was difficult. On bronchoscopic examination through the LMA, the vocal cords could not be visualized in any of these four patients due to vestibular fold collapse. Muscle relaxation did not improve the laryngeal view. Ventilation was impossible in two of the four patients; however, orotracheal intubation was successful. Bronchoscopic intubation via the LMA was not attempted as the glottis could not be visualized. The authors theorized that the presence of the LMA in a narrow, nondistensible hypopharynx may have compressed the larynx and thereby produced glottic collapse.[20]

Ferson et al. reported the use of the Intubating LMA® Fastrach™ (ILMA) in 254 patients with difficult airways, of whom 40 had airway changes related to previous surgery, radiation therapy, or both.[35] In this subset of patients, the authors reported that the correct positioning of the device was more difficult. There were no insertion failures and ventilation was possible in all cases. Bronchoscopic intubation through the ILMA was also successful in all 40 patients. The authors felt that a loss of elasticity due to fibrosis in the neck tissues made positioning of the ILMA more difficult and suggested that bronchoscopic guidance be used when attempting intubation through the ILMA in this group of patients.[35]

Langeron et al. compared the efficacy of blind intubation through the ILMA to bronchoscopic intubation in a group of 100 patients with anticipated difficult intubation undergoing scheduled surgery.[36] In this prospective randomized crossover study, intubation was attempted postinduction either by blind intubation through the ILMA or bronchoscopic intubation through an Ovassapian Airway. In the event of failure of the first technique, the alternative technique was utilized. The first randomly assigned technique failed in seven patients: four in the bronchoscopic group and three in the ILMA group. All were successfully intubated by the alternative technique. In the ILMA group, all three failures occurred in patients who had undergone previous cervical radiotherapy. The operators noted the difficulty in attaining an effective seal and aligning the ILMA with the glottis. This was attributed to nondistensible mucosal and neck tissues. Despite an inadequate seal, the ILMA did prevent oxygen desaturation during intubation attempts. The authors concluded that blind intubation via ILMA could not be recommended in patients with previous cervical radiotherapy.[36]

Siddiqui et al. reported a case of airway rescue using a LMA® Supreme™ in a patient who had undergone oral radiotherapy and who had severe trismus.[37] FMV was difficult. The airway was maintained with the LMA Supreme until an open tracheotomy was performed. Singh et al. similarly reported a case of airway rescue with the Ambu® AuraOnce™ in a postradiotherapy patient who was in respiratory distress.[38] FMV was difficult and intubation by direct laryngoscopy (DL) failed after three attempts. The airway was maintained with the Ambu AuraOnce until a tracheotomy was completed.

Following oral or cervical radiotherapy, FMV may be difficult or impossible.[32] The use of an extraglottic device (EGD) may not be successful due to limited mouth opening or obstruction at the level of the larynx.[35,36] An EGD may prevent oxygen desaturation in emergency situations until a definitive airway can be achieved.[36,38]

Can Endotracheal Intubation by Direct Laryngoscopy Be More Difficult Following Oral or Cervical Radiotherapy?

Trismus, reduced cervical spine extension, and reduced laryngeal mobility due to postradiation fibrosis can make visualization of the glottis by DL difficult or impossible. Fibrotic subcutaneous and submucosal soft tissues lack compliance and may constitute a poorly mobile woody mass that cannot be elevated easily, if at all, on DL. Postirradiation atrophic mucosa is also easily traumatized, and bleeding can readily occur. A thickened edematous epiglottis can obscure glottic visualization, and decreased vocal cord mobility may interfere with glottic cannulation (see Figures 37.4B, 37.6, and 37.7B).

Yaney reported a Cormack-Lehane Grade 3 view with a #3 Macintosh blade following induction of general anesthesia in a patient who had undergone left radical neck dissection and postoperative radiation 10 years back.[39] A "frozen larynx" that was "fibrotic and swollen" was described. Tracheal intubation with a 6.5-mm ID endotracheal tube (ETT) using a #3 Miller blade was difficult but successful.[39]

Reed and Frost reported a case of hypopharyngeal stenosis following cervical radiation.[25] The larynx could not be visualized by DL. Mask ventilation was performed and intubation using a flexible bronchoscope was successful.[25]

In 2012, Iseli et al. reported a series of 152 difficult airway cases associated with head and neck pathology.[40] Intubation techniques included inhalational induction followed by "routine" laryngoscopy (38), vessel dilator cricothyrotomy (44), awake nasotracheal bronchoscopic intubation (68), and awake tracheotomy (2). Of those who had undergone previous radiotherapy, 34 were intubated without difficulty, 5 experienced some difficulty (>3 attempts or >10 minutes of attempted intubation), and 3 required a change of the intubation plan. It is unclear how many of the patients who had radiotherapy underwent DL. One "can't ventilate, can't intubate" patient was "safely allowed to emerge." Radiotherapy was identified as a predictor of airway difficulty.[40]

Delbridge et al. reported 30 consecutive patients who had been treated with head and neck radiation for childhood malignancy who presented for thyroidectomy.[41] Twenty-eight patients underwent straightforward tracheal intubation by DL after induction of general anesthesia but two were unsuccessful. One underwent flexible bronchoscopic intubation under local anesthesia and one who had a Grade 4 laryngeal view had the surgery completed with an LMA.

Arne et al. reported difficult intubation in 12.3% of patients undergoing ENT cancer surgery, although the number of patients who had previous radiotherapy was not specified.[42]

Patients with neck pathology have been identified as having an increased risk of difficult or failed DL.[32,42]

Can Endotracheal Intubation by Video Laryngoscopy or Alternate Intubation Techniques Be More Difficult Following Oral or Cervical Radiotherapy?

Video laryngoscopy of all types (hyperangulated, Macintosh, channeled) has been shown to reduce the risk of failed intubation as compared to Macintosh DL.[43] Successful intubation of a 32-year-old patient who had had previous chemotherapy and radiation for rhabdomyosarcoma of the neck and laryngeal elevation surgery was reported using the PENTAX Airway Scope®.[44] Gupta et al. described successful GlideScope® video laryngoscope (GVL)-assisted nasotracheal intubation using the cuff inflation technique in five patients with oropharyngeal cancer.[45] Mouth opening was limited but greater than 1.8 cm; enough to admit the GVL blade.[45] Successful intubation using the Airtraq® combined with the flexible bronchoscope has also been described in a patient who had a difficult airway subsequent to extensive radiation to the neck.[46] The first attempts with each device alone were unsuccessful, and the authors commented that the combination of both devices overcame their individual limitations.[46] Moon et al. described successful awake GVL intubation in a patient with severe radiation-induced arytenoid swelling who refused awake bronchoscopic intubation.[47]

Despite higher overall first-pass and rescue success rates, video laryngoscopy is not without risk of failure, particularly in patients with a history of oral or cervical radiotherapy. Aziz et al. reviewed 2004 GVL intubations in patients undergoing general anesthesia at two institutions.[48] The authors identified four preoperative predictors significantly associated with failed GVL intubation: neck anatomy, thyromental distance, reduced cervical motion, and institution. Altered neck anatomy due to previous surgery, mass or radiation was found to be the strongest predictor of GVL failure.[48] The authors emphasized the importance of maintaining competency with alternate intubation methods.[48]

Limited mouth opening may preclude rigid bronchoscopic techniques, and flexible bronchoscopic intubation under general anesthesia may be more difficult in the presence of distorted anatomy and decreased mobility of the airway structures. Huitink et al. described awake flexible bronchoscopic intubation in a series of 37 head and neck cancer patients with difficult airways, 29 of whom had chemoradiation.[49] A difficult airway was defined as one in which the airway could not be intubated using conventional laryngoscopy, based on preoperative airway examination.[49] Truong and Truong reported a patient who required bilateral dacryocystorhinostomy and had severe trismus after radiotherapy.[23] The interincisor distance was 9 mm. The first surgery was done following awake nasotracheal intubation, and the second after retromolar bronchoscopic intubation under general anesthesia. Tomioka et al. reported ventilation by face mask under general anesthesia to be easy in a patient who had undergone radiotherapy for a pharyngeal tumor.[50] However, bronchoscopic intubation with a 7.0-mm ID ETT was not possible due to tracheal stenosis, which the authors postulated may have been produced by the radiation therapy.[50]

Langeron et al. reported failed blind intubation through the ILMA in patients who had cervical radiation.[36] However, Ferson et al. reported successful bronchoscopic intubation through the ILMA in patients who had airway changes secondary to radiotherapy.[35]

The light-guided technique using a lightwand is best avoided in the presence of anatomic distortion of the airway.[51] Laryngotracheal abnormality has also been cited as a relative contraindication to retrograde intubation.[52]

Radiation damage to the upper airway may render video laryngoscopy, bronchoscopic intubation, and the use of other advanced intubation techniques more difficult or even impossible. This highlights the importance of a thorough airway exam, a comprehensive and safe airway plan, and maintenance of skill with a few complementary devices.[48]

Can a Front-of-Neck Airway (FONA) Be More Difficult in This Group of Patients?

Radiation-induced subcutaneous fibrosis in the neck can obscure surface anatomical landmarks, obliterate tissue planes, and make a surgical approach to the airway technically challenging (see Figures 37.1 and 37.2). Percutaneous cricothyrotomy may fail in this setting, and open tracheotomy may require more time to complete and be associated with more bleeding.[53] If loss of the airway were to occur during attempts to intubate from above, an emergency FONA may not secure the airway in time. This possibility must be considered when the plan for airway management is made.[32]

What Should Be the Approach to Airway Management in These Patients?

Neck radiation produces a wide spectrum of pathophysiology[32] and airway management of the patient following cervical or oral radiotherapy requires a careful airway assessment. The assessment should focus on the four "dimensions" of airway management as outlined by Murphy et al., and be used to predict potential difficulty with (1) FMV, (2) ventilation using an EGD, (3) laryngoscopy and tracheal intubation, and (4) FONA.[54] When obstructing airway pathology is suspected, the standard airway examination should be enhanced by a review of the patient's most recent CT or MRI scan, and/or performance of awake nasal endoscopy or an oral "awake look" with a video laryngoscope after upper airway topicalization.[55,56]

Each patient and context must be evaluated individually. The increased risk of difficult or impossible FMV,[32] EGD use,[20] laryngoscopy,[33] and surgical airway[32,53] in patients with a history of head and neck radiotherapy should inform this decision-making process. If difficult tracheal intubation is predicted but FMV and EGD use appears viable, then it may be appropriate to manage the airway after induction of anesthesia. In this case, an experienced airway practitioner should perform the intubation, and with a device (e.g., a video laryngoscope) that is likely to maximize first-pass success. If significant difficulty is predicted with more than one of the three modes of ventilation from above (i.e., FMV, EGD use, and tracheal intubation), then awake tracheal intubation should be strongly considered.[57]

Awake intubation with careful upper airway topicalization maintains a wide margin of safety; the patient maintains their own airway patency, protection, and gas exchange.[56,57] If mouth opening is sufficient, a bronchoscope,[56,58] video laryngoscope,[56,59] or a combination of devices can be used to intubate the trachea orally or nasally. Following radiotherapy to the floor of the mouth and/or pharynx, severe trismus may preclude oral intubation techniques, and in this setting awake nasal bronchoscopic intubation may be the most reasonable option.[60] Patient comfort during the procedure may be optimized by positioning them in a sitting or semi-sitting position, and the addition of Heliox may further improve work of breathing if there is evidence of partial airway obstruction.[56]

Despite a good overall safety profile, awake tracheal intubation may fail for a number of reasons. These include nonnavigable anatomy, inadequate airway topicalization, oversedation, lack of patient cooperation, especially in patients with obstructing airway pathology, and complete airway obstruction.[57] Potential causes of complete obstruction in these patients include oversedation and an increase in airflow resistance due to the effects of local anesthetic on airway patency.[61,62] Due to the increased possibility of failed awake tracheal intubation in obstructed patients, the airway practitioner should have an alternate plan in reserve. This plan may involve rapid conversion to a FONA.[57]

Inhalational induction with the maintenance of spontaneous ventilation has been described for the facilitation of tracheal intubation in the setting of obstructing airway pathology.[40,61] However, the functional loss of upper airway tone that occurs with loss of consciousness is exaggerated by sedatives.[63] In combination with an already narrowed airway, this may result in collapse and complete obstruction with inspiration.[64] The 4th National Audit Project (NAP4) of the Royal College of Anaesthetists and the Difficult Airway Society reported 16 patients with head and neck pathology who underwent inhalation induction of anesthesia.[65] In 12 of these patients, spontaneous ventilation became more difficult and oxygen desaturation occurred. In 11 patients, spontaneous ventilation became impossible. These patients developed respiratory distress, airway obstruction, and hypoxemia, and did not rapidly awaken when airway compromise occurred.[65] The audit clearly outlines the hazards of using inhalational induction in adult patients with head and neck pathology. As such, it is not a recommended strategy for these patients.[57]

Patients who have an extremely compromised airway, severe stridor, gross anatomic distortion, or a larynx that cannot be visualized on endoscopy should undergo awake tracheotomy performed under local anesthesia.[56,61]

How Should This Patient's Airway Be Managed?

Previous anesthetic records were available for review. Ten years back, his airway examination was documented as normal for all indices. FMV was described as easy with an oropharyngeal airway (OPA), and a Cormack-Lehane Grade 2 view with percentage of glottic opening (POGO) 10% was obtained with Macintosh DL. The blade size was not described. Seven years later, on assessment for his selective neck dissection, an airway examination revealed a Mallampati III score with severely limited neck extension. FMV was described as easy, and a C-MAC® D-BLADE revealed a Grade 1 view. The anesthesia practitioner deliberately chose the hyperangulated blade based on a prior poor view with the Macintosh blade. There were no issues with EDD advancement in either case.

Three years after selective neck dissection and radiotherapy, he presented with osteoradionecrosis of the clavicle, as described earlier in the chapter. In addition to the routine airway exam, a recent CT scan was reviewed, and the absence of airway obstruction was confirmed. His neck was palpated carefully to assess radiation-induced changes. He was found to have supple, mobile submandibular tissues, and a woody, immobile external larynx (see Figures 37.1 and 37.2). He had noticed no vocal changes since his radiotherapy. Easy FMV was predicted based on previous records and the absence of radiation changes to his submandibular space. Difficult DL was predicted, based on both the previous records and the development of laryngeal induration in the interim. EGD use was thought likely to be successful. FONA was not predicted to be difficult. Due to easily predicted bag-mask ventilation, the anesthesia practitioner deemed it safe to induce the patient and perform tracheal intubation postinduction. They prepared a hyperangulated video laryngoscope (in this case a C-MAC with a D-BLADE) and had a flexible bronchoscope on standby in case of difficulty.

Routine monitoring and IV access were established. The patient was induced in the standard fashion after careful denitrogenation. FMV was easy with an OPA, and a Grade 1 glottic view was easily obtained with hyperangulated video laryngoscopy. The glottic view was then deliberately decreased to Grade 2 for easier ETT passage,[66] and a 7.5-mm ID ETT advanced easily over a stylet. The bronchoscope was not required. Surgery proceeded uneventfully, and the patient was extubated at the end without incident.

POSTINTUBATION CONSIDERATIONS

How Should This Patient Be Extubated?

Severe postextubation laryngeal obstruction due to laryngeal edema has been reported following hepatic resection in a patient who had previously undergone bilateral modified radical neck dissection and radiation therapy.[67] However, laryngeal edema was judged to be unlikely following this relatively brief surgical procedure in which the volume of intravenous fluid administered was small. Furthermore, no evidence of airway obstruction existed preoperatively. If concern exists about pharyngeal or laryngeal edema, an inspection of the pharynx and supraglottic larynx could be carried out by video laryngoscopy prior to emergence. Consideration could also be given to extubation over an 11- or 14-Fr airway exchange catheter, maintaining the tip of the catheter above the carina[57]

SUMMARY

Radiotherapy to the head and neck can produce limited mouth opening, limited cervical spine extension, noncompliant fibrotic soft tissue in the floor of the mouth and pharynx, and alteration of laryngeal anatomy. It is the most significant clinical predictor of impossible FMV[32] and neck mass or radiation is an independent predictor of difficult FMV combined with difficult laryngoscopy.[34] Altered neck anatomy due to previous surgery, mass or radiation is the strongest predictor of GVL failure.[47] DL or video laryngoscopy, EGD use,[20,35,36] bronchoscopic intubation,[50] and performance of a FONA may all be difficult following radiotherapy to the head and neck. Neck radiation changes should be a cause for concern during airway management.[32]

Airway management of the patient following cervical or oral radiotherapy, therefore, requires a careful airway assessment focused on the prediction of difficult FMV, difficult EGD utilization, difficult laryngoscopy and intubation, and difficult FONA. A corresponding airway plan should include safe backup options in case of failure. While complete obstruction has been reported during topicalization and instrumentation of the airway, awake intubation, in general, maintains a wide margin of safety. It is the preferred method when difficulty is predicted with more than one of the three modes of ventilation from above (i.e., FMV, EGD use, and tracheal intubation).[57] If awake intubation is not possible due to severely aberrant or obstructed anatomy, consideration should be given to awake tracheotomy under local anesthesia.

SELF-EVALUATION QUESTIONS

37.1. Which of the following is **NOT** true in the airway management of a patient with a history of radiotherapy to the head and neck?

A. Surgical airway should be uncomplicated.

B. Limited mouth opening may preclude rigid bronchoscopic intubation.

C. Fibrosis of the structures of the floor of the mouth can make direct laryngoscopy difficult.

D. A decrease in vocal cord mobility may interfere with glottic cannulation.

E. In the presence of anatomic distortion of the airway, the light-guided technique using a lightwand is best avoided.

37.2. The most significant clinical predictor of impossible facemask ventilation is:

A. Neck radiation changes

B. Obesity

C. Obstructive sleep apnea

D. Presence of a beard

E. Male sex

37.3. Anatomic and pathophysiologic changes associated with head and neck radiotherapy include:

A. Edema

B. Fibrosis

C. Trismus

D. Xerostomia

E. All of the above

REFERENCES

1. Larson DL. Management of complications of radiotherapy of the head and neck. *Surg Clin North Am.* 1986;66:169-182.
2. Dörr W. Pathogenesis of normal tissue side effects. In: Joiner MC, van der Kogel A, eds. *Basic Clinical Radiobiology.* 5th ed. Boca Raton, FL:CRC Press; 2018:152-170.
3. Wu CH, Hsiao TY, Ko JY, Hsu MM. Dysphagia after radiotherapy: endoscopic examination of swallowing in patients with nasopharyngeal carcinoma. *Ann Otol Rhinol Laryngol.* 2000;109:320-325.
4. Stone HB, Coleman CN, Anscher MS, McBride WH. Effects of radiation on normal tissue: consequences and mechanisms. *Lancet Oncol.* 2003;4:529-536.
5. Trotti A. Toxicity in head and neck cancer: a review of trends and issues. *Int J Radiat Oncol Biol Phys.* 2000;47:1-12.
6. Millender LE. Complications of radiation therapy. In: Eisele DW, Smith RV, eds. *Complications in Head and Neck Surgery.* 2nd ed. Edinburgh:Saunders; 2009:167-179.
7. Parsons J, Mendenhall WM, Million RR. Complications of radiotherapy for head and neck neoplasms. In: Weissler MC, Pillsbury HC, eds. *Complications of Head and Neck Surgery.* New York:Thieme Medical Publishers; 1995:194-229.
8. Cooper JS, Fu K, Marks J, Silverman S. Late effects of radiation therapy in the head and neck region. *Int J Radiat Oncol Biol Phys.* 1995;31:1141-1164.
9. Gaitini LA, Fradis M, Vaida SJ, Somri M, Malatskey SH, Golz A. Pneumomediastinum due to Venturi jet ventilation used during microlaryngeal surgery in a previously neck-irradiated patient. *Ann Otol Rhinol Laryngol.* 2000;109:519-521.
10. Weissler MC. Management of complications resulting from laryngeal cancer treatment. *Otolaryngol Clin North Am.* 1997;30:269-278.
11. Ichimura K, Sugasawa M, Nibu K, Takasago E, Hasezawa K. The significance of arytenoid edema following radiotherapy of laryngeal carcinoma with respect to residual and recurrent tumour. *Auris Nasus Larynx.* 1997;24:391-397.
12. Patterson JM, Hildreth A, Wilson JA. Measuring edema in irradiated head and neck cancer patients. *Ann Otol Rhinol Laryngol.* 2007;116:559-564.
13. Lau DP, Lo YL, Wee J, Tan NG, Low WK. Vocal fold paralysis following radiotherapy for nasopharyngeal carcinoma: laryngeal electromyography findings. *J Voice.* 2003;17:82-87.
14. Francfort JW, Smullens SN, Gallagher JF, Fairman RM. Airway compromise after carotid surgery in patients with cervical irradiation. *J Cardiovasc Surg.* 1989;30:877-81.
15. Rancati T, Schwarz M, Allen AM, et al. Radiation dose-volume effects in the larynx and pharynx. *Int J Radiat Oncol Biol Phys.* 2010;76:S64-S69.
16. Bae JS, Roh JL, Lee SW, et al. Laryngeal edema after radiotherapy in patients with squamous cell carcinomas of the larynx and hypopharynx. *Oral Oncol.* 2012;48:853-858.
17. Dorr W, Hendry JH. Consequential late effects in normal tissues. *Radiother Oncol.* 2001;61:223-231.
18. Denham JW, Hauer-Jensen M. The radiotherapeutic injury–a complex 'wound'. *Radiother Oncol.* 2002;63:129-145.
19. Constine LS, Milano MT, Friedman D, et al. Late effects of cancer treatment on normal tissues. In: Halperin EC, Perez CA, Brady LW, eds. *Perez and Brady's Principles and Practice of Radiation Oncology.* 5th ed. Philadelphia: Wolters Kluwer Health/Lippincott Williams & Wilkins; 2008:320-335.
20. Giraud O, Bourgain JL, Marandas P, Billard V. Limits of laryngeal mask airway in patients after cervical or oral radiotherapy. *Can J Anaesth.* 1997;44:1237-1241.
21. Goldstein M, Maxymiw WG, Cummings BJ, Wood RE. The effects of antitumor irradiation on mandibular opening and mobility: a prospective study of 58 patients. *Oral Surg Oral Med Oral Pathol Oral Radiol Endod.* 1999;88:365-373.
22. Dijkstra PU, Kalk WW, Roodenburg JL. Trismus in head and neck oncology: a systematic review. *Oral Oncol.* 2004;40:879-889.
23. Truong A, Truong DT. Retromolar fibreoptic orotracheal intubation in a patient with severe trismus undergoing nasal surgery. *Can J Anaesth.* 2011;58:460-463.
24. Mittal BB, Pauloski BR, Haraf DJ, et al. Swallowing dysfunction–preventative and rehabilitation strategies in patients with head-and-neck cancers treated with surgery, radiotherapy, and chemotherapy: a critical review. *Int J Radiat Oncol Biol Phys.* 2003;57:1219-1230.
25. Reed AP, Frost EA. Radiation induced hypopharyngeal stenosis masquerading as the larynx: a case report. *Middle East J Anaesthesiol.* 2010;20:731-733.
26. Nageris B, Elidan J, Sichel JY. Aerodigestive tract obstruction as a late complication of radiotherapy. *J Laryngol Otol.* 1995;109:68-69.
27. Stevens MS, Chang A, Simpson CB. Supraglottic stenosis: etiology and treatment of a rare condition. *Ann Otol Rhinol Laryngol.* 2013;122:205-209.
28. Ku PK, Tong MC, Tsang SS, van Hasselt A. Acquired posterior choanal stenosis and atresia: management of this unusual complication after radiotherapy for nasopharyngeal carcinoma. *Am J Otolaryngol.* 2001;22:225-229.
29. Zhou J, Jolly S. Obstructive sleep apnea and fatigue in head and neck cancer patients. *Am J Clin Oncol.* 2015;38:411-414.
30. Sanguineti G, Adapala P, Endres EJ, et al. Dosimetric predictors of laryngeal edema. *Int J Radiat Oncol Biol Phys.* 2007;68:741-749.
31. Rancati T, Fiorino C, Sanguineti G. NTCP modeling of subacute/late laryngeal edema scored by fiberoptic examination. *Int J Radiat Oncol Biol Phys.* 2009;75:915-923.
32. Kheterpal S, Martin L, Shanks AM, Tremper KK. Prediction and outcomes of impossible mask ventilation: a review of 50,000 anesthetics. *Anesthesiology.* 2009;110:891-897.
33. Kheterpal S, Healy D, Aziz MF, et al. Incidence, predictors, and outcome of difficult mask ventilation combined with difficult laryngoscopy: a report from the multicenter perioperative outcomes group. *Anesthesiology.* 2013;119:1360-1369.
34. Kheterpal S, Han R, Tremper KK, et al. Incidence and predictors of difficult and impossible mask ventilation. *Anesthesiology.* 2006;105:885-891.
35. Ferson DZ, Rosenblatt WH, Johansen MJ, Osborn I, Ovassapian A. Use of the intubating LMA-Fastrach in 254 patients with difficult-to-manage airways. *Anesthesiology.* 2001;95:1175-1181.
36. Langeron O, Semjen F, Bourgain JL, Marsac A, Cros AM. Comparison of the intubating laryngeal mask airway with the fiberoptic intubation in anticipated difficult airway management. *Anesthesiology.* 2001;94:968-972.
37. Siddiqui S, Seet E, Chan WY. The use of laryngeal mask airway supreme in rescue airway situation in the critical care unit. *Singapore Med J.* 2014;55:e205-e206.
38. Singh M, Srivastava M, Kapoor D. AMBU-LM aura once® in management of difficult airway in post-radiotherapy oral burns patient admitted in intensive care unit. *J Anaesthesiol Clin Pharmacol.* 2014;30:574-575.
39. Yaney LL. Double-lumen endotracheal tube for one-lung ventilation through a fresh tracheostomy stoma: a case report. *AANA J.* 2007;75:411-415.
40. Iseli TA, Iseli CE, Golden JB, et al. Outcomes of intubation in difficult airways due to head and neck pathology. *Ear Nose Throat J.* 2012;91:E1-E5.
41. Delbridge L, Sutherland J, Somerville H, Steinbeck K, Stevens G. Thyroid surgery and anaesthesia following head and neck irradiation for childhood malignancy. *Aust N Z J Surg.* 2000;70:490-492.
42. Arne J, Descoins P, Fusciardi J, et al. Preoperative assessment for difficult intubation in general and ENT surgery: predictive value of a clinical multivariate risk index. *Br J Anaesth.* 1998;80:140-146.
43. Hansel J, Rogers AM, Lewis SR, Cook TM, Smith AF. Videolaryngoscopy versus direct laryngoscopy for adults undergoing tracheal intubation. *Cochrane Database Syst Rev.* 2022;4:CD011136.
44. Sunohara M, Okada T. An adult case of difficult intubation caused by late complications of radiotherapy for pediatric neck malignancy, as well as a later laryngeal elevation surgery. *Masui.* 2015;64:1269-1272.
45. Gupta N, Garg R, Saini S, Kumar V. GlideScope video laryngoscope-assisted nasotracheal intubation by cuff-inflation technique in head and neck cancer patients. *Br J Anaesth.* 2016;116:559-560.
46. Matioc AA. Use of the Airtraq with a fibreoptic bronchoscope in a difficult intubation outside the operating room. *Can J Anaesth.* 2008;55:561-562.
47. Moon HS, Choi YW, Koh HJ, Chon JY, Park MR. Awake Glidescope® intubation in patients with severe arytenoid swelling after laryngeal surgery with radiation therapy. *Korean J Anesthesiol.* 2013;65:S34-S35.
48. Aziz MF, Healy D, Kheterpal S, Fu RF, Dillman D, Brambrink AM. Routine clinical practice effectiveness of the Glidescope in difficult airway management: an analysis of 2,004 Glidescope intubations, complications, and failures from two institutions. *Anesthesiology.* 2011;114:34-41.

49. Huitink JM, Balm AJ, Keijzer C, Buitelaar DR. Awake fibrecapnic intubation in head and neck cancer patients with difficult airways: new findings and refinements to the technique. *Anaesthesia.* 2007;62:214-219.
50. Tomioka T, Ogawa M, Sawamura S, Hayashida M, Hanaoka K. A case of post-radiation therapy patient with difficulty in intubation unexpected preoperatively. *Masui.* 2003;52:406-408.
51. Scott J, Hung OR. Intubating introducers, stylets, and lighted stylets (Lightwands). In: Hagberg CA, ed. *Benumof and Hagberg's Airway Management.* 3rd ed. Philadelphia, PA: W.B. Saunders; 2013:430-442.
52. Dhara SS. Retrograde tracheal intubation. *Anaesthesia.* 2009;64:1094-1104.
53. Ho AM, Chung DC, To EW, Karmakar MK. Total airway obstsruction during local anesthesia in a non-sedated patient with a compromised airway. *Can J Anaesth.* 2004;51:838-841.
54. Murphy M, Hung O, Launcelott G, Law JA, Morris I. Predicting the difficult laryngoscopic intubation: are we on the right track? *Can J Anaesth.* 2005;52:231-235.
55. Rosenblatt W, Ianus AI, Sukhupragarn W, Fickenscher A, Sasaki C. Preoperative endoscopic airway examination (PEAE) provides superior airway information and may reduce the use of unnecessary awake intubation. *Anesth Analg.* 2011;112:602-607.
56. Law JA, Morris IR, Malpas G. Obstructing pathology of the upper airway in a post-NAP4 world: time to wake up to its optimal management. *Can J Anaesth.* 2017;64:1087-1097.
57. Law JA, Duggan LV, Asselin M, et al. Canadian Airway Focus Group updated consensus-based recommendations for management of the difficult airway: part 2. Planning and implementing safe management of the patient with an anticipated difficult airway. *Can J Anaesth.* 2021;68:1405-1436.
58. El-Boghdadly K, Onwochei DN, Cuddihy J, Ahmad I. A prospective cohort study of awake fibreoptic intubation practice at a tertiary centre. *Anaesthesia.* 2017;72:694-703.
59. Rosenstock CV, Thogersen B, Afshari A, Christensen AL, Eriksen C, Gatke MR. Awake fiberoptic or awake video laryngoscopic tracheal intubation in patients with anticipated difficult airway management: a randomized clinical trial. *Anesthesiology.* 2012;116:1210-1216.
60. Nagarkar R, Kokane G, Wagh A, et al. Airway management techniques in head and neck cancer surgeries: a retrospective analysis. *Oral Maxillofac Surg.* 2019;23:311-315.
61. Mason RA, Fielder CP. The obstructed airway in head and neck surgery. *Anaesthesia.* 1999;54:625-628.
62. Liistro G, Stanescu DC, Veriter C, Rodenstein DO, D'Odemont JP. Upper airway anesthesia induces airflow limitation in awake humans. *Am Rev Respir Dis.* 1992;146:581-585.
63. Maddison KJ, Walsh JH, Shepherd KL, et al. Comparison of collapsibility of the human upper airway during anesthesia and during sleep. *Anesth Analg.* 2020;130:1008-1117.
64. Hillman DR, Platt PR, Eastwood PR. The upper airway during anaesthesia. *Br J Anaesth.* 2003;91:31-39.
65. Patel A, Pearce A, Prady M. Head and neck pathology. In: Cook TM, Woodall N, Frerk C, eds. *4th National Audit Project of the Royal College of Anaesthetists and the Difficult Airway Society Major Complications of Airway Management in the United Kingdom.* London: RCoA; 2011:143-154.
66. Gu Y, Robert J, Kovacs G, et al. A deliberately restricted laryngeal view with the GlideScope video laryngoscope is associated with faster and easier tracheal intubation when compared with a full glottic view: a randomized clinical trial. *Can J Anaesth.* 2016;63:928-937.
67. Burkle CM, Walsh MT, Pryor SG, Kasperbauer JL. Severe postextubation laryngeal obstruction: the role of prior neck dissection and radiation. *Anesth Analg.* 2006;102:322-325.

CHAPTER 38

Airway Management of a Patient in Prone Position

Dennis Drapeau and Orlando R. Hung

CASE PRESENTATION

A 35-year-old intoxicated male 179 cm tall and weighing 110 kg (BMI 34 kg·m^{-2}) presents to the emergency room with a 12-inch hunting knife lodged in his upper thoracic spine after an altercation at a cottage party. Initial examination reveals normal vital signs in the prone position, a reassuring airway and normal screening neurological exam. Initial X-ray studies confirm the knife enters at the level of T3 to T4 and traverses the right side of the spinal canal with the tip of the knife embedded in the T4 vertebral body. The neurosurgeon wishes to take the patient to the operating room for an urgent wound exploration and removal of the foreign body under general anesthesia with careful continuous neurological monitoring throughout the procedure.

INTRODUCTION

What Are Your Concerns When a Patient Is Placed in the Prone Position for a Surgical Procedure?

Proper patient positioning for any medical procedure is an important consideration for a safe and successful outcome. Proper positioning provides for appropriate surgical access and guards against injury due to pressure points and strain on neurological and musculoskeletal structures. The prone position is most commonly required for surgical procedures on the spine, and for selected procedures in neurosurgery, urology, and general surgery. This position is complicated by an increased risk of stretch and pressure injury of nerves, cardiovascular instability, difficulty with ventilation, and problems with providing cardiopulmonary resuscitation[1,2] as compared with the supine position. Airway considerations for patients in the prone position may include difficult access to the airway, migration of the endotracheal tube (ETT) cephalad or caudad with head extension and flexion respectively,[3] changes in ETT cuff pressure,[4] limited ability to reposition the head and neck for face-mask ventilation (FMV), and the potential development of airway edema.[5]

This case presents a challenging situation for airway practitioners: securing the airway in an urgent setting in which the patient cannot be easily positioned supine. Limited information is currently available in the literature to assist the airway practitioner with critical decision-making should they encounter this situation.

AIRWAY CONSIDERATIONS

How Do You Provide Ventilation to a Patient in the Prone Position If Urgently Needed?

Options to manage the airway in a prone patient are similar to those in a supine patient. FMV should be considered the standard and attempted before other measures because the ease of FMV will guide all airway management decisions that follow. However, FMV in the prone patient can be difficult due to limited access to the airway, difficult mask seal due to no occipital support to apply counter pressure to the head,[6] and lack of clinical experience performing FMV in a prone patient. It may be necessary to use a two person FMV technique, with one person achieving a mask seal using both hands, while the second person provides manual ventilation. Provided that a good seal can be maintained between the mask and the patient's face, FMV should be reasonably easy in a patient lying prone as gravity tends to move the tongue away from the posterior pharyngeal wall. The authors would recommend quickly moving to a two person FMV technique (see Chapter 8) and proceeding to alternative methods of ventilation should there be any difficulty obtaining an adequate mask seal.

If FMV is not possible, an extraglottic device (EGD), such as the Laryngeal Mask Airway (LMA®), can be used to provide emergency ventilation and oxygenation for a patient in the prone position. Several reports have evaluated the ease of insertion of LMA devices in the prone position in manikin studies[7,8] as well as for short elective procedures in anesthetized patients.[9–19] Despite these reports, there is still considerable debate in the literature regarding the safe use of EGDs for patients in the prone position.[20–25] Several investigators have reported successful use of EGDs (LMA, LMA®-Supreme™, LMA®-ProSeal™, and others) to regain control of the airway and provide positive-pressure ventilation following ETT dislodgement in the prone position.[26–29] Insertion of the LMA in the prone patient should be attempted using the classic insertion technique recommended for patients in the supine position.[30] Successful insertion of the LMA may actually be easier in the prone position because gravity helps to move the tongue and epiglottis[31] away from the posterior pharyngeal wall and minimizes the risk of down-folding of the epiglottis.

Other EGDs, such as the Combitube®, may be used while the patient is prone, depending on the skill and experience of the practitioner, as well as the available resources. Currently there are no reports in the literature on the successful use of non-LMA-derived EGDs for patients in the prone position. Therefore, the authors do not recommend the use of non-LMA-derived devices in elective airway management situations or as first-line rescue devices in emergency situations.

How Do You Manage a Patient with a Difficult Airway Who Requires Prone Positioning?

Airway management of a patient with a difficult airway who requires surgery in a prone position poses unique challenges for the anesthesia practitioner. These issues can be categorized according to the etiology of the difficult airway: (1) anatomical characteristics making ventilation and/or tracheal intubation difficult and (2) cervical spine instability. If difficult laryngoscopic intubation secondary to anatomical characteristics is predicted (LEMON and CRANE, see Chapter 1), the technique utilized to manage the airway is dependent on whether or not oxygenation can be readily provided (by FMV, EGD, or a surgical airway), aspiration risk, the available resources, as well as the expertise of the practitioner. Once tracheal intubation has been achieved, the ETT must be carefully secured.

The situation becomes more challenging when possible cervical spine instability or spinal cord injury exists. It is generally believed that awake bronchoscopic intubation and prone positioning of the patient prior to induction of anesthesia is ideal, because it allows verification of neurological integrity prior to surgery.[32–34] However, there is no high level of evidence to support this practice. In a retrospective review of 150 patients with cervical spine injury, Suderman and Crosby found no difference in neurological outcomes following tracheal intubation awake or under general anesthesia, with or without in-line cervical spine immobilization[35] (see Chapter 17).

PREPARATION AND PLANS FOR TRACHEAL INTUBATION

What Are the Options for Tracheal Intubation in the Prone Position?

In addition to direct laryngoscopic intubation, alternative intubating techniques can be considered. These include the use of a flexible bronchoscope (FB), an intubating LMA (LMA®-Fastrach™, LMA North America Inc, San Diego, CA), or other EGDs designed to allow intubation through the device, light-guided intubation using the Trachlight™ (Laerdal Medical Corp., Wappingers Falls, New York) and digital intubation. However, there is limited clinical information with regard to the effectiveness and safety of these techniques in patients in prone positions.

Baer performed endotracheal intubation using a direct laryngoscope in the prone position in 200 patients undergoing lumbar surgery.[36] Two failed intubations occurred and these patients were then intubated in the lateral or supine positions, with difficulty.[36] This experience emphasizes the importance of airway assessment and management in the supine position when difficulty is predicted. Komasawa et al. evaluated the utility of a video laryngoscope (Pentax-AWS Airway Scope) for tracheal intubation in different positions in a manikin and found the prone position to be feasible for intubation but it took longer and was subjectively more difficult for the practitioner than the supine position.[37] In a manikin study, Gaszynski found the video laryngoscope (Pentax-AWS Airway Scope) provided shorter time to intubation and caused less pressure on the tongue in the prone position compared to a Macintosh laryngoscope and an Intubrite video laryngoscope.[38] There are several case reports describing airway rescue in prone patients using a FB,[39,40] video laryngoscope,[41] intubating LMA (in a neonate),[42] and flexible bronchoscopy through an LMA device.[29] We caution against attempting intubation through any EGD without flexible bronchoscopy as van Dijck et al. describe a failed study attempting blind intubation through a i-gel® (Intersurgical Ltd, Wokingham, Berkshire, UK) in the prone position.[43] Induction of anesthesia in patients with posterior thoracic injuries in the prone position and subsequent successful tracheal intubation with direct laryngoscopy,[44] flexible bronchoscopic intubation through an i-gel,[45] and an intubating LMA[46,47] have also been reported. We believe that tracheal intubation of patients in the prone position should be reserved for special and rescue situations and for practitioners with the necessary skills and resources. For elective and nonurgent tracheal intubation of patients requiring prone positioning, it would be prudent to secure the airway in the supine position which is most familiar to the airway practitioner.

However, tracheal intubation in the prone position may be necessary if:

1. Ventilation and oxygenation are ineffective using FMV, the LMA, or other EGDs.
2. Ventilation using FMV, the LMA, or other EGDs is adequate but a definitive airway is desired (e.g., prolonged case, risk of aspiration).
3. Transfer of the patient to the supine position is impossible or associated with extreme risk.

Can Tracheal Intubation Be Performed in the Lateral Position?

While transfer of the patient to the supine position would be ideal, it could be difficult to achieve in a timely manner and is not without considerable risk depending on the situation. Therefore, it is desirable to have several alternative approaches for tracheal intubation in this particularly difficult situation.

If it is feasible to place the patient in a lateral position, the left lateral decubitus is preferred by some practitioners for laryngoscopy and intubation, as gravity will help to displace the tongue as well as secretions to the left and facilitate visualization of the glottis.[6] However, others prefer the right lateral decubitus position as the practitioner's left arm has more room to maneuver during the procedure. The tongue can still be easily displaced by the laryngoscope in the right lateral decubitus position. Nathanson et al. found tracheal intubation of a manikin in the lateral position to be more difficult than in the supine position.[48] The ease of intubation increased with each subsequent attempt, indicating that practitioner's experience was a confounding factor.[37,48] An assistant may be necessary to stabilize the head, neck, and body while performing intubation of a patient in the lateral decubitus position.

Blind endotracheal intubation techniques using the intubating LMA (LMA-Fastrach, LMA North America, San Diego) and the lighted stylet have also been described with a patient in the lateral position.[49–51] Practitioner's experience with these intubation techniques will improve the chance of success. However, blind techniques should only be attempted after direct or indirect visualization techniques have failed, especially in trauma patients with the potential for a full stomach and if there is a possibility of anatomic distortion of the airway.

What Are the Options for Positioning This Patient for Induction of General Anesthesia?

This is a complex clinical situation that must take into consideration each of the following prior to developing an appropriate management plan:

1. Urgency of the situation (e.g., presence or absence of respiratory difficulties and hypoxemia)
2. Risk of regurgitation and aspiration (full stomach secondary to drinking at a party)
3. Extent of the patient's spinal injury or other associated injuries (following an altercation at a party)
4. Current hemodynamic status and potential for hemodynamic changes
5. Presence of any neurological compromise and degree of concern for impending neurological compromise
6. Level of the patient's anxiety and willingness to cooperate
7. Position of the patient at presentation

Ultimately, the anesthesia management plan will weigh the risks and benefits of airway interventions and induction of general anesthesia—keeping the patient in his current position with the risks and benefits of repositioning the patient into a potentially more favorable position. If the risk of neurological compromise is deemed to be high, transferring the patient from supine/sitting to prone or prone to supine would be unacceptable. It would be prudent to manage the anesthesia and airway with the patient at or close to his position at presentation. Regardless of the final plan for positioning the patient, careful consideration must be given to securing the equipment, personnel, and resources required to carry out the management plan. Clear and concise communication must be provided to all team members regarding the sequence of steps involved in the management plan (plan A, B, C, and D)

How Would You Position This Patient for Airway Management If He Is Presented in the Sitting Or Upright Position?

If the patient presents to the emergency department in the sitting position with stable neurological and hemodynamic status can be transported to the operating room (OR) in sitting position with sufficient support and care. There are several options for positioning the patient for anesthetic and airway management:

1. His airway can be managed awake with topical anesthesia and the patient can then be turned prone before induction of anesthesia.
2. Two OR tables can be placed side-by-side with a sufficient gap to allow the foreign body to rest between the tables with the patient supine. These OR tables can be adjusted in tandem into an appropriate position (supine, reverse Trendelenburg, semi-sitting, or beach chair) prior to transferring the patient to them (see Figure 38.1). This method may require a third OR table to be present in the room for transferring the patient to the prone position for the surgical procedure after securing the airway and induction of general anesthesia. The length of the foreign body that remains outside of the thorax is a concern as a particularly lengthy foreign body could get caught on one of the OR tables straddling the foreign body while transferring the patient to the prone position.
3. The patient can be transferred to the supine position on an OR table from the sitting position such that the foreign body will lie above the head of the table.

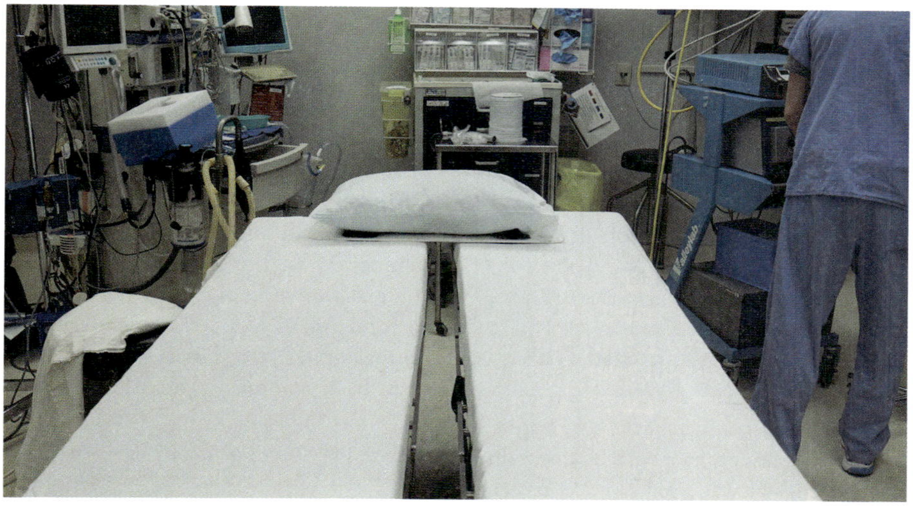

FIGURE 38.1. Two operating tables can be placed side-by-side with a sufficient gap to allow the foreign body to rest between the tables.

With this approach, support of the patient's shoulders and head will be needed as they will also lie above the head of the OR table. This support of the head and shoulders can be achieved with an extra side table, OR table, stretcher, or other device adjusted to the right height (see Figure 38.2).

4. The patient can be transported to the OR in prone position and then transferred to the OR table in the same position. The airway and anesthesia can be managed in the prone position. The risks and benefits of this option will be discussed later in the chapter.
5. The patient can carefully be placed in the lateral position for airway management before being turned into the prone position for the surgical procedure.

How Would You Position This Patient for Airway Management If He Is Presented in the Prone Position?

For the patient with a dorsal foreign body presenting in the prone position, the options are as follows:

1. Carry out airway and anesthetic management with the patient in his current position (prone on a stretcher or bed). Although this option avoids moving or transferring the patient prior to airway management, the patient would still need to be transferred and positioned on the OR table. The authors do not recommend this option.
2. Transfer the patient to the OR table in their final prone position and manage the airway and induction of general

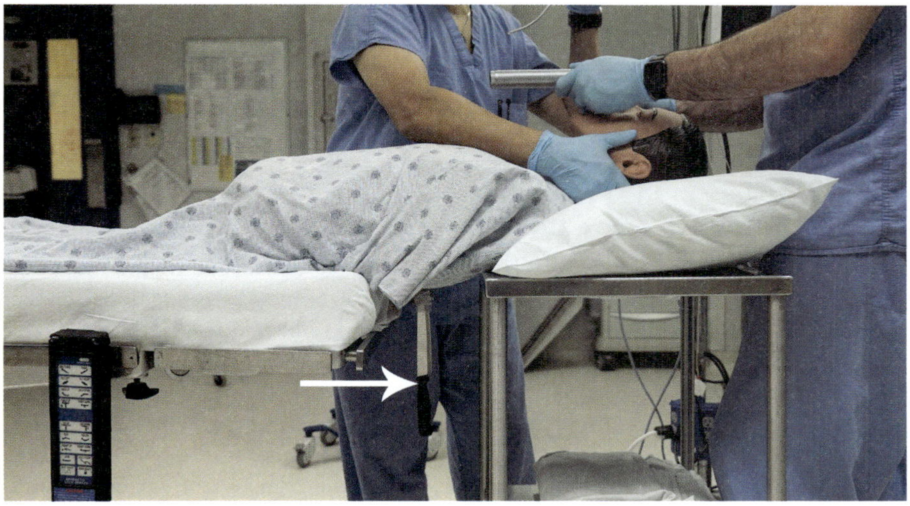

FIGURE 38.2. Using a manikin with a knife in the back (arrow), this figure demonstrates that the patient with a foreign body in the back can be transferred to an operating room table lying supine so that the foreign body will lie above the head of the table and the head and shoulders of the patient resting on an instrument table levelled with the OR table. With this approach, the airway can be secured by any technique familiar to the anesthesia practitioner.

anesthesia in that position. This would allow proper surgical positioning prior to airway management and ensure the patient was neurologically intact prior to induction of anesthesia and the start of the surgical procedure.

3. Arrange OR equipment for anesthetic management in the supine position (see above) and transfer the patient from the prone to supine position for airway management.
4. Turn the patient into the lateral position for airway and anesthetic management (see above).

If the Patient Was Cooperative, Could This Patient's Airway Be Managed Awake?

If the patient was cooperative and could be safely positioned to allow for awake airway management, there are no contraindications to manage this patient's airway awake. For a patient presenting in the sitting position, tracheal intubation could be achieved as described in the previous section. During airway topicalization or awake intubation, it is possible that the patient could change his position by coughing or become agitated and combative. Any patient movement could potentially further impale the foreign body into the spine. Excessive body movement can be minimized by a gentle unhurried airway topicalization technique and by having assistants support the patient's body position during the procedure. Heng et al. studied awake nasotracheal intubation using an FB followed by self-positioning and induction of general anesthesia in 62 patients and found that it was a feasible alternative to routine prone positioning after induction of general anesthesia.[32]

Performing an awake intubation with a patient already in the prone position may be more challenging. Although an OR table could be maneuvered to place the patient in a reverse Trendelenburg/chair position with the patient's head extending over the end of the OR table, it would be difficult to arrange this position with the appropriate bolsters in place. In addition, any patient discomfort while preparing for or during awake intubation could result in patient movement which could result in the patient falling off the OR table. Lastly, most anesthesia practitioners and assistants are unfamiliar with awake intubation in a prone patient and the lack of confidence and preparation may jeopardize the success of the technique and the ability to manage any potential complications.

Can Induction of Anesthesia in the Prone Position Be Safely Performed in This Patient?

There is considerable debate in the literature about the merits of prone positioning and induction of general anesthesia for elective cases. An increasing number of studies, including a substantial number of patients, reported induction of anesthesia in the prone position and the associated complications to be similar to induction of general anesthesia in the supine position. However, extrapolation of this limited evidence to clinical scenarios different from the patient populations and procedures in those reported studies should be done with great caution. All of the reported studies which include induction of general anesthesia in the prone position were carried out in elective patients, the majority of whom were not obese, and always stressed the importance of the need to be able to quickly turn the patient supine should any difficulties present themselves during airway management. Therefore, using currently available evidence, inducing general anesthesia in the prone position for elective surgical patients does not appear to offer the widest margin of safety.

There are several case reports of the induction of general anesthesia and airway management in the prone position for traumatic posterior thoracic injuries.[44,46,47] Agrawal et al. used an inhalation induction followed by tracheal intubation through an Intubating LMA technique for a 25-year-old patient with a normal airway placed in the prone position because of extensive open back wounds.[47] Van Zundert et al. described successful tracheal intubation using direct laryngoscopy in a nonobese patient placed in prone position with a pair of scissors lodged in her spine.[44] Another case report of a patient with a normal airway and a traumatic knife injury to the lumbar spine was managed with induction of anesthesia and intubation in the prone position using an intubating LMA.[46] Gouveia et al. reported a case of penetrating knife wound to the back managed by prone induction of general anesthesia and airway management moving from C-MAC video laryngoscope to a plan B of insertion of i-gel followed by flexible bronchoscopic intubation through the i-gel.[45] Assuming that careful consideration is given to select and prepare the method of airway management, this could be a reasonable management plan if the risks of positioning the patient in a more conventional position for airway management are deemed unacceptably high.

How Can Endotracheal Intubation Be Performed in the Prone Position in the Patient Presented Here?

As stated above, successful tracheal intubation has been reported using a variety of techniques. While the practitioner may be unfamiliar with the awkward prone position, tracheal intubation using an FB can be performed in the prone position with the OR table in a reverse Trendelenburg position and an assistant supporting the patient's head (see Figure 38.3). With an assistant holding the patient's head, tracheal intubation by direct laryngoscopy can also be performed in the prone patient by the airway practitioner who is positioned at the head of the patient facing caudad and uses the right hand to insert the laryngoscope into the pharynx and expose the glottis (Figure 38.4). Operating the laryngoscope with the right hand while the practitioner faces the prone patient allows the laryngoscope blade to displace the tongue in the usual manner—away from the right side of the patient's mouth. The practitioner then uses the left hand to insert the ETT into the trachea. This technique of laryngoscopic intubation in prone patients has been shown to be an effective (99% success rate) and safe.[36] Alternately, direct laryngoscopy and intubation can be performed in a more conventional manner from either side of the patient (Figure 38.5). An assistant can turn the patient's head to the right and elevate the right shoulder slightly to facilitate access to the mouth. The head and neck can also be placed in the familiar sniffing position. The additional concerns with this technique in the patient requiring spinal precautions would make the former

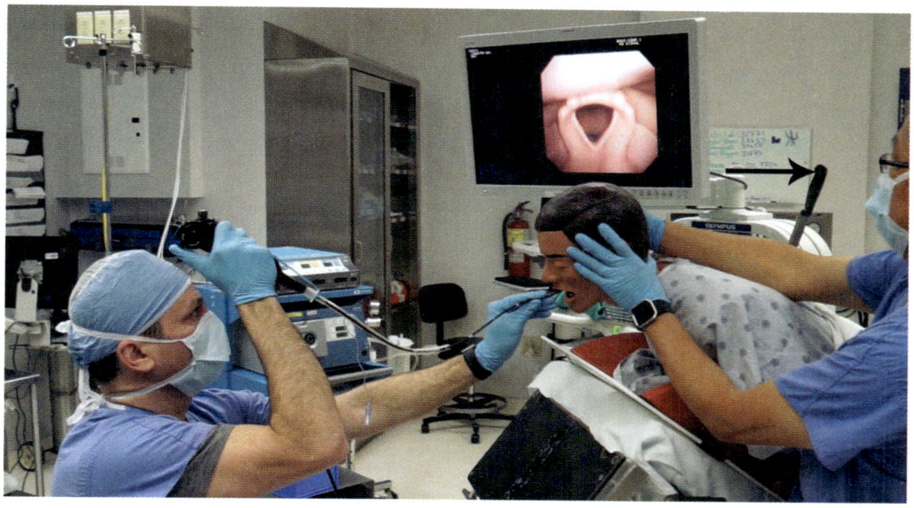

FIGURE 38.3. Bronchoscopic tracheal intubation in a manikin with a knife in the back (arrow) placed in the prone position: Orotracheal intubation using a flexible bronchoscope can be performed in a manikin placed in prone position with the operating room table in a reverse Trendelenburg position and an assistant supporting the manikin's head.

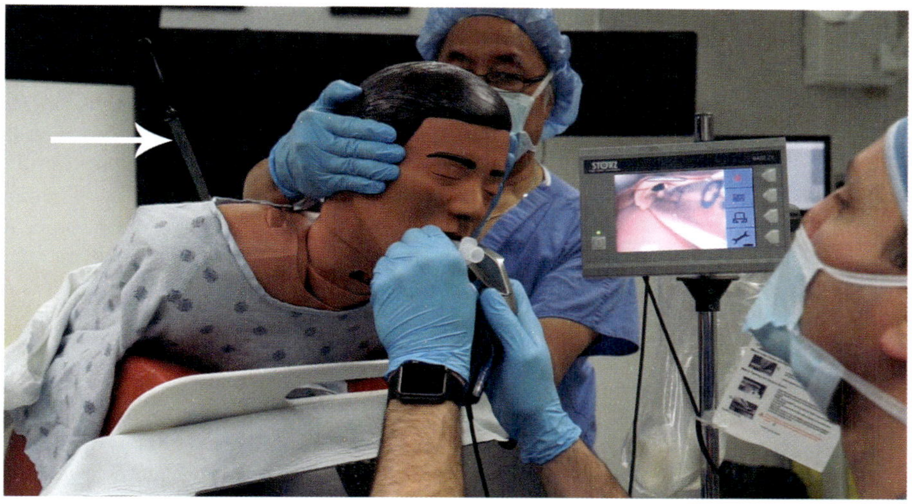

FIGURE 38.4. Laryngoscopic intubation in a manikin with a knife in the back (arrow) placed in the prone position: With the manikin placed in prone position with the operating room table in a reverse Trendelenburg position and with an assistant holding the patient's head, direct laryngoscopic intubation (the CMAC Macintosh blade video laryngoscope is used to show the ETT through the glottis opening) can be performed from the front of the manikin with the right hand holding the laryngoscope.

technique (approaching the airway from the head of the bed) more favorable.

Agrawal et al.[47] described the successful use of the Intubating-LMA (ILMA) for tracheal intubation in a patient in the prone position who presented with injuries precluding supine positioning. The ILMA can provide a conduit through which an ETT can be advanced into the trachea blindly, or with the aid of a lightwand, or the FB (see Chapter 12). However, insertion of an ILMA (as compared to the LMA®-Classic™) can be difficult in the prone position. Alternatively, following successful placement of the LMA-Classic, a FB can be used to facilitate tracheal intubation through the EGD (see section "Can Flexible Bronchoscopic Intubation Be Performed Through Extraglottic Devices?" in Chapter 10). Flexible bronchoscopic-guided intubation can be accomplished by passing a pediatric FB with an ensleeved Aintree Intubation Catheter (AIC, Cook Medical Inc, Bloomington, IN) into the trachea through the "aperture bars" of an in situ LMA-Classic. The bronchoscope and LMA-Classic can then be removed leaving the AIC in the trachea. A cut ETT ≥7.0 mm ID (26 cm) can then be advanced over the AIC (about 50 cm long) into the trachea.

Since the patient was cooperative and the risk of aspiration was high, the anesthesia team decided to perform an awake tracheal intubation using an FB (Plan A) with the patient placed prone on the operating room table (see Figure 38.3). An awake tracheal intubation under direct laryngoscopy in the prone position (see Figure 38.4) would be performed should the flexible bronchoscopic intubation attempt fail (Plan B). The patient

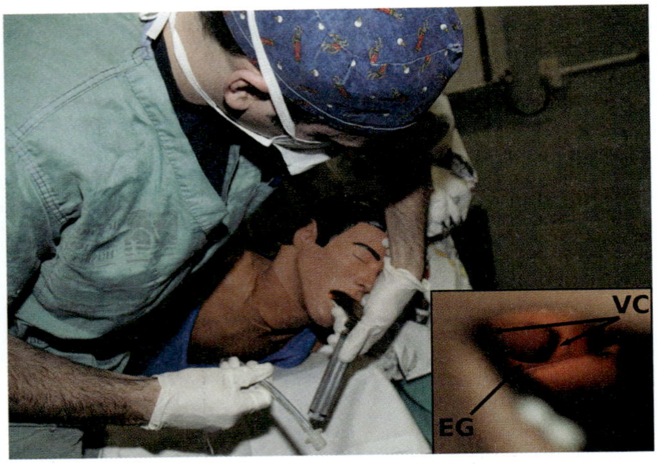

FIGURE 38.5. Laryngoscopic intubation of a manikin placed in the prone position: Laryngoscopic intubation can also be performed from the side (right) of the manikin. The insert shows the laryngoscopic view of this technique. The vocal cords (VC) and the epiglottis (EG) can be visualized easily.

would be placed in the supine position with the foreign body between two OR tables placed side-by-side for airway intervention (Plan C) if both of the techniques were unsuccessful.

POSTINTUBATION AND VENTILATION MANAGEMENT

How Can the Tracheal Tube Be Secured Following Intubation in a Patient with a Beard?

To minimize the risk of ETT dislodgement, it is imperative to secure the ETT properly, particularly for patients in a prone position. The most common method of securing the ETT is to tape it to the face. However, in the presence of facial hair, oils on the skin, perspiration, oropharyngeal secretions, and surgical skin preparation solutions, the adhesive tape may not be effective. Generous use of waterproof tape and the use of multiple attachment points can reinforce the bond to the patient's face. The application of tincture of benzoin to the skin may improve tape adhesiveness. Although adequate taping is required for the prone patient, complete sealing off of the mouth should be avoided, as oropharyngeal secretions should be allowed to drain out. This will minimize pooling of saliva and secretions which may loosen the tape. In addition, the use of an antisialagogue (e.g., glycopyrrolate) may be helpful as a preventive measure to minimize secretions. Placement of a throat pack in the oropharynx or a gauze bite block may also limit the amount of secretions available to disrupt the bond between the tape and the skin. However, the airway practitioner must always be aware of the potential for local pressure injury (e.g., lingual nerve injury) and tongue edema associated with the use of throat packs and bite blocks.[52–55] Patients with facial hair often pose additional problems with securing the airway. For these patients, it may be best to tie the ETT around the neck with an umbilical tape. It is important not to tie the ETT too tightly and thereby obstruct venous return from the head. If the ETT cannot be tied around the neck (e.g., procedures of the cervical spine or posterior fossa craniotomy), other possible options to secure the ETT include: (1) suturing the ETT to the lips; (2) tying the ETT to the upper incisors (if present) or nares; (3) consider using a nasotracheal ETT to facilitate securing the ETT with tape; (4) tie the umbilical tape to the head-pins frame (if it is used) instead of around the neck; and (5) shaving the patient's beard prior to induction of anesthesia.

OTHER CONSIDERATIONS FOR PATIENTS IN THE PRONE POSITION

How Can Airway Edema Be Minimized in a Patient in the Prone Position?

Tissue edema, particularly in dependent areas, can occur in surgical procedures involving significant blood loss and/or fluid shifts. The development of postextubation stridor or airway compromise due to an edematous airway following a surgical procedure in the prone position may require emergency airway interventions. Therefore, all attempts should be made to minimize the development of edema during procedures performed in the prone position. Current fluid management strategies advocate minimizing the amount of intra-operative fluids given during elective surgeries, which is especially prudent in patients requiring surgery in the prone position. Early resuscitation with blood components in the setting of hemorrhage is warranted to minimize the use of crystalloid in order to keep head and neck edema at a minimum. Although the efficacy of this approach has not been scientifically validated, it is our practice to use this approach in order to limit crystalloid use to between 2 and 3 L in total whenever possible.

Venous drainage of the head and neck can be optimized by keeping the head elevated if possible and avoiding compression or "kinking" of jugular veins. If the head must be turned to one side for airway or surgical access, the degree of rotation should be minimized.

How Can Airway Edema Be Assessed and Managed?

The development of edema in the hypopharynx and larynx while in the prone position can produce airway obstruction following extubation. Clinical signs, such as facial, periorbital or conjunctival edema, distended neck veins, and venous congestion of the head, may indicate the presence of upper airway edema. The use of a flexible nasopharyngoscope to assess the extent of airway edema prior to tracheal extubation may be helpful,[56] although there have been no studies to confirm its utility. Antonaglia et al.[57] evaluated postextubation laryngeal edema in ICU patients using a rigid laryngoscope by an otolaryngologist and were able to successfully identify the amount of edema as well as other lesions which would complicate the postextubation course (hematoma, granuloma, ulcers, and arytenoid luxation).

There are no scientifically validated methods to assess the degree of postoperative airway edema or to predict postextubation airway obstruction (see Chapter 31). However, the performance of a leak test prior to extubation in patients with suspected airway edema has been suggested.[58] If the patient is being ventilated by a mechanical ventilator, the leak test measures the decrease in exhaled volume returned to the ventilator following deflation of the ETT cuff. A positive leak test (>110 mL or >10% of the tidal volume) has been shown to indicate that airway patency is sufficient to tolerate extubation without postextubation stridor (PES) (99% specificity, 98% PPV), although a negative leak test is not predictive of the development of PES.[59] The leak test can also be performed by deflating the ETT cuff in a spontaneously breathing patient without ventilator support and then occluding the proximal end of the ETT. The patient is observed for signs of an audible leak or coughing around the ETT. The absence of a leak and/or coughing are positive predictors for PES.[60] Multiple studies have found the leak test to be either helpful for predicting adverse events[61–63] or not,[64–66] but they all suffer from study design flaws. A systematic review which included 16 studies found odds ratios for the cuff-leak test for predicting laryngeal edema and reintubation were 18 and 10.8, respectively.[67] A recent meta-analysis and systematic review of cuff-leak test found pooled sensitivity and specificity of 0.66 and 0.88, respectively,[68] indicating that even patients who pass the cuff-leak test should still be monitored for postextubation stridor.

Laryngeal ultrasound is an emerging method for assessing laryngeal anatomy. Lakhal et al. showed a strong correlation between laryngeal ultrasound and MRI for measuring tracheal diameter at the cricoid ring in 27 young adults.[69] Ding et al. reported a pilot study using a laryngeal ultrasound to predict postextubation stridor in 41 patients.[70] The investigators used real-time ultrasonography to evaluate the air-leak and to determine the relationship between the air column width difference (ACWD) before and after cuff deflation and the development of PES. The results of this study suggest that laryngeal ultrasonography could be a reliable, noninvasive method in the evaluation of laryngeal morphology and airflow through the upper airway. Two recent reports compared ultrasonographic assessment to cuff-leak test for assessing laryngeal edema.[71,72] Sutherasan et al. determined that the ultrasound measurement of ACWD could be a useful tool and had similar sensitivity and specificity (70% and 70%, respectively) and receiver operating characteristic (ROC) curve compared to the cuff-leak test (0.823 vs. 0.840, respectively).[72] Mikaeili et al. demonstrated that both the cuff-leak test and ACWD had poor sensitivity (25% and 50%, respectively), specificity (84% and 54%, respectively) and positive predictive value (both < 20%).[71] Similarly, Bhargava et al. compared ACWD to cuff-leak test and found high sensitivities (91.7% and 92.6%, respectively) and specificities (91.7% and 90.4%, respectively) which resulted in high negative predictive values (>99%) and low positive predictive values (<45%) for both tests.[73] Therefore, airway practitioners should recognize the potential limitations of the application of both of these tests in clinical practice. Interestingly, Antonaglia et al. found that the cuff-leak test correlated with the amount of laryngeal edema as assessed by rigid laryngoscope but not the occurrence of PES.[57] This could explain some of the discrepancy in evaluations of the cuff-leak test and ACWD as tests for laryngeal edema as they relied on PES as a surrogate marker for laryngeal edema.

Other predictors of PES including length of intubation, female gender, body mass index, and ratio of ETT size to laryngeal diameter have also been reported.[59,74] Kwon et al. reported total operative time, and the volume of crystalloid and blood given to be risk factors for delayed extubation.[75]

Even though the patient may have passed the tests for laryngeal edema assessment, if there is clinical evidence of facial and possible airway edema, it would be prudent to perform extubation over an 11-Fr ETT exchange catheter (Cook Critical Care, Bloomington, IN) to provide a means for oxygenation should postextubation airway obstruction occur. For patients failing the leak test, the airway practitioner can perform nasopharyngoscopy, video laryngoscopy and/or laryngeal ultrasound to provide additional information to aid in determining the risk for postextubation problems. If there are still sufficient concerns about airway edema, the authors recommend leaving the ETT in place until the airway edema resolves and a subsequent leak test is satisfactory. Although failing the laryngeal edema tests may not predict postextubation problems with high specificity, using this approach provides for the greatest margin of safety for the patient.

Appropriate treatment of airway edema includes elevation of the head and the use of steroids and diuretics. The efficacy of these measures has not been scientifically validated. Two meta-analyses[76,77] provide a comprehensive review of the effect of steroids on PES and showed that there is evidence to support multiple doses of steroids given 12 to 24 hours prior to extubation in adults for preventing PES in high-risk patients (as determined by the cuff-leak test). The evidence for prophylactic steroids in neonates or children is heterogeneous but shows a trend toward benefit and should be considered for high-risk patients.[77] Steroids may reduce the amount of airway edema and decrease the risk of postextubation airway obstruction; however, evidence supporting a decreased rate of reintubation only exists in the pediatric population.[78–82]

SUMMARY

Airway management in a prone patient presents a unique challenge to all airway practitioners. While the principles of airway management (FMV, use of an EGD, tracheal intubation, and front-of-neck airway) remain unchanged for a patient in any position, oxygenation using these techniques in a prone patient may be difficult and unfamiliar to most airway practitioners. The choice of an airway intervention technique is dependent on the urgency of the clinical status, the available resources, the patient's position, and the skills of the airway practitioner. All airway practitioners must have a strategy to manage a difficult or failed airway in a patient in the prone position. Special attention must be paid to intraoperative fluid management and the assessment of airway edema prior to tracheal extubation in prone patients, particularly for patients undergoing long surgical procedures with significant fluid shifts.

SELF-EVALUATION QUESTIONS

38.1. Which of the following is not an acceptable initial method to provide oxygenation and ventilation to an awake cooperative patient lying prone with a knife in the thoracic spine in the emergency department?

A. Advancing the ETT over a flexible bronchoscope into the trachea

B. Establish a surgical airway

C. Insertion of a Laryngeal Mask Airway

D. Face-mask ventilation (FMV)

E. Intubation through an Intubating LMA

38.2. Following orotracheal intubation, which of the following is NOT an acceptable method of securing the endotracheal tube (ETT) in a patient with facial hair?

A. Tie the ETT around the neck with an umbilical tape.

B. Tie the ETT to the upper incisors.

C. Secure the ETT with a waterproof tape after the application of tincture of benzoin to the face.

D. Shave the patient's beard under general anesthesia.

E. None of the above.

38.3. Which of the following is most reliable in assessing postoperative airway edema in a patient who was placed prone for the procedure?

A. The amount of intraoperative fluid administered to the patient

B. The presence of facial edema

C. The leak test

D. Flexible nasopharyngoscopy

E. None of the above

REFERENCES

1. Anez C, Becerra-Bolanos A, Vives-Lopez A, Rodriguez-Perez A. Cardiopulmonary resuscitation in the prone position in the operating room or in the intensive care unit: a systematic review. *Anesth Analg*. 2021;132:285-292.
2. Barker J, Koeckerling D, West R. A need for prone position CPR guidance for intubated and non-intubated patients during the COVID-19 pandemic. *Resuscitation*. 2020;151:135-136.
3. Minonishi T, Kinoshita H, Hirayama M, et al. The supine-to-prone position change induces modification of endotracheal tube cuff pressure accompanied by tube displacement. *J Clin Anesth*. 2013;25:28-31.
4. Athiraman U, Gupta R, Singh G. Endotracheal cuff pressure changes with change in position in neurosurgical patients. *Int J Crit Illn Inj Sci*. 2015;5:237-241.
5. Jain M, Lal J, Aggrawal D, Sharma J, Singh AK, Bansal T. A Study to evaluate changes in modified mallampati class in patients undergoing spine surgery in prone position. *Cureus*. 2022;14:e25767.
6. Cupitt JM. Induction of anaesthesia in morbidly obese patients. *Br J Anaesth*. 1999;83:964-965.
7. Komasawa N, Ueki R, Fujii A, et al. Comparison of Laryngeal Mask Supreme(R) and Soft Seal(R) for airway management in several positions. *J Anesth*. 2011;25:535-539.
8. Gupta B, Gupta S, Hijam B, Shende P, Rewari V. Comparison of three supraglottic airway devices for airway rescue in the prone position: a manikin-based study. *J Emerg Trauma Shock*. 2015;8:188-192.
9. Taxak S, Gopinath A, Saini S, Bansal T, Ahlawat MS, Bala M. A prospective study to evaluate and compare laryngeal mask airway ProSeal and i-gel airway in the prone position. *Saudi J Anaesth*. 2015;9:446-450.
10. Kang F, Li J, Chai X, Yu J, Zhang H, Tang C. Comparison of the I-gel laryngeal mask airway with the LMA-supreme for airway management in patients undergoing elective lumbar vertebral surgery. *J Neurosurg Anesthesiol*. 2015;27:37-41.
11. Olsen KS, Petersen JT, Pedersen NA, Rovsing L. Self-positioning followed by induction of anaesthesia and insertion of a laryngeal mask airway versus endotracheal intubation and subsequent positioning for spinal surgery in the prone position: a randomised clinical trial. *Eur J Anaesthesiol*. 2014;31:259-265.
12. Lopez AM, Valero R, Hurtado P, Gambus P, Pons M, Anglada T. Comparison of the LMA Supreme with the LMA Proseal for airway management in patients anaesthetized in prone position. *Br J Anaesth*. 2011;107:265-271.
13. Taxak S, Gopinath A. Insertion of the i-gel airway in prone position. *Minerva Anestesiol*. 2010;76:381.
14. Sharma V, Verghese C, McKenna PJ. Prospective audit on the use of the LMA-Supreme for airway management of adult patients undergoing elective orthopaedic surgery in prone position. *Br J Anaesth*. 2010;105:228-232.
15. Lopez AM, Valero R, Brimacombe J. Insertion and use of the LMA Supreme in the prone position. *Anaesthesia*. 2010;65:154-157.
16. Senthil Kumar M, Pandey R, Khanna P. Successful use of I-gel airway in prone position surgery. *Paediatr Anaesth*. 2009;19:176-177.
17. Yano T, Imaizumi T, Uneda C, Nakayama R. Lower intracuff pressure of laryngeal mask airway in the lateral and prone positions compared with that in the supine position. *J Anesth*. 2008;22:312-316.
18. Stevens WC, Mehta PD. Use of the Laryngeal Mask Airway in patients positioned prone for short surgical cases in an ambulatory surgery unit in the United States. *J Clin Anesth*. 2008;20:487-488.
19. Brimacombe JR, Wenzel V, Keller C. The proseal laryngeal mask airway in prone patients: a retrospective audit of 245 patients. *Anaesth Intensive Care*. 2007;35:222-225.
20. Patel A, Clark SR, Schiffmiller M, Schoenberg C, Tewfik G. A survey of practice patterns in the use of laryngeal mask by pediatric anesthesiologists. *Paediatr Anaesth*. 2015;25:1127-1131.
21. Whitacre W, Dieckmann L, Austin PN. An update: use of laryngeal mask airway devices in patients in the prone position. *AANA J*. 2014;82:101-107.
22. Staender S. CON: laryngeal masks must not be used for surgery in the prone position. *Eur J Anaesthesiol*. 2014;31:256-258.
23. Kranke P. Penny wise, pound foolish? Trade-offs when using the laryngeal mask airway for spine surgery in the prone position. *Eur J Anaesthesiol*. 2014;31:249-252.
24. Hinkelbein J. PRO: laryngeal masks can be used for surgery in the prone position. *Eur J Anaesthesiol*. 2014;31:253-255.
25. Abrishami A, Zilberman P, Chung F. Brief review: Airway rescue with insertion of laryngeal mask airway devices with patients in the prone position. *Can J Anaesth*. 2010;57:1014-1020.
26. Dingeman RS, Goumnerova LC, Goobie SM. The use of a laryngeal mask airway for emergent airway management in a prone child. *Anesth Analg*. 2005;100:670-671.
27. Raphael J, Rosenthal-Ganon T, Gozal Y. Emergency airway management with a laryngeal mask airway in a patient placed in the prone position. *J Clin Anesth*. 2004;16:560-561.
28. Brimacombe J, Keller C. An unusual case of airway rescue in the prone position with the ProSeal laryngeal mask airway. *Can J Anaesth*. 2005;52:884.
29. Sohn L, Sawardekar A, Jagannathan N. Airway management options in a prone achondroplastic dwarf with a difficult airway after unintentional tracheal extubation during a wake-up test for spinal fusion: to flip or not to flip? *Can J Anaesth*. 2014;61:741-744.
30. Brain A. Proper technique for insertion of the laryngeal mask. *Anesthesiology*. 1990;73:1053-1054.
31. Ng A, Raitt DG, Smith G. Induction of anesthesia and insertion of a laryngeal mask airway in the prone position for minor surgery. *Anesth Analg*. 2002;94:1194-1108.
32. Heng L, Wang MY, Sun HL, Zhu SS. Awake nasotracheal fiberoptic intubation and self-positioning followed by anesthesia induction in prone patients: a pilot observational study. *Medicine*. 2016;95:e4440.
33. Douglass J, Fraser J, Andrzejowski J. Awake intubation and awake prone positioning of a morbidly obese patient for lumbar spine surgery. *Anaesthesia*. 2014;69:166-169.
34. Malcharek MJ, Rogos B, Watzlawek S, et al. Awake fiberoptic intubation and self-positioning in patients at risk of secondary cervical injury: a pilot study. *J Neurosurg Anesthesiol*. 2012;24:217-221.
35. Suderman VS, Crosby ET, Lui A. Elective oral tracheal intubation in cervical spine-injured adults. *Can J Anaesth*. 1991;38:785-789.
36. Baer K. Is it much more difficult to intubate in prone position? *Lakartidningen*. 1992;89:3657-3660.

37. Komasawa N, Ueki R, Itani M, Nomura H, Nishi SI, Kaminoh Y. Evaluation of tracheal intubation in several positions by the Pentax-AWS Airway Scope: a manikin study. *J Anesth*. 2010;24:908-912.
38. Gaszynski TM. A comparison of a Standard Macintosh Blade Laryngoscope, Pentax-AWS Videolaryngoscope and Intubrite Videolaryngoscope for tracheal intubation in Manikins in sitting and prone positions: a randomized cross-over study. *Diagnostics (Basel)*. 2020;10:603.
39. Hung MH, Fan SZ, Lin CP, Hsu YC, Shih PY, Lee TS. Emergency airway management with fiberoptic intubation in the prone position with a fixed flexed neck. *Anesth Analg*. 2008;107:1704-1706.
40. Kramer DC, Lo JC, Gilad R, Jenkins A 3rd. Fiberoptic scope as a rescue device in an anesthetized patient in the prone position. *Anesth Analg*. 2007;105:890.
41. Gaszynski T. Intubation in prone position using AirTraq Avant videolaryngoscope. *J Clin Monit Comput*. 2019;33:173-174.
42. Jagannathan N, Jagannathan R. Prone insertion of a size 0.5 intubating laryngeal airway overcomes severe upper airway obstruction in an awake neonate with Pierre Robin syndrome. *Can J Anaesth*. 2012;59:1001-1002.
43. van Dijck M, Houweling BM, Koning MV. Blind intubation through an i-gel(R) in the prone position: a prospective cohort study. *Anaesth Intensive Care*. 2020;48:439-443.
44. van Zundert A, Kuczkowski KM, Tijssen F, Weber E. Direct laryngoscopy and endotracheal intubation in the prone position following traumatic thoracic spine injury. *J Anesth*. 2008;22:170-172.
45. Gouveia B, Ferreira L, Sousa M, Fernandes RC. Airway management in prone position: a case of knife injury in the posterior spine. *Oxf Med Case Reports*. 2022;2022(8):omac067.
46. Samantaray A. Tracheal intubation in the prone position with an intubating laryngeal mask airway following posterior spine impaled knife injury. *Saudi J Anaesth*. 2011;5:329-331.
47. Agrawal S, Sharma JP, Jindal P, Sharma UC, Rajan M. Airway management in prone position with an intubating Laryngeal Mask Airway. *J Clin Anesth*. 2007;19:293-295.
48. Nathanson MH, Gajraj NM, Newson CD. Tracheal intubation in a manikin: comparison of supine and left lateral positions. *Br J Anaesth*. 1994;73:690-691.
49. Cheng KI, Chu KS, Chau SW, et al. Lightwand-assisted intubation of patients in the lateral decubitus position. *Anesth Analg*. 2004;99:279-283.
50. Dimitriou V, Voyagis GS, Iatrou C, Brimacombe J. Flexible lightwand-guided intubation using the intubating laryngeal mask airway in the supine, right, and left lateral positions in healthy patients by experienced users. *Anesth Analg*. 2003;96:896-898.
51. Komatsu R, Nagata O, Sessler DI, Ozaki M. The intubating laryngeal mask airway facilitates tracheal intubation in the lateral position. *Anesth Analg*. 2004;98:858-861.
52. Evers KA, Eindhoven GB, Wierda JM. Transient nerve damage following intubation for trans-sphenoidal hypophysectomy. *Can J Anaesth*. 1999;46:1143-1145.
53. Wang KC, Chan WS, Tsai CT, Wu GJ, Chang Y, Tseng HC. Lingual nerve injury following the use of an oropharyngeal airway under endotracheal general anesthesia. *Acta Anaesthesiol Taiwan*. 2006;44:119-122.
54. Panikkar S, Tol G, Siddique I. Iatrogenic bilateral hypoglossal palsy following spinal surgery. *Eur Spine J*. 2018;27:314-317.
55. Walsh A, Peesay T, Newark A, et al. Association of Severe Tongue Edema With Prone Positioning in Patients Intubated for COVID-19. *Laryngoscope*. 2022;132:287-289.
56. Bentsianov BL, Parhiscar A, Azer M, Har-El G. The role of fiberoptic nasopharyngoscopy in the management of the acute airway in angioneurotic edema. *Laryngoscope*. 2000;110:2016-19.
57. Antonaglia V, Vergolini A, Pascotto S, et al. Cuff-leak test predicts the severity of postextubation acute laryngeal lesions: a preliminary study. *Eur J Anaesthesiol*. 2010;27:534-541.
58. Miller RL, Cole RP. Association between reduced cuff leak volume and postextubation stridor. *Chest*. 1996;110:1035-1040.
59. Kriner EJ, Shafazand S, Colice GL. The endotracheal tube cuff-leak test as a predictor for postextubation stridor. *Respir Care*. 2005;50:1632-1638.
60. Maury E, Guglielminotti J, Alzieu M, Qureshi T, Guidet B, Offenstadt G. How to identify patients with no risk for postextubation stridor? *J Crit Care*. 2004;19:23-28.
61. Chung Y-H, Chao T-Y, Chiu C-T, Lin M-C. The cuff-leak test is a simple tool to verify severe laryngeal edema in patients undergoing long-term mechanical ventilation. *Critical Care Medicine*. 2006;34:409-414.
62. Suominen P, Taivainen T, Tuominen N, et al. Optimally fitted tracheal tubes decrease the probability of postextubation adverse events in children undergoing general anesthesia. *Paediatr Anaesth*. 2006;16:641-647.
63. Wang CL, Tsai YH, Huang CC, et al. The role of the cuff leak test in predicting the effects of corticosteroid treatment on postextubation stridor. *Chang Gung Med J*. 2007;30:53-61.
64. Shin SH, Heath K, Reed S, Collins J, Weireter LJ, Britt LD. The cuff leak test is not predictive of successful extubation. *Am Surg*. 2008;74:1182-1185.
65. Suominen PK, Tuominen NA, Salminen JT, et al. The air-leak test is not a good predictor of postextubation adverse events in children undergoing cardiac surgery. *J Cardiothorac Vasc Anesth*. 2007;21:197-202.
66. Wratney AT, Benjamin DK Jr, Slonim AD, He J, Hamel DS, Cheifetz IM. The endotracheal tube air leak test does not predict extubation outcome in critically ill pediatric patients. *Pediatr Crit Care Med*. 2008;9:490-496.
67. Zhou T, Zhang HP, Chen WW, et al. Cuff-leak test for predicting postextubation airway complications: a systematic review. *J Evid Based Med*. 2011;4:242-254.
68. Kuriyama A, Jackson JL, Kamei J. Performance of the cuff leak test in adults in predicting post-extubation airway complications: a systematic review and meta-analysis. *Crit Care*. 2020;24:640.
69. Lakhal K, Delplace X, Cottier JP, et al. The feasibility of ultrasound to assess subglottic diameter. *Anesth Analg*. 2007;104:611-614.
70. Ding LW, Wang HC, Wu HD, Chang CJ, Yang PC. Laryngeal ultrasound: a useful method in predicting post-extubation stridor. A pilot study. *Eur Respir J*. 2006;27:384-389.
71. Mikaeili H, Yazdchi M, Tarzamni MK, Ansarin K, Ghasemzadeh M. Laryngeal ultrasonography versus cuff leak test in predicting postextubation stridor. *J Cardiovasc Thorac Res*. 2014;6:25-28.
72. Sutherasan Y, Theerawit P, Hongphanut T, Kiatboonsri C, Kiatboonsri S. Predicting laryngeal edema in intubated patients by portable intensive care unit ultrasound. *J Crit Care*. 2013;28:675-680.
73. Bhargava T, Kumar A, Bharti A, Khuba S. Comparison of laryngeal ultrasound and cuff leak test to predict post-extubation stridor in total thyroidectomy. *Turk J Anaesthesiol Reanim*. 2021;49:238-243.
74. Erginel S, Ucgun I, Yildirim H, Metintas M, Parspour S. High body mass index and long duration of intubation increase post-extubation stridor in patients with mechanical ventilation. *Tohoku J Exp Med*. 2005;207:125-132.
75. Kwon B, Yoo JU, Furey CG, Rowbottom J, Emery SE. Risk factors for delayed extubation after single-stage, multi-level anterior cervical decompression and posterior fusion. *J Spinal Disord Tech*. 2006;19:389-393.
76. Jaber S, Jung B, Chanques G, Bonnet F, Marret E. Effects of steroids on reintubation and post-extubation stridor in adults: meta-analysis of randomised controlled trials. *Crit Care*. 2009;13:R49.
77. Khemani RG, Randolph A, Markovitz B. Corticosteroids for the prevention and treatment of post-extubation stridor in neonates, children and adults. *Cochrane Database Syst Rev*. 2009:CD001000.
78. Anene O, Meert KL, Uy H, Simpson P, Sarnaik AP. Dexamethasone for the prevention of postextubation airway obstruction: a prospective, randomized, double-blind, placebo-controlled trial. *Crit Care Med*. 1996;24:1666-1669.
79. Darmon JY, Rauss A, Dreyfuss D, et al. Evaluation of risk factors for laryngeal edema after tracheal extubation in adults and its prevention by dexamethasone. A placebo-controlled, double-blind, multicenter study. *Anesthesiology*. 1992;77:245-251.
80. Lukkassen IM, Hassing MB, Markhorst DG. Dexamethasone reduces reintubation rate due to postextubation stridor in a high-risk paediatric population. *Acta Paediatr*. 2006;95:74-76.
81. Markovitz BP, Randolph AG. Corticosteroids for the prevention of reintubation and postextubation stridor in pediatric patients: A meta-analysis. *Pediatr Crit Care Med*. 2002;3:223-226.
82. Meade MO, Guyatt GH, Cook DJ, Sinuff T, Butler R. Trials of corticosteroids to prevent postextubation airway complications. *Chest*. 2001;120:464S-468S.

CHAPTER 39

Lung Separation in the Patient with a Difficult Airway

George W. Kanellakos and Haotian Wang

CASE PRESENTATION

A 45-year-old female presents for a video-assisted thoracoscopic (VATS) left upper lobectomy. She has a history of severe obstructive sleep apnea (OSA) and uses a continuous positive airway pressure (CPAP) machine. She is morbidly obese and her medical history is otherwise unremarkable. Echocardiography reveals normal pulmonary pressure. Her only medication is acetaminophen and she has no allergies.

On examination, she is 150 cm tall and weighs 120 kg (BMI 53 kg·m^{-2}). Vital signs are: BP 140/80 mmHg, HR 69 beats per min and regular, RR 16 breaths per min, temperature 36.9°C, and oxygen saturation is 99% on room air.

Airway examination reveals a Mallampati IV classification, mouth opening of 4 cm, thyromental distance of 4 cm, mandibular mobility of 2 cm, normal cervical spine extension, and full dentition. The chest is clear to auscultation and heart sounds are normal.

ANESTHESIA CONSIDERATIONS

Is This Patient Fit for Anesthesia?

A patient with morbid obesity would be expected to have OSA-related complications, including hypoventilation syndrome and pulmonary hypertension. Her normal echocardiogram is reassuring. Given she is compliant with CPAP therapy, she has no other significant comorbidities and needs no additional preoperative medical optimization.

What Anesthetic Technique Is Required?

General anesthesia is the standard of care for this procedure. Awake VATS has been reported[1,2] but is far from mainstream practice. Lung separation has been requested by the surgeon and is considered essential for successful surgical exposure.

How Can Lung Separation and One-Lung Ventilation (OLV) Be Achieved?

Lung separation and subsequent OLV for thoracic surgery can be achieved by a variety of techniques[3–6] and discussion with the health care team is an essential component in establishing a management plan. Successful lung separation can be dependent on patient factors, the surgical procedure proposed, user familiarity with lung separation equipment, upper airway anatomy, and user knowledge of endoscopic bronchial anatomy. Campos et al.[7] looked at these factors and reported that knowledge of endoscopic bronchial anatomy was the main factor influencing lung separation success among anesthesia practitioners with limited thoracic experience. Emphasis should be placed on how the planned surgical procedure and the patient's existing bronchial anatomy will interact with lung separation devices. A review of endoscopic bronchial anatomy has been published[8] and a Virtual Bronchoscopy simulator can be found online at www.thoracicanesthesia.com or www.pie.med.utoronto.ca/VB.

Double-lumen tubes (DLTs) and bronchial blockers (BB) are considered standard methods of achieving lung separation. Although DLTs have long been considered the gold standard for lung separation, BBs have been shown to provide equivalent surgical exposure when compared to DLTs.[9] The advantages and disadvantages of DLTs and BBs are numerous and well described in the literature.[10–15] A DLT is preferred over BBs when lung isolation is required to protect the nondiseased lung from contamination with blood or pus, in the presence of a bronchopleural or bronchopleural cutaneous fistula, and to perform unilateral pulmonary lavage. A contralateral DLT is preferred when a sleeve resection or lung transplant is performed. However, there are clinical situations in which a DLT may not be the best primary choice. The indications for the use of a BB include the difficult airway, the already intubated patient, the presence of distorted bronchial anatomy, small adults or young children, the presence of a tracheotomy, when nasal intubation or lobar blockade is required, and avoiding the need for a tube exchange.[16] Currently available BBs include the Arndt Wire-Guided Endobronchial Blocker,[17] the Cohen Flexitip Endobronchial Blocker,[18] the Fuji Uniblocker,[19] the Coopdech Endobronchial blocker,[20] and the EZ-blocker.[21]

OLV using a DLT is planned. In the operating room, basic monitors are applied, and a left radial arterial catheter is placed under local anesthesia. Following denitrogenation, general anesthesia is established and face-mask ventilation (FMV) is easily performed. Direct laryngoscopy (DL) with a #4 Macintosh blade reveals a Grade 4 Cormack-Lehane (CL) view (soft palate only).

AIRWAY MANAGEMENT

Is This a "Difficult Airway"?

Predictors of difficult laryngoscopy are well-published in the literature.[22,23] Traditionally, in assessing mouth opening, the Mallampati score, thyromental interval, mandibular protrusion, upper lip bite test, presence and quality of dentition, neck circumference, and cervical flexion and extension have all been used as predictors. Nearly all of them have significant variability in their assessment and individually are poor predictors of a difficult airway.[24,25] Exceptions are large neck circumference, Mallampati score (III or IV), and the upper lip bite test.

The ASA Task Force on Management of the Difficult Airway defines difficult airway as a clinical situation in which a conventionally trained anesthesia practitioner experiences difficulty with FMV, endotracheal intubation, or both.[26,27] The difficult airway can also be defined as one in which an experienced practitioner anticipates or encounters difficulty with any or all of FMV, direct or indirect (e.g., video) laryngoscopy, tracheal intubation, extraglottic device (EGD) use, or surgical airway.[28] Contextual issues such as anticipated safe apnea time, aspiration risk, presence of obstructing pathology, availability of skilled help, and clinical inexperience can also contribute to the degree of difficulty.[29]

DLTs and the Univent tube have been termed "difficult tubes" as they can be more difficult to insert due to their increased outside diameter (OD), shape, lack of a bevel at the tip, and increased overall rigidity which impedes optimal shaping of the tubes.[30,31] The criteria for difficult DLT insertion have not been well-defined. However, difficulty can be encountered in the presence of a CL II (partial glottis) view[32] and it has been shown that placement of a DLT may be challenging in an airway that can be easily intubated with a single-lumen tube (SLT). The Univent is an SLT with an enclosed channel along its concave (anterior) aspect which contains a movable BB.[33] The outside diameter of the Univent is relatively large as compared to a conventional polyvinyl chloride SLT and has increased stiffness and high air-flow resistance.[34,35] It can be problematic to insert in the setting of a difficult intubation and its usefulness in modern practice has been replaced by the newer BB.

Obesity is a predictor of difficult FMV (DMV). DMV has been defined as either mask ventilation that is inadequate to maintain oxygenation saturation SpO_2 >92%, unstable mask ventilation, or mask ventilation requiring two practitioners.[36] In the case presented, mask ventilation has been demonstrated to be easy but DL difficult.

The patient is morbidly obese and therefore positioning should be optimal before induction. This is best achieved by placing the patient in the "head elevated laryngoscopy position" (HELP), which allows for a maximal "safe apnea period" with optimized functional residual capacity.[37,38] Head lift and external laryngeal manipulation should be considered part of the best DL technique. The incidence of Grade 3 or 4 CL view is increased when patient positioning is suboptimal. Despite easy FMV in the case presentation, the patient presents with difficult DL and documentation of the airway as being difficult would be appropriate.

What Are the Options for Airway Management in This Patient?

A patient that presents with a difficult DL and requires OLV should be managed according to the most recent American Society of Anesthesiologists Practice Guidelines for the Management of the Difficult Airway.[27] Emphasis should first be placed on securing an airway. The goal of achieving lung separation or isolation is a secondary priority. The indication[39] and safety of the technique for achieving OLV should be considered. The term "lung separation" refers to a complete anatomical sealing as obtained with a DLT, whereas "lung isolation" refers to a functional sealing as achieved with a BB.[40] Absolute indications for lung separation include massive bleeding or abscess in which the nondiseased lung must be protected from contamination, unilateral air leak from bronchopleural or bronchopleural cutaneous fistula, or unilateral pulmonary lavage for alveolar proteinosis or cystic fibrosis. VATS has been included as an absolute indication for lung isolation.

Airway management options for this case include the placement of an SLT with a BB or the placement of a DLT. If a patient with obesity is positioned appropriately, DL and successful placement of either a DLT or ETT for bronchial blockade should be no different than in a patient without obesity.[41] Historically, a Univent tube would be a popular choice in the management of this patient. If a Univent tube is selected, intubation can be more difficult than with a conventional ETT due to the fixed concavity and its larger OD. With the presence of modern BBs, there are no advantages to placing a Univent tube over a regular SLT. The decision to use an SLT as opposed to a DLT is based on the degree of difficulty anticipated with the more difficult tube, the availability of airway management equipment such as video laryngoscopes, the upper airway anatomy/geometry, endobronchial anatomy, and the expertise of the airway practitioner. The anticipated postoperative clinical course is also relevant, especially if postoperative ventilation is required.

An airway management plan should begin with adequate denitrogenation in order to lower the risk of hypoxemia. This risk can be further reduced by providing apneic oxygenation.[42,43] A blade change can be considered if it is anticipated that a specific anatomic problem can be overcome. Placement of a DLT is best accomplished with a curved blade as it leaves more space in the pharynx through which to pass the relatively bulky DLT. An Eschmann Tracheal Introducer (ETI, commonly known as "bougie") is unlikely to succeed in the presence of a CL Grade 4 view and may produce trauma. As an alternative to DL, intubation could be achieved with flexible bronchoscopy under general anesthesia, assisted with a video laryngoscope[44–46] or intubating through an EGD. Intubation of the unconscious patient using the flexible bronchoscope is a widely accepted technique, although it is considered to be more difficult than when performed in an awake patient. Jaw thrust and tongue traction can be used to open the hypopharynx and facilitate passage of the scope. When performing a flexible bronchoscopic intubation with a DLT, the length of the tube relative to the length of the shaft of the scope limits the maneuverability of the scope.[47] The rigidity of the DLT also makes it more difficult to advance the tube over the scope, though it is possible.

In the setting of predictable difficult DL, awake flexible bronchoscopic intubation has historically been accepted to be the safest means to secure the airway and is still recommended as the preferred technique in the elective setting. However, with the introduction of devices that are proving to be useful in difficult intubation, protocols are changing and video laryngoscopes are challenging bronchoscopy as the first choice for managing these airways.[48–50]

In the event a DLT is chosen, it may require a tube exchange at the end of the procedure. The exchange of a DLT for an SLT is not without risk. Edema, secretions, and trauma from the initial intubation may make reintubation at the end of surgery dangerously difficult and increase the risk of airway trauma and aspiration. In the case presentation, the best airway management choice for the patient would be the placement of an SLT with any of the available BBs. At the end of the case, the BB would be easily removed, allowing for the patient's emergence and extubation to be managed with a familiar, regular SLT.

Retrograde intubation is an option in the clinical scenario presented here if the equipment and expertise are available.[51,52] Intubation with an SLT or airway exchange catheter (AEC) through a laryngeal mask airway (LMA) or an intubating LMA (ILMA) is also an option.[53]

Intubation by transillumination utilizing a lighted-stylet is a nonvisual technique and is not recommended in the presence of pharyngeal masses or anatomic abnormalities of the upper airway.[54] However, successful placement of DLTs using a lighted stylet under general anesthesia in patients with predictors of difficult DL but without airway pathology has been reported.[55–57]

Lastly, there is another DLT that has recently been introduced, the VivaSight-DL with an integrated camera.[58,59] Comparisons to regular DLTs appear to be favorable but their value in a patient with a difficult airway has yet to be established.

In the case presented, intubation was attempted using a C-MAC video laryngoscope with a D-blade. The glottis was visualized but the larynx was extremely anterior and a bougie could not be passed through the glottis because of the acute anterior angle. An ILMA was placed and satisfactory ventilation was achieved. A flexible bronchoscope was passed through the ILMA but the vocal cords could not be identified. The patient was ventilated through the ILMA and awakened after the reversal of muscle relaxation.

What Should Be the Next Steps in This Patient's Management?

The patient requires time-sensitive surgery. She was transported to the Post-Anesthesia Care Unit (PACU) for a period of observation. An explanation of the airway difficulty was provided, an antisialogogue was administered, and the patient was returned to the operating room about 2 hours later for an awake flexible bronchoscopic intubation.

Awake flexible bronchoscopic intubation using an adult bronchoscope and an 8-mm inner diameter (ID) SLT was performed under topical anesthesia. A remifentanil infusion, carefully titrated due to the patient's history of severe OSA, was used to attenuate airway reflexes. The awake intubation was uneventful and was followed by the controlled induction of general anesthesia.

Can Awake Flexible Bronchoscopic Intubation Be Done with a DLT?

Successful awake flexible bronchoscopic intubation with a DLT has been reported by Patane et al.[47] The laryngeal and carinal stimulation produced by the DLT can be intense and profound anesthesia of the airway is required. When the bronchial lumen of a DLT is ensleeved over the bronchoscope, only a short segment of the insertion cord of the scope remains outside the tube and maneuverability is therefore limited. Once the DLT has been placed in the trachea, general anesthesia can be induced before advancing the DLT into the mainstem bronchus under flexible bronchoscopic control. Since modern BB have become available, awake flexible bronchoscopic intubation with a DLT or Univent is rarely performed.

What Are the Options for Lung Separation in This Case Now that an SLT Has Been Placed?

The options for one lung OLV include the use of a BB passed through the SLT or the exchange of the SLT for a DLT using an AEC. When using an AEC, complications[60,61] can be avoided by maintaining visual control utilizing a video laryngoscope.[62,63]

In this case, it was decided to proceed with the placement of a BB and not to exchange the SLT for a DLT. This decision was based on the degree of difficulty anticipated with the tube exchange and the risk associated with this maneuver, as well as the possibility of the requirement for postoperative ventilatory support. A Fuji Uniblocker (Fuji Systems, Tokyo) was chosen and placed uneventfully in the left mainstem bronchus. The cuff was inflated under bronchoscopic control.

The choice of BB is a matter of personal preference. The Fuji Uni-blocker is made of silicone, is 66.5 cm long, and has an angled tip and a spherical high-volume low-pressure cuff (cuff volume of 5-8 mL). The adult blocker is 9 Fr and has a 2-mm lumen. It is maneuvered by rotation in a comparable manner to a bougie. As mentioned earlier, Narayanaswamy et al.[9] compared the Arndt wire-guided BB, the Cohen Flexi-tip BB, the Fuji Uniblocker, and the left DLT in a randomized trial that included 104 patients undergoing left video or open thoracotomy. The three BBs provided surgical exposure equivalent to the left DLT, although the blockers required more time to position and required intraoperative repositioning more often. In a randomized trial that compared the Coopdech blocker, the Arndt, the Univent tube, and the left DLT, Zhong et al.[14] reported that surgical exposure was similar among the groups. The EZ-blocker has a 4-cm bifurcated tip, each limb of which is fitted with a cuff. The blocker is positioned with one cuff in each mainstem bronchus and the cuff on the side to be blocked inflated. Lung collapse using the EZ-blocker has been shown to be equivalent to that achieved with a DLT[64,65] and the Cohen BB.[66]

During the surgery, the left pulmonary artery was disrupted. An emergency thoracotomy was done and Vascular Surgery was called to assist with the case. Six hours after starting the procedure, the artery was patched successfully and the left upper lobe of the lung was removed. The estimated blood loss was 5000 mL. Eight units of packed red blood cells, 1000 mL of plasma, four units of platelets, and 4000 mL of crystalloid were administered. At the end of the case, edema of the face and tongue was evident.

POSTOPERATIVE AIRWAY CONSIDERATIONS

Should This Patient Be Extubated?

Airway edema can occur because of fluid resuscitation and trauma associated with the initial intubation. The presence of airway edema will certainly make reintubation conditions even less favorable than they were at the beginning of the case. In addition, the patient has undergone an extensive surgical procedure and the risk of respiratory failure in the immediate postoperative period is significant. It is clear the patient should not be extubated. Postoperative pain control could be achieved with the placement of a paravertebral catheter.

The BB was deflated and removed but the ETT was left in place. The patient was transported to the intensive care unit (ICU) in stable condition and electively ventilated. Twenty-four hours after the surgery the patient was awake and no longer needed ventilatory support.

How Should the Patient Be Extubated Now?

Whether the patient should be extubated in the ICU or the OR is a matter of clinical judgment and to an extent dependent on the expertise and equipment available. Nasopharyngoscopy could be performed prior to extubation to determine the presence and extent of airway edema. The presence of an air leak around the tube (the leak test) may be reassuring.

Given the degree of difficulty experienced with the intubation, the patient was transported to the OR for extubation. The extubation was performed over an AEC, being careful to match the numbers on the catheter with the numbers on the SLT. A surgeon skilled in the performance of a front-of-neck airway (FONA) was present in the room and the necessary equipment was immediately available. Extubation was uneventful.

OTHER CONSIDERATIONS

If the SLT Had Been Exchanged for a DLT After Induction, How Should This Have Been Done?

Tube exchange should be done utilizing an AEC and under visual control to assist in the guidance of the DLT through the glottis. The AEC should be introduced no further than 24 to 26 cm from the teeth or lips in order to minimize the risk of trauma to the distal trachea and bronchi. Though a minimum length of 70 cm has been identified as sufficient to permit control of the proximal end of the catheter with the DLT ensleeved, an AEC of at least 83 cm in length is recommended for a DLT exchange. A video laryngoscope should be used during tube exchange in either direction: SLT for DLT or DLT for SLT. Tube exchange using an AEC is not without risk. McLean et al.[61] reported a failure rate using the Cook Airway Exchange Catheter of 9.3% for SLT to SLT, 39.9% for SLT to DLT, and 0% for DLT to SLT. The number of cases in which direct or video laryngoscopy was used to assist the exchange was not reported.

If a DLT Had Been Used for Lung Separation, What Constitutes Appropriate Airway Management at the End of the Case? Can the Patient Go to ICU with a DLT in Place?

Intubation was difficult at the start of the case. Given the extent and duration of the surgery and the presence of airway edema, the exchange of the DLT for an SLT at the end of the case could be a highly dangerous maneuver. The view of the glottis was suboptimal with the video laryngoscope at induction and the angle into the larynx was difficult to negotiate. The options then, are to leave the DLT in place, exchange the DLT for an SLT, or perform a tracheotomy. These options are described in detail by Merli et al.[67] in their published "Recommendations for airway control and difficult airway management in thoracic anesthesia and lung separation procedures." If it is anticipated that airway edema will recede in the immediate postoperative period and that prolonged ventilatory support will not be required, tracheotomy is not necessary at this time. Given the intraoperative course, placement of a BB through the SLT was a good decision and avoided the consideration of a risky tube exchange at the end of the case.

A DLT can be used in the critical care setting for OLV or for postoperative two-lung ventilation if tube exchange to an

SLT is too risky. However, ICU medical and nursing staff are less experienced in the management of a DLT. Clinical judgement and personal experience play a role in determining which management option is best. If a DLT is left in an endobronchial position, malposition can occur, particularly if neuromuscular blockade is not employed. The DLT should be withdrawn to the 19 to 20 cm mark such that the endobronchial lumen is above the carina. Both lungs are then ventilated with both lumens with the bronchial cuff deflated. Bronchial toilette is more difficult through a DLT and secretions can be problematic. If required, DLT to ETT exchange can be performed later when clinical conditions improve.

Extubation directly from the DLT can be performed when the conditions of the upper airway and ventilatory function are satisfactory. In this situation, it is recommended that an AEC be maintained inside the tracheal for a short test period. This provides a useful aid for reintubation if clinical conditions deteriorate. If further short-term ventilatory support is anticipated, an SLT can be reinserted over the AEC. For longer-term ventilation, tracheotomy may be more appropriate.

How Should the Airway Have Been Managed If The Surgery Had Been an Emergency and Could Not Be Postponed?

Intubation had failed by DL, GlideScope and flexible bronchoscope through an ILMA. The expertise to perform a retrograde intubation was not available and the likelihood of success was uncertain given the airway assessment. If surgery had been an emergency, a tracheotomy could have been performed under general anesthesia with the patient ventilated via the ILMA. A BB could then be passed through an armored ETT or conventional tracheotomy cannula inserted into the tracheotomy stoma.[68,69] A Fuji Wire-Reinforced ETT, which is longer than a conventional armored ETT and has a short "endobronchial" cuff could also be used but is a tube usually reserved for tracheal resection surgery.[70] A conventional DLT can be inserted through a tracheotomy stoma (size dependent), or a DLT modified for use in tracheotomized patients (e.g., Tracheopart or Naruke tube) could be used.[71–73] A conventional DLT placed through a tracheotomy stoma has been said to be prone to malposition as it is too long relative to the shortened upper airway and the tracheal cuff may be at or proximal to the stoma. Cohen has recommended that a rigid large diameter DLT not be passed through an old tracheotomy stoma. Campos has reported DLTs are the least frequently used devices for OLV in tracheostomized patients and instead recommended the use of an independent BB for these patients.[74]

If a "Can't Intubate, Can't Oxygenate" Situation Had Occurred at Induction, What Should Have Been Done?

If ventilation by a face mask or EGD had become impossible during the failed intubation attempts, emergency cricothyrotomy would have been indicated.

The patient made an uneventful recovery and was discharged home after a week in the hospital.

SUMMARY

Lung separation can be achieved using a DLT, or a BB placed through an SLT. In the setting of a difficult airway, the decision to use a particular device must take into consideration the interaction between the indication for lung separation/isolation, airway anatomy, the anesthesia practitioner's expertise with equipment available, the type of surgery planned, and the anticipated postoperative clinical course. Airway management decisions will depend on whether the difficulty is predicted or unpredicted, the ability to have face-mask-ventilate and whether the surgery is elective or an emergency. In the management of the difficult airway, the priority is to ensure adequate oxygenation and ventilation; OLV becomes a secondary objective. The use of an SLT and an independent BB is frequently the best available option.

SELF-EVALUATION QUESTIONS

39.1. Why have the Univent and Double Lumen tubes been termed "difficult tubes"?

A. Increased external diameter (OD)
B. Increased rigidity
C. Increased rigidity and increased OD
D. None of the above

39.2. Changing an SLT for a double-lumen tube at the end of the case can be difficult due to:

A. Airway edema
B. Intubation trauma
C. Suboptimal head and neck position
D. All the above

39.3. Exchange of an SLT for a DLT should be done:

A. Under visual control
B. With an AEC
C. With an AEC and under visual control
D. None of the above

REFERENCES

1. Kao MC, Lan CH, Huang CJ. Anesthesia for awake video-assisted thoracic surgery. *Acta Anaesthesiol Taiwan*. 2012;50(3):126-130.
2. Zheng H, Hu XF, Jiang GN, Ding JA, Zhu YM. Nonintubated-awake anesthesia for uniportal video-assisted thoracic surgery procedures. *Thorac Surg Clin*. 2017;27(4):399-406.
3. Ashok V, Francis J. A practical approach to adult one-lung ventilation. *BJA Educ*. 2018;18(3):69-74.
4. Falzon D, Alston RP, Coley E, Montgomery K. Lung isolation for thoracic surgery: from inception to evidence-based. *J Cardiothorac Vasc Anesth*. 2017;31(2):678-693.
5. Campos JH. Which device should be considered the best for lung isolation: double-lumen endotracheal tube versus bronchial blockers. *Curr Opin Anaesthesiol*. 2007;20(1):27-31.
6. Brodsky JB, Lemmens HJ. Left double-lumen tubes: clinical experience with 1,170 patients. *J Cardiothorac Vasc Anesth*. 2003;17(3):289-298.
7. Campos JH, Hallam EA, Van Natta T, Kernstine KH. Devices for lung isolation used by anesthesiologists with limited thoracic experience: comparison of double-lumen endotracheal tube, Univent torque control blocker, and Arndt wire-guided endobronchial blocker. *Anesthesiology*. 2006;104(2):261-266.

8. Campos JH. Update on tracheobronchial anatomy and flexible fiberoptic bronchoscopy in thoracic anesthesia. *Curr Opin Anaesthesiol.* 2009; 22(1):4-10.
9. Narayanaswamy M, McRae K, Slinger P, et al. Choosing a lung isolation device for thoracic surgery: a randomized trial of three bronchial blockers versus double-lumen tubes. *Anesth Analg.* 2009;108(4):1097-1101.
10. Campos JH, Massa FC. Is there a better right-sided tube for one-lung ventilation? A comparison of the right-sided double-lumen tube with the single-lumen tube with right-sided enclosed bronchial blocker. *Anesth Analg.* 1998;86(4):696-700.
11. Campos JH, Kernstine KH. A comparison of a left-sided Broncho-Cath with the torque control blocker univent and the wire-guided blocker. *Anesth Analg.* 2003;96(1):283-289.
12. Cohen E. Pro: the new bronchial blockers are preferable to double-lumen tubes for lung isolation. *J Cardiothorac Vasc Anesth.* 2008;22(6): 920-924.
13. Slinger P. Con: the new bronchial blockers are not preferable to double-lumen tubes for lung isolation. *J Cardiothorac Vasc Anesth.* 2008; 22(6):925-929.
14. Zhong T, Wang W, Chen J, Ran L, Story DA. Sore throat or hoarse voice with bronchial blockers or double-lumen tubes for lung isolation: a randomised, prospective trial. *Anaesth Intensive Care.* 2009;37(3):441-446.
15. Kosarek L, Busch E, Abbas A, Falterman J, Nossaman BD. Effective use of bronchial blockers in lung isolation surgery: an analysis of 130 cases. *Ochsner J.* 2013;13(3):389-393.
16. Cohen E. Recommendations for airway control and difficult airway management in thoracic anesthesia and lung separation procedures. Are we ready for the challenge? *Minerva Anestesiol.* 2009;75(1-2):3-5.
17. Arndt GA, DeLessio ST, Kranner PW, Orzepowski W, Ceranski B, Valtysson B. One-lung ventilation when intubation is difficult–presentation of a new endobronchial blocker. *Acta Anaesthesiol Scand.* 1999;43(3):356-358.
18. Cohen E. The Cohen flexitip endobronchial blocker: an alternative to a double lumen tube. *Anesth Analg.* 2005;101(6):1877-1879.
19. Tanabe S, Tanaka A, Nishino T. Experience using an improved bronchial blocker (Phycon TCB bronchial blocker). *Masui.* 2004;53(11):1317-1319.
20. Uzuki M, Kanaya N, Mizuguchi A, et al. One-lung ventilation using a new bronchial blocker in a patient with tracheostomy stoma. *Anesth Analg.* 2003;96(5):1538-1539.
21. Mungroop HE, Wai PT, Morei MN, Loef BG, Epema AH. Lung isolation with a new Y-shaped endobronchial blocking device, the EZ-blocker. *Br J Anaesth.* 2010;104(1):119-120.
22. Vannucci A, Cavallone LF. Bedside predictors of difficult intubation: a systematic review. *Minerva Anestesiol.* 2016;82(1):69-83.
23. Roth D, Pace NL, Lee A, et al. Airway physical examination tests for detection of difficult airway management in apparently normal adult patients. *Cochrane Database Syst Rev.* 2018;5(5):Cd008874.
24. Roth D, Pace NL, Lee A, et al. Bedside tests for predicting difficult airways: an abridged Cochrane diagnostic test accuracy systematic review. *Anaesthesia.* 2019;74(7):915-928.
25. Detsky ME, Jivraj N, Adhikari NK, et al. Will this patient be difficult to intubate? The rational clinical examination systematic review. *JAMA.* 2019;321(5):493-503.
26. Apfelbaum JL, Hagberg CA, Caplan RA, et al. Practice guidelines for management of the difficult airway: an updated report by the American Society of Anesthesiologists Task Force on Management of the Difficult Airway. *Anesthesiology.* 2013;118(2):251-270.
27. Apfelbaum JL, Hagberg CA, Connis RT, et al. American Society of Anesthesiologists Practice Guidelines for Management of the Difficult Airway. *Anesthesiology.* 2022;136(1):31-81.
28. Law JA, Duggan LV, Asselin M, et al. Canadian Airway Focus Group updated consensus-based recommendations for management of the difficult airway: part 1. Difficult airway management encountered in an unconscious patient. *Can J Anaesth.* 2021;68(9):1373-1404.
29. Law JA, Duggan LV, Asselin M, et al. Canadian Airway Focus Group updated consensus-based recommendations for management of the difficult airway: part 2. Planning and implementing safe management of the patient with an anticipated difficult airway. *Can J Anaesth.* 2021;68(9): 1405-1436.
30. Benumof JL. Difficult tubes and difficult airways. *J Cardiothorac Vasc Anesth.* 1998;12(2):131-132.
31. Cohen E, Benumof JL. Lung separation in the patient with a difficult airway. *Curr Opin Anaesthesiol.* 1999;12(1):29-35.
32. Brodsky JB. Lung separation and the difficult airway. *Br J Anaesth.* 2009;103(Suppl 1):i66-75.
33. Inoue H, Shohtsu A, Ogawa J, Kawada S, Koide S. New device for one-lung anesthesia: endotracheal tube with movable blocker. *J Thorac Cardiovasc Surg.* 1982;83(6):940-941.
34. Campos JH. An update on bronchial blockers during lung separation techniques in adults. *Anesth Analg.* 2003;97(5):1266-1274.
35. Slinger PD, Lesiuk L. Flow resistances of disposable double-lumen, single-lumen, and Univent tubes. *J Cardiothorac Vasc Anesth.* 1998;12(2):142-144.
36. Kheterpal S, Healy D, Aziz MF, et al. Incidence, predictors, and outcome of difficult mask ventilation combined with difficult laryngoscopy: a report from the multicenter perioperative outcomes group. *Anesthesiology.* 2013;119(6):1360-1369.
37. Altermatt FR, Muñoz HR, Delfino AE, Cortínez LI. Pre-oxygenation in the obese patient: effects of position on tolerance to apnoea. *Br J Anaesth.* 2005;95(5):706-709.
38. Couture EJ, Provencher S, Somma J, Lellouche F, Marceau S, Bussières JS. Effect of position and positive pressure ventilation on functional residual capacity in morbidly obese patients: a randomized trial. *Can J Anaesth.* 2018;65(5):522-528.
39. Campos J. Lung isolation. In: Slinger P, ed. *Principles and Practice of Anesthesia for Thoracic Surgery.* Springer; 2019:283-309.
40. Szegedi LL, Licker M. Lung isolation versus lung separation: double-lumen tubes. In: Granell Gil M, Şentürk M, eds. *Anesthesia in Thoracic Surgery: Changes of Paradigms.* Springer; 2020:51-63.
41. Campos JH, Hallam EA, Ueda K. Lung isolation in the morbidly obese patient: a comparison of a left-sided double-lumen tracheal tube with the Arndt® wire-guided blocker. *Br J Anaesth.* 2012;109(4):630-635.
42. Pavlov I, Medrano S, Weingart S. Apneic oxygenation reduces the incidence of hypoxemia during emergency intubation: a systematic review and meta-analysis. *Am J Emerg Med.* 2017;35(8):1184-1189.
43. Oliveira JESL, Cabrera D, Barrionuevo P, et al. Effectiveness of apneic oxygenation during intubation: a systematic review and meta-analysis. *Ann Emerg Med.* 2017;70(4):483-494.e11.
44. Aziz MF, Healy D, Kheterpal S, Fu RF, Dillman D, Brambrink AM. Routine clinical practice effectiveness of the Glidescope in difficult airway management: an analysis of 2,004 Glidescope intubations, complications, and failures from two institutions. *Anesthesiology.* 2011;114(1):34-41.
45. Russell T, Slinger P, Roscoe A, McRae K, Van Rensburg A. A randomised controlled trial comparing the GlideScope(®) and the Macintosh laryngoscope for double-lumen endobronchial intubation. *Anaesthesia.* 2013; 68(12):1253-1258.
46. Chen A, Lai HY, Lin PC, Chen TY, Shyr MH. GlideScope-assisted double-lumen endobronchial tube placement in a patient with an unanticipated difficult airway. *J Cardiothorac Vasc Anesth.* 2008;22(1):170-172.
47. Patane PS, Sell BA, Mahla ME. Awake fiberoptic endobronchial intubation. *J Cardiothorac Anesth.* 1990;4(2):229-231.
48. Marco CA, Marco AP. Airway adjuncts. *Emerg Med Clin North Am.* 2008;26(4):1015-1027.
49. Pott LM, Murray WB. Review of video laryngoscopy and rigid fiberoptic laryngoscopy. *Curr Opin Anaesthesiol.* 2008;21(6):750-758.
50. Thong SY, Lim Y. Video and optic laryngoscopy assisted tracheal intubation—the new era. *Anaesth Intensive Care.* 2009;37(2):219-233.
51. Benumof J, Hagberg CA. *Benumof's Airway Management: Principles and Practice.* Elsevier; 2007.
52. Dhara SS. Retrograde tracheal intubation. *Anaesthesia.* 2009;64(10): 1094-1104.
53. Perlin DI, Hannallah MS. Double-lumen tube placement in a patient with a difficult airway. *J Cardiothorac Vasc Anesth.* 1996;10(6):787-788.
54. Hung OR, Stewart RD, Hagberg CA. *Benumof's Airway Management: Principles and Practice.* 2nd ed. Philadelphia, PA: Mosby Inc, 2007, 463-475.
55. O'Connor CJ, O'Connor TA. Use of lighted stylets to facilitate insertion of double-lumen endobronchial tubes in patients with difficult airway anatomy. *J Clin Anesth.* 2006;18(8):616-619.
56. Chen KY, Tsao SL, Lin SK, Wu HS. Double-lumen endobronchial tube intubation in patients with difficult airways using Trachlight and a modified technique. *Anesth Analg.* 2007;105(5):1425-1426.
57. Scanzillo MA, Shulman MS. Lighted stylet for placement of a double-lumen endobronchial tube. *Anesth Analg.* 1995;81(1):205-206.
58. Schuepbach R, Grande B, Camen G, et al. Intubation with VivaSight or conventional left-sided double-lumen tubes: a randomized trial. *Can J Anaesth.* 2015;62(7):762-769.
59. Dean C, Dragnea D, Anwar S, Ong C. The VivaSight-DL double-lumen tube with integrated camera. *Eur J Anaesthesiol.* 2016;33(4):305-308.
60. Thomas V, Neustein SM. Tracheal laceration after the use of an airway exchange catheter for double-lumen tube placement. *J Cardiothorac Vasc Anesth.* 2007;21(5):718-719.
61. McLean S, Lanam CR, Benedict W, Kirkpatrick N, Kheterpal S, Ramachandran SK. Airway exchange failure and complications with the use of the Cook Airway Exchange Catheter®: a single center cohort study of 1177 patients. *Anesth Analg.* 2013;117(6):1325-1327.

62. Hirabayashi Y. GlideScope-assisted endotracheal tube exchange. *J Cardiothorac Vasc Anesth*. 2007;21(5):777.
63. Campos JH. Lung isolation techniques for patients with difficult airway. *Curr Opin Anaesthesiol*. 2010;23(1):12-17.
64. Ruetzler K, Grubhofer G, Schmid W, et al. Randomized clinical trial comparing double-lumen tube and EZ-blocker for single-lung ventilation. *Br J Anaesth*. 2011;106(6):896-902.
65. Mourisse J, Liesveld J, Verhagen A, et al. Efficiency, efficacy, and safety of EZ-blocker compared with left-sided double-lumen tube for one-lung ventilation. *Anesthesiology*. 2013;118(3):550-561.
66. Kus A, Hosten T, Gurkan Y, Gul Akgul A, Solak M, Toker K. A comparison of the EZ-Blocker with a Cohen Flex-Tip blocker for one-lung ventilation. *J Cardiothorac Vasc Anesth*. 2014;28(4):896-899.
67. Merli G, Guarino A, Della Rocca G, et al. Recommendations for airway control and difficult airway management in thoracic anesthesia and lung separation procedures. *Minerva Anestesiol*. 2009;75(1-2):59-96.
68. Campos JH, Kernstine KH. Use of the wire-guided endobronchial blocker for one-lung anesthesia in patients with airway abnormalities. *J Cardiothorac Vasc Anesth*. 2003;17(3):352-354.
69. Tobias JD. Variations on one-lung ventilation. *J Clin Anesth*. 2001;13(1):35-39.
70. McRae K. Tracheal Resection and Reconstruction. In: Slinger P, ed. *Principles and Practice of Anesthesia for Thoracic Surgery*. Springer; 2019:231-248.
71. Brodsky JB, Tobler HG, Mark JB. A double-lumen endobronchial tube for tracheostomies. *Anesthesiology*. 1991;74(2):387-388.
72. Saito T, Naruke T, Carney E, Yokokawa Y, Hiraga K, Carlsson C. New double intrabronchial tube (Naruke tube) for tracheostomized patients. *Anesthesiology*. 1998;89(4):1038-1039.
73. Yaney LL. Double-lumen endotracheal tube for one-lung ventilation through a fresh tracheostomy stoma: a case report. *AANA J*. 2007;75(6):411-415.
74. Campos JH, Musselman ED, Hanada S, Ueda K. lung isolation techniques in patients with early-stage or long-term tracheostomy: a case series report of 70 cases and recommendations. *J Cardiothorac Vasc Anesth*. 2019;33(2):433-439.

CHAPTER 40

Airway Management in an Uncooperative Patient with Down Syndrome with a Perforated Diverticulitis

Mathieu Asselin and François Lemay

CASE PRESENTATION

A 33-year-old female patient with Down syndrome (DS) and moderate intellectual disability presented with a history of vomiting and abdominal pain (Figure 40.1). A perforated diverticulitis was diagnosed in the emergency department (ED).

You first encountered the patient when she was brought to the operating room (OR) during an on-call shift. Shortly after her first bolus of crystalloid fluid, her only intravenous (IV) catheter was inadvertently pulled out. The prepared antibiotics could not yet be administered. Upon arrival, she was not cooperative and did not allow an IV catheter to be reinserted. She did not answer questions. She was lying on her side with her head flexed forward and did not extend her neck when requested nor did she permit you to do so. She appeared to have a short, thick neck. She did not open her mouth as per your request. Her sister, who accompanied her, has been her caregiver for the past 20 years. As far as her sister knew, the patient was healthy, with no known cardiac history and a good functional capacity. As a child, she had two uneventful general anesthetics for dental care. She was on no medication and had no allergies.

On examination, she was 157.5 cm (5 ft 2 in) tall and weighed 96 kg (211 lb). Her body mass index was 38.4 $kg{\cdot}m^{-2}$. Her vital signs have been deteriorating since her arrival. Last vital signs were: heart rate 122 beats per minute, blood pressure 88/54 mmHg, temperature 39.2°C, respiratory rate 28 breaths per minute, and peripheral capillary oxygen saturation (SpO_2) 92% on room air. She was combative and repeatedly removed any supplemental oxygen delivery device. You suspected that she may have aspirated gastric contents.

The patient was thus unable to cooperate and showed features of a potential difficult airway despite limited evaluation. Moreover, she demonstrated signs of sepsis with hemodynamic instability and respiratory compromise due to sepsis and potential aspiration of gastric contents.

The general surgeon planned to attempt a laparoscopic sigmoidectomy. The patient required a general anesthetic with endotracheal intubation.

PATIENT EVALUATION

What Are the Factors That Make Airway Management Challenging in This Situation?

Considering the patient has DS, obesity, and limited airway evaluation, it is anticipated that airway management would be difficult and challenging. The airway practitioner should recognize multiple factors that may further hinder airway management of this patient and be prepared for alternative plans in the event of failure.

First, this patient's physiology has been altered by her sepsis. This will increase cognitive load for the airway practitioner during airway management because of potential hemodynamic instability with induction medications and limited apnea tolerance.

Second, an out-of-hour schedule involves less readily available help than during daily shifts. These considerations must

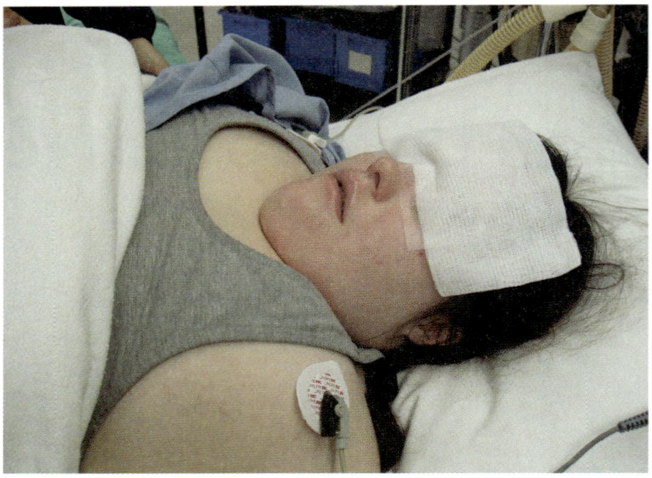

FIGURE 40.1. Patient with Down syndrome admitted to general surgery department with a perforated diverticulitis.

be taken into account in your airway management decisions and can be defined by the concept of context-sensitive airway management (see Chapter 7).

Third, patient's cooperation will be a major issue considering her intellectual disability, pain, sepsis, and anxiety.

How Are Her ABCs?

Regarding the **A**irway, you have no reason to believe she is obstructing at the moment, as there is no snoring nor stridor and you can feel the air coming out of her mouth on the back of your hand. An oxygen mask, nasal prongs, or high-flow nasal cannulas with capnography would be ideal, but she refuses any oxygen delivery on her face.

Regarding **B**reathing, she is tachypneic and her SpO_2 is 92% on room air. She has limited oxygen reserves and will rapidly desaturate if she obstructs or becomes apneic without oxygen being provided by any means.

Her low SpO_2 may be caused by aspiration, as she vomited. It may also be an indication that she is developing an acute respiratory distress syndrome (ARDS) in the course of her sepsis and may be exacerbated by atelectasis as she is breathing at low tidal volumes as she has abdominal pain. She also has obesity (Class II) and is thus expected to have respiratory physiologic changes that will increase her propensity to rapid oxygen desaturation. Moreover, her obesity and facial features carry a risk for obstructive sleep apnea (OSA) which impacts induction and emergence from anesthesia. She will carry ongoing regurgitation and aspiration risk upon extubation. These respiratory risk factors combined with her limited cardiovascular reserve carry a potential need to maintain postoperative mechanical ventilation.

Regarding **C**irculation, hemodynamic instability will need to be addressed concurrently with airway management. The tachycardia and the narrowed pulse pressure suggest intravascular volume depletion related to dehydration and sepsis. Her lack of cooperation, despite being compounded by her intellectual disability, could also be secondary to her sepsis. In this case, the patient is anticipated to be uncooperative on induction and emergence. Her response to sedative hypnotic agents is unpredictable both for sedation and hemodynamic effects.

What About Her Past Medical History?

Patients with DS carry a 50% risk of congenital heart defects. Postnatal echocardiogram is indicated in all patients.[1] It is worth noting that DS patients without structural heart disease may develop valve abnormalities (mitral and aortic valve regurgitation) or pulmonary hypertension later in life.[2] In this patient's case, no previous heart defects or repairs were mentioned, and a good functional capacity was confirmed; thus, no significant heart disease is expected.

There were no additional comorbidities associated with DS found during the patient's preoperative evaluation.[2]

AIRWAY EVALUATION

Employing the Mnemonics Suggested in Chapter 1, Does This Patient Have a Difficult Airway?

Potential difficulties with all modes of oxygenation (face-mask ventilation [FMV], direct laryngoscopy [DL], video laryngoscopy [VL], extraglottic devices [EGDs] and front-of-neck access [FONA]) must be quantified. This will help the practitioner to formulate a precise airway plan.

MOANS-guided airway evaluation for difficult FMV (see section "Difficult FMV: MOANS" in Chapter 1) reveals her obesity as a factor for decreased success for FMV. She may have decreased lung compliance due to her acute respiratory condition. Mask seal may be difficult if she cannot extend her neck, and you cannot evaluate her Mallampati score and jaw protrusion. There is no reason to believe that she has any obstructing lesion. There is no history of snoring, but obesity and DS put her at risk of OSA.

LEMON and CRANE are used to assess the difficulty associated with DL and VL-guided intubation (see sections "Difficult DL Intubation: LEMON" and "Difficult VL Intubation: CRANE" in Chapter 1). When you attempt to evaluate the geometry of her upper airway, you are unable to assess the volume of her mandibular space. This is particularly problematic in a person with DS, as the tongue is relatively large for the volume of the mouth. You cannot determine where her larynx is relative to the base of her tongue. You are unable to evaluate her Mallampati score and her neck mobility. There is no sign of airway obstruction. Obesity is again a risk factor here, and her potential aspiration of gastric content and acute abdomen increase the risk for contamination during VL. There is no recent general anesthesia record to review her Cormack-Lehane grade.

RODS is for difficulties in EGD use (see section "Difficulty with an EGD: "RODS" in Chapter 1). There does not appear to be upper airway obstruction and the airway is neither distorted nor disrupted. Her mouth opening cannot be evaluated at the moment, but collateral history from her sister, such as the capacity to widely open her mouth or difficulty when having dental evaluation, can be obtained. As mentioned earlier, she is obese and decreased lung compliance may militate against successful ventilation with an EGD. Moreover, patients with DS may have subglottic stenosis, further increasing the difficulty to produce adequate tidal volumes with an EGD without increasing positive ventilatory pressure and potential leak with such a device.

Finally, the patient should be assessed for difficult FONA using the mnemonic SHORT (see section "Difficult FONA: SHORT" in Chapter 1). There is no history of prior anterior neck surgery, hematoma, or other overlying process that masks the anatomy. There is no history or evidence of radiation or tumor. Her only risk factor here is her obesity.

According to these mnemonics, she has multiple risk factors for a difficult airway with all modes of oxygenation.

What Concerns Specific to Airway Management Do You Have in Patients with DS?

True incidence of difficult airway management in adult patients with DS is not known. There are some features commonly seen with DS that can increase difficulty with all modes of oxygenation.

Airway obstruction is a frequent feature in patients with DS. There is a prevalence of OSA in about 40% of adult patients with DS.[3] The patient with DS is anatomically predisposed to pharyngeal obstruction due to a relatively narrow nasopharynx and large tongue, among other factors.[4] Lower airway obstruction due to tracheobronchomalacia is a common feature in the pediatric population.[5,6]

Incidence of either acquired or congenital subglottic stenosis is increased in patients with DS compared to the general population.[7–10] This has been attributed, in part, to complications from endotracheal intubation for surgery in early infancy, such as correction of cardiac or gastrointestinal defects.[10] Symptomatic subglottic stenosis is believed to happen in about 3% to 6% of children with DS, which is 10 times higher than in the general population.[5,6] Regurgitation and aspiration in early childhood is also believed to contribute to subglottic stenosis. Patients with DS thus may require an endotracheal tube (ETT) that is smaller than the standard appropriate size.

Patients with pathologic reflux and chronic aspiration episodes are at increased risk of lingual tonsils hypertrophy. This could lead to dramatic bleeding during the approach with a laryngoscopy blade.[11]

Cervical spine subluxation is frequent in patients with DS.[12] Incidence of atlantoaxial instability is reported in about 15% of these patients. However, complications arising during airway management in patients with DS are extremely rare. Asymptomatic patients usually do not need preoperative C-spine imaging, but there should be a high degree of suspicion for atlantoaxial instability. Any patient with neurological symptoms, including, but not limited to, gait difficulties, easy fatigability, and change in bowel and bladder function should be managed as if C-spine instability is present, if not ruled out with proper imaging.[1] The patient's sister denies any symptoms of neck movement limitation or neurological symptoms in this patient.

Intellectual disability is variable in patients with DS and thus cooperation is highly variable. Presence of a caregiver and the use of oral or intranasal premedication are examples of measures that can be implemented to decrease anxiety during techniques such as insertion of an IV catheter or denitrogenation.

MANAGING THE AIRWAY

What Are the Airway Management Options Considering Her IV Catheter Is Gone?

In this scenario, three options are available: induction with inhalation of volatile anesthetics followed by IV access, intramuscular (IM) induction followed by IV access, and further attempts at a vascular access before induction of anesthesia.

The use of inhaled anesthetics to sedate the patient or induce general anesthesia carries a high risk of airway obstruction, oxygen desaturation, and gastric regurgitation. We do not recommend inhalational induction in this clinical case. The 4th National Audit Project of The Royal College of Anaesthetists (NAP4) and the Difficult Airway Society (DAS) data have highlighted that problems may arise even if sedation is carried out with the goal to maintain spontaneous ventilation.[13] Moreover, at the alveolar concentration of volatile agent needed to maintain an adequate depth of anesthesia for endotracheal intubation in adults, vasodilation and potential decrease of cardiac output could lead to profound hypotension in this septic patient. IV access might still be difficult to establish even after inhalational induction, which could limit the potential for rapid vasopressor administration.

Induction dose of IM ketamine can be considered, but its effect will be difficult to predict in this hemodynamically unstable and cognitively impaired patient. Four $mg{\cdot}kg^{-1}$ of ideal body weight IM usually produces reliable sedation and dissociation in approximately 5 minutes.[14–17] Seven $mg{\cdot}kg^{-1}$ (ideal body weight) can be given orally with the expectation that the patient will be dissociated within 20 minutes, at least to the point that an IV can be placed.[17–19] If the degree of cooperation is not sufficient after this dose, half the original dose can be repeated at 20 minutes. Clearly, this is not an option in this case, as apnea and hypotension, although infrequent with ketamine, could still occur in this context and should not be considered as a completely safe option. Again, IV access might still be difficult to establish and delay vasopressor administration.

Therefore, further attempts at a vascular access is the most cautious option left. As mentioned above, sedation of any kind through any route may dramatically impair the patient's unstable hemodynamics and every effort must be taken to improve the situation before managing the airway. The airway practitioner will then be able to concentrate on airway management.

A peripheral IV insertion should be attempted with the help of OR personnel reassuring and gently holding the patient. If this fails, we recommend performing intraosseous (IO) access. IO access is a valuable alternative to implement sedation in a conscious patient, or even to perform induction of anesthesia. If used as a bridge to insertion of an IV catheter, sedation via the

IO route should be kept in a range in which the patient would still protect her airway and minimize the risk of aspiration. IO access has been reported in military and civilian trauma to have a similar success rate for rapid sequence induction (RSI).[20,21] Intramedullary route drains into the central venous system and, as such, the pharmacokinetics of drugs infused through IO are similar to those of IV infusions.[20,22] All medications intended for IV use can be used in an IO. Complication rate is low with IO insertion, and this patient has no contraindications to the insertion of an IO, which can stay in place for up to 24 hours. Various sites can be used such as the proximal humeral site or tibial site. Flow rates depend on the site of insertion, and needle size, and vary among patients. The proximal humerus site usually has faster flow rates than the tibial site. In this case, where collaboration is challenging, the proximal tibial site is the most adequate site of insertion despite inferior flow rates. There is a high variability among studies regarding flow rates at the proximal tibia. In one study, when used with a pressure bag, the 15-gauge tibial site could achieve flow rates of 165 $mL{\cdot}min^{-1}$.[23]

Considering this patient is uncooperative, we do not recommend attempting an awake insertion of a central IV catheter as it would be difficult to perform without risks (vascular trauma, breach in aseptic technique, risk of injury with needle manipulation for the health care worker, etc.). Once the patient is under general anesthesia, a central IV catheter can then be inserted.

With an IV/IO access in place, crystalloids, vasopressors, and antibiotics can be started with the goal of a systolic blood pressure over 100 mmHg and a heart rate below 100 bpm. However, depending on the situation, one must not wait too long to reach specific targets as the definitive treatment in this scenario will consist in proceeding with sigmoidectomy.

What Are the Airway Management Options Now That a Vascular Access Has Been Secured?

With a vascular access in place and improved hemodynamics, now is the time to concentrate on airway management. Considering airway management may be challenging due to the patient's numerous risk factors for difficulty and limited evaluation, an awake intubation is usually the best option (or awake tracheotomy in some cases). However, the lack of cooperation renders this path impractical. This leaves two choices: RSI or spontaneous breathing induction. In either case, oxygen should be delivered with a low-flow or high-flow nasal cannula throughout.

The rationale for maintaining spontaneous ventilation is to theoretically increase the margin of safety in case intubation fails. However, this is not without risks. It takes time to achieve a depth of anesthesia deep enough to intubate the trachea without adverse reactions (airway obstruction, coughing, oxygen desaturation, laryngospasm, etc.). While waiting for a deep anesthetic state, the airway is not secured and the patient cannot protect her airway if vomiting occurs, which is highly possible in this case. On the other hand, it is easier to perform intubation intubate when a neuromuscular blocker is used, less attempts are needed.[24,25]

RSI would provide the fastest way to secure the airway while diminishing the risk of aspiration. Experience from trauma centers supports this approach in potentially difficult airways of uncooperative patients.[26,27] RSI is recommended in uncooperative trauma patients with upper airway burns and in maxillofacial, laryngotracheal, tracheal, and bronchi blunt and penetrative trauma. The R Adams Cowley Shock Trauma Center in Baltimore had a high success rate in uncooperative patients with airway trauma following RSI involving in-line cervical stabilization, a maximum of 3 DL attempts, EGD insertion and FONA by the surgical team when needed. Out of 6088 patients needing airway management within the first hour after arrival, all patients were successfully managed (6008 orotracheal intubations and 21 FONA).[27] As in the case presented here, trauma patients are difficult to assess and examine. Moreover, timely radiographic evaluation is not always possible. In-line stabilization is indicated in trauma as we would do in patients with DS when atlantoaxial instability is a concern.

Delayed sequence induction,[28] in which small doses of sedation are progressively administered to render the patient cooperative with denitrogenation and airway management, is a potential option here. This should be implemented in this case with ketamine, or judicious use of a carefully titrated short-acting medication. Sedation for spontaneously breathing intubation in this situation is not without hazards. The use of sedative-hypnotic agents in large oral or intramuscular dosages may provoke paradoxical excitement, or worse, lead to hypoventilation or apnea. The margin of safety with ketamine is greater than other sedative-hypnotics, such as midazolam, as it preserves ventilatory function, muscle tone, and airway protective reflexes. The disadvantages of ketamine include the risk of laryngospasm, increase in secretions, emergence reactions, and post procedure nausea and vomiting. Apnea, although rare, can also occur with ketamine.[29,30]

Due to her full stomach status, FMV should not be part of plan A, but, if necessary, it should not be avoided. RSI is not synonymous with a contraindication to FMV. It can be performed with low tidal volume and low airway pressures as well as an early neuromuscular blockade. If implemented, FMV should be done with adjuncts such as an oropharyngeal airway and two-handed FMV from the start with limited peak inspiratory pressure to lower gastric insufflation and aspiration risk.

Considering the risk for regurgitation, obesity, and potential for increased ventilation pressure with laparoscopy, an EGD is not a definitive airway device in this case. An EGD (preferably a second-generation EGD with a conduit for tracheal intubation such as LMA-Protector™ [Teleflex, Wayne, PA, USA] or the i-gel® [Intersurgical, Burlington, ON, Canada]) should only be used as a temporary measure when facing a "cannot intubate cannot oxygenate" situation. If successfully inserted, the airway practitioner could then proceed to the STOP AND THINK phase of the Difficult Airway Society or the EXIT STRATEGY phase of the Canadian Airway Focus Group airway management algorithms to assess other management options.[31,32] In this case, the EGD could be used as a bridge to endotracheal intubation or tracheotomy. Indeed, waking the patient up after a successful EGD insertion would not permit a different approach in this case, as awake intubation or awake tracheotomy have already been ruled out.

The potential for gastric regurgitation is likely to render VL intubation difficult. A VL with Macintosh blade in this case should be used as plan A, which would allow both VL and DL in the event of airway soiling.

How Would You Prepare for Airway Management of This Patient?

To prepare for airway management, all equipment should be readily available in the OR or at the bedside. Team members should be briefed about the plan, procedures, and roles. Management will depend on which Plan A is chosen between an awake strategy with delayed sequence induction versus RSI. Preinduction IO/IV access and the importance of improving the patient's hemodynamic parameters before airway management have been discussed above. The patient's sister may be helpful in maintaining reassuring contact with the patient while IO/IV access is established. The neck of the patient should be prepared in as sterile a fashion as the circumstances will allow as soon as possible. The surgeon and OR team should prepare for FONA if needed (double setup).

The following airway devices must be immediately available for use:

- Styletted ETTs of various sizes (5, 6, and 7-mm ID)
- Two suctions with rigid suction handles
- Video laryngoscope with both direct and indirect laryngoscopy capability
- Macintosh laryngoscope with a #3 blade at the ready
- Flexible bronchoscope at the ready
- Different sizes of EGDs (one you are experienced with)
- Supplemental oxygen with either low-flow or high-flow devices

Failure to visualize the airway adequately to intubate with ongoing acceptable oxygen saturations may lead one to resort to Plan B. In the event adequate oxygen saturation cannot be maintained, an EGD must be immediately inserted and the surgical team must be ready, scalpel in hand, to immediately follow with a FONA in case the EGD fails.

How Exactly Was the Airway of This Patient Managed?

The corrugated oxygen tubing was used to provide supplemental oxygen with a blow-by method at 15 L·min^{-1} near her mouth and SpO_2 increased to 96%. Her sister was brought to the OR to help the patient to remain cooperative during vascular access. After a failed IV attempt, an IO access was inserted in her right proximal tibia. Hemodynamic instability was treated with crystalloids and norepinephrine infusion before induction of anesthesia. Small doses of midazolam were given and an airway examination was completed (mouth could be opened and the neck could be extended). Adequate denitrogenation could then be performed. Moreover, there was no risk factor for C-spine instability from collateral history. As no new risk factors for difficult airway management were identified, RSI with ketamine and rocuronium was performed through the IO access. Apneic oxygenation was provided with 15 L·min^{-1} through nasal cannulas while tracheal intubation was achieved with a 7.0-mm ID ETT using a Mac-3 type video laryngoscope. A flexible bronchoscope and EGDs were ready for use in case a combined technique with VL or intubation through EGD would have been necessary. The neck was disinfected by the surgeon and the nurses had FONA equipment prepared. After confirmation of proper tracheal tube placement using continuous waveform capnography (end-tidal CO_2), insertion of a central IV catheter followed, and the use of IO was then discontinued. During sigmoidectomy, the patient needed incremental doses of vasopressors and an increased FiO_2. The patient was thus kept intubated and transferred to the intensive care unit for further management of her septic shock and presumed aspiration.

SUMMARY

This case study serves to illustrate the urgent airway management of an uncooperative, potentially difficult airway patient who has a full stomach, and incipient hemodynamic instability. Time to plan an approach is limited and hindered by the fact that the patient has no IV access. In an emergency, the practitioner must carefully weigh contextual and physiological issues. Adherence to the difficult and failed algorithms is still advised. As always, priority must be given to the most important acute conditions and life-threatening complications.

SELF-EVALUATION QUESTIONS

40.1. Patients with Down syndrome are known to have the following attributes that may lead to failed intubation:

A. Obstructive sleep apnea

B. Large tongue

C. Subglottic stenosis

D. C-spine instability

E. All of the above

40.2. Which statements are true considering intraosseous (IO) access?

A. Rates as high as 165 mL·min^{-1} are possible

B. Any medication can be given through

C. Numerous insertion sites are acceptable

D. Can be kept in place for 24 hours

E. All of the above

40.3. What are the risks associated with spontaneous breathing intubation?

A. Laryngospasm

B. Coughing

C. Oxygen desaturation

D. Obstruction

E. All of the above

SECTION 6

REFERENCES

1. Bull MJ, The Committee on Genetics. Health supervision for children with Down syndrome. *Pediatrics.* 2011;128:393-406.
2. Ostermaier KK. UpToDate - Down syndrome: Clinical features and diagnosis. 2020. https://www.uptodate.com/contents/down-syndrome-clinical-features-and-diagnosis. Accessed on June 7, 2022
3. Hill EA. Obstructive sleep apnoea/hypopnoea syndrome in adults with Down syndrome. *Breathe.* 2016;12:e91-e96.
4. Dahlqvist Å, Rask E, Rosenqvist C-J, et al. Sleep apnea and Down's syndrome. *Acta Oto-Laryngologica.* 2003;123:1094-1097.
5. De Lausnay M, Verhulst S, Boel L, et al. The prevalence of lower airway anomalies in children with Down syndrome compared to controls. *Pediatr Pulmonol.* 2020;55:1259-1263.
6. Hamilton J, Yaneza MMC, Clement WA, Kubba H. The prevalence of airway problems in children with Down's syndrome. *Int J Pediatr Otorhinolaryngol.* 2016;81:1-4.
7. Boseley ME, Link DT, Shott SR, et al. Laryngotracheoplasty for subglottic stenosis in Down syndrome children: the Cincinnati experience. *Int J Pediatr Otorhinolaryngol.* 2001;57:11-15.
8. Mitchell RB, Call E, Kelly J. Diagnosis and therapy for airway obstruction in children with Down syndrome. *Arch Otolaryngol Head Neck Surg.* 2003;129:642.
9. Jacobs IN, Gray RF, Todd NW. Upper airway obstruction in children with Down syndrome. *Arch Otolaryngol Head Neck Surg.* 1996;122:945-950.
10. Miller R, Gray SD, Steven D, Cotton RT, et al. Subglottic stenosis and Down Syndrome. *Am J Otolaryngol.* 1990;11:274-277.
11. Nakazawa K, Ikeda D, Ishikawa S, Makita K. A case of difficult airway due to lingual tonsillar hypertrophy in a patient with downs syndrome. *Anesth Analg.* 2003;97(3):704-705.
12. Hata, T, Todd MM. Cervical Spine considerations when anesthetizing patients with Down syndrome. *Anesthesiology.* 2005;102:680-685.
13. Cook T Woodall, Nick, Frerk, Chris, Royal College of Anaesthetists (Great Britain), Difficult Airway Society (Great Britain). Major complications of airway management in the United Kingdom: report and findings : 4th National Audit Project of the Royal College of Anaesthetists and the Difficult Airway Society : NAP4; 2011.
14. Green SM, Johnson NE. Ketamine sedation for pediatric procedures: Part 2. Review and implications. *Ann Emerg Med.* 1990;19:1033-1046.
15. Green SM, Rothrock SG, Lynch EL, et al. Intramuscular ketamine for pediatric sedation in the emergency department: safety profile in 1,022 cases. *Ann Emerg Med.* 1998;31:688-697.
16. Green SM, Nakamura R, Johnson NE. Ketamine sedation for pediatric procedures: Part 1. A prospective series. *Ann Emerg Med.* 1990;19:1024-1032.
17. Zane R. The morbidly obese patient. In: *Manual of Emergency Airway Management.* 2nd ed. Lippincott Williams and Wilkins; 2004.
18. Younge PA. Sedation for children requiring wound repair: a randomised controlled double blind comparison of oral midazolam and oral ketamine. *Emerg Med J.* 2001;18:30-33.
19. Turhanoglu S, Kararmaz A, Ozylmaz MA, et al. Effects of different doses of oral ketamine for premedication of children. *Eur J Anaesthesiol.* 2003;20:56-60.
20. Barnard EBG, Moy RJ, Kehoe AD, et al. Rapid sequence induction of anaesthesia via the intraosseous route: a prospective observational study. *Emerg Med J.* 2015;32:449-452.
21. Davis J, Bates L. Rapid sequence induction via an intraosseous needle. *J Intensive Care Soc.* 2016;17:178-179.
22. Tobias JD, Ross AK. Intraosseous infusions: a review for the anesthesiologist with a focus on pediatric use. *Anesth Analg.* 2010;110:391-401.
23. Ong MEH, Chan YH, Oh JJ, Ngo AS-Y. An observational, prospective study comparing tibial and humeral intraosseous access using the EZ-IO. *Am J Emerg Med.* 2009;27:8-15.
24. Li J, Murphy-Lavoie H, Bugas C, et al. Complications of emergency intubation with and without paralysis. *Am J Emerg Med.* 1999;17:141-143.
25. Bozeman WP, Kleiner DM, Huggett V. A comparison of rapid-sequence intubation and etomidate-only intubation in the prehospital air medical setting. *Prehosp Emerg Care.* 2006;10:8-13.
26. Mercer SJ, Jones CP, Bridge M, et al. Systematic review of the anaesthetic management of non-iatrogenic acute adult airway trauma. *Br J Anaesth.* 2016;117:i49-i59.
27. Stephens CT, Kahntroff S, Dutton RP. The success of emergency endotracheal intubation in trauma patients: a 10-year experience at a major adult trauma referral center. *Anesth Analg.* 2009;109:866-872.
28. Higgs A, McGrath BA, Goddard C, et al. Guidelines for the management of tracheal intubation in critically ill adults. *Br J Anaesth.* 2018;120:323-352.
29. Driver BE, Reardon RF. Apnea after low-dose ketamine sedation during attempted delayed sequence intubation. *Ann Emerg Med.* 2017;69:34-35.
30. Strayer RJ, Nelson LS. Adverse events associated with ketamine for procedural sedation in adults. *Am J Emerg Med.* 2008;26:985-1028.
31. Frerk C, Mitchell VS, McNarry AF, et al. Difficult Airway Society 2015 guidelines for management of unanticipated difficult intubation in adults. *Br J Anaesth.* 2015;115:827-848.
32. Law JA, Duggan LV, Asselin M, et al. Canadian Airway Focus Group updated consensus-based recommendations for management of the difficult airway: part 1. Difficult airway management encountered in an unconscious patient. *Can J Anesth.* 2021;68:1373-1404.

CHAPTER 41

Airway Management in a Patient with Aspiration of Gastric Content Following Induction of Anesthesia

Kathryn Sparrow and Orlando R. Hung

CASE PRESENTATION

On a Saturday morning, a 42-year-old man presents to the operating room for an urgent cystoscopy to remove a high ureteric stone. He is a smoker and has no known allergies. He has been taking subcutaneous hydromorphone for renal colic for several days as an inpatient, with little relief. He has had numerous uneventful previous cystoscopy and extracorporeal shock wave lithotripsy (ESWL) procedures in the past for nephrolithiasis. His last general anesthetic for a cystoscopy 6 months ago was completed uneventfully after the insertion of an LMA®-Classic™ #5. He has been appropriately fasted for 6 hours when he arrives in the operating room.

The patient's cardiovascular and respiratory examination is unremarkable, his vital signs are stable, and he is afebrile. The urology team does not feel that the patient has urosepsis currently. His BMI is 27.3 kg·m^{-2}. His airway exam is normal with no predictors of difficulties in face-mask ventilation (FMV), use of extraglottic devices (EGDs), tracheal intubation, or surgical airway.

He has a #18-gauge IV catheter in-situ in his left forearm. Following denitrogenation, general anesthesia is induced with midazolam 1 mg IV, fentanyl 50 µg IV, and propofol 250 mg IV. Immediately after propofol administration and as the patient loses consciousness, he complains of pain at the IV site, and bile-colored fluid leaks around the face mask. Projectile vomiting occurs when the face mask is removed. After suctioning the pharynx in the Trendelenburg position, oxygen saturation rapidly decreases to 80%, and there is an audible wheeze. Swelling is noted at the IV site and the gravity feed IV is no longer dripping.

INTRODUCTION

Aspiration of gastric contents is still an important cause of morbidity and mortality associated with airway management. Aspiration was the most common cause of death in anesthesia cases reported to the Fourth National Audit Project—Major complications of airway management in the United Kingdom: Results of the Fourth National Audit Project of the Royal College of Anaesthetists and the Difficult Airway Society (NAP4). This report, published in 2011, illustrated that aspiration is not simply a historical anesthesia complication.[1] Events in which death occurred were associated with significant hypoxemia and brain damage following aspiration.

The incidence of aspiration during anesthesia has been widely estimated, and this is reviewed in Chapter 5. One in five of all NAP4 anesthesia reports described aspiration of gastric contents as a primary or secondary event (17% and 5%, respectively). In addition, many aspiration event survivors had prolonged intensive care stays. Common themes were incomplete assessment of aspiration risk and failure to alter the anesthetic technique when aspiration risk was present.

Great care is taken to discuss preinduction preparation for the prevention of aspiration in airway algorithms, but interestingly, little attention is given to the management of ongoing aspiration in the setting of a CICO difficult airway, and the subsequent management of such events.

This case and chapter will highlight the priorities of: (1) oxygenation; (2) prevention of further pulmonary aspiration of gastric contents; and (3) management of a patient who has experienced an aspiration event in the context of a difficult airway.

Is This Patient at High Risk of Aspiration?

Risk factors for pulmonary aspiration of gastric contents are well described in Chapter 5, with emergency surgery being the most important.[2] Some methods, although not universally accepted, can be used to decrease the risk and minimize complications associated with aspiration.[1,3] These include: (1) performance of regional anesthesia and avoidance of general anesthesia; (2) appropriate preinduction fasting; (3) appropriate nasogastric tube insertion and drainage of gastric contents; (4) premedication with prokinetic medications, antacids, H_2- blockers, and proton pump inhibitors; (5) tracheal intubation; (6) use of rapid sequence intubation or awake intubation when appropriate; and (7) use of a second-generation EGD.

This patient had received many general anesthetics with a first-generation EGD used as the primary airway device with no previously documented complications. It is important to realize that airway management is context-specific, and there may be new patient or situational factors that will require alteration of the anesthetic plan.

Difficult intubation is associated with an increased risk of aspiration. This risk of regurgitation and subsequent aspiration increases exponentially with the number of intubation attempts.[4,5] Coughing or gagging with airway interventions also increases the risk of aspiration,[6–8] and light anesthesia combined with the absence of muscle paralysis when placing the EGD may have placed this patient at an increased risk of aspiration.

The patient had been receiving parenteral opioid medications for several days prior to presenting to the operating room. This is an important risk factor to consider, as opioids have been shown to significantly decrease gastric emptying.[9]

Appropriate patient selection for EGD use is essential. Whereas, it is quite obvious that an alternate method of airway control should be considered in patients at high risk of aspiration, multiple contributing risk factors may create the conditions required for a clinically significant aspiration event. When comparing this case to those reported in NAP4, potential considerations for not using an EGD in this patient would include the culmination of recent opioid use, pain, potential for ileus, and the requirement of the lithotomy position. Given the multitude of risk factors for aspiration,[10] the airway practitioner must determine the level of risk for aspiration when choosing an airway management strategy.

Although EGDs have a documented safety profile in appropriately selected patients and cases, published case reports and series continue to highlight the morbidity and mortality associated with aspiration and EGD use.[11–14]

How Do You Diagnose Aspiration of Gastric Contents?

As reviewed in Chapter 5, a diagnosis of aspiration cannot be made by the presence of gastric material in the oropharynx alone. Given that this patient is now symptomatic with hypoxemia and an audible wheeze, the airway practitioner must have a high index of suspicion for aspiration. This patient requires simultaneous airway management and plans for further treatment of the aspiration event.

Pulmonary aspiration of gastric contents is generally defined as either the presence of bilious secretions or particulate matter in the tracheobronchial tree or, if bronchoscopy is not performed, infiltrates present on a postoperative chest radiograph together with physical examination findings.[2] Sequelae range in severity from mild symptoms, such as hypoxemia, to respiratory failure, acute respiratory distress syndrome (ARDS), cardiovascular collapse, anoxic brain injury, and death.[15] Review of these clinical syndromes in relation to this case will highlight the management of an aspiration event in a patient with a difficult airway.

When this patient vomited on induction, the appropriate measures were taken to prevent further aspiration. The head of the bed was immediately adjusted to a 30-degree Trendelenburg position, and the upper airway was suctioned. Prior to the vomiting, the patient received an induction dose of intravenous propofol, and awakening this symptomatic patient with no definitive airway and ongoing vomiting and aspiration was not a reasonable option. Ideally, the trachea of the patient would be intubated and receive tracheal suctioning before the initiation of positive pressure ventilation.

Aspirated gastric contents, such as fluid or other foreign body material, can cause airway obstruction, laryngospasm, or distal airway closure. This may precipitate hypoxemia, pulmonary edema, reduced lung compliance, bronchospasm, and atelectasis. The clinical consequences will depend on the location of obstruction and the amount and characteristics of the aspirated material. Primary treatment for these events is generally removal of the foreign body and respiratory and cardiovascular support.

Aspiration, and its associated complications, makes the management of an unanticipated difficult airway more challenging. The onset of symptoms associated with aspiration of gastric contents can be rapid, and damage can occur within seconds. First described by Mendelson,[16] chemical pneumonitis can be associated with significant cyanosis and ARDS. Extrapolation from animal studies concluded that aspirate with a pH less than 2.5 and a volume of 25 mL or more correlated with aspiration and resultant pneumonitis.[17] Pathological lung changes evolve rapidly due to the rapid immunological response to the chemical injury. Pulmonary edema, hemorrhage, and consolidation lead to decreased lung compliance, abnormal ventilation-perfusion, and decreased diffusion capacity causing severe hypoxemia. Respiratory support, in the form of mechanical ventilation, is the primary therapeutic approach for these patients.

MANAGEMENT OF GASTRIC ASPIRATION

How Do You Proceed with This Case?

The prevention of pulmonary aspiration of gastric contents is a significant concern for the airway practitioner and focuses prominently in all the difficult airway management algorithms.[18–21] There is, however, no discussion of the steps to follow if regurgitation and aspiration occur during the management of the difficult airway.

Management of the Unanticipated Difficult Airway During Active Aspiration

A call for help and the difficult airway cart is made. Unfortunately, limited assistance is available because it is Saturday. An LMA-Classic #4 was the planned airway for the surgical procedure and equipment and drugs to facilitate tracheal intubation are not ready. In the presence of deteriorating oxygen saturation, the airway practitioner proceeds to use FMV. Unfortunately, the patient's oxygen saturation does not improve from 80% using FMV with an oropharyngeal airway and a fraction of inspired oxygen (FiO_2) 1.0 with a reasonable capnography trace. The decision is made to intubate the trachea for airway protection, bronchoscopic assessment, and suctioning. After a new #18-gauge IV catheter is secured (by the urologist), 100 mg of propofol and 100 mg of succinylcholine are administered, and direct laryngoscopy is performed with the Macintosh #4 laryngoscope. Difficulty is encountered with direct laryngoscopy because of poor head and neck position on the fluoroscopy table. An intubation attempt with the GlideScope also proves difficult, and the oxygen saturation now decreases to 50%. An LMA-Classic #4 is placed with ease, and the oxygen saturation returns to around 85%. A definitive airway is required and the airway practitioner prepares for intubation through the LMA-Classic. Despite suctioning, tracheal intubation using the pediatric flexible bronchoscope (FB) with an ensleeved Aintree catheter (Cook Critical Care, Bloomington, IN) via the LMA-Classic is difficult because of blood and secretions in the airway. Eventually, the tip of the FB is advanced into the trachea and positioned close to carina. The Aintree catheter is advanced to the tip of the bronchoscope and the FB removed. The LMA-Classic is then removed and a cut (at 26 cm) endotracheal tube (ETT) is advanced easily over the Aintree. On manual ventilation through the ETT, no CO_2 is detected and the oxygen saturation rapidly drops to 55%. The ETT is quickly removed, and an LMA-Classic #4 is reinserted. Oxygen saturation improves to 85%.

How Do You Manage the Airway of a "Can't Intubate But Can Barely Oxygenate" Patient Following Gastric Aspiration?

Oxygenation must be the priority while managing a patient with a difficult airway in the setting of aspiration. While an EGD is less than an ideal airway device in a patient who has aspirated gastric contents, it allows the airway practitioner to oxygenate the patient while making preparations for definitive airway management. This is especially important in this case, given that tracheal intubation had not been successful under direct or video laryngoscopy. When reviewing this case, it could be suggested that a second-generation EGD should have been inserted instead of a first-generation EGD. Theoretically, waking up a patient such as this without securing the airway could be considered, but ongoing low-oxygen saturations with episodes of further rapid desaturation and the immediate need for pulmonary toilet and ventilatory support precluded this option. In addition, this patient is at risk to have more regurgitation and aspiration on emergence.

An ENT surgeon is consulted for the performance of a tracheotomy. The tracheotomy is difficult but a #6 Shiley tracheostomy tube (Medtronic, Minneapolis, MN) is successfully placed. The patient's oxygen saturation improves to 95% with manual ventilation and an FiO_2 of 1.0. After communication with the intensive care unit (ICU) attending physician, arrangements are made to transport the patient to the ICU for postoperative monitoring and management.

Is Tracheotomy Necessary for This Patient?

Tracheotomy is commonly performed in critically ill patients who require prolonged mechanical ventilation for acute respiratory failure, neurological insult, and for airway issues.[22] Indications for tracheotomy include upper airway obstruction, requirement of prolonged ventilation, facilitation of weaning from mechanical ventilation, airway protection, and secretion removal. Upper airway obstruction is a less common indication for tracheotomy.

There is limited literature to support best practice in management of a CICO patient who has also aspirated.[23,24] The patient in this case has both acute respiratory distress from the gastric aspiration and inadequate oxygenation through the EGD. The patient's airway is not protected from further aspiration with the currently inserted first-generation EGD. Given the context of this unanticipated CICO situation and the requirement of a definitive airway for mechanical ventilation and airway protection, the decision to perform a tracheotomy was made.

It should be emphasized that the surgical airway cannot be considered "a failure," but rather an alternative method to oxygenate a patient when other methods have failed. A front-of-neck airway (FONA) is one of the four essential methods to provide ventilation and oxygenation; however, airway practitioners are often reluctant to perform a FONA and many may even consider it a failure at critical moments, such as in CICO situations. According to the closed claims analysis report, Peterson et al.[25] reported that two-thirds of the patients who died or had brain damage had a surgical airway or FONA, but the procedure was performed too late. The investigators suggested that "For a surgical airway to be successful as a rescue option, it must be instituted early in the management of the difficult airway. Prompt calls for the appropriate equipment and personnel may save lives." In the well-publicized case of the failed airway management of Elaine Bromiley leading to her death, the Coroner Inquest Report concluded that "*...The management of the 'can't intubate can't ventilate' emergency did not follow the current or any recognised guidance. Too much time was taken trying to intubate the trachea rather than concentrating on ensuring adequate oxygenation. The clinicians became oblivious to the passing of time.... Surgical airway access by either tracheotomy or cricothyrotomy should have been considered and carried out....*"[26]

What Is the Posttracheotomy Care of This Patient?

Safe and effective care for the newly created tracheotomy requires intensive monitoring and care.[27] Given the multiple intubation attempts in this case, ongoing pulmonary toileting, and ventilator support, it is the authors' opinion that this type of patient is best managed in an intensive care or high-dependency unit in the postoperative period.

After securing a surgical airway, discussion with the surgical team is necessary to determine whether or not to proceed with the surgical procedure. In general, elective surgery should be canceled, and emergency surgery should be limited to life and limb-saving procedures. Since the planned procedure is not an emergency, it is postponed until the respiratory status improves. Further management will focus on: (1) immediate respiratory care in the operating room; (2) postoperative respiratory care in a high-dependency unit; (3) fluid therapy and inotropic support as required; (4) coordination of further investigations; (5) consideration of antibiotics; and (6) consideration of other medications, as guided by evidence-based medicine. In addition to adequate sedation and analgesia, initial respiratory care will usually involve mechanical ventilation with FiO_2 1.0 and a lung-protective ventilatory strategy utilizing positive end-expiratory pressure. Bronchoscopy and suctioning via the fresh tracheotomy site must be done carefully, so as not to dislodge the tracheostomy tube. Bronchodilator therapy may also be required.

Careful coordination with the accepting multidisciplinary team will include continuation of mechanical ventilation as required, recognizing that the patient's clinical condition may deteriorate. Prolonged mechanical ventilation may be required. The tracheotomy will provide airway security in this patient with a difficult airway, which is likely to get more difficult secondary to edema and trauma associated with multiple intubation attempts. The patient discussed in the case has now experienced respiratory failure in the setting of aspiration. Careful attention to fluid administration is required. Patients with aspiration may experience pulmonary edema and may develop a systemic inflammatory response syndrome. Inotropic support may be necessary. Placement of an arterial line will facilitate serial blood gas analysis. The clinical course will determine the need for serial chest X-ray evaluation or other diagnostic imaging.

The use of steroids is not recommended for treatment of aspiration. Their efficacy in the critically ill population has not been proven and can adversely affect mortality.[28,29] Prophylactic antibiotic use after an aspiration event will not prevent aspiration pneumonia from occurring, and is not recommended except in specific circumstances.[30] In severely ill patients, empiric use of antibiotics is appropriate. These can be stopped if no infiltrates develop after 48 to 72 hours.

Aspiration pneumonia therapy will generally target bacteria normally found in the upper airways or stomach but will likely be tailored to the clinical scenario and comorbid status of the patient. Complications associated with aspiration include necrotizing pneumonia, lung abscess, or empyema that require appropriate therapies. Appropriate antibiotic therapy will usually be directed by culture and sensitivity results and follow current guidelines.

Although rare, adverse events attributed to tracheotomies do occur. Prevention, early diagnosis, and management of these events are critical. Immediate and early complications include: (1) hemorrhage; (2) infection; (3) subcutaneous emphysema; (4) pneumothorax; (5) tube obstruction; (6) accidental decannulation and loss of the airway; (7) failure of the procedure; (8) air embolism; (9) aspiration; and (10) structural damage to the trachea.[22,31–33] Late complications include: (1) granulation tissue and tracheal stenosis; (2) tracheomalacia; (3) tracheoinnominate artery fistula; (4) tracheoesophageal fistula; and (5) continued aspiration.[34–36]

Recommendations for the optimal management and timing of this patient's decannulation will be made by the multidisciplinary tracheotomy care team.[37] The airway practitioner must ensure that careful communication has occurred with respect to the airway management problems encountered and that the documentation is appropriate.[38] As recommended by NAP4, appropriate monitoring, such as capnography, and a planned emergency response strategy with required equipment readily available is essential in the postoperative management of these challenging patients.

OTHER CONSIDERATIONS

What Is the Swiss Cheese Model in Risk Management?

Chapter 6 provides a detailed discussion of human factors in crisis management. Risk is inherent in the health care environments in which we work.[39] James Reason's Swiss cheese model hypothesizes that while there are many layers of defense that lie between hazards and accidents, there are flaws in each layer that, if aligned, can allow the accident to occur.[40] Errors are seen as consequences of a combination of active failures and latent conditions. In other words, the system produces failures when all individual barrier weaknesses align, permitting "a trajectory of accident opportunity."

Many factors may have contributed to the gastric aspiration and the subsequent difficulties in managing the airway in this patient. These include: (1) the surgical procedure is performed on the weekend with limited resources and assistance; (2) several days of opioid use for pain control prior to surgery may have decreased gastrointestinal motility and delayed gastric emptying; (3) a poorly functioning IV leading to painful injection of propofol and inadequate anesthesia with subsequent vomiting under light anesthesia; (4) improper head and neck position on the fluoroscopy table, making laryngoscopy difficult with both Macintosh and GlideScope laryngoscopes; and (5) reliable and effective airway equipment, such as an FB, is difficult to use in the presence of blood and secretions.

A debrief of this case should review the factors that may have placed this patient at a higher risk of aspiration, patient positioning, preparation of and access to airway equipment, medications, and availability of help.

What Is the Clinical Utility of Perioperative Point-of-Care Gastric Ultrasound?

Point-of-care gastric ultrasound is an emerging diagnostic tool to assess gastric content as part of the perioperative aspiration risk assessment.[41–43] The validity and reliability of point-of-care gastric ultrasound have been evaluated for a variety of patient populations.[44] Although not yet recommended as a standard of practice, the qualification and quantification of gastric contents can assist to define aspiration risk and guide subsequent patient management.[45]

The I-AIM (Indication; Acquisition; Interpretation; Medical management) gastric-ultrasound framework has been developed to visualize and quantify gastric contents and aid in perioperative decision-making when there is known or suspected delayed gastric emptying or the fasting status is unknown.[46]

A low-frequency (1-5 MHz) curved array ultrasound transducer is used with the patient in the supine or right-lateral decubitus position. Sonographic imaging following the I-AIM framework involves sonographic imaging with the transducer in the sagittal plane in the epigastrium. The practitioner sweeps the transducer from the left costal margin, observing for landmarks, including the short axis of the gastric antrum.[44] The practitioner then performs a qualitative assessment to determine if the gastric antrum is empty or contains clear fluid or solid contents. Described stereotypical patterns are demonstrated in Figure 41.1.

Gastric cross-sectional area (CSA) can be calculated. Mathematical modeling studies have been used to correlate gastric CSA and the volume of gastric fluids.[47] Previous studies have shown that the accepted upper limit for gastric secretions or clear fluid in fasted, elective surgical patient is 1.5 $mL \cdot kg^{-1}$.[44,47,48] Point-of-care gastric ultrasound may have limitations in patients who have undergone gastric surgery or have a large hiatal hernia or be inconclusive due to anatomic variations or misinterpretation.[42]

Point-of-care gastric ultrasound has been shown to have a high-sensitivity (1.0), specificity (0.975), positive predictive value (0.976), and negative predictive value (1.0) when practiced by experienced practitioners.[42,49] Point-of-care gastric ultrasound can be a valuable tool, in conjunction with a thorough clinical assessment, to increase safety and airway management plans and to decrease the risk of aspiration of gastric contents.

While point-of-care gastric ultrasound evaluates an important risk, it is important to remember that it is not the only risk of clinically important aspiration.[44] Greater opportunities for training, practice integration, and research are needed. The authors of this chapter invite the reader to review the many excellent and comprehensive reviews and guides on this emerging topic in a variety of patient populations and clinical scenarios.[42,44,46]

What Are the Lessons Learned from This Case?

Great care is taken to discuss preoperative preparation for prevention of aspiration in airway algorithms, but little attention is given to the management of aspiration in the setting of an encountered difficult airway. This paucity of literature is alarming, given the incidence of aspiration and the associated morbidity and mortality.

The webAIRS anesthesia incident reporting database collects clinical incidents in anesthesia from Australia and New Zealand. In 2019, the first 4000 reports were reviewed to evaluate pulmonary aspiration in patients undergoing procedures under general anesthesia or sedation.[50] Evidence of pulmonary aspiration was identified in 121 patients and associated with harm in greater than 50% of the reports. The authors reported

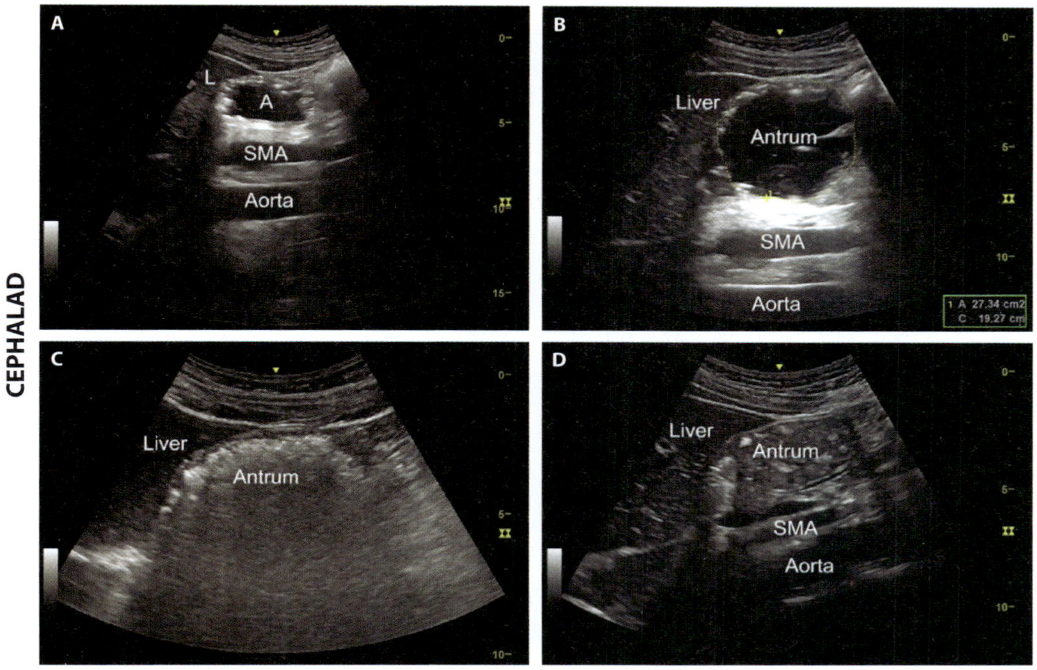

FIGURE 41.1. Ultrasound images of gastric antrum qualitative appearances: **(A)** Gastric antrum containing fluid with air bubbles. **(B)** Gastric antrum containing fluid. A gastric cross-sectional area (CSA) can be calculated in this view. **(C)** and **(D)** Gastric antrum containing solids. (Reproduced with permission from El-Boghdadly K, Wojcikiewicz T, Perlas A. Perioperative point-of-care gastric ultrasound. *BJA Educ.* 2019;19(7):219-226.)

that the most common contributory factors included emergency surgery, delayed gastric emptying, increased body mass index, inadequate depth of anesthesia, and bowel obstruction. There was also a higher incidence of aspiration events during out-of-hours cases. A 2021 Anesthesia Closed Claims Project analysis of pulmonary aspiration of gastric aimed to identify outcomes and patient and process of care risk factors associated with gastric aspiration and revealed similar results.[51] These findings suggest that modifications to preoperative assessment and anesthetic management may lead to improved perioperative outcomes.

The initial presentation of regurgitation and aspiration may include laryngospasm, oxygen desaturation, bronchospasm, respiratory failure, or cardiac arrest. Diagnosis and treatment may be delayed. Rapid recognition and appropriate response are required, and the value of using a structured management approach has been advocated.[52]

There has recently been support in the literature of utilizing head-elevated laryngoscopy position (HELP) to optimize the laryngoscopic view.[53] It is the authors' opinion that in addition to optimizing laryngoscopy success, in the absence of any contraindications to this position, the HELP position may decrease the rate or amount of regurgitated gastric contents that may occur. This may be accomplished with pillows, a wedge, blankets, a commercially available device, or utilizing the bed control on the operating room table. This case highlights the challenges encountered with optimal patient positioning on a fluoroscopy-compatible table. If aspiration occurs in this position, there must be very careful communication with team members regarding the logistics of placing the patient in a head-down position. Airway practitioners and their teams should discuss the risk of aspiration and the ensuing management plans, should this patient safety incident occur, prior to the induction of anesthesia.[50,52] The airway practitioner should consider performing an awake intubation if the patient is felt to be at an unacceptable risk of pulmonary aspiration of gastric contents during the induction of general anesthesia.[18,19] Although limited evidence exists, strategies such as directed suction decontamination approaches[54] and consideration of video laryngoscopy and team-assisted suctioning plans[55] have been suggested.

It is important to ensure that there is clear and accurate documentation of the encountered difficult airway on the patient's medical chart, and that the encountered difficulty and management strategy is communicated to the patient, the patient's family or decision makers, the surgeon, and primary care provider, and a difficult airway letter should be provided. After transporting the patient to ICU, the attending anesthesiologist met with the patient's family to review the difficulties encountered, the aspiration event, and the requirement of a tracheotomy. When the patient was awake and alert in the ICU the next day, the events were reviewed with him.

SUMMARY

Aspiration of gastric contents under general anesthesia still represents a major patient safety concern. The reported mortality associated with aspiration has varied greatly between 1 in 35,000 and 1 in 72,000 patients. Aspiration is an event that many airway practitioners will experience. The principles of managing patients with aspiration of gastric contents include securing the airway to provide mechanical ventilation and oxygenation if needed and pulmonary toileting. Multidisciplinary team management of the patient involving the ICU may be necessary depending on the patient's postaspiration clinical status.

SELF-EVALUATION QUESTIONS

41.1. Which of the following complications is NOT associated with an aspiration event?

A. Laryngospasm

B. Cardiac arrest

C. Anoxic brain injury

D. Hypertension

E. Bronchospasm

41.2. Which of the following is NOT a late complication of aspiration?

A. Tracheal stenosis

B. Tracheoesophageal fistula

C. Increased lower-esophageal sphincter tone

D. Tracheoinominate-artery fistula

E. Tracheomalacia

41.3. All of the following are considered to be acceptable therapy for aspiration events associated with respiratory failure EXCEPT:

A. Steroids

B. Bronchoscopy and suctioning

C. Bronchodilator Therapy

D. Mechanical ventilation with FiO_2 1.0

E. Admission to a high-dependency unit

REFERENCES

1. Cook TM, Woodall N, Frerk C. Major complications of airway management in the UK: results of the Fourth National Audit Project of the Royal College of Anaesthetists and the Difficult Airway Society. Part 1: Anaesthesia. *Br J Anaesth*. 2011;106(5):617-631.
2. Warner MA, Warner ME, Weber JG. Clinical significance of pulmonary aspiration during the perioperative period. *Anesthesiology*. 1993;78(1):56-62.
3. Practice Guidelines for Preoperative Fasting and the Use of Pharmacologic Agents to Reduce the Risk of Pulmonary Aspiration: Application to Healthy Patients Undergoing Elective Procedures. *Anesthesiology*. 2017;126(3):376-393.
4. Sakles JC, Laurin EG, Rantapaa AA, Panacek EA. Airway management in the emergency department: a one-year study of 610 tracheal intubations. *Ann Emerg Med*. 1998;31(3):325-332.
5. Mort TC. Emergency tracheal intubation: complications associated with repeated laryngoscopic attempts. *Anesth Analg*. 2004;99(2):607-613.
6. Kluger MT, Short TG. Aspiration during anaesthesia: a review of 133 cases from the Australian Anaesthetic Incident Monitoring Study (AIMS). *Anaesthesia*. 1999;54(1):19-26.
7. Mellin-Olsen J, Fasting S, Gisvold SE. Routine preoperative gastric emptying is seldom indicated. A study of 85 594 anaesthetics with special focus on aspiration pneumonia. *Acta Anaesthesiol Scand*. 1996;40(10):1184-1188.

8. Olsson GL, Hallen B, Hambraeus-Jonzon K. Aspiration during anaesthesia: a computer-aided study of 185 358 anaesthetics. *Acta Anaesthesiol Scand.* 1986;30(1):84-92.
9. Murphy DB, Sutton JA, Prescott LF, Murphy MB. Opioid-induced delay in gastric emptying. *Anesthesiology.* 1997;87(4):765-770.
10. Asai T. Editorial II: who is at increased risk of pulmonary aspiration? *Br J Anaesth.* 2004;93(4):497-500.
11. Keller C, Brimacombe J, Bittersohl J, Lirk P, von Goedecke A. Aspiration and the laryngeal mask airway: three cases and a review of the literature. *Br J Anaesth.* 2004;93(4):579-582.
12. Cook C, Gande AR. Aspiration and death associated with the use of the laryngeal mask airway. *Br J Anaesth.* 2005;95(3):425-426.
13. Gibbison B, Cook TM, Seller C. Case series: protection from aspiration and failure of protection from aspiration with the i-gel airway. *Br J Anaesth.* 2008;100(3):415-417.
14. Brimacombe JR, Berry A. The incidence of aspiration associated with the laryngeal mask airway: a meta-analysis of published literature. *J Clin Anesth.* 1995;7(4):297-305.
15. Nason KS. Acute Intraoperative pulmonary aspiration. *Thorac Surg Clin.* 2015;25(3):301-307.
16. Mendelson CL. The aspiration of stomach contents into the lungs during obstetric anesthesia. *Am J Obstet Gynecol.* 1946;52(2):191-205.
17. Roberts RB, Shirley MA. Reducing the risk of acid aspiration during cesarean section. *Anesth Analg.* 1974;53(6):859-868.
18. Law JA, Duggan LV, Asselin M, et al. Canadian Airway Focus Group updated consensus-based recommendations for management of the difficult airway: part 1. Difficult airway management encountered in an unconscious patient. *Can J Anesth.* 2021;68(9):1373-1404.
19. Law JA, Duggan LV, Asselin M, et al. Canadian Airway Focus Group updated consensus-based recommendations for management of the difficult airway: part 2. Planning and implementing safe management of the patient with an anticipated difficult airway. *Can J Anesth.* 2021;68(9):1405-1436.
20. Frerk C, Mitchell VS, McNarry AF, et al. Difficult Airway Society 2015 guidelines for management of unanticipated difficult intubation in adults. *Br J Anaesth.* 2015;115(6):827-848.
21. Apfelbaum JL, Hagberg CA, Connis RT, et al. 2022 American Society of Anesthesiologists practice guidelines for management of the difficult airway. *Anesthesiology.* 2022;136(1):31-81.
22. Cheung NH, Napolitano LM. Tracheostomy: epidemiology, indications, timing, technique, and outcomes. *Respir Care.* 2014;59(6):895-919.
23. Janda M, Scheeren TWL, Nöldge-Schomburg GFE. Management of pulmonary aspiration. *Best Pract Res Clin Anaesthesiol.* 2006;20(3):409-427.
24. Ahmed Z, Alalami A, Haupert M, Rajan S, Durgham N, Zestos MM. Airway management for rigid bronchoscopy via a freshly performed tracheostomy in a child with Goldenhar syndrome. *J Clin Anesth.* 2012;24(3):234-237.
25. Peterson GN, Domino KB, Caplan RA, Posner KL, Lee LA, Cheney FW. Management of the difficult airway. *Anesthesiology.* 2005;103(1):33-39.
26. Harmer M. Independent review on the care given to Mrs Elaine Bromiley [Internet]. 2005 Mar [cited July 19, 2022]. https://emcrit.org/wp-content/uploads/ElaineBromileyAnonymousReport.pdf.
27. Brenner MJ, Pandian V, Milliren CE, et al. Global tracheostomy collaborative: data-driven improvements in patient safety through multidisciplinary teamwork, standardisation, education, and patient partnership. *Br J Anaesth.* 2020;125(1):e104-e118.
28. Engelhardt T, Webster NR. Pulmonary aspiration of gastric contents in anaesthesia. *Br J Anaesth.* 1999 Sep;83(3):453-460.
29. Bone RC, Fisher CJ, Clemmer TP, et al. A controlled clinical trial of high-dose methylprednisolone in the treatment of severe sepsis and septic shock. *N Engl J Med.* 1987;317(11):653-658.
30. Johnson JL, Hirsch CS. Aspiration pneumonia: recognizing and managing a potentially growing disorder. *Postgrad Med.* 2003;113(3):99-112.
31. Shah RK, Lander L, Berry JG, Nussenbaum B, Merati A, Roberson DW. Tracheotomy outcomes and complications: a national perspective. *Laryngoscope.* 2012;122(1):25-29.
32. Feller-Kopman D. Acute complications of artificial airways. *Clin Chest Med.* 2003;24(3):445-455.
33. Myers EN, Carrau RL. Early complications of tracheotomy. Incidence and management. *Clin Chest Med.* 1991;12(3):589-595.
34. Halum SL, Ting JY, Plowman EK, et al. A multi-institutional analysis of tracheotomy complications. *Laryngoscope.* 2012;122(1):38-45.
35. Epstein SK. Late complications of tracheostomy. *Respir Care.* 2005;50(4):542-549.
36. Fernandez-Bussy S, Mahajan B, Folch E, Caviedes I, Guerrero J, Majid A. Tracheostomy tube placement: early and late complications. *J Bronchol Interv Pulmonol.* 2015;22(4):357-364.
37. Freeman BD, Morris PE. Tracheostomy practice in adults with acute respiratory failure. *Crit Care Med.* 2012;40(10):2890-2896.
38. McGrath BA, Wallace S. The UK National Tracheostomy Safety Project and the role of speech and language therapists. *Curr Opin Otolaryngol Head Neck Surg.* 2014;22(3):181-187.
39. Vincent C. How to improve patient safety in surgery. *J Health Serv Res Policy.* 2010;15(Suppl 1):40-43.
40. Reason J. Human error: models and management. *BMJ.* 2000;320(7237):768-770.
41. Schwarz SKW, Prabhakar C. What to do when perioperative point-of-care ultrasound shows evidence of a full stomach despite fasting? *Can J Anesth.* 2020;67(7):798-805.
42. El-Boghdadly K, Wojcikiewicz T, Perlas A. Perioperative point-of-care gastric ultrasound. *BJA Educ.* 2019;19(7):219-226.
43. Van de Putte P, Vernieuwe L, Jerjir A, Verschueren L, Tacken M, Perlas A. When fasted is not empty: a retrospective cohort study of gastric content in fasted surgical patients. *Br J Anaesth.* 2017;118(3):363-371.
44. Perlas A, Arzola C, Van de Putte P. Point-of-care gastric ultrasound and aspiration risk assessment: a narrative review. *Can J Anesth.* 2018;65(4):437-448.
45. Perlas A, Chan VWS, Lupu CM, Mitsakakis N, Hanbidge A. Ultrasound assessment of gastric content and volume. Anesthesiology. 2009;111(1):82-89.
46. Perlas A, Van de Putte P, Van Houwe P, Chan VWS. I-AIM framework for point-of-care gastric ultrasound. *Br J Anaesth.* 2016;116(1):7-11.
47. Perlas A, Mitsakakis N, Liu L, et al. Validation of a mathematical model for ultrasound assessment of gastric volume by gastroscopic examination. *Anesth Analg.* 2013;116(2):357-363.
48. Van de Putte P, Perlas A. Ultrasound assessment of gastric content and volume. *Br J Anaesth.* 2014;113(1):12-22.
49. Kruisselbrink R, Gharapetian A, Chaparro LE, et al. Diagnostic accuracy of point-of-care gastric ultrasound. *Anesth Analg.* 2019;128(1):89-95.
50. Kluger MT, Culwick MD, Moore MR, Merry AF. Aspiration during anaesthesia in the first 4000 incidents reported to webAIRS. *Anaesth Intensive Care.* 2019;47(5):442-451.
51. Warner MA, Meyerhoff KL, Warner ME, Posner KL, Stephens L, Domino KB. Pulmonary aspiration of gastric contents: a closed claims analysis. *Anesthesiology.* 2021;135(2):284-291.
52. Kluger M, Visvanathan T, Myburgh J, Westhorpe R. Crisis management during anaesthesia: regurgitation, vomiting, and aspiration. *Qual Saf Health Care.* 2005;14(3):e4.
53. Myatra S. Optimal position for laryngoscopy—time for individualization? *J Anaesthesiol Clin Pharmacol.* 2019;35(3):289.
54. Kovacs G, Sowers N. Airway management in trauma. *Emerg Med Clin North Am.* 2018;36(1):61-84.
55. Turkstra TP, Regan WD. Provider/patient conflict: is it time to reconsider the contraindication for videolaryngoscope use in a bleeding/soiled airway? *Can J Anesth.* 2022;69(1):177-178.

CHAPTER 42

Airway Management for a Patient with Upper Gastrointestinal Bleeding and an Anticipated Difficult Airway

Nate Murray and Michael Aziz

CASE PRESENTATION

A 46-year-old man with a history of nonalcoholic steatohepatitis (NASH) cirrhosis and prior upper gastrointestinal (GI) bleeding presents to the emergency department (ED) with acute onset of hematemesis and melena. His past medical history is significant for obesity with a body mass index of 38 $kg{\cdot}m^{-2}$, obstructive sleep apnea (OSA) for which he declined the use of noninvasive ventilation, diabetes mellitus, and hypertension. He was noted to have ascitic fluid on his most recent liver ultrasound but has never needed large-volume paracentesis. His vital signs demonstrate a sinus tachycardia with a rate of 108 beats per minute and blood pressure of 110/68. He is afebrile and has a mildly delayed peripheral capillary refill. On exam he is an obese man, appears as stated age, in mild distress, and somewhat drowsy. He has a thick neck with palpable, but not visible, laryngeal structures. He has mild retrognathia with a decreased thyromental distance. Examination of his mouth revealed intact dentition, Mallampati IV, and inability to bring the lower incisors above the upper vermillion border.

Discussions are underway between the emergency physician and the gastroenterologist regarding the need for urgent or emergency upper endoscopy for control of a suspected brisk variceal GI hemorrhage. Tracheal intubation is thought to be indicated for either endoscopy or placement of a gastric and esophageal tamponade device. You have been consulted for assistance with airway management and perioperative considerations.

The patient notes that he was once told that his airway was difficult to manage during a prior elective upper endoscopy for variceal surveillance. He recalls that he was given a document regarding the event by the anesthesiology team afterward but does not recall the specifics. Upon perusal of the prior anesthetic records, it appears that the patient developed apnea and oxygen desaturations while undergoing deep sedation with fentanyl, midazolam, and propofol. Face-mask ventilation (FMV) was found to be difficult and two attempts to intubate the trachea via direct laryngoscopy by two different anesthesia practitioners were both unsuccessful. An extraglottic airway device (EGD) was placed as a rescue maneuver and the patient was supported via this device until return of native ventilation at which point the procedure was aborted.

INTRODUCTION

How Urgent Is the Planned Procedure and in Which General Timeframe Should the Airway Be Managed?

Given the presentation of a patient with signs of early shock and altered mentation, the procedure should be considered at least urgent. Given the potential instability of patients with brisk upper GI bleeding, the situation could rapidly progress to emergency if the patient loses the ability to protect his own airway from aspiration. Observational data indicate a higher rate of complications in patients prophylactically intubated for endoscopy.[1] Thus, the decision to intubate would result from the patient's actual clinical status and not from a perceived future benefit. Given the difficulty in predicting the short-term course of the patient's disease, it is imperative that the anesthesia team always maintains readiness to manage the airway. Further, their planning and preparations should be undertaken in such a manner that rescue options remain viable strategies should the primary airway plan become impossible. The choice to preserve or compromise the patient's native respiratory drive and airway protective reflexes is of particular importance in this dynamic situation.

PATIENT MANAGEMENT

What Preoperative Evaluation or Testing Is Needed?

If not already done, the patient should have a basic blood work drawn including a type and screen, complete blood count, and measures of coagulation such as an international normalized ratio. However, if the patient requires emergency airway management, these laboratory investigations should not delay appropriate care. A brief discussion with the patient regarding their exercise tolerance may be beneficial to understand the patient's general cardiovascular risk. However, further cardiovascular risk stratification is not indicated in this situation given the urgency of the procedure.

Should the Patient Undergo Nasogastric Tube Placement Prior to Induction of Anesthesia and Intubation?

Nasogastric tube placement in the setting of upper GI bleeding performs several functions. The most common indication for nasogastric lavage is for diagnosis of upper GI bleeding and in risk stratification of lesions for endoscopy. In this case, the patient has a clinical exam and history consistent with brisk upper GI bleeding (cirrhosis, portal hypertension, and esophageal varices) and so the diagnostic value of nasogastric tube placement is minimal. It is unclear if placement of a nasogastric tube and suction of stomach contents prior to induction reduces the risk of aspiration upon induction of anesthesia in the setting of upper GI bleeding.[2,3]

Should Tracheal Intubation Be Performed Awake?

The patient has several reasons why an awake intubation is the preferred airway management approach if time and patient condition permits. First, their anticipated difficult airway, in conjunction with a history of difficult FMV and failed intubation places them at high risk of developing a "cannot intubate, cannot oxygenate" situation upon induction. Secondly, an awake intubation technique that preserves the patient's native respiratory drive and airway protective reflexes may reduce the risk of aspiration of gastric contents into the lungs should the patient vomit during attempts to secure the airway. Similarly, preservation of the patient's respiratory function may allow more time to consider alternate airway strategies should initial attempts be unsuccessful. These benefits of awake intubation are balanced by the time required to facilitate adequate topicalization of the airway and the level of patient cooperation required by the procedure. Furthermore, airway topicalization may be further impaired in this patient by the presence of blood and secretions in the upper airway. An abrupt decline in the patient's clinical status, such as loss of airway reflexes, diminished level of consciousness, or development of large-volume hematemesis may make an awake intubation technique impossible.

What Methods Should Be Employed to Provide Topical Anesthesia: Pure Awake Technique with Local Only versus Medication-Facilitated "Awake" Intubation?

The appropriate approach to awake intubation depends on many factors including patient cooperation, surgical urgency, and the time available to perform the procedure. In this situation of a hemodynamically unstable patient with an upper GI bleed necessitating urgent airway intervention, the techniques employed to perform awake intubation must be appropriate for an urgent, nonelective procedure. While there are many published explanations of techniques to perform elective awake intubation, in this situation, a more expedient approach is warranted. While little evidence exists comparing techniques for awake intubation, one approach in this situation would be as follows: 0.2 to 0.4 mg of glycopyrrolate is administered IV as an antisialagogue. Meanwhile, the patient is asked to use a gauze sponge to gently dry the oropharynx. Afterward, 5 mL of 4% lidocaine is placed into a nebulizer connected to a nonrebreather oxygen mask and this is nebulized at a low flow rate of 4 to 6 $L{\cdot}min^{-1}$ to create large droplets intended to settle in the oropharynx and hypopharynx. Preparations are made to perform a transcricoid injection of 5 mL of 4% lidocaine. Transcricoid injection of lidocaine achieves several advantageous functions in this situation. First, it is a rapid means of anesthetizing the subglottis without recourse to anatomical or ultrasound-guided injections targeting laryngeal nerves. Secondly, injection through the cricothyroid membrane proves the practitioner's ability to locate and access said membrane in the event of an airway emergency. Third, when front-of-neck airway (FONA) is performed in emergency situations, there exists a tendency for inappropriate delay. This delay is posited by many to be related to cognitive barriers preventing emergency FONA. It has similarly been opined that by either marking the correct site for incision of the cricothyroid membrane with indelible ink or injection of lidocaine through the cricothyroid membrane, the hesitancy to perform an indicated FONA at the time indicated could be ameliorated. Overall, the benefit of this approach is that all aspects may be performed concurrently. While caution is warranted in performing a neck injection in a coagulopathic patient, this technique can be performed with a needle or cannula as small as 22G. At this point, it is likely possible to use a flexible bronchoscope with a loaded endotracheal tube (ETT) and a spray-as-you-go technique without further need of sedating medications. Depending on the comfort of the practitioner with appropriately low dosing of amnestic or sedative medications, these may be a reasonable adjunct to airway topicalization though they should not be a core part of an awake intubation strategy.

Which Route of Intubation (Nasal vs. Oral) Should Be Employed Primarily?

The nasal route for awake intubation may be preferable in this patient because improved alignment with glottic structures is common as the device exits the nasopharynx. Further, topicalization of the nasopharynx is often better tolerated by patients as compared to topicalization of the oropharynx especially if the clinical situation permits predilation of the nasal turbinates with local anesthetic and vasoconstrictors. These benefits should be weighed against the increased risk of epistaxis especially if the patient is known or suspected to have a bleeding diathesis.

If Awake Intubation Is Infeasible, Should Direct or Indirect Visualization of the Glottis Be Chosen as the Primary Technique and What Is the Role of Blind Techniques such as Retrograde Wire Intubation, Blind Nasal Intubation, or Lightwand Intubation?

In situations where visualization of the glottis either directly or indirectly is impaired by contamination of the airway, blind techniques of intubation are often advocated. While there are many case reports of successful use of all of these techniques, they are extremely practitioner dependent and require an increased level of expertise to be employed during emergency situations or as rescue techniques.[4–7]

If Indirect Techniques Are Used, Should Flexible Intubation Scopes or Video Laryngoscopy Be Employed?

Flexible scope techniques are best for abnormal airway anatomy or structurally difficult airways. Video laryngoscopy offers a broader field of view, no minimum ETT size requirements, and the ability to switch ETT sizes without withdrawing the device. Video laryngoscopy may result in faster time to intubation during awake intubation as compared with flexible scopes; however, there is a large variation between devices in the published literature.[8] In addition, there have been several recent reports describing the combined use of flexible scope intubation paired with concurrent video laryngoscopy to both aid navigation of the bronchoscope and manipulating the oropharynx or providing targeted suction of airway contaminants.[9]

If Video Laryngoscopy Is Chosen, Should the Blade Be of Standard Geometry or Hyperangulated?

Often when a video laryngoscope is employed, either by default or as a technique to mitigate an anticipated difficult laryngoscopy, the device employed involves the use of a hyperangulated blade. Such blades do not create a direct line-of-sight between the oropharynx and the glottic inlet. This allows a greater degree of visualization of the glottic inlet when mobilization of the tongue or cervical spine is either impossible or undesirable. The benefit of increased visualization is countered by two issues. First, given the lack of a direct path between oropharynx in the glottis, delivery of the ETT can be difficult, particularly in inexperienced hands. Secondly, the lack of a direct line-of-sight between oropharynx and glottis requires that the optical device at the end of the laryngoscope remain intact, fog-free, and not obscured by either airway structures or contaminants in the airway. Given the ongoing hematemesis and abdominal ascites noted in this patient, it may be quite challenging to keep the lens of the scope free from contamination during the laryngoscopy.

On the other hand, use of standard geometry video laryngoscopy allows somewhat improved visualization of the glottis while also providing the option to perform direct laryngoscopy should the optical device become compromised. While these concerns are reasonable, there are several sources of evidence to indicate that, in fact, video devices are similarly effective as direct laryngoscopes during intubation of the soiled airway.[10,11] Similarly, meta-analyses of duration of intubation have found no strong correlation between time-to-intubation and direct versus indirect laryngoscopy.[12] This is likely indicative of a combination of varying practitioners' familiarity with the devices under investigation and varying device characteristics.[13] Ultimately, the practitioner utilizing an indirect laryngoscope in the setting of a soiled airway should understand the potential for compromise and plan strategies to mitigate this issue should it arise.

Are There Adjunctive Techniques or Devices for Intubation Which Protect Against Aspiration or Facilitate Intubation and How Should the Patient Be Positioned for Induction?

Given this patient's obesity and history of a prior difficult intubation, the patient should be optimally positioned prior to induction if an intubation under general anesthesia is planned. This would include achieving a sniffing position with alignment of the face plane parallel to the ceiling via extension of the atlanto-occipital joint. The tragus of the ear should be elevated above a line continuous with the sternal notch via flexion of the cervical spine (ramping position, see Figure 52.2). In patients with increased intra-abdominal pressure such as obesity, pregnancy, or ascites, as in this case, elevation of the head of the bed or positioning in reverse Trendelenburg has been shown to increase safe apnea time by maximizing the functional residual capacity. Given the patient's history of a difficult intubation, maximizing safe apnea time may be crucial in order to safely secure the airway. On the other hand, there are several resources that advocate for the placement of patients at high risk of aspiration in the Trendelenburg position to facilitate removal of emesis from the oropharynx and decrease the passive flow of regurgitated stomach contents into the lungs and trachea.

Should Cricoid Pressure Be Applied?

Cricoid pressure (CP) has not been shown to decrease the incidence of pulmonary aspiration of gastric contents outside of the small initial studies performed by Dr. Selleck. In large studies evaluating the efficacy of CP, it has been consistently demonstrated that performance of CP does reliably decrease the visualization of the glottic opening.[14] However, both the recent Difficult Airway Society and the Canadian Airway Focus Group guidelines recommend the application of CP in patients with an increased risk of aspiration, and suggest momentarily removal of the CP if it is deemed to be impeding airway intervention or tracheal intubation.[15,16]

Should the Airway Practitioner Place Suction or Obturator Devices into the Esophagus?

Some authors have advocated for the suction-assisted laryngoscopy and decontamination (SALAD) technique.[17] In common parlance, this encompasses everything from rudimentary measures such as placement of a standard Yankauer suction into the esophagus up to proprietary suction devices with large orifices to facilitate evacuation of large particulate emesis.[18] Another technique that has been described is the usage of a large 9.0-mm ID endotracheal tube connected to suction via a meconium aspirator and placed into the esophagus, followed by balloon inflation in an attempt to divert stomach contents from the airway and laryngoscopic field of vision.[19] The relative merits of these techniques are not proven in clinical trials. However, they appear to address important limitations of standard suction techniques in the setting of large volume or large particulate emesis.

Are There Different Considerations Which Should Be Made if Intubation Is Difficult but the Airway Remains Unsoiled?

This patient has a history of successful ventilation with an EGD. If difficulty is encountered in placing an endotracheal tube that is not caused by contamination of the airway with gastric contents, consideration should be made for placing an EGD. This could serve both as a means of oxygenation and ventilation between airway attempts and also be used as a conduit for intubation with a flexible bronchoscope. There remains a role for EGD rescue even in the contaminated airway when difficulty is encountered with both tracheal intubation and FMV.

If the Airway Becomes Soiled, What Techniques or Devices Should Be Employed to Facilitate Intubation and Mitigate Aspiration?

Specialized Suction Catheters

Similar to the above discussion, several devices exist either available for purchase or constructed ad hoc by the practitioner to address the situation. Manikin-based studies generally support that purpose-made large-bore suction devices have higher suction rates and a lower tendency to clog than standard Yankauer rigid suction devices.[18] A discussion of the relative merits is likely less useful than the individual practitioner's consideration of how to address emesis should it occur. That said, in 2010, Weingart and Bhagwan reported their strategy to address flexible bronchoscopic intubation of the difficult soiled airway.[20]

Patient Repositioning

If large volumes of gastric contents are noted in the oropharynx during attempts to secure the airway in anesthetized patients, some resources would advocate immediate placement of the patient into the Trendelenburg position to minimize the passive flow of gastric contents into the trachea. While this technique will likely decrease the amount of passive aspiration of gastric contents, it assumes no positive pressure ventilation is currently occurring. It also likely impairs further attempts at laryngoscopy by placing the practitioner at a disadvantageous viewpoint with respect to the glottis.

Should the Patient be Extubated Following the Procedure?

Extubation of the patient depends greatly on the difficulty encountered in placing the ETT and the individual patient characteristics that influence the predicted postoperative course, especially pulmonary and cognitive function. This said, in general, it is likely safer to keep the patient intubated, with a secure airway, if any doubts exist regarding extubation.

SUMMARY

How Was the Patient's Airway Secured?

The patient's trachea was ultimately intubated awake with a flexible bronchoscope. Despite the recent vomiting, the oropharyngeal airway was dry enough to facilitate topicalization of the upper airway by a nebulized, atomized, and transtracheal injection approach. The patient required minimal sedation prior to securing the airway. Gentle induction of anesthesia commenced, and the surgical procedure was performed uneventfully. The patient was extubated awake over an exchange catheter which was left in place for 30 minutes. While this approach was successful, alternate plans for securing the airway were rehearsed in case of failure of the primary plan.

SELF-EVALUATION QUESTIONS

42.1. During attempts to pharmacologically facilitate an awake intubation, the patient is first noted to be under sedated then progressively bradycardic after repeated dosing. What agent was most likely chosen by the airway team to sedate the patient?

A. Ketamine

B. Remifentanil

C. Dexmedetomidine

D. Propofol

42.2. Which of the following is the most relevant limitation of standard Yankauer suction in a grossly contaminated airway?

A. Low suction force

B. Bulk of the catheter

C. Rigid catheter construction

D. Small suction orifices

42.3. A patient with a history of coronary artery disease, low functional capacity, and moderate COPD presents with an upper GI bleed in need of urgent upper endoscopy. What preoperative testing is required to risk stratify the patient prior to proceeding with the case?

A. Echocardiogram

B. Stress test

C. Pulmonary function

D. None of these

REFERENCES

1. Hayat U, Lee PJ, Ullah H, Sarvepalli S, Lopez R, Vargo JJ. Association of prophylactic endotracheal intubation in critically ill patients with upper GI bleeding and cardiopulmonary unplanned events. *Gastrointest Endosc.* 2017;86(3):500-509.e1.
2. Satiani B, Bonner JT, Stone HH. Factors influencing intraoperative gastric regurgitation: a prospective random study of nasogastric tube drainage. *Arch Surg.* 1978;113(6):721-723.
3. Salem MR, Khorasani A, Saatee S, Crystal GJ, El-Orbany M. Gastric tubes and airway management in patients at risk of aspiration: history, current concepts, and proposal of an algorithm. *Anesth Analg.* 2014;118(3):569-579.
4. Szarpak L. Laryngoscopes for difficult airway scenarios: a comparison of the available devices. *Expert Rev Med Devices.* 2018;15(9):631-643.
5. Sahu S, Agarwal A, Rana A, Lata I. Emergency intubation using a light wand in patients with facial trauma. *J Emerg Trauma Shock.* 2009;2(1):51-53.
6. Fichtner A, Vrtny P, Schaarschmidt F. Ultrasound-guided retrograde emergency intubation: life-saving management of a bleeding airway emergency with unclear anatomical situation. *Anaesthesist.* 2015;64(12):948-952.
7. Weitzel N, Kendall J, Pons P. Blind nasotracheal intubation for patients with penetrating neck trauma. *J Trauma.* 2004;56(5):1097-1101.
8. Alhomary M, Ramadan E, Curran E, Walsh SR. Videolaryngoscopy vs. fibreoptic bronchoscopy for awake tracheal intubation: a systematic review and meta-analysis. *Anaesthesia.* 2018;73(9):1151-1161.
9. Hofmeyr R. Dual endoscopy. OpenAirway. Published June 21, 2018. Accessed December 6, 2021. https://openairway.org/dual-endoscopy/.
10. Sakles JC, Corn GJ, Hollinger P, Arcaris B, Patanwala AE, Mosier JM. The impact of a soiled airway on intubation success in the emergency department when using the GlideScope or the direct laryngoscope. *Acad Emerg Med Off J Soc Acad Emerg Med.* 2017;24(5):628-636.
11. Mihara R, Komasawa N, Matsunami S, Minami T. Comparison of direct and indirect laryngoscopes in vomitus and hematemesis settings: a randomized simulation trial. *BioMed Res Int.* 2015;2015:e806243.
12. Lewis SR, Butler AR, Parker J, Cook TM, Schofield-Robinson OJ, Smith AF. Videolaryngoscopy versus direct laryngoscopy for adult patients requiring tracheal intubation: a Cochrane Systematic Review. *Br J Anaesth.* 2017;119(3):369-383.
13. Pieters BMA, Maas EHA, Knape JTA, van Zundert AAJ. Videolaryngoscopy vs. direct laryngoscopy use by experienced anaesthetists in patients with known difficult airways: a systematic review and meta-analysis. *Anaesthesia.* 2017;72(12):1532-1541.
14. Birenbaum A, Hajage D, Roche S, et al. Effect of cricoid pressure compared with a Sham Procedure in the rapid sequence induction of anesthesia: The IRIS Randomized Clinical Trial. *JAMA Surg.* 2019;154(1):9-17.
15. Frerk C, Mitchell VS, McNarry AF, et al. Difficult Airway Society 2015 guidelines for management of unanticipated difficult intubation in adults. *Br J Anaesth.* Dec 2015;115(6):827-848.
16. Law JA, Duggan LV, Asselin M, et al. Canadian Airway Focus Group updated consensus-based recommendations for management of the difficult airway: part 2. Planning and implementing safe management of the patient with an anticipated difficult airway. *Can J Anaesth.* Sep 2021;68(9):1405-1436.
17. Root CW, Mitchell OJL, Brown R, et al. Suction Assisted Laryngoscopy and Airway Decontamination (SALAD): a technique for improved emergency airway management. *Resusc Plus.* 2020;1-2:100005.
18. Nikolla DA, King B, Heslin A, Carlson JN. Comparison of suction rates between a Standard Yankauer, a commercial large-bore suction device, and a Makeshift Large-Bore Suction Device. *J Emerg Med.* 2021;61(3):265-270.
19. Kei J, Mebust DP. Comparing the effectiveness of a novel suction set-up using an adult endotracheal tube connected to a Meconium Aspirator vs. a traditional Yankauer Suction Instrument. *J Emerg Med.* 2017;52(4):433-437.
20. Weingart SD, Bhagwan SD. A novel set-up to allow suctioning during direct endotracheal and fiberoptic intubation. *J Clin Anesth.* 2011;23(6):518-519.

CHAPTER 43

Management of a Patient with OSA and Retrosternal Multinodular Goiter, Presenting for Total Thyroidectomy

Jinbin Zhang, Edwin Seet, and Orlando R. Hung

CASE PRESENTATION

A 55-year-old female with a BMI of 36 $kg{\cdot}m^{-2}$ presented for total thyroidectomy for a long-standing multinodular goiter. She appeared clinically euthyroid and her thyroid function tests were normal. Although retrosternal extension, mid-tracheal deviation, and compression were demonstrated on the CT scan (Figure 43.1), the patient did not exhibit any compressive symptoms. On preoperative screening using the STOP-Bang questionnaire, the patient was deemed to be at high risk for OSA in view of the presence of loud snoring, daytime sleepiness, history of hypertension, BMI greater than 35 $kg{\cdot}m^{-2}$, and age above 50 years old. She offered the information that she was told "it was difficult to insert a breathing tube" during her previous surgery 10 years ago, but could not recall further details. Airway examination demonstrated mouth opening >5 cm, a short neck but good cervical extension (flexion was limited by the large goiter), Mallampati class IV, large tongue, and thyromental distance of 4 cm. Referral to a sleep physician for sleep study evaluation was offered but the patient declined due to financial reasons. She also adamantly refused awake intubation despite a thorough explanation of the indications. After discussion with the surgeon and patient, the plan was to proceed with the surgery with risk-mitigating strategies in view of patient's refusal for further investigations.

INTRODUCTION

Obstructive sleep apnea (OSA) is the most common sleep-disordered breathing syndrome and is a growing problem with substantial economic costs. The presence of OSA in patients negatively influences postoperative outcomes.[1] Severe perioperative complications (i.e., death and anoxic brain injury) directly related to OSA are being increasingly reported as the central contention of medical malpractice suits, with a substantial medico-legal burden.[2,3] The prevalence of moderate-to-severe OSA among the general population is estimated at 13% in men and 6% in women between the ages of 30 and 70 years, with increased prevalence in the older age group of 50 to 70 years (17% in men, 9% in women). This reflects a substantial relative increase of OSA in the general population from 14% to 55% over the last two decades.[4] The prevalence of OSA in surgical patients is even higher, with a quarter of the surgical population at high risk of OSA.[5–7] Up to 90% of these patients may have undiagnosed OSA, and 40% of them may have moderate-to-severe OSA if subjected to testing by polysomnography (PSG).[6,7]

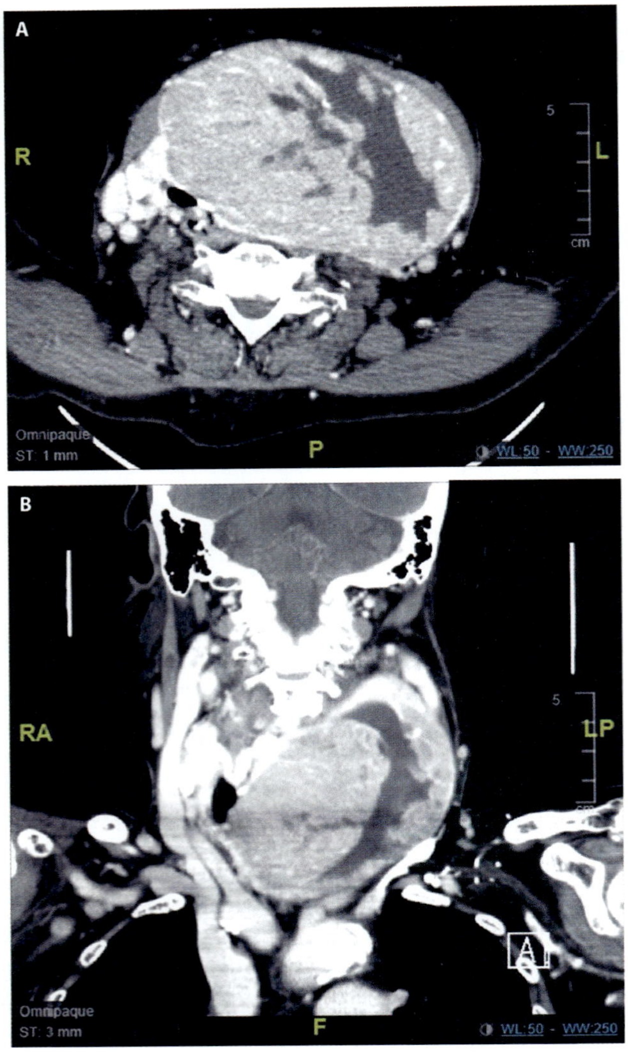

FIGURE 43.1. **(A)** Cross-sectional and **(B)** coronal images of the patient's goiter, showing retrosternal extension, tracheal deviation to the right, and tracheal compression.

What Are the Perioperative Risks of a Patient with OSA?

OSA is an independent predictor of uncontrolled hypertension in patients less than 50 years old. Chronic nocturnal hypoxemia and hypercarbia trigger increased sympathetic activity, and the subsequent hemodynamic stress may lead to cardiovascular diseases through multiple mechanisms.[8] Moderate-to-severe OSA is also associated with multiple medical comorbidities, including metabolic syndrome, obesity, insulin resistance, uncontrolled hypertension, heart failure, arrhythmias, coronary artery disease, and stroke.[8–10] As such, patients with OSA are at increased risk of the following postoperative complications:

1. Cardiovascular complications—atrial fibrillation, myocardial infarction/ischemia, arrhythmia, cardiac arrest
2. Respiratory complications—postoperative oxygen desaturation and hypoxemia (secondary to airway obstruction, opioid-induced central apnea, etc.), acute respiratory distress syndrome (ARDS), aspiration pneumonia, respiratory failure

These result in an increased incidence of postoperative cardiovascular complications, noninvasive ventilation, emergency reintubation, unplanned ICU admission, and mechanical ventilation in both the general and bariatric surgical populations.[11–19] There is also a possible association between OSA and postoperative delirium.[20] Hence, it is imperative to identify patients at risk of OSA preoperatively to allow for adequate optimization and implementation of risk mitigation strategies.

What Is the Pathophysiology of Obstructive Sleep Apnea?

From a morphological perspective, OSA occurs when there is a pharyngeal anatomical imbalance with a capacity limitation of the cervicomaxillomandibular skeletal airway and/or an increase in oropharyngeal soft tissue.[21,22]

In normal subjects, pharyngeal muscle tone decreases during sleep, particularly during rapid-eye movement (REM) sleep. The consequent airway narrowing and increased airflow resistance contribute to hypoventilation and an increase in $PaCO_2$ of 3 to 5 mmHg. This response is exaggerated in patients with sleep-related breathing disorders, including OSA.[23]

OSA is characterized by the closure and collapse of the pharyngeal airspace during sleep. This results in airflow cessation and bouts of hypoxemia and hypercapnia with consequent repeated arousals from sleep. The narrowest part of the airway lies posterior to the soft palate, where the tongue and the soft palate are in close proximity and may be in apposition. The most common site of upper airway obstruction during non-REM sleep is typically located at this point. The posterior movement of the tongue may, in addition, further occlude the retroglossal space in approximately half of the patients with sleep apnea. This segment of the oropharyngeal obstruction may further increase in length during REM sleep when the pharyngeal muscle tone is more suppressed.[23] Recently, a systematic review and meta-analysis demonstrated that tongue base thickness and retroglossal diameter based on ultrasound airway parameters correlated with OSA severity.[24]

Identification of the sites of obstruction during sleep is important in order to guide the implementation of appropriate therapy (e.g., uvulopalatopharyngoplasty, base of tongue surgery, noninvasive positive pressure ventilation, etc.). In addition to obesity, as mentioned above, risk factors for OSA include anatomical factors such as hypertrophied adenoids and tonsils, macroglossia, retrognathia, and micrognathia.

How Is OSA Diagnosed?

Screening tests have been validated to identify patients at risk of OSA, who may then be referred for diagnostic testing. The Society of Anesthesia and Sleep Medicine preoperative guidelines on OSA evaluation recommend that anesthesiologists consider making OSA screening part of standard anesthesia evaluation prior to undergoing a general anesthetic.[2] The Adult Obstructive Sleep Apnea Task Force of the American Academy of Sleep Medicine (AASM) recommends the diagnosis of OSA be based on clinical findings from history, physical examination, and results from objective sleep testing.[25]

The gold standard objective testing for OSA is an in-lab PSG study. However, home testing with portable monitors may be a more suitable and reliable alternative for some patients. The frequency of obstructing events is reported as an apnea-hypopnea index (AHI) or respiratory disturbance index (RDI), in accordance with the *AASM Manual for the Scoring of Sleep and Associated Events*.[26] Apnea is defined as cessation of airflow for at least 10 seconds. Hypopnea occurs where there is reduced airflow with oxygen desaturation of ≥3%, or is associated with arousal. According to the American Academy of Sleep Medicine guidelines, a diagnosis of OSA is confirmed when there are ≥15 obstructive events per hour (apnea, hypopnea, respiratory event-related arousals) on PSG, or ≥5 events per hour in a patient who reports any symptoms such as unintentional sleep episodes during wakefulness, daytime sleepiness, insomnia, loud snoring described by bed partner, or observed obstruction during sleep.[25] Severity of OSA is classified as mild (AHI ≥5 and <15), moderate (AHI 15-30), or severe (AHI >30 events per hour).

Home sleep apnea testing devices may be used to diagnose patients with a high pretest probability of OSA. However, complicated patients, such as those with significant cardiorespiratory disease, neuromuscular disorders, awake or sleep-related hypoventilation, stroke history, chronic opioid use, or severe insomnia are more appropriately referred for formal sleep studies (i.e., PSG).[27]

PREOPERATIVE ASSESSMENT OF PATIENTS WITH KNOWN/SUSPECTED OSA

How Do We Perform a Preoperative Evaluation of a Patient with Known OSA?

A thorough history and physical examination should be performed targeting the symptoms and signs of OSA. Sleep study results should be reviewed to ascertain the severity of OSA.

For patients with a known history of OSA, the following should be identified and optimized:

1. Presence of significant comorbidities such as morbid obesity, obesity hypoventilation syndrome, metabolic syndrome, poorly controlled hypertension, coronary artery disease, arrhythmia, heart failure, cerebrovascular diseases, gastroesophageal reflux disease, and others.
2. Systemic complications of long-standing OSA include hypercarbia, hypoxemia, cor pulmonale, polycythemia, and pulmonary hypertension. The prevalence of pulmonary arterial hypertension in sleep apnea is estimated to be 20% to 34%.[28-31]

A simple bedside observation of a resting oxygen saturation less than 94% on pulse oximetry, in the absence of other possible causes of hypoxemia, may be suspicious for OSA.[32,33] As the degree of pulmonary arterial hypertension associated with OSA is usually mild, the American College of Chest Physicians Guidelines Committee does not recommend routine evaluation for pulmonary hypertension in patients with OSA.[34]

A history of therapies such as surgical treatment, oral appliances, positive airway pressure (PAP) therapy, and hypoglossal nerve stimulation devices (less common) should be identified and documented. PAP therapy includes continuous positive airway pressure (CPAP), bilevel positive airway pressure (BiPAP), and autotitrated positive airway pressure (APAP) therapy. The adequacy of PAP therapy, recommended PAP settings, and compliance of patients to the PAP treatment should be determined. Patients on home PAP therapy should be advised to bring their PAP devices to the medical facility on the day of the general anesthesia for the surgical procedure and to continue with PAP therapy during the perioperative period. Patients who have undergone an anesthetic, and those who have been prescribed alternative therapy such as oral appliances or nasal resistive valves, but have not had a repeat sleep study to document the improvement or resolution of OSA, should be regarded as having a high probability of untreated OSA.[2] Continued use of these appliances in the perioperative setting should be encouraged.[2]

How Do We Perform a Preoperative Evaluation of a Patient with Suspected OSA?

The Society of Anesthesia and Sleep Medicine guidelines recommend the universal screening of preanesthesia patients for OSA[2], as preanesthesia identification of patients at high risk of OSA allows for heightened awareness and the implementation of targeted interventions, which may reduce perioperative complications. Patients suspected clinically to have OSA should be referred for an early preanesthetic evaluation to allow ample time for appropriate referral to a sleep physician and preparation of a perioperative plan. Focused evaluation includes a comprehensive medical record review, patient/family interview, and screening and physical examination. Medical record review should include obtaining a history of a difficult airway, hypertension, other cardiovascular comorbidities, and other congenital/acquired medical conditions. History of observed apnea and snoring offered by the bed partner is useful. Physical examination should include the respiratory, cardiovascular, and neurologic systems. Particular attention should be paid to BMI, evaluation of the airway, and neck circumference. Serum bicarbonate level may be elevated in patients with moderate-to-severe OSA ($HCO_3^- \geq 28$ mmol·L^{-1}) due to renal compensatory mechanisms related to chronic hypercapnia and respiratory acidosis.[35] Baseline oxygen saturation values may be unexpectedly lower than anticipated.[32,33]

Multiple screening tools and questionnaires have been developed to simplify and improve the identification of patients with possible OSA, such as the Berlin Questionnaire,[36] the Sleep Apnea Clinical Score,[37] the ASA checklist,[36] and the STOP-BANG Questionnaire.[38] Effective screening tools are designed with high sensitivity (low false-negative rate) to capture as many suspected cases as possible, recognizing that specificity (high false-positive rate) is often compromised. The STOP-BANG Questionnaire has been identified as possessing the highest sensitivity for predicting moderate-to-severe OSA with high methodological validity.[39]

Developed as a screening tool for OSA in surgical patients, the STOP-BANG questionnaire is easy to administer to patients in a busy clinical setting and has been validated in various populations, including surgical, obese, and morbidly obese patients.[40] It consists of eight questions in a Yes/No format.[38] The acronym STOP-BANG assesses for **S**noring, **T**iredness, **O**bserved apnea,

TABLE 43.1. STOP-Bang Questionnaire

S	**SNORING**	**Do you snore loudly (loud enough to be heard through closed doors or your bed-partner elbows you for snoring at night)?**	**Yes/No**
T	TIRED	Do you often feel tired, fatigued, or sleepy during daytime (such as falling asleep during driving or talking to someone)?	Yes/No
O	OBSERVED	Has anyone observed you stop breathing or choking/gasping during your sleep?	Yes/No
P	PRESSURE	Do you have or are being treated for high blood pressure?	Yes/No
B	BODY MASS INDEX	BMI >35 kg·m^{-2}?	Yes/No
A	AGE	Age >50 years old?	Yes/No
N	NECK CIRCUMFERENCE	Neck size large? (Measured around Adam's apple) For male, is your shirt collar 17 inches/43 cm or larger? For female, is your shirt collar 16 inches/41 cm or larger?	Yes/No
G	GENDER	Male?	Yes/No

Each positive answer is allocated a score of 1.
Low risk of OSA: Yes to 0-2 questions.
Intermediate risk of OSA: Yes to 3-4 questions.
High risk of OSA: Yes to 5-8 questions.
OR Yes to 2 or more of the 4 STOP questions + male gender.
OR Yes to 2 or more of the 4 STOP questions + BMI >35 kg·m^{-2}.
OR Yes to 2 or more of the 4 STOP questions + neck circumference >40 cm.
Reproduced with permission from University Health Network, Toronto, ON, Canada.

high blood **P**ressure, **B**MI >35 kg·m^{-2}, **A**ge > 50 years, **N**eck circumference larger than 40 cm, and male **G**ender (Table 43.1). Each positive answer is allocated a score of 1. Patients are deemed to be at low risk of OSA with a STOP-Bang score of 0-2, at risk of OSA if their STOP-Bang score is ≥3, or at high risk of moderate-to-severe OSA if their score is ≥5.[41] For ease of administration, all items in the STOP-BANG questionnaire are treated equally. However, not all items have an equal predictive weight for OSA.[38,42] A weighted model for the questionnaire may better predict OSA than a linear, equally weighted model.[43] For example, BMI and male gender have been found to carry more weight than neck circumference and age. Further risk stratification via a two-step strategy has been recently proposed for the group of patients with a STOP-BANG score of 3 to 4 (Figure 43.2), in which the subgroup at higher risk of OSA may be identified by examining specific combinations of the STOP-BANG questionnaire. Compared to patients with a nonweighted score of 3 and 4 (any 3 or 4 items positive), the probability of OSA in patients with a STOP score ≥2 + male gender and/or BMI >35 kg·m^{-2} was increased by 64%.[44,45] The addition of serum bicarbonate level

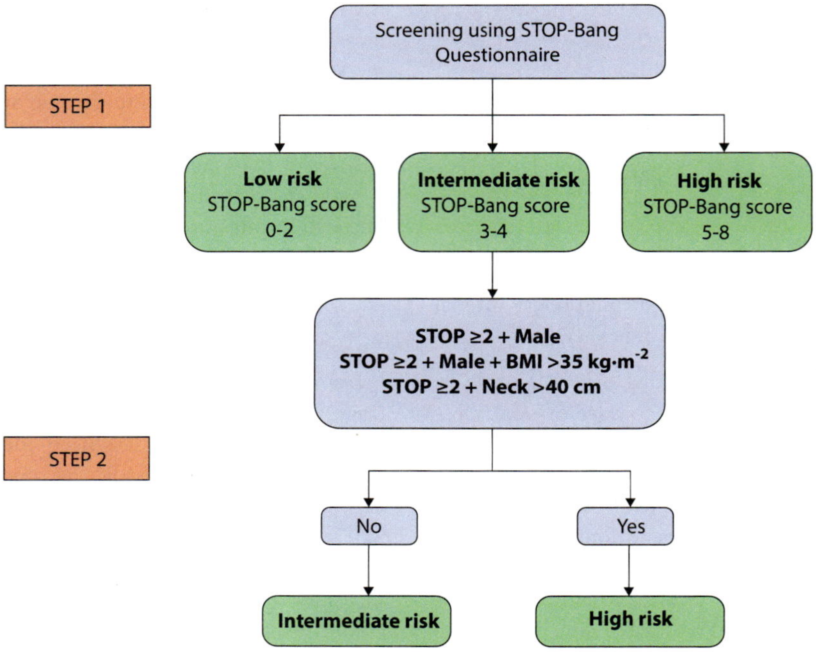

FIGURE 43.2. Suggested flowchart for a two-step OSA screening strategy with the STOP-Bang Questionnaire. (Adapted with permission from Chung F, Abdullah HR, Liao P. STOP-Bang questionnaire: a practical approach to screen for obstructive sleep apnea. *Chest*. 2016;149(3):631-638.)

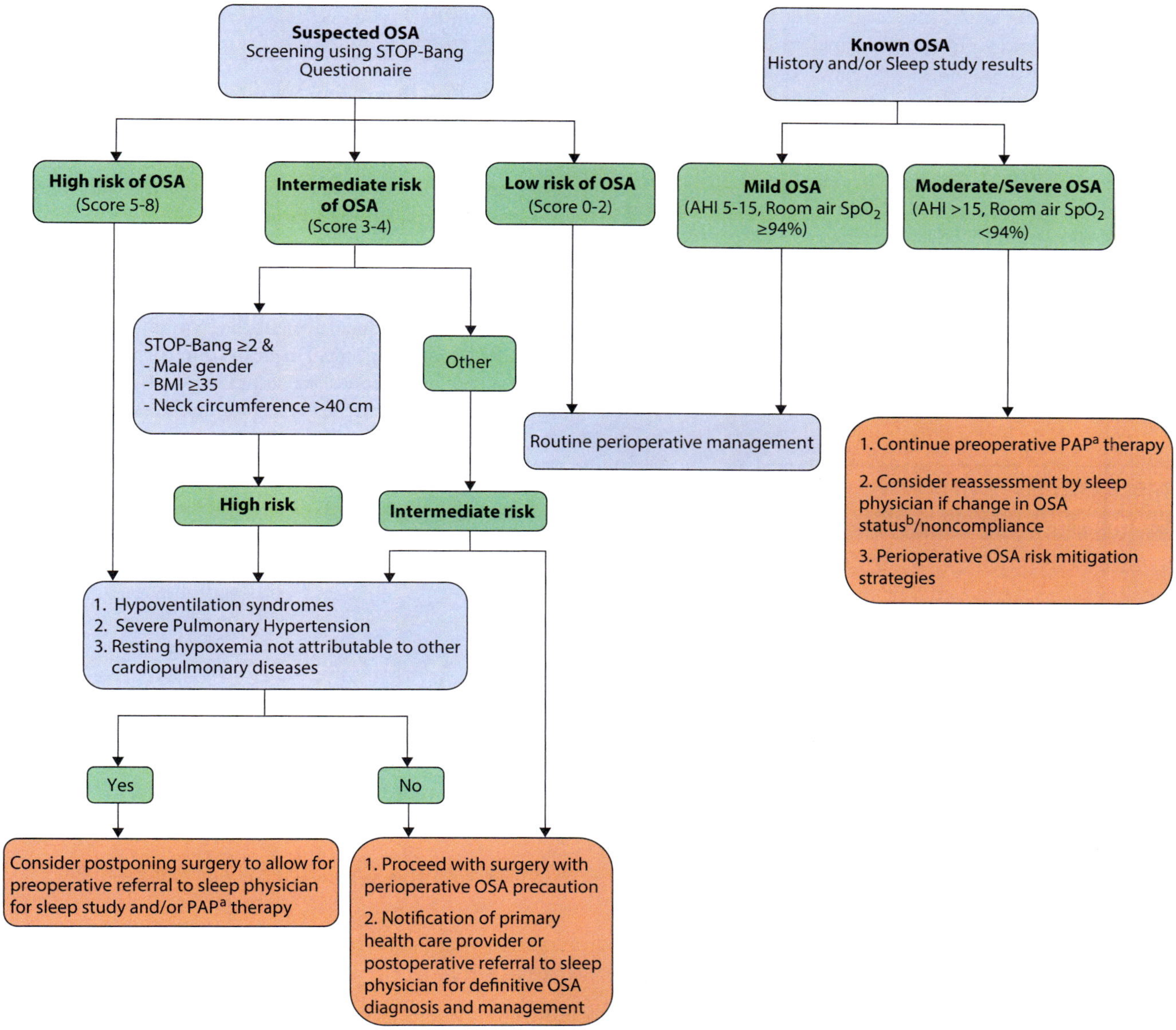

FIGURE 43.3. Preoperative evaluation of patients with known or suspected obstructive sleep apnea. [a]Positive airway pressure (PAP) therapy—includes continuous PAP (CPAP), bilevel PAP (BPAP), and automatically adjusting PAP (APAP). [b]Change in OSA status—recent exacerbation/worsening of OSA symptoms, recent OSA-related surgery, or lost to follow-up. (Modified with permission from Seet E, Chung F. Management of sleep apnea in adults—functional algorithms for the perioperative period: Continuing Professional Development. *Can J Anaesth*. 2010;57(9):849-864.)

(HCO_3^- ≥28 mmol·L^{-1}) further increases the specificity of the STOP-BANG screening in predicting moderate-to-severe OSA.[35] The 2016 guidelines on preoperative screening and assessment of patients with OSA, published by the Society of Anesthesia and Sleep Medicine, suggested that the updated STOP-BANG tool adds clinical value in being an easy method of dichotomous risk stratification of high or low risk of OSA,[2] and that it can guide the need for further assessment and optimization.

Should Surgery Be Cancelled to Allow for the Evaluation of Suspected OSA?

For patients with known OSA, reassessment by their sleep physician prior to an anesthetic should be considered if they have been noncompliant with treatment, defaulted with follow-up, report worsening symptoms, or have undergone a recent therapeutic airway procedure.

There is insufficient evidence to support the cancellation or postponement of anesthesia of patients identified to be at high risk of OSA while awaiting advanced screening techniques such as sleep testing, in the absence of evidence of significant cardiopulmonary disease.[2] To date, evidence is still inconclusive regarding the benefit of PAP therapy in the preoperative setting, as is the duration of therapy needed to reduce perioperative risks in patients with suspected OSA.[46] Hence, the subsequent management of this subset of patients is dependent on various factors: (1) urgency of surgery; (2) invasiveness of the planned procedure; (3) presence of significant systemic diseases (congestive heart failure, atrial fibrillation, refractory hypertension, stroke, pulmonary hypertension, and resting hypoxemia not attributable to other cardiopulmonary disease); (4) presence of hypoventilation syndromes; (5) postoperative opioid requirements; and (6) planned bariatric surgery.[25,47] Taking these factors into consideration, the anesthesia provider and the patient should jointly decide whether to: proceed with an anesthetic and manage the patient based on clinical criteria alone, taking the necessary perioperative OSA precautions with risk mitigation; or to defer the anesthetic to allow time for a referral to a sleep physician, confirmation of diagnosis with a sleep study, and institution of PAP therapy if necessary.[45,47] Figure 43.3 illustrates a comprehensive algorithm for the preoperative evaluation of a patient with known or suspected OSA.

INTRAOPERATIVE MANAGEMENT OF PATIENTS WITH OSA

What Are the Goals of Anesthetic Management of Patients with OSA?

Severe OSA-related perioperative complications (i.e., death and anoxic brain injury) are most commonly due to difficulty in airway management (usually in the form of difficult reintubation after premature extubation), and respiratory arrest in an unmonitored setting.[3] Perianesthetic management of patients with OSA focuses on the rapid restoration of consciousness and baseline cardiorespiratory functions after general anesthesia to minimize adverse outcomes. Risk mitigating strategies in the immediate perianesthetic and postanesthetic periods are summarized in Table 43.2 and include maintaining oxygenation, limiting the use of long-acting

TABLE 43.2. Perioperative Precautions and Risk Mitigation for OSA Patients

Anesthetic Concern	Principles of Management
Premedications	• Avoid sedating premedication
Potential difficult airway (Bag-mask ventilation and intubation)	• Optimal positioning (Head Elevated Laryngoscopy Position), additional "ramping" if patient is obese • Adequate denitrogenation • Consider CPAP denitrogenation • Maintain continuous oxygenation throughout airway manipulation (consider NO DESAT or THRIVE) • Two-handed triple-airway maneuvers • Anticipate difficult airway. Consider awake intubation, use of short-acting muscle relaxants (e.g., succinylcholine or rocuronium with sugammadex for rapid reversal) • Skilled personnel familiar with a specific difficult airway management guideline
Gastroesophageal reflux disease	• Consider proton-pump inhibitors, nonparticulate antacids, rapid sequence induction, and cricoid pressure
Carry-over sedation effects from longer-acting intravenous and volatile anesthetic agents	• Use of propofol/remifentanil for maintenance of anesthesia • Use of insoluble potent volatile agents (Desflurane) • Use of regional blocks as sole anesthetic technique
Opioid-related respiratory depression	• Minimize opioid use • Use of short-acting opioids (remifentanil) • Avoid basal opioid infusion if prescribed patient-controlled analgesia (PCA) • Multimodal, opioid-sparing approach to analgesia (acetaminophen, NSAIDs, COX-II inhibitors, tramadol, ketamine, gabapentin, pregabalin, dexmedetomidine, clonidine) • Consider local or regional anesthesia where appropriate
Excessive sedation in monitored anesthetic care	• Use of capnography for monitoring of ventilation • Avoid long-acting sedatives • Avoid deep sedation. Consider general anesthesia with secured airway
Postextubation airway obstruction	• Verify full reversal of neuromuscular blockade • Extubate only when fully awake and cooperative • Nonsupine position for extubation and recovery • "At-risk" extubation strategies if risk of postextubation airway complications • Resume use of PAP device after surgery

Reproduced with permission from Seet E, Chung F. Management of sleep apnea in adults—functional algorithms for the perioperative period: continuing professional development. *Can J Anaesth.* 2010;57:849-864.

sedative-hypnotics, using short-acting anesthetics for rapid recovery, multimodal analgesia for opioid-sparing effect, performing a safe extubation, and appropriate postoperative disposition.

Is Regional and Local Anesthesia with Sedation Safer Than General Anesthesia?

The use of regional anesthesia may be preferred over general anesthesia[48] as it avoids the need for airway manipulation and the use of sedative-hypnotics and analgesics that impair awakening and postanesthetic neurorespiratory functions. Procedural sedation, including monitored anesthesia care (MAC) is generally safe but patients with OSA may still exhibit increased tendency for oxygen desaturation due to apnea-hypopnea.[1] If moderate sedation is required, continuous oxygen saturation and capnography monitoring are recommended to allow for monitoring of airway patency and ventilation. The use of agents such as low-dose ketamine and dexmedetomidine may confer better safety due to the relative lack of respiratory depressive and upper airway obstructive effects.[49–52] Intravenous propofol and benzodiazepines have a greater propensity for respiratory adverse events during procedural sedation and MAC[49] and dosages should be carefully titrated if their use is unavoidable. However, if deep sedation is required, general anesthesia should be considered as a safer option in view of the high risk of airway obstruction during deep sedation without a secure airway.[47]

Is Obstructive Sleep Apnea Associated with a Difficult Airway?

Patients with OSA often possess features of an anatomically difficult airway due to the presence of a reduced oropharyngeal space from large tongue and collapsible pharyngeal space related to an increase in soft tissue.[24,53] It has been suggested that a history of difficult intubation is associated with a high risk of OSA, and such patients should be screened for signs and symptoms of sleep apnea and PSG considered.[54,55] OSA has been demonstrated to be associated with difficult mask ventilation[56–59] and difficult laryngoscopic intubation.[60–63] Difficult laryngoscopic intubation may occur as often as eight times more frequently in patients with OSA than those without OSA,[61] and there may be a correlation between the **severity** of OSA and difficult laryngoscopic intubation.[64] A recent multicenter observational cohort study suggested that STOP-BANG scores of 3-4 and 5-8 were associated with greater odds of difficult intubation.[64]

Extraglottic devices (EGDs) such as the laryngeal mask airway are effective rescue airway devices in unanticipated difficult intubation. There is little evidence available for OSA being a risk factor for difficult EGD insertion, but large neck circumference may be associated with increased difficulty in laryngeal mask insertion[65] and surgical airway access.

How Should We Prepare for a Difficult Airway?

The 2018 Society of Anesthesia and Sleep Medicine guidelines recommend that a history of known or suspected OSA be considered as an independent predictor for difficult intubation, mask ventilation, or a combination of both.[49] As such, adequate precautions and careful planning for airway management should be taken. Difficult airway adjuncts, difficult airway trolley/cart, and skilled assistants must be available. The airway practitioner should be familiar with difficult airway algorithms and backup plans (based on specific difficult airway management guidelines as recommended by the American Society of Anesthesiologists,[66] the Canadian Airway Focus Group,[67,68] or the Difficult Airway Society[69]) should be communicated to the team prior to the induction of general anesthesia.

Awake tracheal intubation (ATI) should be considered if the patient has a history of, or possesses multiple predictors for a difficult airway. Adequate airway topicalization provides a controlled environment, allowing ATI to be achieved using flexible bronchoscopy, video laryngoscopy, through an EGD (e.g., an LMA-Fastrach), or a combination of techniques.[70]

Maintenance of oxygenation throughout airway manipulation is vital. Adequate denitrogenation increases pulmonary oxygen reserves and delays onset of hypoxemia, hence allowing more time for safe airway management without oxygen desaturation. Denitrogenation is achieved with high flow 100% oxygen for 3 to 5 minutes until the end-tidal oxygen concentration is 90% or more. This can be further facilitated by the use of CPAP at 10 cm H_2O and with the patient propped in a 25-degree head-up position.[69,71–75] Obese patients may require further "ramping" to achieve the optimal alignment for laryngoscopy (*H*ead *E*levated *L*aryngoscopy *P*osition [*HELP*]). This can be achieved by the stacking of blankets or towels, or by using specially designed elevation devices such as the Troop Elevation Pillow (Mercury Medical, Clearwater, FL, USA) (see Figure 51.2).

Gastroesophageal reflux disease (GERD) is commonly associated with OSA.[76] Aspiration prophylaxis can be achieved with preoperative proton-pump inhibitors, nonparticulate antacids, rapid sequence induction, and cricoid pressure. However, if cricoid pressure interferes with bag-mask ventilation and glottis visualization, the cricoid pressure should be reduced or released.[69]

The early use of a video laryngoscope is preferred as the team is able to participate more effectively through shared visualization of the patient's airway, in addition to the benefits of improved glottic view and first-pass success. If a difficult airway is suspected, the use of succinylcholine to achieve muscle paralysis has been considered in the past due to its rapid onset of effect and a short duration of action. However, a larger dose of rocuronium (1.2 $mg{\cdot}kg^{-1}$) may now be preferred due to the rapid onset of muscle paralysis without muscle fasciculation and its paralytic effects can be rapidly antagonized with sugammadex.

Continuous oxygenation using oxygen insufflation via a nasal cannula further increases apnea time during laryngoscopy by utilizing the principle of apneic oxygenation.[77,78] During apnea, oxygen consumption is approximately 250 $mL{\cdot}min^{-1}$. Conversely, only 8 to 20 $mL{\cdot}min^{-1}$ of carbon dioxide diffuses from blood into the alveoli. The differential movement of oxygen and carbon dioxide across the alveolar membrane creates a net negative pressure in the alveoli, generating a mass flow of gas from the pharynx to the alveoli. This bulk flow of gas allows passive oxygenation in the absence of ventilation. By increasing the oxygen flow rate to 15 L·min^{-1} (hence increasing oxygen delivery), ***N***asal ***O***xygen ***D***uring ***E***fforts ***S***ecuring ***a*** ***T***ube (***NO DESAT***) has been demonstrated to extend the apnea time in obese patients and patients with a difficult airway.[78,79] The administration of oxygen should persist throughout the entire duration of airway manipulation. Although high-flow oxygen through a nasal cannula can be uncomfortable due to the desiccating effects on the nasopharyngeal mucosa, it should not cause deleterious effects when used for a short period of time during airway manipulation. Apneic oxygenation using high-flow nasal cannula with humidified high-flow oxygen of up to 70 L·min^{-1} (***T***ransnasal ***H***umidified ***R***apid-***I***nsufflation ***V***entilatory ***E***xchange [***THRIVE***]) is useful in prolonging apnea time during airway manipulation.[80–83] It must, however, be emphasized that a patent airway must be ensured for apneic oxygenation to be effective.

What Is the Anesthetic and Analgesic Strategy for Patients with OSA?

General anesthesia is known to depress central respiratory output to the upper airway dilator muscles and airway reflexes, hence reducing the arousal response to hypoxemia and hypercarbia. Patients with OSA are particularly susceptible to the respiratory depressant effects of sedatives, anesthetics, and opioids, due to their propensity for airway collapse. As such, the anesthesia and analgesia strategy should focus on the prevention of carry-over sedation and opioid effect to minimize postanesthetic respiratory depression and upper airway obstruction.[53] Sedative premedication such as benzodiazepines should be avoided. Short-acting anesthetics (e.g., propofol, desflurane, and remifentanil) are preferred as their short duration of action allows for short duration of action and attenuation of the alerting response to hypoxemia/hypercarbia. As pulmonary hypertension is a known complication of long-standing OSA, triggers for exacerbation of pulmonary arterial pressure elevation, namely, hypoxemia, hypercarbia, acidosis, and hypothermia, should be avoided.

Longer-acting opioids (e.g., morphine, hydromorphone, etc.) are associated with adverse perioperative respiratory events in a dose-dependent fashion[11,84]; hence a multimodal analgesic strategy should be adopted to reduce opioid requirement. An opioid-sparing strategy includes the use of central neuraxial or peripheral nerve blocks, acetaminophen, nonsteroidal anti-inflammatory agents, ketamine, tramadol, and other adjuvants such as anticonvulsants and dexamethasone.[85] Alpha-2 agonists (e.g., clonidine and dexmedetomidine) have been used as opioid-sparing analgesics with reduced respiratory compromise,[86,87] although the potential hemodynamic effects should be taken into consideration.

How Can a Safe Extubation Be Performed?

Planning for extubation is often overlooked, even after a difficult intubation. Premature extubation is associated with difficult reintubation, resulting in serious morbidity and mortality. Extubation is an elective process and should be undertaken after evaluating the risk of postextubation complications.[88] Full reversal of neuromuscular blockade should be achieved. There is currently insufficient evidence to recommend the use of sugammadex over neostigmine in patients with OSA.[49] An objective assessment of neuromuscular recovery using train-of-four monitoring or similar is useful to guide extubation. The patient should be fully conscious with the return of airway protective reflexes, be able to obey commands, and have minimal pain. Propping the patient in a semi-upright position confers better mechanical advantage to respiration. If the patient is assessed to have multiple risk factors (e.g., difficult intubation, severe OSA, obesity, procedure-related issues) that may predispose to airway obstruction following extubation, an "at-risk" extubation strategy should be employed, such as delaying extubation when appropriate, use of a remifentanil technique or an airway exchange catheter (AEC).[88] The use of doxapram, a central respiratory stimulant for rapid restoration of baseline respiratory efforts with improved postoperative recovery outcomes, has been described.[89]

POSTOPERATIVE MANAGEMENT OF PATIENTS WITH OSA

What Is the Postoperative Management Plan for Patients with OSA?

Normal sleep architecture is not restored to baseline until several days after anesthesia and surgery.[90] Risk factors for post-procedure respiratory depression may include: (1) underlying severity of OSA; (2) use of systemic opioids; (3) use of sedatives; (4) site and invasiveness of the procedure. These factors influence the intensity of monitoring required and hence, postprocedural disposition of the patient. The ASA 2014 guidelines stipulate the following management strategies for postprocedure recovery, analgesia, positioning, and oxygenation.[47]

All patients with known or suspected OSA who have undergone general anesthesia should receive supplemental oxygen, and extended monitoring in the Post Anesthesia Care Unit (PACU) with continuous oximetry monitoring. While data are lacking on the optimal duration, the ASA 2006 guidelines recommended prolonged PACU monitoring for 7 hours if respiratory events such as apnea or airway obstruction occur.[91] However, this recommendation is difficult to adhere to and this has since been removed from the 2014 ASA OSA guidelines.[47] A more practical approach would be to prescribe an extended PACU observation for an additional 60 to 120 minutes after the patient has fulfilled the standard PACU discharge criteria.[33] Others have described patient behaviors in the PACU that may portend respiratory complications, which may occur later in the general ward, including recurrent bradypnea, apnea, desaturation, and pain-sedation mismatch.[13]

Multimodal opioid-sparing analgesia techniques should continue into the postoperative phase. If patient-controlled systemic opioids are used, a continuous background infusion should be avoided or used with extreme caution.[47] Postoperative opioid-induced respiratory depression resulting in serious morbidity and mortality has been found to occur usually within 24 hours of anesthesia.[92] Furthermore, low sodium–containing fluids should be used judiciously, bearing in mind the potential for rostral fluid shift and worsening of the OSA by airway narrowing when large volumes of crystalloids are administered.[93]

Supplemental oxygen should be administered to patients who are at increased postoperative risk of OSA until they are able to maintain acceptable room air oxygen saturation. They should also be nursed in a nonsupine (semi-upright +/− lateral) position.[47] It may be beneficial to continue with oxygen therapy while the patient is on parenteral opioids, although it is cautioned that this may increase the duration of apneic episodes, and may delay the detection of hypercapnia and hypoxemia from hypoventilation.[47] PAP therapy should be administered to patients who were using these preanesthesia modalities as soon as possible, unless contraindicated by the procedure (e.g., ENT nasal surgery). Adjustments may be required to compensate for postprocedural changes, such as facial and airway swelling, pharmacotherapy, and respiratory function.[2]

For patients suspected to have OSA with frequent or severe airway obstruction or hypoxemia occurring during postanesthetic monitoring, initiation of PAP therapy may be considered. An open-labeled randomized controlled trial demonstrated beneficial effects of reducing postprocedure AHI and improving oxygenation with the use of autotitrated PAP in these groups of patients.[94]

Upon discharge from PACU, disposition to an unmonitored setting (i.e., unmonitored hospital bed or home) should be avoided if the patient has: (1) undergone a major abdominal, thoracic, neurosurgical, or head and neck surgery[95]; (2) has moderate/severe OSA; (3) is noncompliant with PAP therapy; (4) has significant comorbidities (especially obesity hypoventilation syndrome); (5) has recurrent respiratory events in PACU[13]; or (6) needs postoperative parenteral opioids. Such patients are at high risk of respiratory compromise and should be admitted to a monitored facility with continuous oximetry/ventilation monitoring and the capacity to provide timely intervention if indicated,[95] for example, high-dependency units or intermediate care units.

Can Patients with OSA Be Discharged Home Safely from an Ambulatory Surgery Center?

Careful patient selection is required as management of patients with OSA in an ambulatory setting is potentially challenging. The Society for Ambulatory Anesthesia (SAMBA) has issued a consensus statement on the selection of suitable OSA patients for ambulatory surgery.[96]

Patients with known or suspected OSA can be suitable candidates for ambulatory surgery if the following requirements are met:

1. Well-optimized comorbid medical conditions
2. Minor-to-moderate procedures, where postoperative pain can be well controlled by nonopioid techniques, such as use of local/regional anesthesia, acetaminophen, NSAIDs, and dexamethasone
3. Patients who are able and willing to use PAP therapy after discharge

Patients receiving preoperative PAP therapy should be encouraged to bring their PAP device to the ambulatory care facility. Advice should be given to use their PAP device whenever sleeping, including during daytime for several days postoperatively, as they are at increased risk of apnea until the normal sleep architecture is restored.[90] It is necessary to educate patients and their caregivers on the need for increased vigilance for respiratory complications after discharge and to give clear instructions on seeking medical attention should these occur.

Caution should be exercised if repeated respiratory events are observed in patients with known or suspected OSA in the early postprocedural period.[13] There should be a lower threshold for hospitalization, and ambulatory centers should have transfer arrangements with secondary or tertiary inpatient facilities that have the capacity, equipment, and personnel to manage postoperative OSA-related complications.

WHAT ARE THE ADDITIONAL CONSIDERATIONS FOR MULTINODULAR RETROSTERNAL THYROID GOITER SURGERY?

What Are the Preoperative Airway Concerns for a Retrosternal Goiter (RSG)?

Although slow growing and benign in nature, a large goiter poses potential airway concerns including laryngotracheal deviation and compression, preoperative vocal cord paresis, mediastinal compression by a retrosternal thyroid resulting in superior vena cava (SVC), and lower airway compression. The patient may present with symptoms of aerodigestive tract compression such as dysphagia, dysphonia, and dyspnea on lying supine. Pemberton's sign may be positive: SVC compression at the thoracic inlet when the patient's arms are raised to the sides of the head resulting in facial flushing, congestion, and cyanosis.

Additional examination by flexible nasoendoscopy can ascertain anatomical distortion, position, morphology of the glottic inlet, and baseline vocal cord mobility.[97] Computed tomography (CT) imaging allows for assessment of the extent of retrosternal extension, tracheal deviation, and luminal narrowing. The pattern of tracheal narrowing, presence of luminal wall invasion (suggestive of malignancy), and blood vessel compression can also be examined with CT imaging. It is pertinent to note that CT imaging is performed in the supine position and the static images obtained do not reflect the dynamic changes in airway diameter and patency during respiration.

Does a Large Multinodular Retrosternal Goiter Make Tracheal Intubation Difficult?

The choice of induction technique and airway management is dependent on preexisting airway concerns. Traditional teaching warns of a difficult airway in such patients: difficult mask ventilation and positive pressure ventilation due to tracheal compression; difficult intubation due to anatomical distortion and compression; difficult surgical airway access due to overlying goiter, tracheal deviation, and luminal compression; and difficult extubation due to the risk of tracheomalacia.

Expert opinion on the appropriate airway management of a large RSG differs widely.[98] There is no strong evidence that neuromuscular blockade impedes mask ventilation and positive pressure ventilation. The benign and pliable goiter tissue does not cause fixed annular tracheal stenosis as seen in anterior mediastinal masses. One study demonstrated improved ventilatory dynamics following the administration of neuromuscular blocking agents in patients with laryngotracheal stenosis.[99] There is currently little evidence to suggest that a large RSG in itself is a predictor of difficult intubation. A retrospective review of 60 RSG thyroidectomies[100] recorded an 8% incidence of difficult intubation requiring multiple attempts, but offered no further details. Difficult intubation was encountered in 1.5% of 813 patients with large multinodular goiters in an endemic goiter region.[101] However, in the paper, difficult intubation was loosely defined as three or more attempts or requiring the use of intubation aids. No details on laryngoscopic grade and intubation devices were provided. More recent studies provide little support to the contention that RSG alone causes difficult laryngoscopy. Findlay et al.[102] performed a retrospective review of 334 thyroidectomies, of which 48 were RSG and found no accounts of difficult airway. While 62 patients had tracheal narrowing to <15 mm in diameter, the majority of patients received standard IV induction with no difficulties in mask ventilation and intubation. Gilfillan et al.[103] performed a review of 133 patients with RSG weighing more than 200 g within a single institution and found that although awake flexible bronchoscopic intubation (FBI) was chosen as the primary technique for intubation in 17 patients; only 2 patients possessed additional predictors of difficult airway (ankylosing spondylitis and micrognathia) other than a large goiter. Most patients underwent standard IV induction with neuromuscular blockade and uneventful intubation with Grades 1 and 2 laryngeal views. Awake FBI was abandoned in two patients due to poor tolerance and inhalational induction failed in two patients with resultant desaturation. All four patients were rescued with IV induction, muscle paralysis, and successfully intubated with direct or video laryngoscopy. Difficult mask ventilation was reported in only five patients. A review of a small series of 19 patients[104] with RSG showed easy intubation with Grades 1 and 2 laryngeal view in 18 patients who received standard IV induction with neuromuscular blockade. One intubation failure was reported in a patient who underwent inhalational induction with resultant failed airway and required an emergency tracheotomy. The same patient returned for thyroidectomy 16 months postincident and the airway was secured with FBI. These studies suggest that a large goiter or RSG are not predictors of a difficult airway. The choice of intubation technique should be based on the presence of the usual predictors during bedside assessment.

Is It Necessary to Use Smaller-Sized Tracheal Tubes for Intubation in Patients with Retrosternal Goiter?

There are concerns of difficulty in tracheal tube passage following intubation, due to the presence of tracheal narrowing by the large goiter. However, many studies have demonstrated that the externally compressed trachea can accommodate tracheal tubes much larger than the measured tracheal diameter on CT imaging. In a review by Findlay et al.[102] involving 334 patients who underwent thyroid surgery, tracheal compression was reported in 62 patients with a mean minimum tracheal diameter of 7.6 mm (range 2-15 mm). Of these patients, critical tracheal compression to a diameter of <5 mm was reported in 18. Yet, all patients were intubated successfully with tracheal tubes of 6.0 to 8.0 mm internal diameter (ID), corresponding to outer diameters of 8.2 to 11.0 mm (armored/reinforced tracheal tubes are 0.2-0.3 mm thicker than standard tubes), with no documented difficulties in tube passage. In a series by Dempsey et al.,[104] three patients presented with stridor and narrowed tracheas of 6 to 9.5 mm in diameter on CT imaging. Nonetheless, tracheal tubes of 7.0 to 8.0 mm ID were passed with no difficulties. These findings suggest that the trachea remains distensible in spite of the external compression by the benign goiter.

When Should Awake Flexible Bronchoscopic Intubation Be Chosen as the Primary Technique?

Studies suggest that in view of the benign nature of RSG, IV induction with neuromuscular blockade and laryngoscopy is a safe technique in appropriately experienced hands, for the majority of cases. However, in nonspecialist centers and in the hands of less experienced practitioners, awake FBI remains the technique with the largest margin of safety.[104] As tracheotomy and cricothyrotomy will likely be difficult due to anatomical distortion by the large goiter, awake FBI should also be given due consideration in patients who possess multiple features that may pose difficulties in airway management. Acute intrathyroid hemorrhage, luminal invasion by malignancy, and circumferential tracheal narrowing are additional considerations for awake FBI and the use of smaller-sized tracheal tubes to get beyond the obstruction. If awake FBI is chosen, care must be taken in patients with marked stridor as complete airway obstruction may result during airway topicalization and the insertion of the bronchoscope ("cork in a bottle"). Insertion of a rigid bronchoscope may be necessary if attempts at passing an ETT beyond a mid-lower tracheal obstruction have failed.[105] A rigid bronchoscope also allows for ventilation, tamponade of intratracheal bleeding, and performance of diagnostic and therapeutic procedures.[97]

Should Awake Cardiopulmonary Bypass or Extracorporal Membrane Oxygenation (ECMO) Be Arranged for Large Retrosternal Goiters (See Chapter 45)?

A large RSG poses additional concerns of cardiovascular collapse in the presence of mediastinal vessel compression. For such patients, implementing standby extracorporeal cardiopulmonary bypass has been reported in some cases.[106,107] Notwithstanding these cases, there are no reports in the literature of extreme cardiorespiratory instability related to RSG in adult patients. A cohort study[103] of a thyroid database containing 919 patients with RSG yielded 23 patients with goiters of sizes larger than 400 g, of which none required cardiopulmonary bypass. RSG does not originate within the mediastinum; it arises from the cervical region and extends down into the mediastinum. Hence, it is usually tethered to the neck with less intrathoracic movement and very unlikely to cause cardiorespiratory compromise.

What Are the Other Periprocedural Considerations for Thyroid Surgery?

The use of electrophysiological monitoring of the recurrent laryngeal nerve requires the omission of intraoperative muscle paralysis. Smooth emergence is paramount to reduce the risk of venous congestion, edema, and bleeding. Studies have described the use of EGDs as the intraoperative primary airway of choice,[108,109] or at the end of the surgery to permit a noncoughing emergence and to allow for bronchoscopic examination of the vocal cord mobility.[110] The use of remifentanil is increasingly popular as it obtunds the laryngeal reflexes, reduces the need for muscle relaxants, provides intraoperative analgesia, and allows rapid titration of hemodynamics. However, due to its short duration of action, transitional opioids and local anesthetic infiltration must also be given for postoperative pain relief.

Postoperative complications following thyroid surgery include neck hematoma, recurrent laryngeal nerve palsy, and hypocalcemia. Tracheomalacia following RSG thyroidectomy is extremely uncommon in developed countries with an incidence of 0% to 0.11%.[103] Reintubation may be necessary and may be more complicated and treacherous than the preoperative attempt, due to anatomical distortion and edema.

SUMMARY

To recap, our patient is a middle-aged lady presenting for total thyroidectomy for multinodular goiter. She has a history and features of a difficult airway, suspected OSA, refused a sleep study, and an awake intubation. The anesthetic plan was general anesthesia with muscle paralysis and tracheal intubation using video laryngoscopy, failing which Plan B would be to perform asleep bronchoscopic-assisted intubation.

The patient was positioned using the Troop Elevation Pillow® (Mercury Medical, Clearwater, FL) and denitrogenation was achieved with high flow 100% oxygen for 5 minutes. Nasal cannulas were inserted with constant oxygen insufflation at 5 $L{\cdot}min^{-1}$. General anesthesia was induced using remifentanil, lidocaine, propofol, and rocuronium, recognizing the positive predictors for a difficult airway. Sugammadex was available for immediate reversal of muscle paralysis if necessary. Simultaneously, oxygen flow through the nasal cannula was increased to 15 $L{\cdot}min^{-1}$ in preparation for intubation, and the ability of bag-mask ventilation was confirmed after confirmation of muscle relaxation. A C-MAC D-blade video laryngoscope was used and a Grade 3 view was obtained, improving slightly to reveal the posterior arytenoids with external laryngeal pressure. A 7.5-mm ID electromyogram (EMG) tracheal tube was subsequently railroaded over the bougie with no resistance to tube passage. Tube position confirmed with auscultation and capnography. There was no oxygen desaturation during the tracheal intubation attempt.

Following intubation, the Troop pillow was removed, and the patient was positioned for surgery. Remifentanil infusion was used to avoid the use of muscle relaxants permitting intraoperative recurrent laryngeal nerve monitoring. Surgery was uneventful. The risks of tracheomalacia and postoperative bleeding were deemed to be low. Intraoperative intravenous (IV) acetaminophen, parecoxib, and fentanyl were administered, and the surgeons infiltrated the wound with ropivacaine. Total surgery time was 3 hours. After surgery was concluded, the patient was transferred onto the bed and propped up in a semi-Fowler position. She was allowed to emerge from anesthesia on a background infusion of remifentanil. Once she was awake, able to obey commands, and had satisfactory respiratory efforts, a #11 French airway exchange catheter (AEC) was inserted through the tracheal tube prior to its removal. The patient tolerated the AEC well and the AEC was secured onto her cheek.

The patient was monitored in PACU with the AEC left in-situ. The AEC was removed 2 hours later, when the patient was fully awake with minimal pain, and the risks for airway obstruction were deemed to be low. She was then discharged to an acute care unit with continuous oximetry monitoring. Oral acetaminophen and a COX-II inhibitor were ordered for postoperative analgesia.

SELF-EVALUATION QUESTIONS

43.1. Which of the following findings constitute a diagnosis of severe OSA?

A. STOP-Bang score = 3, AHI <5

B. Day-time sleepiness and observed apnea by spouse

C. STOP-Bang score = 5, AHI = 10

D. STOP-Bang score = 4, AHI = 55

E. STOP-Bang score = 6, AHI <5

43.2. Under which circumstance should the surgery be postponed for a referral to a sleep physician for sleep study?

A. Compliance to PAP therapy

B. STOP-Bang score = 6, history of atrial fibrillation and room air SpO_2 of 92%

C. Patient refusal for further investigations

D. STOP-Bang score = 6, presenting for minor extremity surgery

E. STOP-Bang score = 4, no significant comorbidities

43.3. Which of the following statements on perioperative management of a patient with suspected/known OSA is false?

A. Not all patients with OSA require inpatient admission following surgery.

B. Denitrogenation can be augmented by head-up position and CPAP.

C. Video laryngoscopy can be used as Plan A for intubation.

D. Use of opioids can be reduced with multimodal analgesia.

E. Anxious patients can be premedicated with oral lorazepam.

REFERENCES

1. Opperer M, Cozowicz C, Bugada D, et al. Does obstructive sleep apnea influence perioperative outcome? A qualitative systematic review for the society of anesthesia and sleep medicine task force on preoperative preparation of patients with sleep-disordered breathing. *Anesth Analg.* 2016;122(5):1321-1334.
2. Chung F, Memtsoudis SG, Ramachandran SK, et al. Society of Anesthesia and Sleep Medicine guidelines on preoperative screening and assessment of adult patients with obstructive sleep apnea. *Anesth Analg.* 2016;123(2):452-473.
3. Fouladpour N, Jesudoss R, Bolden N, Shaman Z, Auckley D. Perioperative complications in obstructive sleep apnea patients undergoing surgery: a review of the legal literature. *Anesth Analg.* 2016;122(1):145-151.
4. Peppard PE, Young T, Barnet JH, Palta M, Hagen EW, Hla KM. Increased prevalence of sleep-disordered breathing in adults. *Am J Epidemiol.* 2013; 177(9):1006-1014.
5. Chung F, Ward B, Ho J, Yuan H, Kayumov L, Shapiro C. Preoperative identification of sleep apnea risk in elective surgical patients, using the Berlin questionnaire. *J Clin Anesth.* 2007;19(2):130-134.
6. Finkel KJ, Searleman AC, Tymkew H, et al. Prevalence of undiagnosed obstructive sleep apnea among adult surgical patients in an academic medical center. *Sleep Med.* 2009;10(7):753-758.
7. Singh M, Liao P, Kobah S, Wijeysundera DN, Shapiro C, Chung F. Proportion of surgical patients with undiagnosed obstructive sleep apnoea. *Br J Anaesth.* 2013;110(4):629-636.
8. Somers VK, White DP, Amin R, et al. Sleep apnea and cardiovascular disease: an American Heart Association/American College of Cardiology Foundation Scientific Statement from the American Heart Association Council for High Blood Pressure Research Professional Education Committee, Council on Clinical Cardiology, Stroke Council, and Council on Cardiovascular Nursing. *J Am Coll Cardiol.* 2008;52(8):686-717.
9. Peppard PE, Young T, Palta M, Skatrud J. Prospective study of the association between sleep-disordered breathing and hypertension. *N Engl J Med.* 2000;342(19):1378-1384.
10. Shahar E, Whitney CW, Redline S, et al. Sleep-disordered breathing and cardiovascular disease: cross-sectional results of the Sleep Heart Health Study. *Am J Respir Crit Care Med.* 2001;163(1):19-25.
11. Blake DW, Yew CY, Donnan GB, Williams DL. Postoperative analgesia and respiratory events in patients with symptoms of obstructive sleep apnoea. *Anaesth Intensive Care.* 2009;37(5):720-725.
12. Gaddam S, Gunukula SK, Mador MJ. Post-operative outcomes in adult obstructive sleep apnea patients undergoing non-upper airway surgery: a systematic review and meta-analysis. *Sleep Breath.* 2014;18(3):615-633.
13. Gali B, Whalen FX Jr., Gay PC, et al. Management plan to reduce risks in perioperative care of patients with presumed obstructive sleep apnea syndrome. *J Clin Sleep Med.* 2007;3(6):582-588.
14. Kaw R, Chung F, Pasupuleti V, Mehta J, Gay PC, Hernandez AV. Meta-analysis of the association between obstructive sleep apnoea and postoperative outcome. *Br J Anaesth.* 2012;109(6):897-906.
15. Liao P, Yegneswaran B, Vairavanathan S, Zilberman P, Chung F. Postoperative complications in patients with obstructive sleep apnea: a retrospective matched cohort study. *Can J Anaesth.* 2009;56(11):819-828.
16. Memtsoudis S, Liu SS, Ma Y, et al. Perioperative pulmonary outcomes in patients with sleep apnea after noncardiac surgery. *Anesth Analg.* 2011; 112(1):113-121.
17. Mokhlesi B, Hovda MD, Vekhter B, Arora VM, Chung F, Meltzer DO. Sleep-disordered breathing and postoperative outcomes after bariatric surgery: analysis of the nationwide inpatient sample. *Obes Surg.* 2013;23(11):1842-1851.
18. Mokhlesi B, Hovda MD, Vekhter B, Arora VM, Chung F, Meltzer DO. Sleep-disordered breathing and postoperative outcomes after elective surgery: analysis of the nationwide inpatient sample. *Chest.* 2013;144(3): 903-914.
19. Chan MTV, Wang CY, Seet E, et al. Association of unrecognized obstructive sleep apnea with postoperative cardiovascular events in patients undergoing major noncardiac surgery. *JAMA.* 2019;321(18):1788-1798.
20. Flink BJ, Rivelli SK, Cox EA, et al. Obstructive sleep apnea and incidence of postoperative delirium after elective knee replacement in the nondemented elderly. *Anesthesiology.* 2012;116(4):788-796.
21. Isono S. Obstructive sleep apnea of obese adults: pathophysiology and perioperative airway management. *Anesthesiology.* 2009;110(4):908-921.
22. Solow B, Skov S, Ovesen J, Norup PW, Wildschiodtz G. Airway dimensions and head posture in obstructive sleep apnoea. *Eur J Orthod.* 1996; 18(6):571-579.
23. Horner RL. Pathophysiology of obstructive sleep apnea. *J Cardiopulm Rehabil Prev.* 2008;28(5):289-298.
24. Singh M, Tuteja A, Wong DT, et al. Point-of-care ultrasound for obstructive sleep apnea screening: are we there yet? A systematic review and meta-analysis. *Anesth Analg.* 2019;129(6):1673-1691.
25. Epstein LJ, Kristo D, Strollo PJ Jr., et al. Clinical guideline for the evaluation, management and long-term care of obstructive sleep apnea in adults. *J Clin Sleep Med.* 2009;5(3):263-276.
26. Berry RB, Budhiraja R, Gottlieb DJ, et al. Rules for scoring respiratory events in sleep: update of the 2007 AASM Manual for the Scoring of Sleep and Associated Events. Deliberations of the Sleep Apnea Definitions Task Force of the American Academy of Sleep Medicine. *J Clin Sleep Med.* 2012;8(5):597-619.
27. Kapur VK, Auckley DH, Chowdhuri S, et al. Clinical practice guideline for diagnostic testing for adult obstructive sleep apnea: An American Academy of Sleep Medicine Clinical Practice Guideline. *J Clin Sleep Med.* 2017;13(3):479-504.
28. Alchanatis M, Tourkohoriti G, Kakouros S, Kosmas E, Podaras S, Jordanoglou JB. Daytime pulmonary hypertension in patients with obstructive sleep apnea: the effect of continuous positive airway pressure on pulmonary hemodynamics. *Respiration.* 2001;68(6):566-572.
29. Bady E, Achkar A, Pascal S, Orvoen-Frija E, Laaban JP. Pulmonary arterial hypertension in patients with sleep apnoea syndrome. *Thorax.* 2000;55(11):934-939.
30. Sanner BM, Doberauer C, Konermann M, Sturm A, Zidek W. Pulmonary hypertension in patients with obstructive sleep apnea syndrome. *Arch Intern Med.* 1997;157(21):2483-2487.
31. Yamakawa H, Shiomi T, Sasanabe R, et al. Pulmonary hypertension in patients with severe obstructive sleep apnea. *Psychiatry Clin Neurosci.* 2002;56(3):311-312.
32. Chung F, Zhou L, Liao P. Parameters from preoperative overnight oximetry predict postoperative adverse events. *Minerva Anestesiol.* 2014; 80(10):1084-1095.
33. Seet E, Chung F. Management of sleep apnea in adults—functional algorithms for the perioperative period: continuing professional development. *Can J Anaesth.* 2010;57(9):849-864.
34. Atwood CW Jr., McCrory D, Garcia JG, Abman SH, Ahearn GS. Pulmonary artery hypertension and sleep-disordered breathing: ACCP evidence-based clinical practice guidelines. *Chest.* 2004;126(1 Suppl):72S-77S.
35. Chung F, Chau E, Yang Y, Liao P, Hall R, Mokhlesi B. Serum bicarbonate level improves specificity of STOP-Bang screening for obstructive sleep apnea. *Chest.* 2013;143(5):1284-1293.
36. Chung F, Yegneswaran B, Liao P, et al. Validation of the Berlin questionnaire and American Society of Anesthesiologists checklist as screening tools for obstructive sleep apnea in surgical patients. *Anesthesiology.* 2008;108(5):822-830.
37. Ramachandran SK, Kheterpal S, Consens F, et al. Derivation and validation of a simple perioperative sleep apnea prediction score. *Anesth Analg.* 2010;110(4):1007-1015.
38. Chung F, Yegneswaran B, Liao P, et al. STOP questionnaire: a tool to screen patients for obstructive sleep apnea. *Anesthesiology.* 2008;108(5):812-821.
39. Abrishami A, Khajehdehi A, Chung F. A systematic review of screening questionnaires for obstructive sleep apnea. *Can J Anaesth.* 2010;57(5):423-438.
40. Nagappa M, Liao P, Wong J, et al. Validation of the STOP-Bang Questionnaire as a screening tool for obstructive sleep apnea among different populations: a systematic review and meta-analysis. *PLoS One.* 2015;10(12):e0143697.
41. Chung F, Subramanyam R, Liao P, Sasaki E, Shapiro C, Sun Y. High STOP-Bang score indicates a high probability of obstructive sleep apnoea. *Br J Anaesth.* 2012;108(5):768-775.
42. Ramachandran SK, Josephs LA. A meta-analysis of clinical screening tests for obstructive sleep apnea. *Anesthesiology.* 2009;110(4):928-939.
43. Farney RJ, Walker BS, Farney RM, Snow GL, Walker JM. The STOP-Bang equivalent model and prediction of severity of obstructive sleep apnea: relation to polysomnographic measurements of the apnea/hypopnea index. *J Clin Sleep Med.* 2011;7(5):459-465B.
44. Chung F, Yang Y, Brown R, Liao P. Alternative scoring models of STOP-bang questionnaire improve specificity to detect undiagnosed obstructive sleep apnea. *J Clin Sleep Med.* 2014;10(9):951-958.
45. Chung F, Abdullah HR, Liao P. STOP-Bang questionnaire: a practical approach to screen for obstructive sleep apnea. *Chest.* 2016;149(3):631-638.
46. Chung F, Nagappa M, Singh M, Mokhlesi B. CPAP in the perioperative setting: evidence of support. *Chest.* 2016;149(2):586-597.
47. American Society of Anesthesiologists Task Force on Perioperative Management of patients with obstructive sleep apnea. Practice guidelines for the perioperative management of patients with obstructive sleep apnea: an updated report by the American Society of Anesthesiologists Task Force on Perioperative Management of patients with obstructive sleep apnea. *Anesthesiology.* 2014;120(2):268-286.

48. Memtsoudis SG, Stundner O, Rasul R, et al. Sleep apnea and total joint arthroplasty under various types of anesthesia: a population-based study of perioperative outcomes. *Reg Anesth Pain Med.* 2013;38(4):274-281.
49. Memtsoudis SG, Cozowicz C, Nagappa M, et al. Society of Anesthesia and Sleep Medicine Guideline on Intraoperative Management of Adult Patients With Obstructive Sleep Apnea. *Anesth Analg.* 2018;127(4):967-987.
50. Shin HJ, Kim EY, Hwang JW, Do SH, Na HS. Comparison of upper airway patency in patients with mild obstructive sleep apnea during dexmedetomidine or propofol sedation: a prospective, randomized, controlled trial. *BMC Anesthesiol.* 2018;18(1):120.
51. Murabito P, Serra A, Zappia M, et al. Comparison of genioglossus muscle activity and efficiency of dexmedetomidine or propofol during drug-induced sleep endoscopy in patients with obstructive sleep apnea/hypopnea syndrome. *Eur Rev Med Pharmacol Sci.* 2019;23(1):389-396.
52. Drummond GB. Comparison of sedation with midazolam and ketamine: effects on airway muscle activity. *Br J Anaesth.* 1996;76(5):663-667.
53. Seet E, Nagappa M, Wong DT. Airway management in surgical patients with obstructive sleep apnea. *Anesth Analg.* 2021;132(5):1321-1327.
54. Hiremath AS, Hillman DR, James AL, Noffsinger WJ, Platt PR, Singer SL. Relationship between difficult tracheal intubation and obstructive sleep apnoea. *Br J Anaesth.* 1998;80(5):606-611.
55. Chung F, Yegneswaran B, Herrera F, Shenderey A, Shapiro CM. Patients with difficult intubation may need referral to sleep clinics. *Anesth Analg.* 2008;107(3):915-920.
56. Kheterpal S, Han R, Tremper KK, et al. Incidence and predictors of difficult and impossible mask ventilation. *Anesthesiology.* 2006;105(5):885-891.
57. Kheterpal S, Healy D, Aziz MF, et al. Incidence, predictors, and outcome of difficult mask ventilation combined with difficult laryngoscopy: a report from the multicenter perioperative outcomes group. *Anesthesiology.* 2013; 119(6):1360-1369.
58. Kheterpal S, Martin L, Shanks AM, Tremper KK. Prediction and outcomes of impossible mask ventilation: a review of 50,000 anesthetics. *Anesthesiology.* 2009;110(4):891-897.
59. Shah PN, Sundaram V. Incidence and predictors of difficult mask ventilation and intubation. *J Anaesthesiol Clin Pharmacol.* 2012;28(4):451-455.
60. De Jong A, Molinari N, Pouzeratte Y, et al. Difficult intubation in obese patients: incidence, risk factors, and complications in the operating theatre and in intensive care units. *Br J Anaesth.* 2015;114(2):297-306.
61. Kim JA, Lee JJ. Preoperative predictors of difficult intubation in patients with obstructive sleep apnea syndrome. *Can J Anaesth.* 2006;53(4):393-397.
62. Riad W, Vaez MN, Raveendran R, et al. Neck circumference as a predictor of difficult intubation and difficult mask ventilation in morbidly obese patients: a prospective observational study. *Eur J Anaesthesiol.* 2016; 33(4):244-249.
63. Siyam MA, Benhamou D. Difficult endotracheal intubation in patients with sleep apnea syndrome. *Anesth Analg.* 2002;95(4):1098-1102.
64. Seet E, Chung F, Wang CY, et al. Association of obstructive sleep apnea with difficult intubation: prospective multicenter observational cohort study. *Anesth Analg.* 2021;133(1):196-204.
65. Katsiampoura AD, Killoran PV, Corso RM, Cai C, Hagberg CA, Cattano D. Laryngeal mask placement in a teaching institution: analysis of difficult placements. *F1000Res.* 2015;4:102.
66. Apfelbaum JL, Hagberg CA, Caplan RA, et al. Practice guidelines for management of the difficult airway: an updated report by the American Society of Anesthesiologists Task Force on Management of the Difficult Airsway. *Anesthesiology.* 2013;118(2):251-270.
67. Law JA, Broemling N, Cooper RM, et al. The difficult airway with recommendations for management—part 2—the anticipated difficult airway. *Can J Anaesth.* 2013;60(11):1119-1138.
68. Law JA, Broemling N, Cooper RM, et al. The difficult airway with recommendations for management—part 1—difficult tracheal intubation encountered in an unconscious/induced patient. *Can J Anaesth.* 2013; 60(11):1089-1118.
69. Frerk C, Mitchell VS, McNarry AF, et al. Difficult Airway Society 2015 guidelines for management of unanticipated difficult intubation in adults-dagger. *Br J Anaesth.* 2015;115(6):827-848.
70. Ahmad I, El-Boghdadly K, Bhagrath R, et al. Difficult Airway Society guidelines for awake tracheal intubation (ATI) in adults. *Anaesthesia.* 2020;75(4):509-528.
71. Herriger A, Frascarolo P, Spahn DR, Magnusson L. The effect of positive airway pressure during pre-oxygenation and induction of anaesthesia upon duration of non-hypoxic apnoea. *Anaesthesia.* 2004;59(3):243-247.
72. Delay JM, Sebbane M, Jung B, et al. The effectiveness of noninvasive positive pressure ventilation to enhance preoxygenation in morbidly obese patients: a randomized controlled study. *Anesth Analg.* 2008;107(5):1707-1713.
73. Dixon BJ, Dixon JB, Carden JR, et al. Preoxygenation is more effective in the 25 degrees head-up position than in the supine position in severely obese patients: a randomized controlled study. *Anesthesiology.* 2005;102(6):1110-1115; discussion 5A.
74. Lane S, Saunders D, Schofield A, Padmanabhan R, Hildreth A, Laws D. A prospective, randomised controlled trial comparing the efficacy of pre-oxygenation in the 20 degrees head-up vs supine position. *Anaesthesia.* 2005;60(11):1064-1067.
75. Ramkumar V, Umesh G, Philip FA. Preoxygenation with 20 masculine head-up tilt provides longer duration of non-hypoxic apnea than conventional preoxygenation in non-obese healthy adults. *J Anesth.* 2011;25(2):189-194.
76. Sabate JM, Jouet P, Merrouche M, et al. Gastroesophageal reflux in patients with morbid obesity: a role of obstructive sleep apnea syndrome? *Obes Surg.* 2008;18(11):1479-1484.
77. Ramachandran SK, Cosnowski A, Shanks A, Turner CR. Apneic oxygenation during prolonged laryngoscopy in obese patients: a randomized, controlled trial of nasal oxygen administration. *J Clin Anesth.* 2010; 22(3):164-168.
78. Taha SK, Siddik-Sayyid SM, El-Khatib MF, Dagher CM, Hakki MA, Baraka AS. Nasopharyngeal oxygen insufflation following pre-oxygenation using the four deep breath technique. *Anaesthesia.* 2006;61(5):427-430.
79. Weingart SD, Levitan RM. Preoxygenation and prevention of desaturation during emergency airway management. *Ann Emerg Med.* 2012;59(3):165-175 e1.
80. Miguel-Montanes R, Hajage D, Messika J, et al. Use of high-flow nasal cannula oxygen therapy to prevent desaturation during tracheal intubation of intensive care patients with mild-to-moderate hypoxemia. *Crit Care Med.* 2015;43(3):574-583.
81. Patel A, Nouraei SA. Transnasal Humidified Rapid-Insufflation Ventilatory Exchange (THRIVE): a physiological method of increasing apnoea time in patients with difficult airways. *Anaesthesia.* 2015;70(3):323-329.
82. Wong DT, Yee AJ, Leong SM, Chung F. The effectiveness of apneic oxygenation during tracheal intubation in various clinical settings: a narrative review. *Can J Anaesth.* 2017;64(4):416-427.
83. Oliveira JESL, Cabrera D, Barrionuevo P, et al. Effectiveness of apneic oxygenation during intubation: a systematic review and meta-analysis. *Ann Emerg Med.* 2017;70(4):483-494.e11.
84. Chung F, Liao P, Elsaid H, Shapiro CM, Kang W. Factors associated with postoperative exacerbation of sleep-disordered breathing. *Anesthesiology.* 2014;120(2):299-311.
85. Waldron NH, Jones CA, Gan TJ, Allen TK, Habib AS. Impact of perioperative dexamethasone on postoperative analgesia and side-effects: systematic review and meta-analysis. *Br J Anaesth.* 2013;110(2):191-200.
86. Abdelmageed WM, Elquesny KM, Shabana RI, Abushama HM, Nassar AM. Analgesic properties of a dexmedetomidine infusion after uvulopalatopharyngoplasty in patients with obstructive sleep apnea. *Saudi J Anaesth.* 2011;5(2):150-156.
87. Pawlik MT, Hansen E, Waldhauser D, Selig C, Kuehnel TS. Clonidine premedication in patients with sleep apnea syndrome: a randomized, double-blind, placebo-controlled study. *Anesth Analg.* 2005;101(5):1374-1380.
88. Popat M, Mitchell V, Dravid R, Patel A, Swampillai C, Higgs A. Difficult Airway Society Guidelines for the management of tracheal extubation. *Anaesthesia.* 2012;67(3):318-340.
89. Bamgbade OA. Advantages of doxapram for post-anaesthesia recovery and outcomes in bariatric surgery patients with obstructive sleep apnoea. *Eur J Anaesthesiol.* 2011;28(5):387-388.
90. Chung F, Liao P, Yegneswaran B, Shapiro CM, Kang W. Postoperative changes in sleep-disordered breathing and sleep architecture in patients with obstructive sleep apnea. *Anesthesiology.* 2014;120(2):287-298.
91. Gross JB, Bachenberg KL, Benumof JL, et al. Practice guidelines for the perioperative management of patients with obstructive sleep apnea: a report by the American Society of Anesthesiologists Task Force on Perioperative Management of patients with obstructive sleep apnea. *Anesthesiology.* 2006; 104(5):1081-1093; quiz 117-118.
92. Lee LA, Caplan RA, Stephens LS, et al. Postoperative opioid-induced respiratory depression: a closed claims analysis. *Anesthesiology.* 2015;122(3):659-665.
93. Lam T, Singh M, Yadollahi A, Chung F. Is perioperative fluid and salt balance a contributing factor in postoperative worsening of obstructive sleep apnea? *Anesth Analg.* 2016;122(5):1335-1339.
94. Liao P, Luo Q, Elsaid H, Kang W, Shapiro CM, Chung F. Perioperative auto-titrated continuous positive airway pressure treatment in surgical patients with obstructive sleep apnea: a randomized controlled trial. *Anesthesiology.* 2013;119(4):837-847.
95. Hillman DR, Chung F. Anaesthetic management of sleep-disordered breathing in adults. *Respirology.* 2017;22(2):230-239.
96. Joshi GP, Ankichetty SP, Gan TJ, Chung F. Society for Ambulatory Anesthesia consensus statement on preoperative selection of adult patients with obstructive sleep apnea scheduled for ambulatory surgery. *Anesth Analg.* 2012;115(5):1060-1068.

97. Wong P, Chieh Liew GH, Kothandan H. Anaesthesia for goitre surgery: a review. *Proc Singapore Healthc*. 2015;24(3):165-170.
98. Cook TM, Morgan PJ, Hersch PE. Equal and opposite expert opinion. Airway obstruction caused by a retrosternal thyroid mass: management and prospective international expert opinion. *Anaesthesia*. 2011; 66(9):828-836.
99. Nouraei SA, Giussani DA, Howard DJ, Sandhu GS, Ferguson C, Patel A. Physiological comparison of spontaneous and positive-pressure ventilation in laryngotracheal stenosis. *Br J Anaesth*. 2008;101(3):419-423.
100. Shen WT, Kebebew E, Duh QY, Clark OH. Predictors of airway complications after thyroidectomy for substernal goiter. *Arch Surg*. 2004; 139(6):656-659; discussion 9-60.
101. Agarwal A, Agarwal S, Tewari P, et al. Clinicopathological profile, airway management, and outcome in huge multinodular goiters: an institutional experience from an endemic goiter region. *World J Surg*. 2012;36(4):755-760.
102. Findlay JM, Sadler GP, Bridge H, Mihai R. Post-thyroidectomy tracheomalacia: minimal risk despite significant tracheal compression. *Br J Anaesth*. 2011;106(6):903-906.
103. Gilfillan N, Ball CM, Myles PS, Serpell J, Johnson WR, Paul E. A cohort and database study of airway management in patients undergoing thyroidectomy for retrosternal goitre. *Anaesth Intensive Care*. 2014;42(6):700-708.
104. Dempsey GA, Snell JA, Coathup R, Jones TM. Anaesthesia for massive retrosternal thyroidectomy in a tertiary referral centre. *Br J Anaesth*. 2013;111(4):594-599.
105. Malhotra S, Sodhi V. Anaesthesia for thyroid and parathyroid surgery. *Contin Educ Anaesth Crit Care Pain*. 2007;7:55-58.
106. Tan PC, Esa N. Anesthesia for massive retrosternal goiter with severe intrathoracic tracheal narrowing: the challenges imposed — a case report. *Korean J Anesthesiol*. 2012;62(5):474-478.
107. Wang G, Lin S, Yang L, Wang Z, Sun Z. Surgical management of tracheal compression caused by mediastinal goiter: is extracorporeal circulation requisite? *J Thorac Dis*. 2009;1(1):48-50.
108. Shah EF, Allen JG, Greatorex RA. Use of the laryngeal mask airway in thyroid and parathyroid surgery as an aid to the identification and preservation of the recurrent laryngeal nerves. *Ann R Coll Surg Engl*. 2001;83(5):315-318.
109. Pott L, Swick JT, Stack BC Jr. Assessment of recurrent laryngeal nerve during thyroid surgery with laryngeal mask airway. *Arch Otolaryngol Head Neck Surg*. 2007;133(3):266-269.
110. Tan LZ, An Tan DJ, Seet E. Laryngeal mask airway protector for intubation and extubation in thyroid surgeries: a case report. *Indian J Anaesth*. 2018;62(7):545-548.

CHAPTER 44

Airway Management in a Patient with a Difficult Airway Requiring Microlaryngoscopy, Tracheoscopy, and Pharyngoesophageal Dilation

Jeanette Scott and David Vokes

CASE PRESENTATION

A 17-year-old woman (AB) presents with a 4-year history of dysphagia and is unable to eat solids. She has poor voice with low pitch and stridor at rest and would like these symptoms improved as well.

AB has a complicated airway history. As a neonate, she had a congenital right-sided neck lymphatic malformation (LM) that was surgically excised and then treated with a sclerosing agent. At 1 month of age, a tracheotomy was performed because of airway obstruction secondary to supraglottic swelling. As a child, she had repeated laryngeal procedures with a CO_2 laser. She was decannulated at age 8 after an anterior tracheal augmentation with rib graft.

AB is otherwise well. She is well-nourished, despite her dysphagia, and is an active athlete despite her stridor.

Her anesthetic history postdecannulation includes an uneventful anesthetic using a laryngeal mask airway (LMA®) for nasal surgery performed last year when she was 16 years old.

Nasal endoscopy reveals a small larynx with a relatively large, omega-shaped epiglottis that is fixed in a retroflexed position. She has a supraglottic stenosis, posterior glottic stenosis secondary to interarytenoid scarring, impaired vocal cord motion, circumferential subglottic stenosis, tracheal stenosis, and a pharyngoesophageal stricture (Figure 44.1).

A computerized tomography (CT) scan confirms supraglottic narrowing at the level of the hyoid bone (0.5 cm × 1 cm) (Figure 44.2), a transverse diameter across her vocal cords of 1 cm, infraglottic narrowing measuring 1.5 cm, the transverse diameter of her proximal trachea is 0.8 cm, while her lower trachea and rest of the airways are widely patent and normal.

AB will need multiple laryngeal procedures under general anesthesia to improve her swallowing, voice, and airway. However, her first priority is to be able to eat better, and she presents for microlaryngoscopy, tracheoscopy, and pharyngoesophageal balloon dilation.

PREOPERATIVE ASSESSMENT

What Is a Congenital Lymphatic Malformation?

Congenital LMs are endothelial-lined, lymph-filled cysts caused by an abnormal development of the lymphatic system. Approximately 50% of LMs are in the head and neck area. While fetal LMs detected by ultrasound before 23 weeks of

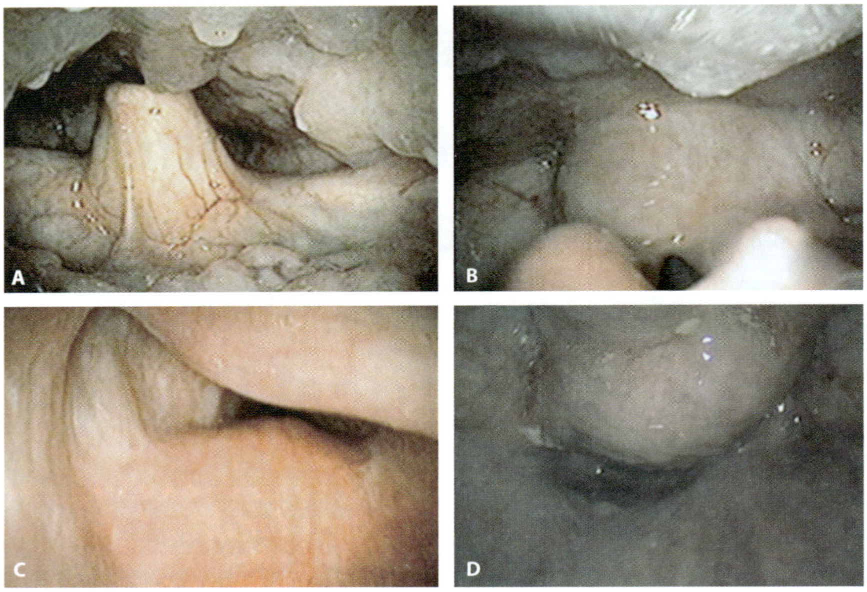

FIGURE 44.1. Flexible laryngoscopic examination findings: **(A)** the valleculae and retroflexed epiglottis; **(B)** the omega-shaped epiglottis; **(B)** and **(C)** the narrow and distorted supraglottic airway; and **(D)** the hypopharynx and postcricoid region of the larynx (larynx is in the upper half of the clinical photograph).

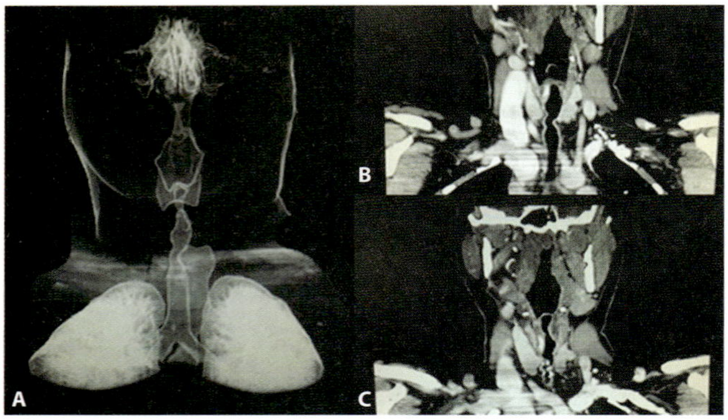

FIGURE 44.2. Preoperative CT Scan of the stenotic airway: **(A)** 3D reconstruction of airway; **(B)** and **(C)** coronal CT images demonstrating numerous sites of airway stenosis.

gestation are associated with karyotypic or genetic abnormalities, LMs appearing after 30 weeks of gestation, as seen in AB's case, tend to be isolated lesions.

Spontaneous regression of these lesions is rare. Without treatment, breathing, swallowing, speech, and cosmesis may be affected. Surgical excision is the mainstay of treatment, although in some cases, anatomical location or local infiltration may make surgical excision difficult and complete excision impossible. Incompletely excised lesions may recur. The injection of sclerosants, laser ablation, or photocoagulation therapies have all been described, with varying degrees of success.

Is This Patient Fit for Anesthesia?

Apart from AB's airway pathology, she is a fit and well 17-year-old. The challenge will be managing her airway safely while providing an unobstructed surgical field.

Define a Difficult Airway

A difficult airway exists when an experienced airway practitioner anticipates or encounters difficulty with any or all of: laryngoscopy or tracheal intubation, face-mask ventilation (FMV), extraglottic airway use, or emergency front-of-neck access (FONA).[1]

Does AB Have a Risk of Difficult Face-Mask Ventilation?

AB has normal facial, dental, nasopharyngeal, and oropharyngeal anatomical structures, the ability to protrude the mandible, and a normal range of neck motion. FMV should not be impeded superior to the level of the larynx.

Her stridor has been slow-onset, over years, and is due to known sites of narrowing of relatively rigid scarred structures. Nasal endoscopy shows that her supraglottic and subglottic stenosis do not narrow further with pressure changes that occur during the respiratory cycle. AB does not have a history of difficulty breathing during sleep.

If her airway is not instrumented, it is likely that AB will be easy to ventilate using a face mask. However, if instrumented, laryngeal edema could cause complete airway obstruction preventing successful FMV.

Does AB Have a Risk of Difficult Extraglottic Device Use?

Despite AB's grossly abnormal larynx, anesthesia with an extraglottic device (EGD) was performed without difficulty just a few months earlier (a reinforced #4 LMA was used) for nasal surgery. For the proposed surgery, a laryngeal mask would completely obstruct the surgical field; however, it could be used as a rescue device if required.

What About the Risk of Difficult Intubation?

AB's larynx would likely not be difficult to visualize under direct (e.g., Macintosh laryngoscope) or indirect laryngoscopy (e.g., video laryngoscope), although the retroflexed infantile epiglottis may obstruct the glottic view.

Owing to the glottic and subglottic stenosis, AB's airway would be a challenge to intubate, if required. The best choice of endotracheal tube (ETT) would probably be a 4.0-mm internal diameter (ID) microlaryngeal tube (MLT, e.g., Mallinckrodt™, Medtronic, Minneapolis, MN or Sheridan LTS Microlaryngeal ETT, Teleflex, Morrisville, NC). Microlaryngeal ETTs differ from their pediatric counterparts of the same ID by possessing a length long enough to be passed through a surgical laryngoscope and an adult-sized cuff (see Figure 44.3). In AB's case, an adult-sized cuff would be necessary to seal her adult-sized trachea distal to her subglottic narrowing. The *external* diameter of a 4.0-mm tube is approximately 5.5 mm depending on the manufacturer and may be a concern. AB's airway is 5.0 mm at its narrowest point. Therefore, endotracheal intubation with the smallest MLT available may cause traumatic injury and swelling with the risk of postextubation airway obstruction.

Does AB Have a Risk of Difficult Front-of-Neck Access?

AB is not keen on any form of FONA due to the psychological experience of having had a tracheostomy as a child. The surgeons are also reluctant, owing to the presence of tracheal stenosis, scar tissue, and previous rib graft. For these reasons, a tracheotomy would be technically challenging, may have consequences for future surgical options, and it would be difficult to decannulate AB, potentially leaving her with a long-term tracheotomy.

What Anesthetic Technique Is Required?

In general, airway management is safest when the patient is awake and able to maintain airway patency, perform gas exchange, and protect themselves from aspiration. Balloon dilation of AB's pharyngoesophageal stricture was first attempted in clinic under local anesthesia but was not well tolerated due to pain. She requests further procedures to be performed under general anesthesia.

Total intravenous anesthesia (TIVA) is preferred by most anesthesia practitioners and surgeons for shared airway procedures. TIVA ensures constant anesthetic administration and avoids the risk of inadvertent inhalation of anesthetic gas by the surgical team when the airway is manipulated. TIVA also permits the use of tubeless oxygenation and ventilation methods, such as apneic oxygenation or narrow-bore ventilating techniques, which best enable exposure of the laryngotracheal surgical field.

In our practice, we administer TIVA using a combination of remifentanil and propofol infusions.

Remifentanil is an ideal drug for TIVA. As a rapid onset/offset opioid, it is both readily titratable and able to provide smooth intraoperative hemodynamic conditions. By blunting the patient's drive to breathe and their response to surgical stimulation, remifentanil may eliminate the need for muscle relaxants. Unlike other opioids, remifentanil maintains a constant context-sensitive half-life and does not accumulate, enabling rapid recovery of respiratory drive and consciousness after prolonged administration. Usual infusion rates are 0.1 to 0.3 $\mu g \cdot kg^{-1} \cdot min^{-1}$.

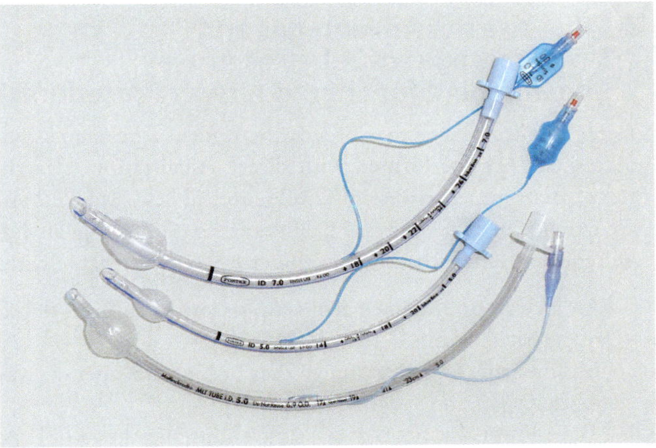

FIGURE 44.3. A size 5.0 microlaryngeal tube (bottom) is longer and has an adult-sized cuff, when compared to the standard size 5.0 mm ID (middle) and standard size 7.0 mm ID (top) endotracheal tube.

AIRWAY MANAGEMENT

Which Airway Management Techniques Best Enable Surgical Access to the Airway?

The mainstay methods of airway management (FMV, EGD use, and endotracheal intubation) would impede the surgeon's access to the surgical field. In AB's case, these airway management modalities are not useful during the surgical procedure, but may be useful for bridging oxygenation or rescue airway techniques.

Possible choices of methods for oxygenation and ventilation during suspension laryngoscopy include:

A. Techniques involving a cuffed tube in the trachea:
   - MLT.
   - Tracheostomy tube.

B. Tubeless techniques:
   - Spontaneous ventilation under generation anesthesia.
   - Intermittent apnea.
   - Transnasal Humidified Rapid-Insufflation Ventilatory Exchange (THRIVE).[2]
   - Extracorporeal membrane oxygenation (ECMO).
   - Narrow-bore oxygenation catheters located above the glottis (supraglottic), through the glottis (subglottic), or through the front-of-neck directly into the trachea (transtracheal); these small-bore catheters are categorized as either <2 mm or <4 mm[3,4] in diameter. Oxygen sources attached to narrow-bore catheters can be attached to either pressure-regulated or flow-regulated oxygenation sources.

CUFFED, WIDE-BORE ENDOTRACHEAL TUBES FOR SHARED AIRWAY SURGERY

What Are the Benefits of Cuffed, Wide-Bore Endotracheal Tubes During Airway Surgery?

Cuffed wide-bore ETTs, including MLTs and standard tracheostomy tubes, connect to conventional anesthesia circuits and ventilators. This enables administration of anesthetic gases and standard positive pressure ventilation techniques. Oxygenation and carbon dioxide clearance will occur via the usual bulk-flow (conventional tidal volume) method of gas exchange with which all anesthesia practitioners are familiar. A cuffed ETT also protects the airway from soiling with surgical debris or gastric contents and protects the surgeon from exhaled gases and blood or debris being blown into the surgical field.

What Are the Characteristics of Microlaryngeal Tubes?

MLTs are oral ETTs of narrow ID designed to allow increased view of the surgical field during laryngeal surgery.

MLTs are available in three sizes, with internal diameters of 4.0, 5.0, or 6.0 mm. Unlike pediatric tubes of the same internal diameter, MLTs have an adult-sized cuff, ensuring that the adult trachea can be sealed to facilitate positive pressure ventilation. MLTs are also longer than their pediatric counterparts, which enables insertion into the airway via a surgeon's suspension laryngoscope if required (see Figures 44.3 and 44.4).

Despite their narrow profile, MLTs will still obscure the posterior glottis and the interarytenoid region. Depending on the pathology, the surgeon may have to lift the MLT anteriorly to improve visualization of the posterior larynx. The subglottis and tracheal airway are also obscured by microlaryngoscopy tubes, making them unsuitable for laryngotracheal work. The laryngeal apertures will also move with ventilation.

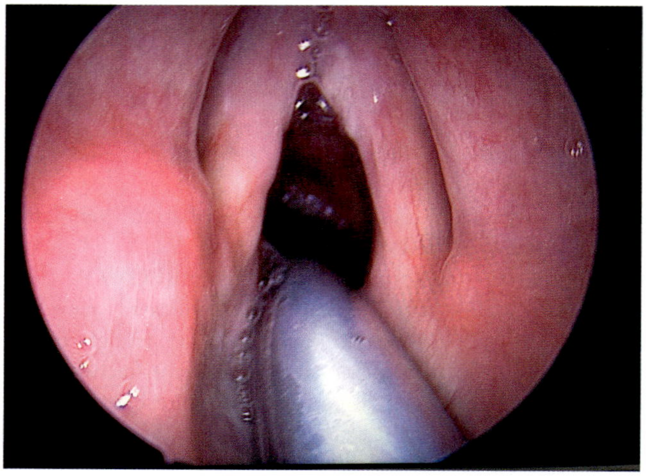

FIGURE 44.4. Despite its narrow profile, a 5.0-mm ID microlaryngeal tube can still obscure the posterior third of the glottis.

Could a Microlaryngeal Tube Be Used in AB's Case?

Physical obstruction by the MLT does not allow assessment of the subglottis and tracheal airway, making them unsuitable for laryngotracheal work and therefore of limited utility in this clinical scenario.

In AB's case, a 4.0-mm ID MLT should be reserved as a possible rescue device.

If endotracheal intubation of AB is required, even with a size 4.0-mm ID MLT, formation of a tracheotomy distal to the subglottic stenosis may be necessary to best ensure airway patency postextubation. This potential outcome should be made explicit both in the patient's written consent and in the discussion of the airway plan prior to initiation of the procedure.

What Are the Advantages of Elective Tracheostomy for Shared Airway Procedures?

Depending on the pathology, a wide-bore tracheostomy tube may be able to provide a cuffed ETT distal to the surgical field. Although clearly an invasive airway technique, for some patients with complicated airways, a tracheotomy is the safest way to manage shared airway procedures, especially in cases at risk of upper airway obstruction under anesthesia. Some patients with complicated upper airways will have tracheotomies for months or years while their upper airway is being managed and improved.

Could an Elective Tracheotomy Be Performed in AB's Case?

As discussed above, neither AB nor the surgical team are keen on any form of FONA. In AB's case, a tracheotomy is best reserved as an alternative, through possible emergency airway rescue option.

TUBELESS AIRWAY MANAGEMENT FOR SHARED AIRWAY SURGERY

What Are the Advantages and Disadvantages of Tubeless Airway Management for Shared Airway Procedures?

From a surgical perspective, procedures under suspension laryngoscopy are best performed with direct visualization (straight line) of an unimpeded and immobile surgical field. Tubeless airway management techniques facilitate these surgical goals but will require the anesthesia practitioner to be comfortable with:

- An airway unprotected from aspiration of surgical debris or gastric contents
- Mechanisms of gas exchange that occur with open-airway oxygenation and ventilation techniques
- The administration of total intravenous anesthesia (TIVA)

Tubeless techniques include:

- Spontaneous ventilation under generation anesthesia
- Intermittent apnea

- THRIVE [2]
- ECMO
- Narrow-bore oxygenation catheters (in supraglottic, subglottic, or FONA locations) with either pressure-regulated or flow-regulated oxygenation devices

TUBELESS AIRWAY MANAGEMENT TECHNIQUES THAT DO NOT REQUIRE NARROW-BORE AIRWAY CANNULAE

What Are the Advantages and Disadvantages of Spontaneous Ventilation Under General Anesthesia During Suspension Laryngoscopy?

Spontaneous ventilation under general anesthesia for suspension laryngoscopy is a technique more commonly used in children than adults. Successful execution of this technique requires a plane of general anesthesia deep enough to blunt laryngeal reflexes and patient movement to stimuli but also maintain regular respiration.

Anesthetic gas (and oxygen) can be delivered via the sideport of a suspension laryngoscope or via a nasopharyngeal or oropharyngeal catheter. Given that the airway is open, gas scavenging is difficult to achieve, and exhaled anesthetic gases will spill toward the surgeon and contaminate the operating room.

TIVA may be a better choice than inhalational anesthesia during suspension laryngoscopy; however, balancing the reliable maintenance of spontaneous respirations with an adequate anesthetic depth requires experience with this technique.

The rapid and shallow pattern of spontaneous ventilation achieved under general anesthesia with propofol may exaggerate dynamic motion of the vocal cords and laryngeal structures, making precision surgery difficult to execute.

Could AB Be Managed with Spontaneous Ventilation?

The exaggerated movement of the laryngeal structures seen during spontaneous ventilation makes this technique undesirable for AB's case. Furthermore, dilation of the pharyngoesophageal segment could lead to reflux of material from the esophagus into the pharynx, which could lead to aspiration.

What Is the "Intermittent Apnea Technique" for Shared Airway Surgery?

The intermittent apnea technique involves the induction of anesthesia, administration of neuromuscular blockers, commencement of TIVA, and application of suspension laryngoscopy followed by intubation of the trachea with a small diameter ETT. This ETT is used to oxygenate and hyperventilate the patient before being removed for short periods of time during which the surgical procedure is performed. The duration of tolerated apnea will be determined by oxygen desaturation and hypercarbia.

Provided the airway is held open (i.e., by the surgical laryngoscope), a patient's apneic window before oxygen desaturation can be considerably extended by continuous flow of oxygen into the nasopharyngeal or oropharynx, for example, with nasal cannula or a shortened ETT placed in the hypopharynx. This is called "apneic oxygenation." Suggested flow rates of 5 to 15 L·min^{-1} have been described.[3] The physiological explanation for this is that oxygen is removed from the alveoli into the bloodstream at a faster rate than carbon dioxide travels in the opposite direction. Consequently, a negative pressure gradient from the lips to the lungs is established, which can be up to 20 cm H_2O pressure. This gradient will continue to draw pharyngeal gas towards the alveoli continuously and oxygenate the patient, provided that there is no airway obstruction.[5]

Could AB Be Managed with Intermittent Apnea Technique?

As discussed earlier, while endotracheal intubation of AB's airway may be possible with a small diameter ETT, doing so risks causing traumatic swelling that could cause postextubation subglottic obstruction. Repeated intubation would be especially undesirable and therefore the intermittent apnea technique is unsuitable in AB's case.

What Is Optiflow™/THRIVE?

Warmed, humidified high-flow nasal oxygen has been used for several years in critical care environments for spontaneously breathing patients with respiratory failure. These devices reduce heat and moisture loss from the airway, are well tolerated, and enable higher flow oxygen (up to 60 L·min^{-1}).[6] If the mouth is closed, a small amount of positive end-expiratory pressure (PEEP) can be achieved, which can stent open upper airways, help reduce atelectasis, and improve gas exchange.

In 2015, Patel and Nouraei first described using Optiflow (Fisher and Paykel Healthcare Ltd, Panmure, Auckland, New Zealand) high-flow nasal oxygen therapy intraoperatively to extend safe apnea time in difficult airway patients having suspension laryngoscopy with complete muscle relaxation.[2] They called this technique Transnasal Humidified Rapid-Insufflation Ventilatory Exchange or "THRIVE."

THRIVE involves warmed, humidified oxygen flowing at rates of 70 to 90 L·min^{-1} via wide-bore nasal cannula during shared airway surgery in an anesthetized, paralyzed patient. This technique has rapidly gained popularity worldwide as it provides an immobile and tubeless surgical field, a prolonged safe apneic time before desaturation (in excess of that achieved with "classical" apneic oxygenation), and some degree of ventilation, as measured by slower than expected rise of carbon dioxide over time.

Fluid modeling at the Fisher and Paykel laboratories has suggested a mechanism for the increased carbon dioxide clearance witnessed during THRIVE. When Optiflow runs at very high flow rates (70 L·min^{-1}), turbulent flow occurs in the pharynx. Cardiac pulsations cause boluses of tracheal gas to be delivered through the cords that are then whisked away by turbulent flow in the pharynx.[7]

Could Optiflow/THRIVE Be Used for AB's Case?

THRIVE would no doubt work temporarily for AB—her normal BMI, young age, and absence of lung pathology are all favorable predictors for sustained oxygenation with THRIVE.

However, when the physiological limitations of THRIVE are reached or airway patency is lost, desaturation can occur rapidly. For all THRIVE cases, reliable backup airway management plans must be ready to be deployed at short notice.

A case series of 105 upper airway endoscopies with THRIVE reported that 95% of the patients could be successfully oxygenated (SpO_2 >92%) for 20 minutes. However, 9.5% of patients desaturated below 92% during at some point during their surgical procedure—around half of these were resolved after simple manipulations to improve airway patency, but the rest required a change in airway management plan to improve oxygenation (e.g., FMV, intubation or insertion of a Hunsaker Mon-Jet tube).[8]

AB's airway is narrowed in multiple locations, including areas with poor line-of-sight. Her procedure has potential for intermittent or sustained airway obstruction caused by surgical manipulation/instrumentation, bleeding, or edema. When using THRIVE, the first sign of clinically relevant airway obstruction is oxygen desaturation. (Patients are apneic during THRIVE so end-tidal capnography cannot be used to give early warning of loss of airway patency.) In addition, THRIVE does not provide enough positive pressure to re-recruit lung units once atelectasis has occurred.

Rescue plans for treating oxygen desaturation while using THRIVE could include oxygenation and lung recruitment via positive pressure with FMV, extraglottic airway device placement, intubation and ventilation with a microlaryngoscopy tube, or emergency FONA. However, in AB's case, there are limitations with each of these, as has been discussed above.

Jet ventilation is often used as a rescue technique for THRIVE cases; however, as will be discussed in a section below, these techniques would be challenging to deploy in AB's case under time pressure, as her anatomy means that there is no direct line-of-sight to the larynx; there are stenoses of the supraglottic, glottic, subglottic, and tracheal portions of the airway; and FONA is challenging owing to the previous tracheal reconstruction.

What Is ECMO?

ECMO is a modified heart-lung machine that can be used for respiratory support in cases of reversible respiratory failure (e.g., acute respiratory distress syndrome) or, more rarely, for cardiac support for severe cardiac failure (see Chapter 15).

ECMO for respiratory indications is usually venovenous (VV)-ECMO, where two large (e.g., 23 Fr) cannulas are placed in large systemic veins. Blood is pumped from one cannula and passed through an oxygenator before being returned to the patient via the other cannula. VV-ECMO can also be achieved using a single dual-lumen catheter. Inserted into the right internal jugular vein, the Avalon© catheter (Marquet Medical Systems, Wayne, NJ) provides for bicaval venous drainage while reinfusing oxygenated blood through the tricuspid valve directly into the heart.

ECMO use requires a medical center with ECMO infrastructure such as surgery, cardiac anesthesia, blood bank, perfusion, and intensive care. Although possible as part of an airway plan, ECMO requires extensive preoperative planning.[9] Case reports[10–13] and small case series[14–17] describe ECMO being used to oxygenate and ventilate patients during surgery for severe airway pathology.

VV-ECMO does not require full heparinization, unlike venoarterial (VA)-ECMO. Life-threatening mechanical complications can still occur, such as air embolism or massive blood loss. Oxygenator or pump failure can be catastrophic. Sepsis and infection are more common in ECMO patients than other ICU patients.[14]

Could ECMO Be Used in AB's Case?

While ECMO should be considered for completeness, most centers currently do not have the multidisciplinary infrastructure to support this modality. However, as this treatment modality becomes more common, it may well be that VV-ECMO may become a more generalizable option for severe airway pathology. In AB's case, the risk of ECMO does not seem to outweigh the benefits when other airway management options are available.

NARROW-BORE AIRWAY CANNULAE AND ASSOCIATED VENTILATION DEVICES

How Is Oxygenation and Ventilation Achieved via a Narrow-Bore Catheter?

Narrow-bore oxygenation catheters can be placed in supraglottic, subglottic, or transtracheal locations[18] (Figure 44.5).

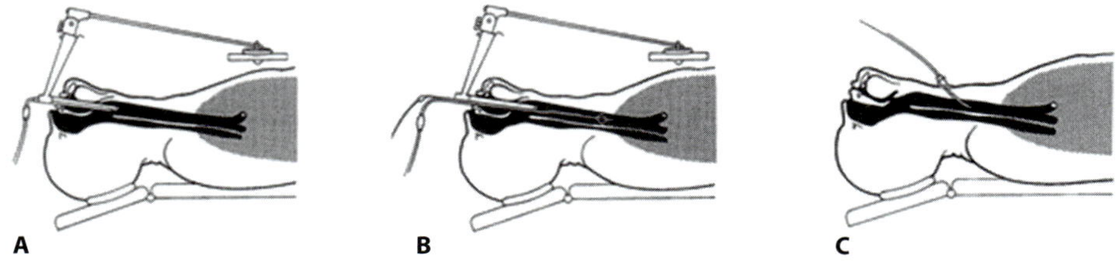

FIGURE 44.5. Oxygenation using narrow-bore catheters during surgical procedures: **(A)** a short supraglottic narrow-bore cannula can be attached to the surgical laryngoscope; **(B)** a Hunsaker Mon-Jet tube is inserted through the surgical laryngoscope and into the trachea as an example of transglottic narrow-bore cannula; **(C)** a kink-resistant transtracheal narrow-bore oxygenation catheter (e.g., Ravussin cannula [VBM]). (Reproduced with permission from Biro P. Jet ventilation for surgical interventions in the upper airway. *Anesthesiol Clin.* 2010;28(3):397-409)

TABLE 44.1. Summary of the Risk of Complications When Using Supraglottic, Translaryngeal, or Transtracheal Narrow-Bore Oxygenation Catheters with Various Oxygenation and Ventilation Devices

		Risk of Complications		
Method of Oxygenation and Ventilation	**Example Device**	**Supraglottic Location**	**Translaryngeal Location (Hunsaker Mon-Jet Tube)**	**Transtracheal Location (Cricothyroid or Transtracheal Catheter)**
Pressure-controlled (jet) low-frequency manual ventilation devices	Manujet III	++	++	+++
Pressure-controlled (jet) high-frequency automated ventilation devices (HPPV)	Monsoon III	+	+	++
Flow-controlled low-frequency manual ventilation devices	Enk oxygen flow modulator	Not described	Not described	? For emergency use during CICO only (rare event, data lacking)
	Ventrain device	Not described	Not described	? Promising concept but data currently lacking

Note: Grades of relative risk: + = small, ++ = moderate, +++ = high, and ? = unknown.

These catheters require high-pressure oxygenation delivery systems to overcome the increased resistance produced by a narrow internal diameter. Careful consideration should also be given to the route of exhalation of gas, as exhalation will not occur through the narrow-bore cannula for most devices. Therefore, with most devices, an open upper airway is required for passive exhalation. Table 44.1 summarizes the risk of complications associated with the use of these catheters.

Jet ventilation can be defined as "the pulsed delivery of volumes of gas from a high-pressure source across small-bore catheters."[19] Jet ventilation devices are pressure-regulated oxygenation devices. They attach directly to hospital wall-pressure oxygen using the disc-index safety system. Broadly speaking, there are low-frequency manual jet ventilators and high-frequency automated jet ventilators.

There are also devices that are driven by regulation of oxygen flow. The Ventrain™ ejector ventilator (Ventinova Medical, Eindhoven, Netherlands) is a flow-driven device that attaches to wall-mounted oxygen flowmeters or the flow regulator on an oxygen cylinder.

The Evone™ (Ventinova Medical, Eindhoven, Netherlands) is a mechanical ventilator that provides both flow-driven ventilation and high-frequency jet ventilation modes.

Although a number of published "home-made" suggestions describe how to attach flow-oxygen to narrow-bore catheters or cannulas, devices without supporting evidence will not be discussed.[20]

What Are the Pressure-Controlled (Jet) Low-Frequency Manual Ventilation Devices and the Problems Associated with Their Uses?

In 1967, Saunders[21] described a high-pressure ventilation device that when attached to a catheter in the proximal end of a surgical laryngoscope enabled oxygenation without obscuring the

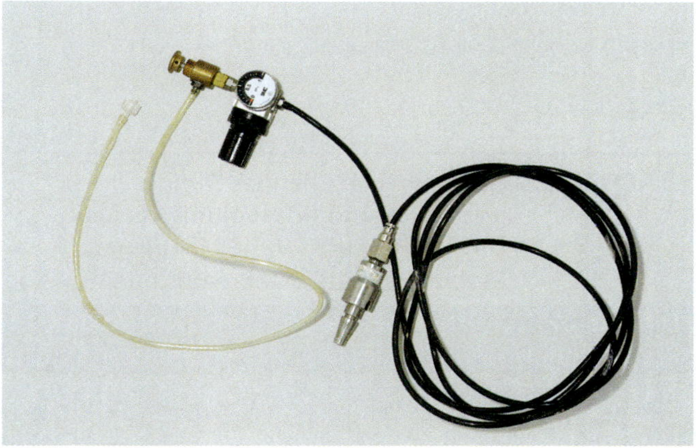

FIGURE 44.6. Sanders jet ventilator.

surgical field. By way of an on/off switch and pressure regulator, Saunders' injector delivered pipeline pressure oxygen (50 psi or 4 atm·bar^{-1}) via a 0.035-in diameter nozzle inside the lumen of the surgical laryngoscope (Figure 44.6). The 100% oxygen high-pressure jet travels down the long axis of the laryngoscope and entrains air to augment the tidal volume and dilute the FiO_2 to 30% to 40%. Vigilant observation of chest wall movement was necessary to judge the duration of manually controlled inspiration and release for passive exhalation.[22]

A more modern hand-controlled high-pressure jet ventilator is the Manujet III (VBM Medizintechnik GmbH, Sulz, Germany) (Figure 44.7). Unlike the Saunders injector, the Manujet's lockable pressure regulator can be adjusted to set the driving pressure between 7 and 50 psi (0.5 and 3.5 bar).

When using low-frequency manual jet ventilators, gas exchange occurs in a similar manner as the more familiar forms of intermittent positive pressure ventilation. It is dependent on tidal volume, respiratory rate, PEEP, and FiO_2.

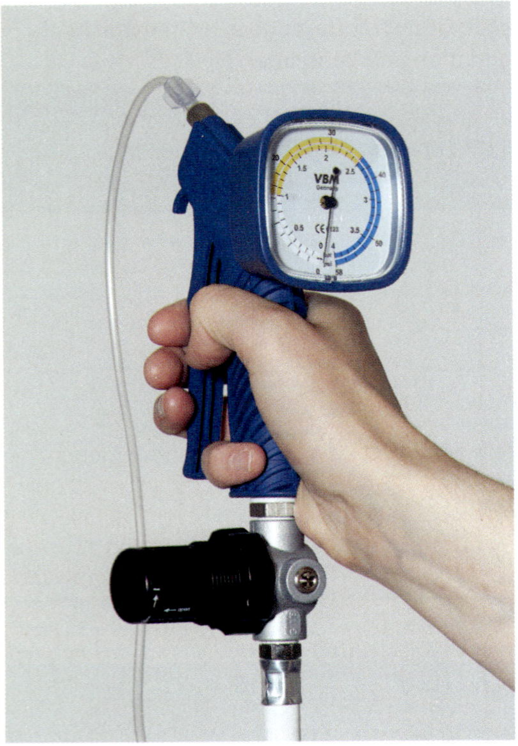

FIGURE 44.7. The Manujet III jet ventilator.

TABLE 44.2. Gas Flow Rate Changes During Inspiration and Tidal Volume Versus Driving Pressure for the Manujet at a Respiratory Rate of 4 Breaths min^{-1}

Driving Pressure (Bar)	Gas Flow (L·min^{-1})	Tidal Volume (mL)
0.5	12.6 ± 1.6	246.0 ± 15.9
1.0	17.4 ± 2.5	304.0 ± 34.9
1.5	23.7 ± 2.9	356.0 ± 25.2
2.0	28.2 ± 4.2	485.3 ± 18.0
2.5	33.9 ± 3.5	626.3 ± 5.5
3.0	37.1 ± 5.8	653.3 ± 50.3

Inspiration time 1 second, oxygen flow 15 L·min^{-1}, tracheal catheter 15 G (2-mm diameter) and 7 cm long, ringed trachea model 15 cm long and 1000 mL "lung" with airways resistance at 5 mbar·L^{-1}·sec^{-1} and lung compliance 30 mbar·mL^{-1}.

Reproduced with permission from Lenfant F, Péan D, Brisard L, et al. Oxygen delivery during transtracheal oxygenation: A comparison of two manual devices. *Anesth Analg*. 2010;111(4):922-924.

The airway is open and not sealed. This, among other factors, leads to a variable tidal volume. Gas flow through the catheter depends upon driving pressure and catheter resistance. The tidal volumes produced by the narrow-bore catheter are therefore determined by these two variables and the practitioner's manual control of inspiratory time[23,24] (see Table 44.2). However, the tidal volume *delivered to the airways* may be more or less than the tidal volume produced by the catheter. Gas delivery is affected by respiratory impedance, entrainment, and spillage from the airway.[19]

- Respiratory impedance is the mechanical restraint of the respiratory system to ventilation changes throughout the respiratory cycle. Its determinants include the elastic properties of the lung tissues and chest wall, and frictional and inertial resistance to gas flow through the airways.
- The high-pressure jet entrains surrounding gas (Venturi effect), resulting in augmentation of the jetted volume and dilution of the fraction of oxygen delivered.
- Gas spillage out of the airway can be considerable. With supraglottic jet ventilation, an unmeasurable amount of gas spills out of the mouth and nares into the atmosphere. With subglottic or transtracheal jet ventilation (TTJV) gas flow is bidirectional with some jetted gas exiting the airway (depending on the degree of upper airway obstruction) instead of moving down the trachea towards areas capable of participating in gas exchange.

In conclusion, the exact tidal volume and FiO_2 delivered to the airways during low-frequency manual jet ventilation is difficult to estimate.[23] The clinical effectiveness and safety of this technique therefore rely on vigilant inspection of chest wall motion and oxygen saturations. Minute ventilation can be monitored by arterial blood gases or transcutaneous carbon dioxide electrodes.

The use of manual jet ventilation has been associated with significant morbidity and mortality. If inhalation is overvigorous and/or appropriate exhalation time is not permitted, or the route of exhalation is temporarily partially or fully occluded, breath-stacking and accumulation of excessive intrathoracic pressures can quickly occur with deleterious respiratory and circulatory consequences. Long expiratory times mitigate the likelihood of barotrauma but decrease minute ventilation and carbon dioxide clearance.

In 2008, a survey identified 65 complications in 36 patients over 5 years that occurred during elective manual jet ventilator use for laryngeal surgery in the United Kingdom. These complications included pneumothorax (15 patients), surgical emphysema (17 patients), pneumomediastinum (5 patients), difficulty ventilating (11 patients), and hypoxia (14 patients), which led to delays in discharge (7 patients), admissions to critical care areas (3 patients), and three deaths.[3]

What Are the Pressure-Controlled (Jet) High-Frequency Automated Ventilation Devices?

High-frequency positive pressure ventilation (HFPPV) for bronchoscopy and laryngeal surgery was first described in the 1970s.[25] It is characterized by automated, high-frequency breaths (60-200 bpm) with tidal volumes that are smaller than anatomical dead space. With lower maximal and mean airway pressures, HFPPV minimizes movement of the laryngotracheal surgical field and minimizes the circulatory effects related to the respiratory cycle.

Like manual jet ventilation, HFPPV can be administered through narrow-bore devices in supraglottic, subglottic, and transtracheal locations.

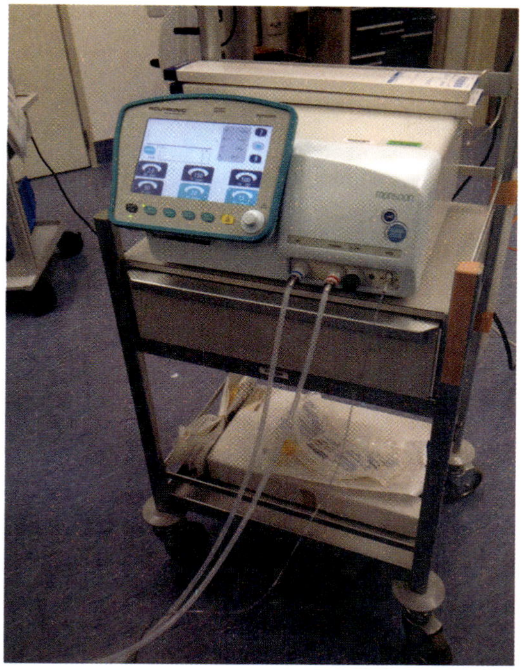

FIGURE 44.8. The Monsoon III (Acutronic) high-frequency jet ventilator.

Unlike manual jet ventilation devices, modern HFPPV machines have a number of safety advantages over the low-frequency manually controlled jet ventilators. These include the ability to accurately set FiO_2, respiratory rate, inspiratory time, driving pressures, and humidification (see Figure 44.8).

If the narrow-bore cannula is placed below the level of the cords, HFPPV machines can also monitor peak and pause airway pressures. If these exceed a preset level, an alarm is triggered and the ventilator automatically shuts off minimizing the risk of barotrauma, a feature that makes them generally safer than manual jet ventilator devices. Normal tidal volume breaths given at set intervals (e.g., every 5 minutes) permit the intermittent determination of end-tidal CO_2.

As HFPPV machines are automated, they free the anesthesia practitioner from controlling each breath enabling their attention to be focused on other anesthesia management tasks.

How Does Gas Exchange Take Place During HFPPV When Tidal Volumes Are Smaller than Anatomical Dead Space?

With such small tidal volumes, the commonly understood bulk-flow method of gas exchange cannot occur to a significant degree during HFPPV. Several alternative methods of gas exchange have been proposed,[26,27] which include:

1. *Direct ventilation of proximal alveoli.* Small tidal volumes may be sufficient to ventilate the alveoli closest to the jet origin via a bulk-flow method of gas exchange.
2. *Convective streaming and augmented molecular diffusion.* Peripheral lung compliance augments the streaming motion achieved during HFPPV to be much greater than what can be achieved by the jet alone. The tracheal jet increases airways pressure, which causes distal airways and alveoli to expand and gas to flow distally. The rapid on-off motion of the jet and variations in airway diameter and compliance cause oscillating asymmetric gas flow, augmenting molecular diffusion between the trachea and alveoli.[27]
3. *Laminar flow with lateral transport by diffusion (Taylor dispersion).* In regions of laminar flow, the parabolic-shaped advancing gas front has the greatest velocity at its center, reducing to zero flow closest to the tracheal walls. Molecules traveling in the higher-velocity areas move laterally to mix with the lower-velocity gas.[28]
4. *Coaxial and bidirectional flow.* In areas of laminar or asymmetric gas flow, bidirectional flow can occur when positive peripheral airway pressure drives expiratory gas to reverse flow direction in lower velocity areas. For example, expiratory gas may travel out of the lung along the tracheal wall while inspiratory gas continues to flow centrally in the other direction.
5. *Pendelluft ("swinging air") ventilation.* Inertance can be defined as the pressure required to overcome the inertia of the respiratory system and cause it to accelerate. At normal respiratory rates, inertance contributes very little to respiratory impedance. However, when respiratory rates exceed those of normal breathing, accelerations become large, and therefore the pressures required to accelerate the tissues and gases of the respiratory system become important. A simple explanation of how high-frequency ventilation causes Pendelluft is that regional differences in inertance, for example, caused by airway diameter, cause lung regions to inflate and deflate out of phase with each other, which results in gas subsequently being passed back and forth between the lung units.[29] More complicated lung modeling that may more accurately explain frequency-related inertance and Pendelluft is beyond the scope of this chapter.
6. *Cardiogenic mixing.* Cardiac pulsations cause airway gas mixing by agitating the surrounding thoracic tissues and enhancing molecular diffusion. This is particularly true in children.
7. *Collateral ventilation* through nonairway connections between neighboring alveoli.

What Are the Flow-Controlled Low-Frequency Manual Ventilation Devices?

Flow-controlled devices enable delivered oxygen volume to be estimated from the set flow-rate and manual control of inspiratory time.[30] For example, if the oxygen-flow meter is set at 15 $L \cdot min^{-1}$, then every second of forward flow from the device will administer 250 mL of oxygen. Dietmar Enk, the designer of the Enk and Ventrain Oxygen Flow Modulators, hoped that this simple concept could reduce the risk of barotrauma when CICO is managed with a transtracheal narrow-bore catheter, especially in cases where the upper airway is completely obstructed (https://soundcloud.com/yaleuniversity/narrow-bore-catheter-ventilation-with-dietmar-enk-md-phd).

What Is the Ventrain?

The Ventrain is a flow-modulated oxygenation device for transtracheal use that is noteworthy because it is the first commercially

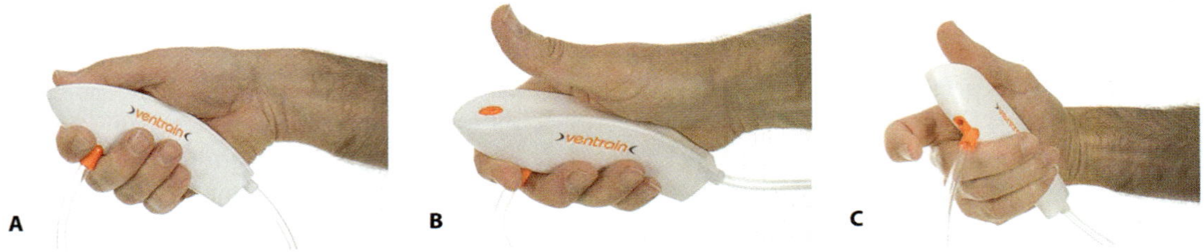

FIGURE 44.9. The Ventrain device: **(A)** occlusion of holes using the thumb and index finger for direct manual control of inhalation; **(B)** Venturi-assisted expiration; and **(C)** the device is open to atmosphere.

available device that actively enables inspiratory and expiratory gas flow through a narrow-bore catheter (see Figure 44.9).

It is a single-use handheld device that attaches to wall or tank oxygen via a standard pressure-compensated flow regulator. With oxygen flow set at 2 to 5 $L \cdot min^{-1}$, the practitioner manually switches between inspiratory and expiratory phases by alternately occluding either one or two purpose-built holes in the handheld device with the index finger and thumb.

If the thumb and index finger are not occluding either device hole, the Ventrain is in equilibrium with the atmosphere, and no oxygen is flowing into the lungs and very little gas is sucked out (Figure 44.9C). If the user's index finger occludes one hole but the user's thumb is free, oxygen flowing into the handheld device is directed away from the airway through an exhaust port (Figure 44.9B). By directing this oxygen flow through a narrowed nozzle, oxygen velocity is increased and, as per the Bernoulli principle, pressure falls. The subatmospheric pressures generated inside the device entrain gas from the attached transtracheal catheter, thereby assisting expiration. When the user's thumb also occludes the other device hole, the exhaust port is closed and oxygen flow is instead directed down the transtracheal catheter (Figure 44.9A).

This method of "expiratory ventilation assistance" (EVA) has two proposed benefits. First, it improves minute ventilation by actively removing end-tidal gas. Second, according to the manufacturer, it "reduces the chance of intrapulmonary pressure build-up and the associated risks of barotrauma and circulatory collapse" (http://www.p3-medical.com/pdf/Ventrain(c)(c)%20 brochure.pdf). Bench and animal studies seem to support both suggested benefits.

A bench study suggests that the Ventrain device is able to achieve minute ventilation of 7.1 $L \cdot min^{-1}$ through a 2-mm ID transtracheal catheter.[31]

Paxian et al. compared transtracheal ventilation with the Ventrain device to the Manujet III in anesthetized pigs with simulated open, partially obstructed, and fully obstructed upper airways.[32] The pigs were hyperoxic in all situations with both devices; however, $PaCO_2$ and airway pressures were consistently lower with the Ventrain device than the Manujet III. Hemodynamic parameters, as measured by mean arterial pressure and central venous pressure, were unremarkable with both devices when the airway was open but were more favorable with Ventrain use compared to the Manujet III when the airway was partially, and especially fully, obstructed.

Berry et al. compared the Ventrain to the Manujet in anesthetized sheep with partially or fully obstructed airways.[33] Like Paxian et al., they discovered that oxygenation was readily achievable with both devices, but the Ventrain produced lower airway pressure and could achieve near-normal minute ventilation.

Despite having been primarily designed for use during CICO emergencies, the Ventrain has been used in a small number of elective situations including oxygenation and ventilation via a cricothyroid needle for a woman with a polyp obstructing the upper airway (https://soundcloud.com/yaleuniversity/narrow-bore-catheter-ventilation-with-dietmar-enk-md-phd, YouTube video). Fearnley et al. describe elective use of the Ventrain attached to a cricothyroid needle in a patient with distorted and partially occluded upper airway anatomy from postradiation scar tissue.[34] Morrison et al. described using the Ventrain attached to a transoral airway exchange catheter for 40 minutes in an anesthetized, paralyzed patient with airway obstruction from advanced vocal cord carcinoma.[35]

While the Ventrain has been used in cases of greater than one-hour duration, clinical utility is probably best with shorter cases. Enk, the device inventor, states, "You need a flexible index finger and a strong thumb to do it for a while" (https://soundcloud.com/yaleuniversity/narrow-bore-catheter-ventilation-with-dietmar-enk-md-phd).

The Ventrain has the potential to revolutionize the role of narrow-bore ventilation but requires good technical understanding and clinical judgment for its proper use.[36] Like all other narrow-bore ventilation devices, overvigorous use of the inspiratory phase will still cause accumulation of intrathoracic volume and therefore pressure. It should not be forgotten that the Ventrain has no pressure release valve and is connected to wall oxygen via a conventional flowmeter.

The Ventrain also poses a new hazard—overvigorous use of the expiratory phase, which could cause very *negative* intrathoracic pressures with respiratory and cardiovascular consequences. Berry et al. reported that when using the Ventrain in a sheep model, he inadvertently achieved subatmospheric pressures of –200 cm H_2O when attempting a 1:1 inspiratory to expiratory ratio, leading him to promote methodical opening of the device to atmospheric pressures during every respiratory cycle (see Figure 44.9C).[33] Enk states that when using the Ventrain, IPPV only occurs "as long as you do not evacuate more gas than has been inflated in advance" (https://soundcloud.com/yaleuniversity/narrow-bore-catheter-ventilation-with-dietmar-enk-md-phd). Without any mechanism for measuring airway pressures, clinical safety is again reliant on vigilant observation of chest rise and fall.

What Is the Evone Mechanical Ventilator?

The Evone is a mechanical ventilator offering a controlled expiration phase (called "flow-controlled ventilation," FCV®) (https://www.ventinovamedical.com/products/). Like the Ventrain, the Evone's FCV mode uses the Bernoulli principle to generate negative pressure within the device, which then actively draws gas out of the patient during the expiration phase.

FCV is a paradigm shift in ventilatory strategy, the strengths and limitations of which are still being studied in a clinical context. With FCV, the practitioner programs FiO_2, inspiration:expiration (I:E) ratio, inspiratory flow rate (e.g., 12 $L{\cdot}min^{-1}$), and peak and minimum airway pressures. After end inspiration, the device maintains a steady expiratory flow rate until the end of the expiration.

FCV certainly has some theoretical advantages, including minimizing mechanical stress on ventilated lungs.[37] Early evidence from animal and human studies suggest that arterial oxygenation and regional lung ventilation may be improved and atelectasis reduced with FCV compared to volume-control ventilation, though comparisons between these ventilation strategies and their effects on arterial blood gases, or respiratory and hemodynamic variables require further study.[38–40]

The Evone ventilator can attach to conventional ETTs, or to narrow proprietary transtracheal (Cricath™) or subglottic (Tritube™) cannulas. It is also capable of a high-frequency ventilation mode, making it an interesting new prospect for the field of laryngeal surgery (https://www.ventinovamedical.com/wp-content/uploads/2021/04/MC031.00-Ventrain-Borchure-EN.pdf).

Describe Supraglottic Jet Ventilation via the Surgical Laryngoscope

As first described by Saunders in 1967, a narrow-bore ventilating cannula can be attached to the lumen of a surgical laryngoscope[21] (see Figure 44.5A). This can then be attached to either a low- or high-frequency jet ventilator. To maximize effective ventilation, minimize spillage out of the mouth, and preventing gastric insufflation, the jet stream should be pointing directly at an unobstructed airway. Given the relatively large distance from the jet to the trachea, some jet spillage will occur and can be accounted for by increasing inspiratory jet pressure. Exhalation can only occur in the pauses between inspiratory phases as the inspiratory jet obstructs exhalation.

The main advantage of this technique is a surgical field free from instrumentation. Secondarily, the jet is also proximal to any airway obstruction—should partial or temporary airway obstruction occur, inspiration is blocked that prevents breath-stacking and barotrauma.

One disadvantage of this technique is that surgical debris, blood, or fumes can be blown into the airway. In addition, supraglottic jet ventilation moves the vocal cords with ventilation.

The high velocity of jetted oxygen will entrain surrounding air into the jet, lowering the received FiO_2. One way to increase the FiO_2 of jetted gas during shared airway surgery is to combine it with THRIVE so the jet will entrain from the enriched oxygen reservoir created by Optiflow high-flow nasal therapy.[41]

Could Supraglottic Jet Ventilation Be Used in AB's case?

This technique is not reliable in AB's case. Her unusual anatomy means that a clear line-of-sight to the larynx is unlikely to be achieved with a surgical laryngoscope. Without line-of-sight, supraglottic jet ventilation cannot be employed because it is associated with a high risk of gastric distension, and inefficient or ineffective ventilation.

Subglottic Jet Ventilation via a Subglottic Catheter (e.g., Hunsaker Mon-Jet tube)

In 1979, Benjamin and Gronow created a 35-cm long, 1-mm ID cuffless catheter designed to be inserted through the vocal cords and used for subglottic jet ventilation.[42] Unlike earlier narrow tubes used for this purpose, the Benjamin Jet Tube had four "petals" at its tip, designed to ensure that the jet is not directed against tracheal mucosa and to minimize the whip-like movement of subglottic catheters that had been observed previously (see Figure 44.5B.)

Characteristics of subglottic ventilation include the blowing of surgical debris, blood, and fumes out of the airway, but toward the surgeon. Because the jet is centered in the airway, exhalation can occur throughout the respiratory cycle.

In 1994, Hunsaker introduced a modified Benjamin Jet Tube.[43] This 35.5-cm long narrow-bore oxygenation catheter has a jet-centering rubber basket surrounding the distal tip. In addition to the 2.7-mm oxygenating lumen, there is a 1-mm port proximal to the basket for monitoring airway pressures and intermittent sampling of end-tidal carbon dioxide. Made of fluoroplastic, the Hunsaker Mon-Jet tube (Figure 44.10) is less flammable than silastic, rubber, or PVC tubes, and is safe to use with a laser.

Hunsaker recommended using his tube with an automated ventilator capable of automated shut-off in the event that monitored intratracheal pressures become raised.[43] Despite this, Orloff et al. reported an 84-patient case series using Hunsaker Mon-Jet tubes with a manual jet ventilation technique without barotrauma.[44] However, in a recent study with 839 cases over 15 years in an academic institution combining the Hunsaker Mon-Jet tube with HFJV, Hu described a complication rate of

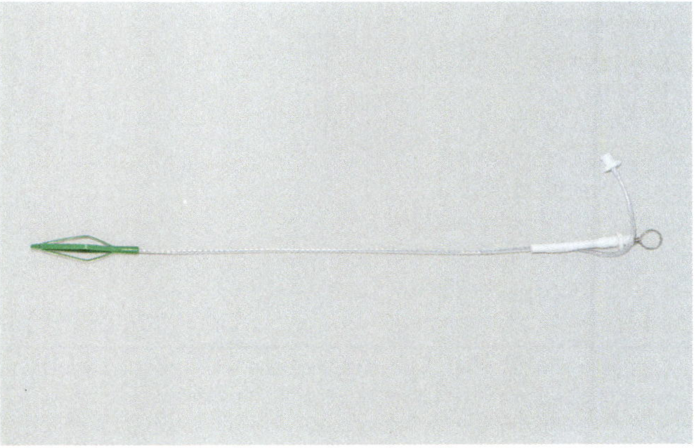

FIGURE 44.10. The Hunsaker Mon-Jet tube.

5.8%. Complications included hypoxemia (3.6%), hypercarbia (2.0%), airway obstruction (0.5%), and barotrauma (0.2%).[45]

Could a Hunsaker Mon-Jet Tube Be Used for AB's Case?

Unlike an MLT, the Hunsaker Mon-Jet tube is likely to be able to be pushed atraumatically past AB's subglottic stenosis.

However, Hunsaker himself cautioned against the use of his tube in cases of *supra*glottic airway obstruction, stating that such cases should be managed with "a large tube with inflatable cuff."[43] The concern is that should the airway become obstructed, jetted gas will have no path of escape.

Successful use of the Hunsaker Mon-Jet tube in AB's case is best performed with a high-frequency jet ventilator capable of measuring intrathoracic pressures with an automatic shut-off should a preset number be exceeded.

What Is the Tritube?

The Tritube is a narrow-lumen, cuffed ETT made by Ventinova Medical B.V. (Eindhoven, Netherlands). With an internal diameter of less than 3 mm and an external diameter of 4.4 mm, it affords less concealment of the laryngeal structures than other models of cuffed ETTs.[46] Benefits of cuffed ETTs include reduced risk of aspiration, improved control of oxygenation and ventilation, and isolation of the patient's respiratory aerosols or secretions from the surgical team.

When the cuff is inflated, the narrow diameter and long length of Tritube provide too much resistance for spontaneous respiration or passive exhalation. The Tritube is not compatible with standard anesthetic ventilators and is only able to be used with either the Ventrain or the Evone ventilator, which both mechanically assist expiration.

Published clinical experience with the Tritube and Evone for laryngeal surgery include case studies,[37,47] a case series,[46,48–50] and a randomized controlled trial that found laryngeal exposure to be more favorable with the Tritube than a size 6.0 microlaryngoscopy tube.[46]

With the cuff deflated, the Tritube can also be used as a subglottic apneic oxygen catheter, or, by applying the jetting mode on the Evone ventilator, a subglottic jet ventilation catheter. By virtue of its narrow diameter, the Tritube with deflated cuff has been reported to be well tolerated when left in-situ during emergence and early recovery from anesthesia.[48]

Describe Jet Ventilation via a Transtracheal Catheter (a Catheter Through the Cricothyroid Membrane or Between Tracheal Rings)

For decades, the use of narrow-bore catheter placed through the cricothyroid membrane and attached to a manually controlled pressure-driven oxygenation device has been advocated for many types of difficult airways, particularly in elective otorhinolaryngological procedures[51] (see Figure 44.5C). Jaquet et al. reported a retrospective case series in which 305 transtracheal cannulas were placed with a 7.5% complication rate (see Table 44.3).[52]

Although advocated for decades as "safe, effective, and simple,"[53] TTJV has been shown in elective otorhinolaryngological surgery to have its share of complications.[3] Settings where complications occur tend to be when manual (vs. high-frequency) ventilation and high-driving pressures are used and end-expiratory pressures are not monitored. Equipment that is not meant for such a purpose (e.g., using intravenous catheters) and lack of endoscopic confirmation of catheter insertion site prior to TTJV have also been associated with complications. As with any high-risk procedure, centers that do not practice this technique regularly, and inexperienced practitioners tend to have higher complication rates.[3]

TABLE 44.3. Incidence of Ventilation-Related Complications During Shared Airway Surgery Depending on the Ventilatory Technique

Event	TTJV	TGJV	AIV	MCV
Minor complications				
Failure[a, b]	3	4	0	0
Mucosal damage[a]	1	0	0	0
Laryngospasm[a]	1	0	5	0
Hemodynamic instability	6	2	0	0
Hypoxemia	2	1	0	0
Myocardial ischemia	1	0	0	0
Cervical emphysema[a]	3	0	0	0
Major complications				
Cervicomediastinal emphysema[a]	1	0	0	0
Pneumothorax[a]	1	1	0	0
Tension pneumothorax[a]	1	0	0	0
Total	20/265 (7.5%)	8/469 (1.7%)	5/359 (1.4%)	0/200 (0%)

AIV, apneic intermittent ventilation; MCV, mechanical controlled ventilation; TGJV, transglottal jet ventilation; TTJV, transtracheal jet ventilation.
[a]Complications directly related to the ventilation procedure.
[b]Failure of insertion of the cannula and failure of ventilation through the cannula.
Reproduced with permission from Jaquet Y, Monnier P, Van Melle G, et al. Complications of different ventilation strategies in endoscopic laryngeal surgery: a 10-year review. *Anesthesiology*. 2006;104(1):52-59.

A recent systematic review showed TTJV in the CICO situation to be associated with a 42% incidence of device failure, 32% incidence of barotrauma, and a total complication rate of 51%.[54] Device failure was associated with the use of manual (vs. automated high-frequency) jetting, intravenous catheters (vs. purpose-made catheters), and "homemade" coupling devices such as three-way stopcocks. The CICO nature of these cases was usually associated with a degree of upper airway obstruction.

If TTJV is performed in AB's case, it is essential that AB maintains a patent upper airway, equipment be purpose-made and not improvised, the location of the catheter confirmed, high-frequency jet ventilation used, and end-expiratory pressure monitored. Centers that do not have these capabilities and do not perform TTJV on a regular basis should use a different technique.

PATIENT MANAGEMENT

How Is the Airway Management Technique Chosen?

After discussion with the surgeon and AB, a Hunsaker Mon-Jet tube with HFPPV was selected to be used during the shared airway procedure. Airway rescue methods (in order of preference) include FMV, #4 laryngeal mask airway (LMA) placement, intubation with a size 4.0-mm ID MLT or, if all of those plans fail, an emergency surgical airway. If AB's airway deteriorates intraoperatively, a tracheotomy may be required.

How Was AB's Airway Managed for Her Surgical Procedure?

The surgical and anesthetic plan was discussed with the patient and consent obtained.

Before the patient arrived in the operating room, a team brief involving surgical, anesthetic, nursing, and technician staff was completed during which the airway management strategy was discussed, and the equipment checked.

On arrival in the operating room, pulse oximetry, noninvasive blood pressure, electrocardiography, and bispectral index EEG monitoring were applied.

Denitrogenation was performed to an end-tidal oxygen concentration of 0.9. General anesthesia was induced and maintained using propofol and remifentanil infusions and muscle paralysis with rocuronium. Dexamethasone was administered to reduce airway swelling.

FMV was easy. Using a Macintosh 3 blade, the glottis was poorly visualized due to supraglottic stenosis and epiglottis retroflexion. Lidocaine (3 mL of 2%) is applied topically to the laryngeal structures.

Control of the airway was handed to the surgeons who employ a suspension laryngoscope to insert the Hunsaker Mon-Jet tube.

A Monsoon© high-frequency jet ventilator was connected to the ventilator port of the Hunsaker Mon-Jet tube (see Figure 44.11). The humidified jet had a driving pressure set at 1.5 bar (750 mmHg or 21.8 psi), a frequency of 150 bpm, and an inspiratory ratio of 0.4. The sampling port on the Hunsaker Mon-Jet tube was connected to the Monsoon for intrathoracic pressure monitoring. Alarms were set at 15 mbar (15.3 CWP) for peak inspiratory pressures and 20 mbar (20.4 CWP) for pause pressures, thereby reducing the risk of breath-stacking and barotrauma by allowing early warning and automated HFPPV shut-off. Automated end-tidal gas sampling was performed by the HFPPV every 5 minutes to test for hypercarbia.

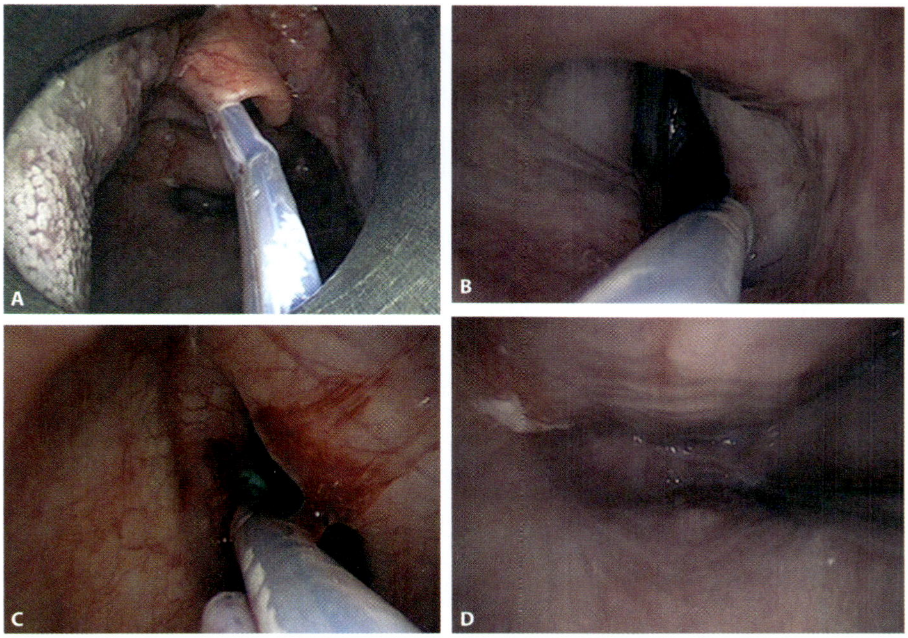

FIGURE 44.11. Endoscopic view of the larynx during the surgical procedure: **(A)** view through the surgical laryngoscope of the supraglottic larynx with the Hunsaker Mon-jet tube in AB's airway; **(B)** the Hunsaker Mon-jet tube passing through the glottis; **(C)** the Hunsaker Mon-jet basket sitting in midtrachea, just distal to AB's tracheal stenosis; and **(D)** AB's pharyngoesophageal segment prior to dilation.

After microlaryngoscopy and tracheoscopy, a Negus anterior commissure laryngoscope was used for pharyngoscopy and pharyngeal dilation was performed.

At the end of the procedure, the surgical equipment was removed and the #4 LMA inserted. TIVA was stopped and the neuromuscular blockade reversed. Spontaneous ventilation resumed, and the patient was placed in the semi-sitting position. AB woke uneventfully and was taken to Post Anesthesia Care Unit for routine postoperative care.

SUMMARY

A symptomatic patient with multiple stenotic lesions of the airway presenting for an endoscopic procedure of the upper airway poses a significant challenge. The mainstay methods of airway management (FMV, EGD use, and tracheal intubation) would be unsuitable as they obstruct the surgical field. While microlaryngeal or tracheostomy tubes may be suitable for some cases, many patients are well managed with "tubeless" airway techniques—these require the anesthesia practitioner to be comfortable with open-airway oxygenation and ventilation techniques and the administration of TIVA. Such techniques could include spontaneous ventilation under anesthesia, intermittent apnea technique, Transnasal Humidified Rapid-Insufflation Ventilatory Exchange (THRIVE), and narrow-bore catheters (in supraglottic, subglottic, or transtracheal locations) using pressure-regulated or flow-regulated oxygenation devices, or ECMO. The anesthesia practitioner and surgeon should together decide upon airway management after careful appraisal of risk versus benefit, the patient's cooperation, available resources, and the expertise of the anesthesia and surgical teams. In addition, before the patient is brought into the operating room, a team brief involving surgical, anesthetic, nursing, and anesthesia assistant staff must be undertaken to discuss the airway management strategy (Plan A, B, and C), and the procedural and rescue airway equipment must be checked.

SELF-EVALUATION QUESTIONS

44.1. Comparing a standard endotracheal tube with a microlaryngeal tube (MLT), which of the following is FALSE?

A. MLT possesses a smaller cuff than a standard adult endotracheal tube.

B. MLT is longer than the standard same-sized endotracheal tube.

C. MLTs are only available in 4.0, 5.0, and 6.0 sizes.

D. MLTs obscure the posterior glottis during suspension laryngoscopy.

44.2. Which of the following is FALSE regarding the Hunsaker Mon-Jet tube?

A. It is capable of monitoring airway pressures.

B. It has a sealed cuff.

C. It is less flammable than standard PVC endotracheal tubes.

D. It is intended for use with jet ventilation.

44.3. Which of the following is TRUE regarding the transtracheal jet ventilation (TTJV)?

A. Manual is safer than high-frequency jet ventilation.

B. It is associated with a high-incidence of complications in elective cases.

C. End-expiratory pressure monitoring is the standard of care.

D. Ventrain is an example of a high-pressure jet ventilation device.

REFERENCES

1. Law JA, Duggan LV, Asselin M, et al. Canadian Airway Focus Group updated consensus-based recommendations for management of the difficult airway: part 1. Difficult airway management encountered in an unconscious patient. *Can J Anesth.* 2021;68:1373-1404.
2. Patel A, Nouraei SR. Transnasal Humidified Rapid-Insufflation Ventilatory Exchange (THRIVE): a physiological method of increasing apnoea time in patients with difficult airways. *Anaesthesia.* 2015;70:323-329.
3. Cook T, Alexander R. Major complications during anaesthesia for elective laryngeal surgery in the UK: a national survey of the use of high-pressure source ventilation. *British J Anaesth.* 2008;101:266-272.
4. Frerk C, Mitchell VS, McNarry AF, et al. Difficult Airway Society 2015 guidelines for management of unanticipated difficult intubation in adults. *Brit J Anaesth.* 2015;115:827-848.
5. Weingart SD, Levitan RM. Preoxygenation and prevention of desaturation during emergency airway management. *Ann Emerg Med.* 2012;59:165-175. e1.
6. Ashraf-Kashani N, Kumar R. High-flow nasal oxygen therapy. *BJA Ed.* 2017;17:63-67.
7. Hermez L, Spence C, Payton M, Nouraei S, Patel A, Barnes T. A physiological study to determine the mechanism of carbon dioxide clearance during apnoea when using transnasal humidified rapid insufflation ventilatory exchange (THRIVE). *Anaesthesia.* 2019;74:441-449.
8. Waters E, Kellner M, Milligan P, Adamson RM, Nixon IJ, McNarry AF. The use of Transnasal Humidified Rapid-Insufflation Ventilatory Exchange (THRIVE) in one hundred and five upper airway endoscopies. A case series. *Clin Otolaryngol.* 2019;44:1115-1119.
9. Sheridan RL, Ryan DP, Fuzaylov G, Nimkin K, Martyn JJ. Case 5-2008: an 18-month-old girl with an advanced neck contracture after a burn. *N Engl J Med.* 2008;358:729-735.
10. Willms DC, Mendez R, Norman V, Chammas JH. Emergency bedside extracorporeal membrane oxygenation for rescue of acute tracheal obstruction. *Respir Care.* 2012;57:646-649.
11. Holliday T, Jackson A. Emergency use of extracorporeal membrane oxygenation for a foreign body obstructing the airway. *Crit Care Resusc.* 2010;12:273-275.
12. Malpas G, Hung O, Gilchrist A, et al. The use of extracorporeal membrane oxygenation in the anticipated difficult airway: a case report and systematic review. *Can J Anesth.* 2018;65:685-697.
13. Keeyapaj W, Alfirevic A. Carinal resection using an airway exchange catheter-assisted venovenous ECMO technique. *Can J Anesth.* 2012;59:1075-1076.
14. Sidebotham D. *Cardiothoracic Critical Care.* Elsevier Health Sciences; 2007.
15. Kim CW, Kim DH, Son BS, Cho JS, Kim YD, Ahn HY. The feasibility of extracorporeal membrane oxygenation in the variant airway problems. *Ann Thorac Cardiovasc Surg.* 2015;21:517-522.
16. Stokes JW, Katsis JM, Gannon WD, et al. Venovenous extracorporeal membrane oxygenation during high-risk airway interventions. *Interactive CardioVasc Thorac Surg.* 2021;33:913-920.
17. Huang S-C, Wu E-T, Chi N-H, et al. Perioperative extracorporeal membrane oxygenation support for critical pediatric airway surgery. *Eur J Pediatr.* 2007;166:1129-1133.
18. Biro P. Jet ventilation for surgical interventions in the upper airway. *Anesthesiol Clin.* 2010;28:397-409.
19. Wiedemann K, Männle C. Anesthesia and gas exchange in tracheal surgery. *Thorac Surg Clin.* 2014;24:13-25.
20. Pandit J, Popat M, Cook T, et al. The Difficult Airway Society 'ADEPT'guidance on selecting airway devices: the basis of a strategy for equipment evaluation. *Anaesthesia.* 2011;66:726-737.

21. Saunders R. Two ventilating attachment for bronchoscopes. *Del Med J.* 1967;39:170-192.
22. Evans E, Biro P, Bedforth N. Jet ventilation. *Continuing Education in Anaesth Crit Care Pain.* 2007;7:2-5.
23. Lenfant F, Péan D, Brisard L, Freysz M, Lejus C. Oxygen delivery during transtracheal oxygenation: a comparison of two manual devices. *Anesth Analg.* 2010;111:922-924.
24. Flint N, Russell W, Thompson J. Comparison of different methods of ventilation via cannula cricothyroidotomy in a trachea–lung model. *Brit J Anaesth.* 2009;103:891-895.
25. Borg U, Eriksson I, Sjöstrand U. High-frequency positive-pressure ventilation (HFPPV): a review based upon its use during bronchoscopy and for laryngoscopy and microlaryngeal surgery under general anesthesia. *Anesth Analg.* 1980;59:594-603.
26. Duval E, Markhorst D, Gemke R, Van Vught A. High-frequency oscillatory ventilation in pediatric patients. *Netherlands J Med.* 2000;56:177-185.
27. Scherer PW, Muller WJ, Raub JB, Haselton FR. Convective mixing mechanisms in high frequency intermittent jet ventilation. *Acta Anaesthesiol Scand.* 1989;33:58-64.
28. Conlon CE. High frequency jet ventilation anaesthesia tutorial of the week 271. ATOTW Weekly. 2012.
29. Greenblatt EE, Butler JP, Venegas JG, Winkler T. Pendelluft in the bronchial tree. *J Appl Physiol.* 2014;117:979-988.
30. Hamaekers A, Borg P, Enk D. Ventrain: an ejector ventilator for emergency use. *Brit J Anaesth.* 2012;108:1017-1021.
31. Hamaekers AE, van der Beek T, Theunissen M, Enk D. Rescue ventilation through a small-bore transtracheal cannula in severe hypoxic pigs using expiratory ventilation assistance. *Anesth Analg.* 2015;120:890.
32. Paxian M, Preussler N, Reinz T, Schlueter A, Gottschall R. Transtracheal ventilation with a novel ejector-based device (Ventrain) in open, partly obstructed, or totally closed upper airways in pigs. *Brit J Anaesth.* 2015;115:308-316.
33. Berry M, Tzeng Y, Marsland C. Percutaneous transtracheal ventilation in an obstructed airway model in post-apnoeic sheep. *Brit J Anaesth.* 2014;113:1039-1045.
34. Fearnley RA, Badiger S, Oakley RJ, Ahmad I. Elective use of the Ventrain for upper airway obstruction during high-frequency jet ventilation. *J Clin Anesth.* 2016;33:233-235.
35. Morrison S, Aerts S, Van Rompaey D, Vanderveken O. Failed awake intubation for critical airway obstruction rescued with the Ventrain device and an Arndt exchange catheter: a case report. *A&A Practice.* 2019;13: 23-26.
36. Noppens R. *Ventilation Through a 'Straw': The Final Answer in a Totally Closed Upper Airway?* Oxford University Press; 2015:168-170.
37. Barnes T, Enk D. Ventilation for low dissipated energy achieved using flow control during both inspiration and expiration. *Trends Anaesth Crit Care.* 2019;24:5-12.
38. Sebrechts T, Morrison SG, Schepens T, Saldien V. Flow-controlled ventilation with the Evone ventilator and Tritube versus volume-controlled ventilation: a clinical cross-over pilot study describing oxygenation, ventilation and haemodynamic variables. *Eur J Anaesthesiol.* 2021;38:209-211.
39. Schmidt J, Wenzel C, Spassov S, et al. Flow-controlled ventilation attenuates lung injury in a porcine model of acute respiratory distress syndrome: a preclinical randomized controlled study. *Critical Care Med.* 2020;48:e241.
40. Schmidt J, Wenzel C, Mahn M, et al. Improved lung recruitment and oxygenation during mandatory ventilation with a new expiratory ventilation assistance device: a controlled interventional trial in healthy pigs. *Eur J Anaesthesiol.* 2018;35:736.
41. Lemay F, Cooper J, Thompson S, Scott J. Combination of transnasal humidified rapid-insufflation ventilatory exchange with high frequency jet ventilation for shared airway surgery. *Can J Anesth.* 2020;67:1264-1265.
42. Benjamin B, Gronow D. A new tube for microlaryngeal surgery. *Anaesth Intensive Care.* 1979;7:258-263.
43. Hunsaker DH. Anesthesia for microlaryngeal surgery: the case for subglottic jet ventilation. *Laryngoscope.* 1994;104:1-30.
44. Orloff LA, Parhizkar N, Ortiz E. The Hunsaker Mon-Jet ventilation tube for microlaryngeal surgery: optimal laryngeal exposure. *Ear Nose Throat J.* 2002;81:390-394.
45. Hu A, Weissbrod PA, Maronian NC, et al. Hunsaker mon-jet tube ventilation: A 15-year experience. *Laryngoscope.* 2012;122:2234-2239.
46. Schmidt J, Günther F, Weber J, et al. Glottic visibility for laryngeal surgery: Tritube vs. microlaryngeal tube: a randomised controlled trial. *Eur J Anaesthesiol.* 2019;36:963.
47. Bailey J, Lee C, Nouraei R, et al. Laryngectomy with a Tritube® and flow-controlled ventilation. *Anaesth Reports.* 2021;9:86-89.
48. Kristensen M, De Wolf M, Rasmussen L. Ventilation via the 2.4 mm internal diameter Tritube® with cuff–new possibilities in airway management. *Acta Anaesthesiol Scand.* 2017;61:580-589.
49. Meulemans J, Jans A, Vermeulen K, Vandommele J, Delaere P, Vander Poorten V. Evone® flow-controlled ventilation during upper airway surgery: a clinical feasibility study and safety assessment. *Front Surg.* 2020;7:6.
50. Ankay Yilbaş A, Melek A, Canbay Ö, Kanbak M. Experience with Tritube and flow-controlled ventilation during airway surgery. 2021.
51. Ross-Anderson DJ, Ferguson C, Patel A. Transtracheal jet ventilation in 50 patients with severe airway compromise and stridor. *Br J Anaesth.* 2011;106:140-144.
52. Jaquet Y, Monnier P, Van Melle G, Ravussin P, Spahn DR, Chollet-Rivier M. Complications of different ventilation strategies in endoscopic laryngeal surgery: a 10-year review. *Anesthesiology.* 2006;104:52-59.
53. Benumof JL, Scheller MS. The importance of transtracheal jet ventilation in the management of the difficult airway. *Anesthesiology.* 1989;71:769-778.
54. Duggan L, Ballantyne Scott B, Law J, Morris I, Murphy M, Griesdale D. Transtracheal jet ventilation in the "can't intubate can't oxygenate" emergency: a systematic review. *Br J Anaesth.* 2016;117(Suppl 1)::i28-i38.

CHAPTER 45

Management of the Impossible Airway

Gemma Malpas and Chang Kim

CASE PRESENTATION

A 77-year-old man presents to the urgent outpatient ORL clinic with difficulty breathing and stridor at rest. He has a high BMI (35 kg·m^{-2}) and a complex cardiac history. He presented to the Emergency Department a week earlier and began a course of prednisone 30 mg for airway swelling. His vital signs are temperature 37°C, heart rate 100 beats per minute, respiratory rate 22 breaths per minute, blood pressure 165/90 mmHg, and oxygen saturation (SpO_2) 95% on room air. The patient is seated, using his accessory muscles respiration with severe stridor.

A computed tomographic (CT) view of the head and neck is performed, which reveals an extensive thyroid carcinoma and a 1 mm opening at the level of the glottis (Figure 45.1). Previous anesthetic records showed a Cormack-Lehane Grade 1 view using a Macintosh laryngoscope. The remainder of his history and investigations were unremarkable.

INTRODUCTION

What Are the Four Fundamental Techniques of Airway Management?

The primary goal of airway management is the provision and maintenance of alveolar oxygenation. Traditionally, there have been four fundamental techniques described that have the ability to provide oxygen under anesthesia. These include face-mask ventilation (FMV), ventilation via an extraglottic device (EGD), an endotracheal tube (ETT), or through front-of-neck access (FONA). FMV involves an airway practitioner holding an appropriately sized face mask over a patient's mouth and nose achieving a seal in which no gas can escape. Oxygen is delivered either via spontaneous ventilation from the patient, or through a ventilatory system (positive pressure generated by a pressurized bag or mechanical ventilator) (see Chapter 8). An EGD is any device that is inserted into the pharynx providing a conduit of gas flow from a ventilatory system to the patient (see Chapter 13). An ETT is defined as any tube that is inserted into the trachea to provide a seal for ventilation directly into the lungs; this is usually inserted under visual guidance, either directly via line-of-sight (see Chapter 9), or indirectly using a video camera-based technique (see Chapters 10 and 11). Finally, FONA is the use of any technique to gain access to the trachea for oxygen delivery. This can include a scalpel technique (scalpel-bougie-tube or open surgical technique) or a cannula-guided technique (see Chapter 14).

Utilizing these four fundamental methods of oxygenation, various organizations have developed and revised guidelines and strategic plans to assist practitioners in making critical decisions when providing oxygenation under challenging situations.[1–4] While these guidelines and strategic plans help in managing patients with a difficult or failed airway, they do not include specific recommendations to manage patients

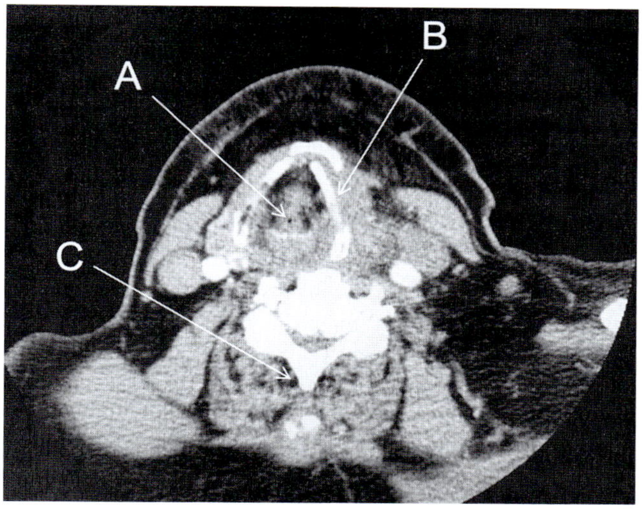

FIGURE 45.1. The computed tomographic view of the head and neck, showing 1-mm internal airway diameter: (**A**) 1-mm subglottic airway; (**B**) left thyroid ala; (**C**) C5 spinous process.

with a critically obstructed airway when all four fundamental techniques of oxygenation are likely to be difficult or failed.

Over recent years, there has been an increase in the use of high-flow nasal cannula (HFNC) oxygen for pre- and intraoperative oxygenation, with particular uptake within airway surgery.[5] This technique involves the placement of Optiflow™ (Fisher & Paykel Healthcare, Auckland, New Zealand) for denitrogenation prior to induction with total intravenous anesthesia (TIVA). Following the onset of apnea, flows are increased to 70 $L{\cdot}min^{-1}$ and maintained throughout the procedure. Similar to the four fundamental techniques of oxygen delivery, this technique requires a patent airway for oxygen delivery.

Define an Impossible Airway

An "impossible airway" is defined as an airway in which all four basic airway techniques are anticipated to be difficult or likely to fail.[3,6] These lesions can be classified as:

1. Supraglottic, with additional or coexisting neck pathology (this can include a wide range of pathologies such as conditions leading to craniofacial deformities with fixed neck flexion through to those with supraglottic cancers and coexisting thyroid masses)
2. At the level of the glottis due to extensive neck pathology
3. Subglottic at a level inaccessible via the neck (tracheal pathology inferior to the suprasternal notch such as critical tracheal stenosis)
4. Intrathoracic (such as compression related to a significant mediastinal mass)

The impossible airway can also include any pathology that prevents insertion of an endotracheal tube or the ability to ventilate the lungs such as tracheal transection, massive hemoptysis, and severe tracheal granulomatosis (Wegener's granulomatosis).

What Is the "Fifth Element" of Oxygenation (Alternative Oxygenation Technique) in Managing Patients with an Impossible Airway?

In addition to oxygen delivery to the lungs via the upper airway, there is an alternative technique commonly used to provide oxygen to the tissues. Cardiopulmonary bypass (CPB), and more recently, extracorporeal membrane oxygenation (ECMO) have been used since the 1970s to provide oxygen when the four fundamental methods of oxygen delivery are anticipated to be impossible.[7] Both CPB and ECMO are methods of extracorporeal life support (ECLS) that focus on oxygenation, carbon dioxide removal, cardiac support, or a combination thereof.[8] CPB is designed for short-term support during various cardiac surgical procedures and is classically instituted via transthoracic cannulation under general anesthesia, whereas ECMO is designed for longer-term support to allow time for intrinsic recovery of the lungs and heart and is instituted using central (intrathoracic) or peripheral access (via cervical or femoral vessels), which can be performed under local anesthesia[9] (see Chapter 15).

ECLS should be considered preemptively in all patients with an "impossible airway" and in cases where a temporary complete airway occlusion is anticipated.[10] ECMO should be initiated prior to general anesthesia in all patients with a critical obstruction of the intrathoracic airways by a mediastinal mass.[10]

What Is ECMO?

Extracorporeal membrane oxygenation (ECMO) is one ECLS entity used for temporary support of patients with respiratory and/or cardiac failure.[8] The components include a centrifugal or impeller pump, a membrane oxygenator, a heat exchanger, heparin-coated polyvinylchloride connecting tubing, and connectors. PVC tubing is heparin coated to enhance biocompatibility and reduce thrombosis. Blood drained from the patient directly enters the pump; therefore, the pump is dependent on the patient's volume status.[11]

How Do You Select the Type of ECMO for Patients with an Impossible Airway?

In a venovenous (VV)-ECMO circuit, the membrane oxygenator is in series with the native lung (Video 31). The improvement in arterial oxygenation in this circuit is due to the increased oxygen saturation of the venous blood flowing through shunt regions of the native lung. The VV-ECMO approach with high flow, even with a very high shunt in the native lung, can provide vital arterial oxygenation. This is the preferred approach for the case presented and for those without a very low cardiac output (or overt cardiac arrest).

The VA-ECMO approach involves the membrane oxygenator in parallel with the native lung. This circuit involves the drainage of venous blood, oxygenation of the blood, and the subsequent return to the aorta through a cannulated artery. In the setting of complete cardiac failure, there is significantly better systemic oxygenation with this technique compared with the

VV-ECMO approach because the artificially oxygenated blood mixes with arterial blood and directly perfuses distal organs.

During airway emergencies, without a compromised cardiac output, the native cardiac output (desaturated blood from the LV) mixes with the blood from the femorally cannulated VA-ECMO, usually in the region of the aortic arch. Accordingly, the coronary arteries, and to a variable degree, the supraaortic vessels are provided with hypoxemic blood.[12] This results in a phenomenon called "differential hypoxia." This only occurs if the arterial cannula is placed peripherally, but not centrally. This can be detected with arterial blood gas collected from the right radial artery.[11]

VV-ECMO is the most common mode in adult respiratory indications.[13,14] Arterial oxygen saturation of more than 80% would be acceptable given that clinical and laboratory evidence of adequate oxygen delivery to the tissues is achieved.[15]

What Patient Factors Would Affect ECMO Cannulation Options?

The most common sites for percutaneous cannulation for establishing peripheral ECMO are femoral artery, femoral vein, or internal jugular vein (IJV). The site and type of cannulas will depend primarily on the method of ECMO technique (VA-ECMO vs. VV-ECMO) and patient factors limiting access to the desired site. It is essential that patient's vascular access and their patency are assessed prior to cannulation. For VV-ECMO, either a double-lumen cannula or two single-lumen cannulas can be used. Double-lumen cannula (e.g., Avalon Elite) is inserted into the right IJV. Its insertion requires transesophageal or image intensifier for correct positioning of the cannula and optimal direction of blood return. Due to this practical limitation, in an emergency airway setting, two single-lumen cannulas are often utilized. Drainage cannula is placed in a femoral vein, and return cannula can either be placed in femoral vein on the other side (fem-fem configuration) or in right IJV (fem-IJ configuration).

PATIENT EVALUATION AND MANAGEMENT OPTIONS

What Are Key Aspects of the Airway Examination in This Situation?

This patient has presented with critical obstruction as a progression of his chronic upper airway pathology. In addition to routine assessments of the airway (see Chapter 1), there is often time to perform advanced airway examinations including MR or CT scan, and flexible nasal endoscopy (FNE). Routine airway examinations will provide information related to the anatomical ease of performing FMV, extraglottic airway insertion, laryngoscopy (direct or indirect), and FONA; however, in patients with critical airway obstruction, they may fail to identify obstructing lesions at or below the level of the glottic opening. These patients require appropriate CT or magnetic resonance imaging (MRI) in addition to FNE to assess the degree and level of obstruction and the availability of the cricothyroid membrane or upper trachea for oxygen delivery.

In this patient, the critical subglottic narrowing was caused by an extensive multifocal papillary thyroid carcinoma involving the entire front of neck, distorting the anatomy, limiting the patient's range of neck movement, and inhibiting their ability to tolerate the supine position.

What Is the Airway Management Plan for This Patient?

The presented case presents problems in all four fundamental methods of oxygen delivery: via FMV, EGD, ETT, and achieving oxygen delivery through FONA. Although this patient has had a previous laryngoscopy documented as a Cormack-Lehane Grade 1 view, the degree of glottic narrowing rendered supraglottic tube passage impossible. Airway management in patients with this degree of obstruction requires assessment for other methods of blood oxygenation, and as such should be assessed for cannula placement for ECMO prior to induction of anesthesia. In addition to the anatomical constraints of airway management, consideration needs to be given to the position of the patient during cannula placement and initiation of anesthesia. With this degree of obstruction, the patient will be most comfortable in the upright position and may become distressed if there is an attempt to lay the patient supine.

Would High-Flow Nasal Oxygenation or Jet Ventilation Be Useful for This Patient?

Increasingly high-flow nasal oxygen (Optiflow) has been used during upper airway surgery, both as a denitrogenation technique and as the sole oxygenation technique during airway surgery. The prerequisite for apneic oxygenation is the presence of a patent airway for delivery of 100% oxygen.[5] For patients with near-complete airway obstruction, high-flow nasal oxygen may provide symptomatic improvement of the airflow limitation and improve oxygen saturations. This method, however, should not be relied upon for the sole mode of oxygenation. Due to the severe nature of the airflow restriction, without respiratory drive, only limited oxygen will reach the alveoli potentially leading to profound hypoxemia.

Occasionally, during surgery for upper airway pathology, particularly vocal cord pathology, jet ventilation is used to maintain oxygenation,[16] with ventilation being maintained through passive expiration. In near complete airway obstruction, however, jet ventilation carries an unacceptably high risk of volutrauma, barotrauma, pneumothorax, hyperventilation, and gastric insufflation.[17]

What Other Patient Factors May Be Relevant in This Situation?

Given the expected difficulty with upper airway oxygen delivery, this patient requires assessment for initiation of ECMO prior to induction of anesthesia. Complex airway cases such as these require immediate consultation with the cardiothoracic team (surgeons and perfusionists) and intensivists, and an appropriate strategy formulated. This patient had a complex cardiac history consisting of coronary artery bypass graft surgery in 2003, with preexisting pacemaker-dependent complete heart block, with subsequent infection at his pacemaker site, requiring removal and replacement with a right infraclavicular pacemaker. Echocardiography in 2015 reported normal biventricular function with no suggestion of elevated pulmonary artery pressures.

In addition to airway examination, the patient should be rapidly assessed for their anesthesia risk. A comprehensive preoperative assessment should be performed consisting of previous anesthesia, medical and surgical history, medication history including allergies and fasting status. Patients with thyroid disease should have thyroid function tests regularly monitored. Ideally, all patients should be euthyroid prior to surgery; however, this isn't always achievable in the acute setting.[18] Abnormal thyroid function tests should be discussed with a perioperative endocrinology specialist and appropriate precautionary measures should be performed.

Patients presenting with critical upper airway obstruction may display signs of superior vena cava (SVC) obstruction. This is indicated by the presence of distended neck veins that do not change with respiration. Pemberton's sign of SVC obstruction may be elicited by asking the patient to raise his arms straight up; if obstruction is present, the patient's face will become blue and engorged. The CT or MRI should also be examined for this complication.

Relevant preoperative assessments and imaging should be reviewed jointly by all team members, prior to formulation of an airway strategy.[19] When an "impossible airway" is encountered, this includes otorhinolaryngologic surgeon, anesthesia practitioner, cardiothoracic surgeon, perfusionist, and intensivist.

What Information Can Be Gained from the CT Neck and What Other Investigations Are Needed for This Patient?

In this situation, a CT of the neck/thorax provides critical information for the management of the airway. In addition to highlighting the degree of tracheal narrowing caused by the thyroid pathology, it also informs us of the level of airway narrowing, and any tracheal deviation or retrosternal extension of the mass. The CT can also give indication of whether the patient has an SVC obstruction caused by the thyroid mass. Patients with obstructing airway pathology should also have the standard airway examination enhanced by a nasal endoscopic evaluation of the upper airway under local anesthesia. Given that this patient has an airway examination suggesting an "impossible airway," the patient should be discussed urgently with the cardiothoracic team, and a CT angiogram should be requested for evaluation of the most appropriate site of ECMO cannulation.

AIRWAY MANAGEMENT OF THE PATIENT

Pending the Decision of Whether and Where to Intubate, How Can the Patient Be Symptomatically Temporized?

Although this patient has presented with advanced airway obstruction that requires immediate intervention, there is time to temporize and optimize the patient prior to invasive airway intervention. Patients presenting with advanced airway obstruction should be immediately admitted to an appropriately monitored unit with continuous blood pressure, heart rate, and pulse oximetry monitoring. IV steroids should be administered to reduce any acute swelling. Heliox (a helium/oxygen blend) via a face mask reduces the patient's work of breathing by reducing the density of the inspired gas, decreasing the resistance to turbulent flow, thereby improving flow of gas to the alveoli. In an acutely hypoxemic patient, there may be limited benefit to the administration of heliox due to the requirement of an increased fraction of inspired oxygen to maintain oxygenation. These patients may experience symptomatic benefits from the use of humidified high-flow nasal oxygen.

How Should Such an Airway Be Approached, and Why?

Safe airway management is dependent on establishing the best airway strategy for any given circumstance considering the experience of the anesthesia practitioner, surgeon, equipment, and team available.[20] In a complex airway case where methods of oxygenation are extremely limited, consultation needs to occur between the anesthesia, otorhinolaryngologic, and cardiothoracic teams. Patients with advanced infraglottic airway disease, limiting FONA should ideally be managed in a tertiary care center where ECMO is available. The absence of a viable plan for "can't intubate can't oxygenate" (CICO) should elevate consideration of awake tracheotomy under local anesthesia as the primary plan or, as in this case, first establishing ECMO under local anesthesia.[21] Airway management should take place in a fully equipped operating room with appropriate personnel available in the room. A clear and concise briefing should occur with all members of the operating room prior to any airway intervention.

How Should We Proceed in This Case?

Preoperative oxygen therapy such as heliox or high-flow nasal oxygen should be continued into the operating room. The patient should be positioned appropriately for optimal airway management, patient comfort, and access to femoral vessels. In this situation, a semirecumbent position provides that compromise. Arterial access for invasive BP monitoring should be placed along with routine monitoring including depth of anesthesia monitoring. Noninvasive near-infrared spectroscopy (NIRS) tissue oximetry, if available, may provide important information regarding cerebral oxygenation.

Following positioning and placement of monitoring, the airway strategy should be communicated to all operating room personnel. As the presented case poses difficulties with FMV, EGD, and tracheal intubation, alternative strategies must be considered. FONA under local anesthesia is also an undesirable option due to the extensive nature of the thyroid carcinoma distorting the anatomy and the inability of the patient to tolerate the supine position. In this circumstance, the safest strategy consists of insertion of ECMO cannulas under local anesthesia and establishing flow. Once established, induction of anesthesia can occur, and this should be administered using TIVA with appropriate depth of anesthesia monitoring, given the inadequacy of gas flow via the tracheal route. Following induction of anesthesia, the anesthesia practitioner can undergo one attempt at tracheal intubation with a standard geometry video-laryngoscope using a styletted microlaryngoscopy tube (MLT). Depending on the view obtained, lack of success at tracheal intubation should be immediately followed with a surgical approach. Either a single attempt at rigid bronchoscopy or immediate progression to surgical tracheotomy through the thyroid carcinoma with supplemental oxygen in the event of failure. Following endotracheal intubation, ECMO can then be rapidly weaned, preventing the need for maintaining therapeutic anticoagulation.

The case presented only required ECMO for the duration of time necessary to achieve a secure airway to directly ventilate the patient's native lungs. Anticoagulation in the form of 5000 IU intravenous heparin was administered prior to cannulation. Following cannulation, the patient was connected to the ECMO circuit and full flow was incrementally instituted. Anesthesia was then induced and maintained with TIVA and neuromuscular blockade. One attempt at direct intraoral tracheal intubation was performed but was unsuccessful because of an inability to advance the tube beyond the solid tumor at the glottic opening. In discussion with the ENT surgeon, it was elected to proceed directly to tracheotomy (foregoing any attempt at rigid bronchoscopy). The tracheotomy, though technically challenging because of the presence of the large anterior obstructive mass, allowed placement of a reinforced 7.0-mm ID ETT. The ECMO was then weaned following which the cannulas were clamped prior to removal. This allowed for the heparin to be reversed using protamine prior to thyroidectomy, laryngectomy, and central lymph node dissection.

OTHER CONSIDERATIONS

Is It Safe to Perform Airway Surgery Under ECMO Without the Use of Anticoagulant?

Patients on ECMO require therapeutic anticoagulation with heparin following arterial and venous cannulation.[22] In order to reduce the incidence of thrombus formation, large doses of heparin are administered to maintain activated clotting times (ACTs) between 180 and 200 seconds. This has obvious implications for airway surgery. Bleeding risk can be minimized during airway surgery using partial heparinization to achieve ACTs between 160 and 180 seconds and heparin-coated tubing to reduce systemic heparin doses.[10] The use of heparin-coated circuits while patients are on VV-ECMO can allow avoidance of systemic anticoagulation as long as the blood flow is maintained at a high enough rate (~2 $L \cdot min^{-1}$). This is not advocated for people needing VA-ECMO. Arterial thrombosis is associated with significant consequences.[11]

What Are the Potential Complications of ECMO?

Long-term ECMO (and long-term intubation) use is associated with significant complications such as hemolysis, circuit thrombosis, infection, and bleeding;[23] many of these being related to the patient's underlying pathology. The reported incidence of complications with ECMO for short periods is low.[7] Compared with VV-ECMO, VA-ECMO is associated with a higher incidence of neurologic events, and major complications such as arterial dissection, pseudoaneurysm formation, or limb ischemia.[24] In cases where ECMO is required to facilitate complex interventions to manage the airway, VV-ECMO may provide adequate oxygenation and ventilation while reducing the potential risk of arterial and neurological complications associated with the use of VA-ECMO.

SUMMARY

In addition to the four fundamental techniques of oxygenation in airway management, alternative strategies should be considered when all methods of oxygenation via the endotracheal route are likely to fail. The use of ECMO in appropriate centers should be considered in patients with severe airway obstruction secondary to anterior neck or tracheal disease. In these cases, ECMO needs to be considered and planned for prior to any alternative airway maneuvers that could result in loss of the existing airway. This approach can provide essential tissue oxygenation while attempts to secure a definitive airway are carried out in a controlled environment.

SELF-EVALUATION QUESTIONS

45.1. Which of the following airway management techniques is contraindicated in near-complete airway obstruction?

A. High-flow nasal oxygen
B. Jet ventilation
C. Inhaled helium-oxygen
D. Face-mask oxygenation
E. Direct laryngoscopy

45.2. Which clinical specialists should be present at induction of the "impossible airway"?

A. Anesthesia
B. Otorhinolaryngologic
C. Cardiothoracic
D. Perfusionists
E. All of the above

45.3. Which of the following statements regarding obstructing airway pathology is TRUE?

A. Topicalization of the upper airway has been known to cause complete loss of airway patency during attempted awake intubation.
B. Inhalational induction allows for a safe wake-up during induction if airway patency is lost.
C. Emergency institution of ECMO is a safe "plan B" for management of the "failed airway."
D. In patients with infraglottic airway obstruction, an awake cricothyroidotomy is a reasonable airway management plan.
E. Lying the patient supine in the "sniffing" position will facilitate safe and easier airway management.

REFERENCES

1. Frerk C, Mitchell VS, McNarry AF, et al. Difficult Airway Society 2015 guidelines for management of unanticipated difficult intubation in adults. *Br J Anaesth*. 2015;115(6):827-848.
2. Law JA, Duggan LV, Asselin M, et al. Canadian Airway Focus Group updated consensus-based recommendations for management of the difficult airway: part 1. Difficult airway management encountered in an unconscious patient. *Can J Anaesth*. 2021;68(9):1373-1404.
3. Law JA, Duggan LV, Asselin M, et al. Canadian Airway Focus Group updated consensus-based recommendations for management of the difficult airway: part 2. Planning and implementing safe management of the patient with an anticipated difficult airway. *Can J Anaesth*. 2021;68(9):1405-1436.
4. Apfelbaum JL, Hagberg CA, Connis RT, et al. 2022 American Society of Anesthesiologists practice guidelines for management of the difficult airway. *Anesthesiology*. 2022;136(1):31-81.
5. Gustafsson IM, Lodenius A, Tunelli J, Ullman J, Jonsson Fagerlund M. Apnoeic oxygenation in adults under general anaesthesia using Transnasal Humidified Rapid-Insufflation Ventilatory Exchange (THRIVE): a physiological study. *Br J Anaesth*. 2017;118(4):610-617.
6. Rosa P Jr, Johnson EA, Barcia PJ. The impossible airway: a plan. *Chest*. 1996;109(6):1649-1650.
7. Malpas G, Hung O, Gilchrist A, et al. The use of extracorporeal membrane oxygenation in the anticipated difficult airway: a case report and systematic review. *Can J Anaesth*. 2018;65(6):685-697.
8. Broman LM, Taccone FS, Lorusso R, et al. The ELSO Maastricht Treaty for ECLS Nomenclature: abbreviations for cannulation configuration in extracorporeal life support. A position paper of the Extracorporeal Life Support Organization. *Crit Care*. 2019;23(1):36.
9. Biscotti M, Yang J, Sonett J, Bacchetta M. Comparison of extracorporeal membrane oxygenation versus cardiopulmonary bypass for lung transplantation. *J Thorac Cardiovasc Surg*. 2014;148(5):2410-2415.
10. Hoetzenecker K, Klepetko W, Keshavjee S, Cypel M. Extracorporeal support in airway surgery. *J Thorac Dis*. 2017;9(7):2108-2117.
11. Vuylsteke A, Brodie D, Combes A, Fowles J, Peek G, eds. *ECMO in the Adult Patient (Core Critical Care)*. Cambridge: Cambridge University Press; 2017.
12. Rupprecht L, Lunz D, Philipp A, Lubnow M, Schmid C. Pitfalls in percutaneous ECMO cannulation. *Heart Lung Vessel*. 2015;7(4):320-326.
13. Combes A, Bacchetta M, Brodie D, Muller T, Pellegrino V. Extracorporeal membrane oxygenation for respiratory failure in adults. *Curr Opin Crit Care*. 2012;18(1):99-104.
14. MacLaren G, Combes A, Bartlett RH. Contemporary extracorporeal membrane oxygenation for adult respiratory failure: life support in the new era. *Intensive Care Med*. 2012;38(2):210-220.
15. Alibrahim OS, Heard CMB. Extracorporeal life support: four decades and counting. *Curr Anesthesiol Rep*. 2017;7(2):168-182.
16. de Wolf MW, Gottschall R, Preussler NP, Paxian M, Enk D. Emergency ventilation with the Ventrain((R)) through an airway exchange catheter in a porcine model of complete upper airway obstruction. *Can J Anaesth*. 2017;64(1):37-44.
17. EH W. The hazards of airway surgery. *South Afr J Anaesth Analg*. 2013;19:52-54.
18. Malhotra S, Sodhi V. Anaesthesia for thyroid and parathyroid surgery. *Continuing Education Anaesth Crit Care Pain*. 2007;7(2):55-58.
19. Cook TM, Woodall N, Frerk C, Fourth National Audit P. Major complications of airway management in the UK: results of the Fourth National Audit Project of the Royal College of Anaesthetists and the Difficult Airway Society. Part 1: anaesthesia. *Br J Anaesth*. 2011;106(5):617-631.
20. Hung O, Murphy M. Context-sensitive airway management. *Anesth Analg*. 2010;110(4):982-983.
21. Law JA, Morris IR, Malpas G. Obstructing pathology of the upper airway in a post-NAP4 world: time to wake up to its optimal management. *Can J Anaesth*. 2017;64(11):1087-1097.
22. Chauhan S, Subin S. Extracorporeal membrane oxygenation, an anesthesiologist's perspective: physiology and principles. Part 1. *Ann Card Anaesth*. 2011;14(3):218-229.
23. Zangrillo A, Landoni G, Biondi-Zoccai G, Greco M, Greco T, Frati G, et al. A meta-analysis of complications and mortality of extracorporeal membrane oxygenation. *Crit Care Resusc*. 2013;15(3):172-178.
24. Hong Y, Jo KW, Lyu J, et al. Use of venovenous extracorporeal membrane oxygenation in central airway obstruction to facilitate interventions leading to definitive airway security. *J Crit Care*. 2013;28(5):669-674.

SECTION 7

AIRWAY MANAGEMENT IN THE PEDIATRIC POPULATION

CHAPTER 46

Unique Airway Issues in the Pediatric Population

Jacob Heninger, Matthew Rowland, and Narasimhan Jagannathan

CASE PRESENTATION

A full-term baby is born with an initial APGAR score of 4. While stimulating the neonate, the neonatologist observes a heart rate less than 100 bpm with poor chest movement, and therefore proceeds to intubate the trachea. After two failed attempts with a Miller 0 and 1 blade, with no clear view of the vocal cords, you are called to help with airway management. The neonate is tachypneic with signs of upper airway obstruction. The oxygen saturation is 88% at 10 minutes with an oral airway and continuous positive airway pressure delivered via a bag valve mask. What are your concerns and how would you manage this child's airway?

THE BASICS

Why Is a Separate Chapter on Pediatrics Important?

Airway and respiratory events are the most common complications in pediatric patients undergoing anesthesia.[1,2] A large prospective observational study looking at over 30,000 anesthetics found the incidence of critical events to be 5.2%, of which 60% were airway management–related events. Laryngospasm and bronchospasm were the most common, with the highest incidence of complications occurring in neonates and infants.[2] These perioperative respiratory events contribute significantly to both morbidity and mortality.[3]

The Pediatric Perioperative Cardiac Arrest (POCA) Registry is a subdivision of the American Society of Anesthesiologists (ASA) Closed Claims Registry dedicated to pediatrics. In the past, 50% of all cardiac arrests documented in the POCA registry were attributed to respiratory causes, with hypoxemia quickly leading to bradycardia and cardiac arrest.[4] Through improvements in technology, cardiac arrest due to difficult or failed airway management has decreased to approximately 25%; however, respiratory causes are still the second most common reason for death and brain damage. The number one cause for death and brain damage is cardiovascular, such as unrecognized hypovolemia.[4]

A multicenter review of children with known difficult airways demonstrated that greater than two attempts at direct laryngoscopy (DL) is associated with a high failure rate and an increased incidence of severe complications.[1] The most common *severe* complication was cardiac arrest occurring in 2% of children. The most common complication overall was hypoxemia. Although children with an ASA status of 3-5 were at higher individual risk of complications, two-thirds of children suffering perioperative death or brain damage were ASA status 1 and 2. Additionally, a review of 1341 healthy infants undergoing routine intubation for elective procedures found a high incidence of multiple laryngoscopy attempts and associated hypoxemia events, underscoring the need for vigilance when caring for *all* pediatric patients.[5]

Adverse respiratory events were more commonly encountered under the care of nonpediatric trained anesthesia practitioners, with 80% of laryngospasm events and 80% of airway obstruction events occurring within this group.[6] Furthermore, the PeDI registry data showed that in difficult pediatric airways, pediatric-trained anesthesia practitioners were more likely to be successful in placement of the endotracheal tube (ETT).[1]

Fortunately, there are more similarities between pediatric and adult airways than differences. The traditional emphasis on the differences likely impairs the performance of an anesthesia practitioner who deals mostly with adults. *When compared to adults, the biggest differences are found in a child less than 2 years old.* For this reason, this age group will be emphasized.

What Is Unique About Pediatric Airway Management?

Variability in equipment sizes, drug dosages, and the propensity of children to be both uncooperative and desaturate quickly can make even the most experienced practitioner wary. A crisis situation is also no time to be calculating drug doses or discovering equipment that is inappropriately sized. Calculating medication doses and equipment sizes is not algorithmic or reflexive and will increase cognitive load. Errors happen: the POCA database estimates 18% of children received wrong drug doses, which contributed to their morbidity and mortality.[7]

Immediate access to dosing and sizing information, including planned and unplanned difficult airway situations, allows the anesthesia practitioner the "mental space" to focus on critical decision-making.[8] The authors enthusiastically support the use of precalculated systems for both drug dosages and equipment sizes. This can be done in a number of ways, such as based on the actual weight, or the length of the child, using a system such as the Broselow-Luten tape (Armstrong Medical, Lincolnshire, IL, USA).[9,10] Other settings have taken the approach of including drug doses in the front of every child's chart.

What Is the Incidence of Difficult Face-Mask Ventilation in Children?

Montreal Children's Hospital reported an incidence of 6.6% for unexpected difficult face-mask ventilation (FMV), requiring additional management techniques to be adequately ventilated in a sample of 484 healthy children aged 0 to 8 years undergoing elective surgery.[11] Difficult FMV was defined as requiring two of the following: application of CPAP >5, use of oral airway, need for two-person ventilation, desaturation <95%, and unanticipated need to increase FiO_2. Age under 1 year and ENT surgery were the only significant risk factors for difficult FMV. Obesity, gender, OSA, and asthma were not associated with difficult FMV. There was an even higher incidence of difficult FMV in the critically ill pediatric population, approaching 10%.[12] A study evaluating FMV in the pediatric population suggested that maintaining adequate ventilation was difficult for many practitioners (19 of the 25 practitioners were anesthesia residents) but this may be improved with feedback mechanisms such as capnography.[13] The incidence of difficult FMV is higher than rates for adult patients, which is reported to be 1.5%.[14] However, some of the variables used to identify difficult FMV (oral airway, CPAP, oxygen desaturation to 90%-95%) are encountered on a daily basis in a pediatric anesthesia practice and usually do not result in any adverse events. Thus, the true incidence of difficult FMV is likely lower than 6.6%.

What Is the Incidence of Difficult Direct Laryngoscopic Intubation in Children?

Difficult direct laryngoscopic intubation rates vary depending on the study but range from 0.25%[15] to as high as 14% in the NICU population.[16] Most papers reported rates from 0.25% to 1.35%[17] with an unanticipated difficult intubation rate from 0.03%[15] to as high as 19%.[1] In a single-center pediatric study with a difficult intubation rate of 0.25% (16/6524), 14 of the difficult intubations were anticipated and none had issues with FMV.[15] Predictors in this study of difficult intubation were narrow inter-incisor distance (93.8%) and mandibular hypoplasia (87.5%).[15] In another single-center study looking at pediatric cardiac patients, the rate was reported as 1.25% (16/1278).[18] This study noted half of the difficult intubation patients were syndromic and the other half had extreme anterior airways and micrognathia.[18] In the largest single-center study over 5 years, the rate of difficult intubation was reported as 1.35% for 11,219 patients undergoing general anesthesia.[17] The Pediatric Difficult Intubation (PeDI) Registry reported similarly low difficult intubation rates of 0.25% to 0.47% in the largest centers.[1] The rate of difficult intubation and unanticipated difficult intubation is much higher in the NICU population with about 14% of intubations being classified as difficult (276/2009 intubations).[16] The most common characteristics were infants less than 32 weeks' gestation or 1500 g.[16] This trend towards more difficult airways is also seen in the PICU population, with a reported incidence of 8.8% (129/1469) requiring more than two attempts.[19] Unanticipated difficult intubation in children is less common than in adults as most difficult airway situations are in children with a syndromic diagnosis or with associated facial features such as micrognathia, maxillary hypoplasia, and macroglossia. Examples of congenital and acquired syndromes associated with difficult intubation in children are listed in Table 46.1.

How Common Is the "Cannot Intubate, Cannot Oxygenate" (CICO) Scenario in Children?

While the exact incidence is unknown, this is a rare event. Children with potentially difficult tracheal intubation are often on easy bag-mask ventilation (BMV), and difficult intubation is usually anticipated. There are exceptions to this generalization. A child with a difficult airway may be detected prenatally and has an associated craniofacial syndrome[20] (Pierre Robin, Goldenhaar, Treacher Collins, Cystic Hygroma, also see Figures 46.1 and 46.2 and Table 46.1). At birth, if the newborn is unable to maintain their airway, a tracheotomy is

TABLE 46.1. Examples of Commonly Encountered Pediatric Syndromes with Airway Implications and Possible Management Techniques

Pierre Robin syndrome
- 1:8000 newborns, variable micrognathia and cleft palate
- Airway improves with age, especially if surgically distracted
- Prone positioning, EGD, elective prone intubation, intubation through an EGD (Figure 46.1)

Mucopolysaccharidosis
- A group of glycosaminoglycan storage diseases, narrow hypopharynx, large tongue, narrow mouth opening, possible atlantoaxial instability
- Airway worsens with increasing age
- Elective tracheotomy, nasal intubation, surgical back-up

Down's syndrome
- 1:1000 newborns, possible cervical spine instability, large tongue, gastroesophageal reflux, and pharyngeal hypotonia
- Straight blade, Eschmann Tracheal Introducer, video device, EGD-assisted flexible fiberoptic bronchoscope intubation

Treacher Collins syndrome
- Micrognathia, ankylosis of the jaw
- Airway worsens with increasing age, despite having mandibular distraction
- EGD, EGD-assisted flexible fiberoptic bronchoscope intubation

Cystic hygroma
- Large tumor of the lymph system of the neck causing pressure on the upper airway and generalized swelling
- Tongue protrudes in an attempt to keep the airway open (Figure 46.2)
- Awake nasal intubation

Juvenile rheumatoid arthritis
- Temporomandibular ankylosis, atlantoaxial and low cervical-spine instability, mandibular hypoplasia, and possible vocal cord fixation
- Awake bronchoscopic intubation, consideration of nasal intubation

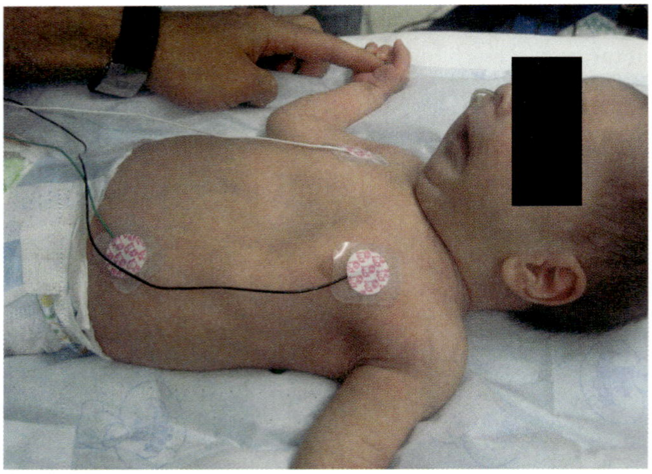

FIGURE 46.1. Pierre Robin neonate. Note the micrognathia and resultant sternal retraction.

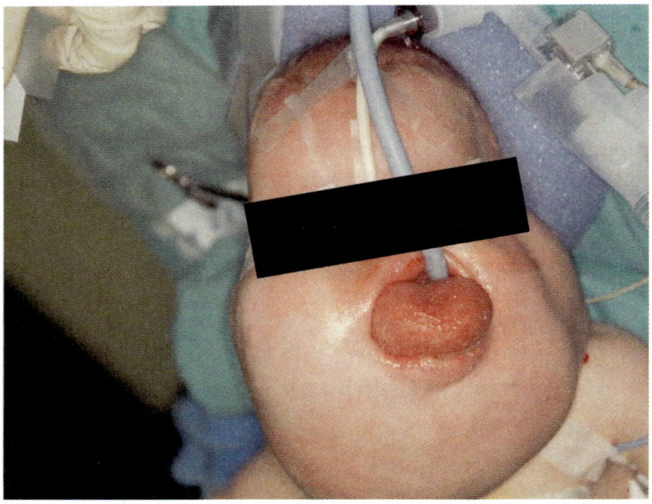

FIGURE 46.2. Congenital cystic hygroma.

placed or an ex-utero intrapartum treatment (EXIT) procedure is performed by an otorhinolaryngologist.[21] If obstruction is mild to moderate, they may undergo procedures to advance their mandible or improve mouth opening during the first few days of life. This is the population that may be at higher risk for a CICO scenario and is unlikely to be encountered by the majority of practicing anesthesia practitioners.

Is There an Airway Algorithm that Specifically Addresses Pediatric Patients?

Yes, guidelines have been developed for the management of difficult airway in children. These guidelines were developed by an expert panel and provide algorithms for difficult FMV, unanticipated difficult tracheal intubation, and a "cannot intubate, cannot oxygenate" scenario. The principles of unanticipated airway management are the same in children and adults; oxygenation and ventilation, not intubation, save lives.[22] Two helpful algorithms for the pediatric difficult airway are outlined by Huang et al. and Krishna et al.[23,24]

ANATOMICAL AND PHYSIOLOGIC DIFFERENCES

What Are the Main Anatomic Differences in the Pediatric Airway?

The pediatric upper airway consists of the nose and mouth leading to the nasopharynx and oropharynx, respectively. These structures are contiguous. The ala of the nose leads to two separate nasal compartments separated by the nasal septum. The lateral wall of each nasal compartment has three scroll-like conchae or turbinate bones. The major air passage lies below the inferior turbinate and is the preferred route for nasal intubation.

The posterior nasal aperture leading to the nasopharynx is called the choanae. Choanal atresia occurs in approximately 1:7000 births; however, only approximately 50% of these babies will have respiratory distress. Although it was once thought that infants are obligate nasal breathers, infants are more accurately described as "preferential" nasal breathers.[25] Infants in respiratory distress will usually cry, raise their soft palate, and become mouth breathers.[26]

From infancy until approximately 2 years of age, the tongue is relatively large surrounded by a small jaw. There is simply not enough space to sweep the tongue to the left of the oral cavity as occurs with DL when employing a curved Macintosh blade in an adult. For this reason, a straight or Miller blade is generally preferred in this age group. This limitation in space in the oropharynx may be improved by using a paraglossal intubation technique, especially in syndromic infants.[27] Of note, this paradigm was questioned with a 2014 study by Passi et al., who found similar rates of optimal laryngeal views in children <2 years old with either a Miller blade lifting the epiglottis or with a MAC blade lifting the tongue base.[28]

The occiput of a small child is much larger than in the adult causing the cervical spine to flex when supine, leading to significant airway obstruction. A shoulder roll allows the cervical spine to stay in neutral position[28,29] aiding in FMV, placement of an extraglottic device, intubation, and very rarely, a surgical airway (Figure 46.3).

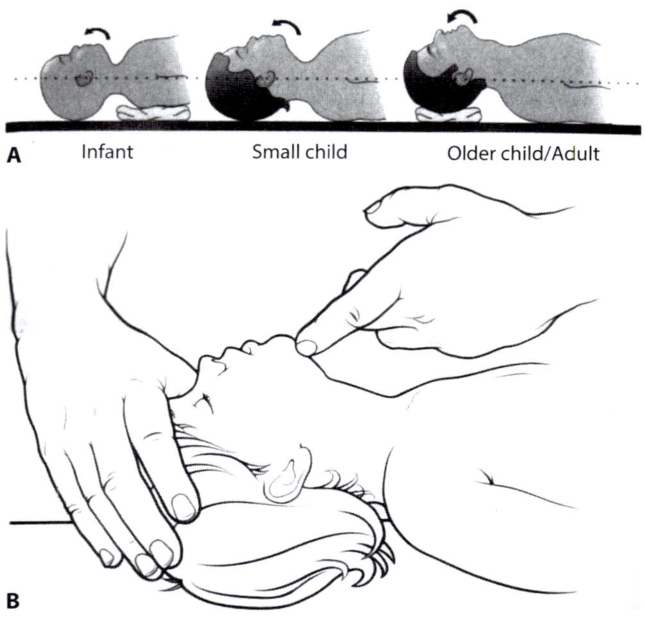

FIGURE 46.3. This figure depicts options to be considered for positioning children of various age groups for BMV and tracheal intubation. (Reproduced with permission from Walls RM, Murphy MF, Luten R, et al. *Manual of Emergency Airway Management*. Philadelphia, PA: Lippincott Williams & Wilkins; 2004.)

What Is the Narrowest Portion of the Infant's Airway?

Traditionally, the airway of a child under 2 years old has been described as "funnel shaped" with the narrowest part being at the level of the cricoid cartilage. However, more recent MRI and CT imaging studies have confirmed that the narrowest portion is in fact the subglottis, which is the same as in adults.[30–32] These studies were performed on children under general anesthesia without a neuromuscular blocker agent (NMBA) and therefore preserved muscle tone. Studies on paralyzed children are still required. A study using video bronchoscopy supported these newer findings as well.[33] However, this does remain a controversial topic, as autopsy specimens continue to suggest that the narrowest portion is the cricoid cartilage.[34] Further, there are limitations with radiographic imaging as the sleep state and anesthetic agents may alter respiratory mechanics and anatomy.[34] Much of the controversy relates to alterations in the airway with the administration of NMBAs. The subglottic region becomes more mobile with NMBAs potentially making the cricoid cartilage area the narrowest or most inflexible portion or area with the most resistance to ETT passage.[35]

Why Do Children Desaturate So Quickly?

As with the anatomy of the airway, the major physiologic differences between adults and children occur in the first 2 years of life.

Young children consume oxygen at two to three times the adult rate (6 mL oxygen·kg^{-1}·min^{-1} vs. 2 mL oxygen·kg^{-1}·min^{-1}), and have a smaller FRC under general anesthetic relative to adults (10-15 mL·kg^{-1} vs. 30 mL·kg^{-1}, respectively). The result is that young children consume their oxygen reserve and desaturate much more quickly than adults.[36]

Although children have tidal volumes similar to adults (7 mL·kg^{-1}), their dead space to tidal volume ratio is larger, leading to proportionately less alveolar ventilation per breath.

In children, an increase in ventilation is primarily achieved by increasing the respiratory rate rather than the depth of each breath.[36] Taken together, this means that respiratory distress in an infant may be subtle and heralded by tachypnea. In turn, because infants and small children have more type 2 respiratory muscle fibers, they are prone to fatigue. By 2 years of age, children have developed a rich supply of type 1 respiratory muscle fibers, which do not fatigue as easily.[36]

Additionally, because the rib cage of young children is highly compliant due to its cartilaginous nature, increased work of breathing doesn't necessarily translate into better alveolar ventilation because the chest wall collapses from the negative inspiratory pressure. The diaphragm is also very compliant[36] leading to a cephalad shift in the face of abdominal distension such as with a bowel obstruction and distension or gastric distension due to FMV. This limits reserve and achievable tidal volume while increasing the work of breathing and reducing FRC.[36] Decompression with a nasogastric tube is recommended to improve ventilation in the setting of gastric distention.

What Are the Effects of Respiratory Acidosis on Children?

Unlike metabolic acidosis, respiratory acidosis is well tolerated in children. Recent trials evaluating high-flow nasal cannula techniques to increase time to oxygen desaturation during intubation attempts have shown that children easily tolerate CO_2 levels of 65 mmHg for up to 10 minutes.[37,38] In the absence of increased intracranial pressure, concurrent metabolic acidosis, or pulmonary hypertension, it is reasonable to assume an $EtCO_2$ of mid-60s will be tolerated. In fact, a case series from 1990 showed five children aged 1 day to 6 months were able to tolerate permissive hypercapnia for 35 minutes to 2 days, with pH values of 6.7 to 7.1. All made a complete neurologic recovery.[39] This is further highlighted by a recent meta-analysis examining the effects of permissive hypercapnia in extremely low-birth-weight infants and their neurodevelopmental outcomes. Permissive hypercapnia was not associated with an increase in cerebral palsy, visual/hearing deficits, or reduced mental or psychomotor developmental scores.[40] Given a child's tolerance for hypercapnia, a more appropriate phrase in the setting of a difficult airway is "can't intubate, can't oxygenate" as opposed to "can't intubate, can't ventilate."

AIRWAY MANAGEMENT

How Do I Assess for a Difficult Airway in Pediatrics?

The mnemonics presented earlier (Chapter 1) with respect to the evaluation of the adult airway for difficulty are: **MOANS** for difficult FMV; **RODS** for difficult extraglottic device (EGD) ventilation; **LEMON** for difficult DL and intubation; and **SHORT** for a difficult front-of-neck airway access (FONA). These mnemonics do not translate directly to small children.

What Is the Role of Neuromuscular Blocking Agent Usage in the Pediatric Difficult Airway?

The first question when managing a difficult airway is whether a child should be awake or asleep. If the child will be put to sleep, the second question is whether muscle relaxants should be used. As a general rule, if a child is dependent on his or her own intrinsic muscle tone to keep an airway open, *don't paralyze*. For example, in infectious disease[41] or foreign body scenarios,[42] the anesthesia practitioner should seriously consider maintaining spontaneous ventilation.

In a 2005 survey of Canadian pediatric anesthesiologists, the majority favored spontaneous ventilation for all difficult airway scenarios they were given except where the airway was shared with a surgeon. Most preferred an inhalational induction technique while maintaining spontaneous ventilation.[43] Due to the risk of laryngospasm in these situations though, IM or IV succinylcholine should be readily available.

However, observational data collected from the PeDI registry found that controlled ventilation, with or without NMBA, was associated with fewer nonsevere complications when compared to spontaneous ventilation.[44] Light anesthesia and resultant airway reactivity were offered as an explanation for these findings.

How Do I Plan for a Difficult Airway? How Does My Planning Change Depending on Whether It Is an Anticipated or Unanticipated Difficult Airway?

An emphasis on oxygenation, as opposed to intubation, prevents task fixation (i.e., repeated attempts at intubation in the setting of poor oxygenation). The PeDI registry exemplified this by showing that 8.5% of patients had 5 or more intubation attempts and that >2 attempts at intubation resulted in more adverse events.[1] Anesthesia practitioners should always have a backup plan in the event that the airway is not able to be secured by traditional DL, and switch to an indirect approach early. Consideration for intubation with flexible bronchoscopy through an EGD in infants less than 1 year of age is supported by the literature[45] and making the first attempt with video laryngoscopy increases success on the first attempt (which always offers the best intubating conditions) when compared to a DL technique.[46] In fact, due to the low success rate of DL in anticipated pediatric difficult airways, this technique offers little advantage compared to video laryngoscopy. Providing supplemental oxygen throughout airway management should also be considered. Apneic oxygenation has been shown in the pediatric population to significantly reduce hypoxemia during intubation. Patients not receiving apneic oxygenation experienced hypoxemia in 50% of cases, while less than 25% had hypoxemia when apneic oxygenation was used.[47]

Planning for the anticipated difficult airway includes communication with all members of the health care team including parents and the child if appropriate. If FONA is a part of that plan, this should be discussed with the parents (and child as appropriate) (Table 46.2).

TABLE 46.2. Management of Anticipated versus Unanticipated Pediatric Difficult Airway

Anticipated
• Parents aware
• Child aware if appropriate age
• Surgeon in room scrubbed and ready with all equipment checked and assembled
• All health care providers aware
• Maintenance and extubation plan in place
• Plan well documented and discussed
Unanticipated
• Can I BMV this patient?
• If not, call for help, two-handed BMV technique
• Consider atropine now
• Consider succinylcholine if appropriate
• Insert an EGD while prepping for front-of-neck airway

AIRWAY DEVICES AND EQUIPMENT

What Size ETT Should I Use in a Child?

Tube sizes are measured in mm of internal diameter (ID) with the external diameter (OD) dependent on the material used and the manufacturer. The smallest uncuffed tube is 2.0-mm ID. The smallest cuffed tube is 2.5-mm ID. Sizes increase by 0.5 mm increments and the OD can vary greatly for the same ID.[48] Because of the large tracheal diameter of the adult airway (20-25 mm), the outer diameter may not be of significance. However, in children with tracheal diameters depending on age,[49] the size of the ETT wall may be a significant consideration. Pediatric ETTs also vary with respect to their beveled end and the presence of a Murphy's eye. Some ETTs have a flexible "beaked" tip that may help in advancing the ETT over a flexible bronchoscope (e.g., Parker Flex-Tip™ Tracheal Tubes, Mercury Medical, Clearwater, FL).

The location and material of the cuff on ETTs will also vary with the manufacturer. Most cuffs are made from polyvinyl chloride (PVC) but can also be made of thinner polyurethane. Polyurethane, such as is seen in the pediatric Microcuff® (Kimberly Clark, Atlanta, USA) has a lower sealing pressure than PVC.[50] An excellent review regarding the various types of pediatric tubes has recently been published by Leong and Black.[48]

The exact size of the tube that ought to be selected for a particular patient can be estimated by several means. Perhaps the best method is to use the length of the patient, such as used in the Broselow-Luten tape. Patient age is also commonly used. The Cole formula[51] originally published in 1957 based on age has been modified to:

Age/4 plus 4

The modified Cole formula was designed to be used for uncuffed tubes. If anything, it underestimates uncuffed tube size. It is recommended that the formula be modified for cuffed tubes to:

(Age/4 plus 4) minus 0.5

Neither the size of the smallest finger of a child nor the size of the external nares estimates ETT size accurately.

We recommend the anesthesia practitioner have the tube size predicted and both a half size larger and smaller immediately available.

Should I Use Cuffed or Uncuffed Endotracheal Tubes?

Cadaveric studies originally described the narrowest part of the pediatric airway as being the cricoid ring. This led to the use of uncuffed tubes because the cricoid ring was thought to provide a snug seal for the tube without the need for a cuff. Practitioners also preferred uncuffed tubes because older cuffed ETTs had high-pressure low-volume cuffs that were associated with ischemic airway mucosal damage and subsequent subglottic stenosis. However, with the increased availability of low-pressure, high-volume ETTs in pediatric sizes, the use of uncuffed tubes has decreased. A 2018 review found that a cuffed tube was chosen 77% of the time[52] and that there was no difference in postoperative respiratory complications between the two types of tubes. A survey sent to members of the Society of Pediatric Anesthesiologist found that the majority routinely used cuffed ETTs in neonates, infants, and children.[53] Those who were less than 5 years from fellowship used cuffed tubes more often than those with more than 20 years' experience, signaling the shift in practice.[53]

A prospective randomized controlled multicenter trial[54] studied the use of uncuffed tubes from various manufacturers and compared them to Microcuff tubes in children under 5 years of age. This study randomized over 2000 children and found the incidence of postoperative croup to be similar.[54] The authors of the study, however, emphasized that cuff pressures need to be monitored. The average cuff pressure was 10.6 cm H_2O, well under the threshold pressure of 25 cm H_2O. This pressure threshold with uncuffed tubes has previously been shown to increase morbidity.[55] It should also be noted that the conclusions drawn from this study might not be valid for cuffed ETTs from other manufacturers with thicker cuff walls, requiring perhaps higher cuff pressures needed to achieve a similar seal.

An interesting finding of this large study was that uncuffed tubes needed to be switched to an alternative size in 30% of patients. Cuffed tubes were switched out for another tube size only 2% of the time.[54] Considering that it has been shown that >2 attempts at DL increase the risk of airway complications,[1] using an appropriately sized cuffed ETT on the first attempt should decrease the number of intubation attempts. In the setting of a difficult airway, preventing the need to switch ETT sizes offers tremendous benefit.

Damage to the airway can occur with both cuffed and uncuffed tubes,[49,50,56,57] and the anesthesia practitioner should reflect and become familiar with the specifics of the ETTs they use in daily practice (e.g., different manufacturers have the cuffs in different positions, and some can herniate onto the vocal cords).

What Are the New Devices Available in Pediatric Sizes for the Management of the Difficult Airway?

Over the past 10 years, a number of new devices have been made available in pediatric sizes for routine, difficult, and failed airway management.

The video laryngoscopes include the GlideScope® (Verathon, Bothwell, Washington), the STORZ™ video laryngoscope (Karl Storz Endoscopy, Tuttlingen, Germany), and the Truview EVO2™ (Truphatek, Netanya, Israel). These devices combine and incorporate video technology into the tip of the laryngoscope blade. This allows images from beyond the tip of the blade to be displayed on video monitors, permitting one to "free hand" the ETT into the trachea. The GlideScope traditionally incorporates a 60-degree angulated distal tip ("hyperangulated" blade) (see Chapter 11). However, more recent pediatric equipment includes standard blades such as a Miller 0 and 1 blade equivalent with a video option. GlideScope use in anticipated difficult airways had an initial success rate of 53% (464/877) and an eventual success rate of 82% (720/877).[46] Furthermore, the device has been updated to allow for easier use with combined airway techniques. The GlideScope® Core™ Advanced Airway Visualization System screen can be split so that half of the screen is video laryngoscopy, while the other half shows the bronchoscope view. The sizes of BFlex™ single-use bronchoscope available for GlideScope are still relatively large (smallest for a 5.0-mm ID cuffed ETT).

The STORZ video laryngoscope comes in a wide variety of sizes appropriate for pediatric intubation with devices matching traditional laryngoscopes and less traditional options like a Macintosh 0 and 1 blade. It also has a hyperangulated "D" blade in some pediatric sizes for anterior airways. In healthy infants <10 kg, the C-MAC® Miller 0 and 1 blades have been shown to produce improved Cormack/Lehane views compared to traditional DL in the hands of experienced pediatric anesthesia practitioners.[58]

The Truview EVO2 is a rigid laryngoscope with an angulated tip that uses a series of prisms to transmit the image from the distal tip to an eyepiece. The tip is angulated 46 degrees anteriorly from the direct line-of-sight, and the device provides a wide-angle magnified view. A new version of this device called the Truview PCD has a video camera and screen that is mounted to a proximal eyepiece, converting it to a video laryngoscope (see Chapter 11). A randomized trial of the Truview PCD compared to the C-MAC and Macintosh blade suggested a better glottic visualization score using the Truview PCD in healthy 10- to 20-kg 1- to 6-year-old patients; however, the time to intubation was slightly longer compared to the C-MAC or Macintosh blades.[59]

The Airtraq™ (Prodol Meditec SA, Vizcaya, Spain) is a novel device that combines a video image with a tube delivery capability. The image provided to the practitioner is a magnified wide-angle view transmitted via a series of mirrors similar to that of a submarine periscope. Once the glottis is viewed, an ETT that has been preloaded into the ETT delivery channel is advanced into the trachea. This is a single-use device with antifogging capability at the distal tip of the blade. There is no need for an external monitor (see Chapter 11). A randomized, controlled trial of 20 infants and 40 children found longer intubation times for children but better laryngeal views for all patients with the Airtraq compared to DL.[60] Another randomized trial showed decreased number of attempts with the Airtraq compared to Macintosh blades in elective surgery for children 2 to 8 years old.[61] A comparison of the Airtraq and STORZ™ video laryngoscope found no difference in the success rate of intubation for 10 children less than 2 years old with a normal airway assessment.[62]

All of the above devices have been used to manage the pediatric difficult airway in case series and case reports.[63–73]

Many of the prospective studies involving the GlideScope[74–76] and STORZ video laryngoscope[77,78] compared to DL show that both these devices provide an improved view of the glottis in children with normal airway anatomy, but require a longer time for intubation. The longer time is probably not significant in clinical practice, and the benefit offered by an improved view likely outweighs the minimal increase in time. It is hypothesized that the longer time is due to inexperience with optical-laryngoscopes compared to DL. Perhaps the most convincing evidence comes from the PeDI database showing similar first-pass success rates of intubation with video laryngoscopes (404 of 786, 51%) compared to flexible bronchoscopic intubations (67 of 114, 59%) in the pediatric population greater than 1-year-old.[45]

Although there are a variety of available blades for use with video laryngoscopes, in the less than 5 kg population, it appears that more traditional shaped blades are more likely to be successful compared to hyperangulated blades. Traditional blades had 51% first-past success and 81% eventual success compared to nontraditional blades with 26% first-past success and 58% eventual success.[79]

Video laryngoscopes may be valuable for inexperienced anesthesia practitioners who encounter an infant with a difficult airway. A study of 30 anesthesia residents attempting to intubate the trachea of an infant with a difficult airway model (airway obstruction and neck immobilization) found higher success rates and shorter intubation times with video laryngoscopy compared to DL.[80]

Is There a Difference Between a Pediatric Flexible Bronchoscope Compared to the Adult Bronchoscope?

Apart from bronchoscope diameter, the answer is NO; there are no material differences between a flexible "pediatric bronchoscope" and an "adult bronchoscope." Generally, a bronchoscope (50-60 cm in length) that is less than 4.0 mm in tip diameter is called a "pediatric bronchoscope." Those larger than 4.0 mm in tip diameter tend to be called adult bronchoscopes.

The flexible bronchoscope remains the cornerstone of pediatric difficult airway management. Technological advances have allowed fiberoptic image transmission to be replaced by CMOS camera technology providing exceptionally high-quality images. These high-definition scopes with a "working channel" or suction channel are limited in size, the smallest being approximately 2.8 mm in tip diameter. Ultra-thin bronchoscopes without a suction channel have a tip diameter of 2.2 to 2.5 mm and are generally used as nasoendoscopes by ENT. The smallest flexible bronchoscope with a suction channel (2.8 mm) has poorer optical quality than the 2.5-mm scope without the suction channel because the channel takes up considerable space at the expense of light and optical fibers.

Which Extraglottic Devices Are Used in Children?

EGDs that are available for use in the pediatric population (below age 2 and <30 kg) include the following (see Chapter 13):

- The LMA family of devices, including the LMA-Classic™, the LMA-ProSeal™, and the LMA-Unique™, LMA-Supreme™ (Teleflex; Triangle Park, NC, USA)
- The air-Q™ (air-Q I™) (Salter Labs, Lake Forest, IL) (Figure 46.4)
- i-gel® (Wokingham, UK)

The Combitube™ and the EasyTube® are available in small adult sizes making them potentially useful for children older than 10 to 12 years. However, these have limited use in the operating room as they are primarily used as rescue devices.

Which Rescue Devices Are Available for Pediatric Patients? Is There an Intubating EGD for Pediatric Patients?

If there is difficulty with FMV, the above-named EGDs constitute the mainstay of nonsurgical rescue airway devices for infants and children <10 years of age. Which EGD is used likely depends on institutional availability. The LMA-ProSeal has been shown to provide a better laryngeal seal pressure than the LMA-Classic,[81,82] and incorporates an esophageal drain tube (the second-generation EGD) and a bite block. This device has been used with greater success when positive pressure ventilation is desired.[83] Other devices used include the CobraPLA™, the King LT/Laryngeal Tube™. Additionally, the i-gel is a second-generation EGD, which is suitable for positive pressure ventilation (Table 46.3).[84,85]

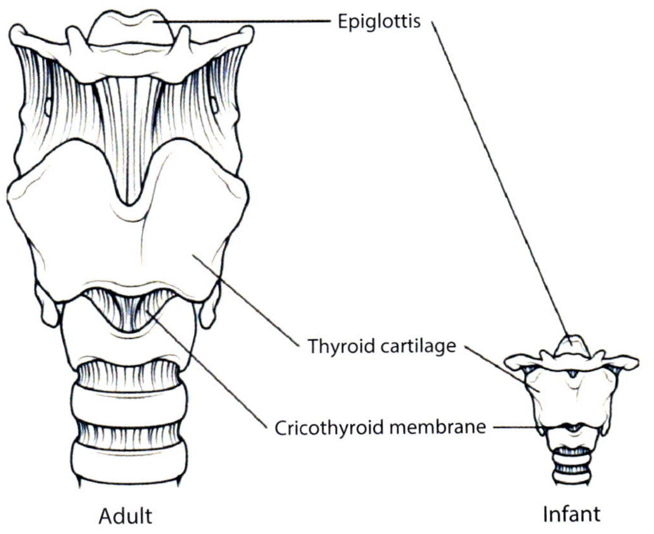

FIGURE 46.4. Size 1.5 air-Q. A total of four pediatric sizes available: 1, 1.5, 2, 2.5. Note the shorter, wider, curved airway tube which is similar in design to the adult LMA-Fastrach. This allows for placement of a cuffed ETT with the ability to easily remove the air-Q after successful tracheal intubation. (Reproduced with permission from Walls RM, Murphy MF, Luten R, et al. *Manual of Emergency Airway Management*. Philadelphia, PA: Lippincott Williams & Wilkins; 2004.)

In addition to EGDs being helpful in patients who are difficult to provide FMV,[22] they have been shown to be used effectively in children with difficult laryngoscopy as an alternative to tracheal intubation.[86]

There is no Fastrach-LMA™ (Intubating LMA) for pediatric patients. The smallest of these devices is a size #3, which is mostly appropriate for children >12 years old.

The air-Q can be utilized as a conduit for tracheal intubation, even in small children. Newer-generation air-Qs overcome many of the prior limitations of intubating through older-generation EGDs.[87] In a 2019 review discussing the "perfect" pediatric EGD, Huang et al. suggest that the air-Q EGD is the "best" device on the market based on its mask design (allows for positive pressure ventilation and facilitates flexible bronchoscopic intubation), airway tube design (short and wide to accommodate a flexible bronchoscope and ETT), and its overall practicality.[88] The air-Q is designed to minimize epiglottic downfolding and its short, wide tube provides a conduit for intubation.

Blind intubation through an EGD is not recommended due to a high incidence of failure (success rate of 15%);[89] however, flexible bronchoscopic intubation through an EGD is considered a highly effective method of securing a difficult airway. This may be the ideal method of intubation for infants with known or presumed difficult airways based on analysis from the PeDI database that showed higher first-attempt success by intubating through an EGD versus video laryngoscopy.[45] Table 46.3 highlights the various difficult airway equipment available for children.

AIRWAY MANAGEMENT ISSUES IN CHILDREN

Can Rapid Sequence Intubation (RSI) Be Employed in Children? If So, How Is It Done and Is It Safe?

When emergency intubation is indicated, RSI should be considered in pediatrics, just as it would be in adults. There should always be a concern for pulmonary aspiration in emergency situations; however, this may be a much rarer event in the pediatric population, with rates around 3 to 4 per 10,000 cases.[90] Although there are no randomized prospective studies, large series from multiple centers support the use of RSI in children and document its safety.[91,92] The sequence of events and drug selection for RSI are no different in children than they are in adults.

Important factors already alluded to must be considered in pediatric patients, especially those younger than 2 years of age. Due to the high oxygen consumption per minute and higher closing capacity in this age group, desaturation can occur very rapidly. In fact, hypoxemia will occur in 26 seconds for a child less than 1 year of age without any denitrogenation and in as little as 6.6 seconds for those less than 1 month old.[93]

For these reasons, some argue for modified RSI techniques. Apneic oxygenation significantly increases desaturation time in pediatric airways allowing for more manipulation time. In one study, apneic oxygenation increased the time for desaturation below 95% from 127 seconds to 202 seconds.[94]

SECTION 7

TABLE 46.3. Devices Available Along with Clinical Advantages and Limitations for the Management of the Difficult Pediatric Airway

Device	Advantages	Limitation
GlideScope	• Wide magnified view • Portable • Antifog camera	• May be difficult to overcome the curve of the blade when placing ETT • May have a suboptimal view in the bleeding airway • Requires moderate degree of mouth opening
Video laryngoscope	• Similar in use to DL • Panoramic view of laryngeal structures	• May have a suboptimal view in the bleeding airway • Requires some degree of mouth opening
Airtraq	• Portable/Disposable • Wide magnified view of laryngeal structures • Antifog camera	• May have a suboptimal view in the bleeding airway • Requires some degree of mouth opening
Flexible bronchoscope	• Use in limited mouth opening: nasal or oral • Can use in conjunction with EGD	• Learning curve • Expensive to clean • Less portable • May have a suboptimal view in the bleeding airway
Shikani Optical Stylet™ *Bonfils Intubation Fiberscope™*	• Use in limited mouth opening • Shikani Optical Stylet is somewhat malleable and can use with an EGD and tailor to patient's anatomy	• Short optical depth of field • No antifog capability • May have a suboptimal view in the bleeding airway
LMA-Classic	• Long history of reliability • Portable • Airway rescue • Conduit for tracheal intubation	• May require use of another visualization device (e.g., flexible bronchoscope) • Requires some degree of mouth opening • Cannot drain the stomach
LMA-ProSeal *LMA-Supreme*	• Same as above • Able to place a drain tube • Can ventilate at higher seal pressures	• May be more difficult to insert than LMA-Classic • Endotracheal intubation through this device more difficult than the LMA-Classic or air-Q • Requires some degree of mouth opening for placement
air-Q	• Portable • Airway rescue • Conduit for tracheal intubation • Designed for tracheal intubation • Evidence base for difficult airways • Stable in small children	• May require use of another visualization device (e.g., flexible bronchoscope) • Requires some degree of mouth opening for placement • Cannot drain the stomach
i-gel	• Stable in small children • Suitable for positive pressure ventilation • Able to place a drain tube • Can ventilate at higher seal pressures	• Requires some degree of mouth opening for placement • Can be used as a conduit for tracheal intubation

Others argue for modified RSI techniques with gentle ventilation (ventilating pressures 10-12 cm H_2O). In a study of 1001 children using gentle ventilating pressure after an RSI, there was noted to be less hypoxemia and desaturation events than previous studies and importantly, no episodes of pulmonary aspiration, although there was one episode of gastric regurgitation.[95]

The idea of not performing a traditional RSI is perhaps best highlighted by a retrospective analysis of 252 pyloric myotomy patients who underwent volatile induction instead of RSI. In this presumed high risk for aspiration population, there were no episodes of aspiration noted.[96]

Is Cricoid Pressure Useful in Children?

Sellick originally described the maneuver as applying external pressure to the cricoid ring to occlude the esophagus to prevent passive regurgitation of stomach contents during RSI.[97] Its success rate in preventing aspiration in adults and children has not been proven. In a 2001 survey of British pediatric anesthesiologists showed perceived benefit of the Sellick maneuver to be quite variable; only 49% would use cricoid pressure in an emergency case even with "known" risk factors (hiatal hernia, reflux, etc.).[98] Cricoid pressure was used more often by general anesthesia practitioners during an emergency case, 60% in infants and 96% in school-aged children.[99] Obviously, the question as to the efficacy of cricoid pressure remains unresolved.[100]

In a recent analysis of the NEAR4KIDs database looking at practice in 35 PICUs, there was no benefit in cricoid pressure to prevent gastric regurgitation. There was a 1.9% (35 of 1819) risk of regurgitation with cricoid pressure and a 1.2% (71 of 6002) risk without cricoid pressure.[101]

What has been shown in children, however, is that the Sellick maneuver is effective in decreasing gastric insufflation during BMV even with ventilation pressures exceeding 40 cm H_2O.[98,102] This is especially important in infants, in whom gastric distention may lead to decreased diaphragmatic excursion, decreased ability to ventilate, and increased risk of aspiration. For this reason, it may be reasonable to apply cricoid pressure during prolonged FMV recognizing that it may hinder one's view of the larynx on DL.[103]

Which NMBAs Should Be Used in Children?

The ideal NMBA varies depending on the clinical situation. Speed of onset, duration of action, and side-effect profile need to be weighed when choosing the appropriate drug.

In elective cases, with adequate denitrogenation and when the onset of action does not need to be less than 60 seconds, a drug with the fewest side effects can be chosen, such as rocuronium in standard doses (0.6-0.8 mg·kg^{-1}), depending on how fast the practitioner wishes for onset time and duration of blockade.

In emergency cases, the ideal drug is one that has a very rapid onset of effect. A short duration of action may also be of benefit in the event one needs to revert to spontaneous ventilation. Succinylcholine is the only depolarizing NMBA agent on the market. It has been available for over 50 years. Both succinylcholine (1.5 mg·kg^{-1}) and rocuronium (1.2 mg·kg^{-1}) produce good intubating conditions in less than 60 seconds in healthy children.[104] Sixty seconds of apnea after effective denitrogenation for 2 minutes may be well tolerated in children including infants undergoing elective intubation;[105] however, this may not be the case in an emergency situation where denitrogenation is suboptimal.[106]

Whether high-dose rocuronium (1.2 mg·kg^{-1}) has a similar onset time as succinylcholine (1.5-2 mg·kg^{-1}) in children remains unclear. A 2015 Cochrane review of the literature evaluating rocuronium versus succinylcholine in RSI, mostly adult studies, found that succinylcholine (1.5-2 mg·kg^{-1}) created superior intubation conditions versus rocuronium at any dose less than 1.2 mg·kg^{-1}. It was concluded that succinylcholine was clinically superior as it has a shorter duration of action.[107] With the introduction of sugammadex as a reversal agent for rocuronium, succinylcholine may not play as pivotal a role in emergency situations.

Although sugammadex has not been approved by the FDA for usage in the pediatric population, numerous studies and reviews have shown sugammadex to be an effective reversal agent of deep rocuronium neuromuscular blockade and well tolerated.[108–110]

Due to its safety and the ability to achieve fast and good intubating conditions with rocuronium, the strategy of using high-dose rocuronium for intubation when needed is acceptable as long as sugammadex is readily available for reversal.

Can I Use Succinylcholine (Suxamethonium) in Children?

Arguably, the drug that has received the most attention in the pediatric anesthesia literature is succinylcholine. In order to understand the indications and concerns, it is important to understand its history.

In December 1993, one manufacturer of the drug identified 36 deaths in young children and adolescents secondary to cardiac arrhythmias/arrest and recommended that the drug should not be used in children. The cardiac arrhythmias/arrest carried a mortality rate that exceeded 50% and were thought to be due to undiagnosed muscular dystrophies, especially Duchenne muscular dystrophy in males less than 8.[111]

The FDA initially recommended the addition of a warning label cautioning that rare hyperkalemic arrest can occur, notably in boys under 8. After further analysis, this warning was upgraded to a *relative contraindication* in children under the age of 16 years.[111] The response from the pediatric anesthesia community was swift: succinylcholine was too important a drug in emergency situations to be taken away altogether. The argument was made that more deaths would occur by NOT giving succinylcholine in life-saving airway securement than would be prevented in rare cases of undiagnosed muscular dystrophies. The FDA downgraded their recommendation to a *warning* in 1994.[112]

In a recent pro-con debate regarding the use of succinylcholine in pediatrics, both debaters agreed that when NMBAs are indicated, *succinylcholine should be reserved for those emergency children where the airway needs to be secured in the fastest means possible*. The debaters also agreed that succinylcholine should not be used in elective pediatric patients.[113]

Furthermore, succinylcholine remains a cornerstone of care of laryngospasm management and should be considered as a definitive management in this clinical scenario. Succinylcholine is frequently used in pediatric anesthesia for this indication.

Should NMBA Be Used in Pediatrics When a Difficult Airway Is Predicted?

It depends on why the airway is predicted to be difficult. If the patency of the airway is reliant on the patient's muscle tone, NMBA is contraindicated. However, if the child's muscle tone is the problem, such as in the case of laryngospasm, NMBA can be required. In the POCA Registry, laryngospasm was the most common reason for airway obstruction.[4]

NMBA may decrease the risk of difficult tracheal intubation.[114] In those clinical situations where the airway needs to be secured quickly, such as in the case of pyloric stenosis or postoperative tonsillar bleed, NMBA may help decrease the time required to intubate the trachea of a patient by improving the laryngeal view. In this situation, the practitioner should use the NMBA with the most rapid onset.

Whichever way is chosen, as previously mentioned, based on a retrospective review of the PeDI database, it appears there are less nonsevere complications in difficult airways when ventilation is controlled (with or without NMBAs) compared to spontaneous ventilation due to a higher risk of laryngospasm and hypoxemia in the spontaneous ventilation group possibly due to light anesthesia.[44]

AIRWAY MANAGEMENT AT VARIOUS AGES

How Do I Intubate the Trachea of a Child Less Than 2 Years Old Using DL?

The larynx is in a more cephalad position near the third cervical vertebrae instead of the fifth cervical vertebrae in the adult. Lying over the laryngeal inlet is a large floppy omega-shaped epiglottis. During DL, it is much easier to lift the epiglottis along with the tongue with a straight or Miller blade than it is to have the tongue follow the blade when compressing the hyoepiglottic ligament in the vallecula with a curved or Macintosh blade. Usually, the posterior third of the tongue will obscure the view of the glottis with a curved blade in the vallecula. Although many authors describe the larynx as "anterior" in the young child, it is actually cephalad, tucked up under the tongue at the angle of the mandible.

Given the acute angle between the oropharynx and the laryngeal inlet, styletted tubes are very helpful for this age group.

Why Is It Difficult to Intubate the Trachea of Micrognathic Infants by DL?

An "anterior" airway may be seen in the setting of micrognathia, such as in the Pierre Robin Sequence (Figure 46.1). In this case, the tongue lies against the posterior oropharyngeal wall causing upper airway obstruction. It is nearly impossible to compress the tongue into the mandibular space, because there isn't any space. A straight or Miller-type blade can be used in a "paraglossal" manner by placing the blade along the buccal mucosa, lifting the epiglottis from the side of the mouth, and avoiding the tongue altogether. The paraglossal technique has been quite successful in this patient population.[27]

Are There Other Alternatives to DL in This Age Group?

Infant and pediatric sizes of the Airtraq, the GlideScope, and the STORZ video laryngoscope are available (approximating a Miller 0 or 1 blade in size). A very good alternative to DL is flexible bronchoscopic intubation through an extraglottic device. The extraglottic device serves as a conduit to direct the bronchoscope to the laryngeal inlet. Further details are provided in the sections below.[115]

Is Blind Nasotracheal Intubation an Option in Children?

Two combined anatomic variations conspire against *blind* nasotracheal intubation in children less than 10 years of age: the presence of nasopharyngeal adenoidal tissue that is frequently enlarged and the acute angle of the higher riding upper airway in the nasopharynx in the child as opposed to the adult.[116]

Adenoidal tissue is often dissected and lodges in the lumen of the nasotracheal tube. The injury may lead to bleeding, hindering visualization. The dissected adenoid tissue, if not recognized and removed, can be forced into the lung leading to obstruction.

While blind techniques are fraught with hazards, video-assisted techniques may be more successful and safer and include:

- An indirect visualization technique using a flexible bronchoscope in small infants and children with small mouth openings[117]
- A nasotracheal tube passed to the oropharynx and placed into the airway with Magill forceps under oral laryngoscopic view using a GlideScope or STORZ video laryngoscope

I Am Planning on Extubating an Infant with a Difficult Airway. Will I Be Able to Extubate Over an Airway Exchange Catheter?

The ASA Difficult Airway Algorithm recommends the use of an airway exchange catheter upon tracheal extubation in adult patients with a difficult airway. This also applies to the pediatric population. Cook Critical Care supplies airway exchange catheters made for ETTs greater than 3-mm ID.

FRONT-OF-NECK AIRWAY ACCESS (FONA) IN CHILDREN (SURGICAL AIRWAYS, CANNULA AIRWAYS, ETC.)

What Is the Appropriate Technique to Obtain Front-of-Neck Airway Access in Children Less Than 8 Years Old?

The need for an emergency FONA in a child of this age is rare, particularly since the introduction of EGDs. A traditional scalpel cricothyrotomy is NOT an option in children less than 8 due to the small size of the cricothyroid membrane; however, a cannula/needle technique may be accommodated even in small infants with appropriate positioning and device selection. A more traditional scalpel cricothyrotomy can be performed in children older than 8. Table 46.4 and Figure 46.5 show the relative sizes and anatomic differences between the adult and infant cricothyroid membranes, respectively.

Although rarely performed in the pediatric population, a practitioner must be able to recognize a "can't intubate, can't ventilate/oxygenate" situation and take the next steps to rectify this situation. In an ideal world, an ENT or general pediatric surgeon would be available to perform the FONA; however, in the situation when these resources are present, airway practitioners must be familiar with the next steps.

Perhaps the easiest method is to rely on a kit-based approach to eliminate decision hesitancy.[118] Due to FONA rarity, there

TABLE 46.4. Relative Sizes of the Cricothyroid Membrane According to Age

Age	<2 years	2 to 8 years	Adult
Cricothyroid membrane dimensions	3 mm × 2.5 mm	10 mm × 8-10 mm	25 mm × 20 mm

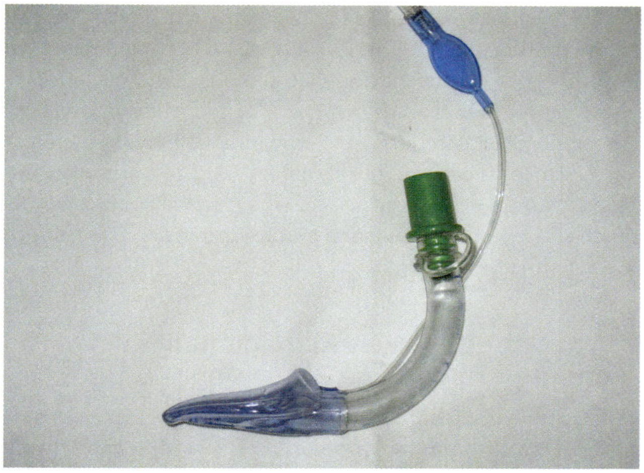

FIGURE 46.5. Adult larynx (left) versus infant larynx (right). Note the difference in size of the cricothyroid membrane. Also see Table 46.4 for dimensions of the cricothyroid membrane in various age groups.

is insufficient evidence to recommend one method or another. Rather, principles such as early recognition, swift decision-making, and patient-focused teamwork are key.

Although a scalpel-based technique is recommended in adults due to possibly higher success rates,[118] this may not be the ideal approach in children due to smaller airway and membrane sizes. In a pediatric model studying anesthesia practitioners using piglets, a scalpel tracheotomy approach was shown to have higher success rates (97% in a 4-minute time frame) than transtracheal cannula-based techniques (65%-68% success within 42 seconds to 69 seconds depending on the device used).[119] However, this is in contrast with a rabbit model study evaluating a scalpel technique compared to the Cook MELKER cricothyroidotomy kit performed under the 1st/2nd tracheal ring, which showed 75% and 100% success, respectively.[120]

Importantly, an airway practitioner can become competent enough to produce acceptable results. Fifty physicians from multiple backgrounds watched an instructional video and then performed scalpel-based tracheotomies on a rabbit model with impressive improvement in technique, time, and complication rate. After 10 attempts, the median time was 55 seconds, had a success rate of 94%, and a complication rate of 14%.[121]

Currently, the Association of Paediatric Anesthetists of Great Britain and Ireland (APAGBI) and Difficult Airway Society (DAS) guidelines recommend a cannula/needle approach at either the level of the cricothyroid membrane or the tracheal membrane in the absence of an ENT specialist.[22] Using a rabbit model to approximate an infant airway, two proceduralists demonstrated a 60% success rate with a cannula approach via a tracheostomy site.[122] In this same model, the QuickTrach Child (a percutaneous device with a 2-mm ID from VBM, Germany) was unsuccessful.[122]

An alternative to a FONA may be rigid laryngoscopy or bronchoscopy, although few nonsurgically trained practitioners have experience with this technique. Rigid techniques are usually immediately available in the OR setting for anticipated difficult airway scenarios, such as foreign body removal or post-tonsillectomy bleed. This approach calls for advance planning with the surgical team and preparation of necessary equipment.

How Do I Perform a Needle Tracheotomy (see also Chapter 14)?

1. A specific needle cricothyrotomy device is connected to a 3-mL saline-filled syringe.
2. The tracheal cartilage is palpated.
3. Air is aspirated via the device into the syringe.
4. The needle from the device is withdrawn.
5. The device is then attached to an ETT adaptor to allow BMV (ETT adaptor size depends on the kit).

Can I Use an Intravenous Catheter as a Needle Cricothyrotomy Device?

The use of an intravenous catheter is not recommended due to a much higher rate of kinking at the skin with resulting obstruction. However, 14-18G devices, depending on patient size, have been used in numerous rabbit models with success.[118]

What Commercially Manufactured Needle Cricothyrotomy Devices Are Available for Children?

Catheters manufactured for this specific task can be seen in Figure 46.6. These are Quicktrach Child (14G) and Baby version (16G) (VBM Laboratories, Germany).[23] These are Teflon©-coated catheters and have been used electively in laryngeal surgery, including children. Another option is the Arndt emergency cricothyrotomy kit (Cook Medical, Bloomington, IN, USA) that can also be placed transtracheally. It has a 3-mm internal diameter and an 18-gauge outer diameter. However, it is relatively long (6 cm) for a small child. The Cook Melkner cricothyroidotomy catheter (Cook Medical, Bloomington, IN,

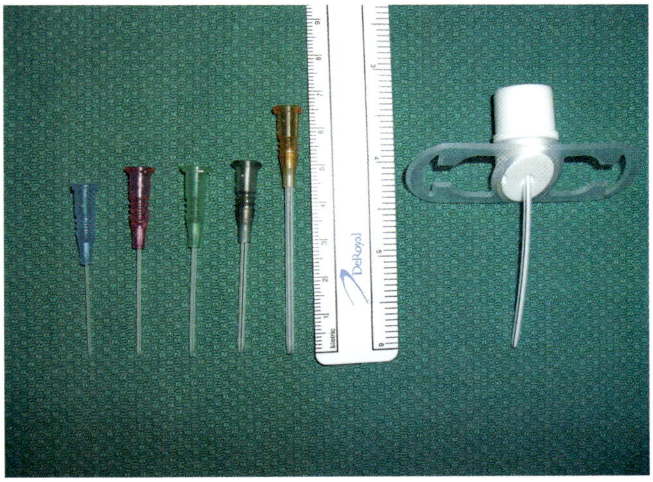

FIGURE 46.6. Ravussin needle tracheotomy catheter.

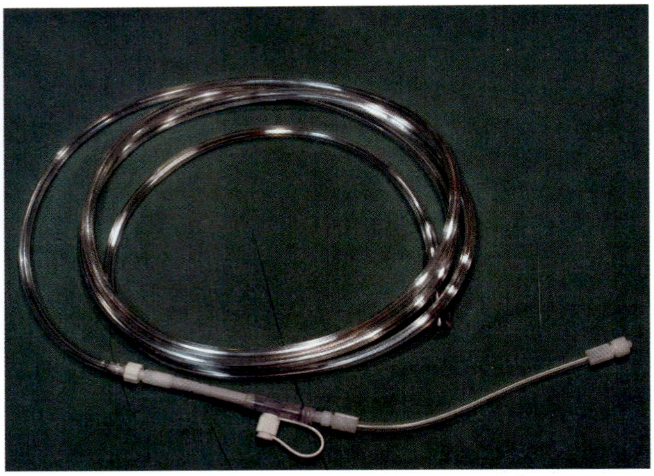

FIGURE 46.7. Enk Oxygen Flow Modulator used in conjunction with an emergency transtracheal catheter when conventional ventilation by mask or endotracheal tube cannot be performed.

USA) was also used in some of the above rabbit models, with an ID size of 3.5 mm and a length of 3.8 cm.

If Needle Tracheotomy Is So Rare in Children, What Oxygen Flow Has Proven to Work and Are There Any Recommendations on How Much Flow to Provide via the Catheter?

The best evidence is in the pig animal model.[123,124] Adequate oxygenation has been demonstrated in the pig model using a low-pressure oxygen supply (i.e., wall-oxygen at 1-15 L·min^{-1}) attached to an Enk Oxygen Flow Regulator (Cook Medical, Figure 46.7). This technique has been shown to provide effective oxygenation for at least 15 minutes.[125,126] A more recent study in rabbits did show a failure to oxygenate some rabbits from an SpO_2 of 75% back to 90% with flow rates at 1 to 15 L·kg^{-1}·min^{-1} but death occurred from barotrauma at a rate of 1.5 L·kg^{-1}·min^{-1}.[127] To date, there are no pediatric case reports or series in the literature using this device.

The two best systems to provide oxygen flow via a cannula are the Enk Oxygen Flow Modulator (Cook Inc, Bloomington, IN, USA) and the Rapid-O2™ insufflator (Meditech Systems Ltd, Shaftesbury, UK). The Enk Oxygen Flow Modulator has five side holes on the device that should all be occluded to deliver appropriate flow during use.[128] The Pediatric Advanced Life Support (PALS course) recommends 100 mL·kg^{-1}·min^{-1}. The Advanced Pediatric Life Support (APLS) course recommends 1 L·min^{-1} per year of age, which has also been recommended based on experimental studies using the Enk Oxygen Flow Modulator.[128]

What About Airway Management in Children Above Age 2?

As stated above, once the child has reached the age of 2, airway management with the exception of size is less "different" than it is before the age of 2. Table 46.5 summarizes airway management issues in older age groups.

SUMMARY

Pediatric airway management engenders fear in most airway practitioners who do not manage children on a daily basis, particularly when the difficult or failed airway is encountered. This fear is compounded by the need to rapidly adjust drug dosages for size and weight, the limited availability of age- and size-specific equipment, and the challenges surrounding surgical airway management in the young child. This chapter is meant to assist such practitioners in accessing rapid reference guides for tackling the difficult pediatric airway.

SELF-EVALUATION QUESTIONS

46.1. Regarding succinylcholine (suxamethonium) use in children under 16 years of age:

A. The FDA defines it as relatively contraindicated.
B. The FDA defines it as contraindicated.
C. The FDA has approved it only in emergency situations.
D. The FDA has warned against its use in various settings.
E. The FDA has never issued any warning regarding its use.

TABLE 46.5. Summary of Airway Management Options in Older Age Groups

Age (years)	2 to 8	8 to 16
Airway Changes	Muscle tone increases, as does the caliber of the aerodigestive tract. The epiglottis becomes firmer and less wide and floppy.	Similar configuration to the adult airway
BMV	Sizing of the mask is the same as in adults	Sizing of the mask is the same as in adults
EGD	LMA-ProSeal, LMA-Classic, LMA-Unique, air-Q	Above 30 kg more options available such as LMA-Fastrach, Combitube, SLIPA™
Direct laryngoscopy	The curved or Macintosh blade becomes more useful	Analogous to the adult
Beyond laryngoscopy	Video laryngoscopes (e.g., GlideScope, flexible bronchoscope)	All airway devices available, just as in adults
Surgical options	Formal tracheotomy or needle tracheotomy	Formal cricothyrotomy, as in adults

46.2. Cuffed endotracheal tubes:

A. Are associated with increased airway injury compared to uncuffed tubes in children less than 2 years.

B. Have not been associated with increased airway injury in children less than 2 years compared to uncuffed tubes.

C. Have to have their cuff pressure measured and maintained at less than 30 cm H_2O.

D. Are not available for children less than 2 years.

E. Should not be used for infants.

46.3. Transtracheal jet ventilation is:

A. An invasive airway option in the ASA difficult airway algorithm.

B. Uses oxygen from a high-pressure source (i.e., pipeline oxygen).

C. Uses oxygen from a high-flow source (i.e., wall oxygen).

D. Is commonly used as a rescue device in children under 8 years of age.

E. Is associated with minimal side effects according to the ASA Closed Claims Studies.

46.4. Which of the following is true regarding rapid sequence intubation (RSI) in children?

A. Rocuronium is the drug of choice.

B. Cricoid pressure improves laryngoscopic grade upon direct laryngoscopy.

C. It is safer in adults versus infants.

D. Cricoid pressure is effective in decreasing gastric insufflation even with ventilation pressures greater than 40 cm H_2O.

E. RSI is contraindicated in neonates.

REFERENCES

1. Fiadjoe JE, Nishisaki A, Jagannathan N, et al. Airway management complications in children with difficult tracheal intubation from the Pediatric Difficult Intubation (PeDI) registry: a prospective cohort analysis. *Lancet Respir Med.* 2016;4:37-48.
2. Habre W., Disma N., Virag K., et al. Incidence of severe critical events in paediatric anaesthesia (APRICOT): a prospective multicentre observational study in 261 hospitals in Europe. *Lancet Respir Med.* 2017;5:412-425.
3. Egbuta C, Mason KP. Recognizing risks and optimizing perioperative care to reduce respiratory complications in the pediatric patient. *J Clin Med.* 2020;9(6):1942.
4. Ramamoorthy C, Haberkern CM, Bhananker SM, et al. Anesthesia-related cardiac arrest in children with heart disease: data from the Pediatric Perioperative Cardiac Arrest (POCA) registry. *Anesth Analg.* 2010;110:1376-1382.
5. Gálvez JA, Acquah S, Ahumada L, et al. Hypoxemia, bradycardia, and multiple laryngoscopy attempts during anesthetic induction in infants: a single-center, retrospective study. *Anesthesiology.* 2019;131(4):830-839.
6. Mamie C, Habre W, Delhumeau C, Barazzone Argiroffo C, Morabia A. Incidence and risk factors of perioperative respiratory adverse events in children undergoing elective surgery. *Pediatr Anesth.* 2004;14(3):218-224.
7. Bhananker SM, Ramamoorthy C, Geiduschek JM, et al. Anesthesia-related cardiac arrest in children: update from the Pediatric Perioperative Cardiac Arrest Registry. *Anesth Analg.* 2007;105:344-350.
8. Marshall S. The use of cognitive aids during emergencies in anesthesia: a review of the literature. *Anesth Analg.* 2013;117:1162-1171.
9. Lubitz DS, Seidel JS, Chameides L, et al. A rapid method for estimating weight and resuscitation drug dosages from length in the pediatric age group. *Ann Emerg Med.* 1988;17:576-581.
10. Luten RC, Wears RL, Broselow J, et al. Length-based endotracheal tube and emergency equipment in pediatrics. *Ann Emerg Med.* 1992;21:900-904.
11. Valois-Gómez T, Oofuvong M, Auer G, et al. Incidence of difficult bag-mask ventilation in children: a prospective observational study. *Paediatr Anaesth.* 2013;23:920-926.
12. Daigle CH, Fiadjoe JE, Laverriere EK, et al. Difficult bag-mask ventilation in critically ill children is independently associated with adverse events. *Crit Care Med.* 2020;48(9):744-752.
13. Becker HJ, Langhan ML. Can providers use clinical skills to assess the adequacy of ventilation in children during bag-valve mask ventilation? *Pediatr Emerg Care.* 2020;36(12):e695-e699.
14. Kheterpal S, Han R, Tremper KK, et al. Incidence and predictors of difficult and impossible mask ventilation. *Anesthesiology.* 2006;105(5):885-891.
15. Tong D, Litman R. The Children"s Hospital of Philadelphia Difficult Intubation Registry (P43). 2007. Available at: http://www2.pedsanesthesia.org/meetings/2007winter/pdfs/P43.pdf.
16. Sawyer T, Foglia EE, Ades A, et al. Incidence, impact and indicators of difficult intubations in the neonatal intensive care unit: a report from the National Emergency Airway Registry for Neonates. *Arch Dis Child Fetal Neonatal Ed.* 2019;104(5):F461-F466.
17. Heinrich S, Birkholz T, Ihmsen H, et al. Incidence and predictors of difficult laryngoscopy in 11,219 pediatric anesthesia procedures. *Paediatr Anaesth.* 2012;22:729-736.
18. Akpek EA, Mutlu H, Kayhan Z. Difficult intubation in pediatric cardiac anesthesia. *J Cardiothorac Vasc Anesth.* 2004;18:610-612.
19. Graciano AL, Tamburro R, Thompson AE, Fiadjoe J, Nadkarni VM, Nishisaki A. Incidence and associated factors of difficult tracheal intubations in pediatric ICUs: a report from National Emergency Airway Registry for Children: NEAR4KIDS. *Intensive Care Med.* 2014;40(11):1659-1669.
20. Nargozian C. The airway in patients with craniofacial abnormalities. *Paediatr Anaesth.* 2004;14:53-59.
21. Bence CM, Wagner AJ. Ex utero intrapartum treatment (EXIT) procedures. *Semin Pediatr Surg.* 2019;28(4):150820.
22. Black AE, Flynn PER, Smith HL, et al. Development of a guideline for the management of the unanticipated difficult airway in pediatric practice. *Paediatr Anaesth.* 2015;25:346-362.
23. Huang AS, Hajduk J, Rim C, Coffield S, Jagannathan N. Focused review on management of the difficult paediatric airway. *Indian J Anaesth.* 2019;63(6):428-436.
24. Krishna S, Bryant J, Tobias J. Management of the difficult airway in the pediatric patient. *J Pediatr Intensive Care.* 2018;07(03):115-125.
25. Bergeson PS, Shaw JC. Are infants really obligatory nasal breathers? *Clin Pediatr (Phila).* 2001;40:567-569.
26. Santillanes G, Gausche-Hill M. Pediatric airway management. *Emerg Med Clin North Am.* 2008;26:961-975, ix.
27. Semjen F, Bordes M, Cros AM. Intubation of infants with Pierre Robin syndrome: the use of the paraglossal approach combined with a gum-elastic bougie in six consecutive cases. *Anaesthesia.* 2008;63(2):147-150.
28. Passi Y, Sathyamoorthy M, Lerman J, et al. Comparison of the laryngoscopy views with the size 1 Miller and Macintosh laryngoscope blades lifting the epiglottis or the base of the tongue in infants and children <2 yr of age. *Br J Anaesth.* 2014;113:869-874.
29. Bingham RM, Proctor LT. Airway management. *Pediatr Clin North Am.* 2008;55:873-886, ix-x.
30. Litman RS, Weissend EE, Shibata D, et al. Developmental changes of laryngeal dimensions in unparalyzed, sedated children. *Anesthesiology.* 2003;98:41-45.
31. Tobias JD. Pediatric airway anatomy may not be what we thought: implications for clinical practice and the use of cuffed endotracheal tubes. *Pediatr Anesth.* 2015;25:9-19.
32. Wani TM, Rafiq M, Talpur S, Soualmi L, Tobias JD. Pediatric upper airway dimensions using three-dimensional computed tomography imaging. *Paediatr Anaesth.* 2017;27(6):604-608.
33. Dalal PG, Murray D, Messner AH, et al. Pediatric laryngeal dimensions: an age-based analysis. *Anesth Analg.* 2009;108:1475-1479.
34. Holzki J, Brown KA, Carroll RG, Coté CJ. The anatomy of the pediatric airway: Has our knowledge changed in 120 years? A review of historic and recent investigations of the anatomy of the pediatric larynx. *Paediatr Anaesth.* 2018;28(1):13-22.
35. Kwon JH, Shin YH, Gil NS, Yeo H, Jeong JS. Analysis of the functionally-narrowest portion of the pediatric upper airway in sedated children. *Med (United States).* 2018;97(27).
36. Neumann RP, Von Ungern-Sternberg BS. The neonatal lung – physiology and ventilation. *Pediatr Anesth.* 2014;24(1):10-21.

SECTION 7

37. Humphreys S., Lee-Archer P., Reyne G., et. al. Transnasal humidified rapid-insufflation ventilatory exchange (THRIVE) in children: a randomized controlled trial. *Br J Anaesth*. 2017;118:232-238.
38. Riva T, Pedersen TH, Seiler S, et al. Transnasal humidified rapid insufflation ventilatory exchange for oxygenation of children during apnea: a prospective randomized controlled trial. *Br J Anaesth*. 2018;120:592-599.
39. Goldstein B, Shannon DC, Todres ID. Supercarbia in children: clinical course and outcome. *Crit Care Med*. 1990;18(2):166-168.
40. Ma J, Ye H. Effects of permissive hypercapnia on pulmonary and neurodevelopmental sequelae in extremely low birth weight infants: a meta-analysis. *Springerplus*. 2016;5(1):764.
41. Jenkins IA, Saunders M. Infections of the airway. *Paediatr Anaesth*. 2009;19(Suppl 1):118-130.
42. Zur KB, Litman RS. Pediatric airway foreign body retrieval: surgical and anesthetic perspectives. *Paediatr Anaesth*. 2009;19(Suppl 1):109-117.
43. Brooks P, Ree R, Rosen D, et al. Canadian pediatric anesthesiologists prefer inhalational anesthesia to manage difficult airways. *Can J Anaesth*. 2005;52:285-290.
44. Garcia-Marcinkiewicz AG, Adams HD, Gurnaney H, et al.; PeDI Collaborative. A retrospective analysis of neuromuscular blocking drug use and ventilation technique on complications in the pediatric difficult intubation registry using propensity score matching. *Anesth Analg*. 2020;131(2):469-479
45. Burjek NE, Nishisaki A, Fiadjoe JE, et al. Videolaryngoscopy versus fiber-optic intubation through a supraglottic airway in children with a difficult airway: an analysis from the Multicenter Pediatric Difficult Intubation Registry. *Anesthesiology*. 2017;127(3):432-440.
46. Park R, Peyton JM, Fiadjoe JE, et al. The efficacy of GlideScope® videolaryngoscopy compared with direct laryngoscopy in children who are difficult to intubate: an analysis from the paediatric difficult intubation registry. *Br J Anaesth*. 2017;119(5):984-992.
47. Vukovic AA, Hanson HR, Murphy SL, Mercurio D, Sheedy CA, Arnold DH. Apneic oxygenation reduces hypoxemia during endotracheal intubation in the pediatric emergency department. *Am J Emerg Med*. 2019;37(1):27-32.
48. Leong L, Black AE. The design of pediatric tracheal tubes. *Paediatr Anaesth*. 2009;19(Suppl 1):38-45.
49. Dullenkopf A, Kretschmar O, Knirsch W, et al. Comparison of tracheal tube cuff diameters with internal transverse diameters of the trachea in children. *Acta Anaesthesiol Scand*. 2006;50:201-205.
50. Dullenkopf A, Schmitz A, Gerber AC, et al. Tracheal sealing characteristics of pediatric cuffed tracheal tubes. *Paediatr Anaesth*. 2004;14:825-830.
51. Cole F. Pediatric formulas for the anesthesiologist. *AMA J Dis Child*. 1957;94:672-673.
52. de Wit M, Peelen LM, van Wolfswinkel L, de Graaff JC. The incidence of postoperative respiratory complications: a retrospective analysis of cuffed vs uncuffed tracheal tubes in children 0-7 years of age. *Paediatr Anaesth*. 2018 Mar;28(3):210-217.
53. Sathyamoorthy M, Lerman J, Okhomina VI, Penman AD. Use of cuffed tracheal tubes in neonates, infants and children: a practice survey of members of the Society of Pediatric Anesthesia. *J Clin Anesth*. 2016;33:266-272.
54. Weiss M, Dullenkopf A, Fischer JE, et al. Prospective randomized controlled multi-centre trial of cuffed or uncuffed endotracheal tubes in small children. *Br J Anaesth*. 2009;103:867-873.
55. Suominen P, Taivainen T, Tuominen N, et al. Optimally fitted tracheal tubes decrease the probability of postextubation adverse events in children undergoing general anesthesia. *Paediatr Anaesth*. 2006;16:641-647.
56. Holzki J, Laschat M, Puder C. Iatrogenic damage to the pediatric airway. Mechanisms and scar development. *Paediatr Anaesth*. 2009;19(Suppl 1):131-146.
57. Holzki J, Laschat M, Puder C. Stridor is not a scientifically valid outcome measure for assessing airway injury. *Paediatr Anaesth*. 2009;19(Suppl 1):180-197.
58. Raimann FJ, Cuca CE, Kern D, et al. Evaluation of the C-MAC Miller video laryngoscope sizes 0 and 1 during tracheal intubation of infants less than 10 kg. *Pediatr Emerg Care*. 2020;36(7):312-316.
59. Singh R, Kumar N, Jain A. A randomised trial to compare Truview PCD®, C-MAC® and Macintosh laryngoscopes in paediatric airway management. *Asian J Anesthesiol*. 2017;55(2):41-44.
60. White MC, Marsh CJ, Beringer RM, et al. A randomised, controlled trial comparing the Airtraq™ optical laryngoscope with conventional laryngoscopy in infants and children. *Anaesthesia*. 2012;67:226-231.
61. Orozco JA, Rojas JL, Medina-Vera AJ. Respuesta hemodinámica y efectividad de la intubación orotraqueal con Airtraq® versus laringoscopio Macintosh en pacientes pediátricos sometidos a cirugía electiva: estudio prospectivo, aleatorizado y ciego. *Rev Esp Anestesiol Reanim*. 2018;65(1): 24-30.
62. Sørensen MK, Holm-Knudsen R. Endotracheal intubation with airtraq® versus storz® videolaryngoscope in children younger than two years - a randomized pilot-study. *BMC Anesthesiol*. 2012;12:7.
63. Aucoin S, Vlatten A, Hackmann T. Difficult airway management with the Bonfils fiberscope in a child with Hurler syndrome. *Paediatr Anaesth*. 2009;19:441-442.
64. Bishop S, Clements P, Kale K, et al. Use of GlideScope Ranger in the management of a child with Treacher Collins syndrome in a developing world setting. *Paediatr Anaesth*. 2009;19:695-696.
65. Caruselli M, Zannini R, Giretti R, et al. Difficult intubation in a small for gestational age newborn by bonfils fiberscope. *Paediatr Anaesth*. 2008;18:990-991.
66. Kim H-J, Kim J-T, Kim H-S, et al. A comparison of GlideScope(®) videolaryngoscopy and direct laryngoscopy for nasotracheal intubation in children. *Paediatr Anaesth*. 2011;21:417-441.
67. Milne AD, Dower AM, Hackmann T. Airway management using the pediatric GlideScope in a child with Goldenhar syndrome and atypical plasma cholinesterase. *Paediatr Anaesth*. 2007;17:484-487.
68. Pfitzner L, Cooper MG, Ho D. The Shikani Seeing Stylet for difficult intubation in children: initial experience. *Anaesth Intensive Care*. 2002;30:462-466.
69. Shukry M, Hanson RD, Koveleskie JR, et al. Management of the difficult pediatric airway with Shikani Optical Stylet. *Paediatr Anaesth*. 2005;15:344-345.
70. Vlatten A, Aucoin S, Gray A, et al. Difficult airway management with the STORZ video laryngoscope in a child with Robin Sequence. *Paediatr Anaesth*. 2009;19:700-701.
71. Vlatten A, Soder C. Airtraq optical laryngoscope intubation in a 5-month-old infant with a difficult airway because of Robin Sequence. *Paediatr Anaesth*. 2009;19:699-700.
72. Xue FS, Liao X, Zhang YM, et al. More maneuvers to facilitate endotracheal intubation using the Bonfils fiberscope in children with difficult airways. *Paediatr Anaesth*. 2009;19:418-419.
73. Xue FS, Zhang YM, Liao X, et al. Measures to decrease failed intubation with the pediatric Bonfils fiberscope by the obscure vision. *Paediatr Anaesth*. 2009;19:419-441.
74. Kim J-T, Na H-S, Bae J-Y, et al. GlideScope video laryngoscope: a randomized clinical trial in 203 paediatric patients. *Br J Anaesth*. 2008;101:531-534.
75. Redel A, Karademir F, Schlitterlau A, et al. Validation of the GlideScope video laryngoscope in pediatric patients. *Paediatr Anaesth*. 2009;19: 667-671.
76. White M, Weale N, Nolan J, et al. Comparison of the Cobalt Glidescope video laryngoscope with conventional laryngoscopy in simulated normal and difficult infant airways. *Paediatr Anaesth*. 2009;19:1108-1112.
77. Fiadjoe JE, Stricker PA, Hackell RS, et al. The efficacy of the Storz Miller 1 video laryngoscope in a simulated infant difficult intubation. *Anesth Analg*. 2009;108:1783-1786.
78. Vlatten A, Aucoin S, Litz S, et al. A comparison of the STORZ video laryngoscope and standard direct laryngoscopy for intubation in the Pediatric airway–a randomized clinical trial. *Paediatr Anaesth*. 2009;19: 1102-1107.
79. Peyton J, Park R, Staffa SJ, et al. A comparison of videolaryngoscopy using standard blades or non-standard blades in children in the Paediatric Difficult Intubation Registry. *Br J Anaesth*. 2021;126(1):331-339.
80. Kalbhenn J, Boelke AK, Steinmann D. Prospective model-based comparison of different laryngoscopes for difficult intubation in infants. *Paediatr Anaesth*. 2012;22:776-780.
81. Lardner DRR, Cox RG, Ewen A, et al. [Comparison of laryngeal mask airway (LMA)- Proseal and the LMA-Classic in ventilated children receiving neuromuscular blockade]. *Can J Anaesth J Can Anesth*. 2008;55: 29-35.
82. Lu PP, Brimacombe J, Yang C, et al. ProSeal versus the Classic laryngeal mask airway for positive pressure ventilation during laparoscopic cholecystectomy. *Br J Anaesth*. 2002;88:824-827.
83. Goldmann K, Roettger C, Wulf H. Use of the ProSeal laryngeal mask airway for pressure-controlled ventilation with and without positive end-expiratory pressure in paediatric patients: a randomized, controlled study. *Br J Anaesth*. 2005;95:831-834.
84. Choi GJ, Kang H, Baek CW, et al. A systematic review and meta-analysis of the i-gel® vs laryngeal mask airway in children. *Anaesthesia*. 2014;69: 1258-1265.
85. Maitra S, Baidya DK, Bhattacharjee S, et al. Evaluation of i-gel(™) airway in children: a meta-analysis. *Paediatr Anaesth*. 2014;24:1072-1079.
86. Jagannathan N, Sequera-Ramos L, Sohn L, et al. Elective use of supraglottic airway devices for primary airway management in children with difficult airways. *Br J Anaesth*. 2014;112:744-748.

87. Jagannathan N, Roth AG, Sohn LE, et al. The new air-Q intubating laryngeal airway for tracheal intubation in children with anticipated difficult airway: a case series. *Paediatr Anaesth*. 2009;19:618-622.
88. Huang AS, Sarver A, Widing A, Hajduk J, Jagannathan N. The design of the perfect pediatric supraglottic airway device. *Pediatr Anesth*. 2020;30:280-287.
89. Kleine-Brueggeney M, Nicolet A, Nabecker S, et al. Blind intubation of anaesthetised children with supraglottic airway devices AmbuAura-i and Air-Q cannot be recommended: a randomised controlled trial. *Eur J Anaesthesiol*. 2015;32:631-639.
90. Engelhardt T. Rapid sequence induction has no use in pediatric anesthesia. *Paediatr Anaesth*. 2015;25(1):5-8.
91. Bledsoe GH, Schexnayder SM. Pediatric rapid sequence intubation: a review. *Pediatr Emerg Care*. 2004;20:339-344.
92. Sakles JC, Laurin EG, Rantapaa AA, et al. Airway management in the emergency department: a one-year study of 610 tracheal intubations. *Ann Emerg Med*. 1998;31:325-332.
93. Hardman JG, Wills JS. The development of hypoxaemia during apnoea in children: a computational modelling investigation. *Br J Anaesth*. 2006;97(4):564-570.
94. Soneru CN, Hurt HF, Petersen TR, Davis DD, Braude DA, Falcon RJ. Apneic nasal oxygenation and safe apnea time during pediatric intubations by learners. *Paediatr Anaesth*. 2019;29(6):628-634.
95. Neuhaus D, Schmitz A, Gerber A, Weiss M. Controlled rapid sequence induction and intubation - an analysis of 1001 children. *Paediatr Anaesth*. 2013;23(8):734-740.
96. Scrimgeour GE, Leather NWF, Perry RS, Pappachan J V., Baldock AJ. Gas induction for pyloromyotomy. *Paediatr Anaesth*. 2015;25(7):677-680.
97. Sellick BA. Cricoid pressure to control regurgitation of stomach contents during induction of anaesthesia. *Lancet Lond Engl*. 1961;2:404-406.
98. Engelhardt T, Strachan L, Johnston G. Aspiration and regurgitation prophylaxis in paediatric anaesthesia. *Paediatr Anaesth*. 2001;11:147-150.
99. Stedeford J, Stoddart P. RSI in pediatric anesthesia - is it used by nonpediatric anesthetists? A survey from south-west England. *Paediatr Anaesth*. 2007;17:235-244.
100. Lerman J. On cricoid pressure: "may the force be with you." *Anesth Analg*. 2009;109:1363-1366.
101. Kojima T, Harwayne-Gidansky I, Shenoi AN, et al. Cricoid pressure during induction for tracheal intubation in critically ill children: a report from National Emergency Airway Registry for Children. *Pediatr Crit Care Med*. 2018;19(6):528-537.
102. Moynihan RJ, Brock-Utne JG, Archer JH, et al. The effect of cricoid pressure on preventing gastric insufflation in infants and children. *Anesthesiology*. 1993;78:652-656.
103. Brock-Utne JG. Is cricoid pressure necessary? *Paediatr Anaesth*. 2002;12:1-4.
104. Cheng CAY, Aun CST, Gin T. Comparison of rocuronium and suxamethonium for rapid tracheal intubation in children. *Paediatr Anaesth*. 2002;12:140-145.
105. Xue FS, Huang YG, Tong SY, et al. A comparative study of early postoperative hypoxemia in infants, children, and adults undergoing elective plastic surgery. *Anesth Analg*. 1996;83:709-715.
106. Weiss M, Gerber AC. Rapid sequence induction in children -- it's not a matter of time! *Paediatr Anaesth*. 2008;18:97-99.
107. Tran DTT, Newton EK, Mount VAH, et al. Rocuronium versus succinylcholine for rapid sequence induction intubation. *Cochrane Database Syst Rev*. 2015;10:CD002788.
108. Gaver RS, Brenn BR, Gartley A, Donahue BS. Retrospective analysis of the safety and efficacy of sugammadex versus neostigmine for the reversal of neuromuscular blockade in children. *Anesth Analg*. 2019;129(4):1124-1129.
109. Liu G, Wang R, Yan Y, Fan L, Xue J, Wang T. The efficacy and safety of sugammadex for reversing postoperative residual neuromuscular blockade in pediatric patients: a systematic review. *Sci Rep*. 2017;7(1):5724.
110. Ozmete O, Bali C, Cok OY, et al. Sugammadex given for rocuronium-induced neuromuscular blockade in infants: a retrospective study. *J Clin Anesth*. 2016;35:497-501.
111. Goudsouzian NG. Recent changes in the package insert for succinylcholine chloride: should this drug be contraindicated for routine use in children and adolescents? (Summary of the discussions of the anesthetic and life support drug advisory meeting of the Food and Drug Administration, FDA building, Rockville, MD, June 9, 1994). *Anesth Analg*. 1995;80:207-208.
112. Morell RC, Berman JM, Royster RI, et al. Revised label regarding use of succinylcholine in children and adolescents. *Anesthesiology*. 1994;80:244-245.
113. Rawicz M, Brandom BW, Wolf A. The place of suxamethonium in pediatric anesthesia. *Paediatr Anaesth*. 2009;19:561-570.
114. Lundstrøm LH, Møller AM, Rosenstock C, et al. Avoidance of neuromuscular blocking agents may increase the risk of difficult tracheal intubation: a cohort study of 103,812 consecutive adult patients recorded in the Danish Anaesthesia Database. *Br J Anaesth*. 2009;103:283-290.
115. Jagannathan N, Kho MF, Kozlowski RJ, et al. Retrospective audit of the air-Q intubating laryngeal airway as a conduit for tracheal intubation in pediatric patients with a difficult airway. *Paediatr Anaesth*. 2011;21:442-447.
116. Walls R, Luten R. *Manual of Emergency Airway Management*. 3rd ed. Philadelphia: LWW; 2008.
117. Holm-Knudsen R, Eriksen K, Rasmussen LS. Using a nasopharyngeal airway during fiberoptic intubation in small children with a difficult airway. *Paediatr Anaesth*. 2005;15:839-845.
118. Sabato SC, Long E. An institutional approach to the management of the "Can't Intubate, Can't Oxygenate" emergency in children. Thomas M, ed. *Pediatr Anesth*. 2016;26(8):784-793.
119. Holm-Knudsen RJ, Rasmussen LS, Charabi B, Bøttger M, Kristensen MS. Emergency airway access in children - transtracheal cannulas and tracheotomy assessed in a porcine model. *Paediatr Anaesth*. 2012;22(12):1159-1165.
120. Prunty SL, Aranda-Palacios A, Heard AM, et al. The "Can't Intubate Can't Oxygenate" scenario in pediatric anesthesia: a comparison of the Melker cricothyroidotomy kit with a scalpel bougie technique. *Paediatr Anaesth*. 2015;25(4):400-404.
121. Ulmer F, Lennertz J, Greif R, Bütikofer L, Theiler L, Riva T. Emergency front of neck access in children: a new learning approach in a rabbit model. *Br J Anaesth*. 2020;125(1):e61-e68.
122. Stacey J, Heard AMB, Chapman G, et al. The "Can't Intubate Can't Oxygenate" scenario in pediatric anesthesia: a comparison of different devices for needle cricothyroidotomy. *Paediatr Anaesth*. 2012;22(12):1155-1158.
123. Holm-Knudsen RJ, Rasmussen LS, Charabi B, et al. Emergency airway access in children–transtracheal cannulas and tracheotomy assessed in a porcine model. *Paediatr Anaesth*. 2012;22:1159-1165.
124. Johansen K, Holm-Knudsen RJ, Charabi B, et al. Cannot ventilate-cannot intubate an infant: surgical tracheotomy or transtracheal cannula? *Paediatr Anaesth*. 2010;20:987-993.
125. Preussler N-P, Schreiber T, Hüter L, et al. Percutaneous transtracheal ventilation: effects of a new oxygen flow modulator on oxygenation and ventilation in pigs compared with a hand triggered emergency jet injector. *Resuscitation*. 2003;56:329-333.
126. Schaefer R, Hueter L, Preussler N-P, et al. Percutaneous transtracheal emergency ventilation with a self-made device in an animal model. *Paediatr Anaesth*. 2007;17:972-976.
127. Lim EHL, Tan AYJ, Sng DDW, Saffari SE, Tan JSK. Transtracheal jet oxygenation: comparing the efficacy and safety of two self-made Y-connector devices with the ENK oxygen flow modulator™ in an infant animal model. *Paediatr Anaesth*. 2019;29(8):799-807.
128. Baker PA, Brown AJ. Experimental adaptation of the Enk oxygen flow modulator for potential pediatric use. *Paediatr Anaesth*. 2009; 19(5):458-463.

CHAPTER 47

Management of 2-Year-Old Child with an Airway Foreign Body

Liane B. Johnson, Brandon D'Souza, Tristan Dumbarton, and Mathew B. Kiberd

CASE PRESENTATION

A 14 kg, 2-year-old boy presents following an aspiration event. The child was playing by a pile of gravel in the backyard and had a significant coughing episode. His parents did some back blows; he then vomited and stabilized. They also did a finger sweep but found nothing. He now continues to cough and is somewhat labored in his breathing.

PATIENT ASSESSMENT

What Are the Initial Clinical Steps in Patient Management?

Initial management of a patient with suspected foreign body aspiration begins with assessment and initial stabilization of ABCs—**A**irway, **B**reathing, **C**irculation. An awake, alert patient without overt airway distress will permit a more complete work-up, while a severely distressed patient with stridor and desaturation will require acute stabilization for transfer to the operating room (OR) for surgical removal of the foreign body. Presenting symptoms following foreign body aspiration are inherently related to the type of object aspirated, the location of the object, and the overall duration of the obstructive event. Obtaining a timely history from the patient's caregivers can provide most of these details, supplemented by a physical exam and investigations.

The practitioner can be lulled into a false sense of (airway) security when the patient is not imminently distressed. The patient must be constantly reassessed and re-evaluated for identification of respiratory change or deterioration. Timely collaborative care involving emergency room personnel, anesthesia practitioners, and the surgical airway management team is critical and should encompass investigations deemed safe based on patient stability, expedited supportive care, and transfer of the patient to the OR to ultimately resolve these tenuous situations.

All patients should be cared for in a high-acuity setting and have their vital signs continuously monitored. Supplemental oxygen may be provided to maximize pathophysiologic stabilization and optimization of the patient's cardiorespiratory status.

What Pathophysiologic Changes Are Seen in a Child That Has Aspirated a Foreign Body?

The pathophysiology of aspiration events is determined mainly by the characteristics of the aspiration event. In particular, the severity and location of airway obstruction, the type, size, and shape of the aspirated object, and the timeline since aspiration are key factors in symptom evolution.

Airway obstruction following foreign body aspiration may be complete or partial, depending on the inherent characteristics of the foreign body relative to the patient's airway diameter.

A **complete airway obstruction** is an emergency, usually associated with profound hypoxemia, subsequent cardiovascular compromise, and leading to cardiorespiratory arrest from asphyxia if left untreated. Mortality from foreign body aspiration has been estimated at 0.43%, with many patients presenting to emergency departments too late to rescue.[1] If a patient presents with vital signs and evidence of complete obstruction, the team is forced to act with their best efforts to gain control of the airway and facilitate the removal or distal displacement of the foreign body.

A partial obstruction in contrast may present with more subtle symptoms such as coughing, focal or diffuse wheezing, and decreased air entry on the affected side. These symptoms may progress over time to drooling, dyspnea, stridor, and respiratory distress due to migration of the foreign body or to local tissue inflammatory response. *It is critical to recognize that while a partial obstruction may permit further investigation and preoperative optimization, a seemingly stable foreign body in the airway may become complete and life-threatening at any time.* Appropriate vigilance is critical for prompt recognition of changes in respiratory status and preparations for swift intervention at a moment's notice.

A foreign body lodged in the lower airway may manifest with different pulmonary findings depending on the type of impaction. Four lower airway obstructive mechanisms have been described: check valve, ball valve, bypass valve, and stop valve.[2]

- A *check valve* implies air can be inhaled, but not exhaled, creating alveolar air trapping and flattening of the ipsilateral diaphragm. It can also lead to cardiovascular compromise from the development of tension physiology, especially with the addition of positive pressure breathing support.
- A *ball valve*, in contrast, allows expiration, but not inspiration of air, creating segmental bronchopulmonary collapse.
- A *bypass valve obstruction* allows partial airflow on both inspiration and expiration around the foreign body, and may not exhibit specific clinical findings.
- A *stop valve* creates complete obstruction to airflow causing airway collapse and consolidation distal to the obstruction.

CASE PRESENTATION CONTINUED

Although this is an unwitnessed event, the history is suggestive of the aspiration of a rock from the gravel pile. Because the patient only has mild respiratory symptoms, the logical assumption is the patient has a partial obstruction from aspirating a non-organic foreign body. Thus, there is time to further optimize the patient and characterize the location of the aspirated material prior to the bronchoscopy. However, as with all foreign body aspirations, this is a dynamic pathophysiologic state that can change if the foreign body migrates in response to coughing, vomiting, crying, or even patient positioning. Monitoring for any signs of decompensation should always be at the forefront of any management strategy.

What Are the Appropriate Investigations for a Foreign Body in the Airway?

Radiologic studies are used as an adjunct to the physical examination in diagnosing suspected aerodigestive foreign bodies. Anteroposterior and lateral chest radiographs, with inspiratory and expiratory views, are helpful tools if the foreign body is opaque, or if there is evidence of bronchial obstruction. Lateral decubitus films are helpful when the patient is unable to cooperate for timed inspiratory/expiratory views. Typical radiologic findings may reveal a foreign body shadow, air trapping, segmental or lobar collapse, or consolidation. Unfortunately, the false negative rate on chest X-ray ranges between 24% and 33% when compared to bronchoscopic findings.[3]

Spiral computed tomography (CT) has shown some benefit when faced with persistent symptoms in pediatric patients with delayed or repeated presentations to the emergency department, especially when the history is atypical or a prior chest X-ray is normal. Fluoroscopy and Cine-CT/functional magnetic resonance imaging (MRI) are of little added benefit when a timely work-up is of the essence, especially if radiographic evidence suggests the presence of a foreign body.[3] Ultimately, the gold standard for diagnosing an aspirated foreign body is rigid bronchoscopy under general anesthesia.[4,5]

PATIENT MANAGEMENT

Do Different Types of Foreign Bodies (Organics, Metals, Plastics, etc.) Influence Patient Management and Outcomes?

Toddlers are at the highest risk for foreign body aspiration because they place encountered objects in their mouths, are more likely to talk, laugh, and run while eating, have incomplete dentition to properly chew, and have relatively immature laryngeal protective reflexes. In North America, the most commonly aspirated organics are nuts (peanut and sunflower seed), meat (chicken, hot dog), popcorn, and carrots. Fatalities are most frequent with hot dogs and other meats, candies, grapes, and peanuts.[6]

Organic matter (nuts, corn, seeds, etc.) and plastics are radiolucent items that are uncommonly visualized on X-ray. Organics must be removed as soon as possible as the diameter of the object will increase over time with the absorption of secretions and moisture. This may convert a stable, partial obstruction to an acute complete obstruction, or obliterate the available space around the foreign body enhancing the complexity of removal. Furthermore, over time the organic matter will become more friable, potentially breaking into multiple pieces, making complete removal very difficult. This increases the risk of airway obstruction and infection in the distal, smaller-generation bronchi.

Additionally, organic matter with natural oils (nuts, bacon, etc.) will create a local inflammatory mucosal response enveloping the foreign body in granulation tissue. This localized tissue reaction begins rapidly after only a few hours of mucosal contact and progresses over time. The development of granulation tissue impedes direct visualization of the foreign body, more readily obstructs distal airflow, and creates bleeding with even minor manipulation, thus further hampering visualization and foreign body removal. Once bleeding from granulation tissue has begun, repeated instillations of dilute epinephrine through the rigid bronchoscope can help briefly diminish the bleeding to assist with further attempts at foreign body retrieval. The bleeding will ultimately stop once the foreign body is removed with its enveloping granulation tissue. If bleeding impedes visualization and risks the safe retrieval of the foreign body, then it may be safest to "rest" the patient for a few days in an intensive care unit where they can receive systemic antibiotics, steroids, aerosolized epinephrine, and positive pressure ventilation before returning to the OR for a second attempt. This treatment will significantly reduce, and possibly eliminate, the associated granulation tissue facilitating foreign body extraction.

Nonorganics, when aspirated, create shape- and size-dependent obstruction and trauma to the airway. Commonly aspirated materials include small plastic toys, pins, marbles, buttons or beads, and rocks or pebbles from playgrounds. Although rocks may have sharp edges and unusual shapes, their weight and bulk lead them to most frequently lodge around the glottis, subglottis, and trachea, occasionally, if small enough, extending down to the small subsegmental bronchi making surgical removal much more challenging. Many other sharp objects, like pins or tacks, will incite very different pathophysiologic changes, sometimes not much more than a persistent cough. These commonly found sharp objects are lighter and have a streamlined shape which generally led to the sharp end embedded in the tracheal mucosa proximally, with the larger blunt end distally located. It is unlikely that pins would cause larger airway obstruction. However, the associated mucosal edema, and/or displacement of the sharp foreign body into the smaller generation bronchi, may then create a risk of airway obstruction.[1]

What Adjunctive Respiratory Therapies Can Be Used to Stabilize the Patient?

All patients should have pulse oximetry and supplemental oxygen may be provided to optimize oxygenation. It is critical to appreciate that to produce symptoms, a foreign body must encroach on 75% of the airway lumen to create turbulent airflow. Respiratory distress or the presence of stridor implies compromise of the airway, and reduction of airflow. The patient's developmental age and parental anxiety will dictate their ability to cooperate when assessing the need for other possible bridging therapies while stabilizing the patient and awaiting transfer to the OR. The initiation of any adjunctive treatment should be under direct clinical observation with cardiorespiratory monitoring to ensure the intervention is beneficial and well tolerated.

Heliox (most commonly 70% helium and 30% oxygen) is an adjunct that can improve oxygenation by maximizing laminar airflow, creating an oxygen gradient in the narrowed airway, thereby decreasing the work of breathing and associated anxiety.[7] The use of heliox serves as a *temporizing measure* in the setting of foreign body aspiration in young children until definitive management can take place. Contemporary heliox setups have a blended system of helium balanced with oxygen, but it should be noted to maximize benefit, the concentration of helium should be over 60%.[8] Heliox must be delivered via closed systems such as non-rebreathing masks, specific custom mechanical ventilators, and high-flow systems.

High-flow nasal oxygen (HFNO) therapy has continued to emerge as a useful tool and may have a role in maintaining oxygenation when challenging airway management is anticipated encounter.[9,10] Transnasal humidified rapid-insufflation ventilatory exchange (THRIVE) or HFNO in the apneic patient has been shown to prolong the safe apnea time during airway management.[10] It can support spontaneous breathing in the anesthetized patient during tubeless airway procedures while reducing the need for interruptions required to perform rescue oxygenation.[10,11] These systems are easily adaptable to also deliver other medical gasses and aerosolized medications.

Aerosolized epinephrine may be an additional means to reducing airway edema, especially at the level of the glottis and subglottis, or in the presence of granulation tissue from an organic foreign body. The use of bronchodilators is considered a relative contraindication until the foreign body is removed from the airway, as its use may cause dislodgement and distal migration of the foreign body by increasing airway caliber. Bronchodilators may, however, be an important adjunct to the pulmonary toilet following foreign body removal.[12]

AIRWAY CONSIDERATIONS

The pediatric foreign body aspiration represents a significant airway challenge to anesthesia providers. Even without a known or predicted difficult anatomic airway, these cases present challenging physiology in a stressful, life-threatening situation. For the occasional pediatric or rural airway practitioner, unfamiliarity with pediatric airways will create an added level of difficulty and complexity. There are several considerations for these cases that can be mitigated with good planning, appropriate resources, and good communication.

A. This is an urgent/emergency condition, with limited time to optimize the patient for surgery. The patient may present in extremis with a very little forewarning to prepare the emergency department or ORs for bronchoscopy. Even if stable upon presentation, there is almost never time to follow fasting guidelines and the patients will be considered "full stomach."
B. The pediatric airway is different from the adult airway in a number of important anatomical ways that impact facemask ventilation and intubation. These differences are marked in neonates and gradually progress to adult-like anatomy as the child approaches the teenage years. The most significant difference is the size of the airways in a child compared to an adult, which, due to Poiseuille's law of flow resistance, means that the smaller diameter airways are exquisitely sensitive to inflammation caused by a foreign body. Added to that are the large occiput that impacts positioning for direct laryngoscopy, an anterior and cephalad larynx, which creates a challenge for direct visualization of the cords, and the need for age- and size-specific airway equipment. Furthermore, given the reduced FRC (even more pronounced with a foreign body), and increased oxygen consumption, the time to desaturation is more rapid in the pediatric patient.
C. Shared airway—emergency bronchoscopy necessitates a collaborative approach to the airway between anesthesia and otolaryngology services. If a rigid bronchoscopy is planned, the patient will often be anesthetized without intubation, and then turned toward the surgeon for bronchoscopy.

A high level of vigilance is necessary for the early identification of obstruction or hypoventilation. Anesthesia practitioners must be familiar with the rigid bronchoscope and how to ventilate through it while the bronchoscopists are removing the foreign body.

ANESTHESIA CONSIDERATIONS

How Would You Approach Induction of Anesthesia in Our Patient with a Foreign Body?

The pillars of anesthetic management in the setting of foreign body aspiration are providing a safe and adequate depth of anesthesia to permit manipulation of the airway without undesirable physiological responses, with balanced cardiorespiratory stability. To achieve these goals, the anesthesia team must weigh the pros and cons of their anesthetic approach based on the anatomic and physiologic parameters of the patient, along with the experience and adeptness of the OR staff. A survey revealed that most anesthesia practitioners attempt to maintain spontaneous ventilation for induction in order to avoid positive pressure ventilation, which in theory, could propagate the foreign body distally or overinflate distal air trapped in the lung.[1]

How one achieves the goal of maintaining spontaneous efforts is a matter of comfort and experience, allowing for both inhalational and intravenous induction techniques.

Sevoflurane is the preferred inhalational agent because it allows for a smooth and rapid induction of general anesthesia while providing some degree of bronchodilation. This is in comparison to other fluorinated agents, known to provoke more airway irritability and less cardiorespiratory stability on induction. However, there are significant drawbacks to volatile anesthetics in the setting of an aspirated foreign body. The time to an adequate depth of anesthesia may be prolonged in the presence of reduced alveolar ventilation secondary to a foreign body. Furthermore, volatile anesthetic delivery will be interrupted frequently, due to airway instrumentation and manipulation. Ventilation challenges and leaks are often countered with higher flows, which compound operative field and environmental pollution.[1,10,13] The difficulty in maintaining and monitoring minimal alveolar concentration (MAC) may result in fluctuations of volatile anesthetic, inadequate depth of anesthesia, suboptimal operative conditions, and the risk of adverse events.

Nitrous oxide should be avoided, as it decreases the percentage of delivered oxygen, encourages atelectasis, and expands air-containing cavities. Expansion of distally trapped air may be of sufficient magnitude to severely compromise pulmonary compliance and generate a pneumothorax.[14]

A common technique blends approaches using an inhalational induction with sevoflurane to maintain spontaneous respiratory efforts transitioning to total intravenous anesthesia (TIVA) for the maintenance phase of the procedure. Some studies suggest a volatile technique improves physiologic conditions and reduces complications while others suggest TIVA's advantages may be preferred because of the reduction of airway reactivity, preservation of hypoxic pulmonary vasoconstriction, improved ciliary function, maintenance of spontaneous ventilation, and reduction of postoperative nausea and vomiting (PONV).[15] Overall, TIVA is more predictable, easily titratable, and allows for a constant depth of anesthesia irrespective of ventilation.[10]

If an IV has already been initiated, it is reasonable to proceed with a TIVA induction with careful titration of infusions to maintain spontaneous breathing. Alternatively, many practitioners may initiate induction with an IV, with the use of topical amethocaine (Ametop, Smith+Nephew, Watford, UK), distractions and assisted holds. TIVA for these cases is most frequently maintained with infusions of propofol, remifentanil, and occasionally dexmedetomidine.[10] Spontaneous breathing can be maintained in pediatric patients with propofol in the range of 200 to 400 $\mu g \cdot kg^{-1} \cdot min^{-1}$, along with remifentanil in the range of 0.05 to 0.2 $\mu g \cdot kg^{-1} \cdot min^{-1}$.[1] A typical TIVA approach entails utilizing infusions of these medications until an adequate depth of anesthesia is achieved. Some advocate for proceeding once the respiratory rate is half of its baseline value.[10] Confirmation of adequate depth may be measured by response to oral airway insertion or laryngoscopy, at which point lidocaine may be applied to the vocal cords.[10]

The main challenge with maintaining a spontaneous breathing technique is that most patients will require some degree of ventilatory assistance during the endoscopic retrieval to optimize tidal volume, improve oxygenation, and reduce hypercapnia. There is emerging evidence that controlled ventilation, despite the theoretical disadvantages, may improve operating conditions, provide better oxygenation and overall ventilation, decrease recovery time, and require less opioid.[1,10] Given the lack of consensus on a management approach, it may be reasonable to consider a dual strategy. By maintaining spontaneous respiration until the airway has been secured and the location of the foreign body has been identified, one can then assess the ease and risks of foreign body retrieval prior to a move to a controlled ventilation technique with muscle relaxation and reversal upon completion. It can be useful to consider this approach if a spontaneous technique has failed and oxygen desaturation remains unresponsive to the usual rescue techniques, then paralysis with a high-dose rocuronium should be considered. Administration of a paralytic in this case may improve ventilation and will give superior surgical conditions for the surgeons while they try to temporize the situation.

The anesthesia practitioner must decide which technique to use to minimize the possibility of patient movement, coughing, and laryngospasm upon airway instrumentation. Ultimately, the choice of anesthetic should be governed by the anesthesia practitioner's clinical experience, expertise with these different techniques, and the individual characteristics of each case.

What Other Pharmacologic Agents May Be Considered?

Intravenous opioids, such as remifentanil and fentanyl, are helpful in suppressing airway reflexes but must be used judiciously to balance their underlying respiratory depressive effects.[14,16] Remifentanil may be particularly attractive for a rapid, atraumatic procedure due to its short half-life.

Dexmedetomidine is a useful adjunct for airway surgery as it provides sedation, maintains spontaneous ventilation, and decreases opiate requirements while reducing emergence agitation.[15]

Topical lidocaine can be sprayed or atomized onto the pharyngeal and laryngeal mucosa and will work synergistically with the anesthetic agents by decreasing the physiologic response to airway instrumentation.

Intravenous dexamethasone, even at a dose of 0.5 mg·kg^{-1} is not a fast-acting strategy but can provide reduction of mucosal edema both from the foreign body and from the airway manipulation for up to 36 hours.[17]

Anticholinergics, such as atropine and glycopyrrolate may help prevent vagally mediated airway responses, such as excessive production of airway secretions, bradycardia, and bronchoconstriction.[14]

Anti-emetics such as ondansetron 0.1 mg·kg^{-1} are often given to assist in the prevention of PONV and frequently given in tandem with other strategies such as TIVA and dexamethasone.

What Are the Anesthetic Options If the Patient Is Uncooperative?

In uncooperative patients, a stormy induction may dislodge the foreign body, hastening the need for emergency intervention.[18] In certain circumstances, oral, nasal, or intramuscular sedation may be considered for smooth induction; however, some patients will react poorly to the administration of the sedation. This may require having all personnel and equipment prepared to intervene if decompensation takes place. *The approach for each case is governed by many factors and the team should consider the safest option for the case presenting to them.*

INTRAOPERATIVE MANAGEMENT

How Do You Perform Rigid Bronchoscopy for Foreign Body Removal?

A complete airway assessment is essential to the planning of the operative foreign body removal while anticipating difficulties encountered therein. Our patient is an otherwise healthy 2-year-old without any medical antecedents. The safest means of removing a potentially sharp-edged foreign body requires that it be securely grasped with optical forceps and then, if possible, ensheathing within the rigid bronchoscope to prevent mucosal trauma along the path of removal. Removal of large tracheal foreign bodies that cannot be partly or fully ensheathed within the rigid bronchoscope is at greater risk of becoming impacted or accidentally dropped from the forceps at the narrower portions of the airway, namely at the level of the glottis or subglottis. Such an event could lead to potential complete airway obstruction. In situations where obstruction is, or becomes, complete, the object may need to be rapidly pushed distally into the right mainstem bronchus so that oxygenation may resume.

It is important to note that the entire airway, pharynx, larynx, trachea, and bilateral first- and second-generation bronchi, must be visualized following removal of the foreign body to ensure the absence of trauma or second airway foreign body, which may be present in up to 5% of cases.[19]

How Do You Provide Oxygenation During Rigid Bronchoscopy?

Provided an appropriately sized bronchoscope is used, rigid bronchoscopy allows for oxygenation and ventilation through the distal opening as well as four small distally placed side ports, equivalent to a Murphy Eye on endotracheal tubes. The anesthesia circuit can be attached to the 15/22 mm ventilation side port of the rigid bronchoscope. Fiberoptic and video technology allows visualization of the airway on a monitor by all members of the OR team. The advent of optical foreign body forceps allows for simultaneous foreign body retrieval and ventilation through the bronchoscope. When using an inhalational anesthetic, the bronchoscope's design helps minimize the loss of anesthetic gases in the OR and helps better maintain the depth of anesthesia. The success rate and the operating time with the use of optical forceps have drastically improved, once again contributing to enhanced patient safety. Depending on the type and shape of the object to be retrieved, a selection of optical foreign body forceps is available.

What Are the Potential Complications and Limitations of Rigid Bronchoscopy?

Anatomic and physiologic complications can arise with the use of rigid bronchoscopy. At-risk structures include dentition, pharynx, cervical spine, larynx, or trachea.

The risks of dental injury would be similar to the risk associated with laryngoscopy; however, an extra precaution is taken with rigid bronchoscopy as a mouth guard is used to protect the upper incisors from chipping, breaking, or avulsing at the root.

Any soft tissue elements in the path of the bronchoscope, such as lips, pharyngeal walls, tonsils, tongue, and vallecular, are at risk of mechanical trauma leading to edema, bleeding, or a hematoma formation. Technical challenges can arise due to patient factors, operator inexperience, or a very difficult foreign body retrieval.

Cervical spine injury can occur from aggressive patient positioning or an underlying disorder, such as atlantoaxial subluxation in children with Trisomy 21.

The larynx and trachea are composed of mucosal-covered cartilaginous structures each with their own susceptibilities to injury, even in experienced hands. The epiglottis can be bruised, malpositioned, folded over, or even torn, and while the arytenoid cartilages are relatively resilient, dislocation is possible. Pediatric vocal cords are an immature bilayer structure until the onset of puberty. This makes them more susceptible to edema with mechanical pressure from repeated transglottic passage of the bronchoscope; however, the vocal cords remain fairly resilient and are rarely torn or avulsed. Although the size of the patient's subglottis dictates the optimal size of the bronchoscope, choosing one too large or torquing and manipulating the bronchoscope can place this area at risk of significant edema, impacting postoperative respiratory status. The posterior tracheal wall is highly elastic and quite forgiving to bronchoscope passage, but a risk of tearing and creation of a tracheoesophageal fistula can happen from the edges of the foreign body itself or, excessive force and instrumentation.

Hemodynamic instability, hypercapnia, or hypoxemia may also occur in association with hypoventilation, dislodgement of the foreign body, or the use of an inappropriately sized bronchoscope. Waveform capnography is unlikely to be continuous and may be absent at times due to the frequent opening of a closed system by the repeated introduction and removal of the telescope for the optical foreign body forceps. The smaller the patient, the smaller the bronchoscope and thus the less space available for insufflation and efflux of gases between the inner walls of the bronchoscope and the telescope.

The use of the rigid bronchoscope in the tracheobronchial tree has limited maneuverability and can only rarely access the secondary bronchi and smaller airways.

What Is the Role of Flexible Bronchoscopy in the Management of Foreign Bodies in the Airway?

The use of flexible bronchoscopy as a primary tool for foreign body removal is not widely practiced but is used with increasing frequency in some centers. Some advocate its use to evaluate the airway prior to foreign body removal by rigid bronchoscopy to allow for localization and planning.[12] It may also be used following retrieval, to ensure that the foreign body has been removed in its entirety and that no other foreign body is found down to the subsegmental bronchi. Lastly, its use may be the sole option in patients with craniofacial or cervical trauma who cannot be properly positioned for rigid endoscopy. A group in Mexico are currently using flexible bronchoscopy in approximately 40% of their pediatric airway foreign body cases, with a 93% success rate.[20]

The flexible bronchoscope can be passed transnasally or transorally, the latter being the preferred approach for foreign body retrieval either through an endotracheal tube, an extraglottic device, or a rigid bronchoscope. Grasping forceps, urologic baskets, and balloon catheters can be placed through the flexible scope's working channel, or fed down the airway alongside the flexible bronchoscope itself.

There are several risks associated with using a flexible bronchoscope for foreign body removal. The foreign body cannot be ensheathed within the flexible bronchoscope and frequently neither can it be passed through the chosen oxygenation conduit (endotracheal tube, laryngeal mask airway [LMA], rigid bronchoscope, etc.), placing the airway at greater risk of injury during foreign body extraction, especially at the level of the subglottis, the larynx, or the pharynx. The size, composition, and presence of sharp edges on the foreign body will increase the complexity of retrieval and the risk of airway injury. The most catastrophic risk is complete airway obstruction and inability to ventilate if the foreign body is dropped or lodged at the level of the glottis on retrieval.

How Is the Foreign Body from This Patient Recovered If It Will Not Pass Through the Glottis?

Because of the size of the patient and the impact of minor edema on airway caliber, it may be impossible to remove the foreign body from whence it came. Even with directed force, the rock may lodge in the subglottis or be unable to pass through the vocal cords leading to complete airway obstruction. In this situation, recognition of the change in circumstance due to space limitation and the risk of creating a complete obstruction makes surgical access to the airway an acceptable option.

If the foreign body still cannot be removed, an open thoracotomy is required. In such cases, a bronchotomy is often necessary to remove the object or even partial lung parenchyma resection.[21] The latter is more commonly seen with an untimely diagnosis of foreign body aspiration and the development of secondary complications.[4] Interestingly, aspirated plastic pen caps have a high propensity for requiring thoracoscopic access for removal, due to a high rate of bronchoscopic extraction failure secondary to their size, shape, and position in the airway.[21,22]

POSTOPERATIVE MANAGEMENT

Is There a Role for Steroids, Epinephrine, Bronchodilators, and Antibiotics in the Postoperative Care of This Patient?

The use of systemic or topical/aerosolized steroids in the postoperative period may be beneficial if mucosal edema and granulation tissue were present in the vicinity of the airway foreign body or anywhere along the respiratory tract that may compromise the airway in the immediate postoperative period. Aerosolized (racemic) epinephrine is rarely needed following easily removed, atraumatic procedures. However, aerosolized epinephrine may be of significant benefit in reducing mucosal edema and scant bleeding in the presence of postoperative stridor following more traumatic foreign body removal. Bronchodilators are used infrequently but may be helpful in the presence of persistent segmental atelectasis in the prolonged presence of a foreign body. Similarly, antibiotics are not used routinely, unless there is evidence of granulation tissue, or suppuration around the foreign body, or in the distal airways.[4]

What Investigative Modalities Are Warranted Postoperatively?

Postoperatively, the patient should be observed upon emergence from anesthesia to ensure that there are no sequelae following foreign body retrievals, such as airway compromise, or respiratory distress. If the object was small and completely removed, with minimal underlying airway edema, the patient may be discharged following a brief period of observation. Difficult retrievals or instability in the operating or recovery room would mandate overnight monitored observation.

A chest X-ray may be considered in the more complex retrieval procedure. If a radiologically confirmed pneumomediastinum is seen postoperatively, clinical symptomatology must be correlated to determine whether further investigation or invasive therapies are warranted. Most commonly there are few signs or symptoms associated with pneumomediastinum, although precordial crepitus and voice change are the most common. Ideally, positive pressure ventilation should be avoided if possible as this may exacerbate the situation.

The patient should be monitored in an intensive care setting where serial chest radiographs would be performed to monitor regression, or progression, of the air trapping. Usually, there is slow resolution over a few days, without significant sequelae.

IN THE CONTEXT OF AIRBORNE DISEASE

The global SARS-CoV-2 pandemic and resulting COVID-19 disease have shifted the focus in health care from one exclusively centered on patient outcomes, to one that includes the health and safety of the health care providers. Nowhere is this more relevant than during aerosol-generating medical procedures (AGMPs), such as intubation or bronchoscopy, necessary for the management of the aspirated foreign body. Preoperative screening and testing are helpful to identify patients who may have communicable SARS-CoV-2, but the patient with a foreign body aspiration requires urgent if not emergency intervention and there may not be time to get test results. These cases will routinely need to proceed regardless of COVID-19 status, which thus necessitates extra caution to ensure health care provider's safety. The use of "airway boxes," plastic bags, other barriers, and interventions to theoretically reduce occupational contamination of aerosolized/droplet nuclei from the patient have been reported but cannot be recommended. These devices have not been sufficiently validated and they represent a deviation from a standard practice, for a high-risk case which can be technically challenging at baseline.[23]

Basic tenets for the provision of AGMPs in patients with diagnosed or presumed COVID-19 include using full personal protective equipment, including fit-tested N95 respirators for all health care providers in the room, paying particular attention to proper donning and doffing and minimizing aerosolization of virus. These steps take time and care, which are directly opposite to the principles of foreign-body airway management, which may be an emergency and time-limited. Health care providers are nonetheless encouraged to take all reasonable steps to protect themselves and their co-workers fully.

How Would We Provide Anesthesia to This Case?

The child was assessed preoperatively, and a thorough history and consent is obtained. Adequate preparations with the team, equipment, and medications are made. The patient is brought into the OR with her parent. Ametop was placed preoperatively over a site with reasonable predicted IV access. With the use of an assisted hold and distractions, an IV is placed without issue. With a SpO_2 monitor attached, 2 $mg{\cdot}kg^{-1}$ of propofol is administered intravenously to begin to induce the child. As she lies down, a mask with 8% of Sevoflurane and 100% of oxygen is held as she breathes spontaneously through an open adjustable pressure-limiting (APL) valve. Infusions of propofol at 200 $\mu g{\cdot}kg^{-1}{\cdot}min^{-1}$ and remifentanil at 0.1 $\mu g{\cdot}kg^{-1}{\cdot}min^{-1}$ are initiated. The administration of volatile agent is chosen to expedite an adequate depth of anesthesia while the plasma concentration of intravenous agents builds, all while maintaining spontaneous respiratory efforts. Once the HR is reduced by 20%, a jaw thrust is attempted. If the child continues to breathe spontaneously, an oral airway is placed. If at this point the child continues to breathe spontaneously and has no hemodynamic response, laryngoscopy is performed, and the vocal cords are sprayed with topical anesthetic. Once again, if the child does not react and continues to breathe spontaneously, the sevoflurane is discontinued, with the FiO_2 of 1.0, propofol and remifentanil infusions continue. Nasal prongs are applied to provide passive oxygenation between airway instrumentation with spontaneous efforts. Subsequently, the bed is turned 90 degrees and the airway is handed over to the surgeon. Anesthetic induction to the maintenance of the child generally takes 5 to 10 minutes with this technique.

For our case, as the surgeon performs laryngoscopy and inserts the rigid bronchoscope, the anesthetic circuit is attached to the rigid bronchoscope and the flow is increased to at least 10 $L{\cdot}min^{-1}$, and the APL valve is set to 30 cm H_2O. If the HR increases more than 10% or the respiratory rate increases, the remifentanil infusion is increased by 0.05 $\mu g{\cdot}kg^{-1}{\cdot}min^{-1}$.

In our case, the rock is carefully endoscopically placed in the right mainstem bronchus, then the airway is secured with a cuffed endotracheal tube. Once the airway is controlled, a temporary tracheotomy is performed through which the rigid bronchoscope is passed to retrieve the rock without as much technical restriction. Primary closure of the tracheotomy must be done judiciously and only if there is minimal airway edema as any coughing or straining could promote an air leak in the neck creating an emerging upper airway obstruction. Once surgical team is closed, the propofol and remifentanil infusions are discontinued, and additional antiemetics are given along with a check to ensure dexamethasone has been administered. At this point, long-acting analgesics are given as required. If the child shows any respiratory distress, adjunctive therapy such as HFNO is considered along with admission to the Pediatric Intensive Care Unit or inpatient ward.

SUMMARY

Airway foreign bodies in children can pose multiple challenges. The task of removing the object requires a team approach for the best possible patient outcome. The size and nature of the aspirated object, its location in the airway, the time elapsed since aspiration, and patient factors such as age and other associated comorbidities, all weigh into the planning of retrieval. Communication, preparation, and practice are the means by which safe outcomes and team success are achieved.

SELF-EVALUATION QUESTIONS

47.1. Which of the following pediatric patient populations has the highest risk for developing a foreign body aspiration event?

A. Neonates

B. Infants

C. Toddlers

D. Grade-schoolers

E. Teenagers

47.2. Which of the following modalities is the gold standard for diagnosing an aspirated foreign body?

A. Chest X-ray

B. Rigid bronchoscopy

C. MRI

D. CT scan

E. Ultrasound

47.3. Surgical removal of an airway foreign body is **NOT** recommended under which of the following circumstances?

A. If the foreign body is sharp, pointed, and embedded in the tracheal or bronchial wall

B. If the foreign body is found in a small inaccessible peripheral bronchus

C. If the foreign body has been present for a prolonged period often for several years

D. If there is significant instability in maintaining control of the airway upon insertion and manipulation of the bronchoscope

E. If the patient also has a concomitant head injury

REFERENCES

1. Fidkowski CW, Zheng H, Firth PG. The anesthetic considerations of tracheobronchial foreign bodies in children: a literature review of 12,979 cases. *Anesth Analg*. 2010;111(4):1016-1025.
2. Chatterji S, Chatterji P. The management of foreign bodies in air passages. *Anaesthesia*. 1972;27(4):390-395.
3. Hong SJ, Goo HW, Roh JL. Utility of spiral and cine CT scans in pediatric patients suspected of aspirating radiolucent foreign bodies. *Otolaryngol Head Neck Surg*. 2008;138(5):576-580.
4. Rovin JD, Rogers BM. Pediatric foreign body aspiration. *Pediatr Rev*. 2000;21:86-90.
5. Gibson SE, Shot SR. Foreign bodies of the upper aerodigestive tract. In: *The Pediatric Airway—An Interdisciplinary Approach*. Philadelphia, PA: JB Lippincott Co; 1995.
6. Altkorn R, Chen X, Milkovich S, et al. Fatal and non-fatal food injuries among children (aged 0–14 years). *Int J Pediatr Otorhinolaryngol*. 2008;72(7):1041-1046.
7. Brown L, Sherwin T, Perez JE, Perez DU. Heliox as a temporizing measure for pediatric foreign body aspiration. *Acad Emerg Med*. 2002;9(4):346-347.
8. McGarvey JM, Pollack CV. Heliox in airway management. *Emerg Med Clin North Am*. 2008;26(4);905-920.
9. Riley RH. Australasian anaesthesia 2017: invited papers and selected continuing education lectures. Australian and New Zealand College of Anaesthetists; 2017.
10. Ridgway R, Dumbarton T, Brown Z. Update on ENT anaesthesia in children. *Anaesth Intensive Care*. 2019;20(1):56-60.
11. Humphreys S, Rosen D, Housden T, Taylor J, Schibler A. Nasal high-flow oxygen delivery in children with abnormal airways. *Paediatr Anaesth*. 2017;27(6):616-620.
12. Midulla F, de Blic J, Barbato A, et al. Flexible endoscopy of paediatric airways. *Eur Respir J*. 2003;22(4):698-708.
13. Zur KB, Litman RS. Pediatric airway foreign body retrieval: surgical and anesthetic perspectives. *Paediatr Anaesth*. 2009;19:109-117.
14. Tan HK, Tan SS. Inhaled foreign bodies in children—anaesthetic considerations. *Singapore Med J*. 2000;41(10):506-510.
15. Lauder GR. Total intravenous anesthesia will supersede inhalational anesthesia in pediatric anesthetic practice. *Paediatr Anaesth*. 2015:25(1):52-64.
16. Litman RS, Ponnuri J, Trogan I. Anesthesia for tracheal or bronchial foreign body removal in children: an analysis of ninety-four cases. *Anesth Analg*. 2000;91(6):1389-1391.
17. Thomas GR, Dave D, Furze A, et al. Managing common otolaryngologic emergencies. *Emerg Med*. 2005;37(5):18-47.
18. Paterson NA. Management of an unusual pediatric difficult airway using ketamine as a sole agent. *Paediatr Anaesth*. 2008;18(8):785-788.
19. McGuirt WF, Holmes KD, Feehs R, Browne JD. Tracheobronchial foreign bodies. *Laryngoscope*. June 1988;98:615-618.
20. Ramirez-Figueroa JL, Gochicoa-Rangel LG, Ramirez-San Juan DH, Vargas MH. Foreign body removal by flexible fiberoptic bronchoscopy in infants and children. *Pediatr Pulmonol*. 2005;40(5):392-397.
21. Marks SC, Marsh BR, Dudgeon DL. Indications for open surgical removal of airway foreign body. *Ann Otol Rhinol Laryngol*. 1993;102(9):690-694.
22. Ulku R, Onen A, Onat S, Ozcelik C. The value of open surgical approaches for aspirated pen caps. *J Pediatr Surg*. 2005;40(11):1780-1783.
23. Kearsley R. Intubation boxes for managing the airway in patients with COVID-19. *Anaesthesia*. 2020;75(7):969.

CHAPTER 48

Management of a Child with a History of Difficult Intubation and Post-Tonsillectomy Bleed

Arnim Vlatten, Holger Gaessler, and Bjoern Hossfeld

CASE PRESENTATION

A 6-year-old boy with Down syndrome is en route to your children's hospital by ambulance with post-tonsillectomy bleeding.

He underwent adenotonsillectomy due to recurrent throat infections under general anesthesia 22 hours earlier. Despite being overweight at 37 kg and enlarged adenoids, he did not suffer from obstructive sleep apnea (OSA) or obstructive sleep-disordered breathing. Prior to his surgery, the child was uncooperative necessitating an inhalational induction. Intravenous access was difficult requiring several attempts and finally was successful in the left saphenous vein. Because of possible atlanto-occipital instability associated with Down syndrome, cervical spine (C-spine) precautions were implemented during airway management. Direct laryngoscopy revealed a Grade 3 Cormack-Lehane (C-L) view of the larynx due to an enlarged tongue. Indirect laryngoscopy was then attempted using the GlideScope which revealed a Grade 1 C-L view. The trachea was intubated with an uncuffed 5.0 mm ID oral Ring Adair Elwyn tube. Adenotonsillectomy was performed uneventfully, and the child was discharged home after an overnight observation period. While at home, the boy ate a tea biscuit, leading to the onset of immediate sharp pain with intraoral bleeding.

The child is in the emergency room sitting on a stretcher and spitting blood frequently into a kidney basin. The child is in moderate distress with the following vital signs: HR 152 bpm, BP 97/57 mmHg. The child does not tolerate nasal prong oxygen and the pulse oximeter reading is 94% on room air. Auscultation of the chest is clear. Examination of the mouth reveals brisk bleeding of the right tonsillar bed. An attempt to start an intravenous line in the right saphenous vein was unsuccessful. However, blood samples are obtained for a complete blood count, coagulation parameters and a cross-match. The child is then transferred to the operating room (OR) for further management.

INTRODUCTION

■ What Is the Incidence, Morbidity, and Mortality of Pediatric Post-Tonsillectomy Bleeding?

Tonsillectomy is one of the most frequently performed surgical procedures in children, with approximately 580,000 pediatric adenotonsillectomies performed annually in the United States.[1] The most common post-tonsillectomy complications are postoperative nausea and vomiting (PONV) and pain. Dehydration may occur in children due to delayed poor oral intake, nausea, and fever. Delayed postoperative bleeding is the most significant complication and is not uncommon.[2,3] Many estimates of the incidence of post-tonsillectomy bleeding exist in the literature, varying widely from 0% to 11.5%.[3] Typically, however, the rate ranges between 0.2% and 4.8%.[4–6] Mortality rates from severe bleeding are rarely reported in the literature. They range from 1 in 10,000[7] in earlier studies to less than

1 in 100,000 in recent publications.[8] Sixty-seven percent of post-tonsillectomy bleeding originates in the tonsillar fossa and 27% in the nasopharynx. There are two major time frames for postoperative bleeding. Most often the bleeding occurs within the first 24 hours after surgery (primary bleeding).[9] Primary bleeding is generally related to surgical technique and the incidence is declining. Twenty-five percent of all post-tonsillectomy occur after 24 hours. Secondary bleeding not related to surgical technique is rare, and of unchanged prevalence over the years.[9] Although it may occur at any time, the average time from tonsillectomy to bleeding is 5.7 to 7.8 days.[9] Infection of the tonsillar bed with clot/eschar sloughing is believed to be the major cause of secondary bleeding. It occurs more commonly in older pediatric patients because the indication in this age group is usually related to recurrent infections rather than airway obstruction, the most common indication for surgery in the younger pediatric age group.[10] Age and history of chronic and recurrent infections requiring a tonsillectomy are shown to be common risk factors for post-tonsillectomy hemorrhage.[10]

PATIENT EVALUATION

What Are the Initial Clinical Steps One Should Take in the Patient with Post-Tonsillectomy Bleeding?

The diagnosis of post-tonsillectomy bleeding is usually made by a focused history and physical examination, evidenced by a blunt or sharp trauma to the oropharynx. An intraoral examination may reveal blood and blood clots. The differential diagnosis includes bleeding tumors of the oropharynx, like hemangiomas.

The child will present with fresh blood in the mouth and frequent swallowing of blood. It is important to emphasize that the amount of blood swallowed may be underestimated. Antiemetic medications may mask or suppress vomiting. It is not uncommon for children to have silent bleeding for prolonged periods with extensive blood loss. The child is often restless, diaphoretic, and pale. The vital signs may show an increased heart rate because of pain and hypovolemia. In awake children, hypotension following blood loss is a very late sign and then indicates significant hypovolemia. The initial assessment and primary survey should focus on airway, breathing, hemodynamic stability, and active bleeding. Intravenous access must be established as soon as possible followed by initial volume resuscitation with crystalloid or colloid solution. A blood sample for baseline hematocrit or hemoglobin is necessary as well as for blood typing and cross-match. Bleeding from the tonsillar bed may initially be controlled using pharyngeal packs and cautery. But children with post-tonsillectomy bleeding should be taken to the OR for exploration and surgical hemostasis. Repeated attempts to stop bleeding on the ward and/or in the emergency department should be avoided, except if exsanguination is imminent.

A questionnaire of children undergoing tonsillectomy with or without postoperative bleeding showed an increased incidence of posttraumatic stress disorder if children were treated on the ward when compared to children treated in the OR.[11]

AIRWAY MANAGEMENT

How Is the Airway Usually Managed in Post-Tonsillectomy Bleeding?

In addition to hypovolemia, patients with post-tonsillectomy bleeding present two major problems related to airway management:

1. *Aspiration:* These patients must be considered to have a full stomach and are at an increased risk for pulmonary aspiration.
2. *Difficult airway:* Blood and blood clots may impair visualization of the glottic opening. Additionally, edema of the oropharynx may have occurred because of surgery or infection. This may lead to altered oropharyngeal and/or laryngeal anatomy.

Because of the risk of aspiration, rapid sequence induction should be considered. The efficacy and use of cricoid pressure in children remain controversial.[12] It is important to remember that cricoid pressure can distort the laryngeal anatomy, potentially worsen the view of the larynx, and can induce vomiting in the partially anesthetized patient.[13] The blood and blood clots in the oropharynx can impair visualization during laryngoscopy or cause obstruction of the placement of the endotracheal tube (ETT) and/or use of the suction apparatus. Therefore, two working suctions are essential. One should be a rigid, large-bore surgical suction and the other mounted with a flexible endotracheal suction catheter. If one becomes blocked with a blood clot, another is readily available. If large amounts of blood clot are present, it may be necessary during the initial laryngoscopy to manually remove them with a finger or gauze. Magill forceps should be available to retrieve clots deeper in the oropharynx. Different-sized curved and straight blades should be available. Different-sized cuffed styletted ETTS, with one size up and down of the calculated size must be prepared. An Eschmann tracheal introducer may be helpful in the presence of a Grade 3 C-L view.[13] If only the epiglottis is visible during laryngoscopy, a chest compression creating air bubbles through the larynx can help to locate the glottic opening.

Indirect laryngoscopy using this class of devices (e.g., GlideScope, STORZ C-MAC, or Airtraq) may be difficult. Blood and secretions may obscure the optical lens, impairing the glottic view. However, this class of devices should be available when difficult direct laryngoscopy is encountered.

Extraglottic devices (e.g., laryngeal mask airway [LMA]) may be an alternative airway device in managing the difficult pediatric airway.[13] It is often used to primarily manage the difficult pediatric airway for adenotonsillectomies. Extraglottic devices are easy to place and may be used as a conduit for a flexible bronchoscopic-guided intubation if required.[13] Use of a laryngeal mask may briefly tamponade the bleeding site, and possibly protects the airway and the optical lens of the bronchoscope. A case report described the successful use of a laryngeal mask for a failed intubation in a post-tonsillectomy bleed.[14]

The use of a flexible bronchoscope alone is not recommended in case of oropharyngeal bleeding. Experts recommend that the practitioner should rely on the alternative techniques with which they have the most experience and skill.[13] An experienced otolaryngologist or other qualified rigid laryngologist/

bronchoscopist should be available prior to anesthetic induction. If direct laryngoscopy fails, a rigid bronchoscope may be useful. Equipment and preparation for a surgical airway are also essential (e.g., tracheotomy tray opened and ready).

What Are the Airway Management Options for This Patient?

This patient presents several issues regarding anesthesia induction and airway management:

- Uncooperative nature of the child
- Aspiration risk
- Difficult venous access
- Potential atlanto-occipital instability
- History of difficult direct laryngoscopy (likely more challenging now due to blood and secretions)

The anesthetic and airway management options for this child need to be considered in light of their respective risks and benefits. The options include the following:

1. *Intravenous induction versus inhalation induction without IV access:* While an inhalation induction with a face mask was performed for his first surgery, a stomach potentially full of blood argues against this approach and favors a rapid sequence induction to minimize the duration of an unprotected airway.
2. *Anesthesia induction with C-Spine precautions versus no C-Spine precaution:* Down syndrome is associated with atlanto-occipital instability in 15% to 20% of children, yet symptomatic atlantoaxial subluxation occurs in only 1%.[15] It can occur in children as young as 4 years of age. The atlanto-occipital instability associated with Down syndrome places him at increased risk for C-spine injury during anesthetic induction and laryngoscopic intubation. Extreme neck extension should be avoided in this child, as children with atlanto-occipital instability may be at risk for quadriplegia.[16] Radiographic findings of C-spine instability in Down syndrome remain controversial.[17] Lateral radiographs of the neck in flexion and extension do not reliably detect atlanto-occipital instability. Old lateral neck radiographs are not available for this child. Since this is an emergency, a radiographic examination is not possible. Therefore, C-spine precautions should be performed.

Is an awake tracheotomy a good option for this child? The awake tracheotomy in an uncooperative child is challenging. While this approach would maintain a protected airway at all times, it is unlikely that this child will tolerate this procedure awake and would be impractical. The plan is to perform an intravenous rapid sequence induction employing indirect laryngoscopy. Preparations for rigid laryngoscopy are in place and the surgeon is also prepared to perform a surgical airway if needed (in this case a triple setup).

What Would You Do If Attempts at Gaining Intravenous Access Fail?

Following the failed attempt to start an intravenous line in the emergency department, the child was brought to the OR. Venous access is crucial for induction and fluid resuscitation. Placement of a central line in the awake child is an option. For internal jugular vein access, the head needs to be rotated increasing the risk associated with atlanto-occipital instability. The subclavian approach has the risk of potentially causing a pneumothorax. An ultrasound-guided femoral vein approach may be a feasible alternative.

Several studies have shown that an intraosseous cannula can be placed rapidly and this line provides excellent access for the administration of medication and fluids.[18] Because of the risk associated with central line placement, an intraosseous cannula was placed without incident in the proximal right tibia. A fluid bolus of 20 $mL{\cdot}kg^{-1}$ was also administered. Atropine 0.1 $mg{\cdot}kg^{-1}$ was administered to reduce additional secretions and mitigate vagal response secondary to laryngoscopy. Routine monitors (pulse oximetry, noninvasive blood pressure, and ECG) were applied prior to the induction of anesthesia.

Discuss the Anesthetic and Airway Management

Concurrent with the placement of an intraosseous cannula, the child was prepared for a rapid sequence induction. The lungs were denitrogenated with 100% FiO_2 for 3 minutes with a face mask that was reasonably tolerated with much cajoling. Considering the possibility of significant hypovolemia, a 50:50 mixture of ketamine and propofol was selected for induction with succinylcholine for neuromuscular blockade. Cricoid pressure during induction was not applied to avoid stimulating vomiting in the already agitated child, and the pressure was applied after the child was deeply anesthetized. The oropharynx was suctioned immediately and several clots were removed with the Magill forceps after anesthesia induction. The brisk bleeding from the right tonsillar bed was noted.

Direct laryngoscopy was not attempted since the initial laryngoscopy revealed a Grade 3 C-L view. Since the oral cavity appeared to be free of clots, indirect laryngoscopy was performed using the GlideScope. Unfortunately, blood obscured the lens of the GlideScope necessitating the removal of the device. Oxygen saturation began to drop below 90% and bag-mask ventilation with cricoid pressure was started with the prompt recovery of oxygen saturation.

Faced with a failed intubation, it was decided to insert an air-Q extraglottic airway device. After thoroughly suctioning the oral cavity under direct laryngoscopy with a rigid catheter, a number 2.5 air-Q was easily inserted. Pressure-controlled ventilation through the air-Q was then initiated. A 5.5 mm ID uncuffed ETT was loaded on a pediatric flexible bronchoscope. Using the air-Q as a conduit, the bronchoscope was advanced into the trachea. Blood and secretions were present in the air-Q and in the trachea but did not obscure the laryngeal view. The ETT was advanced easily over the bronchoscope into the trachea. With a small air leak at 20 cm H_2O airway pressure, it was decided not to change the ETT over an airway exchanger to a cuffed ETT. Since the air-Q did not obscure the surgeon's view, it was decided to leave the air-Q in place and remove it along with the ETT at the conclusion of the procedure. The ENT surgeon cauterized the tonsillar bed, and the artery was successfully ligated.

At the end of the procedure, the air-Q was deflated and an orogastric tube was placed and the stomach was suctioned. The child was taken to the pediatric ICU where the ETT and air-Q were removed one hour later.

OTHER CONSIDERATIONS

What Is the Current Thinking with Respect to the Surgical Management of Post-Tonsillectomy Bleeding?

Life-threatening post-tonsillectomy bleeding requires an aggressive approach to surgical management. Initially, pressure on the bleeding tonsillar fossa with clamped gauze or the index finger may give sufficient time to obtain intravenous access for blood work and cross-match and to provide fluid resuscitation or blood transfusion if indicated. Soaking the gauze with either epinephrine or tranexamic acid or applying topical thrombin or absorbable hemostatic agents will assist with bleeding control.[2] If intraoperative localization of the bleeding source is time-consuming and local treatment is ineffective, ligation of the external carotid artery may be required. This is because an aberrant blood supply to the tonsillar region deriving from the internal carotid artery or the carotid bulb may be present necessitating angiographic embolization of the feeding artery.[19]

Are There Specific Measures to Reduce the Postoperative Morbidity and Mortality of Patients Following Tonsillectomy?

Tonsillectomy Technique

In comparison to the cold knife technique, hot techniques employing bipolar diathermy or coblation are associated with an increased rate of secondary bleeding.[20] The duration, frequency, and surgical extent of these techniques are linked to the amount of damage to the surrounding tissue. This damage leads to deeper zones of local necrosis which is vulnerable to bacteria- and enzyme-containing saliva, and therefore at increased risk of secondary bleeding.[20]

Nonsteroidal Anti-Inflammatory Drugs (NSAIDs)

The concern of increased intraoperative hemorrhage and postoperative bleeding is controversial. An earlier meta-analysis showed an increased risk of reoperation for hemostasis post-tonsillectomy if conventional NSAIDs such as ketorolac/ibuprofen were used for postoperative pain control in children.[21] However, more recent meta-analyses did not find an altered number of perioperative bleeding events in patients receiving NSAIDs for tonsillectomy.[22] A recent clinical practice guideline on tonsillectomy in children strongly recommends the postoperative use of ibuprofen.[3] Postoperative opioids should be used with caution, especially in younger children and/or OSAS.[23]

Effects of PONV

The presence of PONV increases the risk of primary hemorrhage and unexpected postoperative hospital admission. Poorly controlled pain leads to decreased oral intake and dehydration and is one leading cause of delayed hospital discharge or readmission. Dexamethasone has antiemetic properties and its anti-inflammatory effect may decrease postoperative pain in the perioperative setting.[24] A recent clinical practice guideline on tonsillectomy in children strongly recommends a single intraoperative dose of intravenous dexamethasone.[3]

Tonsillectomy as Outpatient Surgery

Tonsillectomies are commonly performed as outpatient procedures. The following list should prompt the need for inpatient admission after tonsillectomy[3,25]:

- Age under 3 years
- Medical conditions that increase surgical and anesthesia risks
- Craniofacial abnormalities
- Abnormal coagulation
- OSA (apnea-hypopnea index > 10, oxygen saturation nadir $<80\%$, or both)
- Acute peritonsillar abscess
- Family conditions that prevent easy and rapid return to a medical facility

Patients should always be observed for a minimum of 6 hours. They should be able to tolerate oral fluids and be pain tolerant prior to discharge. As an alternative to hospital admission, a 23-hour overnight observation period can be considered.

SUMMARY

Post-tonsillectomy bleeding is a rare event, occurring most often within 24 hours following tonsillectomy. However, it may be delayed for up to 14 days postoperatively. The severity of bleeding with the need to ensure a still surgical field makes operative revisions under general anesthesia often necessary. The insidious nature of the bleeding may lead to significant hypovolemia which is often difficult to assess. Intravenous access and fluid resuscitation, with a type and cross-match, are important interventions needed for these children.

Aspiration and a difficult airway are major risks during the induction of anesthesia in patients with post-tonsillectomy bleeding. Rapid sequence induction and tracheal intubation with direct laryngoscopy is the accepted first choice in the management of these children.

An array of alternative pediatric airway management devices (e.g., extraglottic device, video laryngoscope, flexible bronchoscope) must be immediately available. A surgeon experienced in rigid bronchoscopy and establishment of a surgical airway must be present if alternative techniques fail.

SELF-EVALUATION QUESTIONS

48.1. Which of the following airway management techniques would MOST likely be ineffective in managing in a child with post-tonsillectomy bleeding?

A. Direct laryngoscopy

B. Video laryngoscopy

C. Awake intubation using a flexible bronchoscope

D. Supraglottic device with subsequent bronchoscopy-guided endotracheal intubation

SECTION 7

48.2. Which of the following approaches best represents the generally accepted preoperative management in severe post-tonsillectomy bleeding?

A. History and physical, followed by rapid IV access with fluid resuscitation and operative revision under general anesthesia

B. History and physical, followed by rapid IV access with fluid resuscitation and operative revision under sedation without endotracheal intubation to avoid laryngospasm

C. Endotracheal intubation in the emergency room as soon as possible because of the risk of rapid swelling of the oropharynx

D. History and physical, IV access and blood work, and elective operative revision as soon as the 6-hour NPO timeframe is reached because of the risk of aspiration

48.3. Which of the following medications is not recommended in the perioperative setting of tonsillectomy?

A. Propofol

B. Ibuprofen

C. Codeine

D. Sevoflurane

REFERENCES

1. Boss EF, Marsteller JA, Simon AE. Outpatient tonsillectomy in children: demographic and geographic variation in the United States, 2006. *J Pediatr.* 2011;160:814-819.
2. Wal JJ, Tay KY. Postoperative tonsillectomy hemorrhage. *Emerg Med Clin N Am.* 2018;36:415-426.
3. Mitchell RB, Archer SM, Ishman SL, et al. Clinical practice guideline: tonsillectomy in children (update). Executive summary. *Otolaryngol Head Neck Surg.* 2019;160:187-205.
4. Windfuhr JP. Serious complications following tonsillectomy: how frequently are they really? *ORL J Otorhinolaryngol Relat Spec.* 2013;75:166-173.
5. Fields RG, Gencorelli FJ, Litman RS. Anesthestic management of the pediatric bleeding tonsil. *Pediatr Anesth.* 2010;20:982-986.
6. Francis DO, Fonnesbeck C, Sathe N, et al. Postoperative bleeding and associated utilization following tonsillectomy in children: a systematic review and meta-analysis. *Otolaryngol Head Neck Surg.* 2017;156:442-455.
7. Goldman JL, Baugh RF, Davies L, et al. Mortality and major morbidity after tonsillectomy: etiological factors and strategies for prevention. *Laryngoscope.* 2013;123:2544-2553.
8. Rasmussen N. Complications of tonsillectomy and adenoidectomy. *Otolaryngol Clin North Am.* 1987;20:383-390.
9. Windfurh JP, Schloendorff G, Seterhenn AM, et al. Devastating outcome after adenoidectomy and tonsillectomy: ideas for improved prevention and management. *Otolaryngol Head Neck Surg.* 2009;140:191-196.
10. Spektor Z, Saint-Victor S, Kay DJ, et al. Risk factors for pediatric post-tonsillectomy hemorrhage. *Int J Pediatr Otorhinolaryngol.* 2016;79:165-169.
11. Bissonnette B, Dalens BJ. *Pediatric Anesthesia: Principles and Practice.* New York, NY: McGraw-Hill; 2002.
12. Kojima T, Harwayne-Gidansky I, Shenoi A, et al. Cricoid pressure during induction for tracheal intubation in critically children: a report from National Emergency Airway Registry for Children. *Pediatr Crit Care Med.* 2018;19:528-537.
13. Black AE, Flynn PE, Smith HL, Thomas ML, Wilkinson KA. Development of a guideline for the management of the unanticipated difficult airway in pediatric practice. *Paediatr Anesth.* 2015;25:346-362.
14. Lim NL. The use of the laryngeal mask airway in post-tonsillectomy hemorrhage – a case report. *Ann Acad Med.* 2000;29:764-765.
15. Nader-Sepahi A, Casey ATH, Hayward R, Crockard HA, Thompson D. Symptomatic atlantoaxial instability in Down Syndrome. *J Neurosurg.* 2005;103:231-237.
16. Agarwal J, Tandon MS, Singh D, Ganjoo P. Quadriplegia in a child following adenotonsillectomy. *Anesthesia.* 2013;68:523-526.
17. Nakamura N, Inaba Y, Aota Y, et al. New radiological parameters for the assessment of atlantoaxial instability in children with Down syndrome: the normal values and the risk of spinal cord injury. *Bone Joint J.* 2016;98:1704-1710.
18. Whitney R, Langhan M. Vascular access in pediatric patients in the emergency department: types of access, indications, and complications. *Pediatr Emerg Med Pract.* 2017;14:1-20.
19. Windfuhr JP, Schloendorff G, Baburi D, Kremer B. Life-threatening post-tonsillectomy hemorrhage. *Laryngoscope.* 2008;118:1389-1394.
20. Lowe D, Van der Meulen J. Tonsillectomy technique as a risk factor for postoperative hemorrhage. *Lancet.* 2004;364:697-702.
21. Marret E, Flahault A, Samama CM, Bonnet F. Effects of postoperative, non steroidal, anti-inflammatory drugs on bleeding risk after tonsillectomy: meta-analysis of randomized controlled trials. *Anesthesiology.* 2003;98:1497-1502.
22. Riggin L, Ramakrishna DD, Sommer G, Koren A. A 2013 updated systematic review and meta-analysis of 36 randomized controlled trials: no apparent effects of non steroidal anti-inflammatory agents on the risk of bleeding after tonsillectomy. *Clin Otolaryngol.* 2013;38:115-129.
23. Tan GX, Tunkel DE. Control of pain after tonsillectomy in children. A review. *JAMA Otolaryngol Head Neck Surg.* 2017;143:937-942.
24. King A, Elmaranghy C, Lind M, Tobias JD. A review of dexamethasone as an adjunct to adenotonsillectomy in the pediatric population. *J Anesth.* 2020;34:445-452.
25. Lauder G, Emmott A. Confronting the challenges of effective pain management in children following tonsillectomy. *Int J Pediatr Otorhinolaryngol.* 2014;78:1813-1827.

CHAPTER 49

Airway Management in a 6-Year-Old with Pierre Robin Syndrome for Bilateral Inguinal Hernia Repair

Ban C.H. Tsui and Stephanie Pan

CASE PRESENTATION

A 6-year-old child with Pierre Robin sequence (PRS) presents for bilateral inguinal hernia repair. As a newborn, he underwent tongue-lip adhesion surgery for upper airway obstruction and feeding difficulties. The patient's anesthetic record reads, "Anterior larynx. direct laryngoscopy Cormack/Lehane Grade 4 view despite external laryngeal manipulation, with an inability to intubate the trachea." Subsequently, a nasal flexible bronchoscopic intubation was successfully performed. The patient has not had any other surgeries since.

INTRODUCTION

■ What Is Pierre Robin Sequence?

Named for the French dental surgeon who described its symptomatology and management, PRS (also known as Pierre Robin syndrome), is a congenital disorder characterized by a triad of congenital craniofacial anomalies: mandibular hypoplasia, cleft secondary palate, and glossoptosis (rostral displacement of the tongue).[1] Due to this combination of features, PRS is commonly viewed as a classic anticipated difficult airway scenario for pediatric anesthesia practitioners. In half of PRS cases, the positioning of the tongue during development precludes fusion of the maxillary arches, resulting in a broad, U-shaped cleft palate. Changes in the shape of the palate combined with the backward displacement of the tongue cause airway obstruction, respiratory difficulties, sleep apnea, and difficulty swallowing which can lead to chronic hypoxemia, pulmonary hypertension, and failure to thrive. Accurate preprocedural diagnosis is critical to ensure that a child's physical features are not more consistent with another congenital syndrome (e.g., Treacher-Collins syndrome, Stickler syndrome, or velocardiofacial syndrome) since the airway plan will be affected by the presence of associated abnormalities (e.g., congenital heart disease).

Appropriate management of breathing and feeding difficulties in infants with PRS reduces their mortality to less than 5%. Enteral feeding and prone positioning during nursing can improve nutritional intake.[2] Although some respiratory issues are managed without operative intervention, most require surgical intervention.[3] Most commonly, surgery to correct the cleft palate improves airway anatomy and swallowing ability. Tracheotomy is rarely indicated to treat respiratory problems in children with PRS. Mandibular distraction surgery is occasionally required to lengthen the mandible to bring the tongue forward and improve breathing and feeding mechanics. With effective treatment, most PRS individuals undergo normal childhood growth and development and experience healthy, normal adult life.

The craniofacial manifestations of PRS heavily impact an anesthesia practitioner's plans for induction and airway management as tracheal intubation and face-mask ventilation (FMV) are generally difficult. Patients with PRS often require multiple surgeries and general anesthetics. Thus, an effective airway management plan is essential to avoid compounding traumatic events.

What Are Other Congenital or Acquired Abnormalities Associated with Airway Difficulty?

Several congenital syndromes feature head, neck, and cervical spine anomalies that complicate the pediatric airway. These syndromes are summarized in Table 49.1 (see also Table 46.1).[4,5] Other anomalies are instead acquired. Examples of acquired anomalies include temporomandibular joint dysfunction following trauma (e.g., forceps delivery) or inflammation and microstomia from burns and caustic lesions. The following points summarize some issues that an anesthesia practitioner may encounter when attempting FMV or tracheal intubation in patients with malformations that affect airway management. Other sections of this chapter will discuss basic strategies to troubleshoot failed FMV and tracheal intubation. Marraro[6] provides a good resource on congenital and acquired malformations that may contribute to difficult pediatric airway.

TABLE 49.1. Selected Congenital Syndromes and Features Associated with a Difficult Airway

Syndrome	Abnormality
Apert syndrome	• Craniofacial dysostosis • Maxillary hypoplasia
Cockayne syndrome	• Ankylosis (temporomandibular joint) • Protruding incisors
Crouzon syndrome	• Craniofacial dysostosis • Mandibular hypoplasia • Micrognathia (or retrognathia)
Down syndrome (Trisomy 21)	• Atlanto-occipital instability • Pharyngomalacia • Limited cervical mobility • Macroglossia
Freeman-Sheldon syndrome	• Limited cervical mobility • Mandibular hypoplasia • Microstomia
Goldenhar syndrome	• Limited cervical mobility • Mandibular hypoplasia • Microsomia • Palatoschisis
Klippel-Feil syndrome	• Limited cervical mobility • Palatoschisis
Pierre Robin syndrome	• Cleft lip and palate • Glossoptosis • Mandibular hypoplasia • Micrognathia • Palatoschisis
Treacher-Collins syndrome	• Cleft lip and palate • Mandibular hypoplasia • Micrognathia • Maxillary hypoplasia • Palatoschisis • Zygomatic hypoplasia

- Children with craniofacial synostosis have high-arched palates and small nasal passages that lead them to breathe primarily through the mouth. Closing the mouth can cause complete airway occlusion due to the increased resistance to airflow via the small nares.
- In patients with hemifacial hypoplasia or microsomia (Goldenhar syndrome), FMV may be challenging due to the asymmetric fit of the mask over the face. The use of an extraglottic device (EGD) may be beneficial.
- Limited anterior mandibular space relative to the size of the tongue (e.g., PRS, Treacher-Collins syndrome) will make direct laryngoscopy and tracheal intubation difficult. Use of an EGD as a conduit for flexible bronchoscopic-guided intubation may be necessary. Alternatively, a combined technique utilizing video laryngoscopy with a flexible bronchoscope as a stylet can help navigate difficult tracheal intubation without the need to size the bronchoscope through the EGD.
- Tongue hyperplasia with and without mandibular/maxillary hypoplasia can increase the chance of airway obstruction. Curved blades may allow direct laryngoscopy in patients with large tongues (macroglossia), although direct laryngoscopy may be nearly impossible in some patients with mandibular hypoplasia. Since FMV can be challenging to maintain in patients with macroglossia, an oral and/or nasopharyngeal airway may be helpful to maintain airway patency.
- Microstomia (reduced mouth opening) can lead to difficult tracheal intubation difficult, especially with direct laryngoscopy.
- Visualization of the larynx can be challenging when the cervical spine and/or temporomandibular joint movement is limited. Causes of limited cervical spine range of motion can be due to congenital syndromes (e.g., Trisomy 21, Klippel-Feil syndrome), previous cervical spine fusions, trauma, or external soft tissue contractures. In addition to manual in-line stabilization, flexible bronchoscopy and lightwand can be used to facilitate tracheal intubation while minimizing cervical movement.
- Glossopexy, a procedure where the tongue is anchored to the lower lip and mandible to alleviate upper airway obstruction, may be needed in patients with glossoptosis.
- Hunter's syndrome and Hurler's syndrome (congenital mucopolysaccharidosis disorders) are associated with tongue enlargement, soft tissue thickening, and blockage of nasal passages. These patients frequently have a history of snoring. Tracheal intubation by direct laryngoscopy can be challenging because of the large incompressible tongue, which becomes progressively more severe without hematopoietic stem cell transplantation.

In clinical practice, the use of an EGD may be an effective alternative to tracheal intubation for maintaining airway patency, but EGDs are not without risks. Patients susceptible to airway obstruction must receive adequate anesthesia to avoid laryngospasm and bronchospasm. Tracheal intubation options are discussed later in the chapter.

PREPARATIONS FOR AIRWAY MANAGEMENT

How Do You Perform an Airway Assessment on This Patient?

Thorough documentation of the patient's history is essential, especially when diagnosed with an associated difficult airway. Although tracheal intubations in children with PRS tend to become less complicated with increasing age, the anesthesia practitioner should consider previous procedures in which the establishment of an airway was attempted and age-related changes in airway structures since the last airway management. Additionally, current symptoms such as difficulty breathing in certain body positions, recent upper or lower respiratory infections, and obstructive sleep apnea should be recognized and documented.

Systematic tools for airway assessment in adults including MOANS, LEMON, CRANE, RODS, and SHORT as discussed in Chapter 1 may not necessarily be applicable in children.[7] Instead, limited neck extension and flexibility, limited mouth opening, prominent overbite, high arched palate, recessed mandible or micrognathia, shortened thyromental distance, and large tongue size are key factors in predicting the difficulty of intubation in children.[8] Although a physical examination may yield unimpressive findings; one should always be prepared for an unanticipated difficult ventilation and intubation scenario by having appropriate equipment available and ready to use. In general, the physical examination includes the evaluation of:

- Size and shape of the head
- Gross facial features
- Symmetry and size of the mandible
- Tongue size
- The prominence of upper incisors
- Palate shape and anatomy
- Range of motion in the jaw, head, and neck.

It is important to point out that a substantial number of PRS patients present after the neonatal period with issues not related to respiratory failure, including sleep and swallowing problems. A presentation of respiratory failure is predictive of a more severe airway obstruction type and may require a tracheotomy.[9]

Do You Have Any Other Medical Concerns for This Child?

PRS is not associated with congenital cardiac or other major organ involvement in isolation. These patients have usually received general anesthesia early in their life to correct craniofacial abnormalities. However, PRS infants with severe dysphagia or airway obstruction may have recurrent aspiration events and pulmonary hypertension.

What Are the General Principles and Processes for Approaching the Difficult Pediatric Airway?

Comprehensive planning is critical for managing a pediatric patient with a difficult airway. Although the anesthetic plan will be guided primarily by the patient's physical examination and history, the surgical procedure and anesthesia practitioner's experience and familiarity with the available resources will also influence the plan. Since pediatric patients can often have rapid oxygen desaturations in challenging situations, each patient must be evaluated carefully to anticipate potential difficulties and plan for unforeseen issues. The anesthesia practitioner should have sufficient experience with the normal pediatric airway before attempting to deal with a difficult one; additional expertise should be solicited upon suspicion of a difficult airway.

Airway equipment should be prepared ahead of time to deal with both difficult ventilation and intubation scenarios. The patient should be optimally positioned before induction and intubation (i.e., placement of shoulder rolls/bolsters to achieve the "sniffing" position with cervical flexion and atlanto-occipital extension). The induction technique should also be tailored to the specific needs of the patient. Document the anesthetic plan that is discussed with the patient (and their parents) and communicate your plan and concerns to the intraoperative team (both surgeons and nurses) to enhance multidisciplinary awareness and teamwork. The benefits of the planned surgery should always be weighed against the potential risks of the anesthetic management.[10] Table 49.2 lists some key points that should be considered prior to intubating the trachea of a child with a difficult airway.

What Are Appropriate Induction Techniques for Patients with a Difficult Airway?

The primary objectives for induction in a difficult airway situation include maintaining spontaneous ventilation and achieving a plane of anesthesia that will enable airway instrumentation. It is essential to allow sufficient time for visualization of the structures and performance of intubation. A few key considerations are as follows:

- Induction should be smooth and gradual, with the ability to safely abort if alternative plans fail.
- Sedating agents are known to cause loss of airway muscle tone and increase airway resistance. In some cases, premedication with oral midazolam (0.3-0.5 $mg{\cdot}kg^{-1}$, max 20 mg) or intranasal midazolam (0.2-0.3 $mg.kg^{-1}$) can facilitate a smooth induction in an uncooperative or anxious child. The higher range of midazolam may be preferred as lower doses can cause paradoxical agitation in children.
- Glycopyrrolate (oral 20 $\mu g{\cdot}kg^{-1}$ or intravenous [IV]/intramuscular [IM] 4 $\mu g{\cdot}kg^{-1}$, with a maximum of 100 μg) can be used to dry secretions and avoid severe bradycardia during induction. Atropine (oral 30-40 $\mu g{\cdot}kg^{-1}$ or IV/IM 20 $\mu g{\cdot}kg^{-1}$) can be an alternative if glycopyrrolate is not available although glycopyrrolate is preferred due to fewer central nervous system side effects. Either glycopyrrolate or atropine can be given once IV access is secured.
- Since most experts believe that the maintenance of spontaneous ventilation is a top priority, inhalation induction

TABLE 49.2. Considerations for Intubating a Child with a Difficult Airway

Preparation	• Is an appropriate team of health care professionals (e.g., ENT surgeon) available? • Is the equipment required prepared and readily available?
Anesthesia	• Is there an option to perform surgery using regional anesthesia only with light sedation?
Intubation (awake)	• Is there an option to perform bronchoscopic intubation or tracheostomy while the patient is awake?
Intubation (anesthetized)	• Is the ability to maintain spontaneous ventilation possible with ease? • Be aware of any procedures that would eliminate that patient's ability to breathe spontaneously. • Is the IV secured allowing the option of titrating IV agents (e.g., ketamine or propofol/remifentanil) in addition to inhalational agents? • Positive pressure ventilation should only be considered as a last resort.

Adapted with permission from Goldschneider KR, Davidson AJ, Wittkugel EP, et al. *Clinical Pediatric Anesthesia: A Case-Based Handbook*. Oxford: Oxford University Press, 2012.

remains the most popular approach. Still, care must be taken when using inhaled anesthetics, which can cause the risk of apnea, laryngospasm, and loss of airway.[11] Furthermore, this technique can be challenging if the face mask does not have a tight seal on the face. The most commonly used inhalational induction agent is sevoflurane due to its low blood:gas solubility which allows for rapid induction of and emergence from anesthesia, nonpungent odor, lack of irritation to the airway, and minimal end-organ effects.[12] Regardless of the chosen induction route, IV access should be secured prior to any airway instrumentation.

- Alternatively, an IV propofol-remifentanil infusion can be used to induce anesthesia while maintaining spontaneous ventilation. When titrated carefully, greater than 90% of patients will breathe spontaneously with remifentanil 0.05 $\mu g \cdot kg^{-1} \cdot min^{-1}$.[13] Boluses of ketamine (1-2 $mg \cdot kg^{-1}$) can be used to supplement a propofol-remifentanil approach. In practice, a sevoflurane inhaled induction will often commence first followed by a propofol-remifentanil infusion once IV access has been secured. The propofol-remifentanil infusion can then be titrated to an appropriate plane of anesthesia (as any inhaled anesthetic agents are discontinued) for airway management.

What Are the Clinical Strategies for a Challenging Face-Mask Ventilation?

The position and seal of the face mask should be evaluated if FMV is difficult. Repositioning the mask or fingers, changing the mask size or type, and ensuring a continuous circuit can be helpful. Additional considerations include:

- FMV technique should not obstruct the patient's airway. An appropriately sized mask will not compress the nose. The anesthesia practitioner's fingers should be placed along the mandible so as not to compress the submandibular soft tissues.
- If airway obstruction is observed, application of a jaw thrust and placement of an oral and/or nasal airway can improve airway patency. Switching to the lateral decubitus position may help to alleviate the obstruction during FMV but consideration should be given to performing subsequent airway management techniques in the lateral decubitus position versus the supine position. Multiple position changes may not be ideal.
- A chin lift reverses the posterior, gravity-induced displacement of the epiglottis and widens the pharyngeal cavity. One hand is used to lift the inferior border of the mental protuberance to bring the teeth together without protruding the mandible. The thumb and index finger form a C-shape to hold the mask, while the ring finger performs the lift. Large adenoids and tonsils may limit the efficacy of this maneuver in opening the airway.[14]
- A jaw thrust can force the mouth open and requires two hands to pull the mandibular angles upward and anteriorly. This technique is recommended when the chin lift is not successful[15] and can also be used to confirm an adequate depth of anesthesia for EGD insertion.
- Continuous positive airway pressure (CPAP) (e.g., 10 cm H_2O) increases airway volume and area. High airway pressures should be avoided due to resultant insufflation of the stomach, which can lead to increased work of breathing, decreased respiratory compliance, impaired venous return to the heart, and increased aspiration risk.
- An oral airway that is too large may cause obstruction by forcing the epiglottis down over the glottis or may obstruct venous and lymphatic drainage. On the other hand, if the oral airway is too small, it may cause obstruction by pushing the tongue backward. A poorly positioned airway can also induce pressure necrosis of the tongue. The distance between the mouth and the angle of the mandible can be used to estimate the appropriate size of an oral airway.[16]
- If oral airway insertion fails, the use of an EGD (e.g., i-gel, LMA) is an alternative option.

What Are the Clinical Strategies for Difficult Intubation?

In children with anticipated difficult airways, different airway management strategies should be considered in advance to minimize the number of attempts that can lead to upper airway trauma.[4] If the surgery does not require endotracheal intubation, an EGD may be attempted. If EGD placement is suboptimal or contraindicated, direct laryngoscopy or video laryngoscopy may be attempted with either a straight or curved blade. Although intubation of an awake patient (e.g., flexible bronchoscopic intubation) is classically taught as the preferred method for an anticipated difficult intubation, some sedation is often needed in the pediatric population. In rare cases, retrograde intubation or cricothyrotomy may be necessary. In extreme cases, a tracheotomy will be needed, in which case an otorhinolaryngologist should be notified ahead of time.[17]

Figure 49.1 provides an algorithm that can be followed to guide the airway management of a patient with a known difficult airway.

For patients with an unexpected difficult tracheal intubation, the following steps are suggested[4,10,11]:

1. Call for help.
2. Maintain ventilation and oxygenation—if inadequate, refer to the above strategies.
3. Reattempt intubation once the patient's position has been reassessed and optimized (e.g., "sniffing position" with

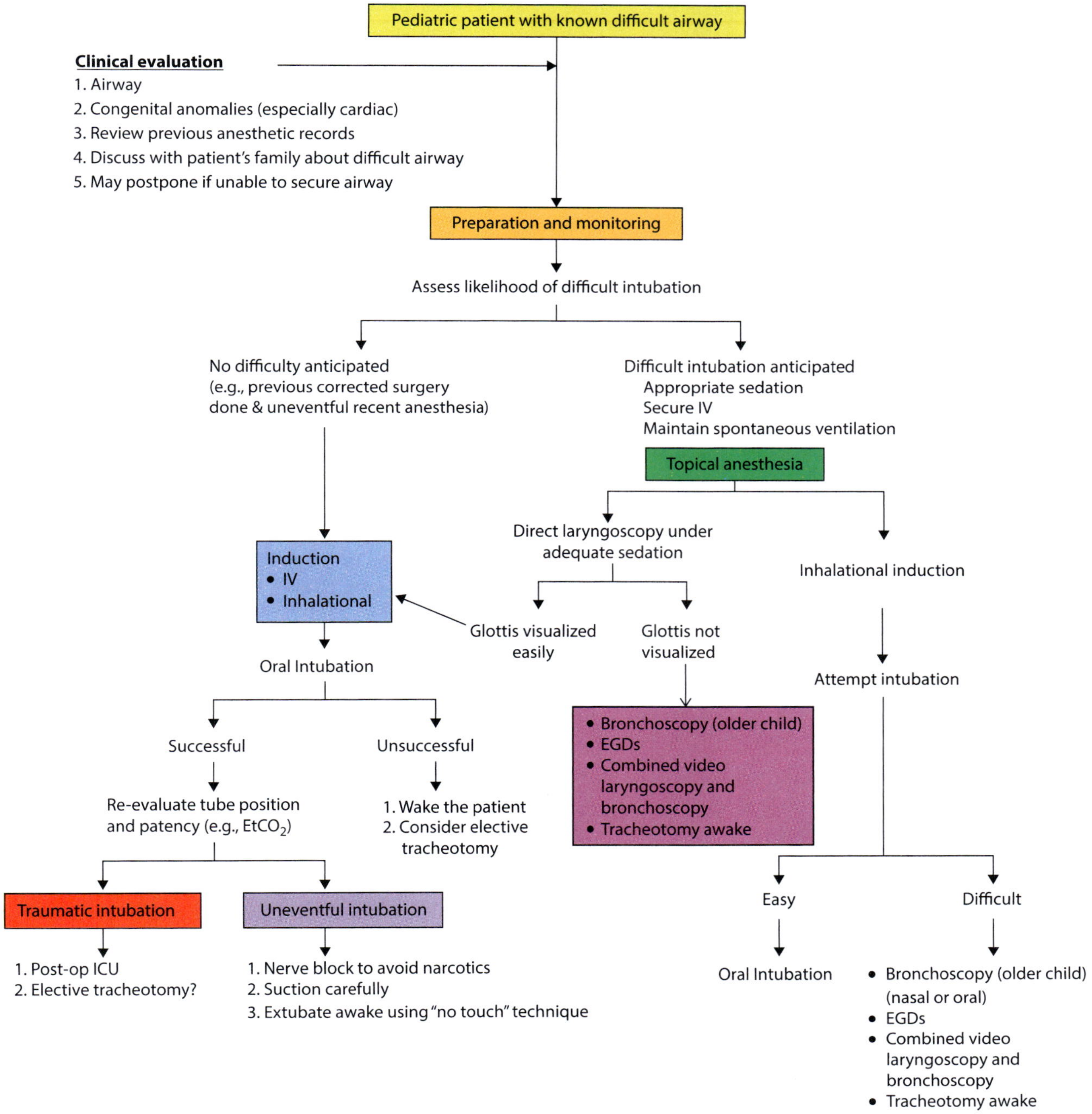

FIGURE 49.1. Algorithm for determining intubation sequence for a child with a known difficult airway.

cervical spine flexion, atlanto-occipital extension). If the initial attempt with direct laryngoscopy was unsuccessful, consider using a different blade or blade size, different intubation equipment (e.g., McCoy levering or video laryngoscope [e.g., GlideScope®]); and/or different intubation technique (e.g., paraglossal[18] or retromolar[19] where the blade is advanced along the lateral pharyngeal wall). External manipulation of the airway (e.g., backward, upward, rightward pressure, or BURP) may improve the laryngeal exposure of an anterior laryngeal view.
4. Place an EGD. Depending on the situation, an EGD may be kept in place (as opposed to intubating the trachea) if adequate oxygenation and ventilation can be maintained and the EGD does not affect the surgical procedure. Otherwise, flexible bronchoscopic intubation through an EGD should be considered.
5. No more than three attempts at intubation should be performed (with no more than two direct laryngoscopy attempts) to minimize morbidity.
6. If multiple failed intubations are encountered, wake the patient up if possible. Otherwise, a tracheotomy or cricothyrotomy may be the fastest option in a "can't ventilate and can't oxygenate" situation.

Equipment for difficult airway cases should include:

- Face masks, nasopharyngeal airways, and oropharyngeal airways in different sizes.
- Two laryngoscope blades of varying lengths and widths. Two laryngoscope handles with optimal light output.
- Tracheal tubes in different sizes with lubricated intubating stylets preloaded.
- EGDs (preferably devices manufactured for tracheal intubation) for airway rescue and for tracheal intubation (e.g., Fastrach-LMA [intubating LMA], Air-Q).
- Other appropriate intubating devices (lightwand [Trachlight™], pediatric Bullard laryngoscope, GlideScope, C-MAC video laryngoscope, infant flexible bronchoscope). All devices should be loaded, tested, and lubricated (where appropriate).
- Surgical tracheotomy tray and uncuffed percutaneous cricothyrotomy set with an otorhinolaryngologist who is either immediately available or, preferably, already present in the room.

Although a detailed description of all airway tools is beyond the scope of this chapter, most devices have been covered and discussed in other chapters. Briefly, the use of alternative laryngoscope blades or modified laryngoscopes (e.g., McCoy laryngoscope, Bullard laryngoscope) may improve the success of securing a difficult airway. EGDs have been used successfully in children as a conduit for endoscopic intubation and should be available in all cases of pediatric airway management, particularly when anticipating any difficulty. Flexible or rigid bronchoscopes may also be used for intubation. A transillumination technique using a lightwand (e.g., Trachlight) may be used when direct laryngoscopy or flexible bronchoscopy has failed. Other devices such as the flexible bronchoscope and video laryngoscopes are discussed in this chapter.

ANESTHESIA MANAGEMENT

What Are the Anesthetic Options for This Child?

At age 6, the patient is well beyond the age at which PRS symptoms present the most significant problems in establishing an airway. At ages 5 to 6, mandibular hypoplasia may be improved but does not completely resolve.[20] Thus, there is still a chance for the anesthesia practitioner to encounter a difficult airway scenario with this patient.

For a 6-year-old child, several options for anesthesia can be considered, all of which have been successfully used in young children:

1. Regional anesthesia with light sedation and without airway intervention.
2. Combined regional and general anesthesia with airway intervention (either EGD placement or tracheal intubation).
3. General anesthesia with tracheal intubation using one of the following methods:
   a. Direct laryngoscopy and intubation.
   b. Flexible bronchoscopic intubation with or without an EGD.
   c. Video laryngoscopic intubation with or without flexible bronchoscopy assistance.
4. Awake intubation before induction of general anesthesia (however, this seldom works in uncooperative children and can be very psychologically traumatizing to a child).

Since the patient is likely too young to be cooperative enough for regional anesthesia alone, general anesthesia with or without regional analgesia is recommended. The flowchart in Figure 49.2 describes alternative anesthetic options based on airway difficulty.

Preparations for Airway Management

The primary goals of the anesthesia practitioner when securing the airway of a pediatric patient include:

1. Maintain adequate spontaneous oxygenation and ventilation.
2. Blunt the airway reflexes to allow for airway manipulation.
3. Minimize hemodynamic responses associated with airway manipulation (e.g., bradycardia and hypertension).
4. Avoid aspiration.
5. Minimize airway trauma.
6. Ensure amnesia followed by rapid recovery of consciousness and airway reflexes.

Any manipulation of the airway should be performed after IV access is secured, which can be done awake or under sedation. If the IV is placed in an awake child, topical EMLA™ cream can be applied to the relevant area 60 to 90 minutes prior to the placement of the IV. Alternatively, analgesia for IV placement can be obtained using buffered lidocaine delivered through a J-tip, a needle-free injection system, for a more immediate effect. EMLA can also provide topical anesthesia when applied to a patient's lower back if regional

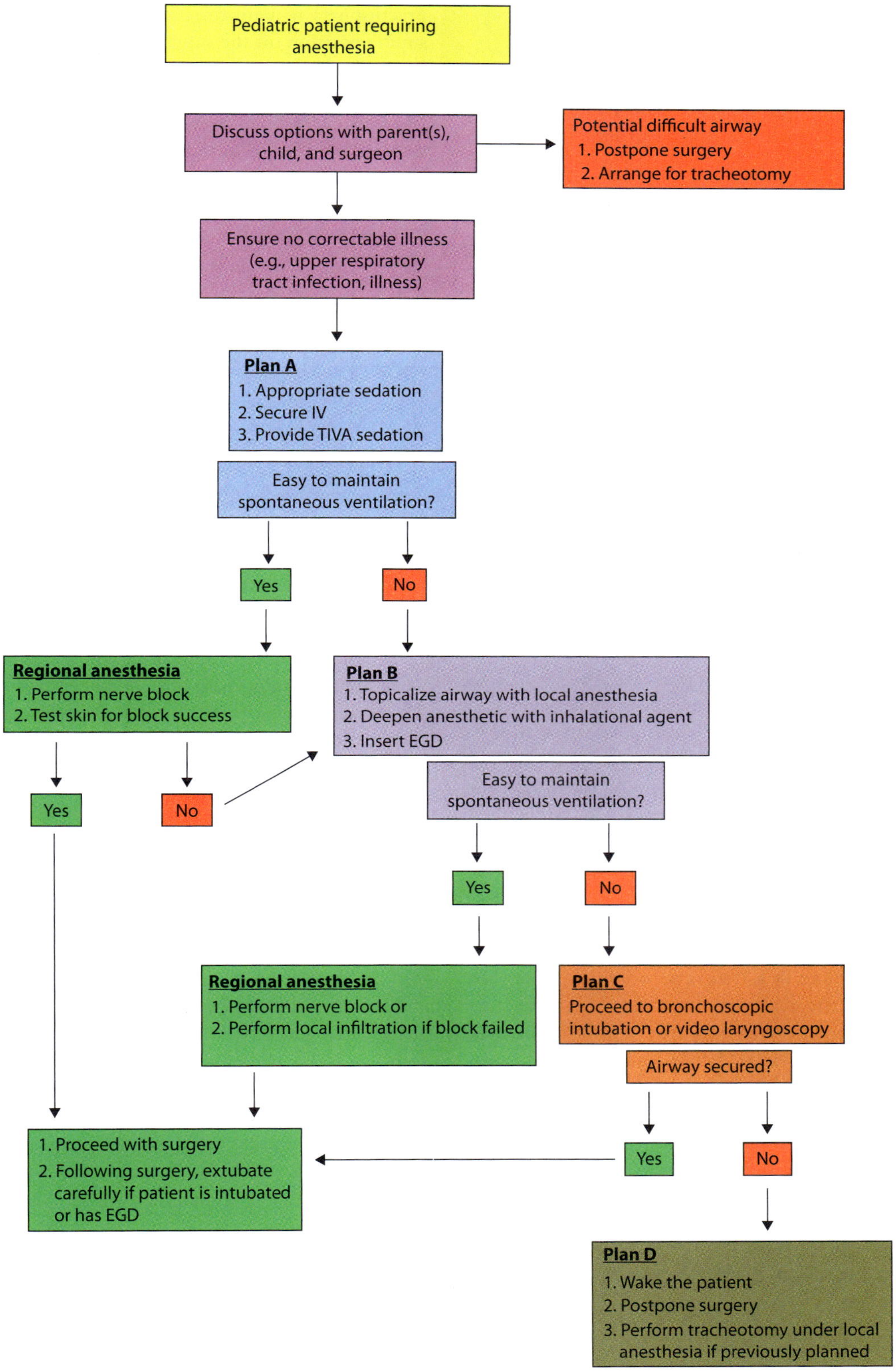

FIGURE 49.2. Options for anesthesia for a pediatric patient undergoing bilateral hernia repair.

anesthesia (caudal epidural or spinal) is considered. If available, a certified child life specialist can be an invaluable resource in helping a child through procedures. Alternatively, virtual reality or distraction using music and videos can also be advantageous.

Prepare all anesthetic and emergency drugs in advance. A difficult airway cart with appropriate equipment should be previously checked and readily on hand. Trained airway assistants should be available, including surgical staff who may be required to obtain a surgical airway if necessary.

What Are the Options for Regional Anesthesia?

For bilateral hernia repair, various regional anesthesia techniques including the ilioinguinal nerve block, the transversus abdominis plane (TAP) block, the quadratus lumborum (QL) block, and the caudal epidural block can be performed. The advantage of the peripheral nerve blocks, such as the ilioinguinal nerve block, TAP block, and QL block, is that the block can be done with the child supine. With less repositioning needed, the risk of dislodging any airway devices present is reduced. Brief descriptions of each block are provided below. Detailed descriptions of these blocks, including landmark and ultrasound-guided approaches, are described elsewhere (see section "Acknowledgments").

For the ilioinguinal nerve block, the patient should be supine. The anterior superior iliac spine (ASIS) and the umbilicus are used as landmarks; the needle insertion site is approximately one patient's fingerbreadth medial and cephalad to the ASIS. Alternatively, a line drawn from the ASIS to the umbilicus is divided into thirds. The needle should be inserted at the lateral third closest to the ASIS. The needle is placed perpendicularly to the skin and a "click" is often felt upon penetration through the internal oblique muscle. After aspiration, 0.3 to 0.5 mL·kg^{-1} of levobupivacaine 0.25%, bupivacaine 0.5%, or ropivacaine 0.5% (up to 3-4 mL) is injected. Another 0.5 to 1 mL of the local anesthetic can be injected subcutaneously to anesthetize the iliohypogastric nerve. Ultrasound can be used to identify the ilioinguinal and iliohypogastric nerves which can be found between the external and internal oblique muscles or between the internal oblique and transversus abdominis muscles, depending on the patient's anatomic variation.

For the TAP and QL blocks, the patient should be in the supine position. Both blocks should be performed under ultrasound guidance to minimize peritoneal or bowel puncture. To perform the TAP block, the ultrasound probe should be placed along the midaxillary line in a transverse orientation between the costal margin and the iliac crest. The three abdominal muscle layers seen from superficial to deep are the external oblique, internal oblique, and transversus abdominis muscles. The needle should be inserted in-plane with the ultrasound. The local anesthetic should be deposited between the internal oblique and transversus abdominis muscles.

Although there are three different types of QL blocks, the lateral QL or QL1 block is the easier one to perform. The ultrasound probe is moved laterally from the view seen in the TAP block such that the lateral border of the quadratus lumborum muscle and the tapering aponeurosis of the transversus abdominis muscle are seen. The needle is typically inserted in-plane from an anterior to posterior approach to avoid injuring the ipsilateral kidney. The local anesthetic is deposited at the tapering of the aponeurosis adjacent to the quadratus lumborum muscle. Commonly used local anesthetics for both the TAP and QL blocks include 0.5 mL·kg^{-1} of levobupivacaine 0.25%, bupivacaine 0.5%, or ropivacaine 0.5% (with a max of 3 mg·kg^{-1} of a local anesthetic to avoid systemic local anesthetic toxicity).

For the caudal block, the patient is placed in the lateral decubitus position (left side down for a right-handed anesthesia practitioner) to perform the block and then returned to the supine position for the surgery. Thus, the airway device should be secured prior to any repositioning, especially in small (<10 kg) children. A local anesthetic agent with rapid onset is preferred to circumvent laryngospasm upon surgical incision. A 1:1 mixture of lidocaine 2% and bupivacaine 0.25% (or ropivacaine 0.2%) 1 mL·kg^{-1} is suitable and will provide adequate block duration. The block duration can be extended by adding preservative-free dexmedetomidine 1 to 2 μg·kg^{-1},[21] clonidine 1 to 2 μg·kg^{-1},[22] or neostigmine 2 to 4 μg·kg^{-1}.[23] The benefits of a caudal block include potential reduction in anesthetic vapor and opioid usage. In addition, if any airway problems arise, there exists a secondary means of providing anesthesia.

Should Anxious Children Receive Premedication?

Some practitioners will advocate for never using a sedating premedication in children with an anticipated difficult airway so as not to compromise ventilation. However, airway secretions are increased in a crying child and an uncooperative child can make both inhalational and IV induction more difficult. All anesthesia practitioners can also appreciate the advantage of being able to connect monitors, apply a face mask, or establish IV access on a calm child in a controlled fashion. Thus, careful use of appropriate premedication anxiolysis with appropriate monitoring (see next section) has the added benefit of creating a more relaxed and therefore safer working environment.

How Should the Child Be Sedated in Preparation for Securing the Airway?

In general, calm children are better equipped to tolerate an inhalational mask induction. In an uncooperative or anxious child, an inhalational mask induction may worsen the child's response and behavior. Apart from extreme circumstances, "gorilla inductions"—in which the patient is forcefully restrained on the operating table with an anesthetic mask clamped over their face[24]—should not be used. Most pediatric anesthesia practitioners find it preferable to administer an anxiolytic prior to induction for an uncooperative child. The anxiolytic dose and route can be adjusted to the child's situation.

Successful sedation is often achieved with oral midazolam 0.5 mg·kg^{-1} dose or ketamine 3 mg·kg^{-1} 30 minutes prior to induction. If using inhalational anesthesia, an anticholinergic (atropine 0.02 mg·kg^{-1} or glycopyrrolate 0.05 mg·kg^{-1}) may also be given to dry secretions and prevent bradycardia. An alternative but less preferable method of sedation is to administer a "stunning" dose of IM ketamine 3 to 7 mg·kg^{-1}. A child with IV access can be sedated with small doses of either IV midazolam, ketamine, or dexmedetomidine.

The IV route has many benefits including easy titration of sedative drugs, avoidance of volatile anesthetic exposure, and reliable access for resuscitative medications. Sedation while maintaining spontaneous respiration can be accomplished with an infusion of propofol with remifentanil (e.g., 100-200 μg·kg^{-1}·min^{-1} of propofol and 0.025-0.075 μg·kg^{-1}·min^{-1}

of remifentanil). Sedatives should be given in small incremental doses only if necessary. Some anesthesia practitioners also use a volatile anesthetic agent, such as sevoflurane, as an adjunct to be administered along with propofol with remifentanil infusion as tolerated.

What Are the Benefits and Risks of Applying Topical Airway Anesthetic?

The goal of airway topicalization is to avoid triggering the airway reflexes upon manipulation of the airway, such as for tracheal intubation with the use of a flexible bronchoscope. Lidocaine is the most often used local anesthetic for airway topicalization due to its quick onset and ease of application through various routes and concentrations (e.g., nebulizer, atomizer, spray, "swish and gargle," soaked cotton pledgets, gel application). Because lidocaine absorption from the highly vascular mucous membranes of the pharynx and trachea is comparable to IV administration, the total amount of lidocaine that can be used should be calculated ahead of time, based on the patient's weight. Failure to do so can cause inadvertent overdoses and local anesthetic systemic toxicity.

Ideally, topicalization should occur preoperatively, but this can be challenging for children in an operative setting. Nebulization is one option, especially if the child is familiar with nebulization used for other medications. Alternatively, lidocaine can be nebulized in-circuit simultaneously with sevoflurane during an inhalational induction.[25]

Another option is spraying the larynx directly after induction of anesthesia through the use of a laryngotracheal atomizer. Although this is the most efficient method, it requires a deep plane of anesthesia and a good view of the larynx, which can be difficult to achieve in a child with a challenging airway.[26]

AIRWAY MANAGEMENT OPTIONS

How Is a Flexible Bronchoscopic Intubation Performed?

Flexible bronchoscopy is a useful option if an EGD cannot be placed easily. Commercially available flexible bronchoscopes come in many sizes including ultra-thin bronchoscopes (2.2-2.5 mm) that allow for endoscopic intubation in infants and neonates. No matter the size of the bronchoscope chosen, all airway equipment should be tested prior to the induction of the patient.

The first step in performing flexible bronchoscopic intubation is airway topicalization. Since a child may not be cooperative with airway topicalization, adequate sedation is often necessary. Both nasal passages should be anesthetized with lidocaine 4%, which can be diluted to 2% with sterile water (not saline) to increase volume. Vasoconstriction can be achieved with the topical administration of oxymetazoline. It is critical to be as gentle as possible when inserting objects into the nasal passages since blood in the airway can hamper or prevent flexible bronchoscopic nasal intubation. Since secretions are difficult to control in younger pediatric patients due to the relatively small suction channel on pediatric and neonatal bronchoscopes, some anesthesia practitioners use low-flow oxygen insufflation to displace secretions. High-flow insufflation can lead to potentially deadly consequences[27] and should be avoided.

Once topical anesthesia of the airway is achieved, adequate oxygenation and deep anesthesia should be maintained to provide sufficient time to obtain optimal visibility during the procedure. Although both the nasal and oral routes can be used to introduce a flexible bronchoscope, the nasal route is generally easier and is particularly useful in patients with limited mouth openings or temporomandibular joint rigidity. The nasal route for intubation is also preferred for some intraoral surgical procedures (e.g., tongue lip adhesion). For both the nasal and oral flexible bronchoscopic intubation approaches, a nasal airway can be inserted into the other nostril as a conduit for oxygen until tracheal intubation is achieved.[28]

If the nasal route is chosen, two different methods can be used to introduce the flexible bronchoscope for tracheal intubation. In the first method, the lubricated nasal endotracheal tube (ETT) is loaded onto the flexible bronchoscope and the bronchoscope is introduced into the nares. A gentle jaw thrust or anterior displacement of the tongue can facilitate visualization of the hypopharynx by elevating the tongue and epiglottis. The bronchoscope is advanced into the nasopharynx until it reaches the vocal folds. The vocal cords are then topicalized using 0.5 to 1 mL of lidocaine 1% or 2% through the side port of the bronchoscope before advancing the bronchoscope into the trachea. Once visualization of the carina is achieved, the ETT is advanced down the length of the bronchoscope. Upon confirmation of the ETT within the trachea, the bronchoscope is removed while leaving the ETT in place.

In the second method, the lubricated ETT is inserted first through the nares such that the ETT tip lies in the upper oropharynx. The flexible bronchoscope is then inserted through the ETT lumen past the larynx and into the trachea while keeping the ETT in place. Similar to the first method, a gentle jaw thrust or anterior displacement of the tongue can aid visualization of the hypopharynx. Lidocaine should also be used to topicalize the vocal cords. Once the bronchoscope is within the trachea, the ETT is then advanced down the length of the bronchoscope. Upon confirmation of the ETT within the trachea, the bronchoscope can be withdrawn. This second approach is often chosen when using a smaller flexible bronchoscope that does not have a suction channel in order to avoid secretions and mucus in the naso- and oropharynx.

If oral flexible bronchoscopic intubation is necessary, several options exist for airway topicalization. Cooperative older children can be coached into gargling a lidocaine solution or having lidocaine jelly gradually applied along the posterior tongue. In some children, spraying lidocaine on the uvula can be an alternative to reduce the gag reflex. However, younger children usually require sedation before any airway topicalization can be performed. Popular methods for oral insertion of a flexible bronchoscope include the use of an EGD (such as the LMA Unique,[29–32] Air-Q, i-gel[33]) or GlideScope where the flexible bronchoscope acts as a flexible stylet for the ETT. Alternatively, if there is good visualization of the hypopharynx with either a gentle jaw thrust or anterior displacement of the tongue, the flexible bronchoscope can be guided into the trachea without the use of any other airway device.

Can a Video Laryngoscope Be Used to Intubate the Trachea of This Patient?

Video laryngoscopes allow a wider field of view and enable the airway practitioner to "see around the corner." Several pediatric models are available such as the GlideScope (Verathon, Bothell, WA, USA) and the C-MAC (Karl Storz, Tuttlingen, Germany). The Airtraq™ (Prodol Meditec S.A., Vizcaya, Spain) is a disposable device that also facilitates ETT insertion.[34] Recently, a simulation study using a Pierre Robin manikin demonstrated that there is no difference in the success rate of the first tracheal intubation attempt when a video laryngoscope or flexible bronchoscope was used.[35]

What If the Flexible Bronchoscope or Video Laryngoscope Is Not Working?

Since this is elective surgery, a tracheotomy is not ideal due to its long-term consequences. Instead, the cause of equipment malfunction should be identified and fixed, or alternative functioning equipment should be available before proceeding with this case. If no appropriate airway equipment is available, then the case should be cancelled and rescheduled. If this case had been urgent or an emergency, and no functioning airway equipment was available, then the option of performing a tracheotomy should be considered by the surgical and anesthesia team and discussed with the family.[36,37] The tracheotomy procedure will be discussed later in the chapter.

POST AIRWAY MANAGEMENT CARE

How Should This Patient Be Managed Following Intubation?

Confirmation of ETT placement within the trachea should be performed with observation of bilateral chest rise, chest auscultation, and most importantly end-tidal CO_2 monitoring. Chest auscultation alone can be misleading and is not recommended especially in younger children. Although end-tidal CO_2 is the gold standard for real-time confirmation of ETT placement, pulmonary ultrasound can also be used to ensure bilateral ventilation through the observation of bilateral lung sliding (Figure 49.3).[38] Once the ETT is confirmed to be in the trachea, it is imperative to secure it well. Skin preparation and use of a commercially available fixation device or adhesive tape on the upper lip should be used to ensure that the tube will not be dislodged.

How Should Extubation Proceed?

The decision as to how to extubate depends on various clinical factors. If FMV and/or tracheal intubation were difficult, the anesthesia practitioner should consider an awake extubation with full reversal of any neuromuscular blockade to ensure return of airway reflexes and spontaneous ventilation.

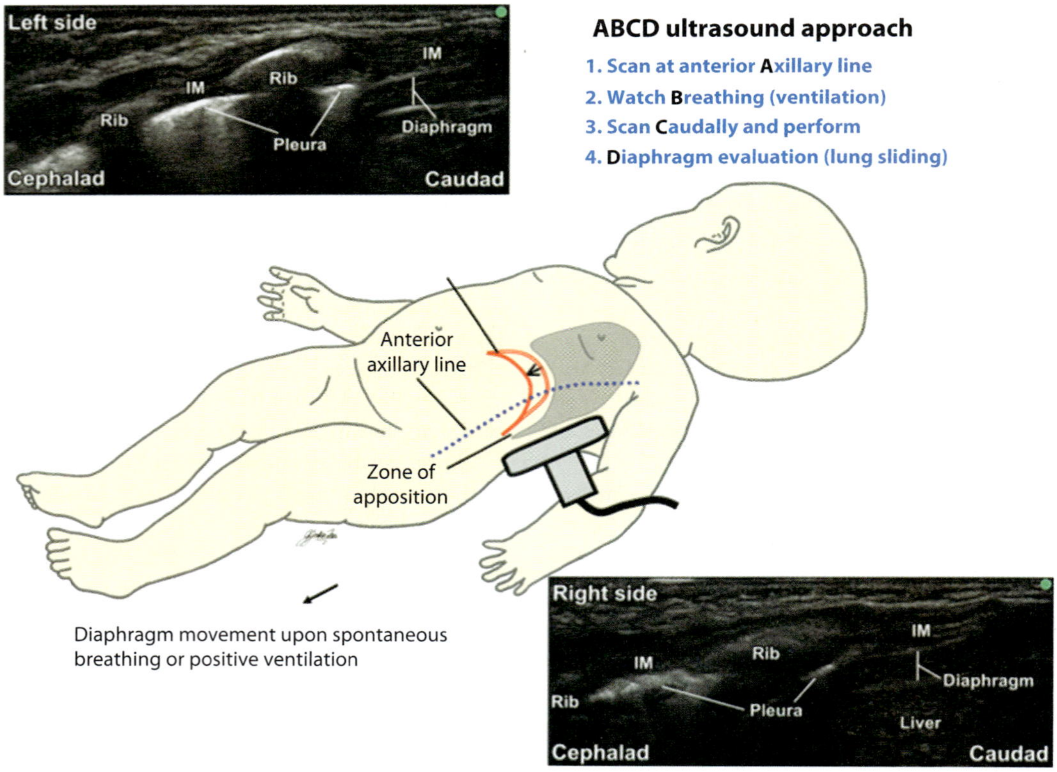

FIGURE 49.3. Ultrasound-based assessment of bilateral ventilation using the ABCD approach. (Reproduced with permission from Tsui BC, Tsui J. ABC diaphragmatic evaluation for neonates. *Paediatr Anaesth.* 2016;26(7):768-769.)

Difficulty during induction or airway management can be a predictor of difficulty during emergence and extubation. Common problems that can be encountered on extubation include airway obstruction, coughing, laryngospasm, bronchospasm, regurgitation, and delirium. Reviewing previous anesthetic notes can help to avoid any past difficulties. Suctioning of the oropharynx is essential to prevent aspiration of any secretions that can cause laryngospasm and bronchospasm, which can make a difficult airway infinitely more challenging. A difficult airway cart or equipment, resuscitation medications, and additional help is recommended prior to extubation of a difficult airway. In adults, keeping an airway exchange catheter in place can be an option in case there is a need for reintubation. However, this is often impractical in smaller children and can lead to laryngospasm and bronchospasm with associated bradycardia.

Some anesthesia practitioners prefer to perform awake extubations using the "no touch" technique.[39] This technique involves careful suctioning of blood and secretions from the pharynx before placing the patient in the lateral (recovery) position while anesthetized. The volatile anesthetic is then discontinued, and the child is not exposed to any further stimulation. Positive ventilation with 100% oxygen is maintained until spontaneous ventilation returns. Tracheal extubation is performed when the patient opens their eyes once the volatile anesthetic has reached minimal levels. Agitation during emergence is not necessarily an appropriate indication to extubate, especially if there are other signs of stage 2 anesthesia since there is a risk of laryngospasm and bronchospasm if premature extubation is attempted.

Following the extubation, the patient should be observed in the postanesthesia care unit or intensive care unit long enough to address any problems associated with postoperative airway obstruction. Opioids should be judiciously used. If opioid-induced respiratory depression occurs, an initial dose of 0.01 $mg{\cdot}kg^{-1}$ naloxone should be given to reverse the effects of the opioid. Nebulized epinephrine can be used to relieve stridor while dexamethasone 0.5 $mg{\cdot}kg^{-1}$ (max of 10-12 mg) may be used to minimize any airway edema. Additionally, humidified oxygen is often administered to ensure that any continued mucus secretions are easily mobilized.

What Are the Management Steps in the Event of Laryngospasm?

Laryngospasm is not uncommon following airway stimulation in a lightly anesthetized patient. It can also be triggered by any secretions that touch the vocal cords and extremely painful stimuli. Laryngospasm usually manifests as strenuous respiratory efforts with rapid oxygen desaturation. It can be complete or partial. In a complete laryngospasm, the glottis is completely closed, and no ventilation is possible. In a partial laryngospasm, stridulous noises can be appreciated in the setting of a partially closed glottis, which allows for some albeit difficult ventilation. Regardless of the type of laryngospasm, early identification and treatment are key.

The best treatment for laryngospasm is prevention. Several pharmacological techniques have been described to avoid laryngospasm including administration of IV lidocaine or magnesium prior to extubation.[40–42] As mentioned above, performing awake extubation using the "no touch" technique can be an effective way to avoid laryngospasm in the first place.[39]

When laryngospasm has occurred, immediately apply positive pressure through FMV and 100% oxygen. If the laryngospasm does not break, deepen the anesthetic using IV agents such as propofol 1 to 2 $mg{\cdot}kg^{-1}$. Because the glottis is closed, inhalational agents will be ineffective in deepening the plane of anesthesia. If the laryngospasm persists, administer succinylcholine 0.25 to 1 $mg{\cdot}kg^{-1}$ IV. In severe laryngospasm that causes bradycardia and hypotension, administer resuscitative techniques and medications to support the cardiovascular system.

An alternative technique to break laryngospasm has been described by Larson.[43] A jaw thrust is performed while applying firm bilateral pressure with the middle fingers at the cephalad portion of the "laryngospasm notch" (also known as the "Larson's point" and is located behind the lobule of the pinna of each ear). The pressure should be directed inwardly toward the base of the skull. Oxygen must be administered when performing the technique.

What If a Tracheotomy Is the Only Option?

The most common indication for pediatric tracheotomy is to provide a stable airway in prolonged respiratory failure or for chronic laryngotracheal lesions.[44] Long-term ventilator dependence may result from chronic upper airway obstruction, trauma, bronchopulmonary dysplasia, or hypotonia secondary to neurological or neuromuscular disorders.[36]

Most pediatric tracheotomies are performed in children under one year of age.[17,36,45] Although tracheotomy can be a life-saving procedure in these children, a tracheotomy is not without significant risks. Overall rates of mortality from tracheotomy complications have declined (ranging between 1.6% and 3.6%),[36,45] largely due to the decreased need for tracheotomy from advances in early treatment options.[36] Ultimately, children with tracheotomies are more likely to die from their primary illness than from tracheotomy-related complications.[36,45]

Emergency tracheotomies are challenging with high mortality rates no matter the age of the child. The airway anatomy is smaller and more difficult to expose, and general anesthesia is almost always necessary for the successful performance of the procedure. As mentioned above, many PRS patients present in late childhood with issues not related to respiratory failure. When respiratory failure is an issue, there is a high likelihood that a child will need a tracheotomy at some point in their medical course.

In clinical practice, tracheotomies are typically performed by pediatric otorhinolaryngologists and not by anesthesia practitioners. Tracheotomies require substantial coordination and communication between the otorhinolaryngologist and anesthesia practitioner to ensure patient safety. A detailed description of the tracheotomy procedure is beyond the scope of this chapter. However, a brief summary is provided as it benefits the anesthesia practitioner to understand the procedure to best tailor the anesthetic and facilitate care coordination with the otorhinolaryngologist.

When feasible, assessment of the airway should be performed by direct microlaryngoscopy and bronchoscopy prior to the tracheotomy. The airway should then be secured with an ETT before tracheotomy is performed. The tracheotomy is usually performed with a horizontal skin incision and vertical tracheal incision involving two to three rings. Careful communication with the otorhinolaryngologist will assist in safely timing the removal of the ETT immediately prior to the insertion of tracheostomy tube. Confirmation of the tracheostomy tube within the tracheal lumen is essential. Tracheostomy tube sutures should remain in place until the tracheostomy tube is changed after approximately 5 to 7 days. Difficult airway equipment should be immediately available in case of accidental removal of the tracheostomy tube within the first week of placement as blind replacement of the tracheostomy tube can create false passages with the inability to ventilate the patient.

SUMMARY

Most pediatric anesthesia practitioners will encounter a patient with a difficult airway at some point in their career. Although one must always be prepared to manage an unanticipated difficult airway, these unexpected events are fortunately very rare in the pediatric population. Key features that predict a potentially difficult airway include facial asymmetry, small or limited mouth opening, glossoptosis, high-arched palate, and mandibular hypoplasia. An experienced assistant and appropriate equipment should be present when managing an anticipated difficult airway. It is prudent to consider postponing the case and preparing for alternate approaches if complications are anticipated. Ideally, spontaneous ventilation should be maintained, and intubation attempts should be minimized to decrease any trauma to the larynx.

The authors recommend Drs. Tsui and Suresh's Pediatric Atlas of Ultrasound and Nerve Stimulation-Guided Regional Anesthesia (New York: Springer; 2016) for additional information regarding the regional anesthesia technique described in this article.

SELF-EVALUATION QUESTIONS

49.1. All of the following features are associated with Pierre Robin sequence **EXCEPT**:

A. Mandibular hypoplasia

B. Cleft secondary palate

C. Glossoptosis

D. Congenital cardiac disease

E. Normal mouth opening

49.2. Which of the following is **TRUE** regarding pediatric difficult airway management?

A. Sedation should be never given to the uncooperative patient.

B. Most practitioners prefer to maintain spontaneous ventilation.

C. Inhalation induction is the only way to maintain spontaneous ventilation.

D. "Can't intubate, can't oxygenate" situations do not occur in the pediatric population.

E. Emergency surgical tracheotomies are easily performed in pediatric patients.

49.3. Which of the following is **TRUE** regarding pediatric difficult airway management?

A. Flexible bronchoscopic intubation is easier via the oral route as compared to the nasal route.

B. When using video laryngoscopes with hyperangulated blade, the blade should be placed in the midline without sweeping the tongue to the side.

C. Extraglottic devices (EGDs) cannot be used as conduits for flexible bronchoscopic intubation.

D. EGDs generally do not seal well in children.

E. Topicalization with local anesthetic of the upper airway is not needed in children who have been anesthetized with general anesthesia.

REFERENCES

1. Cladis F, Kumar A, Grunwaldt L, Otteson T, Ford M, Losee JE. Pierre Robin Sequence: a perioperative review. *Anesth Analg.* 2014;119:400-412.
2. Smith MC, Senders CW. Prognosis of airway obstruction and feeding difficulty in the Robin sequence. *Int J Pediatr Otorhinolaryngol.* 2006;70:319-324.
3. Evans AK, Rahbar R, Rogers GF, Mulliken JB, Volk MS. Robin sequence: a retrospective review of 115 patients. *Int J Pediatr Otorhinolaryngol.* 2006;70:973-980.
4. Infosino A. Pediatric upper airway and congenital anomalies. *Anesthesiol Clin North Am.* 2002;20:747-766.
5. Kundra P, Krishnan H. Airway management in children. *Indian J Anaesth.* 2005;49:300-307.
6. Marraro GA. Difficult Airway. In: Gullo A. Milan, ed. *Anaesthesia, Pain, Intensive Care and Emergency Medicine —A.P.I.C.E.* Springer-Verlag; 2006: 763-778.
7. Finucane BT, Tsui BCH, Santora AH. Pediatric airway management. In: *Principles of Airway Management.* 4th ed. New York: Springer; 2011:415-513.
8. Frei FJ, Ummenhofer W: Difficult intubation in paediatrics. *Paediatr Anaesth.* 1996;6:251-263.
9. Vipulananthan N, Cooper T, Witmans M, El-Hakim H. Primary aerodigestive presentations of Pierre Robin sequence/complex and predictive factors of airway type and management. *Int J Pediatr Otorhinolaryngol.* 2014;78:1726-1730.
10. Walker RW, Ellwood J. The management of difficult intubation in children. *Paediatr Anaesth.* 2009;19(Suppl 1):77-87.
11. Valois T. The Pediatric Difficult Airway, Basics: Anesthesia. In: Astuto M. Milan, ed. *Intensive Care, and Pain in Neonates and Children.* Springer-Verlag; 2009: 31-48.
12. Kandasamy R, Sivalingam P. Use of sevoflurane in difficult airways. *Acta Anaesthesiol Scand.* 2000;44:627-629.
13. Ansermino JM, Brooks P, Rosen D, Vandebeek CA, Reichert C. Spontaneous ventilation with remifentanil in children. *Paediatr Anaesth.* 2005;15:115-121.
14. von Ungern-Sternberg BS, Erb TO, Reber A, Frei FJ. Opening the upper airway–airway maneuvers in pediatric anesthesia. *Paediatr Anaesth.* 2005;15:181-189.
15. Roth B, Magnusson J, Johansson I, Holmberg S, Westrin P. Jaw lift–a simple and effective method to open the airway in children. *Resuscitation.* 1998;39:171-174.
16. Brambrink AM, Braun U. Airway management in infants and children. *Best Pract Res Clin Anaesthesiol.* 2005;19:675-697.
17. Tantinikorn W, Alper CM, Bluestone CD, Casselbrant ML. Outcome in pediatric tracheotomy. *Am J Otolaryngol.* 2003; 24:131-137.

18. Henderson JJ. The use of paraglossal straight blade laryngoscopy in difficult tracheal intubation. *Anaesthesia.* 1997;52:552-560.
19. Saxena KN, Nischal H, Bhardwaj M, Gaba P, Shastry BV. Right molar approach to tracheal intubation in a child with Pierre Robin syndrome, cleft palate, and tongue tie. *Br J Anaesth.* 2008;100:141-142.
20. Cohen SR, Simms C, Burstein FD, Thomsen J. Alternatives to tracheostomy in infants and children with obstructive sleep apnea. *J Pediatr Surg.* 1999;34:182-186.
21. Wang XX, Dai J, Dai L, Guo HJ, Zhou AG, Pan DB. Caudal dexmedetomidine in pediatric caudal anesthesia: a systematic review and meta-analysis of randomized controlled trials. *Medicine.* 2020;99(31):e21397.
22. Klimscha W, Chiari A, Michalek-Sauberer A, et al. The efficacy and safety of a clonidine/bupivacaine combination in caudal blockade for pediatric hernia repair. *Anesth Analg.* 1998;86:54-61.
23. Karaaslan K, Gulcu N, Ozturk H, Sarpkaya A, Colak C, Kocoglu H. Two different doses of caudal neostigmine co-administered with levobupivacaine produces analgesia in children. *Paediatr Anaesth.* 2009;19:487-493.
24. Berry FA. Anesthesia for the child with a difficult airway. In: Berry FA, ed. *Anesthetic Management of Difficult and Routine Pediatric Patients.* 2nd ed. London: Churchill Livingstone; 1990: 167-198.
25. Tsui BC, Cunningham K. Fiberoptic endotracheal intubation after topicalization with in-circuit nebulized lidocaine in a child with a difficult airway. *Anesth Analg.* 2004;98:1286-1288.
26. Beringer R, Skeahan N, Sheppard S, et al. Study to assess the laryngeal and pharyngeal spread of topical local anesthetic administered orally during general anesthesia in children. *Paediatr Anaesth.* 2010; 20: 757-762.
27. Hershey MD, Hannenberg AA. Gastric distention and rupture from oxygen insufflation during fiberoptic intubation. *Anesthesiology.* 1996;85:1479-1480.
28. Evans P. The paediatric airway. In: Calder I, Pearce A, eds. *Core Topics in Airway Management.* 2nd ed. Cambridge: Cambridge University Press; 2005: 193-202.
29. Muraika L, Heyman JS, Shevchenko Y. Fiberoptic tracheal intubation through a laryngeal mask airway in a child with Treacher Collins syndrome. *Anesth Analg.* 2003;97:1298-1299.
30. Johr M, Berger TM. Fiberoptic intubation through the laryngeal mask airway (LMA) as a standardized procedure. *Paediatr Anaesth.* 2004;14:614.
31. Weiss M, Gerber AC, Schmitz A. Continuous ventilation technique for laryngeal mask airway (LMA) removal after fiberoptic intubation in children. *Paediatr Anaesth.* 2004;14:936-940.
32. Yilmaz AS, Gurkan Y, Toker K, Solak M. Laryngeal mask airway-guided fiberoptic tracheal intubation in a 1200-gm infant with difficult airway. *Paediatr Anaesth.* 2005; 15: 1147-1148.
33. Girgis KK, Youssef MM, El Zayyat NS. Comparison of the air-Q intubating laryngeal airway and the cobra perilaryngeal airway as conduits for fiber optic-guided intubation in pediatric patients. *Saudi J Anaesth.* 2014;8 470-476.
34. Redel A, Karademir F, Schlitterlau A, et al. Validation of the GlideScope video laryngoscope in pediatric patients. *Paediatr Anaesth.* 2009;19:667-671.
35. Fiadjoe JE, Hirschfeld M, Wu S, et al. A randomized multi-institutional crossover comparison of the GlideScope® Cobalt Video laryngoscope to the flexible fiberoptic bronchoscope in a Pierre Robin manikin. *Paediatr Anaesth.* 2015;25: 801-806.
36. Carron JD, Derkay CS, Strope GL, Nosonchuk JE, Darrow DH. Pediatric tracheotomies: changing indications and outcomes. *Laryngoscope.* 2000;110:1099-1104.
37. Sculerati N, Gottlieb MD, Zimbler MS, Chibbaro PD, McCarthy JG. Airway management in children with major craniofacial anomalies. *Laryngoscope.* 1998;108:1806-1812.
38. Tsui BC, Tsui J. ABC diaphragmatic evaluation for neonates. *Paediatr Anaesth.* 2016;26(7):768-769.
39. Tsui BC, Wagner A, Cave D, Elliott C, El-Hakim H, Malherbe S. The incidence of laryngospasm with a "no touch" extubation technique after tonsillectomy and adenoidectomy. *Anesth Analg.* 2004;98:327-329.
40. Gulhas N, Durmus M, Demirbilek S, Togal T, Ozturk E, Ersoy MO. The use of magnesium to prevent laryngospasm after tonsillectomy and adenoidectomy: a preliminary study. *Paediatr Anaesth.* 2003;13:43-47.
41. Koc C, Kocaman F, Aygenc E, Ozdem C, Cekic A. The use of preoperative lidocaine to prevent stridor and laryngospasm after tonsillectomy and adenoidectomy. *Otolaryngol Head Neck Surg.* 1998;118:880-882.
42. Mihara T, Uchimoto K, Morita S, Goto T. The efficacy of lidocaine to prevent laryngospasm in children: a systematic review and meta-analysis. *Anaesthesia.* 2014;69(12):1388-1396.
43. Larson CP Jr. Laryngospasm–the best treatment. *Anesthesiology.* 1998;89: 1293-1294.
44. Ozmen S, Ozmen OA, Unal OF. Pediatric tracheotomies: a 37-year experience in 282 children. *Int J Pediatr Otorhinolaryngol.* 2009;73(7):959-961.
45. Mahadevan M, Barber C, Salkeld L, Douglas G, Mills N. Pediatric tracheotomy: 17 year review. *Int J Pediatr Otorhinolaryngol.* 2007;71:1829-1835.

CHAPTER 50

Cannot Intubate and Cannot Oxygenate in an Infant After Induction of Anesthesia

Paul A. Baker and Cédric Sottas

CASE PRESENTATION

A 21-month-old boy with CHARGE syndrome (Figure 50.1) was brought to the operating room for a gastroscopy, echocardiogram, auditory brainstem response (ABR) test, grommets, and examination of his ears and airway under general anesthesia. His medical and surgical history included tracheobronchomalacia, left choanal atresia, a tracheoesophageal fistula (TOF) repair at age 2 days and insertion of a percutaneous endoscopic gastrostomy (PEG). From his past anesthetic history, it was noted that he had difficulty to facemask ventilation (FMV) and that the use of an extraglottic airway (EGD) did not improve his ventilation. It was also found that direct laryngoscopy and tracheal intubation were becoming increasingly difficult with successive procedures. The child was assessed preoperatively and it was reported that he remained clinically unchanged since the previous anesthesia one year ago.

After an inhalation induction with Sevoflurane and oxygen, an intravenous cannula was placed, aided by ultrasound, and a satisfactory airway was achieved with FMV and 20 cm H_2O continuous positive airway pressure (CPAP). An initial attempt at tracheal intubation via direct laryngoscopy revealed a Cormack-Lehane (CL) Grade 3 view of the epiglottis only. Tracheal intubation was unsuccessful. FMV then became impossible. A further attempt at tracheal intubation by direct laryngoscopy was also unsuccessful. In hindsight, a second attempt at tracheal intubation should have been optimized with patient positioning, apneic oxygenation, and included either video laryngoscopy (VL) or flexible bronchoscopy.[1] The choice of VL blade for a child less than 5 kg for optimum efficacy would be a standard Macintosh curved blade. For larger children, it makes no difference whether the blade is hyperangulated or curved Macintosh style.[2]

Rigid bronchoscopy was rapidly performed by an ENT surgeon in an attempt to establish an airway, but this did not provide adequate oxygenation to the patient. In this case, the resulting hypoxemia caused severe bradycardia leading to cardiac arrest which required 15 minutes of cardiopulmonary resuscitation. A needle tracheotomy was attempted and failed. This was followed by an urgent surgical tracheotomy by a surgeon, which was successful in establishing an airway and adequate oxygenation. The tracheotomy consisted of a longitudinal midline scalpel incision through the skin and subcutaneous tissue. Very little blood loss occurred and this was attributed to the cardiac arrest. The midline dissection continued down to the trachea and a midline cut was performed through approximately three tracheal rings providing sufficient space to advance an endotracheal tube (ETT) under direct vision.

All planned procedures were postponed and the child was transferred to the pediatric intensive care unit. He was cooled and remained sedated for 48 hours, after which he was allowed to wake up. Despite the prolonged resuscitation, his neurological function was equivalent to his preoperative state.

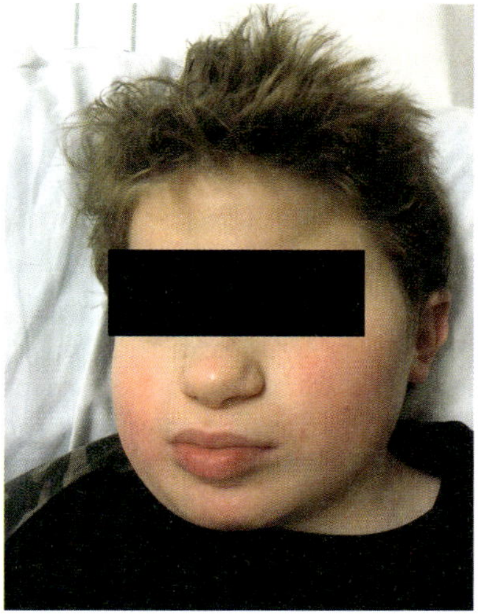

FIGURE 50.1. A patient with CHARGE syndrome.

INTRODUCTION

What Is the CHARGE Syndrome and What Are the Pathological Features?

CHARGE syndrome involves multiple congenital anomalies that can be life-threatening. The acronym CHARGE stands for **C**olobomas of the eye, **H**eart disease, **A**tresia of the choanae, **R**etarded growth or central nervous system anomalies, **G**enital anomalies or hypogonadism, and **E**ar anomalies or deafness.

Features have been further divided into major and minor criteria of the CHARGE syndrome. Major include the classic 4Cs (Choanal atresia, Coloboma, Characteristic ear, and Cranial nerve anomalies). Minor criteria include cardiovascular malformations, genital hypoplasia, cleft lip and palate, TOF, distinctive CHARGE facies, growth deficiency, and developmental delay. The clinical diagnosis is based on the presence of four of the seven features described by the acronym, including at least one major anomaly. None of the components of the CHARGE association is universally present. Occasional associations include renal anomalies (Duplex system, vesicoureteric reflux), spinal anomalies, scoliosis, osteoporosis, and hand, neck, and shoulder anomalies.

CHARGE syndrome is regarded as one of the more common genetic disorders with a birth incidence of up to 1 in 8500.[3] The syndrome involves a midline developmental defect which is thought to arise as a result of embryological arrest during a critical stage of early organogenesis in the second month of gestation.

The genetic basis of the condition remains undiagnosed in one-third of patients, but the remaining two-thirds have heterozygous mutations of the CHD7 gene on the 8q12 chromosome, a member of the chromodomain helicase DNA-binding (CHD) genes, implicated in early embryonic development and responsible for postnatal and prenatal developmental abnormalities. This genetic involvement supports the term "syndrome" rather than "association" for CHARGE.[4] Antenatal suspicion of the condition may arise from ultrasound identification of intrauterine growth retardation, polyhydramnios, and anomalies of the brain and heart. Diagnosis may occur when a neonate presents with feeding difficulties and sleep disturbances including obstructive sleep apnea.

What Are the Causes of Mortality in CHARGE Syndrome?

Given the broad spectrum of diseases associated with CHARGE syndrome, multiple life-threatening conditions can arise throughout life. In the neonatal period, bilateral choanal atresia, complex cardiac disease, esophageal atresia, severe T-cell deficiency, and brain anomalies can cause death. In childhood and adolescence, swallowing problems, gastroesophageal reflux, respiratory aspiration, and postoperative airway events contribute to postneonatal mortality.[5]

What Airway Problems Arise During Anesthesia for Patients with CHARGE Syndrome?

Anesthesia for patients with CHARGE syndrome is associated with significant risk. Difficulty with airway management may arise at multiple levels and tends to increase in severity with age, giving false security from a past history of successful airway management. FMV can be complicated in the presence of micrognathia and midface hypoplasia due to poor seal around the face and the inability to support an open airway. Airway narrowing is the main cause of difficult ventilation, and children with a collapsible upper airway, such as that seen in laryngomalacia, may require CPAP during FMV to stent the airway and increase functional residual capacity. In the absence of choanal atresia, the application of high-flow nasal oxygen (HFNO), combined with mouthpiece oxygen during denitrogenation enhances positive airway pressure.[6] Choanal atresia and stenosis, if bilateral, can cause severe airway obstruction and cyanosis when the mouth is closed, as occurs during breastfeeding. Prior to surgical correction during anesthesia, it is essential to establish an open oral airway. This may require repositioning the patient, an oropharyngeal airway, an EGD or tracheal intubation. Modified "awake" intubation with an EGD is one technique to overcome this problem.[7] Early intervention with a tracheotomy is recommended for these patients to prevent hypoxemic episodes. Positive pressure ventilation through an EGD may also be difficult and relatively contraindicated due to laryngomalacia and tracheomalacia. Distal airway collapse may result in increased airway resistance, causing ventilation pressures to exceed the leak pressure of the EGD. This gives rise to gastric inflation. In this situation, neuromuscular blocking drugs are avoided, spontaneous ventilation is maintained, and a gastric tube will help mitigate gastric inflation.

Micrognathia is associated with difficult laryngoscopy and difficult tracheal intubation (DI). Cleft palate is not associated with increased risk of difficult laryngoscopy or DI. Although there are no specific protective effects from cleft palates during airway management, cleft palates may provide wider nasopharyngeal air spaces. This space may improve the drainage of secretions in those children suffering from cranial nerve dysfunction, poor swallowing, and gastroesophageal reflux. It is also possible that the wider nasopharyngeal air space may create a beneficial large anatomical space and help accommodate EGDs.

What Should Be Done to Prepare This Patient for Anesthesia?

CHARGE syndrome is associated with a broad range of anomalies. These anomalies frequently require surgery and associated airway management. It is essential that children with complex airway problems like CHARGE syndrome are managed in specialist pediatric hospitals.[8] Practitioners responsible for these patients should be experts and experienced in the techniques required for their care. Specialist units, ideally, should include multi-disciplinary teams who work together regularly.

An airway plan helps to formulate strategies to cope with unexpected events: equipment and expertise are assembled to match those strategies. All staff should be briefed preoperatively about the details of the plan and individuals need to be clear about their roles in the overall strategy of patient care. This would occur preoperatively during the team briefing and World Health Organization (WHO) time-out. Various guidelines have been designed for the difficult pediatric airway.[8–10]

MANAGEMENT OF AIRWAY OBSTRUCTION

The management of airway obstruction during pediatric anesthesia depends on the etiology. Weiss and Engelhardt differentiate airway obstruction into two categories: functional airway obstruction and anatomical or mechanical obstruction.[11]

Functional Airway Obstruction

Functional airway obstructions include insufficient anesthesia (rectified by deepening anesthesia with volatile or intravenous agents), laryngospasm (treated with a muscle relaxant), opioid-induced muscle rigidity (treated with a muscle relaxant), and bronchospasm (treated with epinephrine). For an unexpected difficult pediatric airway in a healthy child, FMV will improve with muscle relaxation.

While muscle relaxants can be beneficial for many patients with functional airway obstruction, patients with distal airway obstruction, including tracheomalacia and mediastinal masses, should *not* be paralyzed. If these patients are paralyzed, extrinsic airway compression is exacerbated, diaphragmatic movement is eliminated, large airway compression increases and expiratory flow rates decrease. These patients are treated with spontaneous ventilation and positive airway pressure.

Anatomical or Mechanical Airway Obstruction

Anatomical or mechanical obstructions include poor face-mask technique, obstruction secondary to large tonsils (pharyngeal, adenoid and lingual), obesity associated with obstructive sleep apnea, foreign bodies, regurgitated gastric contents, vomit, secretions, blood, and other unknown reasons. The treatment for these problems is mechanical. The obstruction is usually resolved by basic airway maneuvers including jaw thrust, repositioning of the head and optimum face-mask technique with a two-handed/two-person approach. Airway adjuncts, including oropharyngeal airways and EGDs, are essential items to help relieve upper airway obstruction. Oropharyngeal obstruction may benefit from suction under direct vision or tracheal intubation.

Airway Maneuvers

A review of airway maneuvers in pediatric anesthesia emphasized the value of jaw thrust to determine the depth of anesthesia and to restore airway patency for patients with or without tonsillar hypertrophy. Jaw thrust was found to improve minute ventilation more than chin lift alone or chin lift with CPAP. A combination of jaw thrust and CPAP increased glottic opening and increased minute ventilation.[12]

AIRWAY TECHNIQUES

Can Awake Intubation Be Considered for This Small Child?

An awake intubation technique in children is usually impractical due to poor patient cooperation; however, variants of this technique can be used in neonates and infants. Awake intubation of a neonate with a predicted difficult airway using an EGD is a safe technique for the early establishment of an airway. This technique avoids hypoxemia during induction of anesthesia and has been successfully used in patients with Pierre Robin syndrome and Treacher Collins syndrome.[13] Following the application of local anesthetic, the EGD is inserted and the neonate then receives an inhalation induction, followed by tracheal intubation through the EGD with an ultrathin flexible bronchoscope and an appropriate size ETT.[7]

What Maneuvers or Techniques Can Be Used to Improve the Effectiveness of Face-Mask Ventilation?

FMV is a core skill to maintain oxygenation and ventilation during airway management. Attention to patient and practitioner positioning can improve outcomes. The traditional alignment of the ear to sternal notch for the patient and bed height recommended for tracheal intubation also applies to FMV positioning.[14] An ergonomically optimized arm and body position of the airway practitioner as used in the transverse mandibular technique can help improve ventilation.[15,16] Various alternatives to the original C-E hand grip for single or both hands include the thenar eminence technique or V-E grip and the E-O grip which improves mask seal, particularly with a two-handed technique[17,18] (see Chapter 8).

Are Extraglottic Airway Devices Effective in Pediatric Patients?

Extraglottic devices (EGDs) have multiple applications in the management of pediatric patients with difficult airways. It can be used as a primary airway, a conduit for tracheal intubation, and a rescue ventilation device during resuscitation and for rescue during a failed airway. These devices can be used for extended periods of time for various surgical and medical indications.[19] In the event of neonatal resuscitation, insertion of an EGD has been shown to restore successful resuscitation and ventilation faster than FMV and tracheal intubation.[20]

Absolute contraindications to EGD use include any patient with an increased risk of pulmonary aspiration, airway obstruction beyond the glottis and high airway pressure. Relative contraindications include a partially collapsible lower airway, restricted access to the airway, and inexperience using an EGD.[21]

What Are the Alternative Techniques of Tracheal Intubation in Children with Difficult Laryngoscopy?

Although the incidence of difficult laryngoscopy is lower in children than in adults (1.37 vs. 9%), the incidence of difficult laryngoscopy in infants is significantly higher than in older children (4.7 vs. 0.7%).[21] The incidence of difficult laryngoscopy is doubled in children undergoing cardiac anesthesia, due to the relatively high incidence of concomitant congenital syndromes such as CHARGE syndrome.[22] Difficulty with intubation can change as the child matures. Children with CHARGE syndrome and Treacher Collins syndrome become more difficult to intubate with increasing age, whereas those with Pierre Robin syndrome become easier with age.[23]

Direct laryngoscopy and tracheal intubation, aided by a tracheal introducer (commonly known as "bougie") and optimum external laryngeal manipulation, can be successful in the hands of experienced practitioners. For example, the straight blade paraglossal approach with a bougie was successful for infants with Pierre Robin syndrome.[24] In the event of failure with direct laryngoscopy, alternative options need to be available, including rigid bronchoscopy, flexible bronchoscopy, optical stylet, VL, or front-of-neck airway combined with an apneic oxygenation technique.

Prolonged intubation attempts are associated with hypoxemia and patient awareness.[1,25] Hypoxemia can be avoided by using denitrogenation and apneic oxygenation techniques including low flow (15 $L \cdot min^{-1}$) oxygen, HFNO, buccal oxygen, oxygen via a conduit, and oxygen attached to a laryngoscope.[26] There is a significant increase in patient morbidity following more than two intubation attempts.[1] Small ETTs should be available for unexpected subglottic tracheal stenosis. The Truview® (Truphatek, Netanya, Israel) video laryngoscope has been used successfully to intubate the trachea of patients with unstable necks. Video laryngoscopes are useful devices for tracheal intubation in children, as are optical stylets, and rigid and flexible bronchoscopes.[1]

CANNOT INTUBATE, CANNOT OXYGENATE

The inability to intubate and oxygenate a child can rapidly lead to life-threatening hypoxemia. Lung modelling from Hardman et al. using the Nottingham physiology simulator shows that young children become hypoxemic during apnea earlier than adults; and the younger the child, the earlier the onset of hypoxemia.[27] Unless airway obstruction is quickly reversed, tissue hypoxia ensues, leading to cardiac arrest. Cardiac arrest in neonates is associated with 72% mortality. Numerous barriers have been identified which interfere with re-oxygenation through front-of-neck access (FONA) and potentially lead to lethal delays.

What Are the Barriers That Delay FONA?

Delays in performing FONA can be attributed to organizational and human failures. Inadequate training, supervision, support, and equipment need to be addressed at an organizational level.

Suboptimal treatment, resulting from human factor failings, includes fixation errors, poor communication, distorted situation awareness, inadequate teamwork and poor leadership, task management, and decision-making.

Management of a "cannot intubate, cannot oxygenate" (CICO) crisis may be required only once in an anesthesia practitioner's career. Performing under these circumstances is likely to be an extremely stressful event. Such stress can cause adverse physiological changes to the practitioner, including loss of fine and complex motor skill, cognitive deterioration, perceptual narrowing, and a state of hypervigilance.[28] To cope with this stress and rarity, regular training and preparation is required. Ideally, training should take place under simulated stressful conditions and involve other team members. Training to a standard operating procedure reduces choice, improves reaction time, and helps to decrease the signs and symptoms of extreme stress.

What Are the Options to Restore Oxygenation?

There is a tendency to persist with upper airway maneuvers in the event of a CICO crisis. This leads to airway trauma and delayed re-oxygenation which is a major cause of morbidity and mortality in adult and pediatric airway management. Tracheal intubation attempts should be optimized and conducted by the most expert practitioner available. The number of attempts should be limited to two.[1] A survey of children with difficult tracheal intubation revealed a high failure rate and severe complications after more than two direct laryngoscopy attempts.[1] It is therefore advised to quickly transition to an indirect tracheal intubation technique after two direct laryngoscopy attempts. A similar limit of attempts should apply to EGD and FMV methods. When CICO occurs, a clear declaration of the crisis needs to be made to everybody present. There should be a call for help, and CICO management should immediately unfold. A diagnosis of CICO should be made if the patient cannot be oxygenated despite optimum and limited attempts of FMV, EGD, and tracheal intubation. There are many practice guidelines which recommend what to do next.[9,10]

What Are the Preparations for FONA?

Prior to establishing FONA, paralyze the patient. This treats previously unidentified functional airway obstruction including laryngospasm, opioid-induced muscle rigidity, and insufficient anesthesia. A paralyzed patient is generally easier to ventilate and intubate. Exceptions to muscle relaxation might apply in the presence of a mediastinal mass or distal airway collapse, such as tracheomalacia.

Ensure continuation of 100% oxygen. This can be achieved via a face mask with jaw thrust, HFNO or an EGD. It is rare to have complete upper airway obstruction, and therefore it is possible that some limited flow of oxygen can be achieved, even in a patient where intubation with an EGD or ETT was not possible. Maintaining an open upper airway is also important to assist in the expiration and avoid barotrauma during subsequent emergency subglottic ventilation.

Consider inserting an appropriate-size rigid bronchoscope if the expertise and equipment are available. Intubation with a rigid bronchoscope can be direct or aided with a laryngoscope. Using a paraglossal approach, successful tracheal intubation may be achieved even after failed direct laryngoscopy. This device has numerous advantages: it can be used as a ventilation device to deliver 100% oxygen, with or without a volatile anesthetic agent; it can splint open an obstruction in the airway; it can push an obstructing foreign body beyond the trachea; it can facilitate suctioning; and it can accommodate surgical instruments to remove foreign bodies. Following successful intubation and re-oxygenation with the bronchoscope, a definitive intubation can be achieved with an ETT by inserting an airway exchange catheter, removing the bronchoscope and railroading an appropriate size ETT. In a difficult case involving retrieval of a foreign body, inadequate oxygenation through a rigid bronchoscope was improved by adding HFNO.[29]

What Is the Best Anatomical Location for FONA in a Child?

The age of children ranges from premature neonates to 16-year-olds. This complicates the management of the pediatric CICO situation. The anatomy of an infant airway is structurally different from an adult airway; the size of the infant larynx is approximately one-third of the adult larynx; the infant thyrohyoid membrane is shorter, with the thyroid notch sitting behind the hyoid bone; the thyroid cartilage is rounded, compared to the V-shape of an adult; the infant laryngeal cartilages are softer and more pliable than an adult; the supraglottic and subglottic mucosae are lax in infants, making them predisposed to swelling. The infant larynx is located at the level of the third or fourth cervical vertebra. From age 2, it descends until eventually reaching the adult level of the sixth or seventh vertebra. The high position of the neonatal larynx accounts for the proportionally longer cervical trachea (in neonates there are 10 tracheal rings above the sternal notch, this decreases to 8 for adolescents and 6 for adults). From birth to adolescence, the trachea more than doubles in length, triples in diameter, and increases by six-fold in cross-sectional area.[30]

Locating the cricothyroid membrane (CTM) is challenging in infants where the neck tends to be short and the thyroid cartilage is high and round. In an elective situation, ultrasound can assist identification of the infant CTM, but this is time-consuming and impractical in an emergency.

The small dimensions of the neonatal CTM, the soft pliable laryngeal cartilages with lax subglottic mucosae, and the relatively high position of the larynx in the infant's neck make a front-of-neck approach difficult. These anatomical features make any approach to the CTM very difficult, whether with a cannula or scalpel, even with full neck extension. These factors favor a tracheotomy approach for FONA in infants.

Who Should Perform a FONA Procedure?

The most expert airway practitioner available should perform the FONA procedure. Hopefully, that person will be a skilled pediatric otorhinolaryngologist (ORL) who is specialized in pediatric airway management. If there is no immediate availability of that surgeon, the skilled anesthesia practitioner must be prepared to act. Precious time with a hypoxemic child should not be wasted waiting for a surgeon.

What Should Be Used? Scalpel, Cannula, or Cricothyrotomy Kit?

A CICO event in children is extremely rare. Very few practitioners have ever performed FONA in a child or an adult. There is very little clinical evidence to support any one technique.[31] Randomized trials are ethically impossible and case series in children are not available due to underreporting. Guidelines are largely based on animal studies and expert opinion.

How Can a Scalpel Be Used for FONA in a Child?

Emergency Surgical Tracheotomy

An emergency surgical tracheotomy is favored by many as a rapid, definitive solution for pediatric FONA. Using 10-kg piglet cadaver models, Holm-Knudsen reported a study where anesthesiologists were trained by an ENT surgeon to perform an emergency tracheotomy. The technique consisted of four steps using tools available in the operating room or emergency department. Step 1 required a midline scalpel incision through the skin and subcutaneous tissue. The incision extended from below the thyroid cartilage to the sternal notch to allow blunt digital dissection down to the trachea. Step 2 involved an assistant grasping the wound edges with two towel forceps and exposing the base of the wound. The trachea is identified by blunt digital dissection. In step 3, a third towel forceps is used to hold the trachea immediately below the thyroid cartilage, so as to stabilize the trachea. In step 4, a pair of scissors is used to open the anterior wall of the upper trachea. The sharp tip of the scissors cut distally and longitudinally through two tracheal rings. The final step involved tracheal intubation under direct vision with an ETT. Using this technique, 32 anesthesiologists attempted the tracheotomy and 97% succeeded in a median time of 88 seconds.[32] In this study, there was one failure, two cuts were too deep, hitting laryngeal and tracheal cartilages, and one participant cut six tracheal cartilages, rather than the recommended two.[32]

Given the very rare, but the urgent requirement to competently perform emergency FONA (eFONA), the need for regular training of appropriate medical staff is essential. Using a surgical eFONA technique suitable for children less than 8 years, Ulmer et al. found that pediatric clinicians from different specialty groups could learn eFONA on rabbit cadavers within four attempts and could establish an airway with an overall 94% success in less than 1 minute.[33] An overview of this eFONA technique practiced on rabbit cadavers has been reported with a focus on strategies, structure, and management including a link to an instructional video.[34]

The tracheotomy performed on the child with CHARGE syndrome, reported in this chapter, used only a scalpel and blunt dissection with a finger. A similar technique has been used for many years for FONA of anesthetized pigs during our local airway management training course. An experienced practitioner can open the neck and expose the trachea using a longitudinal midline scalpel incision and blunt digital dissection in less than 30 seconds. This technique involves very little blood loss in a pig.

Surgical tracheotomy can be used as the standard operating procedure for all pediatric age groups. This technique is used in adult airway management by military and civilian groups. It is also recommended as the default procedure if other procedures fail, or if anatomical landmarks cannot be located percutaneously.

Scalpel Bougie Technique

An alternative to a surgical tracheotomy is the scalpel bougie technique. There are several variants of this technique, but the following technique is described in the Difficult Airway Society 2015 guidelines for the management of unanticipated difficult intubation in a paralyzed adult.[35] The practitioner stands on the patient's left side if they are right-handed (and vice versa). The cricoid cartilage is identified with the nondominant hand. A size 10 scalpel blade, held transverse with the dominant hand, is cut through the skin and CTM. The blade is then rotated 90° into a longitudinal plane with the blade directed caudally. The practitioner changes hands and picks up a bougie with their dominant hand while holding the scalpel in their nondominant hand. While keeping the scalpel in a vertical plane, they gently pull it toward themselves to create a triangular opening through which the bougie will be inserted. The bougie is run down the face of the scalpel and directed down the trachea. It is important to keep the scalpel vertical to avoid directing the bougie laterally. The scalpel is removed and a size 6.0-mm internal diameter (ID) ETT is railroaded down the bougie and into the trachea. The bougie is removed from the ETT and the patient is oxygenated and ventilated with a self-inflating ventilation bag or an anesthetic circuit. This provides safe ventilation with a cuffed tube, even in the presence of regurgitation or upper airway obstruction.

In a study using 12 adult human cadavers, three inexperienced anesthesiologists were trained to perform the scalpel bougie technique. Collectively, they were able to complete 34 procedures successfully in a mean time of 37 seconds. There were two failed attempts due to inability to identify the CTM in cadavers with neck circumferences greater than 40 cm. In this situation, the next step would involve a longitudinal neck dissection and a surgical tracheotomy, as described above.[36]

For a scalpel bougie technique, the size of the bougie selected will dictate the size of the ETT. For an adult or child ≥ 12 years, a 6.0 mm ID is the smallest ETT that will accommodate a 14-Fr (4.6 mm outside diameter [OD]) Frova bougie (Cook® Medical, Bloomington, IN, USA). A smaller 8-Fr Frova bougie (2.6 mm OD) can easily accommodate a size 4.0-mm ID ETT. The width of a size 10 scalpel blade is 7 mm which is appropriate for an adult but too wide for an infant or neonate. Scalpel bougie has been studied in 4 kg white rabbits using an 8-Fr Frova bougie, 3.5- to 4.0-mm ID ETT and a size 15 blade.[37] The 15-blade is 4 mm wide and 12 mm long. This blade length is just adequate for the tracheal depth of an 18-month-old child which was measured by ultrasound at 10 mm.[32] Successful intubation was dependent on tracheal level, with 100% through the first level, 62.5% at level 2 and 25% at levels 3 and 4. Posterior wall damage occurred in 50% of attempts on macroscopic inspection.[37]

The dimensions of the adult CTM limit the maximum OD of an ETT to 8.0 mm ID. In a study of adult cadavers in the neutral neck position, the length of the CTM was 10.4 mm (male) and 9.5 mm (female) and the width was 8.2 mm (male) and 6.9 mm (female) between the cricothyroid muscles. The equivalent dimensions in a neonate are 2.6 mm length and 3.0 mm width. It is not advisable to intubate through the CTM in a neonate or infant, due to the difficulty in identifying this landmark, the fragility of the cricoid cartilages, and the small dimensions of the CTM at this age. A tracheotomy is the preferred entry point for neonates and infants.

The end result of a surgical tracheotomy or a scalpel bougie technique is a cuffed ETT which provides a definitive and safe airway, even in the presence of regurgitation or upper airway obstruction. Ventilation through this cuffed ETT is by a low-pressure self-inflating ventilation bag or an anesthetic circuit. The criteria for an ideal FONA technique for CICO are as follows: it should be a straightforward technique which is quick to perform with a high success rate; it should be easy to master with only a few steps; it should protect against aspiration and allow adequate ventilation, regardless of upper airway obstruction.[38] Unlike other recommended FONA solutions, the scalpel technique satisfies these criteria.

What Are the Pros and Cons of a Cannula FONA Technique?

There are only seven cases of emergency pediatric transtracheal needle ventilation reported since 1950. Despite the reported difficulty and complications associated with infant cannula cricothyrotomy, many medical organizations continue to recommend this technique for emergency airway access in children. Cannula cricothyrotomy is promoted by the European Resuscitation Council, the American Heart Association, the Advanced Life Support Group in the United Kingdom, the American Society of Anesthesiologists, the Association of Paediatric Anaesthetists of Great Britain and Ireland, and the Difficult Airway Society.

Like infant cannula cricothyrotomy, cannula tracheotomy is also difficult to perform and is associated with low success and high complication rates, but this may be preferable to a cricothyroid approach for the anatomical reasons already described. Three animal studies have examined the success and complication rates of cannula tracheotomy. Repeated cannulation of rabbit cadaver tracheas using 18G and 14G cannulas resulted in 60% success and posterior tracheal wall perforation in 42% of attempts.[37] Another study used 8-kg euthanized piglets to measure cannula tracheotomy performance by 30 physicians. Eight out of 30 attempts were successful (27%) in a mean time of 68 seconds.[39] In a second study by the same group with 10-kg euthanized piglets, 32 anesthesiologists inserted two different transtracheal cannulas (a jet cannula and a standard intravenous cannula). Success occurred in 65.6% of the jet cannulas in 69 seconds. The intravenous cannula succeeded in 68.8% in 42 seconds. Complication rates were high with 14 tracheal perforations of 27 tracheas inspected. Other complications included translaryngeal catheter insertion, catheter kinking, and failure to cannulate.[32]

What Ventilation Methods Can Be Used Through a Cannula?

Ventilation through a small cannula requires a high-pressure gas source to overcome the resistance of the cannula. Various options have been proposed to manage cannula ventilation. Devices can be divided into flow-regulated volume ventilation and pressure-regulated volume ventilation.[40]

Pressure-regulated devices in the presence of small lung volumes and outflow obstruction can deliver potentially dangerous airway pressures leading to barotrauma and surgical emphysema. Devices such as the Manujet III (VBM Medizintechnik, Sulz, Germany) include pressure ranges on their regulator for different age groups: baby 0 to 1 bar (0-14.5 psi or 0-100 kPa); infant 1 to 2.5 bar (14.5-36.3 psi or 100-250 kPa); adult 2.5 to 4 bar (36.3- 58 psi or 250-400 kPa). It is essential to downregulate prior to use, operating the jet ventilator while holding the cannula and feeling for surgical emphysema. Inspiratory time is kept to a minimum. Start with minimum pressure and increase until chest movement can be seen. The focus should be on the chest, with a goal to restore oxygenation rather than ventilation. Extreme care must be exercised during the use of the jet ventilator, particularly if upper airway obstruction is suspected. Adequate time needs to be allowed for the chest to recoil and expire before giving another breath. Every effort should be used to open the upper airway using jaw thrust or airway adjuncts such as oropharyngeal airways or EGDs. Jet ventilators are associated with a high incidence of complications and are relatively contraindicated for use in neonates, infants, or any other patient with upper airway obstruction.

Flow-regulated volume ventilation includes the Enk oxygen flow modulator (Enk OFM) (Cook Medical Inc; Bloomington, USA) and the Rapid O_2™ insufflator (Meditech Systems Ltd, Shaftesbury, UK). These are both Y-connector variants with equivalent outflow diameters. There is one case report of a Rapid O_2™ insufflator being successfully used clinically in an adult patient with upper airway hemorrhage and obstruction.[41] The Advanced Pediatric Life Support (APLS) guidelines recommend that oxygen flow should be initially set at 1 L·min^{-1} per year of age through a Y-connector. An I:E ratio of 1:4 at a rate of 12 breaths per minute is then recommended. The Enk OFM has been experimentally validated with these settings. Care is required with flows through a flowmeter in excess of 15 L·min^{-1} because of excessive oxygen flow causing the Enk OFM to fail as an on-off device. The Enk OFM is designed with five ventilation holes. All of these holes need to be occluded to achieve inflation during inspiration.[42]

Self-made devices for emergency cannula ventilation are potentially very dangerous. Three-way taps in the oxygen line for ventilation is unsafe due to uncontrolled continuous inflation, even during the expiratory phase. This can rapidly lead to barotrauma because of inadequate expiration through the three-way tap side port. Bag ventilation through a cannula is inadequate to support oxygenation in adults. There is one report of this technique being used successfully in an 11-month-old, 9 kg child, following an emergency 16G cannula cricothyrotomy.[43]

The Ventrain (Dolphys Medical, Eindhoven, The Netherlands) is a flow-regulated oxygen ventilation device which is capable of limiting high intrathoracic pressure by withdrawing inspired gas during the expiratory phase. This occurs due to the Bernoulli principle. The Ventrain is capable of oxygen insufflation and expiratory ventilation assistance (EVA). EVA occurs when the bypass channel of the Ventrain is occluded, creating a subatmospheric pressure (up to −217 cm H_2O) at the side port. Inspiratory flow is controlled by the oxygen flow meter. Negative pressure with the Ventrain requires proximal airway obstruction. To assist EVA in this situation, the upper airway may need artificial obstruction. Safe application of EVA requires practitioner training and an understanding of the mechanism of the Ventrain function. A method for monitoring airway pressure during Ventrain use has been described.[44]

A case report describes the successful use of the Ventrain in an adult patient with near total upper airway obstruction from an exophytic glottis tumor. The patient received an awake elective intubation with a 2-mm cricothyroid cannula prior to successful Ventrain ventilation using EVA. Another two cases refer to neonates where the Ventrain was used to ventilate successfully through an 8-Fr Cook Frova intubating catheter (FIC) using oxygen flows of 4 to 6 L·min^{-1} and respiratory rates of 40 to 100 breaths per minute. In these cases, conventional tracheal intubation failed due to extreme upper airway obstruction. The Frova was used to establish an airway through the vocal cords and the Ventrain was ventilated through the FIC applying EVA.[45]

What Other FONA Devices Exist, and What Are Their Values?

Various large-bore cricothyrotomy kits are available for children, including the pediatric Cook Melker and the Quicktrack Child device.[46] Animal studies have been conducted on both of these airways.[37,47] There is no clinical evidence to suggest these airways perform better than a scalpel technique.

Test lung airway pressures and volumes were measured in a bench study using six trans-tracheal ventilation devices including the Enk oxygen flow modulator, the Rapid O_2 device, the Manujet trans-tracheal jet ventilator, a three-way stop-cock, ventilation from self-inflating ventilation bags, and the Ventrain. Despite the care and controlled conditions to establish consistent outcomes, a large variability in measurements was found, particularly in small test lungs and models with obstructed proximal airways. The Ventrain was the only device to provide oxygen flow without excessive lung volumes and pressures. Self-inflating ventilation bags were inadequate at providing oxygen flow through a cannula.[40]

SUMMARY

The risk of airway complications during anesthesia is heightened for infants and neonates. Within this group, babies with congenital airway anomalies are at particular risk. Careful planning and expertise is required to manage these patients safely.

The need to perform front-of-neck airway access for a child with an obstructed airway is extremely rare. The practitioner placed in the position of managing this life-threatening event will, most likely, feel extremely stressed. Under these conditions, training, support, and a standardized technique are vital ingredients for a successful outcome. Lack of evidence prevents a clear recommendation for the best type of FONA in children. Animal studies and sporadic human cases suggest that a surgical tracheotomy can satisfy the criteria of an ideal emergency airway.

SELF-EVALUATION QUESTIONS

50.1. CHARGE syndrome includes all of the following features EXCEPT:

A. Choanal atresia

B. Trachea-esophageal fistula

C. Cranial nerve anomalies

D. Congenital cataracts

E. Cleft lip

50.2. Prior to embarking on front-of-neck access, perform all of the following EXCEPT:

A. Call for help.

B. Wipe the neck.

C. Administer 100% oxygen.

D. Paralyze the patient.

E. Insert a rigid bronchoscope.

50.3. The following details concerning FONA are correct EXCEPT:

A. A size 15 scalpel is 4 mm wide.

B. The maximum pressure in the Manujet III TTJV baby range is 14.5 psi.

C. A Frova 14-Fr bougie can accommodate a size 5.0-mm ID ETT.

D. The Ventrain creates a subatmospheric pressure up to −217 cm H_2O.

E. The APLS guidelines recommend 4 L/min flow through a Y-connector for a 4-year-old.

REFERENCES

1. Fiadjoe JE, Nishisaki A, Jagannathan N, et al. Airway management complications in children with difficult tracheal intubation from the Pediatric Difficult Intubation (PeDI) registry: a prospective cohort analysis. *Lancet Respir Med.* 2016;4(1):37-48.
2. Peyton J, Park R, Staffa SJ, et al. A comparison of videolaryngoscopy using standard blades or non-standard blades in children in the Paediatric Difficult Intubation Registry. *Br J Anaesth.* 2021;126(1):331-339.
3. Issekutz KA, Graham JM Jr., Prasad C, Smith IM, Blake KD. An epidemiological analysis of CHARGE syndrome: preliminary results from a Canadian study. *Am J Med Genet A.* 2005;133A(3):309-317.
4. Pampal A. CHARGE: an association or a syndrome? *Int J Pediatr Otorhinolaryngol.* 2010;74(7):719-722.
5. Bergman JE, Blake KD, Bakker MK, et al. Death in CHARGE syndrome after the neonatal period. *Clin Genet.* 2010;77(3):232-240.
6. Lyons C, McElwain J, Coughlan MG, et al. Pre-oxygenation with facemask oxygen vs high-flow nasal oxygen vs high-flow nasal oxygen plus mouthpiece: a randomised controlled trial. *Anaesthesia.* 2022;77(1):40-45.
7. Jagannathan N, Truong CT. A simple method to deliver pharyngeal anesthesia in syndromic infants prior to awake insertion of the intubating laryngeal airway. *Can J Anaesth.* 2010;57(12):1138-1139.
8. Engelhardt T, Fiadjoe JE, Weiss M, et al. A framework for the management of the pediatric airway. *Paediatr Anaesth.* 2019;29(10):985-992.
9. Black AE, Flynn PE, Smith HL, Thomas ML, Wilkinson KA. Development of a guideline for the management of the unanticipated difficult airway in pediatric practice. *Paediatr Anaesth.* 2015;25(4):346-362.
10. Weiss M, Engelhardt T. Proposal for the management of the unexpected difficult pediatric airway. *Paediatr Anaesth.* 2010;20(5):454-464.
11. Weiss M, Engelhardt T. Cannot ventilate—paralyze! *Paediatr Anaesth.* 2012;22(12):1147-1149.
12. Von Ungern-Sternberg BS, Erb TO, Reber A, Frei FJ. Opening the upper airway – airway maneuvers in pediatric anesthesia. *Paediatr Anaesth.* 2005; 15(3):181-189.
13. Asai T, Nagata A, Shingu K. Awake tracheal intubation through the laryngeal mask in neonates with upper airway obstruction. *Paediatr Anaesth.* 2008;18(1):77-80.
14. Lee HC, Yun MJ, Hwang JW, Na HS, Kim DH, Park JY. Higher operating tables provide better laryngeal views for tracheal intubation. *Br J Anaesth.* 2014;112(4):749-755.
15. Lemay F, Cooper J. Description of an alternative method for optimal and comfortable two-handed face mask ventilation: the transverse mandibular technique. *Crit Care.* 2020;24(1):267.
16. Bradley WPL, Lyons C. Facemask ventilation. *BJA Education.* 2022; 22(1):5-11.
17. Umesh G, Krishna R, Chaudhuri S, Tim TJ, Shwethapriya R. E-O technique is superior to E-C technique in manikins during single person bag mask ventilation performed by novices. *J Clin Monit Comput.* 2014;28(3):269-273.
18. Fei M, Blair JL, Rice MJ, et al. Comparison of effectiveness of two commonly used two-handed mask ventilation techniques on unconscious apnoeic obese adults. *Br J Anaesth.* 2017;118(4):618-624.
19. Jagannathan N, Sequera-Ramos L, Sohn L, Wallis B, Shertzer A, Schaldenbrand K. Elective use of supraglottic airway devices for primary airway management in children with difficult airways. *Br J Anaesth.* 2014;112(4):742-748.
20. Qureshi MJ, Kumar M. Laryngeal mask airway versus bag-mask ventilation or endotracheal intubation for neonatal resuscitation. *Cochrane Database Syst Rev.* 2018;3:CD003314.
21. Heinrich S, Birkholz T, Ihmsen H, Irouschek A, Ackermann A, Schmidt J. Incidence and predictors of difficult laryngoscopy in 11,219 pediatric anesthesia procedures. *Paediatr Anaesth.* 2012;22(8):729-736.
22. Heinrich S, Birkholz T, Ihmsen H, et al. Incidence and predictors of poor laryngoscopic view in children undergoing pediatric cardiac surgery. *J Cardiothorac Vasc Anesth.* 2013;27(3):516-521.
23. Hosking J, Zoanetti D, Carlyle A, Anderson P, Costi D. Anesthesia for treacher collins syndrome: a review of airway management in 240 pediatric cases. *Paediatr Anaesth.* 2012;22(8):752-758.
24. Semjen F, Bordes M, Cros AM. Intubation of infants with Pierre Robin syndrome: the use of the paraglossal approach combined with a gum-elastic bougie in six consecutive cases. *Anaesthesia.* 2008;63(2):147-150.
25. Lopez U, Habre W, Laurencon M, Haller G, Van der Linden M, Iselin-Chaves IA. Intra-operative awareness in children: the value of an interview adapted to their cognitive abilities. *Anaesthesia.* 2007;62(8):778-789.
26. Miguel-Montanes R, Hajage D, Messika J, et al. Use of high-flow nasal cannula oxygen therapy to prevent desaturation during tracheal intubation of intensive care patients with mild-to-moderate hypoxemia. *Crit Care Med.* 2015;43(3):574-583.
27. Hardman JG, Wills JS. The development of hypoxaemia during apnoea in children: a computational modelling investigation. *Br J Anaesth.* 2006; 97(4):564-570.
28. Siddle BK. *Sharpening the Warrior's Edge: The psychology and science of training.* Millstadt Ill: PPCT Management Systems Inc; 1995.
29. Baker PA, Rankin L. Successful application of optiflow THRIVE to restore oxygenation and facilitate retrieval of an aspirated nut in a severely hypoxic child: a case report. *A A Pract.* 2019;13(4):130-132.

30. Monnier P. Applied surgical anatomy of the larynx and trachea. In: Monnier P, ed. *Pediatric airway surgery*. Springer; 2011:7-29.
31. Graham K, Duggan LV, Baker PA. Pediatric emergency front-of-neck-airway: an update from the airway App. *Trends in Anaesthesia and Critical Care*. 2020;30:e1-e192.
32. Holm-Knudsen RJ, Rasmussen LS, Charabi B, Bøttger M, Kristensen MS. Emergency airway access in children – transtracheal cannulas and tracheotomy assessed in a porcine model. *Paediatr Anaesth*. 2012;22(12):1159-1165.
33. Ulmer F, Lennertz J, Greif R, Butikofer L, Theiler L, Riva T. Emergency front of neck access in children: a new learning approach in a rabbit model. *Br J Anaesth*. 2020;125(1):e61-e68.
34. Berger-Estilita J, Wenzel V, Luedi MM, Riva T. A primer for pediatric emergency front-of-the-neck access. *A A Pract*. 2021;15(4):e01444.
35. Frerk C, Mitchell VS, McNarry AF, et al. Difficult Airway Society 2015 guidelines for management of unanticipated difficult intubation in adults+. *Br J Anaesth*. 2015;115(6):827-848.
36. Baker PA, Fernandez TM, Hamaekers AE, Thompson JM. Parker flex-tip or standard tracheal tube for percutaneous emergency airway access? *Acta anaesthesiologica Scandinavica*. 2013;57(2):165-170.
37. Prunty SL, Aranda-Palacios A, Heard AM, et al. The 'Can't intubate can't oxygenate' scenario in pediatric anesthesia: a comparison of the Melker cricothyroidotomy kit with a scalpel bougie technique. *Paediatr Anaesth*. 2015;25(4):400-404.
38. Hamaekers AE, Henderson JJ. Equipment and strategies for emergency tracheal access in the adult patient. *Anaesthesia*. 2011;66(Suppl 2):65-80.
39. Johansen K, Holm-Knudsen RJ, Charabi B, Kristensen MS, Rasmussen LS. Cannot ventilate-cannot intubate an infant: surgical tracheotomy or transtracheal cannula? *Paediatr Anaesth*. 2010;20(11):987-993.
40. Mann CM, Baker PA, Sainsbury DM, Taylor R. A comparison of cannula insufflation device performance for emergency front of neck airway. *Paediatr Anaesth*. 2021;31(4):482-490.
41. Wexler S, Hall K, Chin RY, Prineas SN. Cannula cricothyroidotomy and rescue oxygenation with the Rapid-O2TM oxygen insufflation device in the management of a can't intubate/can't oxygenate scenario. *Anaesth Intensive Care*. 2018;46(1):97-101.
42. Baker PA, Brown AJ. Experimental adaptation of the Enk oxygen flow modulator for potential pediatric use. *Paediatr Anaesth*. 2009;19(5):458-463.
43. Sandhya VV, Chandra S, Dhanya MR, Velayuden M. Cricothyroidotomy in a pediatric patient with upper airway foreign body. *The Airway Gazette*. 2013;17(2):12.
44. de Wolf M, Enk D, Jagannathan N. Ventilation through small-bore airways in children by implementing active expiration. *Paediatr Anaesth*. 2022;32(2):312-320.
45. Willemsen MG, Noppens R, Mulder AL, Enk D. Ventilation with the Ventrain through a small lumen catheter in the failed paediatric airway: two case reports. *Br J Anaesth*. 2014;112(5):946-947.
46. Sabato SC, Long E. An institutional approach to the management of the 'Can't Intubate, Can't Oxygenate' emergency in children. *Paediatr Anaesth*. 2016;26(8):784-793.
47. Stacey J, Heard AMB, Chapman G, et al. The 'Can't Intubate Can't Oxygenate' scenario in pediatric anesthesia: a comparison of different devices for needle cricothyroidotomy. *Paediatr Anaesth*. 2012;22(12):1155-1158.

CHAPTER 51

A Neonate with a Difficult Airway and Aspiration Risk

Alison Robles, Daniel Thomson, Jacob Heninger, Matthew Rowland, John Hajduk, and Narasimhan Jagannathan

CASE PRESENTATION

A newborn with small bowel obstruction is taken to the operating room for an exploratory laparotomy. You are called to assist with a potentially difficult airway. Initial assessment of the newborn demonstrates a "small chin" and obvious signs of respiratory distress including tachypnea and upper airway obstruction. The baby's oxygen saturation is 91% in the supine position. The primary anesthesia practitioner suggests an "awake" intubation in light of the potential for aspiration and high likelihood of a difficult airway.

BASICS OF THE NEONATAL DIFFICULT AIRWAY

When I See the Patient for the First Time, What Should I Be Looking for?

A thorough assessment of the patient's anatomic features can yield significant information. Features associated with a difficult airway include a narrow inter-incisor distance, restricted head extension, mandibular hypoplasia, midface hypoplasia, macroglossia, and microstomia.[1,2] Furthermore, it is important to determine whether the patient has been diagnosed with any syndromes. One study showed that half of the patients with difficult intubations were diagnosed with a syndrome, and the other half had extremely anterior airways and micrognathia.[3] Another large study identified that micrognathia, a weight less than 10 kg, greater than two tracheal intubation attempts, and three direct laryngoscopy attempts before an indirect technique were independently associated with an increased risk of severe airway complications.[4] It is important to evaluate the patient while lying supine at rest to look for signs of upper airway obstruction, such as paradoxical chest wall movement and/or stridor while observing for any changes in oxygen saturation.

What Are Some of the Most Common Syndromes Associated with a Difficult Airway?

There are several syndromes that are well known to be associated with a difficult airway (see Chapter 46). Each syndrome presents its own functional or anatomic challenge. Classic examples include Pierre Robin sequence (micrognathia), Treacher Collins (mandibular hypoplasia), Goldenhar syndrome (mandibular hypoplasia), Hunter's and Hurler's syndromes (mucopolysaccharidoses) and more.[1] It is important to be familiar with these syndromes as these patients may be at risk for difficult face-mask ventilation (FMV), difficult intubation, or both.[5]

AWAKE INTUBATION BASICS

When Should I Consider Doing an Awake Intubation in a Neonate?

An awake intubation should be strongly considered in a neonate if there is a clinical picture suggestive of difficult FMV, difficult laryngoscopy and intubation, or high aspiration risk with severe upper airway obstruction at rest.[6] Awake patients have the ability to maintain their own life-saving oxygenation and ventilation and are more able to protect themselves from aspiration of regurgitant gastric contents. One airway algorithm to help guide clinical decision-making is listed in Figure 51.1.[7]

What Basic Components Are Needed to Perform an Awake Tracheal Intubation in a Neonate with Airway Obstruction?

Basic components include reliable intravenous access, gastric decompression, and various airway tools readily available for your initial and backup airway plans. The decision to administer anti-sialagogues and/or topicalization of the upper airway must be tailored to each patient scenario. The goals, however, are always the same and these include maintenance of spontaneous ventilation; avoidance of worsening airway obstruction; and an assurance that patients can potentially protect their own airway from aspiration of gastric contents.

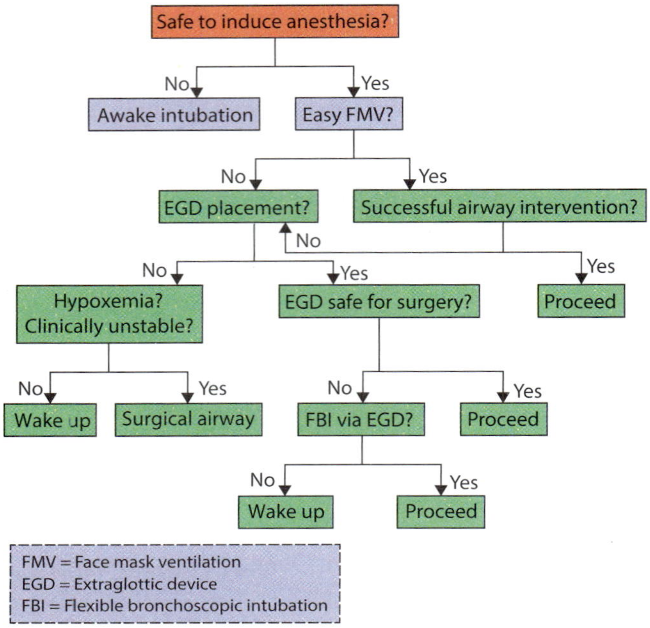

FIGURE 51.1. A useful airway algorithm to help guide clinical decision-making.

TECHNIQUES IN PERFORMING AWAKE INTUBATIONS IN THE NEONATE

What Airway Techniques Are Available to Secure the Airway of an Awake Neonate with a Difficult Airway?

Several techniques have been successfully employed in this scenario.

Direct Laryngoscopy

Consider using a straight blade in the paraglossal/retromolar technique in which the blade enters the side of the mouth along the buccal mucosa and lifts the epiglottis from the side, with the tongue avoided altogether.[8]

Video Laryngoscopy

Commercially available video laryngoscopes for neonatal use include the GlideScope® (Verathon, Bothell, WA, USA) and the pediatric video laryngoscope (Karl Storz, Tuttlingen, Germany). These indirect laryngoscopic devices come in variable sizes but incorporate a camera lens at the distal end of the intubating blade that provides a wider magnified view of the laryngeal inlet. Video laryngoscopy eliminates the need for the practitioner to align multiple axes of the airway and minimizes the need for lifting force or neck manipulation.[9,10] In both difficult and normal pediatric airways, the GlideScope has repeatedly demonstrated a faster time to glottic view, however, required a longer time for successful intubation.[9,11,12] Premature baboon model studies[13] and case reports involving infants with a difficult airway demonstrated that implementation of video laryngoscopy is both feasible and valuable for successful difficult airway management.[14–16]

Flexible Bronchoscopy

This technique remains the "gold standard" for the management of the difficult airway and will be discussed more below.

Would You Attempt Direct Laryngoscopy First in an Anticipated, Yet "Untested" Difficult Airway?

Each practitioner must make this decision based on his or her own expertise, comfort level, and patient factors. However, be aware that persistent attempts with direct laryngoscopy leads to increased complications. Results of the Pediatric Difficult Intubation Registry found that multiple attempts (defined as greater than two) at direct laryngoscopy in pediatric patients with difficult airways were associated with greater rates of failed intubation and severe complications.[4] Severe complications included cardiac arrest, hypoxemia, bronchospasm, esophageal intubation, and severe airway trauma. Additional risk factors for complications include weight < 10 kg and a short thyromental distance (i.e., micrognathia).

Is Flexible Bronchoscopic Intubation the Gold Standard for Difficult Airways in Neonates?

Flexible bronchoscopic intubation is the "gold standard" for tracheal intubation of the pediatric patient with a difficult airway.[5,17,18] The utility of the flexible bronchoscope is derived from its ability to navigate the patient's airway under indirect visualization. Intubation can be achieved through various routes—the mouth, nose, or through an extraglottic airway device. Anatomic reasons for a difficult airway, such as small mouth opening, anterior larynx, and airway masses, can potentially be bypassed with this device.

What Are the Limitations to Flexible Bronchoscopic Intubation?

Limitations include lack of training by the practitioner in using the device, lack of patient cooperation, abnormal airway anatomy, and small amounts of blood and secretions that can easily distort views from its small camera. In order for the device to be a useful airway tool, frequent use and practice are required for the practitioner to maintain a proficient skill level in children.[17–19] In novices, flexible bronchoscopic intubation in children was achieved more quickly through the nasal route than the oral route.[20] Therefore, depending on the expertise of the practitioner, the nasal route should be considered.

What Is Required to Perform an Awake Tracheal Intubation Using a Flexible Bronchoscope in a Free-Handed Manner for a Neonate?

There are multiple flexible bronchoscopic sizes available for neonates. The smallest is 2.2 mm in diameter.[17] The flexible bronchoscopic should be preloaded with an appropriately sized endotracheal tube (ETT) (for a full-term neonate consider using a cuffed 3.0-mm inner diameter [ID] ETT, or smaller). Make sure the scope is white-balanced and examined for proper functioning.

Consider administering medications such as anti-sialagogues or antimuscarinics (in the scenario where the neonate has a vagal response with subsequent bradycardia during intubation). Passive oxygenation can be provided via a nasal cannula or nasal trumpet.

After adequate denitrogenation, an assistant can provide a bilateral jaw thrust and manual tongue traction in order to facilitate entry and passage of the flexible bronchoscope into the oropharynx. To pull the tongue out, consider using sterile gauze or McGill forceps, or stitching the tongue and using the suture to pull and anchor the tongue out.

The scope should be inserted midline. If the anatomy allows, the airway landmarks should be identified as the scope is advanced until the laryngeal inlet is encountered. Once the epiglottis is visualized, the scope should be retroflexed underneath the epiglottis and then subsequently flexed to bring the glottic opening into view.

Alternatively, a nasal flexible bronchoscopic approach may be considered. The nasal approach has the advantage of keeping the bronchoscope relatively midline during tracheal intubation. Prior to nasotracheal intubation, a vasoconstrictor should be instilled into the nares. A thermosoftened ETT should be used to minimize the risk of epistaxis.[21] It has been shown that this approach is faster than the oral bronchoscopic intubation in small children in practitioners inexperienced with using pediatric flexible bronchoscopes.[20]

Each practitioner should decide whether to use induction agents and/or muscle relaxants at this point, with the purpose to minimize laryngeal and pharyngeal reflex activation. However, be aware that optimizing intubation conditions with such medications comes at the cost of ablating the protection of these airway reflexes if the ETT is unable to be passed successfully over the bronchoscope. Conversely, some reports have shown a large proportion of aspiration events can be attributed to a patient coughing or gagging due to inadequate depth of anesthesia and no muscle relaxation.[22]

Once the scope is in the trachea, the ETT should be guided over the bronchoscope into the trachea. Confirmation of tracheal placement and adequate ventilation should be confirmed with the bronchoscope as well as end-tidal capnography.

Why Use an Extraglottic Airway Device as a Conduit for Tracheal Intubation in Neonates?

Multiple studies have shown that extraglottic devices are effective conduits for tracheal intubation in children, and in children with difficult airways.[23–25]

Extraglottic airway devices have a long history of clinical reliability,[26] are usually easy to place, provide the ability to oxygenate and ventilate, and allow for excellent glottic isolation.[27–31] They allow the practitioner to minimize disconnect time from the breathing circuit while providing a conduit for successful tracheal intubation.

How Would You Perform Insertion of an Extraglottic Device in an Awake Neonate? Is Topicalization Necessary?

In patients with difficult airways, the awake placement of an appropriately sized extraglottic device is generally well-tolerated in infants less than 2 months old.[6,32] Case series and reports have described that after extraglottic placement, infants are generally calm or do not demonstrate an increase in crying or distress. Additionally, there is minimal coughing, gagging, or episodes of hypoxemia. In patients demonstrating upper airway obstruction, oxygen saturations improved.[6,27,32]

If the neonate is unable to tolerate the insertion of the device awake, consider topicalization. Lidocaine 2% jelly can be applied manually to the posterior pharynx with a finger, or by an atomizer. Another technique is to inject the lidocaine jelly into a pacifier, create several perforations in the pacifier, and then insert the pacifier into the neonate's mouth. This allows the extrusion of the local anesthetic onto their posterior pharynx. Dosages of local anesthetic must be carefully measured to prevent potential systemic toxicity. Additional cases have performed glossopharyngeal nerve blocks to facilitate placement of extraglottic devices, although this may not be necessary for infants less than 2 months of age.[33]

Difficulty with the insertion of the extraglottic device in an awake neonate may include reflex activation of the airway (bearing down, coughing, laryngospasm, breath holding), or placement of an oversized device. In these instances, these infants may possibly expel the device from their mouth.

Should I Give Any Medications Prior to or During the Intubation Attempt?

Ideally, anesthetic agents and muscle relaxants would be given to produce optimal intubating conditions. These agents would mitigate a stress response, potentially reduce airway trauma, and decrease several physiologic perturbations that may occur with awake intubation. These perturbations include hypertension, bradycardia, tachycardia, hypoxemia, and increased anterior fontanelle pressure and cerebral blood flow.[34,35] It is unclear whether a relatively brief noxious stimulus incurs long-term behavioral effects in neonates.

However, in a known difficult airway situation, it would be prudent to avoid agents that would impair ventilation and oxygenation until the airway is secure. Acute hypertension from intubation may mirror that seen with other noxious stimulation or stressors such as tracheal suction or routine handling. Hemodynamically significant bradycardia secondary to vagal stimulation during awake intubation can be averted by premedication with atropine. Hypoxemia from breath holding may be prevented with supplemental oxygen.

CONSIDERATIONS AND COMPLICATIONS ASSOCIATED WITH AWAKE INTUBATIONS IN THE NEONATE

The Neonate's Oxygen Saturation Falls to 80% When the Flexible Bronchoscope Is Inserted into the Mouth. What Techniques Are Available to Overcome Upper Airway Obstruction Before Tracheal Intubation?

There are several ways to overcome extraglottic obstruction in an awake neonate while providing oxygen. Appropriate placement of an extraglottic device in the hypopharynx bypasses extraglottic obstruction and can both act as a conduit for oxygenation and ventilation and facilitate intubation using a flexible bronchoscope. Additionally, protective airway reflexes are still preserved with the placement of the device. Retrospective studies analyzing the use of extraglottic devices in pediatric patients with difficult airways have generally been favorable, demonstrating successful use in 96% of patients.[23] Extraglottic devices would not be helpful in situations involving glottic or subglottic obstruction.

Another strategy involves inserting a modified nasal trumpet.[36] Once in place, the nasal trumpet is fitted with an adapter that is connected to an oxygen source. The passage of the trumpet can bypass airway obstruction as well as facilitate the addition of supplementary oxygen, and provide nasal CPAP. Another technique to alleviate upper airway obstruction includes placing the patient in prone position.[37] The use of a tongue pull and jaw thrust may also help overcome the obstruction. It is important to emphasize that in all of the above strategies; oxygen should be provided during airway management.

How Would You Perform a Rapid Sequence Intubation Via an Extraglottic Device for a "Full Stomach"?

With established venous access and prior nasogastric stomach decompression, posterior pharyngeal topicalization is performed as described above. Subsequently, an intubating extraglottic device (designed to facilitate tracheal intubation, such as an air-Q® Intubating Laryngeal Airway, SunMed, Grand Rapids, MI) is inserted in the patient awake.[6] Once the extraglottic device is appropriately seated, it is used as a conduit for the flexible bronchoscope preloaded with an ETT. The scope is advanced into the larynx with subsequent tracheal intubation. Consider the administration of induction agents and/or paralysis at this point. An air-Q removal stylet (or another similar size ETT) can be used as a "stabilizer" to facilitate the removal of the extraglottic device (see Chapter 13).

Would You Use a Neuromuscular Blocking Agent Once You Obtained a View of the Glottic Opening with the Flexible Bronchoscope?

The option to proceed with a bronchoscopic-guided intubation via an extraglottic device without neuromuscular blockade is a challenging one. The practitioner risks causing airway trauma, laryngospasm, bronchospasm, aspiration of gastric contents, and potential dislodgment of the tracheal tube. Once adequate visualization of the glottic opening is obtained, an induction agent accompanied by a rapid onset neuromuscular blocker may be administered immediately prior to tracheal intubation to mitigate reflex activation of the airway.[6] Although not yet FDA approved in the pediatric population, a synthetically modified γ-cyclodextrin such as sugammadex has been utilized in the rapid reversal of rocuronium in infants.[38,39] The time from muscle relaxant onset, to securement of the airway with an ETT also risks potential aspiration of gastric contents. If unsure, one should err on the side of preserving spontaneous ventilation until the airway is secured. The decision to use a neuromuscular blocker depends on the clinical situation, and the comfort level of the practitioner performing tracheal intubation.

What Role Can Continuous Oxygenation Play During a Rapid Sequence Intubation?

Due to their increased oxygen consumption relative to their functional residual capacity, in general, oxygen desaturation occurs more quickly in infants compared to older patients. Apneic oxygenation can be utilized to increase the time to oxygen desaturation and facilitate avoidance of rescue oxygenation.[40,41]

How Would You Administer Continuous Oxygenation?

This can be done in several ways. Noninvasively, it can be administered using a nasal cannula or an intubating anesthesia mask. It can also be done more invasively with an EGD using a bronchoscopic adapter, a small oral Ring, Adair, and Elwyn endotracheal tube in the corner of the pharynx, or a modified nasal trumpet connected to a circuit.[42]

When using nasal cannula, one report showed a longer time for oxygen desaturation in patients receiving continuous oxygenation but did not see a difference in those receiving high flows (>2 $L \cdot kg^{-1} \cdot min^{-1}$) versus low flows (0.2 $L \cdot kg^{-1} \cdot min^{-1}$).[43]

What Benefits Would Transnasal Humidified Rapid-Insufflation Ventilatory Exchange (THRIVE) Have over Other Traditional Apneic Oxygenation Delivery Systems?

This mechanism allows for the administration of warm, humidified air at flows much greater than the patient's minute ventilation, allowing for delivery of FiO_2 up to 100%. Additionally, these higher flows can create an insufflating alveolar pressure, providing PEEP, and preventing airway collapse. This method may also mitigate mucosal injury, ciliary dysfunction, and patient discomfort.[40] There is also the potential benefit of the exchange of gases such as CO_2 that has been shown in adults and is uncertain in children and infants.[44]

What Are Potential Barriers to Continuous Oxygenation?

Nasal cannula may interfere with the mask seal and thus the ability to provide FMV. Practitioners unfamiliar with this technique may be uncomfortable with its application. Additionally, while oxygen is being provided, it is uncertain how much gas exchange is occurring. Thus, when used for prolonged periods of time, patients may be susceptible to side effects of hypercapnia such as CO_2 narcosis and arrhythmias.[42]

UTILITY OF GASTRIC ULTRASOUND TO ASSESS FOR ASPIRATION RISK

Are There Any Tests Available to Assess a Patient's Aspiration Risk?

Point-of-care ultrasound has become a popular modality for obtaining clinically useful information. Gastric ultrasound is a noninvasive test that can be used, in conjunction with a complete history and physical examination, to help assess a patient's risk of aspiration when undergoing general anesthesia.[42] The incidence of pulmonary aspiration in the pediatric population is estimated to be 0.04% to 0.1%. This risk is elevated in pediatric patients undergoing urgent or emergency surgery, commonly due to delayed gastric emptying secondary to pain, trauma, congenital disorders, acute abdomen, and medications.[45]

When Is It Appropriate to Use Gastric Ultrasound?

Gastric ultrasound is most useful when there is true clinical uncertainty as to whether a patient has a full stomach. One example would be if there is an uncertain NPO timeline, such as in pediatric patients and patients with cognitive dysfunction or altered mental status. Gastric ultrasound can also be useful in those with comorbidities or physiologic conditions that can delay gastric emptying, such as diabetic gastroparesis, pregnancy, obesity, advanced renal and liver disease, pyloric stenosis, or recent trauma.[46,47]

In this particular case with a neonate having a high risk of aspiration and a potentially difficult airway, gastric ultrasound can provide valuable information regarding a patient's gastric residual volume. Adequate imaging and clinical information can help the anesthesia practitioner decide how to proceed with the induction of anesthesia, and determine whether the risk of pulmonary aspiration is greater than the risk of hypoxemia that could potentially ensue by withholding ventilation due to fear of gastric insufflation.

Describe How to Perform Gastric Ultrasound

Patients are typically examined in both the supine and right lateral decubitus (RLD) positions.[48,49] A low-frequency curved array probe is used for most adults. However, a high-frequency linear array probe can be used in pediatric patients under approximately 40 kg in order to provide greater resolution and obtain better images.[46,47] The ultrasound probe is placed in the sagittal plane of the epigastric region.

Discuss the Basic Principles of Gastric Ultrasound

Gravity will pull gastric contents toward dependent areas of the stomach, in particular the gastric antrum, which is the most amenable portion of the stomach for sonographic evaluation.[45,47] This is due to its consistent, superficial location with favorable windows for sonographic examination.[46] Large quantities of gastric contents can be visualized in the supine position. However, it is more difficult to detect smaller quantities of fluid in this position. In the RLD position, gravitational effects will cause gastric contents to pool in the antrum, allowing the sonographer to detect smaller volumes of gastric fluid that otherwise would not have been visible in the supine position.[47] Numerous studies suggest a positive correlation between the cross-sectional area (CSA) of the gastric antrum and total gastric fluid volume.[45,46,48,50–52] Additionally, the highest correlation between the two is in the RLD position.[46,48,50,52] Gastric volume greater than 1.5 $mL \cdot kg^{-1}$ would suggest a high aspiration risk.[46,47] One study[47] derived the formula below to calculate the gastric volume using ultrasound.

$$\text{Gastric volume (mL)} = -7.8 + (3.5 \times \text{RLD} - \text{CSA}) + (0.127 \times \text{age in months})$$

How Are Gastric Ultrasound Images Interpreted?

Air, liquids, and solids will each have a different echogenicity on ultrasound. Gastric secretions or clear liquids will appear hypoechoic or anechoic, with increasing distention of the antrum as the gastric volume increases. Air or gas bubbles will appear as mobile, punctate echoes. Solids will have a heterogeneous, hyperechoic consistency along with a distended antrum.[48]

In an empty stomach, the antrum will appear small and flat, with juxtaposition of the anterior and posterior walls. The muscular walls will be relatively thick and will give the appearance of a bullseye.[46]

Normal gastric contents and clear liquids will appear hypoechoic on ultrasound. As the volume of gastric fluid increases, the antrum will appear more round and the walls will be thinner and more distended.[46]

A gastric antrum that contains solids will have heterogeneous echogenicity representing different consistencies of consumed particles. The walls of the antrum will become thinner and distended as the volume of contents increases.[47] Immediately following food ingestion, swallowed air will create an air-mucosal interface on the anterior surface of the antrum, giving a "frosted-glass" appearance that will cause artifact posteriorly on ultrasound.[46]

How Is the Antrum Graded Based on Ultrasound Imaging?

The gastric antrum is graded on a scale from 0 to 2. A grade 0 antrum describes an empty stomach in both the supine and RLD positions, which would indicate a low risk for pulmonary aspiration. A grade 1 antrum indicates less than 1.5 $mL{\cdot}kg^{-1}$ of gastric fluid in the RLD position, which also would be designated low risk for aspiration. Grade 2 is if there is greater than 1.5 $mL{\cdot}kg^{-1}$ in any position or if there is any solid matter in the stomach, indicating a high risk for aspiration.[46] A flowchart for gastric ultrasound grading and interpretation is shown in Figure 51.2.

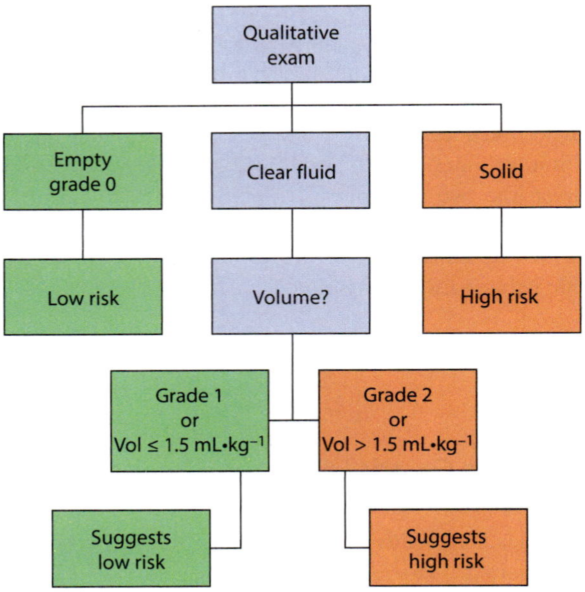

FIGURE 51.2. Flowchart for interpretation of findings and medical decision-making based on gastric point-of-care ultrasound findings. Used with permission from gastricultrasound.org. (Reproduced with permission from Gastric Ultrasound. gastricultrasound.org.)

SUMMARY

Airway management of a newborn with a potentially difficult airway and a high risk of aspiration secondary to a small bowel obstruction poses significant challenges to airway practitioners. Several awake airway management options were discussed. In addition, gastric ultrasound can provide valuable information regarding a patient's gastric residual volume.

SELF-EVALUATION QUESTIONS

51.1. Which of the following are associated with an increased risk of complications during difficult airway management in a child?

A. Body weight less than 10 kg
B. Short thyromental distance
C. Greater than two direct laryngoscopy attempts
D. All of the above

51.2. Which of the following interventions is least likely to improve extraglottic upper airway obstruction during difficult airway management in a neonate with Pierre Robin?

A. Extraglottic device insertion
B. Neck extension
C. Nasal trumpet insertion
D. Prone positioning

51.3. Which of the following is true regarding awake extraglottic device placement in a neonate with a difficult airway?

A. An awake extraglottic device placement is not well-tolerated.
B. An intubating extraglottic device such as an air-Q can be used to facilitate rapid-sequence tracheal intubation.
C. Evidence of extraglottic airway obstruction such as sternal retractions is a contraindication to extraglottic device insertion.
D. Toxicity to local anesthetics precludes the use of topicalization prior to placement of an extraglottic device.

REFERENCES

1. Frei FJ, Ummenhofer W. Difficult intubation in paediatrics. *Paediatr Anaesth.* 1996;6:251-263.
2. Tong DC, Beus J, Litman R. The children's hospital of Philadelphia difficult intubation registry. *Anesthesiology.* 2007;107:A1637.
3. Akpek EA, Mutlu H, Kayhan Z. Difficult intubation in pediatric cardiac anesthesia. *J Cardiothorac Vasc Anesth.* 2004;18:610-612.
4. Fiadjoe JE, Nishisaki A, Jagannathan N, et al. Airway management complications in children with difficult tracheal intubation from the Pediatric Difficult Intubation (PeDI) registry: a prospective cohort analysis. *Lancet Respir Med.* 2016;4:37-48.
5. de Beer D, Bingham R. The child with facial abnormalities. *Curr Opin Anaesthesiol.* 2011;24:282-288.
6. Jagannathan N, Sohn LE, Eidem JM. Use of the air-Q intubating laryngeal airway for rapid-sequence intubation in infants with severe airway obstruction: a case series. *Anaesthesia.* 2013;68:636-638.
7. Huang AS, Hajduk J, Rim C, Coffield S, Jagannathan N. Focused review on management of the difficult paediatric airway. *Indian J Anaesth.* 2019;63:428-436.

8. Saxena KN, Nischal H, Bhardwaj M, Gaba P, Shastry BV. Right molar approach to tracheal intubation in a child with Pierre Robin syndrome, cleft palate, and tongue tie. Br J Anaesth. 2008;100:141-142.
9. Armstrong J, John J, Karsli C. A comparison between the GlideScope Video Laryngoscope and direct laryngoscope in paediatric patients with difficult airways–a pilot study. *Anaesthesia.* 2010;65:353-357.
10. Sun Y, Lu Y, Huang Y, Jiang H. Pediatric video laryngoscope versus direct laryngoscope: a meta-analysis of randomized controlled trials. *Paediatr Anaesth.* 2014;24:1056-1065.
11. Fiadjoe JE, Gurnaney H, Dalesio N, et al. A prospective randomized equivalence trial of the GlideScope Cobalt(R) video laryngoscope to traditional direct laryngoscopy in neonates and infants. *Anesthesiology.* 2012;116:622-628.
12. Lee JH, Park YH, Byon HJ, et al. A comparative trial of the GlideScope(R) video laryngoscope to direct laryngoscope in children with difficult direct laryngoscopy and an evaluation of the effect of blade size. *Anesth Analg.* 2013;117:176-181.
13. Moreira A, Koele-Schmidt L, Leland M, Seidner S, Blanco C. Neonatal intubation with direct laryngoscopy vs videolaryngoscopy: an extremely premature baboon model. *Paediatr Anaesth.* 2014;24:840-844.
14. Lillie EM, Harding L, Thomas M. A new twist in the pediatric difficult airway. *Paediatr Anaesth.* 2015;25:428-430.
15. Trevisanuto D, Fornaro E, Verghese C. The GlideScope video laryngoscope: initial experience in five neonates. *Can J Anaesth.* 2006;53:423-424.
16. Wald SH, Keyes M, Brown A. Pediatric video laryngoscope rescue for a difficult neonatal intubation. *Paediatr Anaesth.* 2008;18:790-792.
17. Sims C, von Ungern-Sternberg BS. The normal and the challenging pediatric airway. *Paediatr Anaesth.* 2012;22:521-526.
18. Sunder RA, Haile DT, Farrell PT, Sharma A. Pediatric airway management: current practices and future directions. *Paediatr Anaesth.* 2012;22:1008-1015.
19. Clarke RC, Gardner AI. Anaesthesia trainees' exposure to airway management in an Australian tertiary adult teaching hospital. *Anaesth Intensive Care.* 2008;36:513-515.
20. Jagannathan N, Sequera-Ramos L, Sohn L, et al. Randomized comparison of experts and trainees with nasal and oral fibreoptic intubation in children less than 2 yr of age. *Br J Anaesth.* 2015;114:290-296.
21. El-Seify ZA, Khattab AM, Shaaban AA, Metwalli OS, Hassan HE, Ajjoub LF. Xylometazoline pretreatment reduces nasotracheal intubation-related epistaxis in paediatric dental surgery. *Br J Anaesth.* 2010;105:501-505.
22. Warner MA, Warner ME, Warner DO, Warner LO, Warner EJ. Perioperative pulmonary aspiration in infants and children. *Anesthesiology.* 1999;90:66-71.
23. Jagannathan N, Sequera-Ramos L, Sohn L, Wallis B, Shertzer A, Schaldenbrand K. Elective use of supraglottic airway devices for primary airway management in children with difficult airways. *Br J Anaesth.* 2014;112:742-748.
24. Jagannathan N, Roth AG, Sohn LE, Pak TY, Amin S, Suresh S. The new air-Q intubating laryngeal airway for tracheal intubation in children with anticipated difficult airway: a case series. *Paediatr Anaesth.* 2009;19:618-622.
25. Jagannathan N, Kho MF, Kozlowski RJ, Sohn LE, Siddiqui A, Wong DT. Retrospective audit of the air-Q intubating laryngeal airway as a conduit for tracheal intubation in pediatric patients with a difficult airway. *Paediatr Anaesth.* 2011;21:422-427.
26. White MC, Cook TM, Stoddart PA. A critique of elective pediatric supraglottic airway devices. *Paediatr Anaesth.* 2009;19(Suppl 1):55-65.
27. Asai T, Nagata A, Shingu K. Awake tracheal intubation through the laryngeal mask in neonates with upper airway obstruction. *Paediatr Anaesth.* 2008;18:77-80.
28. Brain AI, Verghese C, Addy EV, Kapila A. The intubating laryngeal mask. I: Development of a new device for intubation of the trachea. *Br J Anaesth.* 1997;79:699-703.
29. Brain AI, Verghese C, Addy EV, Kapila A, Brimacombe J. The intubating laryngeal mask. II: A preliminary clinical report of a new means of intubating the trachea. *Br J Anaesth.* 1997;79:704-709.
30. Lopez-Gil M, Brimacombe J, Alvarez M. Safety and efficacy of the laryngeal mask airway. A prospective survey of 1400 children. *Anaesthesia.* 1996;51:969-972.
31. Lopez-Gil M, Brimacombe J. The ProSeal laryngeal mask airway in children. *Paediatr Anaesth.* 2005;15:229-234.
32. Markakis DA, Sayson SC, Schreiner MS. Insertion of the laryngeal mask airway in awake infants with the Robin sequence. *Anesth Analg.* 1992;75:822-824.
33. Jagannathan N, Truong CT. A simple method to deliver pharyngeal anesthesia in syndromic infants prior to awake insertion of the intubating laryngeal airway. *Can J Anaesth.* 2010;57:1138-1139.
34. Duncan HP, Zurick NJ, Wolf AR. Should we reconsider awake neonatal intubation? A review of the evidence and treatment strategies. *Paediatr Anaesth.* 2001;11:135-145.
35. Millar C, Bissonnette B. Awake intubation increases intracranial pressure without affecting cerebral blood flow velocity in infants. *Can J Anaesth.* 1994;41:281-287.
36. Holm-Knudsen R, Eriksen K, Rasmussen LS. Using a nasopharyngeal airway during fiberoptic intubation in small children with a difficult airway. *Paediatr Anaesth.* 2005;15:839-845.
37. Jagannathan N, Jagannathan R. Prone insertion of a size 0.5 intubating laryngeal airway overcomes severe upper airway obstruction in an awake neonate with Pierre Robin syndrome. *Can J Anaesth.* 2012;59:1001-1002.
38. Wakimoto M, Burrier C, Tobias JD. Sugammadex for rapid intraoperative reversal of neuromuscular blockade in a neonate. *J Med Cases.* 2018;9.
39. Efune PN, Alex G, Mehta SD. Emergency sugammadex reversal in an 850-G premature infant: a case report. *J Pediatr Pharmacol Ther.* 2021;26:107-110.
40. Humphreys S, Rosen D, Housden T, Taylor J, Schibler A. Nasal high-flow oxygen delivery in children with abnormal airways. *Paediatr Anaesth.* 2017;27:616-620.
41. Kulkarni KS, Dave N, Saran S, Garasia M, Parelkar S. Ultra-modified rapid sequence induction with transnasal humidified rapid insufflation ventilatory exchange: Challenging convention. *Indian J Anaesth.* 2018;62:310-313.
42. Stein ML, Park RS, Kovatsis PG. Emerging trends, techniques, and equipment for airway management in pediatric patients. *Paediatr Anaesth.* 2020;30:269-279.
43. Riva T, Pedersen TH, Seiler S, et al. Transnasal humidified rapid insufflation ventilatory exchange for oxygenation of children during apnoea: a prospective randomised controlled trial. *Br J Anaesth.* 2018;120:592-599.
44. Patel A, Nouraei SA. Transnasal Humidified Rapid-Insufflation Ventilatory Exchange (THRIVE): a physiological method of increasing apnoea time in patients with difficult airways. *Anaesthesia.* 2015;70:323-329.
45. Spencer AO, Walker AM, Yeung AK, et al. Ultrasound assessment of gastric volume in the fasted pediatric patient undergoing upper gastrointestinal endoscopy: development of a predictive model using endoscopically suctioned volumes. *Paediatr Anaesth.* 2015;25:301-308.
46. Perlas A, Arzola C, Van de Putte P. Point-of-care gastric ultrasound and aspiration risk assessment: a narrative review. *Can J Anaesth.* 2018;65:437-448.
47. El-Boghdadly K, Wojcikiewicz T, Perlas A. Perioperative point-of-care gastric ultrasound. *BJA Educ.* 2019;19:219-226.
48. Van de Putte P, Perlas A. Ultrasound assessment of gastric content and volume. *Br J Anaesth.* 2014;113:12-22.
49. Gagey AC, de Queiroz Siqueira M, Monard C, et al. The effect of pre-operative gastric ultrasound examination on the choice of general anaesthetic induction technique for non-elective paediatric surgery. A prospective cohort study. *Anaesthesia.* 2018;73:304-312.
50. Schmitz A, Thomas S, Melanie F, et al. Ultrasonographic gastric antral area and gastric contents volume in children. *Paediatr Anaesth.* 2012;22:144-149.
51. Austin DR, Chang MG, Bittner EA. Use of handheld point-of-care ultrasound in emergency airway management. *Chest.* 2021;159:1155-1165.
52. Gagey AC, de Queiroz Siqueira M, Desgranges FP, Combet S, Naulin C, Chassard D, Bouvet L. Ultrasound assessment of the gastric contents for the guidance of the anaesthetic strategy in infants with hypertrophic pyloric stenosis: a prospective cohort study. *Br J Anaesth.* 2016;116:649-654.

SECTION 8

AIRWAY MANAGEMENT IN OBSTETRICS

CHAPTER 52

What Is Unique About the Obstetrical Airway?

Dolores M. McKeen and Kelly Au

INTRODUCTION

The ability to maintain a patent airway, provide adequate oxygenation, and place an endotracheal tube (ETT) remains a major concern for airway practitioners. Despite many equipment advances and the development of airway algorithms to guide care, management of the obstetric airway is still a cause for concern. Obstetrical anesthesia is a high-risk practice that is replete with medicolegal liability and laden with clinical challenges. In the obstetric service, the practitioner is required to provide safe anesthesia care to the mother and baby, both of whom have unique and demanding anatomical and physiological requirements. The purpose of this chapter is to briefly review the status of maternal morbidity/mortality, highlight the principal reasons that airways of parturients might be difficult to manage, and review current guidelines and algorithms for the management of the obstetrical airway.

Underpinning all discussion is the critical importance of being prepared cognitively for unexpected occurrence and being facile with appropriate emergency airway equipment. Early consultation for anesthesia intervention and airway assessment of obstetric patients at high risk for operative intervention (particularly parturients who may be obese or have advanced maternal age) remain a key preventative pillar of care. Of equal importance, is teamwork between the anesthesia practitioner, the labor and delivery nurses, and the obstetrician. Improved perioperative training of labor and delivery unit support staff (including anesthesia resources for airway management during and after general anesthesia) are important clinical care considerations. Practicing difficult airway scenarios is invaluable. Being unprepared will certainly guarantee failure.

MATERNAL MORBIDITY AND MORTALITY

Discuss the Anesthetic-Related Morbidity and Mortality of Parturients

Women continue to experience preventable pregnancy-related deaths, with airway management being a significant contributor in developed countries.[1–3] These anesthesia-related deaths are particularly catastrophic, because many of these anesthetics are elective, and are administered to young otherwise well mothers.

In 1985, a unique perspective on anesthesia morbidity and mortality was unveiled with the institution of the American Society of Anesthesiologists (ASA) Closed Claims Project database. The data from this project are an accumulation of personal damage insurance claims filed against anesthesiologists and subsequently settled.[4] Of the nearly 6500 cases in the database at that time, 12% were associated with obstetrical anesthesia care, and nearly three-fourths of these claims were associated with cesarean section. Critical events involving the respiratory system were the most common precipitating events in the obstetrical files. Trauma from repeated attempts at intubation was recognized as an issue of particular hazard.

From the ASA Closed Claims Project database of 7328 cases, those associated with obstetric procedures that occurred between 1990 and 2003 were reviewed in 2009. The review revealed 426 cases associated with obstetric anesthesia, with 58% of these claims associated with cesarean section. Maternal deaths and brain injury during this period occurred most frequently with high blocks during regional anesthesia, half of which occurred during placement for a vaginal delivery. While these may be attributable to the change in anesthesia practice and general anesthesia avoidance strategies, failure to detect accidental intrathecal injection resulting in a high block, as well as delayed response to manage associated cardiorespiratory collapse, were major issues. The most common general anesthesia-associated maternal deaths and brain injury claims were due to failed intubation and inadequate treatment of maternal hemorrhage, occurring in equal proportions.[5]

Obstetrical airway catastrophes occur most frequently during emergency cesarean sections. It is often in settings in which regional anesthesia is not an option because of either maternal conditions or severe fetal distress. It is also in these settings that airway evaluation may be particularly hurried and harassed. Overall incidences of obstetrical airway problems are low (7.9%),[6] but appear to be greater than in the nonobstetric patient (2.5%).[7] Face-mask ventilation (FMV) can be difficult or impossible in approximately 0.02% of parturients, an incidence not dissimilar to other surgical populations.[8] Consequences of a failed intubation, however, appear to be greater in the obstetric population.[5,9,10]

There is little prospective evidence, and the literature is unclear, as to the actual incidence of failed intubation under general anesthesia in obstetrical patients. While ranges have been given from one in 283 to one in 2130, a composite incidence of about 0.2%[11] to 0.4%[12] has been suggested. In a 2005 systematic review, Goldszmidt challenged conventional wisdom and examined the evidence as to whether tracheal intubation in the obstetrical population is truly more difficult.[9] In this review, difficult and failed intubation in the obstetric population was found to be rare, and there was no difference in the occurrence of difficult (1-6%) or failed intubation (0-0.7%) compared to general surgical populations.

In 2015, Kinsella et al.[13] reanalyzed over 33 publications in the obstetric anesthesia airway literature from 1970 to 2014, using newly defined failed intubation criteria by McKeen et al. in order to allow for comparability across numerous obstetric airway studies.[14] Using these criteria, their meta-analysis revealed an incidence of failed intubation of 1 in 443 general anesthetics for cesarean delivery (CD), and that number held steady over the time period studied.[13–15] While the actual incidence of difficult airways in the obstetrical population remains unclear, there are concerns that the rates of failed intubation in the obstetric population will increase with declining numbers of women requiring general anesthetics, and the potential loss of skills in managing the airway of an obstetric patient.[12,16–21]

THE PARTURIENT AIRWAY

Why Do Parturients Have More Airway Complications Compared to the General Population?

The parturient is at significantly greater risk for airway complications and possible difficult intubations than her nonpregnant counterpart.[5,10,12,22] A wide range of both anatomical and physiological changes occur during pregnancy, and many of these may impact the airway directly, or indirectly (Table 52.1). Many of the changes are hormonally driven, and the gravid uterus has a significant impact on the respiratory, cardiovascular, and gastrointestinal systems. Finally, there are a number of abnormal pregnancy-related processes that impact heavily on the parturient airway.

TABLE 52.1. Factors Affecting Management of the Parturient Airway

Weight gain (12-20 kg)	• Enlarging gravid uterus • Increasing total body water and interstitial fluid • Increasing blood volume • Deposition of new fat • Enlargement of the breasts
Respiratory system	• Decrease in respiratory reserve volume • Decrease in functional residual capacity (20-30%) • Increased oxygen consumption • More rapid oxygen desaturation
Airway	• Increased oral, nasal, pharyngeal, and tracheal mucosal edema • Vascular engorgement of oral, pharyngeal, and nasal capillaries • Edema of face and neck • Advancement of Mallampati classification with pregnancy • Advancement of Mallampati classification with bearing down during labor
Cardiovascular system	• Inferior caval syndrome (supine hypotensive syndrome) requiring left uterine tilt
Gastrointestinal system	• Steadily increasing intragastric pressure as pregnancy progresses • Decreased lower esophageal sphincter tone due to increasing progesterone • Symptomatic gastroesophageal reflu • Distortion of gastric anatomy • Increased gastric acidity

How Do the Physiological Changes Associated with Pregnancy Impact the Airway of Parturients?

The difficulties in airway management for obstetrical patients may be related to a number of factors:

Weight Gain

During pregnancy, average weight gain can be 12 to 20 kg over the parturient prepregnant weight. This weight gain is related to increases in total body water, interstitial fluid (generalized

CHAPTER 52

body edema), blood volume, deposition of new fat and protein, uterine size and contents, and enlargement of the breasts.

Obesity (BMI>30 kg·m^{-2}) has become much more frequently encountered in the general population over the past decade. FMV is often difficult in obese patients because of reduced chest compliance and increased intra-abdominal pressure. The incidence of partially obliterated oropharyngeal structures in obese parturients is double that of nonobese parturients.[6] In addition, weight gain may create a "short neck (SN)," a large tongue, and large breasts, all of which contribute to difficult laryngoscopy. In the morbidly obese parturient (greater than 140 kg or ~300 lb, BMI ≥ 40 kg·m^{-2}), the risks for diabetes, hypertension, preeclampsia, and primary CD are all increased. There is also a higher incidence of difficult labor resulting in instrumental deliveries, postpartum hemorrhage, or other conditions which may require anesthetic intervention.[23]

Morbidly obese parturients are at increased risk for anesthesia-related complications during CD, and increased risks for failed intubation and gastric aspiration if general anesthesia is required.[24] The cesarean section rate in these patients can exceed 50%, with one-third of attempted tracheal intubations being difficult, and 6% being failures.[25] In the ASA closed claims obstetrical files, damaging events related to the respiratory system were significantly more common among obese (32%) than nonobese (7%) parturients.[26]

Respiratory Changes

Respiratory changes during pregnancy are of special significance to the anesthesia practitioner. Over the course of a normal gestation, the parturient experiences a 30% to 60% increase in oxygen consumption, which induces an increased minute ventilation. Displacement of abdominal contents toward the chest, due to the enlarged uterus, causes a reduction in functional residual capacity (FRC) and premature airway closure, with the widening of the alveolar-arterial oxygen gradient. The FRC begins to decline as early as the fifth month and is reduced to 80% of nonpregnant values by term. This, in combination with an increase in oxygen consumption, leads to exceedingly rapid desaturation with apnea. The tendency toward rapid oxygen desaturation is further aggravated by a decrease in FRC in relation to the supine position and obesity.

As a result of these changes, the oxygenation of the mother and fetus may be compromised.[27] Despite adequate denitrogenation, these physiological changes greatly reduce the time allowable for intubation postinduction.

Airway Changes

Generalized edema may affect the oropharynx and nasopharynx. These changes are aggravated by elevated estrogen levels that stimulate the development of mucosal edema and hypervascularity in the upper airways. Capillary engorgement of the nasal and oropharyngeal mucosa begins early in the first trimester and increases progressively throughout pregnancy. Accordingly, the parturient frequently appears to have symptoms of upper respiratory infection and laryngitis, with nasal congestion and voice changes due to swelling of the false vocal cords and arytenoids. Nasal obstruction from vascularity and edema may complicate FVM.[28]

Numerous case reports suggest that edema of the pharyngeal and laryngeal structures (including vocal cords) may hinder visualization of the cords and passage of an ETT.[29,30] Tongue edema may make a retraction of the tongue into the mandibular space during laryngoscopy difficult. The increased engorgement and vascularity present special challenges in manipulating the nasopharynx (nasal trumpets, nasogastric tubes), or when considering repeated attempts at intubation of the trachea. An ETT one size smaller than might be usual (i.e., 6.0-7.0 mm ID) should be routinely used.

Excessive weight gain, even mild upper respiratory tract infections, preeclampsia, fluid overload, and bearing down can all exacerbate airway edema—potentially leading to a severely compromised airway. The classical Mallampati classification (Samsoon and Young modification) of mouth opening has been reported to advance by one or two classes during pregnancy.[6–15] This has been confirmed by acoustic reflectometry, which measures oropharyngeal volumes, and is likely a surrogate marker for ease of intubation of the trachea. It has demonstrated pharyngeal narrowing in pregnancy and labor, due to edema and an increase in localized fatty tissue volume.[31] The Mallampati score may worsen even further as a consequence of bearing down, and the score may not return to the prelabor state for a further 12 hours postpartum.[32,33] Acoustic reflectometry also revealed decreased volumes both in women after delivery, and in women whose pregnancy was complicated by preeclampsia.[28,33,34]

Cardiovascular Changes

The supine position may result in compression of the aorta and inferior vena cava (or both) by the enlarged pregnant uterus. Compression of the aorta decreases uterine blood flow, impairing fetal oxygenation. Vena caval compression decreases venous return, cardiac output, and ultimately uterine blood flow. A combination of oxygen desaturation and compromised cardiac output is particularly lethal for the pregnant mother and fetus. This situation is further aggravated by obesity. It is therefore imperative that the parturient be positioned with a wedge under the right hip, creating a left lateral displacement of the uterus, away from the great vessels. Unfortunately, such displacement may hinder adequate preoperative airway evaluation and the creation of an optimum position for intubation of the trachea.

Gastrointestinal Changes

The risk of aspiration in the parturient impacts how the anesthesia practitioner approaches and manages the parturient's airway. Several factors increase the risk of aspiration in these patients. While intragastric pressure increases steadily during pregnancy, as the gravid uterus enlarges, a concomitant decrease in lower esophageal sphincter tone occurs as circulating levels of progesterone increase.

The enlarging uterus distorts esophageal and gastric anatomy. The cephalad pressure related to the abdominal uterus decreases the obliquity with which the esophagus contacts the stomach, permitting reflux of gastric contents at lower than usual trans-sphincteric pressures. Gastric emptying appears to be unaffected by pregnancy, though intestinal transit time and gastric acidity are increased. With the onset of labor, gastric emptying slows, and this slowing may be further aggravated by the administration of opioids for labor pain management. Taken together, these gastrointestinal changes mandate that precautions for aspiration of gastric content be taken when a parturient undergoes general anesthesia.

Obstetrical Factors

There are several co-morbid obstetrical factors that may put the parturient at risk for difficulties in airway management and related complications. Gestational hypertension, eclampsia, and preeclampsia aggravate mucosal and interstitial edema.[28] Concomitant proteinuria, with reduced intravascular plasma protein levels, leads to increased edema of the upper airway, an enlarged and less mobile tongue, and soft tissue deposition in the neck.

Preeclampsia is frequently accompanied by coagulopathy and edema, both of which may exaggerate bleeding with repeated attempts at direct laryngoscopy. Airway and laryngeal edema can develop exceedingly rapidly in preeclamptic patients, and neck and face edema, together with dysphonia from uvular edema, should alert the practitioner to the possibility of difficult intubation of the trachea.[35] In these patients, extreme caution should be exercised not only at intubation but at the time of extubation as well.

Maternal knee-chest and left lateral positioning, as part of intrauterine fetal resuscitation for non-reassuring fetal heart tracings, may also limit the ability to conduct adequate preoperative airway evaluation. The impact that all these have on the validity, and the positive and negative predictive values of the preoperative airway assessment, is unknown.

Massive peripartum hemorrhage (e.g., placenta previa, placenta accreta, abruption) and acute fetal distress (e.g., abruption, cord prolapse) are frequently encountered obstetrical emergencies occurring acutely and unannounced. The visual impact of profuse vaginal bleeding, or the slow ominous sound of the tocodynamometer with fetal distress, frequently pushes obstetricians and anesthesia practitioners to urgent general anesthesia, without adequate assessment of the patient's airway. General anesthesia in the obstetric population is most frequently conducted for emergency clinical indications,[36,37] and most airway catastrophes occur when the difficult airway is not recognized before the induction of anesthesia. Indeed, retrospective publications have reported a poor ability to predict difficulty in the obstetrical population, and poor documentation of preoperative airway evaluation.[12,19] Endler et al. found that emergency surgery was implicated in up to 80% of maternal deaths with general anesthesia, and difficult or failed intubation was associated with 4 of 15 deaths.[24]

AIRWAY EVALUATION

■ Why Is It Important to Assess the Airway of Each Parturient?

Ideally, every pregnant patient admitted to the labor and delivery service should have a thorough preanesthetic airway evaluation. In light of this, interdisciplinary education of our obstetric, general practice, midwifery, and nursing colleagues in airway assessment and the risk factors for difficult airways in parturients is imperative. With the always-present risk of acute onset fetal distress, an essential and critical part of airway management is an accurate assessment of the patient's airway.

A detailed discussion of the airway examination and those predictors associated with management difficulties can be found in Chapter 1. Most predictive studies have been conducted on general surgical populations, not parturients. Some 20 factors predicting difficult laryngoscopic intubation have been identified. The obstetrical patient presents unique assessment challenges, often the most important being the pressure of time.

■ How Do You Assess the Airway of a Parturient? What Are the Predictors or Risk Factors of a Difficult Airway for a Parturient?

The increasing use of regional anesthetic techniques for delivery has significantly decreased the opportunity for clinical studies in patients undergoing general anesthesia. While parturients pose many unique airway challenges to anesthesia practitioners, assessment of the pillars of airway management (FMV, the use of extraglottic devices (EGDs), tracheal intubation under direct and indirect laryngoscopy, and establishment of a front-of-neck airway) should not differ from the nonobstetrical population.

Difficult FMV

As discussed, FMV can be difficult to impossible in approximately 0.02% of parturients. However, this incidence is comparable to the general surgical patient.[8] While the mnemonic MOANS (see Chapter 1) is a helpful reminder of the five-patient characteristics associated with difficult FMV,[38] many of these characteristics seldom apply to the obstetrical population. For example, young and healthy pregnant women are typically not older than 55 years of age, or edentulous, and they do not generally have facial hair. Obesity (BMI $\geq$ 30 $kg \cdot m^{-2}$), however, is an important consideration and is becoming increasingly prevalent amongst pregnant women. It is noteworthy that 28% of pregnant patients, and 75% of preeclamptic women, reported snoring compared to 14% of nonpregnant women.[28]

- Difficult direct laryngoscopy and tracheal intubation:

  Chapter 1 discusses in detail the current evidence in assessing the predictors of difficult direct laryngoscopy and intubation (LEMON). DuPont and colleagues conducted one of the early airway studies in the obstetrical population,[39] and reported that the risk of difficult direct laryngoscopic intubation was eight times greater than in the general surgical population. This has since been disputed by Goldszmidt and others.[9,14] Previously published increased rates of difficult and failed intubation in the parturient may in fact be related to anatomic abnormalities unrelated to pregnancy, but rather augmented by emergency conditions, lack of preoperative airway assessment, or differences in intubation experience and expertise.[9]

  The literature suggests a variety of clinical signs that can help determine the degree of difficult direct laryngoscopic intubation (Table 52.2); however, none of these has a high positive predictive value as a single tool, particularly in the obstetrical patient. A number of studies have suggested that, although the presence of risk factors was useful, they were not as reliable as the Mallampati examination. Benumof has

TABLE 52.2. Features of the Airway Examination Useful in Predicting Difficult Laryngoscopy

In the Parturient	• Mallampati class III or IV • Limited thyromental distance • Short thick neck • Limited mouth opening • Prominent incisors

frequently suggested that a patient's relative tongue/pharyngeal size (Mallampati), degree of an atlantooccipital joint extension, and adequacy of the mandibular space provide the practitioner with three easy-to-perform and accurate predictors of difficulty in laryngoscopic intubation.[40]

Rocke et al. conducted one of the sentinel studies specifically looking at the obstetrical population and difficult airway predictors.[6] They prospectively evaluated the airways of 1500 parturients presenting for elective and emergency intubations and found that a highly predictive sign for a difficult airway was a "neutral" to "extension" sternomental distance variation of less than 5 cm. In addition, the authors built a scale of predictive factors showing clearly that the greater the number of abnormal findings, the higher the prediction accuracy for a difficult intubation (Figure 52.1). The associated risk factors included SN, protruding maxillary incisors (PMI), receding mandible (RM), and Mallampati class III and IV. The relative risk of experiencing a difficult intubation in comparison to an uncomplicated Class I airway assessment was as follows: Class II, 3.23; Class III, 7.58; Class IV, 11.3; SN 5.01; RM, 9.71; and PMI, 8.0. Using the probability index for a combination of risk factors, Rocke et al. showed that a combination of either class III or IV, plus PMI, SN, and RM, correlated with a probability of difficult direct laryngoscopy of >90%. It was interesting that neither facial edema nor swollen tongue was associated with difficult laryngoscopic intubation.

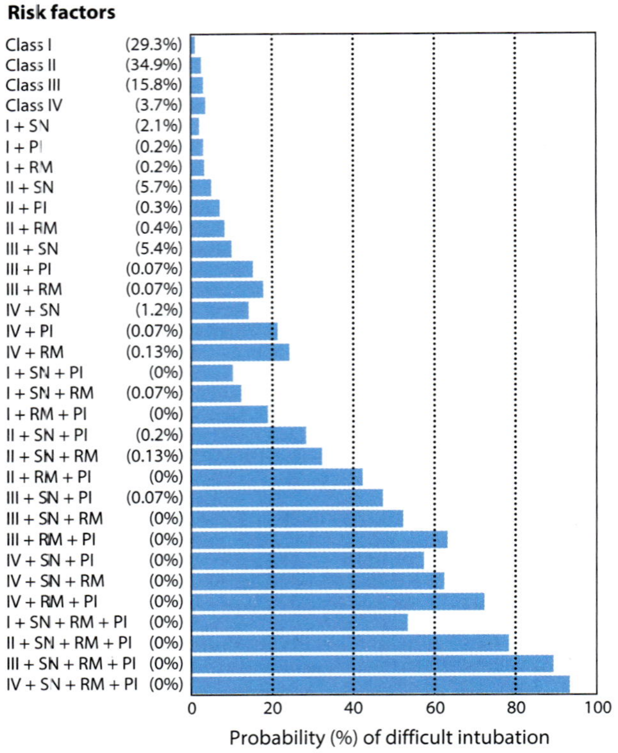

FIGURE 52.1. The probability of experiencing a difficult laryngoscopic intubation for the varying combinations of risk factors and the observed incidence of these combinations. (Reproduced with permission from Rocke D, Murray W, Rout C, et al. Relative risk factors associated with difficult intubation in obstetric anesthesia. *Anesthesiology*. 1992;77(1):67-73.

Overall, the mnemonic LEMON (see Chapter 1) examines almost all the difficult direct laryngoscopic intubation characteristics (with the exception of the PMI) and remains a useful guide for the obstetrical population. Obesity and BMI are not independent predictors of difficult intubation but an increased neck circumference is.[41]

In obstetrical patient, obesity and large pendulous breasts often compound airway problems. It is important that the parturient be assessed in the recumbent position with left uterine displacement. Adjustments in the patient's position should be made before induction of anesthesia, to make intubating conditions easier; but there are limits to the extent that these adjustments can be employed, because of the positioning required to reduce aortocaval compression. In the morbidly obese parturient, elevations (i.e., ramping) (see Figure 52.2) of the thorax, shoulders, and head may be necessary to bring the anatomical axes of the oral, pharyngeal, and laryngeal structures into alignment. Positioning on a ramp and use of a short "stubby" laryngoscope handle may also mitigate the problem of the laryngoscope handle abutting on the patient's chest.

- Difficult indirect laryngoscopy and tracheal intubation using video laryngoscopes:

  While Chapter 1 discusses in detail the current evidence in assessing the predictors of difficult indirect video laryngoscopy and intubation (CRANE), some of the predictors

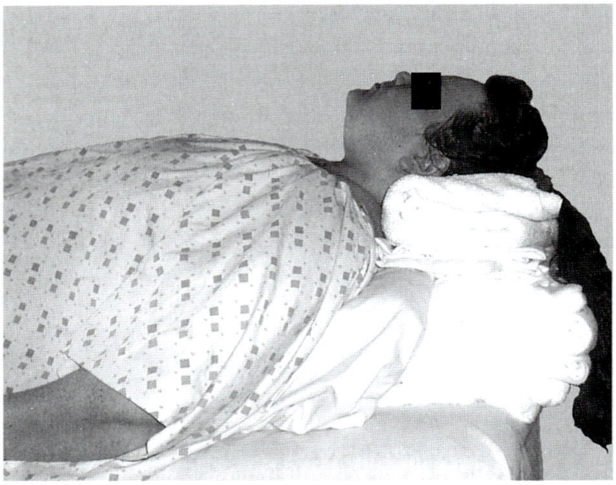

FIGURE 52.2. For induction of general anesthesia, all parturients should be appropriately positioned, e.g., "ramped" as needed to ensure the patient's external auditory meatus is level with the sternal notch. This picture shows a morbidly obese patient lying in a supine position with the shoulder, neck, and head resting on a stacked "ramp" of hospital linen.

(e.g., radiation to the head and neck) may not be applicable to the healthy obstetric population. Furthermore, there are limited clinical information regarding the use of video laryngoscopes in the obstetric population. In a retrospective review with 180 parturients, Aziz et al.[42] showed that video laryngoscopy resulted in 100% (18 out of 18) successful intubations on the first attempt compared to 95% (157 out of 163 patients) with direct laryngoscopy. In a case series involving 27 obstetric patients undergoing general anesthesia, Shonfeld et al.[43] reported that video display from the C-MAC Macintosh blade provided better Cormack-Lehane grade (100% Grade 1 view) compared to standard direct laryngoscopy (52% Grade 1, 44 % Grade 2, and 4% Grade 3 and 4 view). Similarly, in a randomized trial involving 80 obstetric patients, Arici et al.[44] reported that the McGrath Series 5 video laryngoscope provided better views during orotracheal intubation compared to Macintosh laryngoscope, even though the intubation was longer with the video laryngoscope. The Canadian Airway Focus Group recommends the routine primary use of video laryngoscopy in the obstetric population, based on additional mounting evidence in the critical care and emergency literature demonstrating improved first-attempt success, less complications, and fewer esophageal intubations.[15,45]

- Difficulty in the use of EGD:

  The latest iterations of obstetric difficult airway algorithms advocate for even earlier use of an EGD as a part of a failed "Plan A" primary attempt at tracheal intubation. It also advocates that an EGD be used as an important backup maneuver in "Plan B," and serve as a bridging attempt to re-establish gas exchange in a "can't intubate, can't oxygenate" (CICO) setting, while one prepares to perform a surgical airway (i.e., cricothyrotomy, tracheotomy or "front of neck access [FONA]") in parturients. RODS (see Chapter 1) is a mnemonic that is intended to identify patients where the use of an EGD may be difficult.

- Difficult surgical airway:

  While the necessity to perform a surgical airway (i.e., cricothyrotomy) in the obstetric population is exceedingly rare, all parturients requiring a general anesthetic ought to have an assessment of the feasibility of this procedure. The mnemonic SHORT (see Chapter 1) can be used to quickly assess the patient for features that may indicate a difficult cricothyrotomy. In addition, given that the most common complication of this procedure is misplacement due to failure to identify the cricothyroid membrane (CTM),[46] it would seem advisable to identify and mark the CTM ahead of time while in the supine position (at preanesthesia assessment or preinduction) in patients who have risk factors for an anticipated difficult airway.[47] Identification of the CTM using digital palpation is more challenging in females (independent of body habitus) and in obese patients.[48] The use of ultrasound to identify the CTM has greatly improved accuracy, especially on obese patients; and given appropriate training, is potentially an invaluable tool in this setting.[48] Most obstetricians do not have experience in performing a FONA, and it is incumbent upon the anesthesia practitioner to maintain the necessary skills for this procedure despite their infrequent use. It may be prudent to consult with an experienced surgical colleague for assistance when the need for a FONA is anticipated.

  When considering the best technique, studies have shown that the use of a narrow-bore (≤2 mm) cannula technique has the highest failure rate, particularly in obese patients. Greater success is achieved using a wide-bore (≥4 mm) cannula technique (wire-guided Seldinger, or cannula-over trocar technique), with the highest and most consistent success using an open surgical method.[46,49,50]

  While many anesthesiologists are not comfortable with an open technique, the skills required for the rapid four-step cricothyrotomy (palpation, horizontal incision through skin and CTM, retraction of cricoid cartilage with hook [or insertion of a tracheal introducer commonly called a "Bougie"], and insertion of ETT) are easy to master.[46,50] Alternatively, there is an argument for using a 4 cm vertical incision for open cricothyrotomy in patients with a poorly identified CTM.[15] Nonetheless, success depends upon not just having the practical skills, the correct equipment readily available, and trained assistance, but also on timely decision-making. Regardless of the technique used, failure to recognize immediate need (CICO), and reluctance to perform cricothyrotomy (or FONA), can result in disastrous outcomes.[46]

When a Difficult Laryngoscopy Is Anticipated in a Parturient, Is It Useful to Perform an Awake Direct Laryngoscopy (an "Awake Look")?

Awake direct laryngoscopy with a topically anesthetized airway (i.e., an "awake look") has been suggested as a useful assessment tool for the potentially difficult airway prior to induction of anesthesia. However, one must recognize that the airway, as it appears with the patient awake and unparalyzed, might look quite different with the patient under general anesthesia and with muscle paralysis.[51]

CONDUCT OF ANESTHESIA AND TRACHEAL INTUBATION

What Are Necessary Preparations for General Anesthesia for a Parturient?

Several preparations must be made in the labor and delivery suite to ensure safe and expeditious care of the parturient should general anesthesia be required. The operating room table should have a ramp on it at all times (see Figure 52.2). This will prove to be an invaluable aid in optimizing the head position and will help align the oral, pharyngeal, and laryngeal axes in the obese parturient. Furthermore, it will not be problematic in a patient with easy tracheal intubation.

It is important to have all difficult airway equipment in the operating room. It is also important to recognize the importance of having well-trained assistants to help with all aspects of airway management, including rescue devices, as well as the application of cricoid pressure. Because time is often of the essence, and resources are often limited, the practitioner must carefully choose devices with which they are familiar and comfortable, and techniques that can be practiced regularly. Table 52.3 details some of the suggested equipment necessary to manage the difficult airway on the labor floor. A short laryngoscope handle ("stubby") can be particularly helpful. While there are few prospective comparative studies on the obstetric airway and alternative airway equipment success rates, as previously stated, the most important success factor is practitioner familiarity and skills in using the devices.

TABLE 52.3. Equipment Required for Management of Difficult OB Airway

Bed ramp	• Ramping (see Figure 52.2)
Oral airway	• 3 sizes
Intubation guides	• Eschmann™ Tracheal Introducer (Portex Limited, Hythe, UK) • Frova™ Intubation Introducer (Cook Inc, Bloomington, IN, USA) • Lightwand
Endotracheal tubes	• At least three different sized (6.0, 6.5, 7.0 mm ID)
Laryngoscope	• Macintosh #3, 4 • Miller #2, 3 • "Stubby" or short handle on these blades may improve utility
Extraglottic devices (in various sizes)	• LMA-Classic, LMA-Supreme, LMA-Fastrach, North America Inc San Diego, CA • King LTD/LTS-D King Systems, Noblesville, IN • i-gel Intersurgical Ltd, Berkshire, UK • air-Q Cookgas LLC, St Louis, MO • Combitube Kendall-Sheridan, Argyle, NY
Video laryngoscopes, stylets, and indirect scopes	**Video laryngoscopes** • GlideScope, Verathon Medical Canada ULC, Canada • Airtraq, Southmedic Inc, Canada • McGrath Series 5, LMA North America Inc, San Diego, CA • C-MAC, Karl Storz Endoscopy, El Segundo, CA • Pentax AWS, Ambu Inc, Burnie, MD • King Vision, King Systems, Noblesville, IN • CoPilot VL Magaw Medical, Fort Worth, T **Video stylet** • Bonfils, Karl Storz Endoscopy Retromolar access • Shikani, Clarus Medical, St Paul, MN **Indirect scopes (rigid)** • UpsherScope, The Upsher Laryngoscope Corporation, Foster City, CA
Flexible bronchoscope	• Adult and pediatric sizes
Cricothyrotomy kit	• Percutaneous or open

All obstetric patients requiring general anesthesia must receive aspiration prophylaxis (nonparticulate antacid, H_2 blocker, and a prokinetic).[52] Induction should be in rapid sequence fashion (RSI), including the application of cricoid pressure. However, conventional teaching for obstetric RSI is being challenged. It has been shown that even when correctly applied, cricoid pressure may not always be completely effective.[53] Consideration for discontinuation of cricoid pressure is recommended should difficulty with FMV, laryngoscopy, or EGD insertion be encountered. The airway practitioner should consider gentle FMV ($<$20 cm H_2O) while awaiting the onset of paralysis, and 15 L·min^{-1} oxygen flow via nasal cannulas or high-flow nasal oxygen (HFNO) (along with mask denitrogenation as described in the following text), to maintain apneic oxygenation and prevention of arterial oxygen desaturation during intubation attempts.[15,54–56]

Because the pregnant patient is at increased risk for hypoxemia, even during short periods of apnea, it is especially important that adequate denitrogenation with 100% oxygen prior to the induction of general anesthesia is performed. Various techniques for denitrogenation have been advocated. Norris and Dewan observed that 3 minutes of denitrogenation, and the four-breath denitrogenation technique, resulted in similar measurements of PaO_2 in pregnant women undergoing rapid sequence induction of general anesthesia for cesarean section.[27] If the tidal volume is large, and the respiratory rate is high, denitrogenation may need to be only 1 minute in duration. However, this 1 minute can be one of the most important minutes of the induction and should not be further shortened.

Describe an Appropriate Algorithm for a Difficult/Failed Intubation in a Parturient

The difficult airway algorithm in the parturient is significantly different from that used in the operating room for nonobstetrical surgical patients. In general, the differences focus on the presence or absence of fetal distress. There are now several algorithms available to address obstetric-specific considerations, and to guide airway management and patient care.[15,52]

Frequently, general anesthetics on the labor and delivery service are required in patients with whom the anesthesia practitioner has little or no foreknowledge. In addition, the environment is often volatile, with considerable pressure to proceed with an emergency induction, because fetal viability is in question and fetal rescue is required. In such an event, it is imperative that the practitioner has a simple, clear algorithm to follow when a difficult airway is encountered. Equally important is that the practitioner regularly practices this algorithm with the labor and delivery personnel and that they are familiar with the airway devices that might be employed in an emergency.

Anticipated Difficult Airway

When the anesthesia practitioner anticipates a difficult airway, a regional anesthetic technique may be preferable (Table 52.4). However, there are numerous conditions that may preclude the use of regional anesthesia. When regional anesthesia is not

TABLE 52.4. Important Points for Managing the Anticipated Difficult Obstetrical Airway

Identify parturients at high risk for operative intervention
Obesity
Advanced maternal age
Non-reassuring fetal or maternal conditions
Detailed discussions with the obstetrician concerning delivery plan
Crash' induction is not an option
Speak to patient and family early in labor
Identify the cricothyroid membrane (CTM) ahead of time
Persist with regional techniques
Awake look or intubation if necessary—using a flexible bronchoscope
Wishful thinking is a poor anesthetic plan—know that your regional technique is working

TABLE 52.5. Important Points for Managing the Unanticipated Difficult Obstetrical Airway

Thorough and careful airway evaluations	• know your predictors—which ones work for you
Strategy for intubating the difficult airway	• pick your algorithm ahead of time
Make basic preparations for the difficult airway	• keep it simple • pick your equipment ahead of time (LMA-Classic, LMA-Supreme, LMA-Fastrach, Eschmann Tracheal Introducer, Combitube, cricothyrotomy kit) and know your skill sets. • communication: share your concerns early • know your team: who can help you or provide skilled assistance • practice, multidisciplinary simulation where possible and more practice

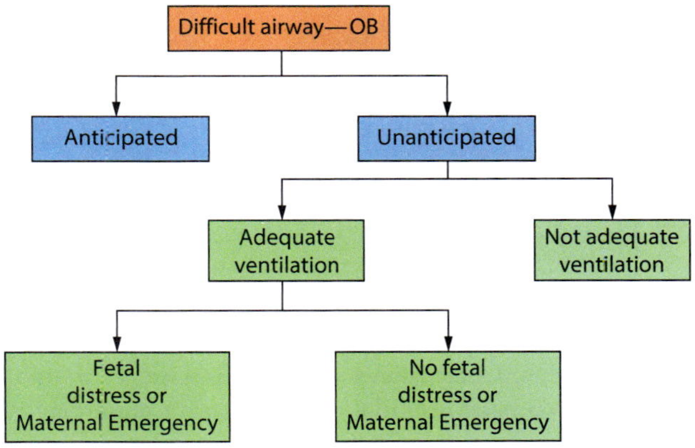

FIGURE 52.3. Basic decision points for the difficult airway algorithm in the obstetrical patient.

possible, one of the first things that must occur is a thorough discussion with the obstetrician, the patient, the patient's family, and nurses, pointing out any airway management concerns that the anesthesia practitioner has. In some circumstances, the anesthesia practitioner ought to make it clear that the patient's airway management cannot be hurried, implying that a decision to go to surgery may need to be made earlier rather than later. The hope is that anesthesia practitioner is not pushed into a general anesthetic when more deliberate planning may have permitted a regional technique.

In those instances when regional anesthesia is contraindicated, an anticipated difficult airway is recognized, and time permits, an awake look or awake tracheal intubation (ATI) should be employed. Flexible bronchoscopy (FB) has become the method most frequently used. The specifics of this technique can be found in Chapter 10. However, there are several points that should be reiterated for the obstetric patient. Because the parturient airway is often edematous, and engorged, topicalization of the upper airway can frequently be difficult and requires considerable patience. A drying agent is necessary, and aspiration prophylaxis must be initiated prior to the application of topical anesthesia. One should not hesitate to sedate the mother as needed.

There are a host of specialized fiberoptic or video laryngoscope blades and handles (e.g., GlideScope, Storz C-MAC Video laryngoscope), each with individualized light sources, or fiberoptic bundles ending at various distances into the oral pharynx (see Chapter 11). Considerable effort is needed to maintain these in working condition, and considerable practice is necessary to become skilled in their use. Certainly, for the anticipated difficult airway in which time and technical assistance will be available, these devices may be useful. However, in general, time and assistance are perpetually in short supply for labor and delivery services.

Unanticipated Difficult Airway

Table 52.5 lists several important points to remember in managing an unanticipated difficult obstetrical airway. Figures 52.3 and 52.4 are algorithms one might choose to use in the event of an unanticipated failed tracheal intubation in an obstetrical patient.[15] Figure 52.3 simplifies the critical points in the management of an obstetrical patient requiring general anesthesia: anticipated versus unanticipated; adequate ventilation versus inadequate ventilation; fetal/maternal emergency versus non-emergency scenario.

Failed Primary Attempt at Intubation Encountered in an Induced/Unconscious Parturient

The Canadian Airway Focus Group recommends the primary use of video laryngoscopy to facilitate tracheal intubation of the parturient.[15]

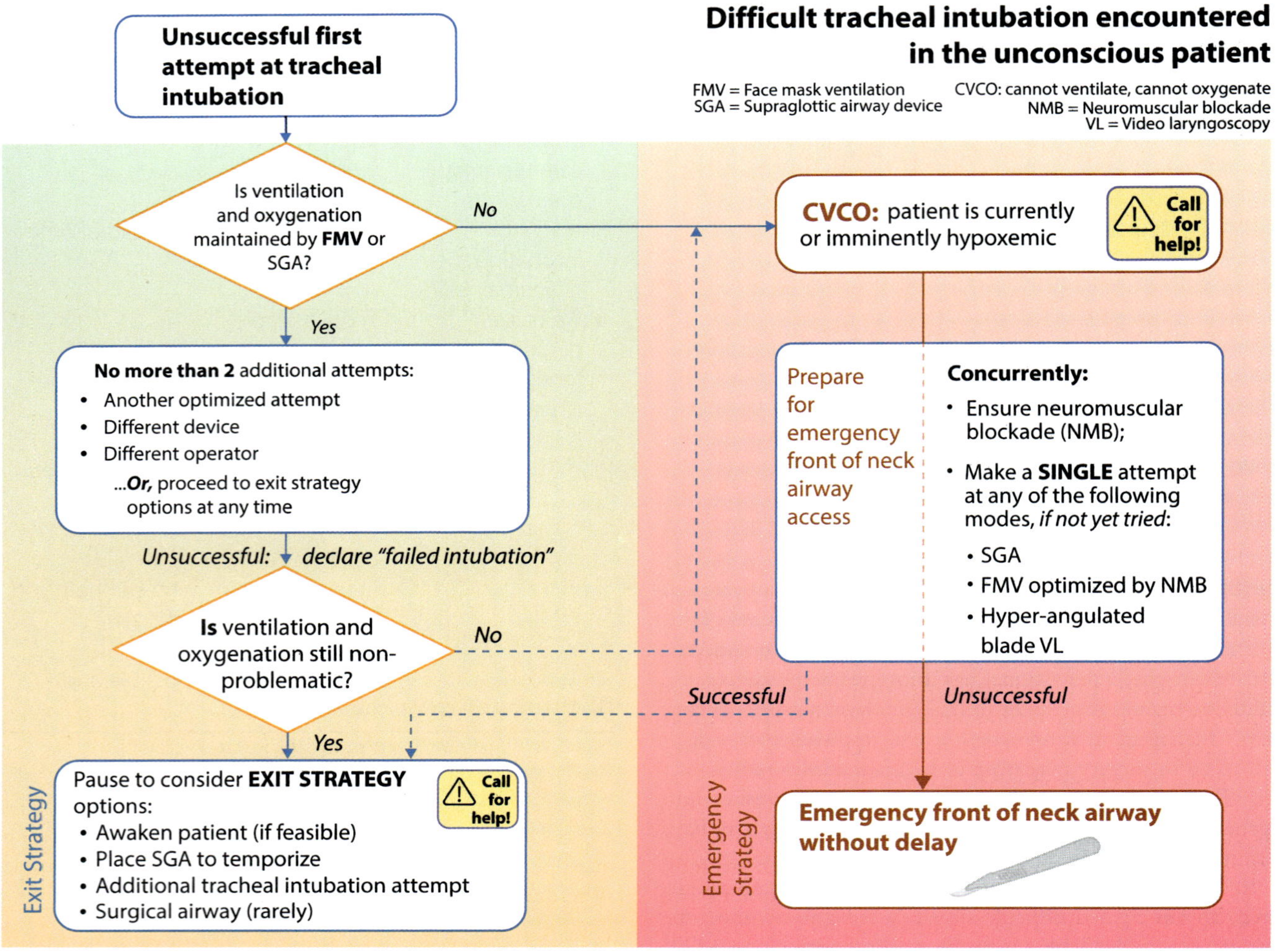

FIGURE 52.4. Flow diagram: difficult tracheal intubation encountered in the unconscious patient. (Reproduced with permission from Law JA, Duggan LV, Asselin M, et al. Canadian Airway Focus Group updated consensus-based recommendations for management of the difficult airway: part 1. Difficult airway management encountered in an unconscious patient. *Can J Anaesth.* 2021;68(9):1373-1404.)

The anesthesia practitioner should consider 15 L·min^{-1} oxygen flow via nasal cannulas or HFNO with mask denitrogenation, to maintain bulk flow of oxygen during intubation attempts.[15,56] Airway adjuncts (i.e., Eschmann Tracheal Introducer [ETI], oropharyngeal [OPA] airways) should be immediately available and ramped positioning used for all cases.

If despite an optimized technique, the first attempt at tracheal intubation is not successful, FMV should be started immediately, and skilled help summoned. Cricoid pressure should be maintained, and FMV conducted with the lowest insufflation pressure (<20 cm H_2O) possible.[15,57,58] Consider prophylactic OPA insertion to help achieve this goal, modifications including a two-handed mask hold with jaw thrust, and incremental release of cricoid pressure may be required. EGD (preferably a second-generation EGD) placement should be considered if the primary intubation attempt (Plan A) fails and difficulty with FMV is encountered.

If oxygenation is satisfactory by either FMV or EGD, a second tracheal intubation attempt is not considered mandatory. It should only be considered if the practitioner feels, based on clinical observations at the initial attempt, that there may be a success if a different technique (e.g., a different device or different, more experienced practitioner) is utilized, or that the first attempt was not optimized (ramping or adequate neuromuscular relaxation was not achieved). Repeated prolonged attempts without changing the primary approach or technique are recognized as contributing to poor outcomes.[59]

Exit Strategy—Failed Tracheal Intubation in the Oxygenated Parturient with NO Fetal or Maternal Emergency

If tracheal intubation has failed and further intubation attempts have a low probability of success, the urgency of the situation should be assessed. In the case of no emergency and FMV easily maintaining oxygenation, allowing the parturient to emerge from general anesthesia would be an appropriate exit strategy. If FMV becomes difficult, an EGD should be placed to assist oxygenation while awaiting emergence from anesthesia. The use of a second-generation EGD with gastric venting should be considered. This period of emergence with an unprotected airway is potentially a high-risk time for maternal regurgitation and pulmonary aspiration; thus, patient stimulation should be minimized and vigilance is mandatory.[59,60] At this point, a decision can be made to revisit regional anesthesia (if not contraindicated) or proceed with an ATI for general anesthesia. While there have been numerous reports of successful safe use of various first- and second-generation EGDs in elective, fasted CD patients; in an unplanned, failed airway, continuation of CD with a rescued EGD airway in a nonemergency scenario is still not recommended.[61]

Exit Strategy—Failed Tracheal Intubation in the Oxygenated Parturient WITH Fetal or Maternal Emergency

If a persistent fetal or maternal emergency exists following failed tracheal intubation in the adequately oxygenated parturient, CD and/or maternal resuscitation can proceed with a face mask or EGD ventilation. Cricoid pressure should be released for EGD insertion, as the likelihood of successful placement is improved. In this situation, where there are critical fetal or maternal conditions, further attempts at tracheal intubation are contraindicated, and it would be impractical to allow the mother to awaken.

Proceeding with CD under FVM, or EGD ventilation, in an emergency, requires close communication with the perioperative team. This decision is influenced by numerous factors that are constantly evolving, often time-pressured, and under extremely challenging high-stakes clinical situations.[52,62] Maternal and fetal issues, and airway difficulties, may only be appreciated by the practitioner in the immediate clinical context (stridor, obesity, full stomach, absence of reflux prophylaxis, etc.). Human factors, clinical experience, and challenging environments must all be considered in the ability to adhere to algorithms and guidelines. The obstetrician should understand that, under these circumstances, an expeditious surgical delivery is desired, with a generous surgical incision, possible use of vacuum extraction at the time of delivery, avoidance of fundal pressure, and avoidance of exteriorization of the uterus. In the presence of fetal distress, and all these issues considered, the emergency CD procedure can be completed with FVM or EGD ventilation.

Once the fetus has been delivered and any maternal emergency is stabilized, an exit strategy either with or without a secured airway (e.g., Intubating Laryngeal Mask Airway [LMA] or flexible bronchoscopic intubation through an EGD) should be considered. If an ETT is to be placed and conditions permit, the surgery should be halted while the airway is secured, with optimized patient positioning and obstructing drapes moved. During tracheal intubation, the maintenance of adequate depth of general anesthesia, together with the use of neuromuscular blockade, must be considered.

Emergency Strategy—Failed Intubation, Oxygenation NOT Possible with Face-Mask or EGD Ventilation

In a CICO scenario, with complete inability to oxygenate the patient. the parturient will undergo rapid oxygen desaturation resulting in both maternal and fetal compromise. The default is now to an "emergency strategy," with an immediate need for a surgical airway i.e., cricothyrotomy, or other FONA, with a concurrent parallel attempt at oxygenation with an EGD if not already tried. If successful, the parturient is re-oxygenated (via EGD or cuffed cricothyrotomy) and CD should proceed and further resuscitation if the maternal emergency continues. If these strategies are unsuccessful, planning for respiratory arrest and perimortum CD needs to occur.

The Canadian Airway Focus Group, in its summary of recommendations for difficult airway management, has suggested that consideration could be made for the administration or redosing of a neuromuscular blocking agent to address possible laryngospasm and to facilitate FMV in the management of CICO scenario in the unconscious patient.[15] While there is little published evidence to support or refute this recommendation, it may also be considered in the obstetric CICO population.

Along these same lines, sugammadex, a cyclodextrin capable of rapid reversal of profound nondepolarizing neuromuscular blockade, is now widely available. This drug, however, will only be helpful where resumption of spontaneous ventilation will alleviate the CICO situation.[54,55] This strategy offers the possibility of rapid recovery of a failed airway when awakening the patient is a viable option (i.e., cesarean section for noncritical fetal indications). In obstetrics, this is usually not the case in critical maternal events, such as hemorrhage, or critical fetal events.

Emergence and Extubation

Reviews of maternal mortality trends and statistics from both the United States and the United Kingdom indicate a shift in many airway catastrophes from the induction of general anesthesia to the postpartum period, i.e., at emergence, in the post anesthesia care unit, or in the event of postpartum surgical procedures.[59,60] As previously mentioned, this period of emergence is potentially a high-risk time for maternal regurgitation and pulmonary aspiration, and a heightened vigilance is clearly required.[22] Perioperative standards of care as they pertain to general anesthesia recovery, should be applied to the postpartum surgical population.

SUMMARY

Difficult or failed intubation remains a major contributor to maternal morbidity and mortality during obstetrical emergencies. Careful preanesthetic evaluation focusing on the parturients airway should identify patients at risk for difficult airway management. Early communication with the obstetricians, regular review and practice of a formal difficult airway algorithm, and facility with current difficult airway devices should mitigate some of the risks of injuries to parturients when a failed intubation does occur.

SELF-EVALUATION QUESTIONS

52.1. With respect to maternal morbidity and mortality, which of the following is **FALSE**?

A. The incidence of airway problems is greater in obstetric patients than in nonobstetric patients.

B. In the 1985 ASA Closed Claims Project database, most of the obstetric anesthesia-related claims were associated with inadequate labor analgesia.

C. Obstetrical airway catastrophes occur most frequently when cesarean sections are emergent.

D. Face-mask ventilation can be difficult or impossible in approximately 0.02% of parturients.

52.2. Concerning the obstetrical airway, which of the following is **FALSE**?

A. The combination of Mallampati Class III or IV, protruding maxillary incisors, short neck, and receding mandible correlates to a probability of difficult direct laryngoscopy of > 90% in parturients.

B. Mallampati classification of the oropharyngeal space can advance during labor.

C. The use of ultrasound to identify the cricothyroid membrane (CTM) has improved accuracy in female and obese patients.

D. An "awake look" will simulate the appearance of the airway under general anesthesia.

52.3. Considering the difficult airway algorithm in the parturient, which of the following is **TRUE**?

A. The first intubation attempt should be optimized using ramped positioning and a video laryngoscope.

B. High-flow nasal oxygen (HFNO) can be used as an effective method of denitrogenation and apneic oxygenation.

C. In an elective cesarean delivery (CD) scenario, if a failed intubation is rescued with an extraglottic device (EGD), it is recommended to continue the CD with the application of cricoid pressure.

D. In an emergency CD scenario, if a "can't intubate, can't oxygenate" (CICO) situation is rescued with front-of-neck access (FONA), sugammadex should be administered and the patient should be awakened.

REFERENCES

1. Cantwell R, Clutton-Brock T, Cooper G, et al. Saving Mothers' Lives: reviewing maternal deaths to make motherhood safer: 2006-2008. The eighth report of the confidential enquiries into maternal deaths in the United Kingdom. *BJOG*. 2011;118(Suppl 1):1-203.
2. Joseph KS, Liu S, Rouleau J, et al. Severe maternal morbidity in Canada, 2003 to 2007: surveillance using routine hospitalization data and ICD-10CA codes. *J Obstet Gynaecol Can*. 2010;32:837-846.
3. Mhyre JM, Riesner MN, Polley LS, Naughton NN. A series of anesthesia-related maternal deaths in Michigan, 1985-2003. *Anesthesiology*. 2007;106:1096-1104.
4. Ross BK. ASA closed claims in obstetrics: lessons learned. *Anesthesiol Clin North Am*. 2003;21:183-197.
5. Davies JM, Posner KL, Lee LA, Cheney FW, Domino KB. Liability associated with obstetric anesthesia: a closed claims analysis. *Anesthesiology*. 2009;110:131-139.
6. Rocke DA, Murray WB, Rout CC, Gouws E. Relative risk analysis of factors associated with difficult intubation in obstetric anesthesia. *Anesthesiology*. 1992;77:67-73.
7. Rose DK, Cohen MM. The airway: problems and predictions in 18,500 patients. *Can J Anaesth*. 1994;41:372-383.
8. Benumof JL. Difficult laryngoscopy: obtaining the best view. *Can J Anaesth*. 1994;41:361-365.
9. Goldszmidt E. Principles and practices of obstetric airway management. *Anesthesiol Clin*. 2008;26:109-125.
10. Munnur U, Suresh MS. Airway problems in pregnancy. *Crit Care Clin*. 2004;20:617-642.
11. Davies JM, Weeks S, Crone LA, Pavlin E. Difficult intubation in the parturient. *Can J Anaesth*. 1989;36:668-674.
12. Hawthorne L, Wilson R, Lyons G, Dresner M. Failed intubation revisited: 17-yr experience in a teaching maternity unit. *Br J Anaesth*. 1996;76:680-684.
13. Kinsella SM, Winton AL, Mushambi MC, et al. Failed tracheal intubation during obstetric general anaesthesia: a literature review. *Int J Obstet Anesth*. 2015;24:356-374.
14. McKeen DM, George RB, O'Connell CM, et al. Difficult and failed intubation: Incident rates and maternal, obstetrical, and anesthetic predictors. *Can J Anaesth*. 2011;58:514-524.
15. Law JA, Duggan LV, Asselin M, et al. Canadian Airway Focus Group updated consensus-based recommendations for management of the difficult airway: part 1. Difficult airway management encountered in an unconscious patient. *Can J Anaesth*. 2021;68:1373-1404.
16. Cook TM. Failed intubation in obstetric anaesthesia. *Anaesthesia*. 2006;61:605-606.
17. Cooper G, Reynolds F. The drive for regional anaesthesia for elective caesarean section has gone too far. *Int J Obstet Anesth*. 2002;11:289-295.
18. Cormack RS. Failed intubation in obstetric anaesthesia. *Anaesthesia*. 2006;61:505-506.
19. Jenkins JG. Failed intubation during obstetric anaesthesia. *Br J Anaesth*. 1996;77:698.
20. Lipman S, Carvalho B, Brock-Utne J. The demise of general anesthesia in obstetrics revisited: prescription for a cure. *Int J Obstet Anesth*. 2005;14:2-4.
21. Saravanakumar K, Cooper GM. Failed intubation in obstetrics: has the incidence changed recently? *Br J Anaesth*. 2005;94:690.
22. Wong CA. Saving mothers' lives: the 2006-2008 anaesthesia perspective. *Br J Anaesth*. 2011;107:119-122.
23. Cedergren MI. Maternal morbid obesity and the risk of adverse pregnancy outcome. *Obstet Gynecol*. 2004;103:219-224.
24. Endler GC, Mariona FG, Sokol RJ, Stevenson LB. Anesthesia-related maternal mortality in Michigan, 1972 to 1984. *Am J Obstet Gynecol*. 1988;159:187-193.
25. Hood DD, Dewan DM. Anesthetic and obstetric outcome in morbidly obese parturients. *Anesthesiology*. 1993;79:1210-1218.
26. Chadwick HS. Obstetric Anesthesia closed claims update II. *ASA Newsletter*. 1999;63(6):12-15.
27. Norris MC, Dewan DM. Preoxygenation for cesarean section: a comparison of two techniques. *Anesthesiology*. 1985;62:827-829.
28. Izci B, Riha RL, Martin SE, et al. The upper airway in pregnancy and pre-eclampsia. *Am J Respir Crit Care Med*. 2003;167:137-140.
29. Dobb G. Laryngeal oedema complicating obstetric anaesthesia. *Anaesthesia*. 1978;33:839-840.
30. Jouppila R, Jouppila P, Hollmen A. Laryngeal oedema as an obstetric anaesthesia complication: case reports. *Acta Anaesthesiologica Scandinavica*. 1980;24:97-98.
31. Leboulanger N, Louvet N, Rigouzzo A, et al. Pregnancy is associated with a decrease in pharyngeal but not tracheal or laryngeal cross-sectional area: a pilot study using the acoustic reflection method. *Int J Obstet Anesth*. 2014;23:35-39.
32. Farcon EL, Kim MH, Marx GF. Changing Mallampati score during labour. *Can J Anaesth*. 1994;41:50-51.
33. Kodali BS, Chandrasekhar S, Bulich LN, Topulos GP, Datta S. Airway changes during labor and delivery. *Anesthesiology*. 2008;108:357-362.
34. Bhavani-Shankar K, Bulich L, Kafiluddir R, et al. Does labor and delivery induce airway changes? *Anesthesiology*. 2001;93:A1035.
35. Perlow JH, Kirz DS. Severe preeclampsia presenting as dysphonia secondary to uvular edema. A case report. *J Reprod Med*. 1990;35:1059-1062.
36. McDonnell NJ, Paech MJ, Clavisi OM, Scott KL. Difficult and failed intubation in obstetric anaesthesia: an observational study of airway management and complications associated with general anaesthesia for caesarean section. *Int J Obstet Anesth*. 2008;17:292-297.
37. Tsen LC, Pitner R, Camann WR. General anesthesia for cesarean section at a tertiary care hospital 1990-1995: indications and implications. *Int J Obstet Anesth*. 1998;7:147-152.
38. Langeron O, Masso E, Huraux C, et al. Prediction of difficult mask ventilation. *Anesthesiology*. 2000;92:1229-1236.
39. Dupont X, Hamza J, Jullien P, Narchi P. Risk factors associated with difficult airway in normotensive parturients. *Anesthesiology*. 1990;73:A999.
40. Benumof JL. Management of the difficult adult airway. With special emphasis on awake tracheal intubation. *Anesthesiology*. 1991;75:1087-1110.
41. Brodsky JB, Lemmens HJ, Brock-Utne JG, Vierra M, Saidman LJ. Morbid obesity and tracheal intubation. *Anesth Analg*. 2002;94:732-736.
42. Aziz MF, Kim D, Mako J, Hand K, Brambrink AM. A retrospective study of the performance of video laryngoscopy in an obstetric unit. *Anesth Analg*. 2012;115:904-906.

43. Shonfeld A, Gray K, Lucas N, et al. Video laryngoscopy in obstetric anesthesia. *J Obstet Anaesth Crit Care*. 2012;2:53.
44. Arici S, Karaman S, Dogru S, et al. The McGrath Series 5 video laryngoscope versus the Macintosh laryngoscope: a randomized trial in obstetric patients. *Turk J Med Sci*. 2014;44:387-392.
45. De Jong A, Molinari N, Conseil M, et al. Video laryngoscopy versus direct laryngoscopy for orotracheal intubation in the intensive care unit: a systematic review and meta-analysis. *Intensive Care Med*. 2014;40:629-639.
46. Hamaekers AE, Henderson JJ. Equipment and strategies for emergency tracheal access in the adult patient. *Anaesthesia*. 2011;66(Suppl 2):65-80.
47. Preston R. Management of the obstetric airway—time for a paradigm shift (or two)? *Int J Obstet Anesth*. 2015;24:293-296.
48. You-Ten KE, Desai D, Postonogova T, Siddiqui N. Accuracy of conventional digital palpation and ultrasound of the cricothyroid membrane in obese women in labour. *Anaesthesia*. 2015;70:1230-1234.
49. Cook TM, Woodall N, Frerk C. Major complications of airway management in the UK: results of the Fourth National Audit Project of the Royal College of Anaesthetists and the Difficult Airway Society. Part 1: Anaesthesia. *Br J Anaesth*. 2011;106:617-631.
50. Kristensen MS, Teoh WH, Baker PA. Percutaneous emergency airway access; prevention, preparation, technique and training. *Br J Anaesth*. 2015;114:357-361.
51. Sivarajan M, Fink BR. The position and the state of the larynx during general anesthesia and muscle paralysis. *Anesthesiology*. 1990;72:439-442.
52. Mushambi MC, Kinsella SM, Popat M, et al. Obstetric Anaesthetists' Association and Difficult Airway Society guidelines for the management of difficult and failed tracheal intubation in obstetrics. *Anaesthesia*. 2015;70:1286-1306.
53. Brimacombe JR, Berry AM. Cricoid pressure. *Can J Anaesth*. 1997;44:414-425.
54. Frerk C, Mitchell VS, McNarry AF, et al. Difficult Airway Society 2015 guidelines for management of unanticipated difficult intubation in adults. *Br J Anaesth*. 2015;115:827-848.
55. Sharp LM, Levy DM. Rapid sequence induction in obstetrics revisited. *Curr Opin Anaesthesiol*. 2009;22:357-361.
56. Phillips S, Subair S, Husain T, Sultan P. Apnoeic oxygenation during maternal cardiac arrest in a parturient with extreme obesity. *Int J Obstet Anesth*. 2017;29:88-90.
57. Henderson JJ, Popat MT, Latto IP, Pearce AC. Difficult Airway Society guidelines for management of the unanticipated difficult intubation. *Anaesthesia*. 2004;59:675-694.
58. Matioc AA, Olson J. Use of the Laryngeal Tube in two unexpected difficult airway situations: lingual tonsillar hyperplasia and morbid obesity. *Can J Anaesth*. 2004;51:1018-1121.
59. Hawkins JL, Chang J, Palmer SK, Gibbs CP, Callaghan WM. Anesthesia-related maternal mortality in the United States: 1979-2002. *Obstet Gynecol*. 2011;117:69-74.
60. McClure JH, Cooper GM, Clutton-Brock TH. Saving mothers' lives: reviewing maternal deaths to make motherhood safer: 2006-2008: a review. *Br J Anaesth*. 2011;107:127-132.
61. Han TH, Brimacombe J, Lee EJ, Yang HS. The laryngeal mask airway is effective (and probably safe) in selected healthy parturients for elective Cesarean section: a prospective study of 1067 cases. *Can J Anaesth*. 2001;48:1117-1121.
62. Rucklidge MW, Yentis SM. Obstetric difficult airway guidelines—decision-making in critical situations. *Anaesthesia*. 2015;70:1221-1225.

CHAPTER 53

Airway Management of the Obstetrical Patient with an Anticipated Difficult Airway

Ana Sjaus and Leo Fares

CASE PRESENTATION

A 38-year-old woman, gravida 2 para 0, currently at 35 weeks' gestation, presents for induction of labor due to worsening preeclampsia, marked by persistent headache and worsening laboratory indices of hepatic and renal function.

A review of her medical history reveals that the patient has been living with morbid obesity, essential hypertension, and obstructive sleep apnea. The weight gain has accelerated during pregnancy.

Several years earlier, she underwent diagnostic laparoscopy complicated by deep vein thrombosis. The anesthetic record is not available; however, the patient recalls having a "sore throat" for several days after the procedure.

On admission to labor and delivery, her blood pressure is 156/98, heart rate is regular at 92 beats per minute, and her oxygen saturation is 95% on room air. The airway examination shows a prominent dorsocervical fat pad and large neck. Examination of the airway identifies Mallampati Class IV oropharynx, 3 cm mouth opening, 1 cm thyromental distance, minimal mandibular protrusion, and restricted range of motion in the cervical spine. Her BMI is 50.8 kg·m^{-2} (133 kg). The current medications are antihypertensives, intravenous magnesium sulfate, and dalteparin, 5000 U every 8 hours (last given 2 hours prior to induction of labor). Her platelet count is 70,000 $\times$ 10^{9}/L.

The patient makes rapid progress and is offered intravenous patient-controlled analgesia. After 8 hours of labor and 2.5 hours of unsuccessful expulsive efforts, the patient is tired and the fetal heart trace is class 2. As fetal position is not amenable to assisted vaginal delivery, a decision is made to proceed with cesarean section.

PATIENT CONSIDERATIONS

What Is the Impact of Anatomic and Physiologic Changes of Pregnancy on Airway Management?

Pregnancy has profound effects on the respiratory, cardiovascular, and gastrointestinal systems.[1–3] The incidence of complicated airway instrumentation in pregnancy is around 10 times higher than in the general population.[4] A number of physiologic and anatomic changes compound the risks of intubation.

1. Pregnant patients can exhibit rapid desaturation and decreased apneic oxygenation time upon induction of anesthesia. A recent multicenter cohort study found that up to 20% of parturients who had general anesthesia suffered hypoxemia (10% had severe hypoxemia).[5] This is thought to be due to a combination of increased metabolic oxygen requirement, decreased functional residual capacity, and a higher lung closing volume.
2. During face-mask ventilation (FMV), higher positive pressure may be required to achieve adequate tidal volume. This is due to increased intra-abdominal pressure and decreased chest wall compliance from breast tissue hypertrophy.

3. Breast enlargement can hinder laryngoscope insertion.
4. Increased mucosal vascularity and edema can compromise airway patency and increase friability of mucosal surfaces. Snoring and nose bleeds are common in pregnancy as is new or worsening obstructive sleep apnea.
5. The risk of passive regurgitation of gastric contents during airway management is increased.[1] Displacement of the diaphragm and higher progesterone levels diminish the lower esophageal sphincter tone and lead to gastroesophageal reflux during pregnancy. During labor, gastric transit time is prolonged and gastric volume is increased.

These anatomic and physiologic changes can be further exacerbated by excessive weight gain, pregnancy-related pathology, and intrapartum events.

Why Does Preeclampsia Complicate Airway Management?

Preeclampsia is a hypertensive disorder of pregnancy that complicates between 2% and 8% of all births. The pathophysiology of preeclampsia is characterized by a complex interplay between placental development and genetic and immunologic factors that lead to placental and maternal end-organ dysfunction.[6] Clinical manifestations, in addition to maternal hypertension, may include headaches, visual disturbances, hyperreflexia, epigastric pain, worsening edema, and oliguria. Antihypertensives, magnesium sulfate infusion, restriction of fluid intake, and restriction of physical activity are used to attenuate systemic progression, and to prevent eclampsia. Evidence of worsening end-organ involvement is indication for delivery.

This patient has preeclampsia with severe features marked by central nervous system dysfunction (persistent headache), thrombocytopenia (platelet count $<100,000 \times 10^9/L$), and renal dysfunction.

Preeclampsia affects airway anatomy and airway management strategies. Increased systemic vascular resistance, cardiac output, and capillary permeability are present in the majority of patients with preeclampsia. When combined with decreased intravascular oncotic pressure due to proteinuria, airway edema and mucosal friability are exacerbated. The same factors increase the risk of pulmonary edema, which further worsens oxygenation and pulmonary mechanics, doubling the risk of hypoxemia.[7] Additionally, patients with preeclampsia have exaggerated hemodynamic response to laryngoscopy. Uncontrolled hypertension at the time of intubation can increase the risk of cerebral hemorrhage, particularly in patients with cerebral edema, encephalopathy, and coagulopathy. Suppressing this response requires additional measures that may be in conflict with the goals of rapid sequence induction (RSI).

What Preexisting Comorbidities Require Special Consideration When It Comes to Airway Management in a Parturient?

Any preexisting condition associated with difficult airway management may elevate the risks to the parturient. Craniofacial deformities, cervical spine fusion, airway tumors, and severe cardiopulmonary diseases should all trigger early prenatal consultation with an anesthesia practitioner.

Morbid obesity is an independent risk factor for both difficult FMV and difficult laryngoscopy.[8] In addition, features commonly associated with obesity are predictors of difficulty with extraglottic airway device (EGD) insertion, and front-of-neck airway (FONA) access. In addition to a high risk of preeclampsia, hypertension, gestational diabetes, and thromboembolism, morbidly obese parturients suffer increased rates of obstetric complications including stillbirth, fetal distress, failed labor induction, operative delivery, and postpartum hemorrhage.[8] Many of these complications require emergency operative management making timely identification of airway risks and planning of anesthetic management a crucial determinant of patient safety.

Does Being in Labor Impact the Airway?

During labor, particularly the second stage, markers of difficult airway have been found to increase by at least one Mallampati airway classification grade in over 30% of parturients.[9]

Several factors contribute to these changes. Prolonged intravenous fluid administration and oxytocin infusion, with its antidiuretic effect, contribute to significant fluid retention. Valsalva maneuvers during expulsive efforts of the second stage, in concert with increased interstitial fluid, can further worsen airway edema.

Further, maternal metabolic oxygen demand increases in active labor, which decreases apneic oxygenation time and increases the risk of hypoxemia.

What Predictors of Difficulty and Potential Complications of Airway Management Can Be Identified in This Patient?

This patient's risk factors include preeclampsia, morbid obesity, and obstructive sleep apnea. In addition, several other associated risks of complicated airway management are found on physical examination (small mouth opening, full dentition, and decreased mandibular mobility).

She is at an increased risk of difficult FMV, aspiration of gastric contents, airway bleeding, and failed intubation. In addition, she is at a significant risk of rapid oxygen desaturation, prolonged hypoxemia, and uncontrolled hypertension with laryngoscopy. FONA as a rescue in the event of a "can't ventilate can't oxygenate" (CICO) situation is expected to be difficult.

AIRWAY MANAGEMENT FOR A PARTURIENT WITH AN ANTICIPATED DIFFICULT AIRWAY

When Should Difficult Airway Management Be Discussed with the Patient and the Multidisciplinary Team?

Despite the numerous advances in airway management, the incidence of failed airway in pregnant patients has remained stable for the past 20 years (~2.5/100,000). Difficult intubation has not been anticipated in over 50% of cases.[10]

The CICO scenario occurs in 5% to 25% of failed intubations, with an estimated airway-related mortality at ~2 per 100,000 of general anesthetics.[10] In addition to maternal and pregnancy-related factors, human and systems factors have been implicated in leading to higher rates of complicated airways in obstetrics.[2,11]

Although the classical predictors of difficult laryngoscopy (such as Mallampati grade) perform poorly in the obstetric population,[12] airway assessment should be performed for every parturient under anesthetic care. Predictors of difficult FMV, FONA, or even oral piercings can be identified in advance. The more recently investigated markers of airway difficulty such as neck circumference, chest circumference-thyromental distance ratio, height-thyromental distance ratio, and pregnancy weight gain and sonographic measurements, were found to improve specificity and sensitivity of bedside airway assessment.[12] While evidence for these novel markers is evolving, the most rational approach is to use multiple predictors concurrently.

It is important to proactively identify all parturients with known or predicted difficult airway, and anesthesiology consultation should be initiated as early as possible. Considerations should include medical comorbidities, obstetrical plan, and risk factors for operative delivery. The patients' understanding of the role of neuraxial analgesia, and their attitudes toward it should be explored, given the fact that neuraxial techniques decrease the need for general anesthesia during labor and delivery. Any contraindications must be identified and a contingency plan considered. Facility and time-of-day availability of equipment and expertise must be taken into account. In extreme cases, where availability of specialized equipment or expertise cannot be guaranteed, consideration of elective cesarean delivery may be warranted at a time when optimal conditions can be guaranteed.[13,14]

At admission to the birthing unit for a laboring parturient, initial and regular reassessments are essential in preparing for an advanced airway requirement. Multidisciplinary planning, timely communication, and shared decision making, are necessary to ensure appropriate management and informed parturient consent. The possible scenarios should be discussed for these patients, and early epidural placement undertaken, should that be the optimum choice in a given patient.

Which Anesthetic Technique Is Preferred in Patients with the Anticipated Difficult Airway?

Neuraxial anesthesia reduces, but does not eliminate, the need for airway intervention in parturients with an anticipated difficult airway.[15] Spinal, epidural, and combined techniques are all highly effective and reliable in managing labor pain, and providing surgical anesthesia for operative delivery. However, general anesthesia may be required due to the failure of, or contraindication to, a neuraxial technique (e.g., coagulopathy), or other considerations.[14] In addition, some of the factors that complicate airway management also pose difficulties with neuraxial procedures. In these regards, morbid obesity is the most common issue, and skeletal abnormalities are associated with conditions such as ankylosing spondylitis, surgically stabilized spinal injuries, and congenital syndromes. Furthermore, even when a neuraxial technique is successful, other developments and complications may require an airway intervention, and this should be considered in the anesthetic plan.

In the case that is presented, airway management is predicted to be difficult and at high risk of complications. As per current guidelines, neuraxial anesthesia may be considered for patients with thrombocytopenia (between 50 and 70,000 $\times$ 10^9) if the benefits of neuraxial anesthesia in minimizing the risks of general anesthetic significantly outweigh the risk of spinal hematoma.[16] However, neuraxial instrumentation is contraindicated at this time, in this patient, due to recent administration of low-molecular-weight heparin.[17] Although unlikely in this case, the option to delay delivery until neuraxial anesthetic is no longer contraindicated should be discussed with the obstetrician.

How Should the Parturient Be Prepared for Airway Management?

The risk of aspiration of gastric contents can be mitigated by restriction of oral intake and administration of an H_2 blocker, a motility agent (metoclopramide), and a nonparticulate antacid (sodium citrate) prior to induction of anesthesia.[18]

Meticulous positioning for airway management involves ramping up the head of the bed to 20 to 30 degrees, or until tragus of the ear is above the level of the sternum (see Figure 52.2). Left uterine displacement can be achieved by placing a right hip wedge. In addition to facilitating airway opening maneuvers during FMV and optimizing glottic visualization during laryngoscopy, this position improves functional residual capacity and decreases the risk of aspiration in the event of regurgitation of gastric contents. Access for FONA is also improved by this ramped position, and advance marking of surface landmarks should be considered in cases when "double set-up" is planned.

Denitrogenation prolongs apneic oxygenation time in obstetric patients who are otherwise expected to have oxygen desaturation quickly during intubation. The current recommendation is to achieve target end-expiratory oxygen fraction of >90% prior to induction of general anesthesia even in emergency cesarean deliveries.[2] This is best done by using an FiO_2 of 1.0 at >10 L·min^{-1} flows via a tight-fitting face mask for at least 3 minutes of vital capacity breathing. Alternative methods, such as high-flow nasal oxygen (HFNO), have been recommended for denitrogenation and during intubation to extend the apneic oxygenation time.[2] More recent investigations in obstetric patients showed that HFNO as the sole method is not reliable when compared to standard denitrogenation by face mask.[19,20]

Topical anesthesia of the airway is required if the plan includes awake endotracheal intubation. In the obstetric population, this may be most appropriate with a relaxed, cooperative patient undergoing general anesthesia for elective indications in a controlled environment. Alternatively, based on the difficult airway algorithm, awake techniques of sedation can still be considered following emergence after a failed intubation attempt.[2] Pretreatment with glycopyrrolate and judicious use of sedation are advised if this is feasible.

What Specific Techniques and Equipment Are Recommended in the Management of a Parturient with Obesity, Preeclampsia, and Additional Predictors of Difficult Airway?

Once committed to general anesthesia, the team should confirm that the applicable cognitive aides are available and, ideally, review the algorithm prior to the procedure. The principles of management, regardless of which technique or adjunct is used, should prioritize the overarching goal of maintaining maternal and fetal oxygenation at every junction. These include meticulous denitrogenation, gentle positive pressure ventilation with cricoid pressure, and EGD insertion following a failed intubation attempt. Both pulse oximetry and continuous capnography should be used to confirm the adequacy of these techniques. The information gained during the first attempt should be used to guide the second as persistence with the same technique has the potential to cause harm. The team must be prepared to efficiently act on decisions, such as the pre-established exit strategy after failed attempts, FONA, and perimortem delivery. Help should be called early, as repeat attempts should be minimized and performed by increasingly skilled personnel.[21]

In the presented semi-urgent case, predicted difficulty in multiple aspects of airway management should prompt consideration of awake tracheal intubation. Various airway topicalization techniques have been described in pregnant patients, without evidence to support a specific recommendation, except to provide supplemental oxygen by face mask, standard nasal cannula, or HFNO.[1,13] As airway topicalization diminishes protective airway reflexes, oropharyngeal suction must be available to manage airway secretions.

The positioning should ensure adequate airway opening and head elevation from the outset.[2] A serious consideration should be given to a "double set-up," when predictors of both difficult laryngoscopy and difficult FMV are present. FONA is more difficult in female, obese patients, and in pregnancy. Point-of-care ultrasound may be helpful to mark the cricothyroid membrane prior to airway intervention.

As the airway is expected to be edematous and narrowed, a flexible bronchoscope of a caliber that can accommodate smaller diameter endotracheal tubes (6.0-6.5 mm ID) should be prepared. Due to the risk of bleeding, nasal intubation is generally avoided. Video-laryngoscopes (VL) have become first-line intubation devices in difficult airways and rescue adjuncts after failed intubation attempts.[22] VL with a hyperangulated or MAC blade, and a range of sizes of stylet endotracheal tubes (ETTs) can be used to guide awake intubation.[13] Alternative reported approaches include awake direct laryngoscopy (DL) and EGD-guided awake intubation.[13] Awake look with VL or DL requires oropharyngeal topicalization and can confirm visualization of the glottis prior to induction. While this may provide comfort to the anesthesia practitioner, VL view after the patient is paralyzed may not correlate with a prior awake look. A backup plan should be discussed with the team in advance, as proceeding with induction of anesthesia, following failure of an awake technique, exposes the patient to significant risks.

If securing the airway after induction of anesthesia is thought to be more appropriate, either DL or VL may be used as the intubation technique of choice.[23] Evolving evidence supports the use of VL in obstetrics as the first-line and a rescue technique.[22]

An appropriately sized EGD should be immediately available and prepared for use. In the difficult obstetrical airway algorithm, EGD is used after failed intubation as a rescue device after a failed attempt, as a bridge to definitive management, or as an exit strategy.[2,21] Increasingly, if EGD can be used to oxygenate and ventilate, it is left in place as the definitive airway for the duration of the case.[24] Second-generation devices (LMA-ProSeal™, LMA-Supreme™, i-gel®) are recommended in obstetrics with good evidence of safety and effectiveness.[25–27] In addition to providing a patent airway and ability to proceed with surgery, the EGD can serve as a conduit for tracheal intubation both directly (small diameter ETT over a flexible bronchoscope) and indirectly[26] (Aintree Intubation Catheter [Cook Medical, Bloomington, IN] over which an ETT is subsequently "railroaded" through an LMA-Classic™).

The selection of appropriate pharmacological adjuncts will ensure adequate intubating conditions that minimize the risks of prolonged hypoxemia, airway trauma, and intraoperative awareness. Propofol is recommended for induction of general anesthesia owing to its familiarity, availability, and safety in obstetrics.[1,5] Its short duration of action allows for rapid emergence in the event of failed intubation, but may require repeat administration to prevent awareness if the airway is not quickly secured. Classically, succinylcholine is administered as a part of the RSI; however, high-dose rocuronium (1.2 $mg \cdot kg^{-1}$) is increasingly used in obstetric airway management, especially when sugammadex reversal is immediately available (see Chapter 4). It is important to note that the reliability of the latter approach in restoring the airway patency, and spontaneous ventilation in "can't intubate, can't oxygenate" (CICO) situations, has not been confirmed with sufficient degree of certainty.

In patients with preeclampsia, laryngoscopy can provoke uncontrolled hypertension. While airway topicalization can be expected to attenuate the response, additional agents should be available during awake and asleep airway management. Preemptive short-acting opioids, adrenergic blockers, or nitrates, may be administered for suppression of a hypertensive response in the absence of topical airway anesthesia. Prolonged neuromuscular blockade has been reported as an interaction between intravenous magnesium sulfate and nondepolarizing muscle relaxants. Despite the case reports of recurarization following sugammadex reversal in parturients with concurrent magnesium sulfate infusion,[28–31] an ex-vivo study, and a randomized controlled trial in nonobstetric patients, found that magnesium does not attenuate the effectiveness or duration of sugammadex reversal. Quantitative monitoring of neuromuscular blockade should be used as per best practice guidelines.

How Should Failed Intubation Be Managed in This Case?

If the first attempt at intubation fails, the priority is to maintain oxygenation. Failed awake intubation requires consideration of maternal and neonatal status, and the reasons for failure. The necessity of proceeding with cesarean section has to be assessed against the risks of further awake attempts, induction of general anesthesia, or deferring until neuraxial anesthetic can be performed. Additional topical anesthetic may be administered if the amount of local anesthetic used has not exceeded the maximum dose allowed (see Chapter 3) and patient is stable and appears to tolerate another awake attempt.

If the parturient is under general anesthesia, apneic oxygenation (5-15 $L{\cdot}min^{-1}$ by nasal prongs or HFNO) can be used during laryngoscopy, and additional anesthetic administered to prevent awareness. FMV with insufflation pressure of <20 mmHg should be used to maintain oxygenation between the attempts.[2]

Additional personnel should be called to help. A second attempt using alternative equipment (i.e., VL), a modified view (i.e., releasing cricoid pressure), or by a more experienced anesthesia practitioner should be considered. Cricoid pressure can be released if it interferes with visualization of the glottis during laryngoscopy to facilitate insertion of EGD, or if it is found to impede FMV. A third attempt at intubation should be considered by a more experienced colleague, if present. If failure at tracheal intubation persists at this point, an emergency should be verbalized to the operating room and oxygenation maintained. Options for proceeding depend on the status of the mother and the fetus.[2]

If the maternal and fetal clinical situation is reassuring and stable, the mother can be allowed to emerge from general anesthesia, with adequate reversal of neuromuscular blockade and continued airway support to maintain oxygenation. Once awake, a neuraxial anesthetic approach can be reassessed, or an awake flexible bronchoscopic intubation can be considered.

If there is maternal and/or fetal instability, and the clinical situation is an emergency, an EGD should be inserted as the rescue device and used to facilitate cesarean delivery, preferably a second-generation EGD with an esophageal drainage port allowing for decompression of gastric contents.[26] While the continuation of cesarean section with a well-fitting EGD in place seems safe, there is little evidence to guide its use after delivery in morbidly obese patients following failed intubation. If EGD is providing effective oxygenation and ventilation, it can be closely monitored, or used as a conduit for tracheal intubation over a flexible bronchoscope, keeping in mind that any additional airway instrumentation may result in further airway edema and the loss of oxygenation provided by the EGD.

When failed tracheal intubation occurs, and ventilation and oxygenation by either face mask or EGD cannot be achieved, the parturient has entered a CICO situation. A CICO scenario occurs in 5% to 28% of failed intubations.[32,33] This emergency must be vocalized to the room and additional personnel, ideally proficient in FONA, must be called immediately. Further deterioration of oxygenation is certain unless a FONA is established without delay. Adequate neuromuscular blockade should be confirmed, and one last attempt made at face mask, EGD placement, or VL technique, while concurrently preparing for a FONA via cricothyrotomy (see section "The Airway Management Algorithms" for more detail). Once placement of an ETT has been verified, the cesarean delivery may proceed.

POSTINTUBATION CARE OF A PARTURIENT WITH A DIFFICULT AIRWAY

Planning for safe extubation is a crucial aspect of airway management in a parturient. It is important to recognize that airway instrumentation, intravenous fluid administration, supine position, and surgical stress can adversely impact postextubation airway patency and decrease the prospects of successful reintubation in the event that extubation fails.

Individual factors will vary depending on the clinical context and the patient. However, general principles for extubation would include ensuring the patient is awake, alert, and responsive. They should be free of any residual neuromuscular blockade and provided supplemental oxygen throughout.

The anesthesia practitioner should be prepared to reintubate and ensure the appropriate medication, equipment, and personnel are available. If there is a concern regarding airway edema postextubation, it may be prudent to examine the airway prior to emergence. This can be done by direct, indirect, or flexible nasopharyngoscopy, deflating the cuff and checking for a leak around the ETT, or placing an airway exchange catheter to help facilitate reintubation prior to withdrawing the ETT.

If there are any doubts around neurologic status, level of sedation, or airway patency postextubation, it may be prudent to transfer the parturient to a critical care unit for ongoing ventilatory support and assessment. If extubation is delayed due to airway edema, steroid administration and diuresis may be indicated. Extended postextubation monitoring, oxygen supplementation, and positive pressure support (CPAP or BIPAP) may prevent adverse postextubation events in a parturient with difficult airway, following anesthetic for operative delivery.

SUMMARY

Pregnant patients are at higher risk of complications due to difficult and failed airway management than the general population. In cases where additional predictors of difficulty are identified, careful consideration of obstetric and anesthetic concerns, and meticulous management can minimize the potential for airway-related morbidity and mortality. Timely identification, prenatal planning, and counseling toward early labor epidural should be standard measures to minimize the risk of emergency airway management.

Teamwork, communication, and crisis leadership are essential components of airway management when difficulty is anticipated. Whether general anesthesia is required electively or in an emergency, the airway can be complicated by factors such as preeclampsia, morbid obesity, prolonged labor induction, and prolonged second stage. Depending on the circumstances, maternal condition, and fetal stability, awake intubation using either flexible bronchoscope or VL may be the choice in select cases when patients are stable, cooperative, and can tolerate airway topicalization.

Most often, obstetrical difficult airway is managed through the use of RSI. Airway double setup for FONA can minimize the time to oxygenation, if a CICO situation is encountered, and should be a part of advance preparation. Aspiration prophylaxis, careful positioning, adequate denitrogenation, and gentle FMV in the presence of cricoid pressure can mitigate the expected rapid oxygen desaturation and afford the time for intubation using advanced airway adjuncts. The choice of pharmacological agents should be guided by reducing the time interval between induction of anesthesia and intubation. A second-generation EGD can be used as a bridge to intubation, or maintained for the duration of the case. Another consideration is the availability of reversal agents and the ability to wake the patient up should the intubation fail. A failed airway plan should be reviewed prior to induction of anesthesia and an appropriate exit strategy clearly defined.

Postintubation care requires careful consideration based on the specific circumstances of the case. These may involve delayed extubation, diuresis to minimize airway edema, and extended postextubation monitoring.

SELF-EVALUATION QUESTIONS

53.1. Which physiologic change seen in healthy pregnancy can impact airway management in parturients?

A. Decreased upper esophageal sphincter tone.

B. Increased residual volume and functional residual capacity.

C. Decreased gastric emptying time.

D. Breast tissue hypertrophy.

E. All of the listed changes impact airway management.

53.2. Which of the following explains the rationale for recommending early epidural placement to a parturient presenting with the BMI of >60 $kg{\cdot}m^{-2}$ and predictors of difficult airway?

A. Because her risk of requiring operative delivery is increased, having an epidural in place would decrease the need for emergency general anesthetic which in her case would carry a high risk of airway complications.

B. If she needs an emergency delivery because of fetal distress and does not already have an epidural, an emergency anesthetic (general or regional) would be challenging, take additional time, and likely delay the delivery potentially compromising the neonate.

C. Early epidural decreases the risk of general anesthesia for mother and fetus because it is placed when labor pain is not yet interfering with proper positioning, with plenty of time to do the procedure and to confirm that the epidural is working well.

D. Epidural analgesia in patients with obesity is safe, eliminates the risks of other labor analgesia, minimizes the need for general anesthetic and, to maximize the potential benefits, it should be placed early.

E. All of the above statements would be good reasons to recommend early epidural.

53.3. Concerning airway assessment in obstetric patients, which of the following is **TRUE**?

A. Because bedside examination has poor predictive value for difficult laryngoscopy, routine airway examination is only necessary in obstetric patients with morbid obesity or preeclampsia.

B. Airway changes occur in pregnancy up until the onset of labor.

C. Airway examination predicts majority of difficult intubations in obstetrics.

D. Preeclampsia is the main risk factor for airway edema during labor.

E. Assessment of maternal and fetal condition and availability of equipment and personnel should be considered in addition to examination of airway anatomy.

53.4. Which of the following adjuncts should be used as first-line for awake intubation following topicalization of the airway in parturient with micrognathia requiring cesarean delivery under general anesthesia?

A. Direct laryngoscope with MAC 3 blade

B. Flexible bronchoscope with 7.5 to 8.0-mm ID orotracheal tube

C. Flexible bronchoscope with 6.0 to 6.5-mm ID orotracheal tube

D. Aintree intubating catheter

E. Endotracheal tube exchange catheter to railroad a 6.0 to 6.5-mm ID orotracheal tube over

53.5. Which of the following describes the currently recommended procedure for denitrogenation in a spontaneously breathing parturient with predicted difficult airway undergoing induction of general anesthesia?

A. High-flow nasal oxygenation for at least 3 minutes.

B. Standard nasal cannula with 100% oxygen at 5 to 15 $L{\cdot}min^{-1}$ for 10 minutes or until expired fraction of O_2 of >90% is achieved.

C. Non-rebreather oxygen face mask with 100% oxygen at 5 to 15 $L{\cdot}min^{-1}$ for three vital capacity breaths.

D. Non-rebreather oxygen face mask with 100% oxygen at 5 to 15 $L{\cdot}min^{-1}$ for 3 minutes.

E. Tight fitting face mask with 100% oxygen at 10 to 15 $L{\cdot}min^{-1}$ and vital capacity breathing until expired fraction of O_2 of >90% is achieved.

53.6. Your first attempt at intubation using VL under general anesthesia in a parturient with severe preeclampsia and fetal distress has failed. Which of the following would present a departure from the most appropriate course of action at this time?

A. Continue gentle positive pressure ventilation with 100% oxygen.

B. Call for a more experienced colleague.

C. Ask for ultrasound to landmark for front-of-neck airway.

D. Administer an additional dose of anesthetic to prevent awareness.

E. Ask the assistant to remove cricoid pressure.

53.7. Which of the following should be included in preparing for airway management after induction of anesthesia in an unstable patient with a known difficult airway?

A. Video-laryngoscope.

B. Airway "double set-up."

C. A second-generation EGD prepared for use.

D. 100% oxygen by standard nasal cannula at 5 to 15 L·min^{-1} to prolong apneic oxygenation.

E. All of the listed options are essential in the safe airway management of this patient.

REFERENCES

1. Patel S, Wali A. Airway management of the obstetric patient. *Curr Anesthesiol Rep*. 2020;10:350-360.
2. Mushambi MC, Kinsella SM, Popat M, et al. Obstetric Anaesthetists' Association and Difficult Airway Society guidelines for the management of difficult and failed tracheal intubation in obstetrics. *Anaesth*. 2015;70(11):1286-1306.
3. Delgado C, Ring L, Mushambi MC. General anaesthesia in obstetrics. *BJA Educ*. 2020;20(6):201.
4. Preston R, Jee R. Obstetric airway management. *Int Anesthesiol Clin*. 2014;52(2):1-28.
5. Bonnet MP, Mercier FJ, Vicaut E, Galand A, Keita H, et al. Incidence and risk factors for maternal hypoxaemia during induction of general anaesthesia for non-elective caesarean section: a prospective multicentre study. *Br J Anaesth*. 2020;125(1):e81-e87.
6. Magee LA, Pels A, Helewa M, et al. Diagnosis, evaluation, and management of the hypertensive disorders of pregnancy: executive summary. *JOGC*. 2014;36(5):416-438.
7. Smit MI, du Toit L, Dyer RA, et al. Hypoxaemia during tracheal intubation in patients with hypertensive disorders of pregnancy: analysis of data from an obstetric airway management registry. *Int J Obstet Anesth*. 2021;45:41-48.
8. Taylor CR, Dominguez JE, Habib AS. Obesity and obstetric anesthesia: current insights. *Local Reg Anesth*. 2019;12:111-124.
9. Ahuja P, Jain D, Bhardwaj N, Jain K, Gainder S, Kang M. Airway changes following labor and delivery in preeclamptic parturients: a prospective case control study. *Int J Obstet Anesth*. 2018;33:17-22.
10. Kinsella SM, Winton AL, Mushambi MC, et al. Failed tracheal intubation during obstetric general anaesthesia: a literature review. *Int J Obstet Anesth*. 2015;24(4):356-374.
11. Preston R. Management of the obstetric airway—time for a paradigm shift (or two)? *Int J Obstet Anesth*. 2015;24(4):293-296.
12. Jarraya A, Choura D, Mejdoub Y, Kammoun M, Grati F. New predictors of difficult intubation in obstetric patients: A prospective observational study. *Trends Anaesth*. 2019;24:22-25.
13. Mushambi MC, Athanassoglou V, Kinsella SM. Anticipated difficult airway during obstetric general anaesthesia: narrative literature review and management recommendations. *Anaesth*. 2020;75(7):945-961.
14. McGuire B, Lucas DN. Planning the obstetric airway. *Anaesth*. 2020;75(7): 852-855.
15. Ring L, Landau R, Delgado C. The current role of general anesthesia for cesarean delivery. *Current Anesth Rep*. 2021;1-10.
16. Bauer ME, Arendt K, Beilin Y, et al. The society for obstetric Anesthesia and Perinatology interdisciplinary consensus statement on neuraxial procedures in obstetric patients with thrombocytopenia. *Anesth Analg*. 2021;132(6):1531-1544.
17. Leffert L, Butwick A, Carvalho B, et al. The Society for Obstetric Anesthesia and Perinatology consensus statement on the anesthetic management of pregnant and postpartum women receiving thromboprophylaxis or higher dose anticoagulants. *Anesth Analg*. 2018;126(3):928-944.
18. Practice Guidelines for Obstetric Anesthesia: An Updated Report by the American Society of Anesthesiologists Task Force on Obstetric Anesthesia and the Society for Obstetric Anesthesia and Perinatology. *Anesthesiology*. 2016;124:270-300.
19. Shippam W, Preston R, Douglas J, Taylor J, Albert A, et al. High-flow nasal oxygen vs. standard flow-rate facemask pre-oxygenation in pregnant patients: a randomised physiological study. *Anaesth*. 2019;74(4): 450-456.
20. Au K, Shippam W, Taylor J, Albert A, Chau A. Determining the effective pre-oxygenation interval in obstetric patients using high-flow nasal oxygen and standard flow rate facemask: a biased-coin up–down sequential allocation trial. *Anaesth*. 2020;75(5):609-616.
21. Law JA, Duggan LV, Asselin M, et al. Canadian Airway Focus Group. Canadian Airway Focus Group updated consensus-based recommendations for management of the difficult airway: part 2. Planning and implementing safe management of the patient with an anticipated difficult airway. *Can J Anaesth*. 2021;68:1405-1436.
22. Howle R, Onwochei D, Harrison SL, Desai N. Comparison of videolaryngoscopy and direct laryngoscopy for tracheal intubation in obstetrics: a mixed-methods systematic review and meta-analysis. *Can J Anaesth*. 2021;68:546-565.
23. Scott-Brown S, Russell R. Video laryngoscopes and the obstetric airway. *IJOA*. 2015;24(2):137-146.
24. Lim MJ, Tan HS, Tan CW, et al. The effects of labor on airway outcomes with Supreme™ laryngeal mask in women undergoing cesarean delivery under general anesthesia: a cohort study. *BMC Anesthesiol*. 2020;20:213.
25. Yao WY, Li SY, Yuan YJ, et al. Comparison of Supreme laryngeal mask airway versus endotracheal intubation for airway management during general anesthesia for cesarean section: a randomized controlled trial. *BMC Anesthesiol*. 2019;19:123.
26. Wong P, Sng BL, Lim WY. Rescue supraglottic airway devices at caesarean delivery: what are the options to consider? *Int J Obstet Anesth*. 2020;42:65-75.
27. Tan HS, Li SY, Yao WY, et al. Association of Mallampati scoring on airway outcomes in women undergoing general anesthesia with Supreme™ laryngeal mask airway in cesarean section. *BMC Anesthesiol*. 2019;19:122.
28. Unterbuchner C, Ziegleder R, Graf B, et al. Magnesium-induced recurarisation after reversal of rocuronium-induced neuromuscular block with sugammadex. *Acta Anaesthesiol*. 2015;59(4):536-540.
29. Fábián ÁI, Csernoch V, Tassonyi E, Fedor M, Fülesdi B. The effect of magnesium on the reversal of rocuronium-induced neuromuscular block with sugammadex: an ex vivo laboratory study. *BMC Anesthesiol*. 2019;19(1):1-8.
30. Moriwaki K, Kayashima K. Prolonged neuromuscular blockade and insufficient reversal after sugammadex administration in cesarean section under general anesthesia: a case report. *JA Clinical Reports*. 2019;5(1):1-4.
31. Germano Filho PA, Cavalcanti IL, Barrucand L, Verçosa N. Effect of magnesium sulphate on sugammadex reversal time for neuromuscular blockade: a randomised controlled study. *Anaesth*. 2015;70(8):956-961.
32. Odor PM, Bampoe S, Moonesinghe SR, et al. General anaesthetic and airway management practice for obstetric surgery in England: a prospective, multicentre observational study. *Anaesth*. 2021;76(4):460-471.
33. Kinsella SM, Winton AL, Mushambi MC, et al. Failed tracheal intubation during obstetric general anaesthesia: a literature review. *Int J Obstet Anesth*. 2015;24(4):356-374.

CHAPTER 54

Unanticipated Difficult Airway in an Obstetrical Patient Requiring an Emergency Cesarean Section

Christina Ratto and Holly A. Muir

CASE PRESENTATION

A 25-year-old primigravida at 39 weeks gestational age presents to the labor and delivery floor with ruptured membranes and frequent uterine contractions. She does not want to have epidural analgesia because of a story she heard about an epidural complication suffered by one of her distant relatives. After 14 hours of labor augmented with oxytocin, and now 2 hours of pushing, she is urgently taken to the operating room for emergency cesarean section because of prolonged late decelerations. She weighs 253 lbs (115 kg) and is 5′3″ (160 cm) tall, giving her a BMI of approximately 45 $kg{\cdot}m^{-2}$. Airway examination on admission revealed a Mallampati II and a thyromental distance of 4 cm. She has full neck extension with normal dentition and a normal mouth opening. On arrival in the operating room, her Mallampati score is now assessed to be a grade III. She has large gravid breasts. Her blood pressure is 128/68 mmHg, heart rate 100 beats per minute (bpm), respiratory rate 20 breaths per minute, and SaO_2 of 99% on a 100% oxygen via a non-rebreather face mask. On arrival in the operating room, the fetal heart rate is 80 bpm.

ANESTHETIC CONSIDERATIONS

What Are the Anesthetic Options for Cesarean Section in This Patient?

An emergency cesarean section is mandated to deliver a fetus with persistent bradycardia (late decelerations) while minimizing potential/preventable risks to the mother. Anesthesia risk factors for airway management in this patient include her BMI (45 $kg{\cdot}m^{-2}$), potential for airway edema after 2 hours of pushing, infusion of oxytocin, and enlarged breasts. Although regional anesthesia has become the standard of anesthetic care for operative delivery in obstetrics,[1] this patient has refused the regional approach.

The concerns for emergency cesarean section under general anesthesia include securing the airway, minimizing the risk of aspiration, reducing the sympathetic response to laryngoscopy and intubation, ensuring adequate fluid resuscitation, and the potential for blood loss due to volatile agent-induced uterine atony. With respect to the first of these concerns, all labor and delivery facilities must have a difficult airway cart and contingency plans for failed laryngoscopic intubation.[1]

AIRWAY CONSIDERATIONS

What Are the Airway Considerations in Pregnant Women?

Pregnancy is associated with fluid retention and weight gain.[2] Mallampati classes III and IV airways seem to be more prevalent in parturients at the beginning of labor (28%) than in the general adult population (7%-17%), suggesting that an increase in tongue volume may be one of the physiologic changes of a normal pregnancy.[3] Structurally, the pharyngeal airway is surrounded by soft tissues (such as the tongue and soft palate), which are enclosed by bony structures (such as the mandible and spine). The size of the airway space is determined by the balance between the bony enclosure space and soft tissue volume when the tone of pharyngeal muscles is attenuated or eliminated by general anesthetics and muscle relaxants. Pharyngeal edema, presumably due to fluid retention during pregnancy, and pharyngeal swelling, which develops acutely during labor, increase the soft tissue volume surrounding the airway, thus narrowing the pharyngeal airway in parturients.[2] Many have hypothesized that changes in airway anatomy in the parturient include such factors as weight gain during pregnancy, fluid administration during labor, and the length of the first and second stages of labor.

Boutonnet et al. reported an increase in the incidence of Mallampati classes III and IV airways beginning in the eighth month of pregnancy, extending throughout labor, and not fully reversed for up to 48 hours after delivery.[4] Moreover, these changes occurred irrespective of any increase in body weight, duration of first and second stages of labor, or volume of IV fluid administered. In their study, they observed patients at four time points: 8 months of gestation (not in labor); when the epidural was placed; 20 minutes after delivery; and 48 hours after delivery. They found no changes in Mallampati score in 38.8% of their patients. However, in the remaining women, significant changes were observed in the interval between the first nonlaboring assessment at 8 months, at the time of placement of the epidural, and between placing the epidural and delivery. Figure 54.1 illustrates their findings of a progressive increase in Mallampati classes III and IV airways.

Similar results were observed by Kodali et al.[5] As with the Boutonnet et al. study,[4] no correlation was observed between airway changes during labor and duration of labor, or quantity of fluids administered during labor.

Research related to the pathophysiology of upper airway obstruction has revealed a significant reduction of lung volume in patients with pharyngeal narrowing.[6] Obese parturients are prone to develop progressively narrower pharyngeal airways due to increased soft tissue volume surrounding the pharyngeal

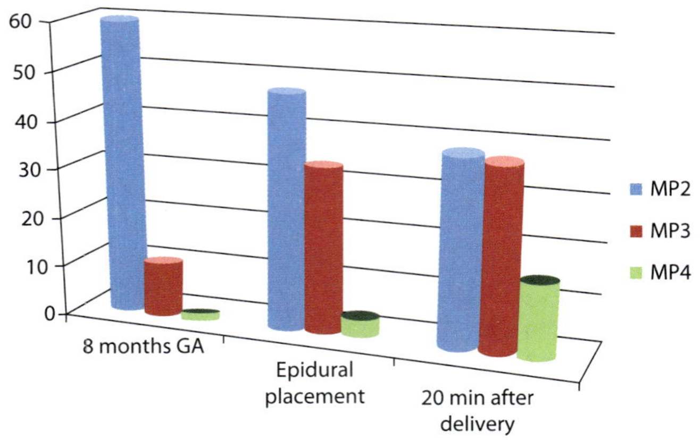

FIGURE 54.1. Progression of Mallampati changes seen from late pregnancy to delivery. (Data from Boutonnet M, Faitot V, Katz A, et al. Mallampati class changes during pregnancy, labour, and after delivery: can these be predicted? *Br J Anaesth*. 2010;104(1):67-70.)

airway, and lung volume reduction during general anesthesia is known to be more prominent and prolonged in obese patients. The assumption is that FRC is decreased, further contributing to the more rapid oxygen desaturation following induction seen in these patients.

The assessment of the pregnant patient must specifically address features that increase the risk of difficult laryngoscopic intubation, including receding mandible, limited mouth opening, short neck, limited neck movement, high Mallampati grade (III and IV), etc. Taken together, these features are known to increase the likelihood of a difficult laryngoscopic intubation.[7] Using the airway assessment strategies as described in Chapter 1 (MOANS, LEMON, CRANE, RODS, and SHORT), this patient's airway assessment suggests possible difficult face-mask ventilation (FMV), difficult direct and indirect (video) laryngoscopy, difficult use of extraglottic devices (EGD), and difficult front-of-neck access (FONA).

The standard of care in obstetrical anesthesia demands that the airway of this patient be secured in such a manner that the risk of aspiration is minimized, leaving the airway practitioner with two choices in this case: rapid sequence induction (RSI); or an awake technique. An awake technique reduces the risk of a failed airway in an anesthetized and paralyzed patient. The decision to perform an awake intubation technique, rather than an RSI, should be on the basis of clinical findings and the experience of the practitioner. In either case, contingency plans (Plans B and C) must be in place in the event that these techniques fail. One of the contingency plans must be a FONA, or cricothyrotomy.

CONDUCT OF ANESTHESIA

How Should the Anesthetic Be Conducted in This Patient?

Aspiration prophylaxis using oral 0.3 M sodium citrate (30 mL), and intravenous ranitidine 50 mg (± metoclopramide 10 mg) should be given, following the placement of an intravenous catheter. Appropriate intravenous anesthesia induction agents (propofol 2 mg·kg^{-1}), or thiopentone 3 to 4 mg·kg^{-1}, and succinylcholine 1.5 mg·kg^{-1} are prepared. A designated assistant, with experience in applying cricoid pressure during the RSI, must be available if an awake technique is not employed.

The patient is placed in a left tilt (at least 15 degrees) to minimize the risk of aortocaval compression (supine hypotensive syndrome). In addition, the thorax, shoulders, neck, and head of this morbidly obese parturient should be elevated (ramping) to bring the anatomical axes of the oral, pharyngeal, and laryngeal structures into alignment (see Figure 52.2). Evidence suggests that placing the patient in a 20- to 30-degree head-up position improves ventilation and denitrogenation, reduces interference with laryngoscope insertion by large breasts, improves the view at laryngoscopy, and may reduce gastroesophageal reflux.[8] A polio handle (short handle) laryngoscope may facilitate blade insertion in the case of large breasts. Alternatively, an assistant may be designated to retract the breasts caudally during laryngoscopy.

In all circumstances, a difficult airway cart with appropriate airway devices must be immediately available. Denitrogenation is crucial. Though some have noted that modified shorter-duration denitrogenation techniques may suffice and be effective,[9,10] standard techniques and durations are recommended. The addition of high-flow nasal oxygen (10-15 $L \cdot min^{-1}$) for the duration of the induction/intubation sequence can maintain good oxygenation in an apneic patient for a prolonged period of time and should be considered for all pregnant women at induction of anesthesia[11] (see Chapter 8).

Following an RSI with cricoid pressure, direct laryngoscopy using a #3 Macintosh blade reveals a Cormack/Lehane (C/L) Grade IV view (only the hard palate is visible). A second attempt at laryngoscopy using a #3 Miller blade also fails to reveal any identifiable glottic structures, despite laryngeal manipulation. Following the second attempt at laryngoscopic intubation, the patient's O_2 saturation falls to 85%, her heart rate is 120 bpm, and her BP is 180/120 mmHg.

What Does One Do If One Cannot Visualize the Cords on Second Attempt of Laryngoscopy?

There should be no delay in summoning additional assistance and informing all team members of the gravity of the situation. It is necessary to analyze why the attempts were unsuccessful by recalling the six factors that affect the success of the attempt: the practitioner, optimum head and neck position, optimum paralysis, best external laryngeal manipulation, type of laryngoscope blade, and length of blade (see Chapter 9).

Various laryngoscope blades, rigid fiberoptic laryngoscopes, and video laryngoscopes (with modified curved and straight blades) can be considered if the practitioner possesses a degree of expertise in their use. Improperly applied cricoid pressure can make visualization of the glottic opening more difficult, necessitating guidance by the practitioner. The use of cricoid pressure has become a source of controversy; however, to date, it remains as a recommendation in most obstetric difficult airway algorithms.[12] Other external laryngeal manipulation or repositioning of the head and neck can also help improve the laryngeal view such as backward, upward, and right side pressure (BURP) on the thyroid cartilage. Additionally, an Eschmann Tracheal Introducer (commonly known as a "bougie") or stylet can help identify the cricoid cartilage, but blind placement increases the risk of additional airway trauma. The "bougie" is useful if the epiglottis can be visualized, otherwise, it has a limited role. In the environment of a rapidly developing crisis, and a glottis that is difficult to visualize, a flexible bronchoscopic intubation would likely be inappropriate.

How Does One Apply the Failed Airway Algorithm in This Situation?

The rapid oxygen desaturation after the second intubation attempt is likely related to the decrease in functional residual capacity (FRC) and increase in O_2 consumption (basal metabolic rate) seen in the gravid state.[13] This patient's respiratory reserve is further compromised by her obesity and supine positioning. In addition, repeated attempts at intubation are likely going to lead to upper airway trauma, particularly in the parturient, in which the airway is edematous and the submucosal capillaries are fragile.

Because of these factors, and in the face of unacceptable oxygen saturations after the second attempt, it is imprudent to proceed to a third laryngoscopic attempt without first attempting FMV with cricoid pressure. Adopting a Failed Airway Algorithm approach at this point must be considered. If FMV is effective, provided the fetal distress has resolved, one should consider waking the patient up and proceeding with an awake technique to secure the airway (see Chapter 52).

In the presence of fetal distress, if FMV is effective with cricoid pressure, a decision should be made about proceeding. Factors to be considered in this decision include: the availability of extra assistance, the expected duration of the surgery, the skill of the obstetrician, the availability of equipment and skill to execute a definitive plan for securing the airway, and an assessment of the potential intraoperative complication this patient may pose (such as hemorrhage). A plan must be in place for securing the airway if a decision is made to proceed. If FMV is unsuccessful, even by easing the cricoid pressure, a rescue device should be placed.

The ASA Difficult Airway Algorithm[14] recommends that a laryngeal mask airway (LMA) be inserted as a rescue device for ventilation and oxygenation in a "can't ventilate, can't oxygenate" (CICO) situation. Failing that, the ASA algorithm recommends a FONA. It is the opinion of the authors and editors that a sequential approach in an airway emergency is imprudent, and a concurrent approach is advocated (see section "Failed Airway Algorithm" in Chapter 2).

The choice of which EGD is best in the CICO situation with a failed FMV has not been formally studied and remains subjective on the basis of availability of the EGD and the comfort and familiarity of the practitioner with the device. As the parturient has an increased aspiration risk, a second-generation device with an esophageal vent such as an LMA-ProSeal™ or a disposable LMA-Supreme™ (see Chapter 13) may be a more appropriate rescue device, as long as the practitioner is familiar with its placement. Anecdotal reports have demonstrated success with its use in similar circumstances with better seating and ventilation, and a reduced risk of aspiration related to the venting of contents through the gastric port.[15,16] The disadvantage of these devices is the inability to employ the device as an intubation conduit for securing the airway with an endotracheal tube (ETT). In contrast, an intubating LMA (ILMA; e.g., LMA-Fastrack, LMA-Protector™, i-gel®, Cook ILA, or Air-Q)[17] can facilitate tracheal intubation using a flexible bronchoscope (FB),[18] or a lightwand device.[19] The use of a flexible bronchoscope allows visualization of the cords, facilitating the placement of the ETT under indirect vision and avoiding potential trauma from a blind technique.

Placement of an EGD may be hindered by cricoid pressure. It has been suggested that relaxing cricoid pressure, briefly, may allow higher placement success rates.[20,21] Cricoid pressure has also been shown to reduce tidal volumes and increase airway pressures.[22] These difficulties have served to highlight recent studies questioning the efficacy of cricoid pressure in the prevention of aspiration and its hindrance in airway management.[23,24] Others, however, have not demonstrated such disadvantages.[25]

The current recommendations[26] and the rationale for them are presented in Chapter 2.

If One Is Successful in Providing Ventilation and Oxygenation with an EGD, Should One Proceed with the Cesarean Section?

When an airway cannot be secured with an ETT, EGDs are effective rescue aids. Following the insertion of the device, proper placement should be confirmed by end-tidal CO_2 ($ETCO_2$) detection, an unobstructed $ETCO_2$ trace pattern (if continuous capnography is employed), and adequate chest and abdominal excursion during ventilation.

While EGDs have been shown to be effective and safe in providing ventilation and oxygenation to healthy, nonobese, fasted parturients for elective cesarean section,[27] it is generally accepted that they should be used only as an emergency device for airway management in the parturient when tracheal intubation is unexpectedly difficult.[28] The decision to proceed with cesarean section in this circumstance should be on the basis of a risk–benefit assessment of the effectiveness of oxygenation, the condition of the fetus, the ability to expedite the delivery of the fetus, and ultimately, the safety of the parturient (context-sensitive). The Canadian Airway Focus Group publication has provided guidance consistent with these recommendations.[26]

Actions that may lead to regurgitation and aspiration must be minimized if one proceeds with an EGD as the airway. Coughing related to light anesthesia may lead to regurgitation and must be avoided. High intragastric pressure and incompetence of the lower esophageal sphincter likewise predispose to regurgitation. There is evidence that gastric insufflation leading to elevated intragastric pressure is reduced by the application of cricoid pressure,[29,30] and the avoidance of increased intragastric pressure may permit ventilation of the patient at lower peak airway pressures.[31] Finally, the obstetrician should be advised to minimize fundal pressure, if possible, during delivery of the baby.[32]

Should there be a serious doubt with regard to the safety of the mother in regard to difficult airway scenario options, the parturient should be awakened, despite the presence of fetal distress. An alternative means of intubation (such as a flexible bronchoscopic technique), or of anesthesia (regional or local anesthesia), should then be undertaken.

When Should One Proceed with a Surgical Airway? Who Should Do It? What Equipment Should Be Immediately Available on the Labor Unit?

A FONA in a parturient is performed when the patient cannot be ventilated or oxygenated (CICO, a failed airway). Clinically, the oxygen saturation declines rapidly due to an increased metabolic rate and a diminished FRC in the pregnant woman. Delay in recognizing a CICO failed airway contributes to adverse outcomes and increased maternal mortality.[33] Surgical and nursing support must be immediately available to assist as necessary.

Equipment for performing cricothyrotomy should be available in all maternity suites, and their use should be regularly reviewed. Chapter 14 provides a detailed description of the commercial kit recommended and the techniques of cricothyrotomy. In the situation that cricothyrotomy is unsuccessful, an additional technique for improving and maintaining oxygenation is ECMO cannulation. Unfortunately, the initiation of ECMO takes time and it would not be a useful emergency rescue oxygenation technique.

It should be emphasized that recognizing the potential for a difficult airway, avoiding delay in recognizing the CICO situation, and regularly practicing a failed intubation drill all contribute to improved outcomes. Although both surgical and anesthesia practitioners should be conversant with this procedure, the onus is on the anesthesia practitioner to perform the procedure if indicated. With the risk of the failed airway being 10 times more common in the parturient than in the general surgical population, it is mandatory that those who provide anesthesia care in the labor ward be trained in the use of these devices and techniques.[34]

POSTOPERATIVE CONSIDERATIONS

Having Secured the Airway, How Does One Manage This Patient Postoperatively?

The likelihood of successful extubation is on the basis of several factors and guided by the condition of the patient's airway, but must err on the side of caution. In situations in which airway edema is anticipated to increase, such as significant fluid resuscitation or an already edematous airway from trauma during intubation attempts, the prudent course is to ventilate the patient for 12 to 24 hours postoperatively in a 15- to 30-degree head-up position.

Consideration should also be given to the effect of residual sedatives, or the likely need for further sedatives or analgesics, in the postoperative period. The pharyngeal airway is a collapsible tube and its patency is regulated by upper airway dilating muscles. Increase in the dilating muscle activity acts to maintain the narrowed pharyngeal airway in awake patients with obstructive sleep apnea, and similar neural mechanisms presumably compensate for the progressive narrowing of the upper airway in parturients. Preservation of these neural regulatory mechanisms is, therefore, crucial for parturients with a high Mallampati class. General anesthesia, sedation, and residual anesthetic agents impede these neural compensatory mechanisms.

A trial of extubation may only be attempted if the patient is fully awake, neuromuscular blocking agents fully reversed, and preparations are in place for immediate reintubation. ETT exchange catheters may be placed through the tracheal tube prior to its removal to serve as a reintubation guide should it be required. The patient usually tolerates these small diameter devices reasonably well. These devices have a hollow lumen, providing limited gas insufflation capacity if reintubation over the catheter proves difficult or impossible. Employing a laryngoscope to straighten the angle of approach aids tracheal tube placement over an exchange catheter, as do smaller tracheal tubes that are less likely to impinge on the laryngeal structures. Increasing obstruction, significant respiratory effort, or increasing $PaCO_2$ are early indications of extubation failure.

SUMMARY

The incidence of the CICO failed airway is more than 10-fold in the parturient at term compared to the general surgical population. The obstetrical anesthesia practitioner must be prepared to manage the difficult and failed airway. Regular rehearsal of a failed airway plan of action along with the obstetric anesthesia team maintaining skills in the use of a rescue device (e.g., the intubating LMA) and ensuring that surgical airway devices are immediately available are essential components of that preparation.

SELF-EVALUATION QUESTIONS

54.1. Which of the following is **TRUE** with regard to the use of an LMA for the parturient undergoing the cesarean section under general anesthesia?

A. LMA can be used as a rescue device in a parturient with a failed airway undergoing emergency cesarean section.

B. LMA has been shown to be effective and safe in providing ventilation for all parturients undergoing cesarean section.

C. There are no data to support the use of LMA for any parturient undergoing cesarean section.

D. The LMA has been shown to be effective and safe in providing ventilation for obese parturients undergoing cesarean section.

E. Use of LMA is associated with a reduced risk of aspiration for parturients undergoing cesarean section.

54.2. What should the anesthesia practitioner do if the vocal cords cannot be seen after two attempts at laryngoscopy in a parturient requiring an emergency cesarean section for placenta previa associated with exsanguinating hemorrhage?

A. Awaken the patient and perform an awake fiberoptic intubation.

B. Awaken the patient and perform the cesarean section under regional anesthesia.

C. Immediate cricothyrotomy.

D. Ventilation using FMV or an EGD while maintaining cricoid pressure, and if oxygenation is unsatisfactory, proceed with the emergency surgical airway.

E. Reposition the head and neck of the parturient to facilitate further attempts of laryngoscopy.

54.3. Which of the following is a reasonable approach to minimize the risk of regurgitation and aspiration in a healthy parturient undergoing emergency cesarean section?

A. Preoperative oral administration of 0.3 M sodium citrate (30 mL)

B. Preoperative IV administration of ranitidine

C. Preoperative IV administration of metoclopramide

D. A designated assistant with experience in applying cricoid pressure during the rapid sequence intubation

E. All of the above

REFERENCES

1. Kuczkowski KM, Reisner LS, Benumof JL. Airway problems and new solutions for the obstetric patient. *J Clin Anesth.* 2003;15:552-563.
2. Pilkington S, Carli F, Dakin MJ, et al. Increase in Mallampati score during pregnancy. *Br J Anaesth.* 1995;74:638-642.
3. Watanabe T, Isono S, Tanaka A, Tanzawa H, Nishino T. Contribution of body habitus and craniofacial characteristics to segmental closing pressures of the passive pharynx in patients with sleep-disordered breathing. *Am J Respir Crit Care Med.* 2002;165:260-265.
4. Boutonnet M, Faitot V, Katz A, Salomon L, Keita H. Mallampati class changes during pregnancy, labour, and after delivery: can these be predicted? *Br J Anaesth.* 2010;104:67-70.
5. Kodali BS, Chandrasekhar S, Bulich LN, Topulos GP, Datta S. Airway changes during labor and delivery. *Anesthesiology.* 2008;108:357-362.
6. Tagaito Y, Isono S, Remmers JE, Tanaka A, Nishino T. Lung volume and collapsibility of the passive pharynx in patients with sleep-disordered breathing. *J Appl Physiol.* 2007;103:1379-1385.
7. Rocke DA, Murray WB, Rout CC, Gouws E. Relative risk analysis of factors associated with difficult intubation in obstetric anesthesia. *Anesthesiology.* 1992;77:67-73.
8. Lane S, Saunders D, Schofield A, Padmanabhan R, Hildreth A, Laws D. A prospective, randomised controlled trial comparing the efficacy of pre-oxygenation in the 20 degrees head-up vs supine position. *Anaesthesia.* 2005;60:1064-1067.
9. Baraka A, Haroun-Bizri S, Khoury S, Chehab IR. Single vital capacity breath for preoxygenation. *Can J Anaesth.* 2000;47:1144-1146.
10. Nimmagadda U, Chiravuri SD, Salem MR, et al. Preoxygenation with tidal volume and deep breathing techniques: the impact of duration of breathing and fresh gas flow. *Anesth Analg.* 2001;92:1337-1341.
11. Weingart SD, Levitan RM. Preoxygenation and prevention of desaturation during emergency airway management. *Ann Emerg Med.* 2012;59: 165-175 e1.
12. Mushambi MC, Kinsella SM, Popat M, et al. Obstetric Anaesthetists' Association and Difficult Airway Society guidelines for the management of difficult and failed tracheal intubation in obstetrics. *Anaesthesia.* 2015;70:1286-1306.
13. Russell IF, Chambers WA. Closing volume in normal pregnancy. *Br J Anaesth.* 1981;53:1043-1047.
14. Apfelbaum JL, Hagberg CA, Connis RT, et al. 2022 American society of anesthesiologists practice guidelines for management of the difficult airway. *Anesthesiology.* 2022;136(1):31-81.
15. Awan R, Nolan JP, Cook TM. Use of a ProSeal laryngeal mask airway for airway maintenance during emergency Caesarean section after failed tracheal intubation. *Br J Anaesth.* 2004;92:144-146.
16. Keller C, Brimacombe J, Lirk P, Puhringer F. Failed obstetric tracheal intubation and postoperative respiratory support with the ProSeal laryngeal mask airway. *Anesth Analg.* 2004;98:1467-1470, table of contents.
17. Minville V, N'Guyen L, Coustet B, Fourcade O, Samii K. Difficult airway in obstetric using Ilma-Fastrach. *Anesth Analg.* 2004;99:1873.
18. Joo HS, Rose DK. The intubating laryngeal mask airway with and without fiberoptic guidance. *Anesth Analg.* 1999;88:662-666.
19. Fan KH, Hung OR, Agro F. A comparative study of tracheal intubation using an intubating laryngeal mask (Fastrach) alone or together with a lightwand (Trachlight). *J Clin Anesth.* 2000;12:581-585.
20. Aoyama K, Takenaka I, Sata T, Shigematsu A. Cricoid pressure impedes positioning and ventilation through the laryngeal mask airway. *Can J Anaesth.* 1996;43:1035-1040.
21. Harry RM, Nolan JP. The use of cricoid pressure with the intubating laryngeal mask. *Anaesthesia.* 1999;54:656-659.
22. Hocking G, Roberts FL, Thew ME. Airway obstruction with cricoid pressure and lateral tilt. *Anaesthesia.* 2001;56:825-828.
23. Jackson SH. Efficacy and safety of cricoid pressure needs scientific validation. *Anesthesiology.* 1996;84:751-752.
24. Janda M, Vagts DA, Noldge-Schomburg GF. Cricoid pressure—safety necessity or unnecessary risk?. *Anaesthesiol Reanim.* 2004;29:4-7.
25. Brimacombe JR, Berry AM. Cricoid pressure. *Can J Anaesth.* 1997;44:414-425.

26. Law JA, Duggan LV, Asselin M, et al. The Difficult Airway with Consensus-Based Recommendations for Management. Part 1. Difficult Airway Management Encountered in an Unconscious Patient. *Can J Anesth.* 2021;68: 1373-1404.
27. Han TH, Brimacombe J, Lee EJ, Yang HS. The laryngeal mask airway is effective (and probably safe) in selected healthy parturients for elective Cesarean section: a prospective study of 1067 cases. *Can J Anaesth.* 2001;48: 1117-1121.
28. Preston R. The evolving role of the laryngeal mask airway in obstetrics. *Can J Anaesth.* 2001;48:1061-1065.
29. Asai T, Barclay K, McBeth C, Vaughan RS. Cricoid pressure applied after placement of the laryngeal mask prevents gastric insufflation but inhibits ventilation. *Br J Anaesth.* 1996;76:772-776.
30. Lawes EG, Campbell I, Mercer D. Inflation pressure, gastric insufflation and rapid sequence induction. *Br J Anaesth.* 1987;59:315-318.
31. Moynihan RJ, Brock-Utne JG, Archer JH, Feld LH, Kreitzman TR. The effect of cricoid pressure on preventing gastric insufflation in infants and children. *Anesthesiology.* 1993;78:652-656.
32. Hartsilver EL, Vanner RG, Bewley J, Clayton T. Gastric pressure during emergency caesarean section under general anaesthesia. *Br J Anaesth.* 1999;82:752-754.
33. Walls RM. Management of the difficult airway in the trauma patient. *Emerg Med Clin North Am.* 1998;16:45-61.
34. Samsoon GL, Young JR. Difficult tracheal intubation: a retrospective study. *Anaesthesia.* 1987;42:487-490.

CHAPTER 55

Airway Management in the Pregnant Trauma Victim

Christina Ratto and Holly A. Muir

CASE PRESENTATION

A 35-year-old pregnant woman, approximately 36 weeks gestation, is admitted to the emergency department (ED) following a motor vehicle crash. She has a closed head injury, bilateral femoral fractures, and possible abdominal trauma. Her Glasgow Coma Scale (GCS) score is 5: she does not open her eyes (1); there is no audible vocalization (1); and she is showing decorticate rigidity (3). Her heart rate is 135 beats per minute, blood pressure is 85/40 mmHg, and respiratory rate is 40 breaths per minute and shallow. Fetal heart rate (FHR) is 110 beats per minute. Her oxygen saturation (SaO_2) is 90% on a non-rebreathing oxygen mask. A cervical collar is in place and Thomas splints are being applied to both legs.

INITIAL ASSESSMENT OF THE PATIENT

What Are the Immediate Evaluation and Management Priorities in This Patient?

Initial evaluation and management priorities for the near-term parturient are no different than any other trauma victim—assessment of airway, breathing, and circulation (ABCs), followed by a secondary survey, including assessment of the abdomen and fetus.

Unique considerations related to the pregnancy, such as supine hypotensive syndrome and the significant capillary engorgement of the nasal and oropharyngeal mucosa, may impact positioning, hemodynamics, and airway management.[1]

Immediate attention is directed to the airway. Her GCS and oxygen saturations mandate endotracheal intubation and ventilation. She is not a crash airway, and therefore, there is time for an airway evaluation utilizing the MOANS, LEMON, CRANE, RODS, and SHORT mnemonics (see Chapter 1). In this particular patient, difficulty should be anticipated and an approach as suggested in the Difficult Airway Algorithm (see Chapter 2) adopted; recognizing that parturients at term have a substantially elevated risk of aspiration, particularly in this circumstance where protective airway reflexes are compromised and the patient is not responding to commands.

Following airway management, attention is directed to an assessment of breathing. Her lung fields must be evaluated for presence, equality, and quality of breath sounds. This evaluation, coupled with a stat portable chest X-ray, may uncover a pneumothorax and/or hemothorax that may require treatment.

In pregnancy, minute ventilation is normally increased by approximately 45%, largely through an increase in tidal volume. This increased minute ventilation results in a fall in $PaCO_2$ to approximately 30 mmHg. Therefore, one should initially (moderately and empirically) hyperventilate this patient. Ventilation may be guided by arterial blood gases, once resuscitation has been established.

Pregnant women should be considered to have a full stomach after 18 weeks gestation. There is an increase in gastric acid production, which results in both an increase in gastric fluid volume and a decrease in pH. Coupled with a decrease in the competency of the lower esophageal sphincter, the risk of reflux is greatly enhanced. The most effective protection against aspiration in this situation is the presence of a cuffed endotracheal tube (ETT) in the trachea.

The final step of the primary survey is directed toward the evaluation and management of circulation. This patient is hypotensive. Attention should be given to volume resuscitation and positioning to minimize supine hypotensive syndrome (or aortocaval compression syndrome). A wedge should be placed under the right hip to create 30 degrees of left uterine displacement. This will reduce aortocaval compression and improve systemic and placental perfusion.[2] Large-bore IV cannulas and fluids must be initiated as the parturient can lose 30% of her blood volume before demonstrating cardiovascular changes.[3] There is a strong correlation between hypotension and negative outcomes after a brain injury for both the mother and the fetus. Relative anemia (approximately 11 g·dL^{-1} or 6.9 mmol·L^{-1}), related to an increased blood volume, is a physiologic response to pregnancy. In a healthy near-term parturient, blood pressure may remain at near normal values until greater than 1000 mL of blood loss occurs. In addition to the usual sources of blood loss in a trauma victim, the uterus can be a source of significant hemorrhage. For example, both placental and uterine abruption may be associated with blunt abdominal trauma, such as a seat belt injury.

Having addressed the primary ABCs, attention can now be turned to the secondary survey, focusing on her head injury, her abdomen, stabilization of her fractures, and her fetus. Her GCS of less than 7 indicates a significant head injury and she is at risk of further decompensation at any time. Securing an airway in a timely fashion may be critical in limiting hypoxic brain injury, and avoiding elevations in intracranial pressure (ICP) related to elevations of $PaCO_2$.[4]

AIRWAY CONSIDERATIONS

What Is Unique About Managing the Airway Urgently in a Patient with a Traumatic Brain Injury, Who Also Happens to Be a Near-Term Parturient?

As discussed above, the practitioner must deal with multiple concerns. The patient has features suggestive of difficult intubation, specifically, difficult face-mask ventilation (FMV) and difficult extraglottic device (EGD) use. A secondary concern is suspicion of blunt chest trauma. Acute severe head injury and the risk of aspiration mandate a need for rapid and atraumatic intubation, guided by the principles of airway evaluation and management articulated in Chapter 2. The practitioner has time to call for help and a difficult airway cart, since the SaO_2 is acceptable (while borderline), and the FHR is normal. The airway practitioner should begin denitrogenation quickly, using high-flow oxygen and a non-rebreather facemask.

Assisted ventilation may be required, but care should be taken to avoid gastric insufflation. The rapid respiratory rate makes this a challenge. If the practitioner is not confident that tracheal intubation will be successful in their hands, or that the ability to provide gas exchange using FMV or EGD will be successful following induction and paralysis, an "awake look" with a laryngoscope (direct laryngoscopy [DL] or indirect (video) laryngoscopy [VL]) will influence the decision either to proceed with a rapid sequence induction (RSI), or move directly to a surgical airway. The need to maintain in-line stabilization of the C-spine may also influence this decision.

Should RSI be selected in the setting of a patient with acute severe head injury, the administration of pretreatment agents to attenuate rise in ICP may be prudent (see Chapter 17). The selection of an induction agent and the dose employed will be guided by the degree of hemodynamic stability, and in this case, is likely to be etomidate at a reduced dose (e.g., 0.2 mg·kg^{-1}). The dose of the neuromuscular blocker, such as succinylcholine, is never modified and is 1.5 mg·kg^{-1}.

Alternatively, an "awake look" with a DL or VL to determine suitability for tracheal intubation may be performed. This patient has a GCS of 5 and may not require sedation (e.g., etomidate titration). However, patients with acute severe head injury may present with a clenched jaw, prohibiting an awake look. If this occurs, the only options are RSI or cricothyrotomy.

Medications and tools for induction of anesthesia and muscle paralysis must be prepared prior to attempting to secure the airway. A selection of intubation and rescue airway devices familiar to the airway practitioner must also be prepared. In this case, laryngoscopic intubation is judged to be highly likely (Plan A). Plan B is to use an EGD, preferably one that permits intubation through it (e.g., LMA-Fastrach or LMA-Evo), and Plan C is a front-of-neck access (FONA) in the event that both fail.

Following denitrogenation with 100% oxygen via a face mask and the application of nasal cannula oxygen at 10 to 15 L·min^{-1}, induction and paralytic medications are administered. An experienced assistant should apply cricoid pressure, and a second assistant should maintain manual in-line stabilization of the neck. The trachea is successfully intubated on this first attempt using a video laryngoscope with the hyperangulated blade (C-MAC D-Blade), and after detection of end-tidal carbon dioxide confirms tracheal placement, the ETT is secured. An orogastric tube may be placed to remove gastric contents in order to reduce the risk of aspiration.

As a cautionary note, despite the advances that are continuously made in airway management, the incidence of failed or difficult airway in an obstetrical population remains higher than that seen in the general population. An Australian multiinstitution audit conducted to assess the practice of general anesthesia for cesarean section confirmed an incidence of failed intubation of 1:274, and difficult intubation of 1:30.[5] These numbers are generally quoted in the literature.

The reason why intubation is more difficult in pregnancy is controversial. Some have argued that the difficulty is self-imposed: by anxiety related to the urgency of situation; inexperienced anesthesia practitioners performing the procedure; a lack of opportunity to practice skills; and as a consequence of the prevalence of regional anesthesia in obstetrics.[6,7] Regardless of the reasons, the potential loss of an airway with resulting hypoxemia and increased possibility of aspiration place the mother's and her fetus' life at risk.

In our case, the status of an unclear C-spine carries additional risk of injury if a difficult intubation is encountered.

If, on assessment of this mother, there is any element of doubt about one's ability to efficiently and safely place a tracheal tube, a strong argument can be made for a FONA (without paralysis or sedation) by a skilled practitioner. She may well need a tracheotomy for prolonged ventilation at any rate.

How Would You Secure the Airway If There Are Three Attempts at Laryngoscopic Intubation?

Help and a difficult airway cart, if not already present, should be summoned. While maintaining cricoid pressure, ventilation should be provided by FMV with 100% oxygen. Gradual relaxation of cricoid pressure may be indicated if it is felt to hinder the ability to ventilate. If, at any point, the ability to maintain oxygen saturation is lost, an immediate FONA is indicated. As preparations for the FONA are underway, an EGD (preferably an intubating LMA such as the LMA-Evo) can be inserted. Should this reestablish adequate oxygenation, tracheal intubation through the intubating LMA can be considered. Oxygen desaturation and hypotension are associated with poor outcomes in patients with acute severe head injury.

What Specific Concerns Related to the Airway Do You Have If This Patient Needs to Be Transported to the Radiology Suite for Diagnostic Imaging?

This patient will require ongoing sedation, paralysis, and mechanical ventilation during transport to maintain oxygenation and to keep her $PaCO_2$ within her physiologic range (between 30 and 32 mmHg). Although hypocapnia has traditionally been considered an important part of management of traumatic brain injury (increased ICP) in pregnancy, a reduction in $PaCO_2$ below 30 mmHg can be associated with a harmful reduction in uterine and cerebral blood flow, which compromises fetal perfusion.[8] Following the acute resuscitation phase, $PaCO_2$ levels should be monitored continuously by capnometry/capnography, or periodically by arterial blood gas sampling.

The ETT should be properly secured as movement from stretchers to radiology tables increases the risk of accidental extubation. In addition, appropriate equipment and personnel to manage reintubation should be immediately available, including drugs (both induction agents and neuromuscular blocking drugs), laryngoscopes, ETTs, and rescue devices (including an Eschmann Tracheal Introducer [commonly known as a "bougie"] and an EGD).

Are the Use of Sedating Drugs and Muscle Relaxants Safe in Pregnancy?

The duration of action of agents such as vecuronium and rocuronium may be prolonged in the pregnant patient. Therefore, in *nonresuscitation situations*, dosing should be titrated using a neuromuscular function monitor.[9] Although small amounts of nondepolarizing muscle relaxants are known to cross the placenta to the fetus when administered as a bolus, there are no reports of adverse fetal effects. The fetal effects of prolonged (greater than 24 hours) neuromuscular blocking drug administration to the mother are unknown. It has been shown that the fetal/maternal ratio of vecuronium increases significantly with prolonged induction to delivery times.[10] In a scenario such as this, personnel must be prepared to either ventilate using a face mask, or intubate the trachea of a neonate should the need arise.

All patients intubated during an emergency resuscitation ought to receive sufficient sedation and muscle relaxation to facilitate mechanical ventilation and attenuate the stress responses (increased airway resistance, ICP, blood pressure, and heart rate). This is particularly important in patients with increased ICP, such as this patient. Drug selection in pregnancy is somewhat problematic as few of the available drugs are approved for use in parturients. Although the key teratogenic period is from 31 to 71 days postconception, fetal brain and organ development continue throughout gestation, rendering them susceptible to adverse effects of agents administered to the mother.

The prevailing wisdom in the decision-making process is to bear in mind that the general health and well-being of the fetus is *entirely* dependent on the survival and well-being of the mother. As a general principle, drugs with a known "safe" history of use in pregnancy, such as thiopental and fentanyl, can be used. There is a growing body of evidence that propofol is also safe, although the experience is substantially less than those for thiopental and fentanyl. The fact that propofol is commonly used in the care of adult patients with neurotrauma would suggest its favorable application in this case. Despite traditional cautions regarding the possible teratogenic effects of benzodiazepines, evidence indicates that these agents are not proven teratogens.[11] The safety of etomidate in pregnancy has not been established. The drug crosses the placenta and has been shown to produce a fall in serum cortisol in the fetus lasting for about 6 hours. The significance of this finding is unclear. The selection of etomidate in this case was driven by the considerable hemodynamic instability noted in the mother. By and large, there is little evidence that a single dose of any currently available IV induction agent is harmful to the fetus.

OTHER CONSIDERATIONS

What Fetal Monitoring Is Required in This Situation?

Fetal monitoring during trauma resuscitation is often challenging because of limited access to the abdomen. Continuous fetal monitoring is possible from about 18 weeks' gestational age, although it is technically difficult to perform transabdominally early in gestation. FHR variability as an indicator of fetal well-being is usually not established until 25 to 27 weeks of gestation. Additionally, sedating agents affect FHR variability, further limiting its usefulness.[12] Therefore, persistent and marked fetal bradycardia may be the only true indicator of fetal distress in early pregnancy, or in pregnant patients receiving sedating medications.

Blunt or penetrating abdominal trauma places the fetus directly at risk due to the potential for placental abruption or uterine hypoperfusion related to maternal hemodynamic instability.

As indicated above, it is reasonable to use continuous fetal monitoring in a pregnant trauma victim if it is physically possible. This assumes that personnel skilled in FHR trace readings are available and a plan to deliver the fetus is executed if there is evidence of fetal compromise. The American College of Obstetricians and Gynecologists supports a position of individualizing the use of monitoring in these situations, as a team approach to optimize the safety of both the mother and the fetus.[13] After 35 weeks' gestation, delivery results in minimal morbidity to the fetus.

What Findings Would Lead to a Decision to Expedite the Delivery of the Fetus?

Evaluation of the pregnant trauma victim involves the evaluation of two patients: the mother and the fetus. Assessment and stabilization of the mother is always the first priority. Occasionally, the resuscitation of the mother requires the delivery of the fetus. The classic example is during maternal cardiac arrest. If the fetus is older than 23 weeks and if it has not been possible to resuscitate the mother after 4 minutes of cardiopulmonary resuscitation (CPR), the fetus should be delivered by emergency cesarean section. This is done to improve fetal outcome and the effectiveness of maternal CPR by removing any aortocaval compression.

In cases where the mother is hemodynamically unstable secondary to hemorrhage and possible placental abruption, delivery of the fetus may be necessary as part of maternal resuscitation. Immediate induction of anesthesia with airway management is mandated.

A more common scenario is that of a hemodynamically stable mother with a fetus demonstrating signs of terminal fetal distress (severe fetal bradycardia). This situation parallels any other emergency cesarean section for fetal distress. As in all situations where anesthesia induction agents and muscle relaxants are used, plans (Plan A, B, and C) must be in place for management of the potential failed intubation.

SUMMARY

The management of trauma in a parturient often provides significant challenges for practitioners. The physiologic changes of pregnancy must be considered when one interprets vital signs, response to resuscitative maneuvers, and laboratory investigations in these trauma victims. The fetus adds a second dimension to the resuscitation, although maternal well-being and safety should remain the primary concern.

The benefit of left uterine displacement as part of the resuscitation must be recognized. Airway protection is a critical part of management as these patients are at higher risk of aspiration due to the physiologic and mechanical changes of pregnancy. The value of airway management algorithms in crisis situations, such as the resuscitation of the parturient, cannot be overemphasized.

SELF-EVALUATION QUESTIONS

55.1. Which of the following anesthetic induction agents has been shown in clinical trials to be safe for a pregnant patient?

A. Etomidate
B. Propofol
C. Thiopental
D. Ketamine
E. None of the above

55.2. During a rapid sequence induction for an emergency cesarean section, you are neither able to intubate nor oxygenate the patient. Which of the following is NOT an appropriate course of action?

A. Repeating laryngoscopy and intubation
B. Ventilation using Combitube™
C. Immediate preparations for cricothyrotomy
D. Ventilation using an LMA
E. Relaxing cricoid pressure to determine if FMV can be improved

55.3. Which of the following is NOT an indication to deliver the fetus in a trauma victim who is 37 weeks pregnant?

A. To aid in the resuscitation of the mother, the fetus must be delivered in an expeditious fashion.
B. Maternal cardiac arrest.
C. Hemodynamically stable mother and the fetus is showing signs of terminal fetal distress with severe fetal bradycardia.
D. The mother is hemodynamically unstable secondary to hemorrhage and placental abruption.
E. Maternal respiratory arrest.

REFERENCES

1. Leontic EA. Respiratory disease in pregnancy. *Med Clin North Am.* 1977;61:111-128.
2. Camann WR, Ostheimer GW. Physiological adaptations during pregnancy. *Int Anesthesiol Clin.* 1990;28:2-10.
3. ACOG educational bulletin. Obstetric aspects of trauma management. Number 251, September 1998 (replaces Number 151, January 1991, and Number 161, November 1991). American College of Obstetricians and Gynecologists. *Int J Gynaecol Obstet.* 1999;64:87-94.
4. Gelb AW, Manninen PH, Mezon BJ, Lee RJ, Durward QJ. The anaesthetist and the head-injured patient. *Can Anaesth Soc J.* 1984;31:98-108.
5. McDonnell NJ, Paech MJ, Clavisi OM, Scott KL. Difficult and failed intubation in obstetric anaesthesia: an observational study of airway management and complications associated with general anaesthesia for caesarean section. *Int J Obstet Anesth.* 2008;17:292-297.
6. Djabatey EA, Barclay PM. Difficult and failed intubation in 3430 obstetric general anaesthetics. *Anaesthesia.* 2009;64:1168-1171.
7. Goldszmidt E. Principles and practices of obstetric airway management. *Anesthesiol Clin.* 2008;26:109-125, vii.
8. Morishima HO, Daniel SS, Adamsons K Jr., James LS. Effects of positive pressure ventilation of the mother upon the acid-base state of the fetus. *Am J Obstet Gynecol.* 1965;93:269-273.
9. Khuenl-Brady KS, Koller J, Mair P, Puhringer F, Mitterschiffthaler G. Comparison of vecuronium- and atracurium-induced neuromuscular blockade in postpartum and nonpregnant patients. *Anesth Analg.* 1991;72:110-113.
10. Iwama H, Kaneko T, Tobishima S, Komatsu T, Watanabe K, Akutsu H. Time dependency of the ratio of umbilical vein/maternal artery concentrations of vecuronium in caesarean section. *Acta Anaesthesiol Scand.* 1999;43:9-12.
11. Sheppard T. *Catalog of Teratogenic Agents.* 7th edn. ed. Baltimore, MD: John Hopkins University Press; 1992.
12. Immer-Bansi A, Immer FF, Henle S, Sporri S, Petersen-Felix S. Unnecessary emergency caesarean section due to silent CTG during anaesthesia? *Br J Anaesth.* 2001;87:791-793.
13. ACOG Committee on Obstetric Practice. ACOG Committee Opinion Number 284, August 2003: Nonobstetric surgery in pregnancy. *Obstet Gynecol* 2003;102:431.

CHAPTER 56

Appendicitis in Pregnancy

Allana Munro, Brendan E. Morgan, and Ronald B. George

CASE PRESENTATION

A 20-year-old female, G1P0 at 17 weeks' gestation, presents to the emergency department complaining of right-sided abdominal pain. The pain began 10 hours ago accompanied by nausea and two episodes of vomiting. The patient is afebrile and has a blood pressure of 130/72 mmHg. Her heart rate is 86 beats per minute (bpm) and respiratory rate is 20 breaths per minute. She weighs 198 lb (90 kg) and is 5 ft 7 in (169 cm) in height, with a body mass index (BMI) of 31 $kg \cdot m^{-2}$. She admits to right-sided tenderness to palpation, localized to the inguinal region. After ultrasonography by an obstetrician, the cause of pain is felt not to be related to pregnancy. The general surgery service is consulted, and it is their opinion that the patient has appendicitis and will require a laparoscopic appendectomy.

The parturient has had an unremarkable pregnancy thus far and has no medical comorbidities or allergies. She is a nonsmoker and does not consume alcohol. She takes prenatal vitamins, but no prescription medications. She has had no prior anesthetics and has no family history of anesthesia-related problems. Physical examination of her heart and lungs is unremarkable. There are no physical abnormalities of her spine. Her airway examination reveals a Mallampati Class IV airway with limited mouth opening. She has a normal range of motion of her cervical spine, full dentition, and minimal mandibular protrusion. The thyromental distance is 5 cm and the hyomental distance is 3 cm.

INTRODUCTION

What Is the Incidence of Appendicitis in Pregnancy?

The incidence of acute appendicitis in pregnancy has been reported between 1:1000 and 1:1500,[1–5] which is similar to the incidence in nonpregnant women of childbearing age.[6] Appendicitis is the most common nonobstetrical cause of acute abdomen in the parturient, and appendectomy is the most common nonobstetrical surgical procedure performed during pregnancy.[7] Relative incidence varies throughout pregnancy, ranging from 19% to 36% during the first trimester, 27% to 60% during the second trimester, and 15% to 33% during the third trimester of pregnancy.[8] While pregnancy does not appear to increase the risk of appendicitis, the anatomic and physiologic changes that accompany pregnancy may obscure the diagnosis.[9] Perforation and complicated acute appendicitis may be more prevalent in pregnant patients than in the nonpregnant population,[9,10] though some recent studies dispute this notion.[11,12] The risk of appendiceal perforation ranges from 11% to 43%,[5,10–13] and increases with advanced gestation and delay in diagnosis.[13,14]

Parturients with appendicitis are at increased risk of perinatal morbidity and mortality. Historically, premature delivery occurred at a rate of 15% to 45%, although a recent, large population study demonstrated an incidence of 4% to 11%.[12] The rate of fetal loss for simple and complex appendectomies is 2% and 6%, respectively,[12] which is much lower than what had been historically found in smaller studies.[15] The risk of maternal mortality is minimal, and the decrease in morbidity and mortality may be attributed to the use of advanced antibiotics, close perioperative monitoring, multidisciplinary case involvement, and improved perioperative management.[16]

How Is Appendicitis Diagnosed During Pregnancy?

Anatomic and physiologic changes accompanying pregnancy and labor (such as the gravid uterus, physiologic leukocytosis, and nausea and vomiting) may make the diagnosis of appendicitis challenging by confounding clinical signs and diagnostic tests. While delayed recognition increases risk of perforation, preterm delivery, and fetal demise, multiple studies have also shown that appendicitis can also be "overdiagnosed" in obstetrical patients. The rate of negative appendectomy is significantly higher in obstetrical patients (9-31%) than for nonpregnant women of childbearing age (3-18%).[8,10,12,17] Unfortunately, unnecessary surgery for a negative appendectomy confers a higher risk of premature delivery and fetal demise than an appendectomy for simple appendicitis.[12,17]

A recent study demonstrated that the clinical presentation of acute appendicitis is similar among pregnant and nonpregnant women of reproductive age.[11] Despite the appendix being pushed superiorly and laterally with advancing gestation,[18] right lower quadrant pain, located at McBurney's point, remains the most common symptom of appendicitis for patients in all trimesters of pregnancy,[19] and it is the presenting complaint for 85% of pregnant patients with acute appendicitis.[20] Furthermore, the Alvarado Score, a validated diagnostic tool used for assessing patients with suspected appendicitis, performs with similar efficacy in pregnant and nonpregnant patients.[21]

Due to its availability and safety profile, ultrasound is the modality of choice for diagnostic imaging of the appendix in pregnancy. It may be useful for identifying a normal appendix and ruling out other causes of abdominal pain in pregnancy.[22] Unfortunately, due to the size of the gravid uterus, it may be difficult to localize the appendix during the third trimester.[23]

Despite its routine use, ultrasound has only been found to have a sensitivity of 46.1% for diagnosing appendicitis in pregnancy.[23] In the event of an inconclusive ultrasound exam, computed tomography (CT) and magnetic resonance imaging (MRI) are both options. CT is widely available and effective in the diagnosis of appendicitis in pregnancy, with a reported sensitivity of 85.7% and specificity of 97.4%.[24] While, with modifications, fetal radiation exposure with a helical CT scan is less than 3 mGy, well below the 30 mGy limit considered a risk for carcinogenesis.[25] However, concern about fetal radiation exposure has limited the use of CT. Comparatively, a meta-analysis evaluating the use of MRI for diagnosing appendicitis during pregnancy reported a sensitivity of 94% and a specificity of 97%.[26] In pregnancy, gadolinium is not routinely administered due to theoretical fetal safety concerns, as contrast agents have been shown to cross the placenta.[27] Length of time to access MRI may be a limitation, and the diagnostic benefit must be weighed against the risk of appendiceal rupture. Because of its superior safety profile and diagnostic performance, MRI has become the diagnostic modality of choice when ultrasound evaluation of appendicitis during pregnancy is inconclusive.[26–28] However, if MRI is not immediately available, CT is a reasonable and effective imaging modality in the face of an unclear ultrasound diagnosis.

What Are the Options for Managing Appendicitis in Pregnancy?

Traditionally, acute appendicitis has been treated with surgical appendectomy combined with intravenous antibiotics.[29] Recently, conservative management with only antibiotics has been suggested for nonpregnant patients with acute appendicitis.[30,31] A meta-analysis suggested that antibiotics are both effective and safe as primary treatment for patients with uncomplicated acute appendicitis.[31] While this nonsurgical option has not been fully evaluated in the pregnant population, there are reports describing successful management of acute, uncomplicated appendicitis in pregnancy with conservative antibiotic treatment.[5,29,32] However, to date, medical management of uncomplicated acute appendicitis in pregnant patients is not advised because of a likely higher rate of peritonitis, fetal demise, shock, and venous thromboembolism, as compared to surgical management.[5,33] Therefore, the majority of parturients continue to be managed with a surgical approach.

There are two surgical options for removing the appendix. Appendectomy can be performed via an exploratory laparotomy (open technique) or laparoscopic technique. A population-based cohort study from 2003 to 2010 evaluating perinatal outcomes in pregnant patients with appendicitis found that 60.3% of patients were managed by laparotomy, 30.7% were managed by laparoscopy, and 9.1% were managed medically.[34] However, in a 20-year Danish population-based prevalence study of obstetric and nonobstetric surgery during pregnancy, the proportion of appendectomies conducted laparoscopically has increased relative to laparotomy in all trimesters (4.2-79.2%).[35]

There is debate around the optimal surgical approach; however, laparoscopic appendectomy is now suggested as a standard approach for pregnant patients.[36,37] The cited advantages of the open technique include better direct visualization, decreased operating room costs, and reduced fetal exposure to carbon dioxide. In addition, an open appendectomy is an established and safe operation, with acceptable morbidity and low mortality rates.[16]

Studies have shown that laparoscopy is also safe and effective, with very low rates of preterm delivery and, in most series, no reports of fetal demise.[38–40] The advantages of the laparoscopic technique include fewer wound infections, reduced postoperative pain and opioid use, reduced uterine handling, early return of gastrointestinal function, reduced risk of ileus, earlier ambulation, and shorter hospital stay. The disadvantages of laparoscopic technique include potential uterine or fetal injury, reduced cardiac output and uterine blood flow, preterm labor, and fetal acidosis.[40–42] There is mixed evidence regarding outcomes in laparoscopy compared to laparotomy. In a recent meta-analysis of 21 studies of 6276 patients, laparoscopy was associated with an increased risk of fetal loss without a difference in any other postoperative or obstetric outcomes.[43] However, a recent large retrospective cohort study of 6018 pregnant patients found laparoscopy was associated with a lower risk of fetal adverse events, such as stillbirth and premature labor; lower incidence of blood transfusion; shorter operative time; and shorter stay in hospital. Laparoscopic appendectomy is considered safe during any trimester; however, pregnant patients should receive venous thromboembolism prophylaxis due to a risk of venous stasis secondary to carbon dioxide pneumoperitoneum.[40] Other obstetrical outcomes, such as Apgar score at one minute after delivery, birth weight, preterm birth rates, and surgical outcomes, such as wound infection rates, intraoperative duration, and postoperative hospital stay duration did not differ between operative approaches in a recent metaanalysis.[44]

How Does Laparoscopy Impact Physiology in the Pregnant Patient?

The physiologic changes accompanying the pregnant state are reviewed in detail in standard obstetric anesthesia texts. Under normal circumstances, the creation of the pneumoperitoneum will impact cardiovascular and respiratory physiology.[40] Carbon dioxide insufflation of the peritoneal cavity will initially increase venous return as intravascular blood volume is augmented by compression of the splanchnic vasculature. The result is an increase in cardiac output and arterial blood pressure. Sympathetic nervous system activation due to carbon dioxide absorption causes an increase in systemic vascular resistance.[45] As intra-abdominal pressure increases beyond 15 mmHg, venous return will then decrease due to compression of the vena cava leading to a reduction in cardiac output and hypotension. Intra-abdominal pressures should be limited to 10 to 15 mmHg.[40] Pressures of 15 mmHg have been used without increasing adverse outcomes to the patient or the fetus.[38] Insufflation may also result in bradyarrhythmia due to vagal effects from peritoneal stretching, or tachyarrhythmia due to sympathetic activation and hypercarbia. Aortocaval compression secondary to pregnancy may be exacerbated by the elevated intra-abdominal pressure and may compromise uterine and placental perfusion. Patients should be positioned with left uterine displacement to maximize uterine perfusion. The pneumoperitoneum decreases pulmonary and thoracic compliance and increases peak inspiratory pressures. Elevation of the diaphragm further reduces the functional residual capacity, possibly leading to hypoxemia.[40] Carbon dioxide absorption may produce respiratory acidosis. These changes may lead to fetal compromise as a result of hypotension, hypoxemia, and fetal acidosis. Other sources of respiratory complications include subcutaneous emphysema, pneumothorax, endobronchial intubation, and gas embolism.

ANESTHETIC MANAGEMENT

What Are the Anesthetic Options for Laparoscopic Appendectomy?

General and regional anesthesia are both anesthetic options for laparoscopic procedures in the nonparturient patient.[45] Regional anesthesia for laparoscopy, such as epidural or spinal techniques, are not recommended in pregnancy. The pneumoperitoneum may increase intra-abdominal pressures causing the gravid uterus to compromise spontaneous ventilation leading to hypercarbia and hypoxemia, and increase the risk of regurgitation and aspiration.[41] In addition, diaphragmatic irritation due to carbon dioxide insufflation can produce shoulder tip pain, necessitating supplementation with sedatives and analgesics. Therefore, general anesthesia with endotracheal intubation may be a better choice to provide a secure airway. In addition, general anesthesia permits controlled ventilation to avoid hypercarbia and hypoxemia and allows the use of muscle relaxants to facilitate surgery.

What Are Your Concerns in Giving a General Anesthetic to a 17-Week Pregnant Patient?

A recent, large Danish registry-based cohort study examining nonobstetric abdominal surgery during pregnancy found that, when compared to pregnant patients who did not require surgery, nonobstetric surgery conferred an increased hazard ratio for small-for-gestational age, preterm birth, and miscarriage (1.3, 2.1-2.8, and 3.1, respectively).[46]

Surgery should be done at an institution with neonatal and pediatric services and where an obstetric care provider with cesarean delivery privileges is readily available.[47]

Special considerations must be given to the well-being and the safety of the fetus. To address the concern of drugs administered to females during pregnancy, the US Federal Drug Administration (FDA) published the classification of drugs for teratogenic risk in 1994.[48] In general, anesthetic drugs and muscle relaxants fall into the category "C" group, for which risks cannot be ruled out. However, in the clinical doses that are commonly administered, most anesthetic agents, including volatile agents, nitrous oxide, propofol, opioids, benzodiazepines, and muscle relaxants are likely to be safe to use.[49] The Committee on Obstetric Practice American Society of Anesthesiologists opinion on nonobstetric surgery during pregnancy states that no currently used anesthetic agents have teratogenic effects in humans when using standard concentrations at any gestational age.[47] They suggest there is no evidence that in utero human exposure to anesthetic or sedative drugs affects the developing fetal brain. Additionally, there is no animal data to support an effect on the fetus when exposures are limited to less than 3 hours.[47] Pregnant patients may require reduced doses, with propofol requirements dropping by 8% and volatile agent requirements decreasing by up to 30%.[50]

Pregnancy causes anatomical and physiological changes that have implications for this case. The complete list of these changes is extensively documented[51] and should be considered in keeping with the gestational age of the fetus. Some of the significant physiological alterations include a baseline respiratory alkalosis, rapid desaturation due to decreased functional residual volume, increased cardiac output, decreased systemic vascular resistance, risk of thromboembolism or coagulopathy, and anemia.[51]

Finally, there needs to be special and careful consideration of the management of the airway in the pregnant patient. Compared to the general population, the incidence of difficult or failed intubation is higher in obstetrical patients, in part due to anatomic and physiologic changes during pregnancy, including airway edema and decreased functional residual capacity.[52] While the changes become more pronounced with increasing gestational age, they should be considered in all pregnant patients.

Should Fetal Monitoring Be Used During the Procedure for This Patient?

According to the 2019 American Society of Anesthesiologists (ASA) and American College of Obstetricians and Gynecologists (ACOG) joint statement on nonobstetric surgery during pregnancy, physicians should "obtain obstetric consultation before performing nonobstetric surgery and some invasive procedures (e.g., cardiac catheterization, colonoscopy), because obstetricians are uniquely qualified to discuss aspects of maternal physiology and anatomy that may affect intraoperative maternal-fetal well-being." While fetal monitoring practices will vary based on institutional protocols, the ASA/ACOG guidelines recommend fetal heart rate (FHR) monitoring intraoperatively for viable fetuses, provided that it does not interfere with surgical access or impact case management. Regardless of gestational age, a pre- and postoperative FHR should be recorded. Moreover, "if the fetus is considered previable, it is generally sufficient to ascertain the fetal heart rate by Doppler before and after the procedure."[47]

The definition of fetal viability is problematic. However, the majority of consensus statements and clinical practice consider 24 weeks gestational age to be the standard limit.[53,54] In this case, 17 weeks is considered previable and it would be sufficient to check FHR by Doppler before and after the surgical procedure.

AIRWAY MANAGEMENT

How Do You Assess the Airway of This Patient?

Airway evaluation should focus on identifying patient characteristics predictive of difficulty in bag-mask ventilation, use of extraglottic devices (EGDs), performance of direct laryngoscopy and endotracheal intubation, and ease of achievement of a surgical airway.

The mnemonic MOANS (see section "Difficult BMV: MOANS" in Chapter 1) is used to identify predictors of ease of ventilation. This patient has at least two predictors of difficulty in ventilation. She is obese and she has a Mallampati Class IV airway.

Of the four predictors of difficulty in use of an EGD identified by the mnemonic RODS (see section "Difficult Use of an EGD: RODS" in Chapter 1), this patient has two predictors of difficulty. She has restricted mouth opening and decreased thoracic compliance due to her obesity and the gravid uterus.

The mnemonics LEMON and CRANE (see sections "Difficult DL Intubation: LEMON" and "Difficult VL Intubation: CRANE" in Chapter 1) are used to identify features, which would make direct and indirect laryngoscopy and intubation difficult. This patient demonstrates a limited mouth opening and a Mallampati Class IV airway. Restricted mouth opening may also limit the ability to utilize rigid and semi-rigid fiberoptic devices, and video laryngoscopy for tracheal intubation.

The mnemonic SHORT (see section "Difficult Cricothyrotomy: SHORT" in Chapter 1) describes features that might make a surgical airway a challenge. Apart from obesity, this patient has no other features suggesting difficulty with a surgical airway that would be encountered if needed.

What Preparations Should Be Made Prior to Surgery?

Obstetric difficult airway guidelines, such as those jointly published by the Obstetric Anaesthetists' Association (OAA) and Difficult Airway Society (DAS), include an algorithm to support a safe approach to general anesthesia in the obstetric patient.[55] This algorithm emphasizes preoperative preparation, including an airway assessment, adequate fasting and antacid prophylaxis, and intrauterine fetal resuscitation when appropriate.[55] Furthermore, as the anatomic and physiologic changes of pregnancy can confer a difficult airway, the OAA/DAS recommend that a video laryngoscope be immediately available for all obstetric general anesthetics. Checklists specific to obstetric anesthesia are available and can be utilized to ensure the preoperative conditions have been optimized.[56]

A thorough history and physical examination of the patient must be completed prior to entry into the operating room. Specific information regarding previous anesthesia experiences and airway management should be elicited, and previous anesthesia records procured. A thorough airway exam should ensue to establish a plan for airway management, which should include backup alternatives in the face of difficulty. It is recommended that anesthesia practitioner have a preformulated strategy for intubation of the difficult airway, as repeated conventional intubation attempts may contribute to patient morbidity.[55] In this case, the patient has limited mouth opening. The interincisor distance should be assessed to determine the potential utility of various devices and techniques available to the anesthesia practitioner.

The operating room should be prepared, and anesthesia equipment checked. This includes ensuring there is a complete anesthesia circuit, appropriately sized face masks, and a functioning end-tidal carbon dioxide monitor; and that suction is available and working. Nasal prongs should be available for pre-induction oxygenation.

In light of the previously mentioned predictors, a difficult airway should be anticipated. Although a recent meta-analysis found no difference in first pass success and time to intubation between direct laryngoscopy and video laryngoscopy in pregnant patients without a difficult airway, subanalysis of patients with difficult airway found that video laryngoscopes were more likely to be used on the initial attempt or were required as a rescue technique.[52] These findings support the OAA/DAS assertion that a video laryngoscope should be immediately available and, in this case, in the operating room. If using a direct laryngoscope, consider using a shorter, "stubby" handle to facilitate easier insertion of the blade into the mouth, especially if the patient is obese or has large breasts. Smaller-sized (e.g., 6.5- and 7.0-mm ID) endotracheal tubes (ETTs) should be available. Additionally, a stylet should be preloaded into the ETT and a bougie should be readily available. A difficult airway cart should be brought into the operating room and appropriately trained assistants should be available.

The patient may be at risk for gastrointestinal stasis, reflux, and aspiration. The patient should be fasted, if possible. Gastric emptying in the nonlaboring pregnant patient is the same as in the nonpregnant patient;[57] therefore, perioperative fasting guidelines for elective surgery for pregnant patients are similar to those for nonpregnant patients.[58] Preoperative gastric ultrasound is gaining recognition as a useful method to quantify gastric contents, and it may add valuable information in pregnant patients. A standardized framework of the technique has been proposed in nonpregnant patients.[59] In the pregnant patient, the general principles remain the same, but technical challenges arise due to the gravid uterus.

The prophylactic use of prokinetic drugs, antacids, H2-receptor antagonists, and proton pump inhibitors (PPI) aims to reduce the volume and increase the pH of gastric contents and minimize the risk of regurgitation and aspiration. Once intravenous (IV) access is established, the patient should receive acid aspiration prophylaxis.

Metoclopramide 10 mg IV can be used as a prokinetic to enhance gastric emptying. H2-receptor antagonists, such as ranitidine (50 mg IV or 150 mg orally) and famotidine (20 mg IV), administered before surgery, are associated with higher gastric pH. These should be administered in a timely manner as they require 30 to 120 minutes after IV and oral administration, respectively, to be maximally effective.[60] A PPI (e.g., pantoprazole 40 mg IV) may be an adequate substitute for H2 blockers. Nonparticulate antacids, such as sodium citrate (30 mL orally), increase gastric pH immediately and for approximately one hour, and therefore should be administered shortly before induction of general anesthesia.[61]

The operating table should be prepared, with a ramp to position the patient in anticipation of a difficult airway. In addition, care should be taken to ensure that the patient is positioned appropriately on the operating table with left uterine displacement.

How Should the Airway of This Patient Be Managed?

The specific technique and devices used for airway management under any circumstances should be predicated on the results of the patient's airway assessment, and the anesthesia practitioner's skill, proficiency, and confidence with various devices and techniques. Despite the variety of techniques available to secure the airway, there are choices that would be unsafe in light of this patient's airway assessment. For example, a rapid sequence induction (RSI) followed by direct laryngoscopy would likely be a poor choice for this patient in whom difficulty should be anticipated. The patient's airway should be secured prior to induction of general anesthesia. An antisialagogue should be administered in preparation for awake airway management. The patient's airway will need to be anesthetized with topical anesthetics. Specific details regarding the technique of topicalization of the airway may be found in Chapter 3. Nasal prongs for oxygen delivery during the procedure should be considered, especially if anxiolytics are used with the procedure.

While flexible bronchoscopic intubation will be the usual technique of choice for this patient, there are numerous alternative techniques and devices that may be used to secure the airway awake. The decision will be based on the availability of equipment, the interincisor distance, and the skills of the airway practitioner.

Retrograde intubation is a simple technique that could be used for this patient with mild sedation. Retrograde intubation has been used numerous times in patients with very limited mouth opening[62–64] and has been thoroughly reviewed recently (see Chapter 12).[65,66] The advantages of retrograde intubation are shorter procedural time compared to an awake fiberoptic technique, and it is less invasive than cricothyrotomy. Injury to larynx, trachea or esophagus, hematoma, failed intubation, subcutaneous emphysema, pneumomediastinum, and infection are possible complications.[64] In this patient, however, it may be difficult to adequately locate the landmarks for a cricothyroid membrane puncture as a result of her obesity. The technique is not practiced regularly because it is felt to be outdated in this advanced airway management era.

Rigid and semi-rigid optical stylets represent another option in airway management. They offer benefits in restricted mouth opening and may also be used for retromolar intubation. The essential advantage that an intubation stylet represents is its small compact dimension, which enables successful tracheal intubation, even in an insufficiently opened mouth.[67] There are several fiberoptic intubating stylets available (see Chapter 11). These stylets can be used together with either direct laryngoscopy, or with a jaw thrust, to improve visualization. Most of these devices vary in diameter between 5 mm and 6 mm and can accommodate 5.5 mm ID and larger ETTs. Shikani[68] performed five awake intubations of the trachea using the Shikani Optical Scope®. Several studies have assessed the Bonfils stylet as a device for awake tracheal intubation in patients with predicted difficult airway.[69,70] The Bonfils Retromolar Fiberscope® was used by Corbanese and Possamai[71] to successfully carry out awake intubation of the trachea in 29 of 30 patients with difficult airways. Intubation with the Bonfils intubating fiberscope in 33 awake patients with predicted difficult intubation undergoing ear, nose, and throat surgery was successful in most patients (93.9%).[69] Awake intubation with either retromolar Bonfils or GlideScope found that both devices can be successfully used in morbidly obese patients with expected difficult airways. However, the Bonfils intubating fiberscope was more tolerated by patients.[70]

Several other fiberoptic intubating stylets have been used successfully to carry out awake intubations of the trachea in patients with difficult airways or small mouth opening.[72–75] LaToyaMason[76] reported the successful use of an optical lighted stylet in the setting of difficult airway management in pregnancy under general anesthesia. The authors used a Levitan® optical stylet, with a preloaded tracheal tube, to intubate the trachea of a patient with a Grade IIIB laryngoscopic view, after an initial failed intubation.[76]

Video laryngoscopes are easier to use and more amenable to use by anesthesiologists inexperienced with awake bronchoscopic intubation.[77] However, it must be remembered that all of the optical stylets and video laryngoscopes share the disadvantage of fogging, and require some antifogging maneuver prior to their use. In addition, as any blood or secretions in the airway will obscure the view, it is highly recommended that the oropharynx be suctioned prior to the insertion of these devices.

Rigid fiberoptic laryngoscopes and video laryngoscopes, such as the Bullard laryngoscope®, UpsherScope®, WuScope®, GlideScope®, and C-MAC® may be useful in this patient. A full review of these devices is presented in Chapter 11. Cohn and Zornow[78] performed awake intubations using the Bullard laryngoscope in eight patients at risk for neurological injury and requiring awake intubation of the trachea. However, none of the patients were specifically reported to have a limited mouth opening. The Bullard laryngoscope has a spatula-like blade, which may be useful in patients with limited mouth opening. Due to its "low" profile blade, it may be possible to carry out laryngoscopy with an interincisor distance of as little as 6 mm. However, it may prove to be difficult to insert or manipulate an ETT of 6 mm ID or larger size. The WuScope, due to its design, requires an interincisor distance of at least 20 mm to adequately accommodate the scope and ETT combination.[79] The use of the GlideScope for difficult airway management has increased in recent years. It has been used for awake intubation of the trachea in patients with a difficult airway,[80,81] and as an adjunct for an awake bronchoscopic intubation.[81] The GlideScope provides an improved view of the laryngeal inlet and has been shown to have a high rate of intubation success. The newer model has a 14.5 mm blade flange profile which may be useful in this patient. The C-MAC Video-Stylet—with its small diameter and flexible tip—offers an effective alternative. The successful use of the C-MAC Video-Stylet to secure the airway in a patient with minimal mouth opening due to the side effects of previous neck surgery and radiation therapy has been described.[82]

There is limited published data on the use of rigid and video laryngoscopes for awake intubation in pregnancy. Kariya et al.[83] described two successful cases where intraoperative awake tracheal intubation was completed using the Airway Scope®, a video laryngoscope, during cesarean section. The Airway Scope was chosen to assist with the potentially difficult intubation of the pregnant patient and avoid the hemodynamic compromise of general anesthesia.[83] Another report describes using a C-MAC video laryngoscope with D-blade in a patient with spondylothoracic dysostosis for a cesarean delivery. The technique was successful despite the patient having a short neck with limited extension and a Mallampati Class IV airway.[84]

While numerous options to secure the airway of patients with an anticipated difficult laryngoscopic intubation have been discussed, the use of these devices in obstetrical patients is limited. However, it is the authors' preference to perform an awake bronchoscopic intubation in this patient. Successful awake intubation will depend on satisfactory topical anesthesia of pharyngeal and laryngeal structures. Airway edema that accompanies the pregnant state may pose a challenge to topicalization and considerable patience may be required. Specific details of the techniques of topicalization and bronchoscopic intubation are discussed in Chapters 3 and 10.

What Is the Plan for Extubation of This Patient's Trachea Following Appendectomy?

No difficult airway management plan is considered complete without a predefined strategy for the safe and successful extubation of the patient's trachea following the completion of the procedure. Almost a third of all adverse airway events associated with anesthesia occurred at the end of surgery and in recovery in the United Kingdom's fourth National Audit Project (NAP4) analysis.[85] Extubation of the trachea in the obstetric patient should follow routine guidance as provided by a difficult airway guideline.[55] In this case, one must assure that all muscle relaxants have been reversed and the patient is fully awake, following commands, and able to protect their airway prior to extubation. It is important to remember that physiologic changes in pregnancy may modify the pharmacologic and pharmacokinetic profile of some drugs, including neuromuscular blocking drugs. In a study of pancuronium and vecuronium in patients undergoing cesarean delivery, a shorter elimination half-life and a higher total body clearance of both drugs was observed when compared with nonpregnant patients.[86] However, as rocuronium is the most commonly used nondepolarizing neuromuscular blocker for RSI, the consequence of prolonged neuromuscular blockade in pregnancy is most likely negated by the use of sugammadex. While the effect of pregnancy on volume of distribution of sugammadex is unknown, the effectiveness of rocuronium block reversal in parturients has been consistently reported.[87] Sugammadex reversal of rocuronium appears to be effective and safe in parturients at the end of surgery. Reported dosing strategies include 2 to 4 $mg{\cdot}kg^{-1}$ and repeat 2 $mg{\cdot}kg^{-1}$ doses repeated at 3-minute intervals based on evoked response to neuromuscular stimulator monitoring.[88] All equipment required for reintubation should be ready and available at the time of extubation. The patient should be extubated in the operating room where access to equipment and medications is assured.

SUMMARY

Although the use of general anesthesia in obstetric patients has been declining, it may still be required for open or laparoscopic appendectomies. Parturients presenting for nonobstetric surgery may have potential difficult airways. Airway management plans must be designed and formulated based on a thorough airway examination. Familiarity with devices and techniques is gained through regular review and practice, and anesthesia practitioners must become facile with a number of options for airway management. Patients with limited mouth opening present an additional challenge, but there are various options for securing the airway. The final management plan should depend on the airway evaluation of the patient, the available resources, and the skill set of the anesthesia practitioner.

SELF-EVALUATION QUESTIONS

56.1. Which of the following is true about appendicitis in pregnancy?

A. It occurs rarely during pregnancy.

B. It is predominantly a condition of the first trimester.

C. Delay in diagnosis increases risk of morbidity and mortality.

D. Laparoscopic procedures are contraindicated during pregnancy.

56.2. Appropriate aspiration prophylaxis for a parturient undergoing nonobstetrical surgery may include all the following, EXCEPT:

A. Metoclopramide 10 mg IV

B. Ranitidine 50 mg IV

C. Sodium citrate 30 mL orally

D. Dexamethasone 10 mg IV

56.3. Which is true in managing the airway of patients with a limited mouth opening?

A. Patients with limited mouth opening can usually be intubated via direct laryngoscopy postinduction of general anesthesia.

B. Degree of mouth opening will determine which device or technique may be useful in securing the airway.

C. Any device can be used for this patient population.

D. Awake bronchoscopic intubation is the only technique to secure the airway in this patient population.

REFERENCES

1. Wittich AC, DeSantis RA, Lockrow EG. Appendectomy during pregnancy: a survey of two army medical activities. *Mil Med.* 1999;164(10):671-674.
2. Kort B, Katz VL, Watson WJ. The effect of nonobstetric operation during pregnancy. *Surg Gynecol Obstet.* 1993;177(4):371-376.
3. Mazze RI, Källén B. Appendectomy during pregnancy: a Swedish registry study of 778 cases. *Obstet Gynecol.* 1991;77(6):835-840.
4. Kave M, Parooie F, Salarzaei M. Pregnancy and appendicitis: a systematic review and meta-analysis on the clinical use of MRI in diagnosis of appendicitis in pregnant women. *World J Emerg Surg.* 2019;14:37.
5. Abbasi N, Patenaude V, Abenhaim HA. Management and outcomes of acute appendicitis in pregnancy-population-based study of over 7000 cases. *BJOG.* 2014;121(12):1509-1514.
6. Addiss DG, Shaffer N, Fowler BS, Tauxe RV. The epidemiology of appendicitis and appendectomy in the United States. *Am J Epidemiol.* 1990;132(5):910-925.
7. Augustin G, Majerovic M. Non-obstetrical acute abdomen during pregnancy. *Eur J Obstet Gynecol Reprod Biol.* 2007;131(1):4-12.
8. Pastore PA, Loomis DM, Sauret J. Appendicitis in pregnancy. *J Am Board Fam Med.* 2006;19(6):621-626.
9. Tracey M, Fletcher HS. Appendicitis in pregnancy. *Am Surg.* 2000;66(6):555-559; discussion 559-560.
10. Vasileiou G, Eid AI, Qian S, et al. Appendicitis in pregnancy: a post-hoc analysis of an EAST multicenter study. *Surg Infect (Larchmt).* 2020;21(3):205-211.
11. Segev L, Segev Y, Rayman S, Nissan A, Sadot E. Acute Appendicitis During Pregnancy: different from the nonpregnant state? *World J Surg.* 2017;41(1):75-81.
12. McGory ML, Zingmond DS, Tillou A, Hiatt JR, Ko CY, Cryer HM. Negative appendectomy in pregnant women is associated with a substantial risk of fetal loss. *J Am Coll Surg.* 2007;205(4):534-540.
13. Borst AR. Acute appendicitis: pregnancy complicates this diagnosis. *JAAPA.* 2007;20(12):36-38, 41.
14. Bickell NA, Aufses AH Jr., Rojas M, Bodian C. How time affects the risk of rupture in appendicitis. *J Am Coll Surg.* 2006;202(3):401-406.
15. Babaknia A, Parsa H, Woodruff JD. Appendicitis during pregnancy. *Obstet Gynecol.* 1977;50(1):40-44.
16. Wilasrusmee C, Sukrat B, McEvoy M, Attia J, Thakkinstian A. Systematic review and meta-analysis of safety of laparoscopic versus open appendicectomy for suspected appendicitis in pregnancy. *Br J Surg.* 2012;99(11):1470-1478.
17. Ito K, Ito H, Whang EE, Tavakkolizadeh A. Appendectomy in pregnancy: evaluation of the risks of a negative appendectomy. *Am J Surg.* 2012;203(2):145-150.
18. House JB, Bourne CL, Seymour HM, Brewer KL. Location of the appendix in the gravid patient. *J Emerg Med.* 2014;46(5):741-744.
19. Mourad J, Elliott JP, Erickson L, Lisboa L. Appendicitis in pregnancy: new information that contradicts long-held clinical beliefs. *Am J Obstet Gynecol.* 2000;182(5):1027-1029.
20. Mahmoodian S. Appendicitis complicating pregnancy. *South Med J.* 1992;85(1):19-24.
21. Tatli F, Yucel Y, Gozeneli O, et al. The Alvarado Score is accurate in pregnancy: a retrospective case-control study. *Eur J Trauma Emerg Surg.* 2019;45(3):411-416.
22. Smith MP, Katz DS, Lalani T, et al. ACR Appropriateness Criteria® Right Lower Quadrant Pain--Suspected Appendicitis. *Ultrasound Q.* 2015;31(2):85-91.
23. Shetty MK, Garrett NM, Carpenter WS, Shah YP, Roberts C. Abdominal computed tomography during pregnancy for suspected appendicitis: a 5-year experience at a maternity hospital. *Semin Ultrasound CT MR.* 2010;31(1):8-13.
24. Basaran A, Basaran M. Diagnosis of acute appendicitis during pregnancy: a systematic review. *Obstet Gynecol Surv.* 2009;64(7):481-488; quiz 499.
25. Long SS, Long C, Lai H, Macura KJ. Imaging strategies for right lower quadrant pain in pregnancy. *AJR Am J Roentgenol.* 2011;196(1):4-12.
26. Duke E, Kalb B, Arif-Tiwari H, et al. A systematic review and meta-analysis of diagnostic performance of MRI for evaluation of acute appendicitis. *AJR Am J Roentgenol.* 2016;206(3):508-517.
27. Kanal E, Barkovich AJ, Bell C, et al. ACR guidance document on MR safe practices: 2013. *J Magn Reson Imaging.* 2013;37(3):501-530.
28. Kinner S, Repplinger MD, Pickhardt PJ, Reeder SB. Contrast-enhanced abdominal MRI for suspected appendicitis: how we do it. *Am J Roentgenol.* 2016;207(1):49-57.
29. Yefet E, Romano S, Chazan B, Nachum Z. Successful treatment of acute uncomplicated appendicitis in pregnancy with intravenous antibiotics. *Eur J Obstet Gynecol Reprod Biol.* 2013;169(1):121-122.
30. Vons C, Barry C, Maitre S, et al. Amoxicillin plus clavulanic acid versus appendicectomy for treatment of acute uncomplicated appendicitis: an open-label, non-inferiority, randomised controlled trial. *Lancet.* 2011;377(9777):1573-1579.
31. Varadhan KK, Neal KR, Lobo DN. Safety and efficacy of antibiotics compared with appendicectomy for treatment of uncomplicated acute appendicitis: meta-analysis of randomised controlled trials. *BMJ.* 2012;344:e2156.
32. Carstens AK, Fensby L, Penninga L. Nonoperative treatment of appendicitis during pregnancy in a remote area. *AJP Rep.* 2018;8(1):e37-e38.
33. Cheng HT, Wang YC, Lo HC, et al. Laparoscopic appendectomy versus open appendectomy in pregnancy: a population-based analysis of maternal outcome. *Surg Endosc.* 2015;29(6):1394-1399.
34. Abbasi N, Patenaude V, Abenhaim HA. Evaluation of obstetrical and fetal outcomes in pregnancies complicated by acute appendicitis. *Arch Gynecol Obstet.* 2014;290(4):661-667.
35. Rasmussen AS, Christiansen CF, Uldbjerg N, Nørgaard M. Obstetric and non-obstetric surgery during pregnancy: A 20-year Danish population-based prevalence study. *BMJ Open.* 2019;9(5):e028136.
36. Gök AFK, Soydaş Y, Bayraktar A, et al. Laparoscopic versus open appendectomy in pregnancy: a single center experience. *Ulus Travma Acil Cerrahi Derg.* 2018;24(6):552-556.
37. Gorter RR, Eker HH, Gorter-Stam MA, et al. Diagnosis and management of acute appendicitis. EAES consensus development conference 2015. *Surg Endosc.* 2016;30(11):4668-4690.
38. Rollins MD, Chan KJ, Price RR. Laparoscopy for appendicitis and cholelithiasis during pregnancy: a new standard of care. *Surg Endosc.* 2004;18(2):237-241.
39. Sadot E, Telem DA, Arora M, Butala P, Nguyen SQ, Divino CM. Laparoscopy: a safe approach to appendicitis during pregnancy. *Surg Endosc.* 2010;24(2):383-389.
40. Pearl JP, Price RR, Tonkin AE, Richardson WS, Stefanidis D. SAGES guidelines for the use of laparoscopy during pregnancy. *Surg Endosc.* 2017;31(10):3767-3782.

41. Kirshtein B, Perry ZH, Avinoach E, Mizrahi S, Lantsberg L. Safety of laparoscopic appendectomy during pregnancy. *World J Surg*. 2009;33(3):475-480.
42. Kuczkowski KM. Laparoscopic procedures during pregnancy and the risks of anesthesia: what does an obstetrician need to know? *Arch Gynecol Obstet*. 2007;276(3):201-209.
43. Frountzas M, Nikolaou C, Stergios K, Kontzoglou K, Toutouzas K, Pergialiotis V. Is the laparoscopic approach a safe choice for the management of acute appendicitis in pregnant women? A meta-analysis of observational studies. *Ann R Coll Surg Engl*. 2019;101(4):235-248.
44. Shigemi D, Aso S, Matsui H, Fushimi K, Yasunaga H. Safety of laparoscopic surgery for benign diseases during pregnancy: a nationwide retrospective cohort study. *J Minim Invasive Gynecol*. 2019;26(3):501-506.
45. Gerges FJ, Kanazi GE, Jabbour-Khoury SI. Anesthesia for laparoscopy: a review. *J Clin Anesth*. 2006;18(1):67-78.
46. Rasmussen AS, Christiansen CF, Ulrichsen SP, Uldbjerg N, Nørgaard M. Non-obstetric abdominal surgery during pregnancy and birth outcomes: a Danish registry-based cohort study. *Acta Obstet Gynecol Scand*. 2020;99(4):469-476.
47. ACOG Committee Opinion No. 775: Nonobstetric surgery during pregnancy. *Obstet Gynecol*. 2019;133(4):e285-e286.
48. FDA classification of drugs for teratogenic risk. Teratology Society Public Affairs Committee. *Teratology*. 1994;49(6):446-447.
49. MA R. Anesthesia for the pregnant patient undergoing surgery. *ASA Refresher Course in Anesthesiology*. 2009.
50. Okeagu CN, Anandi P, Gennuso S, et al. Clinical management of the pregnant patient undergoing non-obstetric surgery: review of guidelines. *Best Pract Res Clin Anaesthesiol*. 2020;34(2):269-281.
51. Vasco Ramirez M, Valencia GC. Anesthesia for nonobstetric surgery in pregnancy. *Clin Obstet Gynecol*. 2020;63(2):351-363.
52. Howle R, Onwochei D, Harrison SL, Desai N. Comparison of videolaryngoscopy and direct laryngoscopy for tracheal intubation in obstetrics: a mixed-methods systematic review and meta-analysis. *Can J Anaesth*. 2021;68(4):546-565.
53. Ladhani NNN, Chari RS, Dunn MS, Jones G, Shah P, Barrett JFR. No. 347-Obstetric management at borderline viability. *J Obstet Gynaecol Can*. 2017;39(9):781-791.
54. Vavasseur C, Foran A, Murphy JF. Consensus statements on the borderlands of neonatal viability: from uncertainty to grey areas. *Ir Med J*. 2007;100(8):561-564.
55. Mushambi MC, Kinsella SM, Popat M, et al. Obstetric Anaesthetists' Association and Difficult Airway Society guidelines for the management of difficult and failed tracheal intubation in obstetrics. *Anaesthesia*. 2015;70(11):1286-1306.
56. Wittenberg MD, Vaughan DJ, Lucas DN. A novel airway checklist for obstetric general anaesthesia. *Int J Obstet Anesth*. 2013;22(3):264-265.
57. Macfie AG, Magides AD, Richmond MN, Reilly CS. Gastric emptying in pregnancy. *Br J Anaesth*. 1991;67(1):54-57.
58. Practice guidelines for preoperative fasting and the use of pharmacologic agents to reduce the risk of pulmonary aspiration: application to healthy patients undergoing elective procedures: an updated report by the American Society of Anesthesiologists Task Force on preoperative fasting and the use of pharmacologic agents to reduce the risk of pulmonary aspiration. *Anesthesiology*. 2017;126(3):376-393.
59. Perlas A, Van de Putte P, Van Houwe P, Chan VW. I-AIM framework for point-of-care gastric ultrasound. *Br J Anaesth*. 2016;116(1):7-11.
60. Rout CC, Rocke DA, Gouws E. Intravenous ranitidine reduces the risk of acid aspiration of gastric contents at emergency cesarean section. *Anesth Analg*. 1993;76(1):156-161.
61. Dewan DM, Floyd HM, Thistlewood JM, Bogard TD, Spielman FJ. Sodium citrate pretreatment in elective cesarean section patients. *Anesth Analg*. 1985;64(1):34-37.
62. Bhattacharya P, Biswas BK, Baniwal S. Retrieval of a retrograde catheter using suction, in patients who cannot open their mouths. *Br J Anaesth*. 2004;92(6):888-901.
63. Biswas BK, Bhattacharyya P, Joshi S, Tuladhar UR, Baniwal S. Fluoroscope-aided retrograde placement of guidewire for tracheal intubation in patients with limited mouth opening. *Br J Anaesth*. 2005;94(1):128-131.
64. Reena, Rastogi V. Limited mouth opening: retrograde intubation revisited. *Saudi J Anaesth*. 2018;12(2):349-351.
65. Burbulys D, Kiai K. Retrograde intubation. *Emerg Med Clin North Am*. 2008;26(4):1029-1041, x.
66. Dhara SS. Retrograde tracheal intubation. *Anaesthesia*. 2009;64(10): 1094-1104.
67. Matek J, Kolek F, Klementova O, Michalek P, Vymazal T. Optical devices in tracheal intubation-state of the art in 2020. *Diagnostics (Basel)*. 2021;11(3):575.
68. Shikani AH. New "seeing" stylet-scope and method for the management of the difficult airway. *Otolaryngol Head Neck Surg*. 1999;120(1):113-116.
69. Mazères JE, Lefranc A, Cropet C, et al. Evaluation of the bonfils intubating fibrescope for predicted difficult intubation in awake patients with ear, nose and throat cancer. *Eur J Anaesthesiol*. 2011;28(9):646-650.
70. Nassar M, Zanaty OM, Ibrahim M. Bonfils fiberscope vs GlideScope for awake intubation in morbidly obese patients with expected difficult airways. *J Clin Anesth*. 2016;32:101-105.
71. Corbanese U, Possamai C. Awake intubation with the Bonfils fibrescope in patients with difficult airway. *Eur J Anaesthesiol*. 2009;26(10):837-841.
72. Abramson SI, Holmes AA, Hagberg CA. Awake insertion of the Bonfils Retromolar Intubation Fiberscope in five patients with anticipated difficult airways. *Anesth Analg*. 2008;106(4):1215-1217, table of contents.
73. Hamada T, Morokura N, Suzuki Y, Katori K, Yamamoto S, Higa K. [Orotracheal intubation using a StyletScope in a patient to avoid neck recurvation]. *Masui*. 2001;50(5):519-520.
74. He N, Xue FS, Xu YC, Liao X, Xu XZ. Awake orotracheal intubation under airway topical anesthesia using the Bonfils in patients with a predicted difficult airway. *Can J Anaesth*. 2008;55(12):881-882.
75. Nagashima M, Saito T, Takahata O, Sengoku K, Iwasaki H. [Orotracheal intubation using a StyletScope in a patient with restricted opening of the mouth]. *Masui*. 2002;51(7):775-776.
76. LaToya Mason C. Difficult airway management using the Levitan optical stylet in an emergency cesarean delivery. *J Anesth Clin Res*. 2014;5(4). doi:10.4172/2155-6148.1000399.
77. Gaszynska E, Gaszynski T. The King Vision™ video laryngoscope for awake intubation: series of cases and literature review. *Ther Clin Risk Manag*. 2014;10:475-478.
78. Cohn AI, Zornow MH. Awake endotracheal intubation in patients with cervical spine disease: a comparison of the Bullard laryngoscope and the fiberoptic bronchoscope. *Anesth Analg*. 1995;81(6):1283-1286.
79. Smith CE, Sidhu TS, Lever J, Pinchak AB. The complexity of tracheal intubation using rigid fiberoptic laryngoscopy (WuScope). *Anesth Analg*. 1999;89(1):236-239.
80. Doyle DJ. Awake intubation using the GlideScope video laryngoscope: initial experience in four cases. *Can J Anaesth*. 2004;51(5):520-521.
81. Xue FS, Li CW, Zhang GH, et al. GlideScope-assisted awake fibreoptic intubation: initial experience in 13 patients. *Anaesthesia*. 2006;61(10):1014-1015.
82. Pius J, Ioanidis K, Noppens RR. Use of the Novel C-MAC video stylet in a case of predicted difficult intubation: a case report. *A A Pract*. 2019;13(3):88-90.
83. Kariya N, Kimura K, Iwasaki R, Ueki R, Tatara T, Tashiro C. Intraoperative awake tracheal intubation using the Airway Scope™ in caesarean section. *Anaesth Intensive Care*. 2013;41(3):390-392.
84. Zbeidy R, Torres Buendia N, Souki FG. Anaesthetic management of a parturient with spondylothoracic dysostosis. *BMJ Case Rep*. 2020;13(1):e232964.
85. Cook TM, Woodall N, Frerk C. Major complications of airway management in the UK: results of the Fourth National Audit Project of the Royal College of Anaesthetists and the Difficult Airway Society. Part 1: anaesthesia. *Br J Anaesth*. 2011;106(5):617-631.
86. Dailey PA, Fisher DM, Shnider SM, et al. Pharmacokinetics, placental transfer, and neonatal effects of vecuronium and pancuronium administered during cesarean section. *Anesthesiology*. 1984;60(6):569-574.
87. Richardson MG, Raymond BL. Sugammadex administration in pregnant women and in women of reproductive potential: a narrative review. *Anesth Analg*. 2020;130(6):1628-1637.
88. Stourac P, Adamus M, Seidlova D, et al. Low-dose or high-dose rocuronium reversed with neostigmine or sugammadex for cesarean delivery anesthesia: a randomized controlled noninferiority trial of time to tracheal intubation and extubation. *Anesth Analg*. 2016;122(5):1536-1545.

SECTION 9

AIRWAY MANAGEMENT IN UNIQUE ENVIRONMENT

CHAPTER 57

Unique Challenges of Ectopic Airway Management

Michael F. Murphy

CASE PRESENTATION

A 42-year-old obese man is undergoing renal dialysis in a hospital dialysis unit when he suddenly suffers a cardiac arrest. He is a diabetic with a history of cerebrovascular disease, peripheral vascular disease, and angina. He is a nonsmoker. He had no premonitory symptoms.

You are called to manage his airway. When you arrive on the scene, you see a cyanotic male looking older than his stated age, reclining at 45 degrees in a dialysis chair. He is still connected to a dialysis machine via a vascular shunt in his left arm. The head of the chair, which is not on wheels, is against the wall. A dialysis technician is straddling the patient performing cardiopulmonary resuscitation and a nurse is delivering ineffective face-mask ventilation (FMV) from the right side of the patient. You are informed that he receives dialysis three times a week. His *dry weight* is 188 kg (414 lb).

The crash cart has arrived, containing both oral and nasal airways, endotracheal tubes, a laryngoscope handle, and #3 and #4 Macintosh blades. There is an intubating stylet as well. This is the third time this year you have been called to this unit. Unfortunately, the equipment you prefer to use for airway management is *never* available in the dialysis unit, despite continuous reminders that you prefer a Miller blade.

INTRODUCTION

What Is Meant by the Term "Ectopic" Airway Management?

Anesthesia practitioners, emergency physicians, intensivists, hospitalists, and other health care providers with airway management expertise often become involved in emergency and urgent airway management outside of their usual operating room (OR) milieu. This is referred to as "ectopic" airway management.

It is important not to conflate this term with nonoperating room anesthesia (NORA), also called "ectopic anesthesia." While there is an overlap in terms of the immediate availability of devices, medications, assistance, and focus of ancillary staff, the challenges of NORA are substantially more complex.

What Are the Common Examples of Ectopic Venues?

There are several areas of a hospital where it should be *anticipated* that emergency airway management will be required occasionally, or even perhaps regularly. These include but are not exclusive to:

- Postanesthetic care unit (PACU).
- Diagnostic imaging locations where emergency and intensive care unit (ICU) patients are taken; particularly computed tomography (CT) scan, magnetic resonance imaging (MRI), ultrasound, and angiography units.
- Units where procedural sedation is undertaken:
  - Endoscopy
  - Invasive cardiology

- Interventional imaging
- Pediatric clinics, such as dentistry, ophthalmology, electroencephalogram (EEG), otorhinolaryngology, and others
- Lithotripsy
- Cardiac stress testing facilities
- Medical and surgical inpatient units
- Obstetrical delivery suites

Outpatient clinics, medical offices, and nonpatient care areas (e.g., cafeterias, residences, waiting rooms, administrative offices, and the areas immediately external to the health care facility) are occasionally the site of an airway emergency.

AIRWAY MANAGEMENT CHALLENGES

What Are the Unique Challenges of Ectopic Airway Management?

Managing a difficult airway is always anxiety provoking and somewhat dysphoric. Most ectopic airway management is difficult for a variety of reasons: some are related to the patient's airway anatomy; others to the patient's condition; and some are unique to the situation. The result is performance anxiety that may lead to less-than-optimal performance. Consider the following unique challenges inherent in managing the ectopic airway:

- Medicolegal risk
- Consistency and availability of airway kits/carts and medications
- Unfamiliar environment
- Unknown patient medical conditions
- Assistants unfamiliar with airway management
- Emotionally charged environment, stressed response
- Postintubation management

What Are the Medicolegal Risks Associated with Ectopic Airway Management?

Ectopic airway management is associated with an element of medicolegal risk in the event of a poor outcome. Peterson et al.[1] published an update of the *Management of the Difficult Airway: A Closed Claims Analysis* in 2005. Out of 179 claims for difficult airway management, 86 (48%) were from events occurring from 1985 to 1992 and 93 (52%) were from events occurring from 1993 to 1999. Most claims for difficult airway management (156 out of 179 or 87%) involved perioperative care and 23 claims (13%) involved ectopic locations. Out of these 23 cases of airway management *misadventures* outside the OR environment, 25% involved endotracheal tube change, and nearly half were not related to surgical procedures. Reintubation on the ward or ICU some time after a surgical procedure was related to neck swelling with respiratory distress. The procedures included cervical fusion (n = 3), total thyroidectomy (n = 1), intraoral/pharyngeal procedures (n = 2), and fluid extravasation from a central catheter (n = 1). The reality of medicolegal risk associated with airway management continues. Crosby et al. in a Canadian Closed Claims analysis published in 2021 found that 54% of cases were outside of the OR.[2]

The typical scenario coming to litigation has the following features:

- The patient is unknown to the airway practitioner.
- It is an emergency situation:
  - Which is emotionally charged and chaotic.
  - In which events preceding the airway emergency are unclear.
  - In which the amount of information about the patient is limited.
  - In which action is needed immediately.
  - With a difficult airway (e.g., post-thyroidectomy in PACU; patient in a halo jacket).
  - In which evaluation of the airway for difficulty is inadequate.
  - In which paralytic agents are inappropriately given.
  - In which the management strategy is poorly thought out and executed, leading to a failed airway.

The fact that the airway practitioner is thrust into an emotionally charged and unfamiliar environment provides little if any legal protection or indemnification. Furthermore, the defense of *lack of familiarity* or *lack of desired equipment* may be discredited. This is particularly so if it can be established that emergency airway management is *expected* to occur from time to time in that unit *and* that the individual charged with airway management in such situations (i.e., you) *knew or ought to have known* that they might be summoned to do so.

Part of the solution to this problem is in the realm of *prevention* by establishing policies and procedures with respect to the availability of airway management equipment and its maintenance in areas where it is predictable that emergency or urgent airway intervention will occasionally be required. This requires that the disciplines involved take ownership of this issue and communicate with each other, and among themselves, about the specifics of such policies that will ensure safe, and hopefully litigation-free, ectopic airway management.[3]

What Airway Equipment or Carts Should Be Available in These Ectopic Facilities?

Airways are managed virtually every day in the ORs, emergency departments (EDs), and ICUs of most hospitals. These units ordinarily assemble routine and rescue airway management equipment into varying configurations of storage units where they are checked regularly (e.g., daily or with shift change) for availability and function, and are easily accessed in an emergency. Routine and difficult/failed airway equipment may be arranged in separate drawers in the storage areas of the same cart (e.g., EDs and ICUs); or sometimes in different carts (e.g., the OR's difficult airway cart, see Chapter 63). The literature, albeit limited, provides little guidance as to what ought to be stocked in these *carts*, or alternatively in a *carry out* kit that the practitioner takes along to an airway management event.[4]

The equipment on the carts is typically determined by the consensus among the airway practitioners or staff who respond to manage an airway emergency in these units. The equipment should be arranged in a consistent fashion such that the drawers always contain the same airway equipment. This site-to-site consistency is particularly important when large specialty groups cover several facilities. Such consistency will likely avoid wasting valuable time to find the proper airway equipment in an emergency situation. Chapter 63 addresses the policy and content aspects of difficult airway carts in operating suites, EDs, and ICUs.

In areas of the hospital where airway management may be required on a regular basis, or patients are placed at risk for respiratory failure, it is recommended that routine and rescue airway management equipment be immediately available. Furthermore, the storage of this equipment should be consistent from area to area, and the equipment should be checked for inventory and function daily.

Carry out emergency airway satchels that can be quickly retrieved and carried to the site of an airway emergency are used by some practitioners and departments (see Chapter 63).[4] The same issues arise with these kits as with permanent on-site carts, including:

- Consistent location of kits to permit rapid retrieval.
- Contain both routine and rescue devices.
- Organized consistently to permit rapid access to the desired equipment.
- Regular inspections to ensure that the kits are complete and replenished after each use.
- Daily inspections of each kit to ensure proper function of all devices.

Some areas may have unique needs that require special equipment.[5] The most common example is an area serving pediatric patients. Some areas of a health care facility may see this population from time to time, while others may not.[5]

What Are the Challenges Associated with Managing the Airway in the Ectopic Environment?

Leaving the comfort of one's usual environment and venturing into unfamiliar territory should not hinder appropriate airway management. Practitioners who may be summoned to ectopic areas to manage airways should familiarize themselves with the staff, the equipment, and the storage systems *before* the emergency arises. Participating in the decisions as to what is stored, where it is stored, and how it is maintained (i.e., policy) is only reasonable.

The scene on arrival is generally chaotic, emotionally charged, and boisterous. As there are substantial expectations placed on the responding airway practitioner, it is critical that the airway practitioner does not participate in or inflame the chaos, which fosters bad airway management decisions (see Chapter 6).

Why Is Airway Management in an Ectopic Location More Challenging?

Patients requiring airway management in these ectopic locations are generally not known to the airway practitioners. Most of these patients are not prepared for airway management (e.g., often have a full stomach with a higher risk of regurgitation and aspiration). Furthermore, airway assessment is often hurried and incomplete. Thus, the formulation of a rational and well-thought-out airway management plan is unlikely. As indicated previously, the single most important factor leading to a failed airway is failure to properly assess a patient and predict a difficult airway.[6] Consequently, it is more common to encounter a *difficult airway* in an ectopic environment.[7]

What Are the Challenges Faced by the Practitioners Managing These Patients' Airways in Ectopic Locations?

Emergency airway management presenting in PACU (e.g., post-thyroidectomy bleed) may be quite different from those occurring in the CT scanner (e.g., pediatric patients). Airway practitioners have varying skills and few have expertise in managing all types of situations.

In addition, unlike the situation in the OR, PACU, ICU, or ED, airway management assistants in these ectopic locations may be unfamiliar with even the basic needs of the airway practitioner. Maneuvers, such as cricoid pressure, external laryngeal manipulation (BURP), head lift, use of a tracheal introducer (commonly called "bougie"), using an extraglottic device (EGD), or even passing the endotracheal tube correctly to the airway practitioner, may not be fully understood.

To minimize these difficulties, institutions should provide basic airway training to both airway practitioners and assistants to manage the airways of patients that present in various ectopic locations.

How Should the Airway Be Managed in Ectopic Locations?

The following simple rules of engagement may be helpful:

- Remain calm and take control of the scene.
- Speak firmly and give clear instructions to assistants without shouting.
- If patient behavior management is not an issue, managing oxygenation and ventilation or gas exchange must be achieved quickly:
  - Move to the head of the patient to confirm or establish airway patency, ventilation, and oxygenation.
  - If positive pressure ventilation is indicated, take over FMV and avoid aggressive ventilation (i.e., avoid high-frequency, large tidal volume, and high airway pressure). Consider use of a PEEP valve.
  - Insert an oropharyngeal airway and two nasopharyngeal airways if needed.
  - If this fails, and the patient will tolerate it inserting an EGD (e.g., LMA) is reasonable.
  - Gather your wits and composure as you establish adequate gas exchange.
- While maintaining gas exchange, it is important to evaluate the airway and formulate a plan.
  - Formally evaluate the airway using the mnemonics described in Chapter 1 (i.e., with MOANS, LEMON, RODS, CRANE, SHORT).

- Identify and communicate to the room Plans A, B, and C (including a plan for failed intubation and failed oxygenation) and assemble the required equipment and drugs.
- Avoid muscle paralysis if the ability to maintain ventilation or gas exchange once the patient is paralyzed is uncertain.
- Optimize conditions—invest time to properly position the patient at the head of the bed, elevate the bed to the proper height, and place the patient's head and neck in the appropriate (i.e., *sniffing*) position.

- Use nasal prong oxygen at 10 to 15 L·min^{-1} to supply supplemental oxygen during the airway management process.
  - Execute the plan in a deliberate and controlled manner.

When faced with inadequate equipment (or skills) in an ectopic location, it is important to think of alternatives:

- Call for assistance if available. A colleague or an assistant can contribute with suggestions, expertise, and more importantly, moral support.
- Does the patient really need tracheal intubation *right now* or will an FMV or an EGD suffice until additional equipment or expertise arrives?
- Are there any other options (e.g., blind nasal intubation)?
- Consider titration of intravenous haloperidol and/or ketamine, and avoid succinylcholine, if the patient's behavior hinders adequate management of ventilation and oxygenation.

Finally, Mort compared the outcomes of patients undergoing emergency tracheal intubation in his institution before and after the application of the American Society of Anesthesiologists (ASA) guidelines.[8] The rate of cardiac arrest during emergency intubation was reduced by 50%.

POSTINTUBATION CONSIDERATION

What Should Be Done Following Tracheal Intubation in Ectopic Locations?

While confirmation of tracheal intubation is critical following intubation, proper equipment (capnometry, capnography, or an esophageal detection device [EDD] self-inflating bulb) may not be available. This important equipment, together with hemodynamic monitors such as a blood pressure cuff and pulse oximetry, should be stocked in ectopic locations where airway management may be required or should be called for if they are not available. Ensure that the airway device (e.g., ETT, EGD, etc.) is secured properly. Longer-term neuromuscular blockade with accompanying sedation may be necessary to facilitate mechanical ventilation and ensure that the patient does not self-extubate. Ensure that appropriate mechanical ventilation parameters are established if indicated.

Following airway management in these unusual environments, it is essential to document the following elements:

- Any evaluation that indicates that the airway might be difficult.
- Ensure that the resuscitation record or nurses' notes accurately record the time you were summoned, arrived, completed key interventions, etc.
- Ensure that drug doses are accurately recorded.
- Document the airway management, and the intratracheal verification methods employed (end-tidal carbon dioxide detection is the standard of care).

If significant difficulty with airway management had been encountered, clinician-to-clinician communication is warranted when the patient leaves for another care area.

SUMMARY

Let's revisit the case. Poor planning and anticipation of a difficult airway in a setting where airway emergencies had occurred in the past led to a situation where face-mask ventilation (FMV) adjuncts, alternatives to FMV, such as an EGD, and alternatives to direct laryngoscopic intubation, such as video-laryngoscopy were unavailable. The patient's airway could not be managed, and the patient died.

A legal action ensued where the facility and the anesthesia practitioner involved were found liable for not having available the equipment necessary to manage such an airway. The court criticized the practitioner because the practitioner knew or ought to have known that the airway management kit on the unit was deficient having been called to this very unit in the past and having found the airway management kit was indeed deficient.

To minimize the risk, adverse outcome, and the anxiety associated with airway management of patients in an ectopic environment, it is important to:

- Participate in crafting hospital and departmental policies regarding airway management equipment in areas where you are called to manage them (see Chapter 63).[4]
- Familiarize yourself with different hospital units and their staff.
- Minimize the chaos.
- Assess the airway and formulate airway strategies quickly.
- Call for assistance early.
- Avoid paralyzing the patient if the ability to artificially maintain postparalysis gas exchange is uncertain.
- Document the airway management episode.

SELF-EVALUATION QUESTIONS

57.1. Ectopic airway management is associated with measurable medicolegal risk. Of the closed claims related to difficult airway management in the ASA Closed Claims Database between 1985 and 1999, the approximate percentage of those occurring at an ectopic location is:

A. 2%

B. 5%

C. 15%

D. 25%

E. 43%

57.2. The most important factor related to successfully managing an airway in an ectopic location is:

A. Getting there quickly.

B. Making it clear that you are the most skilled airway practitioner at the scene.

C. You have familiarized yourself with the equipment that will be available to you beforehand.

D. That you speak in a low voice to avoid fanning the flames of anxiety.

E. That you paralyze the patient quickly to enhance your success rate.

57.3. All of the following are associated with ectopic airway management EXCEPT:

A. Chaos is the norm.

B. Failure rates are higher in locations where you usually work.

C. Policies with respect to airway management equipment maintenance are the norm.

D. Good help is usually present at the scene.

E. The person who performs the intubation is responsible to see that it is secured in place.

REFERENCES

1. Peterson GN, Domino KB, Caplan RA, Posner KL, Lee LA, Cheney FW. Management of the difficult airway: a closed claims analysis. *Anesthesiology.* 2005;103(1):33-39.
2. Crosby ET, Duggan LV, Finestone PJ, Liu R, De Gorter R, Calder LA. Anesthesiology airway-related medicolegal cases from the Canadian Medical Protection Association. *Can J Anaesth.* 2021;68(2):183-195.
3. Mark LJ, Herzer KR, Cover R, et al. Difficult airway response team: a novel quality improvement program for managing hospital-wide airway emergencies. *Anesth Analg.* 2015;121(1):127-139.
4. Apfelbaum JL, Hagberg CA, Connis RT, et al. American Society of Anesthesiologists Practice Guidelines for management of the difficult airway. *Anesthesiology.* 2022;136(1):31-81.
5. Calder A, Hegarty M, Davies K, von Ungern-Sternberg BS. The difficult airway trolley in pediatric anesthesia: an international survey of experience and training. *Paediatr Anaesth.* 2012;22(12):1150-1154.
6. Caplan RA, Benumof JL, Berry FA, et al. Practice Guidelines for Management of the Difficultl Airway. *Anesthesiology.* 1993;78:597-602.
7. Sakles JC, Douglas MJK, Hypes CD, Patanwala AE, Mosier JM. Management of patients with predicted difficult airways in an academic emergency department. *J Emerg Med.* 2017;53(2):163-171.
8. Mort TC. The incidence and risk factors for cardiac arrest during emergency tracheal intubation: a justification for incorporating the ASA Guidelines in the remote location. *J Clin Anesth.* 2004;16(7):508-516.

CHAPTER 58

Airway Management of the Patient with a Neck Hematoma

Mallory Garza and Konstantin Lorenz

CASE PRESENTATION

A 49-year-old female has been recovering in the postanesthetic care unit (PACU) for the last 4 hours. She has a slowly expanding neck hematoma following an uneventful left carotid endarterectomy under general anesthesia. Subtle neck swelling was noticed shortly after her arrival, and a cooling pressure pack has been placed on the surgical site. One hour earlier, she was noted to have difficulty in swallowing. She has since been noted to have increased respiratory efforts and does not want to lie flat. Vascular surgery has been informed and has booked her for urgent wound exploration and evacuation of hematoma. Her medical history included hypertension and type II diabetes. She is a nonsmoker. She was noted preoperatively to have reassuring airway anatomy. Her prior airway management was documented as easy bag-mask ventilation (BMV) without an oropharyngeal airway (OPA), and a Cormack–Lehane (C/L)[1] Grade 1 view with direct laryngoscopy using a Macintosh #4 blade. The trachea was easily intubated with a 7.5-mm internal diameter (ID) endotracheal tube (ETT).

In PACU, she is now sitting upright with a non-rebreathing facemask. Although restless, she is rational and complaining of dyspnea, dysphagia, and neck pain. Her blood pressure is 195/95 mmHg, heart rate is 105 beats per minute, respiratory rate is 28 breaths per minute, and her SpO_2 is 94%. She is becoming audibly stridulous. Under a blood-stained dressing, the left side of her neck looks visibly enlarged and discolored. The patient is 5′3″ (164 cm) in height and weighs 172 lb (78 kg). She has adequate vascular access. The OR is being prepared for her return.

PATIENT EVALUATION AND MANAGEMENT OPTIONS

In What Ways Might This Patient Present Difficulty with Airway Management? What Are the Key Aspects of the Airway Examination in This Situation?

This is an urgent situation. The patient must be quickly assessed, and decisions made. Although some patients with neck hematomas may be managed with watchful expectancy, case reports attest to the difficulty in predicting if, or when, these individuals will go on to sudden and catastrophic airway obstruction.[2–4] As part of the patient's evaluation, a formal airway examination should be performed, seeking predictors of difficulty in all aspects of airway management.[5] Even though the patient's anatomy presented no difficulty with airway management earlier that day, the presence of a neck hematoma changes everything. With evidence of obstructing pathology in the airway (as manifested by stridor, neck swelling, and the patient's dyspnea and agitation), difficulty can now be anticipated with BMV, direct and indirect laryngoscopy, tracheal intubation, use of an extraglottic device (EGD), and open cricothyrotomy, as external landmarks become shifted or indistinct.

Although situational acuity will often preclude diagnostic imaging of the patient presenting with obstructing pathology, if patient cooperation allows, useful information may be obtained by performing nasopharyngoscopy immediately before an attempt at securing the airway.[6,7] This is generally well tolerated, and can provide information about any lateral displacement of the larynx, the degree of perilaryngeal edema, and the location and size of an obstructing mass that may impede laryngoscopy, flexible bronchoscopy, tracheal intubation, and successful EGD placement.

What Other Patient Factors May Be Relevant in This Situation?

With predicted difficulty in all aspects of airway management limiting options in this patient, an awake approach to securing the airway is preferable. However, for awake airway interventions, patient cooperation is generally needed. Patient cooperation may be lost as hypoxemia occurs or as the patient panics, with progressive airway lumen narrowing and worsening dyspnea.

All of the above speak to the need for early identification of the need for reintubation, while cooperation is retained. Sedating a less cooperative patient with a tenuous airway is hazardous, and may precipitate complete airway obstruction.[8,9] Other patient comorbidities will assume secondary importance in comparison with the gravity of threatened loss of the airway.

What Are the Causes of Airway Obstruction in a Patient with a Postsurgical Neck Hematoma?

Neck hematomas tend to originate from venous or capillary sources more often than arterial bleeding.[10–12] Although arterial bleeds may present earlier or more quickly,[11] neck hematomas arising from a venous or capillary source can be insidious and just as devastating in their ability to cause airway obstruction. The following mechanisms may contribute to the development of symptomatic airway obstruction in the patient with a neck hematoma:

1. *Physical pressure effect.* The presence of a hematoma in the neck can mechanically displace the laryngeal inlet away from the midline position.[3,11,13–15] In addition, the lumen of the pharynx can be physically compressed by a hematoma, as it is unprotected by a bony or cartilaginous framework.[16] Accordingly, it follows that some authors have considered significant compression of the larynx and trachea by a hematoma to be unlikely, due to their rigid cartilaginous structures.[17,18] However, in a human cadaver study, Thakur and colleagues[19] found that a mean pressure of only 136 mmHg (i.e., within physiologic range) completely collapsed the trachea when applied in an oblique direction. In addition, even if the cartilaginous framework remains intact, the posterior, membranous portion of the trachea may be significantly compressed by a hematoma.[20] Case reports have indeed been published that include CT scan images of significant tracheal compression by hematomas.[21,22] Bukht and Langford[23] have described a case in which an adult patient with a neck hematoma was intubated (with difficulty) with a 5-mm ID ETT. No leak was apparent even without ETT cuff inflation; however, upon subsequent release of the hematoma, a large leak immediately developed. Such reports and studies suggest that physical compression of the trachea or larynx can indeed occur with a neck hematoma, in addition to lateral displacement.
2. *The development of perilaryngeal edema.* This is a consistent feature in case reports of patients with neck hematomas,[2–4,11,13,21,23–29] and is often out of proportion to any degree of externally visible neck swelling or discoloration. Most authors agree that this is due to interference with normal venous and/or lymphatic[30] drainage by both the neck hematoma itself and blood tracking into interstitial tissue, away from the site of the original hematoma.[3,18,21,24,31,32] Release of tissue inflammatory mediators may also contribute.[31,33] At direct laryngoscopy, the resulting edema is variously described as "swollen supraglottic mucosal folds,"[3,11] or a "watery, pale swelling of the mucosa,"[18,24] which in many cases substantially obscures the glottic opening. Interestingly, some published case reports have documented the development of similar perilaryngeal edema after neck surgery, even without an obvious hematoma.[11,34]
3. *Blood dissection along tissue planes in the neck.* The parapharyngeal space is contiguous medially with the retropharyngeal space,[20] which in turn extends from the skull base to the upper mediastinum.[35] The parapharyngeal space also communicates anteriorly with pretracheal and submandibular spaces, and subcutaneous tissues.[35] Blood from a neck hematoma in any of these areas can thus spread remotely from its initial location to further compromise the airway. Retropharyngeal collections of blood are often manifested symptomatically by neck pain, dysphagia, or odynophagia, in addition to hoarseness and dyspnea.[32] Retropharyngeal hematomas can cause airway obstruction by compression of the arytenoid cartilages, which may in turn adduct the vocal cords.[36] In addition, retropharyngeal swelling can render direct laryngoscopy more difficult by shifting the laryngeal inlet anteriorly and, as it can be a large, dark mass, a retropharyngeal hematoma can absorb light from the laryngoscope, worsening visibility.[37]

It should be noted that, although the surgical incision should be reopened immediately in the patient in respiratory extremis, edema and remotely tracking blood will not remit promptly upon evacuation of clot, accounting for the variable success of this step in alleviating the patient's symptoms.

Three other factors can also potentially contribute to postoperative airway compromise in patients undergoing routine head and neck surgery:

1. Large volumes of fluid administered intraoperatively can exacerbate airway edema.
2. Simply undergoing certain operations in the head and neck region may transiently cause narrowing of the upper airway, even in the absence of a neck hematoma. Carmichael and colleagues demonstrated a significant loss (up to 32%) of airway volume after routine carotid endarterectomy, greatest in the region of the hyoid, but also present at the level of the arytenoids and cricoid ring.[33,38]

3. Neck surgery can result in transient palsies to cranial nerves (IX–XII),[39,40] due to direct injury during dissection, retractor pressure, or other causes.[41] If unilateral, such palsies may be asymptomatic; however, particularly in patients with a history of previous neck surgery, or presenting for staged bilateral procedures (e.g., carotid endarterectomies), bilateral nerve damage can result in complete airway obstruction. Vocal cord palsy can result from damage to the vagal trunk or its recurrent laryngeal branches, while bilateral hypoglossal nerve palsies can result in airway obstruction from loss of innervation to the intrinsic muscles of the tongue and pharyngeal musculature.[40] One final point to note in the patient undergoing staged bilateral carotid endarterectomies is that ablation of the carotid bodies bilaterally can result in loss of the ventilatory response to hypoxemia.[42]

MANAGING THE AIRWAY

Pending the Decision of Whether and Where to Reintubate, How Can the Patient Be Symptomatically Temporized?

It should be reiterated that patients with partial airway obstruction are unpredictable in when, where, and if they will go on to complete airway obstruction. Indeed, some case reports document a decision to conservatively manage neck hematoma patients by observation, only to be confronted with sudden and catastrophic airway obstruction some hours later.[2,3] In addition, patients going on to complete airway obstruction in this setting can do so without first developing the physical sign of stridor.[2,4,11] It follows that nursing staff and airway practitioners must be educated to recognize the early signs of impending obstruction from a neck hematoma (or airway edema from any cause), including subtle voice changes and hoarseness, with later progression to agitation, dyspnea, and eventually stridor. Stridor, a late sign of airway compromise, is variously considered to be a sign of an extrathoracic airway narrowed by 50%,[43] or to a diameter of 4 mm or less.[44] The patient in the presented case should be assumed to be near respiratory extremis. Once compromising airway edema from a cause such as a neck hematoma is suspected, the wound must be fully opened, plans formulated for securing the airway, and surgical re-exploration initiated.

To temporize a case such as this in the short term (e.g., while organizing a return to the OR, or while obtaining equipment for reintubation), a number of maneuvers can be undertaken:

1. Fully open the wound. Some,[23,45] but not all,[11,24–26,46] case reports document rapid clinical improvement following this maneuver. While a significant hematoma mass may be decompressed immediately, associated laryngeal edema and/or blood tracking remotely from the hematoma site will resolve more slowly. Clinical judgment dictates where and when to open the neck wound: the patient in respiratory extremis should have it opened immediately, while others may be safely managed upon returning to the more controlled conditions of the OR, especially desirable if an arterial origin is suspected. In general, any attempt at tracheal intubation should be preceded by release of the neck wound, whether in or out of the OR. This directive should be tempered by clinical judgment: for example, if a breach of the arteriotomy site is suspected after carotid endarterectomy (based on a history of a rapid-onset neck swelling), the management should parallel that recommended for the patient with penetrating neck trauma, in whom the possible presence of damaged major vessels mandates securing the airway by tracheal intubation prior to neck exploration.
2. The head of the bed should be elevated, anywhere from 30 degrees to fully sitting,[47] to promote venous drainage and improve the mechanics of breathing. The patient with significant airway compromise will most likely naturally wish to assume the sitting position.
3. Helium and oxygen (Heliox) can be administered. Heliox, a mixture of helium gas with oxygen, is less dense than air or pure oxygen. With its lower density, a helium-oxygen mixture minimizes the work of breathing by converting some or all of the turbulent flow (through and distal to a critically narrowed airway) to more laminar flow.[48–50] Heliox is available in different oxygen/helium dilutions from 20/80 to 40/60. To maximize its clinical effect, the mixture with the highest concentration of helium should be used that is consistent with adequate oxygenation. Improved flow with Heliox can lead to larger tidal volumes and less alveolar shunting, sometimes resulting in improved oxygenation.[50–53] In addition, as a patient breathes more easily with alleviation of dyspnea-associated anxiety, the lessened negative inspiratory pressure applied to the obstructed area may result in less airway collapse, thus actually improving the degree of obstruction.[50] Therefore, Heliox use in the patient with a critically narrowed airway can provide significant symptomatic relief, in turn potentially improving patient cooperation. In the setting of a neck hematoma, however, it should be assumed that Heliox has no definitive therapeutic effect and is strictly a temporizing agent.
4. The use of epinephrine aerosols[54] and systemic steroids (e.g., dexamethasone) has been described for upper airway edema; however, there is no published evidence of their short-term efficacy in the setting of neck hematoma-induced airway compromise.

Should the Trachea of This Patient Be Intubated in the PACU or in the OR? How Do You Decide?

The short answer is that the patient with a neck hematoma is ideally reintubated in the clean, controlled conditions of the OR, with the immediate availability of surgical equipment and staff for an "airway double setup" (Table 58.1) and immediate access to difficult airway equipment and expert help. Although the OR offers the option of an inhalational induction of anesthesia, if required, the 4th National Audit Project (NAP4) report of airway-related morbidity and mortality from the United Kingdom reported a significant failure rate with this technique.[55] Ultimately, the decision about reintubation

TABLE 58.1. The Airway Double Setup

The Airway Double Setup
Definition
The presence of equipment and personnel for the purpose of moving rapidly to front-of-neck airway access, should an attempted oral or nasal tracheal intubation result in a failed airway situation.
Rationale
Attempted oral or nasal tracheal intubation in the patient with an advanced degree of pathologic airway obstruction can result in complete loss of the airway during the attempt. If the patient cannot be oxygenated with BMV, and intubation with direct or video laryngoscopy fails, rapid tracheotomy or OPEN cricothyrotomy is needed to avoid a hypoxemic cardiac arrest.
Preparation
The following conditions should be met:
Personnel: scrubbed/gowned scrub nurse; circulating nurse; scrubbed/gowned surgeon in addition to anesthesia staff;
Equipment: surgical instruments for a tracheotomy or an OPEN cricothyrotomy (see Chapter 14).
An ultrasound should also be available;
Patient: in position of comfort; cricothyroid membrane identified (e.g., by external palpation or with ultrasound); overlying skin marked, disinfected, and possibly infiltrated with local anesthetic.
Execution
Tracheotomy or open cricothyrotomy commences as soon as a failed airway and CICO is declared. Generally, a single attempt at EGD placement is warranted before putting knife to skin;
Consider this!
Some patients with obstructing pathology may have marked submandibular swelling, as part of their disease process, that extends down to, and obscures, landmarks of the cricothyroid membrane. As this may preclude easy and rapid open cricothyrotomy, the safety margin provided by the airway double setup is diminished. As such, it may be an indication that the primary technique of choice should be awake tracheotomy under local anesthesia, rather than attempted oral or nasal tracheal intubation.

on-the-spot versus a return to the OR will be tempered by the following factors:

1. Is the patient *in extremis*? If so, the airway should be secured on the spot.
2. If the patient is becoming increasingly dyspneic, is the rate of decline such that a return to the OR may be safely undertaken?
3. How far is the OR from the patient's present location and is the OR located on the same floor as the PACU?
4. If the patient's airway obstructs during transport to the OR, would it be possible to bag-mask ventilate the patient? The extensive upper airway edema accompanying most neck hematomas is likely to make BMV impossible once the patient has an obstructed airway.

How Should Such an Airway Be Approached, and Why?

Patients with significant narrowing of the airway due to pathological processes are in a dangerous situation. Onset of dyspnea, and then stridor, suggests critical airway narrowing, and in the setting of a neck hematoma should generally be regarded as signs of impending complete airway obstruction. In this patient, the airway assessment has suggested the potential for difficulty with BMV, direct and indirect (video) laryngoscopic intubation, EGD rescue ventilation, and a front-of-neck airway access (FONA). If time and the patient's clinical condition permit, evaluation of the upper airway may be obtained with nasopharyngoscopy. Following the application of topical nasal anesthesia, a flexible nasopharyngoscope is inserted through the nose to permit the evaluation of the glottis and surrounding structures, for the degree of edema and deviation of the larynx. In one study of 138 patients with head and neck pathology presenting for elective surgery, preoperative nasopharyngoscopy resulted in a change in planned airway management in 26% of cases.[7] "Awake look" direct[56] or video laryngoscopy may also provide useful information. Regardless, careful consideration must occur on how best to proceed. A number of options exist:

1. *Local or regional anesthesia.* One published case series in the surgical literature documents hematoma evacuation in eight patients under local anesthesia with no morbidity, which contrasted significantly with the 57% complication rate in seven other patients done under general anesthesia.[10] Hematoma evacuation and exploration using local, regional (or no) anesthesia may be feasible before the patient is significantly short of breath and is still able to cooperate.[47] However, regional anesthesia (e.g., superficial cervical blockade) may be difficult to perform, if an enlarging hematoma obscures anatomic landmarks.[11]
2. *Awake open cricothyrotomy or tracheotomy under local anesthesia.* Some authorities suggest that patients with advanced degrees of obstructing airway pathology, particularly those with lesions of sufficient size to preclude passage of even a small ETT, should have their airways secured with awake tracheotomy under local anesthesia.[43,57] In expert hands, and with patient cooperation, this is a procedure that can be done relatively quickly and painlessly. Technical difficulty can be encountered if midline landmarks are shifted laterally or are obscured by an expanding hematoma. In addition, airway edema can also occur internally at the level of the cricoid ring, potentially impacting the ease of open cricothyrotomy.[33]
3. *Awake oral or nasal (translaryngeal) intubation.* Awake translaryngeal intubation (via oral or nasal routes) confers the advantage of having a breathing patient who is maintaining and protecting the airway and would be the method of choice by many experts in this situation. In the setting of a neck hematoma, distorted anatomy can be anticipated (see section "What Are the Causes of Airway Obstruction in a Patient with a Postsurgical Neck Hematoma?" in this chapter).

In the awake patient, movement of swollen mucosal folds with inspiration and expiration, and the location of bubbles during expiration, may help locate the laryngeal inlet. An attempted awake intubation from above must, however, confer a high probability of success, in order to outweigh the risk of loss of the airway during the attempt (which can happen even in expert hands).[9,35] The NAP4 study reported on 23 patients with head and neck pathology who were intubated with a flexible bronchoscopic technique. The attempt failed in 14, and of those, 4 had been attempted in the awake patient.[55] Special attention should be given to topical airway anesthesia (see section "Local Anesthesia of the Airway" in Chapter 3, and the section "Although Awake Intubation is Considered the Gold Standard, Why Did the Patient Obstruct During Application of Topical Airway Anesthesia?" below). A high level of situation awareness, good flexible bronchoscopic equipment, and experienced hands are necessary.[11,58] Alternatively, direct laryngoscopy and video laryngoscopy have also been described for awake intubations.[12,59,60]

4. *Inhalational induction*. An inhalational induction has been espoused, in a number of reports, as an option to facilitate intubation of a patient with a neck hematoma.[11,30,35,43] However, during an inhalational induction, while spontaneous ventilatory efforts may continue, it must be appreciated that volatile anesthetics have deleterious effects on upper airway tone and patency similar to those of intravenously administered sedatives.[6,61] While the inhalational induction may be considered for the patient unable to cooperate with an awake intubation or tracheotomy, an airway double setup should be arranged, the neck wound should be opened before induction of anesthesia, and close attention should be paid to maximizing airway patency as the patient loses consciousness (Table 58.2). Inhalational inductions in the setting of neck hematomas, in published case reports, have been successful in some cases, although often prolonged or difficult.[3,11,24,35] More recently, data from the NAP4 study suggests that in the setting of obstructing pathology, this technique can and does fail. In 27 patients with head and neck pathology undergoing inhalational induction, there was no compromise to spontaneous ventilation in only 4 patients, some compromise with oxygen desaturation in 12, and in 11 patients ventilation became impossible, either before or after laryngoscopy attempts.[55] At this time, inhalational induction cannot be condoned as the primary technique to facilitate reintubation in these patients, unless a lack of patient cooperation precludes an awake technique.
5. *Intravenous (IV) induction*. For the cooperative patient, unless asymptomatic, and in whom an awake internal airway assessment has been ruled out for significant edema or laryngeal displacement, this route *cannot be recommended* as the method of choice to facilitate tracheal intubation with obstructing airway pathology due to a neck hematoma. IV induction of anesthesia, with or without muscle relaxant administration, is fraught with hazard in this setting, with case reports attesting to the lack of any identifiable landmarks at direct laryngoscopy,[3,62] often in conjunction with the inability to bag-mask ventilate the patient.[11,55,62]

TABLE 58.2. Strategies to Help Maximize Upper Airway Patency During Difficult Inhalational Inductions

1. Maintain the patient in a sitting or semi-sitting position.
2. Keep the head and upper C-spine extended and lower C-spine flexed, to maintain longitudinal traction on the upper airway, thus decreasing its collapsibility.[61]
3. Apply a jaw thrust to increase retropalatal and retrolingual airway caliber.[61]
4. Through a nostril already topically anesthetized, insert a nasopharyngeal airway to help overcome approximation of the soft palate to the posterior pharyngeal wall, while the patient is still too light to tolerate an OPA.[43]
5. Application of CPAP during the inhalational induction may help to splint open collapsible supraglottic structures.

How Should We Proceed in This Case?

Our Plan A here is for an awake tracheal intubation with a flexible bronchoscope under topical airway anesthesia, a viable option if good equipment and expertise is available with the flexible bronchoscope, and if patient cooperation can be enlisted. In the event of an uncooperative patient, an inhalational induction could be considered. If the patient were to obstruct during attempted awake intubation and a failed airway situation ensued, Plan B would be rapid conversion to an open cricothyrotomy.[63,64]

How Will You Prepare for the Awake Intubation?

In the OR, an airway double setup should be readied (Table 58.1), with scrubbed surgical staff and equipment available for urgent tracheotomy or open cricothyrotomy. The difficult airway cart should be in the room. IV access should be assured, monitors applied, and the patient positioned in his position of comfort (often sitting). The cricothyroid membrane should be identified, marked, and disinfectant solution applied to the anterior neck. If not already done, and if deemed appropriate, all layers[65,66] of the surgical incision should be opened and any easily accessible clot removed. Psychological preparation should be undertaken with confident reassurance that successful intubation will totally alleviate the patient's dyspnea, while at the same time emphasizing the need for cooperation. If Heliox had been applied, it should be interrupted for only brief periods during application of topical airway anesthesia. Topical airway anesthetic agents and techniques have been addressed elsewhere (see Chapter 3). Systemic sedation should be avoided, if at all possible. An adult flexible bronchoscope (e.g., 6.2 mm OD) should be loaded with a small (e.g., 7 mm ID) ETT. An assistant can apply gentle tongue traction.

It is worth noting that even experienced anesthesia practitioners frequently fail to correctly locate the external landmark of the cricothyroid membrane. Studies with volunteer subjects have demonstrated an average success of less than 30% to 40% across gender and body habitus.[67–69] With neck anatomy altered by a neck hematoma, an even lower success rate ought to be anticipated. If time permits, ultrasound may be of use in identifying the location of the cricothyroid membrane, as part of the airway double setup.

What Can You Expect During the Awake Flexible Bronchoscopic Intubation?

Awake flexible bronchoscopic intubation of the patient with extensive upper airway edema due to a neck hematoma differs substantially from that in a patient without obstructing pathology. In the patient with no obstructing pathology, navigation of the bronchoscope can proceed from landmark to landmark in the upper airway, for example, from uvula to base of tongue, to epiglottis, then to and through the glottis. In the patient with upper airway edema, both the epiglottis and glottic opening may be obscured by "clouds" of edematous tissue. This leaves tissue movement and the suggestion of an opening (e.g., bubbles on expiration) as the only indications of the path to the vocal cords. As this happens, the bronchoscope is advanced in a slow and controlled fashion toward the opening or bubbles. During inspiration, edematous tissues may be sucked together, obscuring the opening. It is important to have the bronchoscope remain motionless in the airway during this phase, simply waiting for the view to reappear during the next expiration prior to resuming scope advancement. Often in this setting, one simply continues navigating toward the opening suggested by movement, until the cords suddenly appear in front of the scope.

As the only landmarks leading to the airway after the uvula, the presence of both movement and bubbles on expiration are crucial clues. This is one reason why it is critical to avoid ablation of spontaneous respiration in these patients.

It should also be noted that a neck hematoma can significantly displace the larynx to the left or right of its expected midline location. This can be anticipated, prior to beginning the bronchoscopic intubation, by examining the front of the neck, looking or feeling for the location of the thyroid cartilage, or performing an internal airway evaluation by nasopharyngoscopy or oral video laryngoscopy, under local anesthesia.

During Application of Topical Airway Anesthesia, the Patient's Airway Obstructs—What Should You Do Now?

If the patient's airway obstructs, common sense should prevail. One should do what one would always do to ventilate the apneic patient: attempt an airway-opening maneuver and perform BMV, using a two-person technique. An oropharyngeal or nasopharyngeal airway may be used, depending on the patient's level of consciousness. PEEP should be applied during BMV to help stent open collapsed tissues and ease any laryngospasm.[6,61,70]

What If BMV Fails? Should a Front-of-Neck Airway Access (FONA) Be Performed?

A failed airway situation has been defined as the inability to maintain adequate oxygen saturation with BMV, *and* failure to intubate on at least one occasion (see section "The Failed Airway Algorithm" in Chapter 2). A single attempt at direct or video laryngoscopic intubation should be made. If this is unsuccessful, a failed airway is declared, and the default response becomes a tracheotomy or open (scalpel) cricothyrotomy.[63,64]

At Direct Laryngoscopy, Only Extensive Edematous Mucosa Is Seen, Along with the Tip of the Epiglottis, Deviated to the Right

If the patient is already unconscious from hypoxemia, it is worth performing a single chest compression during laryngoscopy, in order to see if a bubble is produced, indicating the entrance to the airway. With or without a bubble, a tracheal tube introducer, or small styleted ETT, can be blindly placed where the glottic opening would be expected to be, beneath the epiglottis. If this single attempt fails, however, the default maneuver is to proceed to a FONA in order to maximize the chances of salvaging a bad situation. Unfortunately, and all too frequently, the decision to proceed with a FONA is made too late to salvage the patient.

What Is the Role, If Any, of an EGD Such as a Laryngeal Mask Airway?

An EGD such as a laryngeal mask airway (LMA) may fail to oxygenate the patient in this setting as (1) correct seating in the pharynx may be difficult due to retropharyngeal swelling or a displaced laryngeal inlet and (2) even if correctly seated, extensive edema at or above the level of the cords may preclude effective ventilation. However, several centers have reported successful oxygenation of patients with LMAs in failed airway situations due to neck hematomas,[25,26,46,62,71,72] or other obstructing pathology.[73,74] This may occur as the EGD bypasses more proximal edematous and obstructs soft tissues, allowing positive pressure ventilation from a position immediately in front of the laryngeal inlet. While the correct response in the failed airway "can't intubate, can't oxygenate" (CICO) situation is a FONA, it is worth a single attempt at EGD insertion while preparations are underway to proceed with a FONA.[64]

Although Awake Intubation Is Considered the Gold Standard, Why Did the Patient's Airway Obstruct During Application of Topical Airway Anesthesia?

Loss of the airway during application of topical airway anesthesia,[70,74,75] or attempted awake oral or nasal endoscopic intubation,[9,46,55,76] in the patient with a neck hematoma or other obstructing pathology is well described. Apart from the natural progression of the disease process, this may occur for a number of reasons:

1. *Systemically administered sedative agents* may provoke sudden and total obstruction.[9,61]
2. *Laryngospasm* during the airway topicalization process,[43,74,77] particularly in the patient with deeper sedation.
3. *Patient panic.* As the dyspneic patient desperately tries to inspire, the high negative inspiratory pressure applied to an already narrowed, collapsible upper airway may contribute to complete collapse.[77,78]
4. *Direct effect of local anesthetic agents on upper airway mechanoreceptors.* The existence of laryngeal and supralaryngeal pressure and stretch receptors has been hypothesized as being responsible for maintaining airway patency, by responding to

negative intraluminal airway pressure via increasing neural and muscular activity[79,80] (see Chapter 3). The activity of such receptors can be affected or abolished by application of topical airway anesthesia.[79,80] This in turn can significantly affect inspiratory flow, even in normal individuals. Pulmonary function studies in healthy volunteers have demonstrated a significant reduction in maximal,[81] peak, and forced[82] inspiratory flow rates following topical airway anesthesia. Studies of the sleep-apnea population in whom topical airway anesthesia has been applied have also shown worsening of obstructive parameters. This is an underappreciated side effect of topical airway anesthesia, and in the patient with a tenuous airway, may be an important phenomenon to consider. It does not preclude proceeding with awake oral or nasal tracheal intubation with topical airway anesthesia, but does underscore the need for planning and an airway double setup. In addition, in any patient with significant obstructing airway pathology, awake tracheotomy or open cricothyrotomy should be considered as a primary technique.

OTHER CONSIDERATIONS

How Should the Postoperative Disposition of a Patient Reintubated for a Neck Hematoma Be Managed?

Although the immediate mechanical compression of the airway caused by the hematoma may be relieved after surgical re-exploration and/or evacuation of hematoma, other mechanisms of airway compromise, for example, perilaryngeal edema and blood dissection along tissue planes, may take longer to resolve. Caution must prevail, and consideration should be given to keeping the patient intubated and ventilated for a period of time (e.g., 24 hours) in an intensive care setting. The patient should be nursed head-up to promote venous drainage, and consideration can be given to administering steroids. Admittedly, many randomized controlled trials looking at the effect of steroid administration on upper airway[38] and laryngeal edema,[83] postextubation stridor,[84] or airway-related delayed extubation[85] in adults have failed to demonstrate a beneficial effect. Results of studies in the pediatric setting have been mixed.[86,87] Future studies looking at alternative doses, dosing intervals, or specific subpopulations may yet identify a beneficial effect of steroid administration.

What Criteria Should Be Met Prior to Extubation?

Prior to extubation of the patient intubated for airway pathology such as a neck hematoma, an attempt should be made to evaluate both the caliber of the subglottic airway and the condition of the laryngeal inlet, in addition to the usual extubation criteria. Traditionally, the presence of a "cuff leak" has been sought as a reassuring sign of an airway patent enough to withstand extubation, although a systematic review and meta-analysis of studies has concluded that "the presence of a detectable leak has a low predictive value, and (after extubation) does not rule out the occurrence of upper airway obstruction, or the need for reintubation."[88] Thus, instead of, or in addition to a cuff-leak test, a visual evaluation of the larynx, usually with nasopharyngoscopy or oral video laryngoscopy, should be undertaken, looking for:

- The appropriate midline location of the laryngeal inlet
- The absence of significant perilaryngeal edema
- Appropriate bilateral vocal cord movement[41]

Returning to the OR for extubation should be considered, and extubation over an airway exchange catheter is advisable.

What Other Situations or Types of Surgery Incur the Risk of Neck Hematomas? Are There Any Risk Factors or Preventive Measures That Can Be Undertaken?

Any surgery of the head, neck, and thorax can lead to airway compromising hematomas and swelling. Common examples include carotid endarterectomy,[11,89,90] parathyroid and thyroid surgery,[18,24,91] and anterior cervical discectomy/fusion (ACDF),[45,92] with most reported series suggesting a neck hematoma incidence of 1% to 8%.[12,89,93–99] Case reports have also identified central line insertion[2,4,13,14,21,29,100,101] and stellate ganglion blocks[28,102] in the development of life-threatening neck hematomas. Spontaneous bleeds resulting in neck hematomas have also occurred, in both anticoagulated and nonanticoagulated patients.[15,32,35,103–107] Blunt trauma has been contributory in some, often resulting in retropharyngeal hematomas.[108–113] Neck hematoma has also been reported after endovascular carotid revascularization[114] and transesophageal echocardiography.[115]

Risk factors for the development of postoperative hematomas following carotid artery and other head and neck surgeries include:

- Antiplatelet agents (particularly clopidogrel)[3,11,89,116,117];
- Male sex[116,117];
- Black race[117];
- Four or more comorbidities[117];
- Failure to reverse intraoperatively administered heparin[31,90,118,119];
- The use of a vein graft[120] or shunt[119]
- Conversion from a regional to a general anesthetic technique[89]
- Significant intraoperative hypotension[119]
- Postoperative hypertension (e.g., systolic blood pressure of >200 mmHg)[3,11,31,89,90]

This latter underscores the importance of aggressive control of hemodynamics in a high-dependency care environment postoperatively. A multicenter study on neck hematoma after thyroid surgery identified use of a drain, Grave's disease, benign pathology, and the use of antiplatelet medication as risk factors.[91] Surgical drains have not demonstrated a benefit in the prevention of postoperative neck hematomas following thyroidectomy[66,91,99,121] or carotid endarterectomy.

How Does a Neck Hematoma Affect the Patient's Prognosis?

The occurrence of a postsurgical neck hematoma in the patient undergoing carotid endarterectomy increases the risk of stroke or death 2.5- to 4-fold.[96,122] Some of this morbidity and mortality may be related to postoperative airway compromise.

SUMMARY

Once airway compromise from any cause has been identified, the postsurgical patient should be observed in a high-dependency nursing unit. A decision on definitive airway management should occur early, while patient cooperation allows the option of awake tracheal intubation. More information on how to proceed most safely with reintubation can be obtained with an internal airway exam (e.g., nasopharyngoscopy), if the patient's condition permits. Awake intubation in the patient with obstructing pathology should always occur with the "airway double setup," availability of equipment, and personnel to allow an emergency tracheotomy or open cricothyrotomy. Inhalational induction in the patient with obstructing pathology is hazardous and should not be considered as a primary technique. Regardless of technique, reintubation should generally be preceded by a release of the surgical incision.

CHECKLIST

1. Formulate a plan with the surgical team (airway plan, location, temporization, double setup).
2. With patient in sitting or semi-sitting position, consider Heliox to temporize the patient's stridor and respiratory distress (epinephrine nebulizers/steroids have a delayed effect).
3. If the patient is in extremis, discuss reopening wound with surgeon.
4. Perform a nasopharyngoscopy if the patient is cooperative to better assess supraglottic/glottic structures.
5. Consider your options: (a) local or regional anesthesia; (b) awake open cricothyrotomy or tracheotomy under local anesthesia; (c) awake oral or nasal intubation; and (d) inhalation induction. Have a difficult airway cart set up in the room with surgeons prepared with a double setup.
6. Awake nasal or tracheal intubation is preferred if the patient is cooperative. If the patient is not cooperative, consider inhalation induction. Be aware that both options have a high risk of provoking sudden airway collapse due to local topicalization or volatile effects.
7. If the patient obstructs: Optimize your BMV techniques. It is reasonable to try one attempt at intubation.
8. If these fail, place an EGD (e.g., LMA) and proceed quickly to a FONA.
9. Disposition to ICU is recommended. Review criteria for a planned extubation.

SELF-EVALUATION QUESTIONS

58.1. Recognizing that no method of intubation can be guaranteed 100% complication free, which of the following approaches to securing the airway is LEAST safe in the patient with a neck hematoma?

A. Awake intubation with topical airway anesthesia
B. Rapid-sequence intubation with induction agent and muscle relaxant
C. Local or regional anesthesia for evacuation of hematoma and no intubation
D. Inhalational induction
E. Awake tracheostomy under local anesthesia

58.2. In the patient with obstructing airway pathology such as a neck hematoma, which of the following is the LEAST safe option to help symptomatically temporize the patient while preparing for intubation?

A. Use sedative agents to alleviate patient anxiety.
B. If patient oxygenation permits, use Heliox to help to decrease the work of breathing.
C. Have the patient in the sitting or semi-sitting position.
D. Administer racemic epinephrine via aerosol.
E. Give intravenous steroids to help counteract any inflammatory component.

58.3. In the patient with obstructing airway pathology such as a neck hematoma, which of the following airway management techniques would be (at least relatively) contraindicated?

A. Direct laryngoscopy and intubation
B. Placement of a laryngeal mask airway
C. Blind ETT passage through an intubating laryngeal mask airway (Fastrach®)
D. Awake intubation with a flexible bronchoscope
E. Bag-mask ventilation with an oropharyngeal airway

REFERENCES

1. Cormack RS, Lehane J. Difficult tracheal intubation in obstetrics. *Anaesthesia*. 1984;39:1105-1111.
2. Digby S. Fatal respiratory obstruction following insertion of a central venous line. *Anaesthesia*. 1994;49:1013-1014.
3. Munro FJ, Makin AP, Reid J. Airway problems after carotid endarterectomy. *Br J Anaesth*. 1996;76:156-159.
4. Randalls B, Toomey PJ. Laryngeal oedema from a neck haematoma. A complication of internal jugular vein cannulation. *Anaesthesia*. 1990;45:850-852.
5. Murphy M, Hung O, Launcelott G, Law JA, Morris I. Predicting the difficult laryngoscopic intubation: are we on the right track? *Can J Anaesth*. 2005;52:231-235.
6. Patel A, Pearce A. Progress in management of the obstructed airway. *Anaesthesia*. 2011;66(Suppl 2):93-100.
7. Rosenblatt W, Ianus AI, Sukhupragarn W, Fickenscher A, Sasaki C. Preoperative endoscopic airway examination (PEAE) provides superior airway information and may reduce the use of unnecessary awake intubation. *Anesth Analg*. 2011;112:602-607.
8. Byard RW, Gilbert JD. Narcotic administration and stenosing lesions of the upper airway – a potentially lethal combination. *J Clin Forensic Med*. 2005;12:29-31.
9. McGuire G, el-Beheiry H. Complete upper airway obstruction during awake fibreoptic intubation in patients with unstable cervical spine fractures. *Can J Anaesth*. 1999;46:176-178.
10. Kunkel JM, Gomez ER, Spebar MJ, Delgado RJ, Jarstfer BS, Collins GJ. Wound hematomas after carotid endarterectomy. *Am J Surg*. 1984;148:844-847.
11. O'Sullivan JC, Wells DG, Wells GR. Difficult airway management with neck swelling after carotid endarterectomy. *Anaesth Intensive Care*. 1986;14:460-464.
12. Shakespeare WA, Lanier WL, Perkins WJ, Pasternak JJ. Airway management in patients who develop neck hematomas after carotid endarterectomy. *Anesth Analg*. 2010;110:588-593.

13. Lo WK, Chong JL. Neck haematoma and airway obstruction in a pre-eclamptic patient: a complication of internal jugular vein cannulation. *Anaesth Intensive Care*. 1997;25:423-425.
14. Smurthwaite GJ, Letheren MJ. Airway obstruction after trans-jugular liver biopsy: anaesthetic management. *Br J Anaesth*. 1995;75:102-104.
15. Stenner M, Helmstaedter V, Spuentrup E, Quante G, Huettenbrink KB. Cervical hemorrhage due to spontaneous rupture of the superior thyroid artery: case report and review of the literature. *Head Neck*. 2010;32:1277-1281.
16. Quick E, Byard RW. Postoperative cervical soft tissue hemorrhage with acute upper airway obstruction. *J Forensic Sci*. 2013;58(Suppl 1): S264-S266.
17. Carr ER, Benjamin E. In vitro study investigating post neck surgery haematoma airway obstruction. *J Laryngol Otol*. 2009;123:662-665.
18. Hare R. Respiratory obstruction after thyroidectomy. *Anaesthesia*. 1982;37:1136.
19. Thakur NA, McDonnell M, Paller D, Palumbo M. Wound hematoma after anterior cervical spine surgery: in vitro study of the pathophysiology of airway obstruction. *Am J Orthop*. 2013;42:E35-E37.
20. Paleri V, Maroju RS, Ali MS, Ruckley RW. Spontaneous retro- and parapharyngeal haematoma caused by intrathyroid bleed. *J Laryngol Otol*. 2002;116:854-858.
21. Kua JS, Tan IK. Airway obstruction following internal jugular vein cannulation. *Anaesthesia*. 1997;52:776-780.
22. Thomas MD, Torres A, Garcia-Polo J, Gavilan C. Life-threatening cervico-mediastinal haematoma after carotid sinus massage. *J Laryngol Otol*. 1991;105:381-383.
23. Bukht D, Langford RM. Airway obstruction after surgery in the neck. *Anaesthesia*. 1983;38:389-390.
24. Bexton MD, Radford R. An unusual cause of respiratory obstruction after thyroidectomy. *Anaesthesia*. 1982;37:596.
25. Ebrahimy DM, Behnaz M, Khorasanizadeh SH, Kouzekanani HNG. Airway management in a case of expanding neck hematoma after carotid endarterectomy. *Novel Biomed*. 2018;6:199-201.
26. Gerasimov M, Lee B, Bittner EA. Postoperative Anterior Neck Hematoma (ANH): timely intervention is vital. *APSF Newsletter*. 2021;36:44-47.
27. Knoblanche GE. Respiratory obstruction due to haematoma following internal jugular vein cannulation. *Anaesth Intensive Care*. 1979;7:286.
28. Uchida T, Nakao S, Morimoto M, Iwamoto T. Serious cervical hematoma after stellate ganglion block. *J Anesth*. 2015;29:321.
29. Wu PJ, Chau SW, Lu IC, Hsu HT, Cheng KI. Delayed airway obstruction after internal jugular venous catheterization in a patient with anticoagulant therapy. *Case Rep Anesthesiol*. 2011;2011:359867.
30. Wells DG, Zelcer J, Wells GR, Sherman GP. A theoretical mechanism for massive supraglottic swelling following carotid endarterectomy. *Aust N Z J Surg*. 1988;58:979-981.
31. Holdsworth RJ, McCollum PT. Acute laryngeal oedema following carotid endarterectomy. *J Cardiovasc Surg*. 1994;35:249-251.
32. Inokuchi G, Kurita N, Baba M, Hata Y, Okuno T. Retropharyngeal hematoma from parathyroid hemorrhage in a hemodialysis patient. *Auris Nasus Larynx*. 2012;39:527-530.
33. Carmichael FJ, McGuire GP, Wong DT, Crofts S, Sharma S, Montanera W. Computed tomographic analysis of airway dimensions after carotid endarterectomy. *Anesth Analg* 1996;83:12-17.
34. Wade JS. Cecil Joll Lecture, 1979. Respiratory obstruction in thyroid surgery. *Ann R Coll Surg Engl*. 1980;62:15-24.
35. Ahmed J, Philpott J, Lew-Gor S, Blunt D. Airway obstruction: a rare complication of thrombolytic therapy. *J Laryngol Otol*. 2005;119:819-821.
36. Field JR, DeSaussure RL. Retropharyngeal hemorrhage with respiratory obstruction following angiography. *J Neurosurg*. 1965;22:610-611.
37. Myssiorek D, Shalmi C. Traumatic retropharyngeal hematoma. *Arch Otolaryngol Head Neck Surg*. 1989:115:1130-1132.
38. Hughes R, McGuire G, Montanera W, Wong D, Carmichael FJ. Upper airway edema after carotid endarterectomy: the effect of steroid administration. *Anesth Analg*. 1997;84:475-478.
39. Itobi E, Sutherland AD, Whinney D, Davies JN. Acute airway obstruction complicating unilateral carotid endarterectomy. *Eur J Vasc Endovasc Surg*. 2005;30:152-153.
40. Spiekermann BF, Stone DJ, Bogdonoff DL, Yemen TA. Airway management in neuroanaesthesia. *Can J Anaesth*. 1996;43:820-834.
41. Tyers MR, Cronin K. Airway obstruction following second operation for carotid endarterectomy. *Anaesth Intensive Care*. 1986;14:314-316.
42. Wade JG, Larson CP Jr., Hickey RF, Ehrenfeld WK, Severinghaus JW. Effect of carotid endarterectomy on carotid chemoreceptor and baroreceptor function in man. *N Engl J Med*. 1970;282:823-829.
43. Mason RA, Fielder CP. The obstructed airway in head and neck surgery. *Anaesthesia*. 1999;54:625-628.
44. Donlon J. Jr. *Anesthetic and Airway Management of Laryngoscopy and Bronchoscopy*. St. Louis: Mosby; 1996.
45. Roy SP. Acute postoperative neck hematoma. *Am J Emerg Med*. 1999;17: 308-309.
46. Martin R, Girouard Y, Cote DJ. Use of a laryngeal mask in acute airway obstruction after carotid endarterectomy. *Can J Anaesth*. 2002;49:890.
47. Dixon JL, Snyder SK, Lairmore TC, Jupiter D, Govednik C, Hendricks JC. A novel method for the management of post-thyroidectomy or parathyroidectomy hematoma: a single-institution experience after over 4,000 central neck operations. *World J Surg*. 2014;38:1262-1267.
48. Hashemian SM, Fallahian F. The use of heliox in critical care. *Int J Crit Illn Inj Sci*. 2014;4:138-142.
49. Hessan H, Houck J, Harvey H. Airway obstruction due to lymphoma of the larynx and trachea. *Laryngoscope*. 1988;98:176-180.
50. Ho AM, Dion PW, Karmakar MK, Chung DC, Tay BA. Use of heliox in critical upper airway obstruction. Physical and physiologic considerations in choosing the optimal helium:oxygen mix. *Resuscitation*. 2002;52:297-300.
51. Khanlou H, Eiger G. Safety and efficacy of heliox as a treatment for upper airway obstruction due to radiation-induced laryngeal dysfunction. *Heart Lung*. 2001;30:146-147.
52. Moraa I, Sturman N, McGuire T, van Driel ML. Heliox for croup in children. *Cochrane Database Syst Rev*. 2013;12:CD006822.
53. Riley RH, Raper GD, Newman MA. Helium-oxygen and cardiopulmonary bypass standby in anaesthesia for tracheal stenosis. *Anaesth Intensive Care*. 1994;22:710-713.
54. MacDonnell SP, Timmins AC, Watson JD. Adrenaline administered via a nebulizer in adult patients with upper airway obstruction. *Anaesthesia*. 1995;50:35-36.
55. Patel A, Pearce A, Pracy P. Head and neck pathology. In: Cook T, Woodall N, Frerk C, eds. *4th National Audit Project of the Royal College of Anaesthetists and the Difficult Airway Society. Major complications of airway management in the United Kingdom. London: RCoA*; 2011:143-154.
56. Gupta S, Macneil R, Bryson G. Laryngoscopy in conscious patients with remifentanil: how useful is an "awake look"? *J Clin Anesth*. 2012;24:19-24.
57. Goldberg D, Bhatti N. Management of the impaired airway in the adult. In: *Cummings, ed. Otolaryngology, Head and Neck Surgery*. 4th ed. Philadelphia, PA: Elsevier, Mosby; 2005:2441-2453.
58. Ovassapian A, Tuncbilek M, Weitzel EK, Joshi CW. Airway management in adult patients with deep neck infections: a case series and review of the literature. *Anesth Analg*. 2005;100:585-589.
59. Moore A, Schricker T. Awake videolaryngoscopy versus fiberoptic bronchoscopy. *Curr Opin Anaesthesiol*. 2019;32:764-768.
60. Rosenstock CV, Thogersen B, Afshari A, Christensen AL, Eriksen C, Gatke MR. Awake fiberoptic or awake video laryngoscopic tracheal intubation in patients with anticipated difficult airway management: a randomized clinical trial. *Anesthesiology*. 2012;116:1210-1216.
61. Hillman DR, Platt PR, Eastwood PR. The upper airway during anaesthesia. *Br J Anaesth*. 2003;91:31-39.
62. Augoustides JG, Groff BE, Mann DG, Johansson JS. Difficult airway management after carotid endarterectomy: utility and limitations of the Laryngeal Mask Airway. *J Clin Anesth*. 2007;19:218-221.
63. Apfelbaum JL, Hagberg CA, Caplan RA, et al. Practice guidelines for management of the difficult airway: an updated report by the American Society of Anesthesiologists Task Force on management of the difficult airway. *Anesthesiology*. 2013;118:251-270.
64. Law JA, Duggan LV, Asselin M, et al. Canadian Airway Focus Group updated consensus-based recommendations for management of the difficult airway: part 1. Difficult airway management encountered in an unconscious patient. *Can J Anaesth*. 2021;68:1373-1404.
65. Pelizzo MR, Toniato A, Piotto A, Bernante P, Pagetta C, Bernardi C. Prevention and treatment of intra- and post-operative complications in thyroid surgery. *Ann Ital Chir*. 2001;72:273-276.
66. Shandilya M, Kieran S, Walshe P, Timon C. Cervical haematoma after thyroid surgery: management and prevention. *Irish Med J*. 2006;99: 266-268.
67. Aslani A, Ng SC, Hurley M, McCarthy KF, McNicholas M, McCaul CL. Accuracy of identification of the cricothyroid membrane in female subjects using palpation: an observational study. *Anesth Analg*. 2012;114:987-992.
68. Elliott DS, Baker PA, Scott MR, Birch CW, Thompson JM. Accuracy of surface landmark identification for cannula cricothyroidotomy. *Anaesthesia*. 2010;65:889-894.
69. Lamb A, Zhang J, Hung O, et al. Accuracy of identifying the cricothyroid membrane by anesthesia trainees and staff in a Canadian institution. *Can J Anaesth*. 2015;62:495-503.
70. Calder I, Koh K. Cervical haematoma and airway obstruction. *Br J Anaesth*. 1996;76:888-889.

71. Jones DA, Geraghty IF. Emergency management of upper airway obstruction due to a rapidly expanding haematoma in the neck. *Br J Hosp Med.* 1995;53:589-590.
72. Ozyuvaci E, Akyol O, Erden DV, Vatansever SD, Yilmaz GD, Toprak N. Upper airway obstruction due to retropharyngeal haematoma after posterior cervical spine surgery. *Anaesth Intensive Care.* 2011;39:768-770.
73. King CJ, Davey AJ, Chandradeva K. Emergency use of the laryngeal mask airway in severe upper airway obstruction caused by supraglottic oedema. *Br J Anaesth.* 1995;75:785-786.
74. Shaw IC, Welchew EA, Harrison BJ, Michael S. Complete airway obstruction during awake fibreoptic intubation. *Anaesthesia.* 1997;52:582-585.
75. White MC, Reynolds F. Sudden airway obstruction following inhalation drug abuse. *Br J Anaesth.* 1999;82:808.
76. Wulf H, Brinkmann G, Rautenberg M. Management of the difficult airway. A case of failed fiberoptic intubation. *Acta Anaesthesiol Scand.* 1997;41:1080-1082.
77. Ho AM, Chung DC, To EW, Karmakar MK. Total airway obstruction during local anesthesia in a non-sedated patient with a compromised airway. *Can J Anaesth.* 2004;51:838-841.
78. Shiratori T, Hara K, Ando N. Acute airway obstruction secondary to retropharyngeal hematoma. *J Anesth.* 2003;17:46-48.
79. Berry RB, McNellis MI, Kouchi K, Light RW. Upper airway anesthesia reduces phasic genioglossus activity during sleep apnea. *Am J Respir Crit Care Med.* 1997;156:127-132.
80. Horner RL, Innes JA, Holden HB, Guz A. Afferent pathway(s) for pharyngeal dilator reflex to negative pressure in man: a study using upper airway anaesthesia. *J Physiol.* 1991;436:31-44.
81. Liistro G, Stanescu DC, Veriter C, Rodenstein DO, D'Odemont JP. Upper airway anesthesia induces airflow limitation in awake humans. *Am Rev Respir Dis.* 1992;146:581-585.
82. Kuna ST, Woodson GE, Sant'Ambrogio G. Effect of laryngeal anesthesia on pulmonary function testing in normal subjects. *Am Rev Respir Dis.* 1988;137:656-661.
83. Darmon JY, Rauss A, Dreyfuss D, et al. Evaluation of risk factors for laryngeal edema after tracheal extubation in adults and its prevention by dexamethasone. A placebo-controlled, double-blind, multicenter study. *Anesthesiology.* 1992;77:245-251.
84. Ho LI, Harn HJ, Lien TC, Hu PY, Wang JH. Postextubation laryngeal edema in adults. Risk factor evaluation and prevention by hydrocortisone. *Intensive Care Med.* 1996;22:933-936.
85. Emery SE, Akhavan S, Miller P, et al. Steroids and risk factors for airway compromise in multilevel cervical corpectomy patients: a prospective, randomized, double-blind study. *Spine (Phila Pa 1976).* 2009;34:229-232.
86. Anene O, Meert KL, Uy H, Simpson P, Sarnaik AP. Dexamethasone for the prevention of postextubation airway obstruction: a prospective, randomized, double-blind, placebo-controlled trial. *Crit Care Med.* 1996;24:1666-1669.
87. Tellez DW, Galvis AG, Storgion SA, Amer HN, Hoseyni M, Deakers TW. Dexamethasone in the prevention of postextubation stridor in children. *J Pediatr.* 1991;118:289-294.
88. Ochoa ME, Marin Mdel C, Frutos-Vivar F, et al. Cuff-leak test for the diagnosis of upper airway obstruction in adults: a systematic review and meta-analysis. *Intensive Care Med.* 2009;35:1171-1179.
89. Morales Gisbert SM, Sala Almonacil VA, Zaragoza Garcia JM, Genoves Gasco B, Gomez Palones FJ, Ortiz Monzon E. Predictors of cervical bleeding after carotid endarterectomy. *Ann Vasc Surg.* 2014;28:366-374.
90. Nunn DB. Carotid endarterectomy: an analysis of 234 operative cases. *Ann Surg.* 1975;182:733-738.
91. Campbell MJ, McCoy KL, Shen WT, et al. A multi-institutional international study of risk factors for hematoma after thyroidectomy. *Surgery.* 2013;154:1283-1289; discussion 9-91.
92. Yu NH, Jahng TA, Kim CH, Chung CK. Life-threatening late hemorrhage due to superior thyroid artery dissection after anterior cervical discectomy and fusion. *Spine (Phila Pa 1976).* 2010;35:E739-E742.
93. Assadian A, Knobl P, Hubl W, et al. Safety and efficacy of intravenous enoxaparin for carotid endarterectomy: a prospective randomized pilot trial. *J Vasc Surg.* 2008;47:537-542.
94. Bertalanffy H, Eggert HR. Complications of anterior cervical discectomy without fusion in 450 consecutive patients. *Acta Neurochirurgica.* 1989;99:41-50.
95. Fountas KN, Kapsalaki EZ, Nikolakakos LG, et al. Anterior cervical discectomy and fusion associated complications. *Spine (Phila Pa 1976).* 2007;32:2310-2317.
96. Greenstein AJ, Chassin MR, Wang J, et al. Association between minor and major surgical complications after carotid endarterectomy: results of the New York Carotid Artery Surgery study. *J Vasc Surg.* 2007;46:1138-1144; discussion 45-46.
97. Lee HS, Lee BJ, Kim SW, et al. Patterns of post-thyroidectomy hemorrhage. *Clin Exp Otorhinolaryngol.* 2009;2:72-77.
98. Liu JT, Briner RP, Friedman JA. Comparison of inpatient vs. outpatient anterior cervical discectomy and fusion: a retrospective case series. *BMC Surg.* 2009;9:3.
99. Sanabria A, Carvalho AL, Silver CE, et al. Routine drainage after thyroid surgery: a meta-analysis. *J Surg Oncol.* 2007;96:273-280.
100. Barbara DW, Smith BC, Lynch JJ. Neck hematoma complicating endotracheal extubation. *Can J Anaesth.* 2014;61:676-677.
101. Guilbert MC, Elkouri S, Bracco D, et al. Arterial trauma during central venous catheter insertion: case series, review and proposed algorithm. *J Vasc Surg.* 2008;48:918-925; discussion 25.
102. Higa K, Hirata K, Hirota K, Nitahara K, Shono S. Retropharyngeal hematoma after stellate ganglion block: Analysis of 27 patients reported in the literature. *Anesthesiology.* 2006;105:1238-1245; discussion 5A-6A.
103. Akoglu E, Seyfeli E, Akoglu S, Karazincir S, Okuyucu S, Dagli AS. Retropharyngeal hematoma as a complication of anticoagulation therapy. *Ear Nose Throat J.* 2008;87:156-159.
104. Fujiwara T, Kuriyama A, Shimizu T. A woman with sudden-onset facial oedema. *Emerg Med J.* 2013;30:985.
105. Getnick GS, Lin SJ, Raviv JR, Walsh WE, Altman KW. Lingual hematoma and heparin-induced thrombocytopenia: a case report. *Ear Nose Throat J.* 2008;87:163-165.
106. Kirkham L, Homewood J, Brook P. Case of the month: a case of airway obstruction following tenecteplase administration. *Emerg Med J.* 2006;23:815-816.
107. Pazardzhikliev DD, Yovchev IP, Zhelev DD. Neck hematoma caused by spontaneous common carotid artery rupture. *Laryngoscope.* 2008;118:684-686.
108. Iizuka S, Morita S, Otsuka H, et al. Sudden asphyxia caused by retropharyngeal hematoma after blunt thyrocervical artery injury. *J Emerg Med.* 2012;43:451-456.
109. Keogh IJ, Rowley H, Russell J. Critical airway compromise caused by neck haematoma. *Clin Otolaryngol Allied Sci.* 2002;27:244-245.
110. Lin JY, Wang CH, Huang TW. Traumatic retropharyngeal hematoma: case report. *Auris Nasus Larynx.* 2007;34:423-425.
111. Lin M, Sinclair C. Retropharyngeal haematoma: an unusual cause of airway obstruction. *J Surg Case Rep.* 2011;2011:5.
112. Pfeiffer J, Ridder GJ. An elderly woman with increasing dyspnoea after a fall. *Emerg Med J.* 2011;28:806-808.
113. Senel AC, Gunduz AK. Retropharyngeal hematoma secondary to minor blunt neck trauma: case report. *Rev Bras Anestesiol.* 2012;62:731-735.
114. Grandhi R, Gande A, Zwagerman NT, Jankowitz BT. Facial and neck hematoma after carotid artery stenting: an uncommon misadventure in endovascular carotid revascularization. *J Neurointerv Surg.* 2014;6:e39.
115. Ottaviani F, Schindler A, Mozzanica F, Peri A, Rezzonico S, Turiel M. Surgical management of a life-threatening retro-pharyngeal haematoma following trans-oesophageal echocardiography. *Acta Otorhinolaryngol Ital.* 2011;31:39-42.
116. Fan C, Zhou X, Su G, et al. Risk factors for neck hematoma requiring surgical re-intervention after thyroidectomy: a systematic review and meta-analysis. *BMC Surg.* 2019;19:98.
117. Shah-Becker S, Greenleaf EK, Boltz MM, Hollenbeak CS, Goyal N. Neck hematoma after major head and neck surgery: Risk factors, costs, and resource utilization. *Head Neck.* 2018;40:1219-1227.
118. Dellagrammaticas D, Lewis SC, Gough MJ. Is heparin reversal with protamine after carotid endarterectomy dangerous? *Eur J Vasc Endovasc Surg.* 2008;36:41-44.
119. Self DD, Bryson GL, Sullivan PJ. Risk factors for post-carotid endarterectomy hematoma formation. *Can J Anaesth.* 1999;46:635-640.
120. Tawes RL Jr., Treiman RL. Vein patch rupture after carotid endarterectomy: a survey of the Western Vascular Society members. *Ann Vasc Surg.* 1991;5:71-73.
121. Youssef F, Jenkins MP, Dawson KJ, Berger L, Myint F, Hamilton G. The value of suction wound drain after carotid and femoral artery surgery: a randomised trial using duplex assessment of the volume of post-operative haematoma. *Eur J Vasc Endovasc Surg.* 2005;29:162-166.
122. Ferguson GG, Eliasziw M, Barr HW, et al. The North American Symptomatic Carotid Endarterectomy Trial: surgical results in 1415 patients. *Stroke.* 1999;30:1751-1758.

CHAPTER 59

Airway Management Under Combat Situations

Bjoern Hossfeld, Matthias Helm, Arnim Vlatten, and Christopher Hung

CASE PRESENTATION

A unit of a 14-person, 6-vehicle military convoy is moving through a remote village of a combat zone. As the convoy pulls out on the open road at the end of that village, an improvised explosive device (IED) explodes under the second vehicle, manned with two soldiers. Intensive sniper fire follows, and the rest of the convoy is busily engaged in suppressing it. The nonarmored disabled vehicle is right side up and not on fire. You are the medic of the unit, and you are in an armored vehicle, next to the demolished vehicle with the two victims. As you arrive at the vehicle, you find two casualties: Casualty #1 is the driver of the vehicle. He sustained bilateral mid-thigh traumatic amputations and a penetrating injury of the pelvis and the abdomen. Furthermore, there is a large open head wound in which mangled gray matter is clearly visible. There are no vital signs—he is obviously dead. Casualty #2 is the front-seat passenger. He sustained a below-knee amputation of his left leg with heavy arterial bleeding from the stump, and multiple injuries to the left face. He has significant soft-tissue trauma, the mandibula is visible, and obviously comminuted fractured. You note moderate bleeding from the left face injury. The soldier is conscious and has a good radial pulse but the airway seems compromised due to disrupted airway anatomy (maxillofacial trauma) and bleeding into the airway.

INTRODUCTION

Prehospital trauma care on the battlefield varies in many respects from prehospital trauma care as practiced in the civilian setting. Firstly, these traumas are involved in different causes, types, and severity of the injuries. In addition, these cases are often associated with the threat of hostile fire, working in the dark without using bright light, multiple casualties, limited medical equipment, and prolonged evacuation times. Therefore, treatment guidelines developed for the civilian setting do not necessarily work well in the military setting.

Using the US Mortality Trauma Registry of the Armed Forces Medical Examiner Service, Eastridge et al.[1] reported that there were 4596 battlefield fatalities in Operation Iraqi Freedom and Operation Enduring Freedom (Afghanistan) from October 2001 to June 2011. Majority of all injury mortality (87.3%, n = 4013) occurred in the prehospital environment. Of the prehospital deaths, 24.3% (n = 976) were deemed potentially survivable. Historically, airway compromise represents the third leading cause of potentially preventable death on the battlefield, behind hemorrhage and tension pneumothorax.[2] In a retrospective review of 982 autopsies of US military personnel who died in combat in Iraq and Afghanistan between 2003 and 2006, Mabry et al.[3] reported that 18 cases (1.8% of the total deaths) were found to have airway compromise as the likely mechanism of death. These include penetrating trauma to the face or neck, which were accompanied by significant hemorrhage, leading to death from airway compromise. While cricothyrotomy were attempted, the procedure failed in all instances in this series of cases. It is unknown whether cricothyrotomy failure was related to the reluctance of providers to perform it, the lack of proper equipment and training, or a tactical situation that precluded immediate lifesaving care.

The need for reconsideration of trauma care guidelines in the tactical setting has long been recognized.[4–6] The Tactical Combat Casualty Care (TCCC) project was initiated by the US Naval Special Warfare Command in 1993, and later continued by the US Special Operations Command (USSOCOM). Within the framework of this project, a bundle of tactically appropriate battlefield trauma care guidelines were developed.[7] These TCCC guidelines combine "good medicine" with "small-unit tactics."

TCCC has three goals for trauma care in the tactical setting: (1) prevent additional casualties; (2) treat the casualty; and (3) complete the mission. In order to achieve these goals, TCCC is divided into three phases:

- Care Under Fire
- Tactical Field Care
- Tactical Evacuation Care

TCCC is performing the correct intervention at the correct time in the continuum of field care (Figure 59.1). In the "*Care Under Fire*" phase, medical personnel and casualties are under effective hostile fire and tactical considerations predominate. The medical care is limited to extremity hemorrhage control with tourniquets if the patient is unable to apply self-aid. In the "*Tactical Field Care*" phase, more extensive medical care can be provided, because there is no direct hostile fire. In the "*Tactical Evacuation Care*" phase, the casualties are transported (air, ground, or sea) to a medical facility with the opportunity to provide additional medical personnel and equipment to further increase the level of care. The TCCC guidelines will be updated periodically by the Committee on Tactical Combat Casualty Care (CoTCCC). Furthermore, the TCCC guidelines are currently adapted into civilian Tactical Emergency Medical Service (TEMS) systems.

TCCC was introduced in the Canadian Forces (CF) first to their Special Operation Forces in 1999 and to the conventional forces before the initial deployment of Canadian soldiers to Kandahar/Afghanistan in 2002. During the Afghan war, the CF gained substantial experience delivering TCCC to wounded soldiers on the battlefield. Compared to past conflicts, this conflict has seen a dramatic reduction in the number of soldiers killed from combat wounds.[8,9] Savage et al.[10] conclude in their publication on lessons learned from the Afghan war that *"though this success is multifactorial, the determination and resolve of CF leadership to develop and deliver comprehensive, multileveled TCCC packages to soldiers and medics is a significant reason for that and has unquestionably saved the lives of Canadian, Coalition and Afghan Security Forces."*

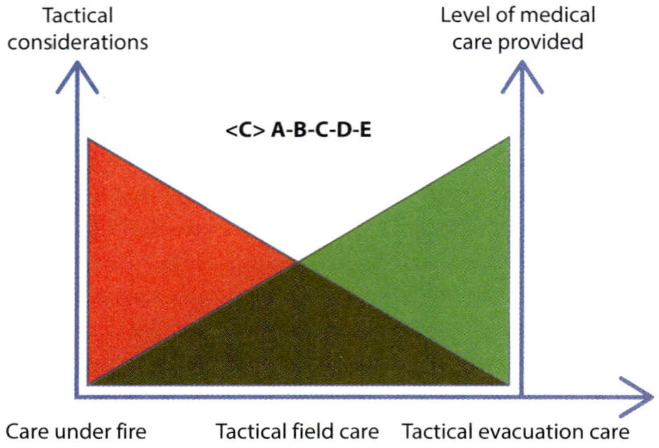

FIGURE 59.1. TCCC performs the correct intervention at the correct time in the continuum of field care. The closer you are to the "kill zone," the more tactical considerations predominate—the farther away you are to the kill zone the higher is the level of medical care provided.

ASSESSMENT OF THE PATIENT

What Are the Considerations According to the Tactical Combat Casualty Care (TCCC) Guidelines?

Care Under Fire Phase

According to the TCCC guidelines, during the *Care Under Fire* phase, the casualty and responders are under effective hostile fire and limited medical care should be attempted. The major considerations during this phase of care are the following:

- Suppression of hostile fire to prevent further casualties
- Moving the casualty to a safe position
- Treatment of immediate life-threatening hemorrhage

Casualty treatment during the *Care Under Fire* phase is complicated by several tactical factors[11]: First, the medical equipment available for care is limited to that, which is carried by the individual soldier and rescuer. Second, the unit's personnel will be engaged with hostile forces and, especially in small-unit engagements, will not be available to assist with casualty treatment and evacuation. Third, the tactical situation prevents the medic or medical provider from performing a detailed examination or definitive treatment of casualties.

Defensive Actions

It is commonly said that "the best medicine on the battlefield is fire superiority." It is the best way to prevent risk of injury to other personnel or additional injuries to the casualty. As soon as the rescuer is directed or able, their first major objective is to keep the casualty from sustaining additional injuries. The casualty is directed to move to cover and apply self-aid, if able. If the casualty is responsive but not able to move, the casualty must be dragged or carried by rescuers to a safe position.

Hemorrhage Control

Extremity hemorrhage is the most frequent cause of preventable battlefield deaths.[12] Because of their effectiveness at hemorrhage control and the speed with which they can be applied, tourniquets are the best option for temporary control of life-threatening extremity hemorrhage in the tactical environment.[13] During the *Care Under Fire* phase, "hasty tourniquets" are applied as proximal on the injured extremity as possible and over the uniform.

Based on the experience of combat medics on the battlefield of Iraq and Afghanistan, the use of hemostatic agents was reconsidered and is not recommended for this phase of care. The requirement to hold direct pressure on the bleeding site after application of a hemostatic agent for at least 3 to 5 minutes was felt to be tactically infeasible when the casualty and the responder are under effective hostile fire. Once under cover, a hemostatic agent can be a highly effective option in life-threatening nonextremity wounds.

Airway

No immediate management of the airway should be anticipated at this point because of the need to move the casualty to cover as quickly as possible.[7] The time, equipment, and positioning required to manage an impaired airway expose the casualty and the rescuer to increased risk. Rescuers should defer airway management until the *Tactical Field Care* phase, when the casualty and the rescuer are safe from hostile fire.

Tactical Field Care Phase

Once the casualty and the rescuer are no longer under effective hostile fire, *Tactical Field Care* is the care rendered to the casualty. The *Tactical Field Care* phase is characterized by the following:[11]

- The risk from hostile fire has been reduced, but still exists.
- The medical equipment available is still limited by what has been brought into the field by mission personnel.
- The time for treatment is highly variable. Time prior to evacuation can range from a few minutes to many hours.

The medical care provided during this phase is directed toward more in-depth evaluation and treatment of the casualty, focusing on those conditions not addressed during the *Care Under Fire* phase of treatment. While the casualty and the rescuer are now in a somewhat less hazardous situation, evaluation and treatment are still dictated by the tactical situation, which may change quickly.

Altered Mental Status

The casualty with an altered mental status has to be disarmed immediately. An armed combatant with an altered mental status is a significant risk to themself and those in their unit. Main reasons for an altered mental status are traumatic brain injury (TBI), pain, shock, and analgesic medication.

Bleeding

In the *Tactical Field Care* phase, hemorrhage control includes addressing any significant bleeding sites not previously controlled:

- If not already done, use a tourniquet to control life-threatening external hemorrhage that is anatomically amenable to tourniquet application.
- For compressible hemorrhage not amenable to tourniquet, use pressure dressings supplemented by hemostatic agents.
- Reassess prior tourniquet application. If required, transition to a "deliberate tourniquet" (placed 2 inches proximal to the injury and against the skin) in the *Tactical Field Care* phase.

Airway Management

In this phase of care, initial management to the evaluation and treatment of the casualty's airway once all hemorrhage problems have been addressed is of utmost importance. Intervention should proceed from the least invasive procedure to the most invasive:

- Unconscious casualties should have their airways opened with the chin lift or jaw thrust maneuver.
- In unconscious patients with spontaneous breathing, no airway obstruction, and no suspected skull fractures, use the nasopharyngeal airway (NPA).
- Unconscious patients are placed in the semiprone recovery position to help prevent aspiration.
- Allow conscious patients with maxillofacial trauma to assume whatever position that allows them to breathe most easily including sitting upright if able.
- If an airway obstruction develops or persists despite the use of an NPA, a more definitive airway will be required. In these cases, front-of-neck access (surgical airway) is preferable to tracheal intubation in the tactical setting. The reasons for this recommendation are: (1) Most corpsmen and medics are inexperienced in the technique of tracheal intubation (on a live casualty or even a cadaver). (2) Tracheal intubation techniques entail the use of white light in the laryngoscope, which may be tactically compromising.[13] (3) Tracheal intubation may be extremely difficult in patients with maxillofacial injury.[14] (4) An esophageal intubation may be unrecognized more easily in the tactical setting.

Breathing

The next aspect of casualty care in the *Tactical Field Care* phase is the treatment of any breathing problems, especially the development of either an open pneumothorax (PTX) or a tension PTX:

- All penetrating chest wounds should be treated as an open PTX by applying an occlusive material to cover the defect and securing it in place. There are numerous commercial chest seals available. The casualty should be monitored for the development of a tension PTX.
- Consider tension PTX in a casualty with progressive respiratory distress and known or suspected torso trauma. Decompress the chest on the side of the injury with a 14-gauge needle of appropriate length (min. 8 cm) / catheter unit inserted in the second intercostal space at the midclavicular line (needle thoracostomy).

Vascular Access and Fluid Resuscitation

Individuals in shock and requiring fluid resuscitation or those who need intravenous medications should have an IV started. In contrast to the civilian practice (two large-bore intravenous catheters), an 18-gauge catheter is preferred in the field because of ease of cannulation. If IV access is not obtainable, the intraosseous (IO) route should be used.[13,15] IO devices for sternal access should be preferred, because the majority of injuries are penetrating lower extremity injuries, and especially in military personnel, the trunk often is protected by body armor.

Fluid resuscitation during the *Tactical Field Care* phase is significantly different than in the civilian prehospital setting: limited time for thorough fluid resuscitation due to the tactical situation; limited availability of fluids carried by the combat medic; and limited diagnostic tools to monitor fluid resuscitation and shock. Therefore, fluid resuscitation should be provided in this phase only to those casualties exhibiting signs of shock and/or severe TBI. An altered mental status (in the absence of head injury) and/or weak or absent peripheral pulses may assume that the casualty is in shock. The optimal resuscitation fluid and regimen for use in combat casualties remains a topic of great interest in military medical research. Approximately 1000 mL of Lactated Ringer's solution should be given, and/or whole blood depending on recommendations of national practice. In casualties with both shock and TBI, fluid resuscitation should be administered until radial pulse is restored, which corresponds to a systolic BP of approximately 70 mmHg.

Hypothermia Prevention

Combat casualties are at high risk for accidental hypothermia (core body temperature below 35°C). It is more prevalent in combat trauma than it was previously realized, and it independently contributes to overall mortality.[16] Therefore, prevention of heat loss should start as soon as the tactical situation permits. Wet clothing should be replaced with dry clothes (if possible) and the casualty should be wrapped in a Blizzard™ emergency blanket. To add an element of active rewarming, the Ready-Heat™ emergency blanket should be applied to the casualty's torso (not directly to the skin) inside the emergency blanket.

Monitoring

Pulse oximetry should be available as an adjunct to clinical monitoring.

Pain Management

All casualties in pain should be given analgesia. The type and route of medication is dependent upon whether the casualty is conscious, hemodynamically stable, still able to fight, and if vascular access has been obtained. Because of increasing the risk of bleeding, analgesic medications that adversely affect platelet function should not be used.[7] If the casualty is conscious and still able to fight, oral pain medication that will not alter their level of consciousness should be given. For mild to moderate pain, the COX-2-inhibitor meloxicam is recommended.[17] For severe pain, opioid analgesia should be used: If vascular access is present, morphine sulfate remains the "gold standard." If vascular access is not established, oral transmucosal fentanyl citrate is recommended.

Eye Trauma

In case of suspected penetrating eye trauma, a rapid field test of visual acuity should be performed. A useful field quantification is (from best to worse): (1) able to read print, (2) can count the number of fingers held up, (3) can see motion, and (4) can see light. A rigid shield should be taped over the injured eye and an oral antibiotic (recommended is moxifloxacin) should be given to prevent infection inside the eye.

Tactical Evacuation Care (TACEVAC) Phase

In this phase, the casualty is being prepared for transport or has been picked up from the battlefield by an aircraft (rotary and/or fixed wing), vehicle, or boat for transportation to a higher echelon of care, and additional medical equipment and personnel is provided. This allows for an enhanced level of medical care compared to *Care Under Fire* and *Tactical Field Care*.

Airway

Airway management during the TACEVAC phase follows the same principles as during the *Tactical Field Care* phase:

- Positioning and airway adjuncts are the initial management options. However, if the management of an impaired airway is exceedingly difficult during this phase, a more definitive airway might be obtained if sufficient equipment and provider's expertise are available. Possible airway management options may include:
  - Extraglottic airway devices, such as laryngeal mask airway (LMA), or the laryngeal tube (LT).
  - Tracheal intubation, preferred using a video laryngoscopy (VL), if the equipment is available and the care provider has the appropriate expertise.
  - Cricothyrotomy is still an appropriate option when an NPA is not effective and when the equipment for more advanced airway techniques (extraglottic airway devices and tracheal intubation) is not available and/or the care provider lacks the appropriate expertise.

Breathing

In a casualty with progressive respiratory distress and known or suspected torso trauma, a tension PTX should be considered. Treat tension PTX with needle decompression. If no improvement and/or a long-term transport is anticipated (even if the initial needle decompression was successful), consider chest tube insertion. Oxygen is an adjunct that may be present on TACEVAC. Most combat casualties do not require supplemental oxygen. Oxygen administration may be of benefit for casualties with:

- Low oxygen saturation (pulse oximetry)
- Injuries associated with impaired oxygenation
- Unconsciousness
- TBI (maintain oxygen saturation >90%)
- Shock
- At high altitude

Bleeding

During the TCEVAC phase, a thorough examination for additional wounds should be performed and the adequacy of hemorrhage control measures previously employed must be reassessed. The same principles of hemorrhage control should be employed including the use of tourniquets and hemostatic adjuncts.

Fluid Resuscitation

During the TACEVAC phase, additional options in fluid resuscitation may be possible. Fluid resuscitation should be continued in casualties in shock and/or with TBI. If indicated and available, continue fluid resuscitation with packed red blood cells (PRBCs), or Lactated Ringer's solution.

Hypothermia Prevention

Hypothermia prevention/treatment becomes paramount during the TACEVAC phase, especially if the casualty is evacuated in a helicopter (open doors for the fire power provided by the door gunner). Continue to follow the hypothermia prevention principles of the *Tactical Field Care* phase.

Monitoring

Casualty assessment might be difficult during the TACEVAC phase due to high noise and vibration levels (inside a vehicle or helicopter), and the need to avoid visible lights at night for tactical safety reasons. Therefore, an extended electronic monitoring should be applied to the casualty, capable to monitor blood pressure, heart rate, pulse oximetry, and end-tidal carbon dioxide.

All other aspects of care during the TACEVAC phase are identical to those during the *Tactical Field Care* phase.

MANAGEMENT OF THIS PATIENT

How Is the Casualty Managed?

While the rest of the convoy is providing suppressive fire, the medic applies a Combat Application Tourniquet (C-A-T®) to the left thigh over the uniform to control the extremity hemorrhage caused by below-knee amputation in the front seat passenger. This is the most important life-saving intervention in *Care Under Fire* and is the *only* medical care rendered before the casualty is moved to cover. The soldier is conscious and has a good radial pulse, but he is unable to move because of his below-knee amputation.

Despite signs of a compromised airway, *no immediate airway management* is anticipated at this point, because of the need to move the casualty to cover as quickly as possible, thereby minimizing the risk to the casualty and the rescuer!

Because the rest of the convoy is busy in engaging and suppressing hostile fire, you decide to drag the casualty out of the nonarmored disabled vehicle and carry him in a one-person technique called Hawes Carry (Figure 59.2), over a short distance to the next armored vehicle of the convoy. The advantage of this method is that it limits the number of people exposed to hostile fire. Furthermore, the casualty is in a more "upright and leaning forward" position so that blood may drain out instead of down into the airway. The disadvantage of this method is that it is not the fastest way to move a casualty with less control and it is more difficult for the rescuer. The fastest method for moving is dragging along the long axis of the body by two rescuers. If the mental status of this casualty would be altered, an alternative method for moving would be the so-called SEAL Team THREE Carry (Figure 59.3): It is fast and has the same advantages regarding airway and breathing like the Hawes Carry, but it needs a second rescuer. Once arrived at the armored vehicle, the casualty's status is communicated to the team leader. The team leader commands the convoy to sortie and moves as fast as possible to a safer compound two miles ahead of the point of attack. After a few minutes, all vehicles reach the compound without further critical incident.

While the rest of the convoy establishes a secure perimeter, you continue to take care of the wounded soldier. In a rapid initial assessment for life-threatening conditions, you find the following:

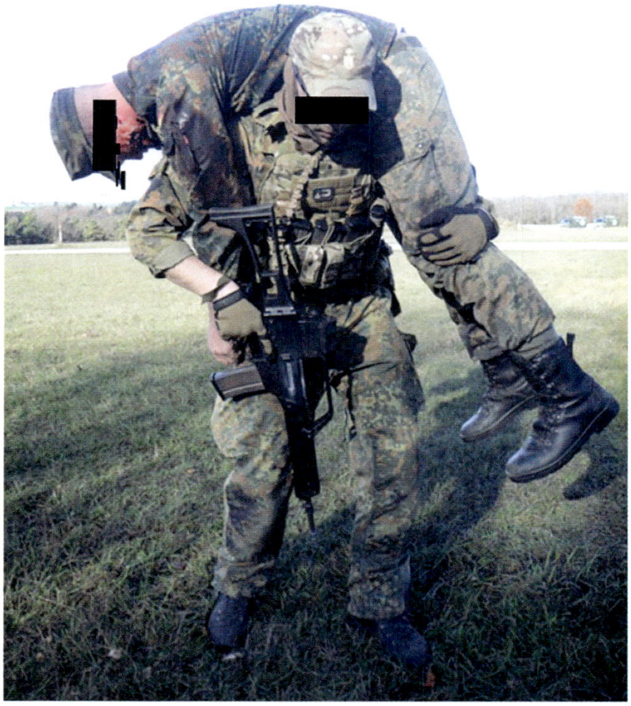

FIGURE 59.2. One person carry technique which is called Hawes Carry to carry casualties over a short distance (training scenario).

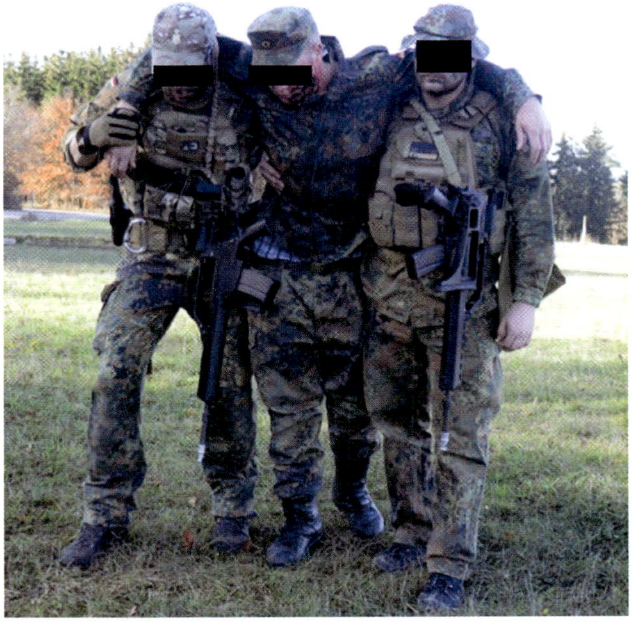

FIGURE 59.3. Two-person carry technique for moving a casualty, the so-called SEAL Team THREE (training scenario).

- Blast injury
  - Below-knee amputation of left leg; previously heavy arterial bleeding still sufficiently stopped by applied tourniquet.

- Significant soft-tissue trauma to the left face with obviously comminuted fractured mandible; moderate bleeding from the left face injury.
- No other wounds seen.

While "critical" external bleeding appears controlled (sufficiently applied tourniquet) and still with a good radial pulse, the patient's airway appears compromised due to the disrupted airway anatomy caused by maxillofacial trauma and bleeding into the airway. The patient is still conscious and cooperative. Therefore, the casualty is asked to get into a "sitting up and leaning forward" position so that the blood drains out of the mouth instead of down into the airway (Figure 59.4). This procedure provides an acceptable airway. Furthermore, the patient shows no signs of respiratory distress. The oxygen saturation, measured by pulse oximetry, is 95%. To control the moderate external bleeding from soft-tissue trauma to the left face, a hemostatic dressing (CELOX Gauze™) is applied over the bleeding site. After 3 minutes of sustained direct pressure to the bleeding site, a pressure dressing is applied to cover the wound and the agent and to maintain a degree of pressure. There is still a slight intraoral bleeding.

Because of severe pain caused by the underlying injury pattern and the tourniquet application, an 18-gauge IV is established and 100 mg of ketamine sulfate is administered. The same dose is repeated after 10 minutes because of inadequate pain relief. To prevent the risk of nausea and vomiting, 4 mg Ondansetron IV is administered intravenously.

To prevent hypothermia, a Ready-Heat blanket is applied to the casualty's torso and the patient is wrapped in a Blizzard survival blanket. According to the tactical situation and the urgency of the movement of this patient, the tactical leader of the convoy calls for air evacuation. The team leader is informed that a medevac helicopter will be on scene in 20 minutes.

While documenting the casualty's injuries and the care rendered on the TCCC Casualty Card, you notice that the patient is not able to maintain a "sitting up and leaning forward" position anymore. Furthermore, the mental status of the patient is progressively altered, while the slight intraoral bleeding is still present. You decide to place the patient in a semiprone recovery position to prevent aspiration of blood due to intraoral bleeding. In view of the impending TECEVAC by helicopter, you decide to initiate a more definitive airway. You follow the TCCC recommendations and perform a cricothyrotomy (conventional anatomical-surgical preparation technique), insert a 6.0-mm endotracheal tube and confirm proper placement by lung auscultation. Following cricothyrotomy, the casualty is ventilated with a bag connected to the tube. In Figure 59.5, a training scenario situation during a TCCC training at the Federal Armed Forces Medical Center Ulm, Germany, using the conventional surgical cricothyroidotomy technique in a mannequin is shown. The recently introduced cricothyroidotomy set used by the German Armed Forces Medical Corps is shown in Figure 59.6.

The insertion of an extraglottic airway device such as the LT or laryngeal mask may not be appropriate in this case, because of persistent intraoral bleeding due to the intraoral soft-tissue trauma, the fractured mandible, and the subsequent risk of (silent) blood aspiration. Similarly, tracheal intubation may be difficult to accomplish even in the hands of a more experienced paramedical personnel and under less austere conditions.

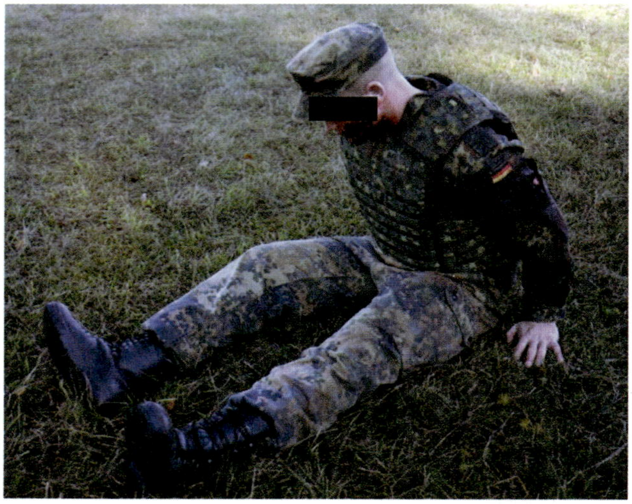

FIGURE 59.4. The "sitting up and leaning forward" position (training scenario).

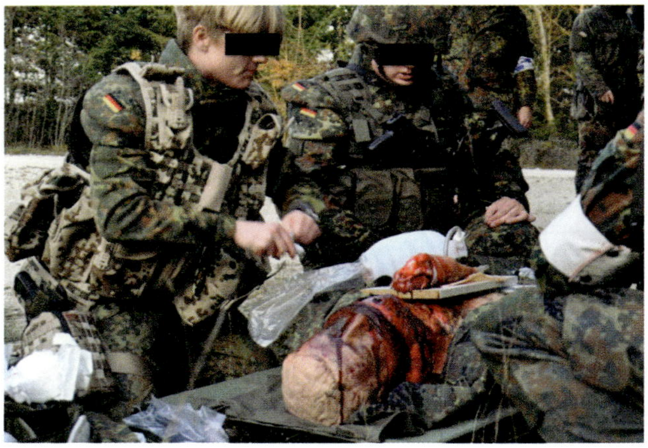

FIGURE 59.5. Surgicric II cricothyrotomy set (VBM; Sulz am Neckar—Germany) used by the German Armed Forces Medical Corps for conventional anatomical surgical preparation technique.

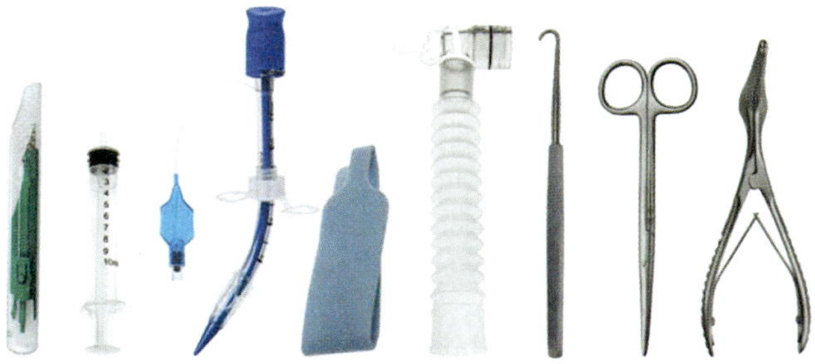

FIGURE 59.6. A training scenario situation during a TCCC training at the Federal Armed Forces Medical Center Ulm, Germany, using the conventional surgical cricothyroidotomy technique in a mannequin.

The medevac helicopter lands on time at the scene in a secure landing zone. The tactical situation and time allow for an extended patient handover. To provide for continued good assessment of the casualty's status during transport, an electronic monitoring is placed, which comprises of 3-lead ECG (sinus rhythm), heart rate (80 beats per min), noninvasive automatic blood pressure measurement (120/80 mmHg), pulse oximetry (SpO_2: 96%), and capnography (end-tidal CO_2: 35 mmHg). In addition, the patient is connected to a mechanical before transportation. Anesthesia is maintained by IV midazolam and fentanyl. With the exception of the minor intraoral bleeding, all bleeding sources are under control and the patient remains hemodynamically stable. To stop the intraoral bleeding, the oral cavity is packed with a wound bandage.

After 5 minutes ground time, the medevac helicopter leaves the scene for a 20-minute flight to the next Combat Support hospital. The flight proceeds without any incident.

SUMMARY

Prehospital trauma care on the battlefield varies in many respects from prehospital trauma care as practiced in the civilian setting. Therefore, the military setting needs its own guidelines: the TCCC concept. It combines "good medicine" with "small-unit tactics" and has three goals: prevention of additional casualties, casualty treatment, and mission completion. It is divided into three phases: *Care Under Fire*, *Tactical Field Care*, and *Tactical Evacuation Care*. The closer one is to a hostile threat, the more tactical considerations predominate—the farther away one is to a hostile threat, the higher is the level of medical care provided.

SELF-EVALUATION QUESTIONS

59.1. What of the following is NOT a goal for trauma care in the tactical setting according to the TCCC principles?

A. Treat the casualty.

B. Apply the same quality of medical care as practiced in the civilian setting.

C. Prevent additional casualties.

D. Stop mission.

E. Complete mission.

59.2. What is the most important medical measure in a combat situation during the *Care Under Fire* phase?

A. Initiate an IV and start fluid resuscitation.

B. Application of a hemostatic agent in compressible hemorrhage not amenable to tourniquet.

C. Perform endotracheal intubation in casualties with altered mental status.

D. Pain therapy by administering Aspirin.

E. Control life-threatening extremity hemorrhage by tourniquet application.

59.3. What is NOT the preferable airway management measure in the *Tactical Field Care* phase?

A. Chin lift or jaw thrust maneuver in unconscious casualties.

B. The use of a NPA if an airway obstruction persists in unconscious patients.

C. Tracheal intubation.

D. Placing unconscious patients with spontaneous breathing in a semiprone position.

E. Perform cricothyrotomy when NPA is not effective.

REFERENCES

1. Eastridge BJ, Mabry RL, Seguin P, et al. Death on the battlefield (2001-2011): implications for the future of combat casualty care. *J Trauma Acute Care Surg.* 2012;73:S431-S437.
2. Bellamy R. How people die in ground combat? Presented to the Joint Health Services Support Vision 2010 Working Group. 1996.
3. Mabry RL, Edens JW, Pearse L, Kelly JF, Harke H. Fatal airway injuries during Operation Enduring Freedom and Operation Iraqi Freedom. *Prehosp Emerg Care.* 2010;14:272-277.
4. Baker MS. Advanced trauma life support: is it adequate stand-alone training for military medicine? *Mil Med.* 1994;159:587-590.
5. Bellamy RF. How shall we train for combat casualty care? *Mil Med.* 1987;152:617-621.
6. Heiskell LE, Carmona RH. Tactical emergency medical services: an emerging subspecialty of emergency medicine. *Ann Emerg Med.* 1994;23:778-785.
7. Butler FK Jr, Hagmann J, Butler EG. Tactical combat casualty care in special operations. *Mil Med.* 1996;161(Suppl):3-16.
8. Eastridge BJ, Jenkins D, Flaherty S, Schiller H, Holcomb JB. Trauma system development in a theater of war: Experiences from Operation Iraqi Freedom and Operation Enduring Freedom. *J Trauma.* 2006;61:1366-1372; discussion 72-73.
9. Holcomb JB, Stansbury LG, Champion HR, Wade C, Bellamy RF. Understanding combat casualty care statistics. *J Trauma.* 2006;60:397-401.
10. Savage E, Forestier C, Withers N, Tien H, Pannell D. Tactical combat casualty care in the Canadian Forces: lessons learned from the Afghan war. *Can J Surg.* 2011;54:S118-S123.
11. Tactical Combat Casualty Care (TCCC) Guidelines for Medical Personnel. 2021.
12. Maughon JS. An inquiry into the nature of wounds resulting in killed in action in Vietnam. *Mil Med.* 1970;135:8-13.
13. Butler FK Jr, Holcomb JB, Giebner SD, McSwain NE, Bagian J. Tactical combat casualty care 2007: evolving concepts and battlefield experience. *Mil Med.* 2007;172:1-19.
14. Zajtchuk R, Jenkins DP, RF B. Office of the Surgeon General at TMM Publications; 1991.
15. Dubick MA, Holcomb JB. A review of intraosseous vascular access: current status and military application. *Mil Med.* 2000;165:552-559.
16. Arthurs Z, Cuadrado D, Beekley A, et al. The impact of hypothermia on trauma care at the 31st combat support hospital. *Am J Surg.* 2006;191:610-614.
17. Kotwal RS, O'Connor KC, Johnson TR, Mosely DS, Meyer DE, Holcomb JB. A novel pain management strategy for combat casualty care. *Ann Emerg Med.* 2004;44:121-127.

CHAPTER 60

Airway Management in Austere Environments

Batgombo Natsagdorj, David Pescod, Rachael Pescod, Paulin R. Banguti, Haydn Perndt, and Thomas J. Coonan

CASE PRESENTATION

As an anesthesia practitioner, you are part of a short-term volunteer surgical program in a low-income country (LIC). The team includes a plastic reconstructive surgeon and two nurses. Your mandate is to collaborate with local health care providers to deliver surgical treatment to people who otherwise could not access the procedures. Some surgical infrastructure exists at the local hospital; however, there is a significant shortage of both personnel and equipment needed to provide safe anesthetic care. But importantly, there is capacity for basic ongoing postoperative care by local health providers after the departure of the surgical team.

Just a few days after arrival, an otherwise healthy 22-year-old woman presents with facial burns following a domestic cooking accident. The World Health Organization (WHO) describes burns worldwide as a "serious public health problem" with an estimated 265,000 deaths annually. Over 96% of fire fatalities occur in low- and middle-income countries (LMICs) with millions more suffering permanent disfigurement. This young patient can no longer close her eyes effectively because of worsening contractures; corneal ulcers are developing, and she is becoming blind. The surgeon states that she can perform some small split skin grafts that will save her sight (Figure 60.1).

On examination, the patient has some perioral scarring, limited mouth opening, and a full set of healthy teeth.

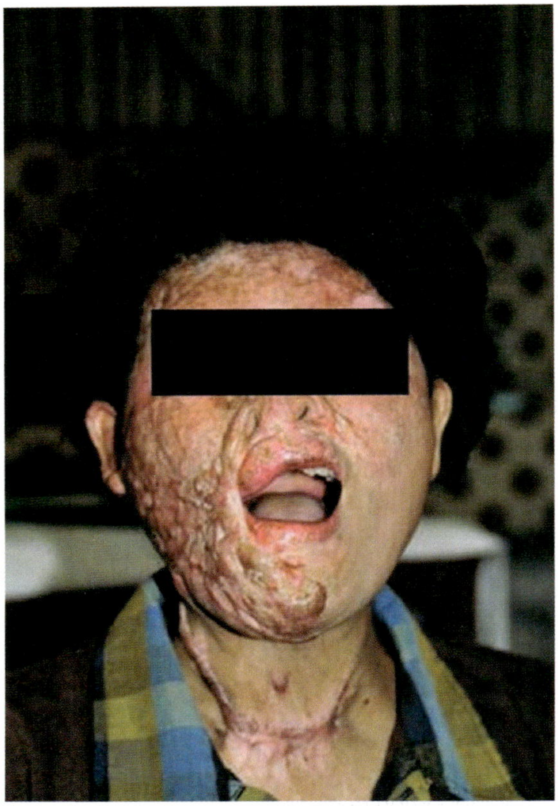

FIGURE 60.1. Twenty-two-year-old woman with burn contractures.

Her Mallampati score is III, and she has a normal thyromental distance and normal neck extension. There is some scarring over her anterior neck, but you can easily palpate airway structures.

INTRODUCTION

In high-income countries (HICs), about 1:50 general anesthesia cases will present difficult tracheal intubation, 1:75 will result in a failed intubation, and a failure to intubate and to ventilate will occur in 1:1000 to 1:12,000 anesthetics. In this regard, airway management may be particularly challenging in obstetrical anesthesia (see Chapters 1 and 52). Although the principles of airway management are similar worldwide, the anesthesia practitioner in the LIC can expect to face challenges, both unrelated and related, to airway anatomy (Table 60.1). A variety of difficult conditions can be encountered, often in later stages of evolution, and often presenting greater challenges. Diseases and conditions less familiar to the average practitioner can also be expected. Pediatric and obstetrical patients make up a higher proportion of anesthetic practice in an LIC.

What Are the Risks Inherent in Airway Management in Austere Environments?

Fifty years of intense commitment has greatly reduced avoidable anesthesia-related mortality in wealthy countries to a rate of about 1/56,000 anesthetics (1/180,000 when anesthesia is the sole cause of mortality and morbidity), and airway misadventure is no longer the primary reason for seriously adverse outcomes.[1,2] In 2011, the 4th National Audit Project of the Royal College of Anaesthetists and the Difficult Airway Society (NAP4) reported an incidence of airway-related death and brain damage of only 7 per million general anesthetics in the United Kingdom.[3] Training in airway management has advanced, guidelines and standards have been introduced, technology has evolved immensely, and a culture of safety is in place.[4,5] Sadly, such benefits have been largely restricted to the few who live in relatively privileged societies. Published mortality due to airway misadventure in less-resourced areas can vary from 100 to 1000 times greater than that in affluent societies.[6–9] Indeed, in one report, the avoidable mortality from airway-related causes was 1/183 anesthetics.[9] Obstetric anesthesia is a particular risk in this regard.[10]

The challenges facing developing countries are far more profound than the unavailability of the latest aids for tracheal intubation. Many barriers to improving difficult airway management exist in LICs, including minimal education and training on the difficult airway for local physician and nonphysician practitioners. Additional factors involve limited functional advanced airway equipment and safety monitoring, unpredictable access to essential medicines (including oxygen), and a lack of emphasis on vigilance, sustainable organizational structure, and modern systems of quality review.[11] One major priority, universal pulse oximetry, is still often lacking in 77,000 operating rooms globally,[12] but so too are vigorous educational support, mentorship, and team building.

TABLE 60.1. Expected Developing Country Conditions with the Potential for Difficult Airway Management

- Familiar conditions, but more advanced:
  - Obstetric—eclampsia
  - Goiter—high incidence, related to dietary deficiency
  - Head and neck infections and tumors
  - Quinsy
  - Dental abscess
- Less familiar conditions:
  - Severe uncorrected head/neck burn contractures
  - Uncorrected congenital defects
  - Cancrum Oris ("Noma")
  - Ameloblastoma
  - Late presentations of obstructing tumors
  - Temporomandibular ankylosis
- Higher proportion of pediatric and obstetric anesthesia practice

AIRWAY EQUIPMENT IN AUSTERE ENVIRONMENTS

What Are the Equipment Considerations for Difficult Airway Management in the Developing World?

Aggressive attention to the needs of the developing world has been paid by the international anesthesia community since 1989,[13] and a series of standards have evolved.[5,14] Sadly, most of the first referral hospitals in many countries are challenged to meet even the basic standards of the World Federation of Societies of Anaesthesia (WFSA). Appropriate low-resource strategies, equipment, and approaches must be considered, and local input from government, hospital systems, and on-the-ground practitioners must be considered and included.[15]

Nomenclature around hospital classification is not universal. The WHO uses three levels (1-3) to categorize health care facilities. The Lancet Commission on Global Surgery (LCoGS) and the Disease Control Priorities (DCP-3) both also refer to three levels of facility, which approximately align with the WHO levels; however, they have different naming systems. In 2018, the WFSA and WHO released The International Standards for a Safe Practice of Anesthesia.[16] They are "intended to provide guidance and assistance to anesthesia providers, their professional organizations, hospital and facility administrators, and governments for maintaining and improving the quality and safety of anesthesia care."

WHO Level 1 Facilities: Small Hospital/Health Center (LCoGS: Primary Health Center, DCP3: Community Facility and Health Care Center)

Level 1 facilities are expected by the World Health Organization (WHO) to provide emergency and basic surgery, resuscitation, stabilization, and vaginal delivery.[17] It must be emphasized that, in LICs, there are frequently only nonphysician practitioners, many of whom have limited training and very few advanced skills. Airway management in these settings should be trained for and provided by a team of the most skilled individuals. General anesthesia in these settings should be avoided whenever possible, but this is often not possible. Indeed, it may not be possible to refer a seriously ill patient to a higher-level treatment center. In many environments, the compressed gases are expensive, the supply unreliable, and frequently unavailable. Under such circumstances, oxygen concentrators, ketamine, and draw-over anesthesia offer significant advantages.[18] WHO level 1 facilities providing surgery and anesthesia should comply with the *highly recommended* standards of the WHO-WFSA International Standards for a Safe Practice of Anesthesia (Tables 60.2 and 60.3). Once again, it must be recognized that these medications and equipment may not be available.[15]

WHO Level 2 Facilities: District or Provincial Hospitals (LCoGS: First-Level Hospital, DCP3: First-Level Hospital)

WHO level 2 facilities generally have 100 to 300 beds and are adequately equipped for major and minor operations. They undertake the bellwether procedures of cesarean section, laparotomy, and treatment of open fractures, which do not require a high level of specialization and technology.[17] Provision of the bellwether procedures is indicative of a surgical system that is advanced enough to perform most other surgical procedures. While there may be an expectation that there will be at least one trained anesthesiologist, one or more trained surgeons, obstetricians, visiting specialists, district medical officers, senior clinical officers, nurses, and midwives, in some countries WHO level 2 facilities will still lack physician anesthesia practitioners, and anesthesia care will be delivered by clinical officers and nurse anesthetists. Additional drugs and equipment (Tables 60.4 and 60.5) are expected to be available

TABLE 60.2. *Highly Recommended* Medications and Intravenous Fluids[16]

- Oxygen
- Ketamine
- Lidocaine 1%, 2%, or bupivacaine
- Diazepam or midazolam
- Morphine
- Epinephrine
- Atropine
- Dextrose (for neonates)
- 0.9% Normal saline
- Acetaminophen
- Nonsteroidal anti-inflammatory medicine
- Magnesium

TABLE 60.3. *Highly Recommended* Equipment[16]

- Tilting table
- Supply of oxygen
- Oropharyngeal airways
- Face masks both adult and pediatric
- Laryngoscopes with adult and pediatric blades
- Endotracheal tubes for adults and pediatrics
- Intubation aids (e.g., Magill forceps, bougie, stylet)
- Suction devices and catheters
- Equipment for IV infusions
- Equipment for spinal and regional blocks
- Stethoscope
- Access to a defibrillator
- Pulse oximeter
- Carbon dioxide detector
- Noninvasive blood pressure monitors with adult/pediatric cuffs

TABLE 60.4. *Recommended* Additional Medications and Intravenous Fluids WHO Level 2 Facility[16]

- Thiopental or propofol
- Succinylcholine
- Neostigmine
- Appropriate nondepolarizing muscle relaxants
- Inhalational anesthetics
- Furosemide
- Hydralazine
- Amiodarone
- Salbutamol
- Ephedrine, metaraminol, norepinephrine, or phenylephrine
- Hydrocortisone
- Mannitol,
- Plasmalyte
- Calcium gluconate (or chloride)

TABLE 60.5. *Recommended* Additional Facilities and Equipment WHO Level 2 Facilities[16]

- System for delivering inhalation anesthesia (draw-over or plenum)
- For plenum systems:
  - Inspired oxygen concentration monitor
  - Antihypoxic device
  - System to prevent misconnection of gas sources
  - Automated ventilator with disconnect alarm
- IV pressure infusion bag
- Device for IV fluid warming
- Continuous wave capnography
- Electrocardiogram
- Temperature monitoring
- Peripheral neuromuscular transmission monitor

to supplement those in WHO level 1 facilities, but these also might not, in fact, be available.[15,19]

WHO Level 3 Facilities: Referral Hospital (LCoGS: Higher-Level Secondary or Tertiary Hospital, DCP3: Second- and Third-Level Hospital)

WHO level 3 facilities usually have the capacity to undertake subspecialty and more complex surgery with intensive care availability. They act as a hub for system-wide clinical, education, and research support.[17] Personnel include surgical, anesthesia, and critical care subspecialists. The WHO-WFSA International Guidelines clearly define required medications and equipment for such referral centers,[5] but once again, such prescriptions are well beyond the reach for many LICs.

What Equipment Should Volunteers Travelling to LICs Bring with Them?

There is a variance in the needs for practice in an austere environment, depending on the nature of the mission. Anesthesiologists should be prepared to work in WHO level 2 facilities and on rare occasions WHO level 1 facilities. Longer-term teaching missions generally involve educating local practitioners to use equipment already present (or easily obtained) and maintained in the specific environment. In contrast, in the case of short-term service missions, a traveling team arrives to directly provide medical care, and airway equipment is generally transported in and out with the team.[20] Regardless of duration, all surgical missions should include a structured educational component. True capacity-building can only occur with committed long-term education that has been crafted in collaboration with the host surgical team.

Airway Equipment and an Associated Consideration for Longer-Term/Teaching Missions

A fundamental premise of longer-term missions is to teach and use airway equipment that is "locally sustainable." A locally sustainable device is defined as one that is already present in the environment or can readily be obtained. In addition, it must be easily disinfected and should be simple to maintain or repair if broken. If electronically powered, the device should have a reliable power source, batteries or otherwise, and in this context, it must be stressed that electrical power (and compressed gases) are often unreliable in disadvantaged countries. Generally, equipment must be reusable, and it must be assumed that any "single-use" items will be reused.

Even if a device can be obtained and maintained, other factors must be considered. Introducing devices that are difficult to use, or with complex storage or disinfection needs, should be discouraged. Donation of equipment that is fragile or requires frequent servicing (e.g., a flexible bronchoscope with a video tower), while well meaning, can be counterproductive in an austere environment. If such a device is presented, it helps to designate one local practitioner as champion for the product, charged with responsibility for ensuring it is used, cleaned, and stored appropriately. Any equipment donated should be accompanied with structured education and ongoing support.

Equipment Considerations for Short-Term Surgical Missions

Airway equipment considerations differ for a short-term surgical mission (Table 60.6). Under these conditions, routine and difficult airway equipment is transported by the team, such equipment being limited only by its portability and durability. This "kit" should ideally be available in adult and pediatric versions, given the high occurrence of pediatric cases. If battery-powered, sufficient batteries should also be available for the equipment, and disinfection requirements should be straightforward. Thankfully, portable oximetry and capnography units (ideally combined) are now quite affordable. If logistics permit, disposable equipment would be of value. It is the responsibility of the individual anesthetist to check that the "kit" is adequate. Additionally, the anesthetists should always provide

TABLE 60.6. Sample Airway Equipment for a Short-Term Service Mission

Equipment

Highly recommended:

- Adult and pediatric self-inflating bag
- Eschmann tracheal introducers/gum elastic bougie, adult and child
- Front of neck access kit (cricothyroidotomy)
- Preferred rescue airway device, adult and pediatric
- Portable, battery-powered pulse oximeters/capnograph
- Tongue depressor, 5% lidocaine ointment, atomizer, 4% lidocaine

Recommended:

- Range of oropharyngeal airways
- Range of nasopharyngeal airways
- Range of face masks
- Two laryngoscopes with preferred blades, bulbs, batteries, battery charger
- Range of tracheal tubes and stylets
- A lighted-stylet
- Magill forceps
- Adult and pediatric reservoir bags
- Tracheal Tube Exchange Catheter
- Video laryngoscope
- EGDs–full range of sizes
- Precordial stethoscope
- Peripheral Nerve Stimulator
- Pasteurization equipment—silicon sieve, food thermometer
- Cleaning devices—pipe cleaners, little scrubbing brush
- Multipurpose tool, tape

Medications

- Neostigmine, glycopyrrolate, salbutamol, 5% lidocaine paste, 10% lidocaine spray with nozzles, 4% lidocaine solution, atomizer, tongue depressor

CHAPTER 60

their own *highly recommended* airway equipment (Table 60.6). This equipment is essential for airway rescue and may not be available in the country. A tongue depressor, 5% lidocaine ointment (not gel), an atomizer, and 4% aqueous lidocaine are also listed as highly recommended. These are the components of one approach to awake tracheal intubation (ATI) and may not be available in the country. If the appropriate equipment/drugs are not available in the country, substituting available alternatives (shortcuts) is not evidence-based and is likely to result in failure.

The selection of airway equipment is not simply acquiring the most advanced equipment available. Sophisticated airway equipment is usually not required for most patients. Paradoxically, the most sophisticated airway equipment could decrease patient safety. Anesthetists on short-term surgical missions, in addition to recognizing their own level of airway expertise and the expertise of the surgical team, must also be very aware of the paucity of equipment, drugs, and perioperative support in the austere and unfamiliar environment in which they will be working. Sophisticated airway equipment may create a sense of safety for the anesthetist, which is not supported by the perioperative environment.

What Is the Present Status of Short-Term Surgical Missions (STSM)?

Recent data (DCP3) suggest that, overall, short-term surgical missions may be less cost-effective, and have additional limitations (such as follow-up and complication management) when compared to other options—such as Self-Contained Mobile Surgical Platforms and Specialty Surgical Hospitals. The best STSMs promote collaboration, continuity, and sustainability. They should be guided by in-country partners and incorporated into the long-term planning of the LIC such that the STSM plan to include their phasing out as local capacity is developed. STSMs should always provide structured education, practice to a standard of care equivalent to that in their home countries, and be culturally competent and respectful. At least until 2030, when it is anticipated that surgical care will reach improved levels in many LMICs, they play a critical, life-sustaining role in environments in which other sources of surgical care are lacking.[21,22] In the interim, STSMs should strive to plan, deliver, and evaluate programs.

What Can Be Done to Disinfect Equipment in an Austere Environment?

Sterilization and disinfection methods in some resource-poor countries[23] may require modification due to inconsistencies in the quality of equipment, processing, and monitoring of effectiveness. Predictably, admirable ingenuity can often be seen in the methods of steam/sterilization, pasteurization, and affordable chemical disinfection. Familiar technologies such as automatic processors, pasteurizers, STERIS™ systems, and ethylene oxide may not be found. In some situations, high-level disinfection (HLD) may need to be accepted rather than sterilization. Fortuitously, the HLD process kills all vegetative microorganisms, mycobacteria, lipid and nonlipid viruses, fungal spores, and some bacterial spores. It lags sterilization only in regard to the destruction of spores and protozoa with cysts, a problem not usually associated with airway management equipment. The WHO lists respiratory equipment as being of intermediate (semicritical) risk requiring only HLD.[24] The routine for HLD should be clean, rinse, dry, process, and protect.

Effective cleaning and preparation are a prerequisite for all modalities of disinfection and sterilization. Effective cleaning decreases bioburden by 80%. Items should be washed with a neutral detergent in water at 50°C to 60°C. Too high a temperature coagulates protein, making it difficult to remove. Enzymatic cleaners are helpful, and tube brushes/pipe cleaners are indispensable. Items need to be rinsed with sterile water at 40°C to 50°C and (ideally) dried in cabinets at 65°C to 70°C. Organic matter or residual moisture from the cleaning process can dilute or inactivate the active ingredients in the HLD and can interfere with direct contact to the device surfaces.[24]

Pasteurization is the immersion of equipment in water at 70°C to 75°C for 30 minutes and, while water does boil at a lower temperature at altitude, this is not a practical issue. An oven thermometer is a useful piece of kit.

Chlorine-based agents are effective high-level disinfectants at a minimum concentration of 1000 ppm available chlorine on a clean surface and are the primary disinfectant in LICs.[25] In addition, indirect transmission through contaminated surfaces (fomites) is an important component of outbreaks of viral respiratory and enteric diseases, such as COVID-19 virus,[26] and chlorine-based surface disinfection is a significant part of prevention and control strategies in response to infectious disease outbreaks. Several chloride compounds are available including sodium hypochlorite (NaOCl), sodium dichloroisocyanurate (NaDCC), and calcium hypochlorite (HTH). NaOCl, also known as household bleach, is ubiquitously available. It is a pH-stabilized liquid at concentrations of 3% to 6%, with a shelf-life of at least one month. NaDCC and HTH are both available as powders. They all act by inhibition of enzymatic reactions, denaturation of proteins, and inactivation of nucleic acids; however, they are corrosive on prolonged contact (>30 minutes) or if used at incorrect concentrations. Hypochlorites are irritating to the mucous membranes of the skin, eyes, and lungs. Their stability is affected by heat, increased pH, and ultraviolet radiation. Once diluted, hypochlorite solution should be prepared daily and kept in opaque containers. They must be kept below 25°C.[24]

Glutaraldehyde is both a sterilizing and HLD agent. A 2% concentration at an alkaline pH for 12 to 30 minutes of exposure is recommended for HLD. Glutaraldehyde acts by causing alkylation of cellular components that alter the protein synthesis of DNA and RNA.[24] It is generally advised that glutaraldehyde not be used on equipment that might contact tissues, though this has been common in the past—after thorough washing. Glutaraldehyde has an advantage of being noncorrosive of metals. However, glutaraldehyde vapors can be toxic, and contact can generate allergic reactions. Workers using glutaraldehyde should do so in well-ventilated environments. Glutaraldehyde should not be discarded in a general sewage system.

Alcohols (70%-90%) are intermediate to low-level disinfectants that act by dissolving the cell membrane.[24] **Chlorhexidine** (a bisbiguanide) will often be used as a skin disinfectant and is sometimes used as a general disinfectant, commonly in association with 70% alcohol and Cetrimide (a quaternary ammonium compound). Its efficacy as a high-level disinfectant is not well documented.[27]

Hydrogen peroxide is a very useful general disinfectant, especially when activated, but not widely available in LICs. It destroys microorganisms by producing destructive hydroxyl free radicals that attack membrane lipids and essential cell components. HLD requires immersion in 6% solution for 30 minutes; however, hydrogen peroxide is an oxidant for metal articles.[24]

Formaldehyde (40%) produces inactivation of microorganisms by affecting nucleic acid synthesis. Due to its hazardous health effects, its use should be discouraged.[24]

A sampling of common practice guidelines can be found in Tables 60.7 to 60.11, and an excellent guide in improving standards in sterile services across health care facilities worldwide is referenced.[24]

TABLE 60.7. Organism Responsiveness

Sterilization: *Bacillus subtilis*, *Clostridium sporogenes*, *Clostridium difficile*
High-Level Disinfection: *Mycobacterium tuberculosis*
Intermediate-Level Disinfection: Poliovirus, Coxsackie virus, Rhinovirus.
Low-Level Disinfection: *Staphylococcus*, *Pseudomonas aeruginosa*, *E. coli*, *Salmonella* spp., enveloped viruses Hepatitis B&C, HIV, CMV, Herpes, RSV, etc.

TABLE 60.8. Recommended Equipment Management in Austere Environments

1. Single-use bacterial filters are now standard issue for many missions.
2. Rubber reusable and plastic single-use tubing should be decontaminated and cleaned. After drying, rubber tubing can be autoclaved or pasteurized. Plastic tubing cannot be autoclaved and should be disinfected, ideally with pasteurization.
3. Ambu® or Heidbrink® valves must be decontaminated, cleaned, and pasteurized after each patient when a filter is not used. Ambu valves can be autoclaved.
4. Face masks, Guedel® airways, Yankaur® suctions are decontaminated, cleaned, and autoclaved (rubber, metal) or pasteurized (rubber, metal, or plastic). Metal laryngoscope blades may be autoclaved (with the bulb removed) or pasteurized.

TABLE 60.9. Equipment for Pasteurization

- A large pan of water
- A silicon sieve that can be suspended in the pan
- A candy or oven thermometer

TABLE 60.10. Management of Consumable Anesthetic Equipment in Austere Environments

- Single-use tracheal tubes are to be used as single use if supplies are sufficient. If in short supply, they can be decontaminated and pasteurized. Practitioners are cautioned against the use of chemical disinfection for equipment that will be placed in the airway. If a practitioner decides to proceed in this manner, great care is required to ensure that disinfectant solution is removed.
- Reusable rubber tubes are to be decontaminated, cleaned, autoclaved, or pasteurized.
- Reusable Laryngeal Mask Airways (LMA-Classic) are to be decontaminated, cleaned and autoclaved, or pasteurized, between each patient.

TABLE 60.11. Disinfection Options in Austere Environments

- Items should be decontaminated and thoroughly cleaned.
- Pasteurization is almost always the method of choice for anesthesia equipment.
- Items should be left for 30 minutes in solution. Glutaraldehyde solution is satisfactory for this purpose, but another solution (e.g., bleach) may be used if more appropriate for the program. Chlorhexidine/Cetrimide solutions in 70% alcohol are also commonly used.
- Hypochlorite (bleach) minimum concentration to eliminate mycobacteria on a clean surface is 0.1% for 10 minutes:
  - Corrodes metal and may destroy adhesives with prolonged soaking.
  - Wash thoroughly.
  - Diluted bleach must be maintained at less than 25°C.

Difficult Airway Management in an Austere Environment

Should a Patient with a Very Difficult Airway Be Managed Electively in an Austere Environment at All?

Deplorably, there is no shortage of very difficult airway anatomy in LICs. Patients are forced to present late when their surgical disease is extreme. Based on the density of operating theatres alone, it is estimated that at least 2 billion people lack access to surgery.[28] In 2015, The Lancet Commission of Global Surgery report highlighted that 4.8 billion people do not have access to safe, affordable surgical care when needed.[29] If presented with such a case, Table 60.12 is a planning approach that should be considered. Though essential, the availability of airway equipment has purposefully been listed last. For a service mission with defined objectives, a very high-acuity case may fall outside the team's capabilities (e.g., due to extreme airway considerations or

SECTION 9

TABLE 60.12. Planning for a Difficult Airway

- Would you undertake this case in your home hospital?
- What is the intraoperative and postoperative support (blood, ICU/HDU, ward care/monitoring, managing emergency complications)?
- Anesthetic experience/capability of other team members/local team
- Long-term outcome for a patient
- Caseload/mix presenting
- Long-term outcome for you and your team
- Equipment available

the anticipated significant need for blood products). Even if the case may be possible from a surgical and anesthetic perspective, postoperative requirements may exceed available facilities (e.g., the lack of an intensive-care unit with ventilators, or suction and humidification for postoperative management of a patient with a fresh tracheotomy, or physiotherapy and rehabilitation). Ward care/monitoring may be very limited, and there may be no or very limited capability to manage emergency complications. Sadly, when time is limited, other patients may present safer options that will have long-term benefit. It is also entirely possible that a team will be inappropriately blamed for a bad outcome, with severe consequences for further engagement with health systems by a community. Dishearteningly, declining surgery may be the only realistic decision. Especially with children, it may be possible to arrange care, through aid organizations, in a more favorable environment.

Can the Surgical Procedure Be Done with Local or Regional Anesthesia?

Utilizing regional or local anesthesia may allow a procedure to proceed without airway manipulation. In addition, local anesthesia could also allow for surgical revision of difficult airway anatomy, permitting safer induction of general anesthesia (e.g., the partial release of a neck burn contracture). Though unusual in HICs, an awake tracheotomy is a very safe method of securing the airway and should be discussed with the surgeon and patient.

If General Anesthesia Is Required, Can the Airway Be Safely Secured Postinduction?

The guiding principles of the ASA difficult airway algorithm (see Chapter 2) are still applicable (with some modification) in resource-poor countries, despite the common absence of flexible bronchoscopy and newer airway adjuncts. Though novel approaches have been suggested,[30–33] embarking on unpracticed and unfamiliar techniques in austere, unsupported environments, in the presence of extreme airway disease, should not be attempted. Awake intubation offers greater safety. Prior to the advent of flexible bronchoscopic intubation, awake blind nasal, and retrograde intubation were practicable techniques; however, contemporary anesthetists do not have the opportunity to acquire and maintain these skills. In contrast, ATI with local anesthesia/sedation is a technique that is appropriate in austere environments, which can be appropriately learnt and practiced in HICs.

ATI has a high success rate with low risk and can be performed with standard anesthesia equipment. It should be performed as an elective procedure; it is not a good choice of emergency airway management when intubation fails. It can be performed using direct or video laryngoscopy. The choice of technique will depend on the availability of equipment, anesthesia provider experience, and patient factors. The key to success is establishing (and testing) effective topicalization. Supplemental oxygen should be administered, and sedation managed with care. Sedation should not be used as a substitute for inadequate topicalizations. It is safer to take more time than give more sedation. Numerous methods of topicalization/local anesthesia have been described (e.g., nerve block, nebulization, mucosal atomization, and spray as you go). The Difficult Airway Society have recently published their guidelines for ATI.[34] Though there is insufficient evidence to recommend any individual technique for topicalization, invasive techniques (glossopharyngeal and superior laryngeal nerve blocks) are not recommended. The maximum dose of lignocaine for any technique should not exceed 9 $mg{\cdot}kg^{-1}$ lean body weight. In LIC, ketamine (0.2-0.5 $mg{\cdot}kg^{-1}$ IV) is available to facilitate ATI.

Notwithstanding skill and equipment challenges, a lack of patient cooperation due to age, and language barriers may militate against the option of successful awake intubation in the patient with a difficult airway.

Anesthesia induction and pharmacologic paralysis in a patient with significant predictors of difficult direct laryngoscopy mandates thorough assessment of all modes of ventilation (i.e., ease of successful bag-mask ventilation, ease of placement of an extraglottic device [EGD], ease of endotracheal intubation, and the ease of successfully undertaking front-of-neck access [surgical airway]). The airway plan should include only a primary technique and a plan for rescue oxygenation, usually via an EGD. It also should be borne in mind that, while a case planned with endotracheal intubation might be able to be managed with an EGD (at least in an emergency), it is generally unwise to rely on an EGD in an elective procedure in which the capacity to place a tracheal tube is in doubt. The seating of an EGD may fail with adjustments in position, and an EGD doesn't protect against reflux and aspiration. A rescue airway plan must remain for rescue.

Once again, it must be stressed that considerable judgment is required across the spectrum of clinical circumstances. In general, caution must be advised in elective situations.

PATIENT MANAGEMENT

Are There Likely to Be Difficulties with Face-Mask Ventilation (FMV) in This Patient?

There is thick facial scarring around the patient's mouth, and producing a seal with a face mask may be difficult. There is a compromise of lower jaw protrusion, most likely related to facial scarring. Mouth opening is decreased, but adequate for the placement of an oropharyngeal airway. The patient has a full set of teeth, normal thyromandibular distance, and normal neck extension. She is not obese, and there is no suggestion of obstructive sleep apnea (OSA). Provided that a mask can be fitted, it is likely that adequate FMV can be accomplished. However, a two-hand and two-person FMV may be necessary (see Chapter 8).

Are There Likely to Be Difficulties in Placement of an EGD in This Patient?

The patient's mouth opening is assessed at 2 cm, adequate for most EGDs. There is no evidence of airway obstruction or deviation. The patient has good neck extension and there is no lung stiffness. Unlike children who are still growing, it is unlikely that the external burns have significantly altered the oropharyngeal anatomy. It is likely that an EGD can be satisfactorily seated in this patient.

If in doubt, a device such as a laryngeal mask airway (LMA) can be inserted awake, under topical local anesthetic only, in motivated patients. Once the airway is established, induction of anesthesia can proceed.

Careful consideration needs to be given to the risk of relying on EGD for prolonged cases or those with risk of intraoperative surgical complications.

Are There Likely to Be Difficulties with Laryngoscopy and Orotracheal Intubation in This Patient?

The patient's Mallampati score of III and her less-than-normal jaw protrusion are not reassuring, but usually compatible with successful intubation of the trachea. The normal thyromandibular distance is reassuring, as is her normal cervical spine extension. A simple adjuvant, such as a tracheal introducer or tracheal tube stylet should be adequate.

Would Cricothyrotomy Be Feasible in This Patient?

The neck scaring appears to be close to the cricothyroid membrane but the membrane is easily palpable. Major blood vessels are unlikely to be inadvertently damaged, as neck anatomy does not appear grossly distorted.

What Coexisting Medical Problems Can Be Anticipated in This Patient?

Often, large burns contractures are likely to have compromised nutrition and general conditioning. In addition, if a substantial part of the chest was involved with the burn, scarring and contracture of the chest will significantly reduce the compliance of the lungs (restrictive pulmonary dysfunction).[35] Large burns contractures also can have excessive bleeding and prolonged surgery. These are not issues in this case.

What Was Done in This Case?

A feasibility assessment was performed. Equipment for skin harvesting was available, and as the area requiring grafting was limited, the need for blood products was judged unlikely. Local medical and nursing expertise was deemed capable of taking on postoperative care. An interpreter was found and the patient consented. Advanced airway equipment, such as a flexible bronchoscope or video laryngoscope, was not available.

An operating room team meeting was held. The entire team was very motivated to perform this simple operation to prevent this women's blindness. The anesthetic plan for the potentially difficult airway was discussed and roles allocated. The risk that the anesthetic might have turned out to be more complex than hoped for was discussed. The possibility that the surgery might not have been able to be performed was raised, should the anesthetic risk have been (unexpectedly) found to be too high.

The patient was taken to the operating room accompanied by an interpreter, and intravenous access was obtained. Monitoring included pulse oximetry, end-tidal carbon dioxide analysis, automated noninvasive blood pressure, and electrocardiogram.

A range of face masks were assessed. A round silicone pediatric size #2 mask was found to be soft enough to conform to the facial scarring and to make a firm seal around the young woman's small mouth (Figure 60.1). The lungs of the patient were denitrogenated with oxygen and a hypnotic low dose of propofol was given. FMV was attempted and proved successful. A further dose of propofol was given and a direct laryngoscopy using a size 3 Macintosh laryngoscope blade was performed. This demonstrated a Cormack-Lehane grade IIb view of the glottis (see Chapter 1) without muscle relaxant. This confirmed that in the event of an EGD failure, oral intubation of the trachea under direct vision would be possible. A common phrase in anesthesia: "Plan for the worst and hope for the best" is particularly pertinent in this environment, and establishing that this woman's trachea can indeed be intubated is important before embarking on surgery. A size 3 LMA was inserted and the anesthesia and surgery proceeded uneventfully. Other options that could have been considered included an inhalational induction with a volatile anesthetic agent to keep the patient spontaneously breathing throughout the surgery. Intubating the patient's airway using a muscle relaxant, following the initial quick direct laryngoscopy, was another option.

In low- and middle-income countries, airway issues from burn contractures can be much more extreme than described in this case. Consider the patient in Figure 60.2, it is natural for health professionals to want to do everything in their power to

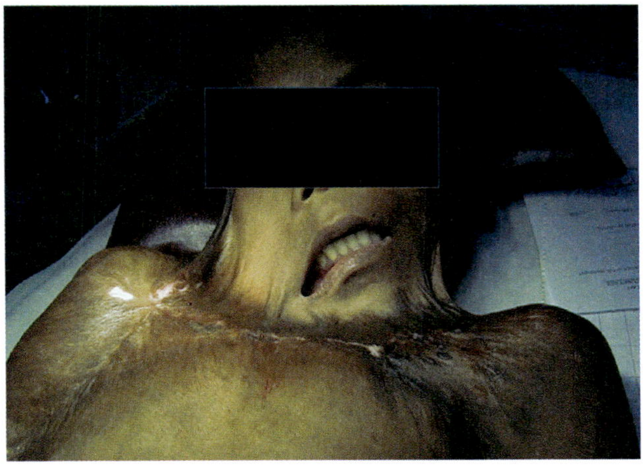

FIGURE 60.2. A 12-year-old boy with severe burn contractures.

help a patient. In an austere environment, it is psychologically easy to take large risks in an attempt to improve these patients' lives. It is described that the worst of these neck contractures can be relieved with ketamine alone. In practice, the fixed neck flexion caused by the contracture does not improve as much as predicted, because of the concurrent musculoskeletal shortening and stiffness. It is possible to do these cases by simply relying on an LMA, but the masks often do not sit well when a patient's head is flexed and rotated. Indeed, many anesthesia practitioners would prefer that a patient's airway was secured before embarking on surgery of the head and neck region, especially in an environment in which assistance was less than predictable.

Consider, for example, the situation in which an LMA was chosen. The surgeon has been working for 2 hours around the neck of the patient in Figure 60.2, and there is another hour away from completing the neck skin graft. The patient is hypotensive from blood loss and the LMA, which has never been ideal, now appears to have moved and the end-tidal carbon dioxide trace disappears. One is unlikely to be able to intubate the trachea of this patient orally, and surgical airway rescue is impossible because of the scarring. Converting to FMV is likely to fail. Ketamine-facilitated ATI, with the plan of canceling surgery if unsuccessful, may be a safer choice of airway management for many difficult airways.

The consequences of a catastrophic airway complication to this patient, the family, you and your team, the local staff and hospital, and your organization cannot be overemphasized when considering whether or not to attempt anesthesia in these difficult airway cases with limited resources.

SUMMARY

Airway management in the austere environment of many resource-poor countries can be challenging on many fronts: the advanced state of the diseases and injuries encountered, equipment availability, limited access to essential medicines, and insufficient local hospital infrastructure and staffing. The practitioner teaching or practicing in these conditions must be resourceful and sensitive to local culture and conditions. As difficult as it may be to accept, there may be cases better not done in these circumstances. Cases presenting with difficult airway considerations should be approached bearing in mind the limitations of both intra- and postoperative resources.

SELF-EVALUATION QUESTIONS

60.1. Which of the following is not included in WHO guidelines for district hospitals in all countries?

A. Pulse oximetry

B. Capnography

C. Flexible bronchoscope

D. Tracheal introducer (commonly known as "bougies")

E. Oxygen analyzers

60.2. In purchasing airway equipment for poorly resourced countries, which of the following is least relevant at this time?

A. Cost of compressed gases

B. Ease of maintenance

C. Unreliability of electrical power

D. Uniformity of international standards

E. Cost of equipment

60.3. Which of the following is not a disinfection option for airway equipment in developing countries?[2]

A. Autoclaving

B. Ethylene oxide

C. Bleach

D. Chlorhexidine/cetrimide

E. Boiling

REFERENCES

1. Mackay P, Cousins M. Safety in anaesthesia. *Anaesth Intensive Care.* 2006;34(3):303-304.
2. Bainbridge D, Martin J, Arango M, Cheng D; Evidence-based Peri-operative Clinical Outcomes Research Group. Perioperative and anaesthetic-related mortality in developed and developing countries: a systematic review and meta-analysis. *Lancet.* 2012;380(9847):1075-1081.
3. Cook TM, Woodall N, Frerk C. Major complications of airway management in the UK: results of the 4th National Audit Project of the Royal College of Anaesthetists and the Difficult Airway Society. Part 1: Anaesthesia. *Br J Anaesth.* 2011;106:617-631.
4. Eichorn JH. Prevention of intraoperative anesthesia accidents and related severe injury through safety monitoring. *Anesthesiology.* 1989;70:572-577.
5. Merry AF, Cooper JB, Soyannwo O, Wilson IH, Eichhorn JH. International standards for a safe practice of anesthesia 2010. *Can J Anaesth.* 2010;57(11):1027-1034.
6. Hansen D, Gausi SC, Merikebu M. Anaesthesia in Malawi: complications and deaths. *Trop Doct.* 2000;30(3):146-149.
7. Heywood AJ, Wilson IH, Sinclair JR. Perioperative mortality in Zambia. *Ann R Coll Surg Engl.* 1989;71(6):354-358.
8. McKenzie AG. Mortality associated with anaesthesia at Zimbabwean teaching hospitals. *S Afr Med J.* 1996;86(4):338-342.
9. Ouro-Bang'na Maman AF, Tomta K, Ahouangbevi S, Chobli M. Deaths associated with anaesthesia in Togo, West Africa. *Trop Doct.* 2005;35(4):220-222.
10. Vasdev GM, Harrison BA, Keegan MT, Burkle CM. Management of the difficult and failed airway in obstetric anesthesia. *J Anesth.* 2008;22(1):38-48.
11. Dubowitz G. Global health and global anesthesia. *Int Anesthesiol Clin.* 2010;48(2):39-46.
12. Funk LM, Weiser TG, Berry WR, et al. Global operating theatre distribution and pulse oximetry supply: an estimation from reported data. *Lancet.* 2010;376(9746):1055-1061.
13. Eichorn JH. Prevention of intraoperative anesthesia accidents and related severe injury through safety monitoring. *Anesthesiology.* 1989;70:572-577.
14. Merry AF, Barraclough BH. The WHO surgical safety checklist. *Med J Aust.* 2010;192(11):631-632.
15. McQueen KA, Coonan T, Ottaway A, et al. The bare minimum: the reality of global anaesthesia and patient safety. *World J Surg.* 2015;39:2153-2160.
16. Gelb AW, Morriss WW, Johnson W, et al. World Health Organization-World Federation of Societies of Anaesthesiologists (WHO-WFSA) international standards for a safe practice of anesthesia. *Can J Anesth.* 2018;65;698-708.
17. McCord C, Kruk ME, Mock CN, et al. Organization of essential services and the role of first-level hospitals. In: Debas HT, Donkor P, Gawande A, Jamison DT, Kruk ME, Mock CN, eds. *Essential Surgery: Disease Control Priorities, Third Edition (Volume 1).* Washington, DC: The International Bank for Reconstruction and Development/The World Bank; 2015.

18. Dobson M. Surgical care at the district hospital. *World Health Organization*. 2003.
19. Hodges SC, Mijumbi C, Okello M, McCormick BA, Walker IA, Wilson IH. Anaesthesia services in developing countries: defining the problems. *Anaesthesia*. 2007;62(1):4-11.
20. Hodges SC, Hodges AM. A protocol for safe anesthesia for cleft lip and palate surgery in developing countries. *Anaesthesia*. 2000;55(5):436-441.
21. Shrime MG, Sleemi A, Ravilla TD. Charitable platforms in global surgery: a systematic review of their effectiveness, cost-effectiveness, sustainability, and role training. *World J Surg*. 2015;39(1):10-20.
22. Shrime MG, Sleemi A, Ravilla TD. Specialized surgical platforms. In: Debas HT, Donkor P, Gawande A, Jamison DT, Kruk ME, Mock CN, eds. *Essential Surgery: Disease Control Priorities, Third Edition (Volume 1)*. Washington, DC: The International Bank for Reconstruction and Development/The World Bank; 2015.
23. Guideline for Disinfection and Sterilization in Healthcare Facilities. http://www.cdc.gov/hicpac/Disinfection_Sterilization/2_approach.html.
24. World Health Organisation and Pan American Health Organisation. *Decontamination and Reprocessing of Medical Devices for Health-Care Facilities. Secondary Decontamination and Reprocessing of Medical Devices for Health-Care Facilities*. WHO; 2016.
25. Gallandat K, Kolus RC, Julian TR, Lantagne DS. A systematic review of chlorine-based surface disinfection efficacy to inform recommendations for low-resource outbreak settings. *Am J Infect Control*. 2021;49(1):90-103.
26. Ong SWX, Tan YK, Chia PY, et al. Air, surface environmental, and personal protective equipment contamination by severe acute respiratory syndrome coronavirus 2 (SARS-CoV-2) from a symptomatic patient. *JAMA*. 2020;323(16):1610-1612.
27. http://www.cfsph.iastate.edu/Disinfection/.../CharacteristicsSelected Disinfectant.
28. Funk LM, Weiser TG, Berry WR, et al. Global operating theatre distribution and pulse oximetry supply: an estimation from reported data. *Lancet*. 2010;376:1055-1061.
29. Meara JG, Leather AJ, Hagander L, et al. Global Surgery 2030: evidence and solutions for achieving health, welfare, and economic development. *Lancet*. 2015;386(9993):569-624.
30. Dahra SS. Aids to tracheal intubation. *World Anaesth Update Anaesth*. 2003;17:8-13.
31. Wilson IH, Kopf A. Prediction and management of difficult tracheal intubation. *World Anaesth Update Anaesth*. 1998;9:37-45.
32. Arora MK, Karamchandani K, Trikha A. Use of a gum elastic bougie to facilitate blind nasotracheal intubation in children: a series of three cases. *Anaesthesia*. 2006;61(3):291-294.
33. Metz S, Beattie C. A modified nasal trumpet to facilitate fibreoptic intubation. *Br J Anaesth*. 2003;90(3):388-391.
34. Ahmad I, El-Boghdadly K, Bhagrath R, et al. Difficult Airway Society guidelines for awake tracheal intubation (ATI) in adults. *Anaesthesia*. 2020;75:509-528.
35. Mlcak R, Desai MH, Robinson E, Nichols R, Herndon DN. Lung function following thermal injury in children: an 8-year follow up. *Burns*. 1998;24(3):213-216.

CHAPTER 61

Respiratory Management in the Magnetic Resonance Imaging Suite

Richard D. Roda and Andrew D. Milne

CASE PRESENTATION

Mr. S is a 52-year-old entrepreneur in the waste management industry. He weighs 119 kg, is 175 cm tall (BMI of 38.9 kg·m^{-2}), and is being investigated for "dizzy spells." His medical problem list includes obesity, untreated hypertension, and possible obstructive sleep apnea (OSA) (based on his wife's observation that "sometimes he just stops breathing" at night). A previous attempt at a magnetic resonance imaging (MRI) scan was unsuccessful because Mr. S, startled by the onset of the loud noises made by the MRI machine, panicked and tried to get out of the MRI scanner. Upon further questioning, he admits to extreme claustrophobia, possibly the result of a protracted period of time spent in a car trunk as a child.

On this occasion, the MRI team decides that Mr. S might be more cooperative with pharmacologic assistance and to this end has given him 5 mg of IV midazolam (Versed®). Unknown to the clinical team, just before arriving at the MRI suite, Mr. S had also taken 6 mg of his wife's lorazepam (Ativan®) to help reduce his considerable anxiety. For the scan, a pulse oximeter and nasal capnograph are used to monitor respiration. Oxygen is administered by nasal prongs at 3 L·min^{-1}.

About 10 minutes into the MRI scan, the pulse oximeter alarm activates, drawing attention to an oxygen saturation reading of 81%. The pulse oximeter waveform quality appears to be good. However, no waveform can be obtained from the capnograph. Since Mr. S is deep inside the MRI machine, it is difficult to visually assess his respiratory status. You are urgently summoned to the MRI suite by the radiology team to help manage this patient.

INTRODUCTION

Discuss the Physics of Magnetic Resonance Imaging

A basic understanding of how MRI works is important for both medical management and the safety of both patients and medical personnel in the MRI suite. In simple terms, MRI systems use high-strength magnetic fields and radio waves to generate images based on interactions between the generated magnetic fields and hydrogen molecules in the tissues being imaged. More specifically, static magnetic fields generated by an MRI scanner interact with small fields generated by atomic nuclei. Some nuclei develop a magnetic dipole moment when subject to this field, deflected at a slight angle to the static magnetic field. These nuclei also "wobble" about the direction of the magnetic field much like a spinning "top" at what is known as the precession frequency, which is proportional to the magnetic field strength. When a variable magnetic field is applied at the precessional frequency, more nuclei move from a lower to a higher energy state. When the variable field is removed, they relax, emitting energy at the same precessional frequency which is then detected by a receiving coil in the scanner. Medical-grade MRI scanners are typically tuned to interact with hydrogen and water, while the receiving coils detect energy in the radiofrequency (RF) range. Thus, images are generated by small spatial gradient (variable) field perturbations that localize individual tissues which then emit RF signals detected by the receiving coil and reconstructed with a computer in 3D space.

Why Do We Have Different Types of Scanners?

Modern MRI scanners typically use static field strengths from 0.5 to 3 Tesla (T) with many research machines now producing 4 T. Most diagnostic scanners operate at 1.5 T. For perspective, 1 Tesla = 10,000 Gauss (G), and the earth's magnetic field is approximately 0.5 G. A cylindrical bore at the center of the scanner is surrounded by a superconducting solenoid housed in liquid helium. Field strength is strongest within the bore of the scanner and expressed in Tesla. Fringe fields extend outward from the scanner with the shape dictated in part by the magnet design and by shielding, typically expressed in Gauss[1,2] (Figure 61.1).

Intraoperative MRI (iMRI) systems are a more recent tool for both diagnostic and therapeutic interventions. They can be used for preoperative functional brain mapping of eloquent brain areas as well as for real-time brain mapping for invasive neurosurgical procedures. Examples include monitoring progressive changes in the lesion and surrounding tissue, or updating brain mapping by accounting for brain shift after opening up the dura.[2]

What Are the MRI Suite Zones?

The MRI suite is organized into four concentric "zones" corresponding to the increasing level of hazard (Figure 61.2). Zone I includes all remaining zones within and is the area where patients and health care providers must gain access to the MRI suite. It is generally publicly accessible. Zone II is a controlled area restricting access to Zone III. Patients are interviewed and checked in here and under the supervision of MRI personnel. Zone II must have a ferrous metal detector as well as a 1000-G handheld magnet to screen equipment and patients entering the MRI suite. Zone III requires completed screening from Zone II of all personnel and patients as any contraindicated equipment and devices may interact with the MRI static and time-varying magnetic fields causing serious injury or death. Zone IV is contained within Zone III and is the room containing the MRI magnet itself. Zone IV is heavily restricted and under full supervision by MRI suite personnel.[3] Entrances to all zones should be appropriately labeled and controlled, and it is in Zone III and IV where the anesthesia practitioner must consider the safety restrictions of the MRI magnetic fields when formulating an anesthetic plan.

What Are the Hazards Intrinsic to the MRI Suite?

The physics of MRI dictates the identification of unique patient and equipment considerations when managing cases in the MRI suite. Not only can the strong magnetic fields directly affect patient physiology such as vestibular function, hearing, and interaction with ferromagnetic prostheses, but they also create numerous safety concerns with how and what equipment is used. Electronic interference leading to equipment malfunction, metallic projectiles from strong magnetic fields, and limited patient access are a few examples and represent occupational health and safety concerns that must be identified and mitigated. As long as these hazards are understood and appreciated, the anesthesia practitioner can safely provide anesthesia even within Zone VI of the MRI suite while image requisition is taking place.

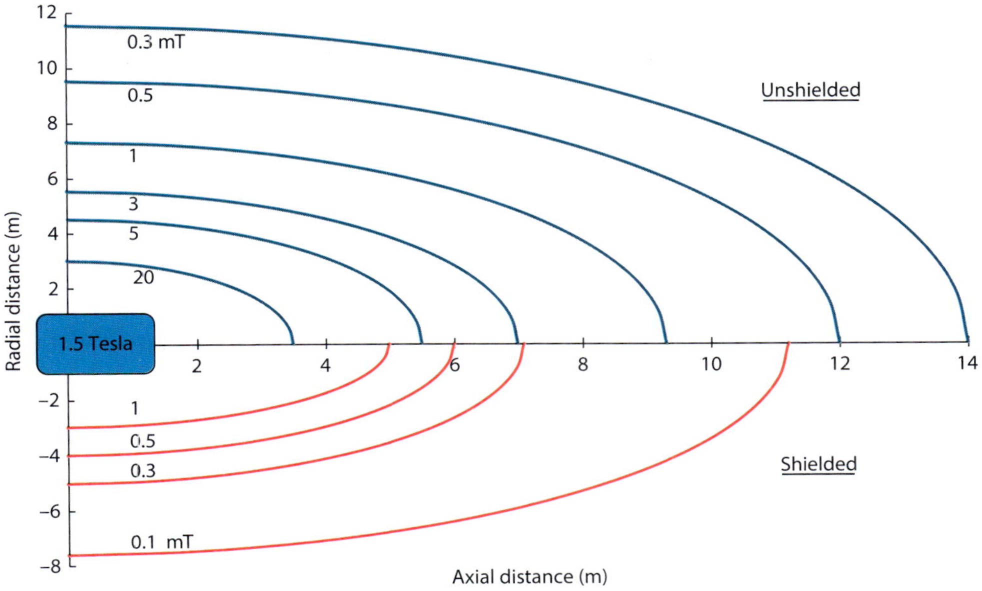

FIGURE 61.1. Unshielded and passively shielded field strength contours from a 1.5-T MRI extending radially and axially from magnet bore. (Reproduced with permission from Bushberg J, Seibert J, Leidholdt E, et al. *The Essential Physics of Medical Imaging*, 2nd ed. Philadelphia, PA: Lippincott Williams & Wilkins; 2002.)

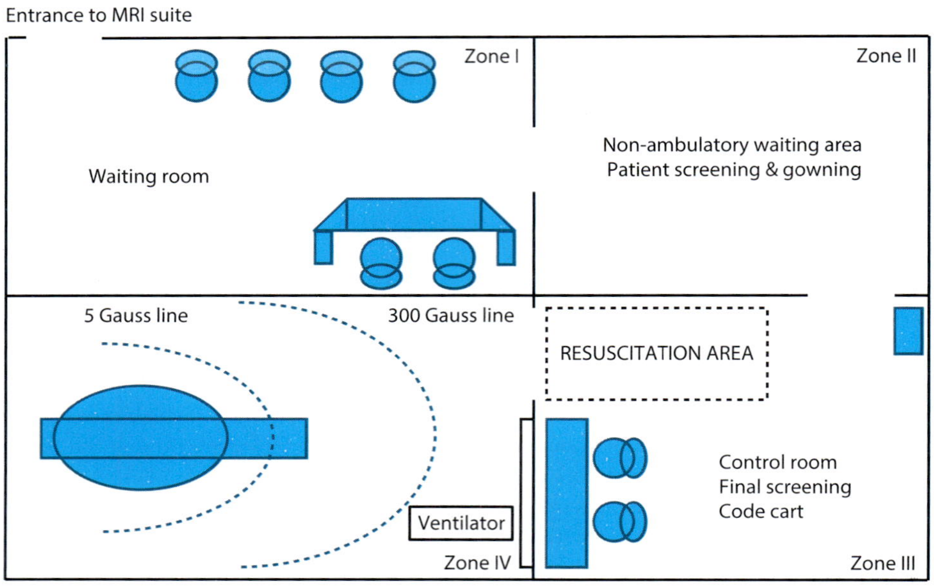

FIGURE 61.2. Diagram illustrating the four zones of the MRI suite. All patients and staff must enter through Zone I and undergo appropriate screening in Zone II before entering Zones III and IV. Certain MRI conditional equipment may enter Zone IV but must be outside the appropriate 5- or 300-G contour as designated by magnetic screening or the manufacturer. A predetermined location in Zone III must be readily available to move the patient in the event of emergency such as a cardiopulmonary collapse.

What Is the Static Magnetic Field and How Does It Affect Patients and Health Care Workers?

MRI scanners employ a static magnetic field within Zone 1 that may always be on between cases. Within the 30-G field line, any ferromagnetic objects may be drawn toward the center of the bore as well as experience a torque in order to line up with the magnetic field. It should be common practice to fully screen patients and staff before passing through the 5-G contour (marked on the floor of Zone 1) of the static field.[1] These fields may interact directly with patients and health care workers as well as with surrounding objects and equipment. Occupational health surveys of factory workers in a 1.0- and 1.5-T MRI magnet manufacturing facility reported transient symptoms of headache (27%), vertigo (22%), and metallic taste (11%). Median magnetic field exposure time for these symptoms was as short as 20 minutes.[4]

Displacement, twisting, or migration of ferromagnetic aneurysm clips with the magnet field in the MRI suite[5] has resulted in fatal outcomes in prior case reports in the literature. Specific metal alloys containing alpha-phase iron such as in stainless steel have been implicated in reacting with strong magnetic fields. A recent literature review discussed the evolution of aneurysm clips toward MRI compatibility; however, current recommendations assume contraindication if there is any doubt about compatibility.[6]

The dangers of these strong magnetic fields in the MRI suite cannot be understated. In July of 2001, a 6-year-old child undergoing MRI suffered a skull fracture and intracranial hemorrhage from a projectile oxygen tank that had errantly been brought into the room. The child had received more sedation than necessary and became bradypneic. The anesthesia practitioner noted that there was no flow through the wall oxygen supply, and while technologists sought a solution, a nurse handed the anesthesia practitioner an oxygen tank. They brought this tank into the MRI suite, and it was drawn with great force toward the magnet bore, hitting the child and causing the skull fracture. He passed away two days later from this injury.[7,8] There are multiple case reports of such accidents or near misses during the last two decades.[5,7,9–12]

Screening of equipment for ferromagnetic materials may be performed onsite with hand-held rare earth magnets of 1000 G or greater. They can be used to detect even weakly ferromagnetic equipment by assessing if there is any perceptible force interaction between the rare earth magnet and equipment being tested. However, equipment with no apparent ferromagnetic material after magnetic screening may still pose a threat. Zimmer et al.[10] describe a case report of a young boy under general anesthesia who underwent an abdominal MRI. A portable sevoflurane vaporizer was brought into the MRI suite and subsequently was attracted to the magnet. Two individuals were able to deflect the trajectory of the vaporizer so that it struck the MRI gantry and not the child within the magnet bore. Although an emergency quench of the magnet was considered (described below), the vaporizer was ultimately removed with the help of three individuals. A strong handheld magnet showed no attraction to the vaporizer. However, when investigated further it did contain small amounts of ferromagnetic material within the temperature compensation module. Similar to the principle stated above regarding aneurysm clips, any equipment with unknown MRI compatibility should be considered dangerous until its safety has been definitively confirmed.

What Are Time-Varying Magnetic Field Gradients?

Low-amplitude magnetic fields that vary throughout the MRI imaging sequence can interact with equipment and the patient.

These fields can induce current in a coiled wire, such as with ECG leads, creating current and heat strong enough to cause tissue burns.[1] These fields have also been shown to stimulate peripheral nerve and muscle cells.[1] Humans, mice, and zebrafish have all demonstrated behaviors implicating peripheral vestibular stimulation while subject to strong static and changing magnetic fields. One such theory involves a Lorentz force interacting with natural ionic currents flowing within the inner ear endolymph to vestibular hair cells sufficient to displace semicircular canal cupula and induce vertigo and horizontal nystagmus in humans and mice.[13] Another theory implicates electromagnetic induction, where currents can be induced within the body by changing magnetic fields directly stimulating neural tissue.[13] Even transient visual disturbances described as flashes of light called phosphenes have been reported in research grade (4-7 T) scanners.[13] At present there is no evidence to suggest these sensory effects are harmful to the patient. However, there are case reports of acute vertigo experiences by anesthesia practitioners even in 3-T MRI scanners.[14]

What Is the Acoustic Noise Associated with the MRI Scanner?

Noise generated with the switching of gradient fields is usually above 85 dB within the MRI suite. Exposure to these noise levels can contribute to hearing loss for both staff and patients (awake or under general anesthesia) and ear protection is necessary.[1] Additionally, the noise can be a distraction from monitor alarms and during emergency situations, inhibiting communication between staff.

What Is the Radiofrequency (RF) Heating?

Power dissipation from the strong radio transmitter can interact with patients' tissues leading to increases in temperature and having the potential to burn the patient. Although the RF power of the MRI is monitored, other environmental factors can contribute to temperature changes, such as ambient temperature, airflow, humidity, and clothing.[1] Additionally, any conductive metal material can rapidly increase in temperature causing burns on the patient. Case reports implicate induced thermal burns from circular metal implants, tattoos, deep brain stimulators, halo pins, ECG leads, coiled wiring, and transdermal patches. Studies have shown temperatures as high as 63°C can be achieved. These burns can be dramatic, and have, for example, resulted in full-thickness burns leading to amputation in a child.[9]

What Is Helium Escape/Quench?

In extreme situations that require an emergency magnetic field shut down, a process called a quench can be performed. The superconductor that maintains the static magnetic field is housed in approximately 1000 L of liquid helium near absolute zero. During a quench, this helium is rapidly vaporized and expands, rapidly disabling the magnet with subsequent dissipation of the magnetic field. All MRI suites should be designed to rapidly vent the helium vapor; however, if there is a failure or blockage of the vented vapors then a hypoxic mixture can result within the magnet bore. Oxygen sensors and backup venting strategies should also be in place.[1] Extra oxygen face masks or nasal prongs compatible with the suite should be available to connect to MRI safe wall oxygen or tanks outside Zone IV in the event the patient or other personnel are subjected to this hypoxic environment. It should be noted that a magnet quench can very easily cause damage to the magnet coil and it can take on the order of weeks to months before the MRI is ready for imaging. As such, the decision to quench should not be taken lightly but is necessary when patient safety is at risk.

While there are few case reports on MRI quenches, one incident led to a quench when a clinician carried an oxygen cylinder into Zone IV to treat hypoxemia in an overly sedated patient.[11] Another involved a failed quench when a replacement oxygen H-cylinder was brought into Zone IV without adequate screening or signage.[12] In both cases, the cylinders became projectiles, causing damage to the MRI machine, and in the latter case, the patient suffered severe facial fractures. These cases highlight the importance of having MRI-compatible supplemental oxygen strategies for patients in Zone IV. Current American Society of Anesthesiology guidelines additionally recommend available supplemental oxygen for health care providers, helium venting strategies, and a plan for removal of the patient from Zone IV, in the event of an initiated quench.[3]

ANESTHESIA AND PATIENT CONSIDERATIONS

What Are the Equipment Considerations for the MRI Suite?

The nature of how equipment interacts with the static and time-varying magnetic fields generated by the magnet coils dictates safety and compatibility in the MRI suite. Equipment is broadly categorized into physiologic monitors, invasive monitors, intubation equipment, and oxygenation and ventilation equipment.[3] For each category, equipment is further stratified between "Acceptable," "Unacceptable," and "Cautionary" with regards to safety in the MRI suite. It is important to note that even "MRI acceptable" equipment may only be rated for use up to a maximum magnetic field strength. Other 'Cautionary' equipment may only be suitable for use in Zone III. It is up to the anesthesia practitioner and radiology department to be knowledgeable in the limitations of the equipment stocked and available for use in the MRI suite.[3] A broader reference on equipment and monitoring is available in the Practice Advisory on Anesthetic Care for Magnetic Resonance Imaging by the American Society of Anesthesiologists, revised in 2015[3]; however, the focus of this chapter will be on airway equipment and management.

What Precautions Are Necessary for the Monitors Used for Anesthesia Care?

Considerations for safe monitoring include the use of MRI conditional/acceptable monitors in Zone III and IV respectively and the ability for remote monitoring from Zone III. Monitoring should be consistent with the American Society of Anesthesiology standards and it is expected the anesthesia practitioner will be familiar with the limitations of available monitors. Notably, care should be taken as inadvertently coiled wires may induce burns in the patient by the static and time-varying magnetic fields.[3] Seemingly harmless equipment such as ECG electrodes can cause burns and imaging artifacts. There are numerous MRI-compatible wireless monitoring technologies available in the market that also include appropriate filtering of signal noise due to the MRI scanner itself. Wired technologies typically require a RF radiation filter in order to be passed from Zone III to IV. The bottom line is that it is important that anesthesia practitioners know what is and is not safe at their institution and plan accordingly.

What Airway Equipment Are Compatible for Use in the MRI Unit?

Airway management within the MRI suite is complicated by:

1. Limited accessibility to the patient's airway
2. Difficulty in visual and auditory assessments

While literature is sparse in assessing the management of airway emergencies in the MRI suite, most would agree that preparation and planning are critically important for the anesthesia practitioner. If there are concerns about potential airway compromise during the scanning procedure in the MRI unit (a duration typically ranged between 15 and 90 minutes) particularly in a patient who is morbidly obese and is not cooperative, it may be more prudent to secure the airway with an endotracheal tube than employing sedation or use of a laryngeal mask airway. If more advanced airway techniques are required (e.g., flexible bronchoscopic intubation or video laryngoscopy) then airway management should be performed outside Zone IV (such as in the operating room) with the appropriate equipment and support. Backup MRI conditional/acceptable airway equipment must be functional and available at all times, including suction.[3]

Most airway equipment available has not been specifically designed for the MRI suite. Effects can be divided into two categories: (1) safety of equipment in MRI environment in avoiding projectile behavior or causing thermal burns and (2) actual functioning of equipment once in MRI environment. While conventional laryngoscopes contain a substantial amount of ferromagnetic material, there are laryngoscopes available that are acceptable and designed for 3.0-T magnet environments. The Airtraq Avant® (Mercury Medical, Clearwater, FL, USA) is designated as MRI compatible, allowing for an angulated view of the glottis without aligning the oropharyngeal axes of the airway much like with video laryngoscopy. MRI safe laryngeal masks can be obtained and extraglottic devices such as the cuffless i-gel™ (Intersurgical, Burlington, ON, Canada) has been used in the pediatric population.[15] Although MRI-compatible, seemingly benign equipment such as endotracheal tubes and laryngeal mask airways contain metallic springs in the balloon cuff valve. While the amount of ferromagnetic material may not be sufficient to cause direct harm to the patient, there have been case reports of misdiagnoses due to imaging quality interference from pilot balloon metallic springs.[16,17] The Ambu® AuraOnce™ Disposable Laryngeal Mask (Ambu Inc, Columbia, MD, USA) and i-gel airway were both associated with better image quality, while conversely, prominent artifacts were seen with LMA-ProSeal™ (Teleflex Medical, Morrisville, NC, USA).[18] Generally speaking, current video laryngoscopes and flexible bronchoscopes are not Zone IV MRI compatible, subject to interference and projectile risk. Testing magnets are typically available in the MRI suite if there is doubt.

When inhalational or total intravenous anesthesia is used, MRI conditional vaporizer-ventilators or intravenous pumps from Zone III are required.[3] Long ventilator circuits or intravenous tubing passed through a waveguide must be used and which can result in larger time constants when changing the depth of anesthesia. A waveguide is typically a brass tube entering the shielded enclosure of Zone IV that allows passage of any lines containing fluid (e.g., ventilation circuit, IV tubing) while reflecting RF radiation back into Zone IV and effectively shielding the surrounding zones of the MRI suite. Bolus injections can also be used in either Zone III or IV, but again care must be taken given the limited access to the patient. Notably, MRI acceptable ventilators and anesthesia machines do exist for use within Zone IV, typically with gauss limits governing distance from the center of the magnet bore.

In the event of emergency such as respiratory or circulatory arrest, calling for help, initiating cardiopulmonary resuscitation if indicated, and moving the patient from Zone IV are crucial. A safe predetermined location containing appropriate resuscitation equipment for advanced cardiac life support should be designated ahead of time.[3] Nonoperating room anesthesia (NORA) poses further unique challenges as these environments often are unfamiliar to the anesthesia practitioner, equipment and drugs may need to be brought to the suite, and support personnel in the event of an emergency may be far away.[19]

What Are the Patient Considerations for the MRI Suite?

The patient population typically seen in the MRI suite can be categorized into two broad categories. The first is elective walk-in and semielective inpatients. The second is critically ill patients. The approach to each patient can vary significantly for a given MR study. Within these categories, further patient considerations include children, people living with intellectual disability, claustrophobia, and anxiety.

MRI may take up to 10 minutes per image to acquire and studies typically consist of multiple image sequences. Any movement can create significant distortion requiring reacquisition of the imaging. Awake patients within the magnet bore are subject to noise and immobility which creates a claustrophobic environment. Management options include the patient being fully awake, judicious sedation (with reversal agents such as naloxone and flumazenil readily available), or in the case of severe phobias or anxiety discontinuing the study until anesthesia support is available should a general anesthetic be required.

Much of the time, elective and semielective patients opt for sedation. A careful preoperative assessment is necessary including fasting status, any history of OSA symptoms, and a focused cardiorespiratory and airway examination, paying particular attention to how sedation may be tolerated. Although MRI is considered nonstimulating when compared to other procedures, the noisy environment may dictate substantial sedation. Equally important is the risk of laryngospasm with light anesthesia due to the sudden loud noises and other nonpainful stimuli within the MRI suite. Hypoventilation, apnea, or airway obstruction are primary concerns in this case. Patient characteristics such as OSA, obesity, and other airway pathologies may make patients more sensitive to sedative medications. Patients who are uncooperative, such as children and those with intellectual disability, may endanger the success of the MRI study, which may necessitate a general anesthetic to obtain optimal imaging. These considerations should be weighed with the challenges of the patient's airway, patient poor access, and direct observation.

Choice of drug used for sedation may vary and should be tailored to the pharmacokinetic and pharmacodynamic effects for each patient. For the MRI environment, an ideal sedative agent is short-acting, easy to titrate, has minimal potential to cause hypoventilation, and has a short recovery time (see Chapter 4). Propofol has been used and exhibits some of the qualities above. Midazolam, ketamine, propofol, and combinations of these medications may all be used in both adult and pediatric populations for procedural sedation.[20]

Dexmedetomidine is a relatively novel alpha-2 adrenergic agonist medication with sedative properties ideal for procedural sedation. These effects act by activation of specific transmembrane alpha-2 adrenergic receptors throughout the central nervous system (CNS). The potential lies in the maintenance of respiratory drive during infusion while providing sedation, anxiolysis, and analgesia. Deleterious hemodynamic effects exist, primarily during initial loading bolus, including hypotension and bradycardia.[20] Furthermore, it must be delivered via infusion pump which can present its own challenges in the MRI suite as described previously. Dexmedetomidine has already been used in awake craniotomies with functional brain mapping and intraoperative MRI.[21]

Critically ill patients pose a different challenge. Typically, the airway is already secured as they tend to arrive from critical care services. These patients may require sedation, vasoactive infusions, and ventilation. As discussed previously, the anesthesia practitioner must develop a plan keeping in mind the additional equipment requirements and MRI compatibility including any other pumps, lines, tubes, or monitors the patient may have in situ from the critical care unit. Hand-bag ventilation may be used in certain situations; however, substantial ventilator support with high airway pressures and peak end-expiratory pressure may be beyond the capabilities of what is available for respiratory equipment in the MRI suite. A computed tomography (CT) scan may be a reasonable alternative and allow for safer mechanical ventilation and should be part of the discussion with the radiology service. Having infusion pumps with long lines passed through the waveguide into Zone IV primed and available ensures minimal disruption of drug delivery. The clinical utility of the MRI scan must be weighed against the clinical acuity and stability of the patient.

There are unique patient considerations obtained from past medical history pertinent to anesthetic management in the MRI suite that are common to elective, semielective, and critically ill patients. Electronic implanted devices such as pacemakers, implanted cardio defibrillators, deep brain stimulators, spinal cord/peripheral nerve stimulators, and other patient implants such as aneurysm clips, coronary stents, prosthetic heart valves, orthodontic appliances, and orthopedic implants all pose a risk to the patient and MRI staff. The underlying principle of ferromagnetism explains much of the hazards associated with these devices and has been explained in the foregoing narrative. Additionally, pacemakers and implanted cardio defibrillators may suffer from interference causing malfunction of the sensing, pacing, and response capabilities of these devices. Newer models of these devices have been tested and deemed MRI compatible for certain field strengths. A conservative approach by radiology and anesthesiology services is necessary to ensure patient safety. If the response to MRI is unknown, delaying or canceling the study, or the use of an alternative diagnostic tool such as a CT scan should be considered.

■ Are There Guidelines for Anesthetic Management in the MRI Suite?

The American Society of Anesthesiologists Task Force on Anesthetic Care for Magnetic Imaging released a Practice Advisory in 2009 on anesthetic care of MRI. This practice advisory was updated in March of 2015.[3] The more recent advisory contains updated evidence since 2009. This includes new evidence on Food and Drug Administration (FDA) approved MRI-compatible conditional implantable cardiac pacing generators and lead systems. An additional guideline was published by the Association of Anaesthetists and the Neuro Anaesthesia and Critical Care Society of Great Britain and Ireland in 2019.[22] This guideline focuses on the importance of anesthesiologist leadership, proper MRI safe education for all involved staff members, and use of safety protocols such as MRI safe checklists in conjunction with the World Health Organization (WHO) checklist.

AIRWAY MANAGEMENT

■ How Do You Manage the Hypoxemia of This Patient in the MRI Suite?

Mr. S is an example of a patient seen increasingly more commonly: the obese patient with probable undiagnosed OSA. His uncontrolled hypertension is likely in part due to the progression of his OSA. As the anesthesia practitioner on-call, you arrive at the suite through Zones I and II being mindful to remove any items containing ferromagnetic material once in Zone III. This includes stethoscopes, cellphones/pagers, pens, wallets, and even some shoes. Scanning the monitors, you obtain a brief history with vitals (heart rate 74 bpm, respiratory rate 5 breaths per minute, oxygen saturation now 78%) while simultaneously diagnosing and treating for hypoxemia. Given the history, the most likely diagnosis is hypoventilation secondary to excessive sedation from midazolam combined with his self-medication at home with lorazepam. While initiating therapy it is important to keep alternative differential diagnoses of hypoxemia, such as deceased FiO_2, alternative causes of hypoventilation (e.g., stroke), and pathologies leading to V/Q mismatch, shunt, or diffusion defects.

The unique challenges with this case include limited patient access and avoiding intrinsic hazards of the MRI suite magnet. Mr. S is currently deep within the magnet bore and his airway and head cannot be visualized so it is impossible to immediately assess if he is making respiratory efforts or if he is even awake. Direct assessment is necessary given the acuity and degree of his hypoxemia. Since only plethysmography and capnography monitoring were initially employed, an assessment of the remainder of his vital signs such as blood pressure is necessary. It should be noted that the ASA guidelines for anesthetic care in the MRI suite make no specific recommendations on blood pressure monitoring during MRI; however, monitoring should be consistent with ASA "Standards for Basic Anesthesia Monitoring." At this point, if not already done so, the gantry should be retracted to remove the patient from the magnet bore.

A call is made for additional help from screened MRI personnel. You enter Zone IV after having been screened for ferromagnetic material. The importance of this screening cannot be more emphasized. A paperclip or hairpin can reach a terminal velocity of 40 miles per hour[23] within Zone IV, causing serious harm to patients and staff.

Larger objects can cause significant damage to patients and staff if one rushes into Zone IV with MRI-contraindicated equipment. This was clearly described earlier in the chapter in a similar situation of hypoxemia, resulting in the death of a young child. Upon assessing Mr. S on the retracted gantry, he responds minimally to sternal rub with GCS 8. He is making respiratory efforts but is obstructing with no effective ventilation and no CO_2 trace from his CO_2 nasal prongs. His airway obstruction is only minimally relieved by applying a jaw thrust maneuver, but SpO_2 remains in the low 80s range.

Airway equipment that is readily available and safe for Zone IV include oropharyngeal airways, portable manual bag-mask ventilation system, such as Ambu Bag, and laryngeal mask airways. Note that although oxygen tanks are generally contraindicated within Zone IV, oxygen tubing may be passed from wall oxygen for face-mask ventilation. One may not be able to rely on obtaining MRI acceptable direct laryngoscopes, suction, or other equipment to intubate within Zone IV, especially within a short time frame. Nevertheless, it should be common practice to include MRI-acceptable direct laryngoscopes as part of the airway management kit in the MRI suite.

While a nurse goes to retrieve flumazenil for benzodiazepine reversal, Mr. S tolerates an oropharyngeal airway. Portable face-mask ventilation with oxygen tubing attached to the wall oxygen proves difficult, even with two-hand and two-person technique, and you still cannot reliably ventilate Mr. S. His oxygen saturation remains at 85% with good plethysmographic trace. In accordance with preestablished protocols, using an MRI-acceptable stretcher outside the 5-G line, you move Mr. S with help from staff onto the stretcher and promptly moved him to a predesignated area in Zone III for further management. It should be noted that not all MRI suites are the same and some may not have all MRI-compatible equipment, so it is important to determine what can and cannot be used ahead of time prior to the imaging study. Within Zone III, basic airway equipment is available and may be used safely. At this time, full cardiorespiratory monitoring is available from a dedicated MRI suite code blue cart outside Zone IV, including blood pressure, 3-lead electrocardiography, plethysmography, and portable capnography. You insert a size #5 LMA-Supreme™ without any difficulties and obtain a good seal. Ventilation appears to be adequate with good quantitative carbon dioxide waveform displayed on the portable monitor. His oxygen saturation is now 97% with 15 $L \cdot min^{-1}$ of oxygen. At this point, the nurse arrives with flumazenil, and Mr. S rouses shortly after intravenous administration of two doses of 0.2 mg of flumazenil.

Although the outcome, in this case, was favorable, it is important to recognize that if two-handed face-mask ventilation and the use of laryngeal mask airway (LMA) were unsuccessful, the anesthesia practitioner should have made arrangements for further airway intervention. In the event, the LMA did not provide adequate seal and oxygenation/ventilation, a more definitive airway would be required, such as tracheal intubation. Calling for basic airway equipment early, including direct laryngoscope with an appropriate Macintosh blade, a variety of endotracheal tube sizes, stylet, airway suction device, syringe, a tracheal introducer (also known as "bougie"), induction drugs, and portable ventilation device such as Ambu Bag with oxygen source, is prudent. Based on airway examination, calling early for advanced airway adjuncts such as a portable video laryngoscope with hyperangulated blade may be necessary.

If flumazenil did not resolve Mr. S' apnea or was unavailable, and the LMA was insufficient for oxygenation/ventilation, then tracheal intubation may be indicated. Considering his airway exam, the patient should be optimally positioned in the "sniffing position" and ramped appropriately for his body habitus in preparation for securing a definitive airway. Given that we are unable to denitrogenate well and must assume a full stomach, an rapid sequence intubation (RSI) is indicated. It is important to consider the conflict of a full stomach requiring RSI versus predicted successful laryngoscopic intubation if the airway examination is unfavorable. In such cases an awake technique may be prudent, acknowledging the risk of aspiration.

This case highlights two important points when working within the MRI suite: (1) being cognizant of equipment limitations in managing the airway in Zone IV with the "always on" MRI magnet and (2) knowing how to expeditiously gain access to the patient's head and airway from the magnet bore for further assessment. Planning should consider whether the airway could be managed in Zone IV with the equipment available or whether induction in Zone III with advanced airway equipment such as a video-laryngoscope or a flexible bronchoscope is necessary. Identifying when to remove the patient from Zone IV for more definitive airway management is aided by your initial assessment and by having predetermined protocols and areas within Zone III for emergency patient transport. Not all MRI suites have these protocols in place and the onus is on the anesthesia practitioner to liaise with MRI staff and the radiology department ahead of time to ensure prompt management of unstable patients can be safely instituted. As such, anesthesia department should be involved with the stocking of appropriate equipment for airway and anesthetic management, including MRI-compatible anesthesia workstations.

How Would You Manage the Anticipated Difficult Airway in the MRI Suite?

The MRI suite poses additional risks for the anticipated difficult airway. The MRI suite is typically in a remote location in the hospital away from the main operating rooms. Additional special airway equipment and help from other anesthesia staff may not be readily available and thus additional forward planning is necessary. The layout of the MRI suite must ensure that advanced airway equipment (video laryngoscope or flexible bronchoscope) may be used in Zone III to control the airway without interference or safety hazard from the MRI magnetic field. Once the airway is secured and the patient is moved to the MRI magnet bore in Zone IV, access to the airway is limited, and the anesthesia practitioner must be vigilant in monitoring. Transfer will require MRI-safe bag-valve ventilation until hooked up to a ventilator either MRI-safe in Zone IV or with an extended circuit from Zone III. Vaporizers in Zone III with the elongated circuit or total intravenous anesthesia with long extension tubing through a wave guide from Zone III may be used for the maintenance of anesthetic. Otherwise, algorithms for approaching the anticipated difficult airway are described by Law et al.[24] as well as in Chapter 2 and should be utilized bearing in mind the additional restrictions or limitations of the MRI suite.

SUMMARY

Unique considerations for anesthetic care in the MRI suite are summarized in Table 61.1. While this may not be exhaustive for each situation, it gives the anesthesia practitioner guidance to formulate an airway management plan. This should include a designated safe location outside Zone IV not only for the management of anticipated difficult airway but also as a part of a predetermined action plan in the event of a cardiopulmonary collapse. Understanding patient factors and how they interact with the potential hazards, limitations, and equipment incompatibility concerns of the MRI suite is critical for safe anesthetic management.

TABLE 61.1. Summary of Considerations for Anesthetic Care in the MRI Suite

Procedural Factors	Patient Factors
• Intrinsic hazards of MRI • Equipment compatibility/safety • Poor patient access and visualization • Low stimulus procedure • Nonoperating room anesthesia	• MRI incompatible implants • Critically Ill vs. Elective/Semielective • Pediatric patients • Patients with intellectual disability • Anxiety/Claustrophobia

SELF-EVALUATION QUESTIONS

61.1. Which of the following is **NOT** a known hazard in the MRI suite?

A. Patients with implanted ferromagnetic objects like aneurysm clips
B. Patients with pacemakers
C. The endotracheal tube
D. Stethoscopes
E. Portable sevoflurane vaporizer

61.2. What airway equipment may be used safely in an MRI suite?

A. Laryngeal mask airway
B. Any video laryngoscope
C. Flexible bronchoscope
D. Macintosh laryngoscope
E. Bullard laryngoscope

61.3. TRUE or FALSE, the time-varying magnet field generated by the MRI system can directly cause serious burns to patients during imaging studies.

A. TRUE
B. FALSE

REFERENCES

1. Reddy U, White MJ, Wilson SR. Anaesthesia for magnetic resonance imaging. *Contin Educ Anaesth. Crit Care Pain*. 2012;12(3):140-144.
2. Bergese SD, Puente EG. Anesthesia in the intraoperative MRI environment. *Neurosurg Clin N Am*. 2009;20(2):155-162.
3. American Society of Anesthesiologists. Practice advisory on anesthetic care for magnetic resonance imaging. *Anesthesiology*. 2015;122(3):495-520.
4. De Vocht F, Van Drooge H, Engels H, Kromhout H.Exposure, health complaints and cognitive performance among employees of an MRI scanners manufacturing department. *J Magn Reson Imaging*. 2006;23(2):197-204.
5. Klucznik R, Carrier D, Pyka R, Haid R. Placement of a ferromagnetic intracerebral aneurysm clip in a magnetic field with a fatal outcome. *Radiology*. 1993;187(3):855-856.
6. McFadden JT. Magnetic resonance imaging and aneurysm clips. *J Neurosurg*. 2012;117(1):1-11.
7. Landrigan C. Preventable deaths and injuries during magnetic resonance imaging. *N Engl J Med*. 2001;345(13):1000-1001.
8. Gilk T, Latino RJ. MRI safety 10 years later. *Patient Saf Qual Healthc*. 2011. http://psqh.com/mri-safety-10-years-later.
9. Haik J, Daniel S, Tessone A, Orenstein A, Winkler E. MRI induced fourth-degree burn in an extremity, leading to amputation. *Burns*. 2009;35(2): 294-296.
10. Zimmer C, Janssen M, Treschan T, Peters J. Near-miss accident during magnetic resonance imaging by a "flying sevoflurane vaporizer" due to ferromagnetism undetectable by handheld magnet. *Anesthesiology*. 2004;100: 1329-1330.
11. Chaljub G, Kramer LA, Johnson RF 3rd, Singh H, Crow WN. Projectile cylinder accidents resulting from the presence of ferromagnetic nitrous oxide or oxygen tanks in the MR suite. *AJR Am J Roentgenol*. 2001;177(1):27-30.
12. Colletti PM. Size "H" oxygen cylinder: accidental MR projectile at 1.5 Tesla. *J Magn Reson Imaging*. 2004;19(1):141-143.
13. Ward BK, Roberts DC, Della Santina CC, Carey JP, Zee DS. Vestibular stimulation by magnetic fields. *Ann N Y Acad Sci*. 2015;1343(1):69-79.
14. Gorlin A, Hoxworth JM, Pavlicek W, Thunberg CA, Seamans D. Acute vertigo in an anesthesia provider during exposure to a 3T MRI scanner. *Med Devices*. 2015;8:161-166.
15. Susheela T, Bhardwaj M, Gopinath A. The i-gel™ —A promising airway device for magnetic resonance imaging suite. *J Anaesthesiol Clin Pharmacol*. 2012;28(2):263-264.

16. Schiebee T, Patel A, Davidson M. Laryngeal mask airway (LMA) artifact resulting in MRI misdiagnosis. *Pediatr Radiol.* 2008;38:328-330.
17. Langton J, Wilson I, Fell D. Use of laryngeal mask airway during magnetic resonance imaging. *Anaesthesia.* 1992;47:532.
18. Zaballos M, Bastida E, del Castillo T, de Villoria J, Jimenez C. In vitro study of the magnetic resonance imaging artifacts of six supraglottic airway devices. *Anaesthesia.* 2010;65(6):569-572.
19. Walls JD, Weiss MS. Safety in non-operating room anesthesia (NORA). *APSF Newsl Off J Anesth Patient Saf Found.* 2019;34(1):3-21. www.apsf.org.
20. Tobias J, Leder M. Procedural sedation: a review of sedative agents, monitoring, and management of complications. *Saudi J Anaesth.* 2011;5(4):395-410.
21. Sim E, Tan T. Awake craniotomy with intraoperative MRI: description of a sedation technique using remifentanil and dexmedetomidine. *Proc Singapore Healthc.* 2014;23(3):257-264.
22. Wilson SR, Shinde S, Appleby I, et al. Guidelines for the safe provision of anaesthesia in magnetic resonance units 2019: Guidelines from the Association of Anaesthetists and the Neuro Anaesthesia and Critical Care Society of Great Britain and Ireland. *Anaesthesia.* 2019;74(5):638-650.
23. Capizzani R. *Strategic Outcomes Practice Technical Advisory Bulletin: Magnetic Resonance Imaging Hazards and Safety Guidlines.* Willis HRH; 2009. http://www.willis.com/documents/publications/Services/Claims_Management/MRI_Safety_August_2009_V6.pdf.
24. Law JA, Duggan LV., Asselin M, et al. Canadian Airway Focus Group updated consensus-based recommendations for management of the difficult airway: Part 2. Planning and implementing safe management of the patient with an anticipated difficult airway. *Can J Anesth.* 2021;68(9):1405-1436.

CHAPTER 62

Postobstructive Pulmonary Edema (POPE)

Franziska Miller and Matthew G. Simms

CASE PRESENTATION

Your next patient on the orthopedic wait list is a 26-year-old man scheduled to have an intramedullary tibial nail open reduction internal fixation (ORIF) after colliding with two other players playing recreational hockey 36 hours ago. His past medical history includes a 5 pack-year history of smoking. As for his past surgical history, he underwent an anterior cruciate ligament (ACL) repair two years ago secondary to a football injury. His only medication consists of subcutaneous hydromorphone on the floor for pain. Laboratory investigations are normal. He weighs 220 lbs (100 kg) and is 6′0″ (183 cm) tall; body mass index (BMI) is 29.9 kg·m^{-2}. Preoperative airway examination reveals normal mouth opening with full set of teeth, a thyromental span of 4 cm, and good jaw protrusion. He demonstrates a modified Mallampati score of II and has a normal cervical range of motion. The rest of his physical examination is unremarkable. He has been fasting since midnight.

Following appropriate positioning and denitrogenation, the induction is performed using midazolam, fentanyl, propofol, and rocuronium. Direct laryngoscopy using a Macintosh #4 blade reveals a Cormack-Lehane (C-L)[1] Grade 2 view. The trachea is successfully intubated using an 8.0-mm internal diameter (ID) endotracheal tube (ETT). General anesthesia is maintained with sevoflurane. After the airway is secured, three stacks of gauze are rolled up and inserted into the mouth as a bite block. Over the course of the case, several doses of hydromorphone are given for analgesia. Additional doses of rocuronium are also given for muscle relaxation. Two and a half liters of Ringer's lactate are given during the 2-hour procedure. On emergence, residual neuromuscular blockade is fully reversed.

At this time, the patient starts to cough and buck on the ventilator. He then proceeds to spit out the gauze bite block and subsequently bites down on the ETT. For a period of approximately 60 seconds, no gas exchange occurs, even with attempted assisted manual ventilation via the anesthetic circuit. Although respiratory efforts continue, no CO_2 trace is apparent during the episode. Oxygen saturation falls to 78% before his jaw relaxes somewhat, allowing assisted, then spontaneous ventilation to resume. At this point, the patient is extubated. Shortly after extubation, he begins to cough up frothy, pink fluid without either retching or vomiting. His oxygen saturation, which had been 97% on a simple oxygen face mask immediately postextubation, drops to 85%.

INTRODUCTION

■ What Is Postobstructive Pulmonary Edema (POPE)?

Postobstructive pulmonary edema (POPE) is characterized by the sudden onset of pulmonary edema of varying severity following vigorous inspiratory efforts against an obstructed upper airway. It most often occurs in a patient with no intrinsic cardiac, neurologic, or pulmonary disease. POPE usually presents with dyspnea, tachypnea, hypoxemia and a cough productive of pink, frothy sputum. After confirming that the obstruction has been relieved, treatment of POPE is usually symptomatic, and varies from simple application of supplemental oxygen to intubation with mechanical ventilation and application of positive end-expiratory pressure (PEEP). The condition usually resolves within 24 to 48 hours and most patients suffer no long-term sequelae.

Pulmonary edema following acute upper airway obstruction was first described in children in 1973.[2] A few years later, Oswalt described a number of cases of respiratory distress and pulmonary congestion following episodes of severe acute upper airway obstruction in otherwise healthy patients.[3] Since then, numerous case reports and case series have been published on this phenomenon.

What Synonyms Have Been Used to Refer to POPE?

Many synonyms appear in the literature to describe this process. These include the following:

- Negative pressure pulmonary edema[4–12]
- Postlaryngospasm pulmonary edema[13]
- Laryngospasm-induced pulmonary edema[7,14,15]
- Postextubation pulmonary edema[16,17]
- Noncardiogenic pulmonary edema[4]
- Athletic pulmonary edema[7]

What Are the Two Types of POPE?

Two types of POPE have been described.[18] They present with similar clinical pictures, and most likely have similar pathophysiologies:

- **POPE type I:** This typically occurs shortly after relief of an episode of acute upper airway obstruction from any cause, e.g., laryngospasm.
- **POPE type II:** POPE type II occurs after relief of a chronic upper airway obstruction, caused by conditions such as chronic tonsillar hypertrophy, laryngeal tumor, goiter, or bilateral vocal cord paralysis.[4]

The remainder of this chapter refers mainly to POPE type I, as this is most commonly encountered in anesthetic and airway management practice.

INCIDENCE, ETIOLOGY, AND PATHOPHYSIOLOGY

What Is the Incidence of POPE?

The incidence of POPE has been estimated at 0.5 to 1.0 case per thousand surgical patients.[6,19] Of patients who have experienced or required intervention for an episode of acute upper airway obstruction, published figures suggest a 5% to 10% incidence of progression to POPE.[8,19,20] POPE occurs most often in younger adults and children, most with ASA 1 and 2 status.[5,6] Young, athletic males are strongly represented in case series,[17,21] possibly because their well-developed musculature enables them to develop stronger inspiratory efforts against the upper airway obstruction, with resultant highly negative intrathoracic pressures. Most cases occur following tracheal extubation.[6]

What Predisposes to the Occurrence of POPE?

In the adult population, the most common cause of POPE is postextubation laryngospasm,[17,22] while in children younger than 10, most cases follow upper airway obstruction from croup, epiglottitis[5,20] and to a lesser extent, laryngospasm. However, POPE following vigorous attempts to inspire against upper airway obstruction has been reported from many other causes, including biting down and occluding the lumen of ETTs[9,23] and laryngeal mask airways (LMAs).[11,12] POPE has also been reported following upper airway obstruction from hanging, strangulation,[3,9] foreign body aspiration,[24,25] laryngeal tumor,[5] hematoma, goiter,[9,26] obstructive sleep apnea,[27] bilateral vocal cord paralysis,[28] and direct suctioning of both ETTs[29] and chest tubes.[30] Unilateral POPE has also been described in a lung occluded by an accidental mainstem bronchus intubation of the contralateral lung.[31]

What Is the Pathophysiology of POPE?

The clinical and laboratory manifestations of POPE probably reflect its multifactorial pathophysiology and various degrees of severity. The two proposed mechanisms of edema formation relate to (a) consequences of the highly negative intrathoracic pressure generated during an episode of complete upper airway obstruction (the Mueller maneuver),[20,22,25] and (b) the hyperadrenergic response to airway obstruction and hypoxia[5,16,18] (Figure 62.1). The following are probable contributory mechanisms:

1. *Negative pressure transfer to the pulmonary alveoli and interstitium* affects Starling forces by creating a gradient that favors transudation of fluid out of the pulmonary capillaries to the interstitium.[4,24] Once the capacity of pulmonary lymphatics to remove fluid from the interstitium is exceeded, leakage of fluid occurs into the alveolar space.[16,32,33]
2. *Enhanced venous return to the right heart and pulmonary arteries* results from the generated negative intrathoracic pressure[4–6,22,24] and is compounded by central blood redistribution from the hyperadrenergic state caused by significant hypoxemia, anxiety, and hypercarbia.[5,9,16,22,24,32,34] Higher pulmonary arteriolar and capillary bed blood volumes and hydrostatic pressures further favor fluid transudation from capillary to interstitium.[8]
3. *Impeded outflow from the pulmonary capillary bed* occurs as left-sided pressures rise from (a) decreased stroke volume resulting from increased systemic vascular resistance[6,24,32,34]; (b) decreased left ventricular (LV) diastolic compliance (from right ventricular distension); and (c) depression of myocardial contractility, from hypoxia and acidosis.[9]
4. *Hypoxic pulmonary vasoconstriction* directly contributes to increases in pulmonary capillary pressures.[5,16]

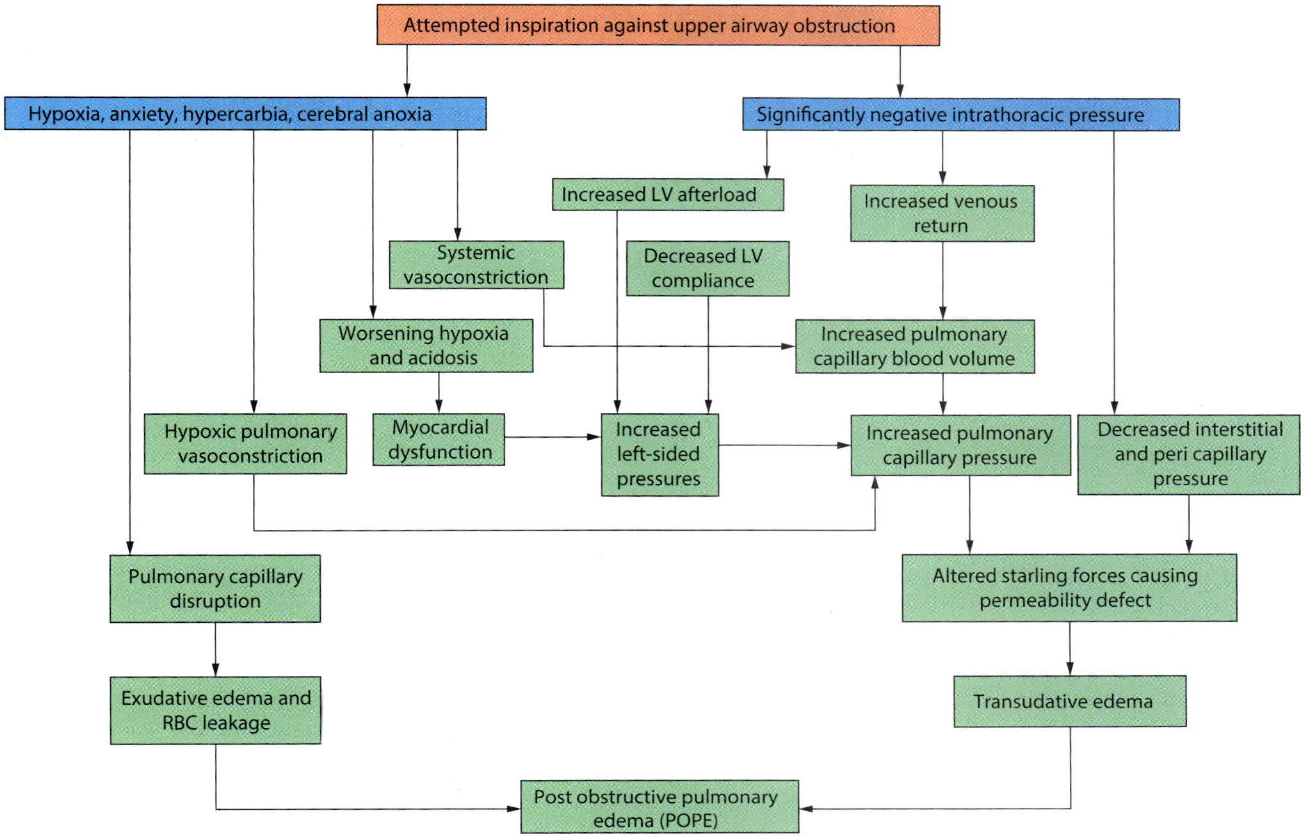

FIGURE 62.1. Pathophysiology of postobstructive pulmonary edema.

5. *Disruption of the alveolar-capillary membrane* ("stress failure")[35] and its barrier function can eventually occur from damage to the capillary endothelium by increased pulmonary capillary volume and pressures. In addition, particularly with prolonged hypoxia,[24] the hyperadrenergic state can directly contribute to further membrane disruption.[4,6] Such disruption can be manifested by the leakage of both protein-rich exudative and hemorrhagic fluid.

POPE has a spectrum of clinical presentations. It is likely that in most cases, with intact pulmonary capillaries, simple alteration in Starling forces result in the transudative production of low-protein edema fluid.[34] Fremont and his group looked retrospectively at a series of 341 patients intubated for pulmonary edema and identified ten individuals who had POPE as the etiology. Analysis of the edema fluid of this subset of patients, looking at the edema fluid/plasma protein ratio and its rate of clearance, strongly suggested a transudative, hydrostatic mechanism in most of the patients.[36]

However, higher negative intrathoracic pressures, coupled with a hyperadrenergic response, may result in ultrastructural changes in the capillary endothelial barrier, allowing the escape of exudative edema, as documented in some case reports.[28,37] Extreme cases result in breaks in the alveolar-capillary membrane, allowing red blood cell leakage, and possibly frank hemorrhage. Chest radiographs in this latter situation may show an alveolar pattern of edema, in contrast to the more interstitial pattern typical of transudative edema.[7] That case reports differ in their reporting of transudative and exudative edema, or primarily interstitial or alveolar patterns of edema on chest radiography probably reflects the varying degrees of severity of the obstructive episode causing the POPE.

Why Does POPE Appear Only After the Relief of Upper Airway Obstruction?

Type I POPE generally appears shortly after the relief of an acute upper airway obstruction. In many cases, this is a fixed obstruction, such as laryngospasm or an occluded ETT. Profoundly negative intrathoracic pressures generated during attempted inspiration (Mueller maneuvers) may be balanced during attempted expiration against the same fixed obstruction (i.e., a Valsalva maneuver), akin to an "auto-PEEP" phenomenon. It may be that this PEEP-like effect during attempted expiration is somewhat protective by limiting the transcapillary pressure gradient. On relief of the obstruction, pulmonary edema becomes manifest[5,6,24] with the sudden transient drop in mean airway pressure,[8] together with the increase in venous return and pulmonary hydrostatic pressure.[7,32]

In Type II POPE, the chronic variety, usually associated with variable obstruction favors the Mueller maneuver in that more obstruction occurs during attempted inspiration than expiration. In this situation, the generated negative intrathoracic pressure is counteracted by more modest levels of PEEP. Although still somewhat protective against the development of pulmonary edema,[38] published reports document abnormal

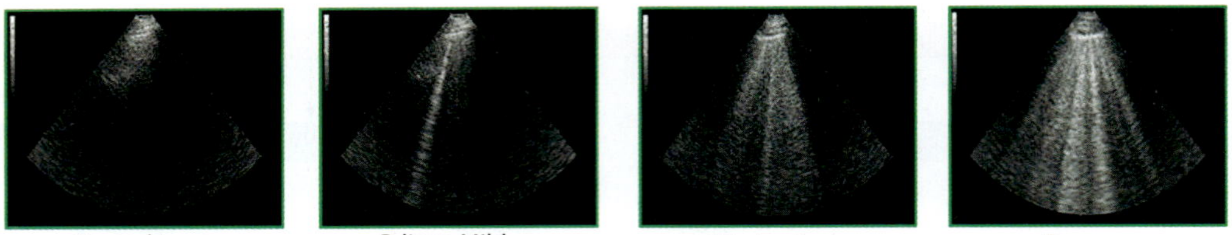

FIGURE 62.2. Lung ultrasound assessment of extravascular lung water (EVLW) by B-lines: The normal lung is black (no signal); the abnormal wet lung with interstitial pulmonary edema is black and white (with some B-lines departing from the pleural line); and the lung with alveolar pulmonary edema is white (confluent B-lines in a fully echogenic lung). (Reproduced with permission from Picano E, Pellikka PA. Ultrasound of extravascular lung water: a new standard for pulmonary congestion. *Eur Heart J.* 2016:37(27):2097-2104.)

A-a gradients and radiographic evidence of pulmonary edema *before* relief of chronic upper airway obstructions.[5,6,24] Following the relief of both Type I and Type II obstructions, it is likely that altered capillary permeability, previously occult interstitial edema,[38] and LV dysfunction[24] contribute to the development of POPE in spite of now-normal lung volumes and pressures.

DIAGNOSIS AND INVESTIGATIONS

What Are the Presenting Symptoms and Signs of POPE?

The patient with POPE often presents within minutes[5,22] after the relief of an episode of upper airway obstruction characterized by vigorous inspiratory efforts without significant air movement.[16,34] The initial presentation is often with dyspnea,[8] tachypnea,[24,39,40] agitation,[8,21,34] and cough[11,21,22] producing pink, frothy fluid.[3,4,8,9,22,34,41] In addition to hypoxemia,[7,39] the patient is also often tachycardic[14,34] and hypertensive.[34] Other patients have presented with frank hemoptysis,[9,12,19,23,42] although this is less frequent. Residual partial obstruction may be present in this population, manifested by stridor[8,11,16,21,43] or intercostal and subcostal retractions.[21,24,44] On auscultation, most patients have rales,[12,16,22,24,40,41] sometimes with associated rhonchi.[3,14,22,25,34,40]

What Are the Results of Investigations Typically Performed on the Patient with POPE?

- *Invasive monitoring* of central venous pressure (CVP) or pulmonary artery pressure (PAP) is rarely undertaken in the patient recognized to have POPE. However, when reported, pressures, including CVP[3,22] and pulmonary capillary wedge pressures (PCWP)[5,22,45,46] have generally been normal, while PAPs have been normal or only slightly elevated.[22]
- *Chest radiographs* of the patient with POPE often show signs of edema with either an alveolar (airspace consolidation)[5,16,19,44] or interstitial (perihilar haze, perivascular or peribronchial cuffing, and Kerley lines)[3,4,6,25] pattern, or both.[7,24,39] Most often the edema distribution is predominantly central and bilateral, although asymmetrical[34] or even unilateral distributions have been reported.[7,11,19] Heart size is generally normal.[7,19,24] Vascular pedicle width in one series was found to be above normal, suggesting an increase in central blood volume.[7]
- Ultrasound examination is a reliable diagnostic tool to identify pulmonary edema, with a sensitivity of 92.3% and a specificity of 91.7%.[47] Advantages of ultrasound over chest radiographs include improved portability of ultrasound over the X-ray machine, and the ability of real-time examination without exposing the patient to radiation.[48,49] In addition, ultrasound examination of the lung is a skill easily acquired, with a learning curve of roughly 10 examinations, and is fast to perform, requiring less than 3 minutes.[49] On ultrasound, pulmonary edema can be diagnosed utilizing lung comets or better known as B-lines, which are defined as vertical reverberations likely originating from water-thickened interlobular septa and fanning out from the pleura.[49] A common protocol utilized for the lung examination using ultrasound is the Bedside Lung Ultrasound in an Emergency (BLUE) protocol.[50]

The number of B-lines found on ultrasound has been correlated with invasive evaluation of extravascular lung water utilizing the gold standard of wet/dry ratio by gravimetric method postmortem (see Figure 62.2).[47] The number of B-lines in the anterolateral chest scan with a cardiac, convex, or linear probe can be translated into a severity score of extravascular lung water (see Table 62.1).[47]

Nonetheless, it is important to remember that there is some inter-observer variation of B-lines on ultrasound. Some research has been conducted on algorithm-based signal-processing methods but further studies are required.[51] Another caveat is that B-lines can occur in a variety of clinical scenarios. Utilizing both convex and linear probes as part of an examination can provide additional information for an accurate diagnosis. Convex probes can identify alveolar-interstitial syndromes, while the linear probe can further characterize these syndromes

TABLE 62.1. Severity score of extravascular lung water

Score	Number of B-lines	Extravascular Lung Water
0	≤5	Absent
1	6-15	Mild
2	16-30	Moderate
3	>30	Severe

by looking at areas of subpleural consolidation or the appearance of the pleural line diagnosis.[52]

- *High-resolution CT scans* of the chest have shown findings of ground-glass opacities, peribronchial cuffing, and interlobular septal thickening, typical of interstitial pulmonary edema.[25,42] Others have shown diffuse patchy lobular airspace disease.[24]
- *Bronchoscopy* performed on patients with POPE has shown punctate bleeding lesions in both trachea and mainstem bronchi[43] or more generalized blood staining of the tracheobronchial tree.[23,34] Bronchial-alveolar lavage (BAL) in one report revealed a progressively bloody return, consistent with alveolar hemorrhage,[34] while in a second report, BAL produced clear returns.[25]
- No specific *electrocardiogram (ECG) pattern* has been reported in the POPE patient population. When reported, ECG findings have been uniformly normal.

Should the Patient Presenting with POPE Be Referred for Echocardiography?

Most case reports and case series of patients experiencing POPE have documented rapid resolution of the episode with no long-term sequelae and no special cardiac work-up performed. Echocardiograms have generally been normal.[9,16,19,25,26,34,42,53,54] One exception was a case series of 6 patients who had experienced POPE, all of whom had echocardiograms. In this small retrospective series, abnormalities were detected in 50% of the cases: one patient had hypertrophic cardiomyopathy, and the other two had pulmonary and tricuspid valvular insufficiency.[4] However, in the absence of other recognized indications, the current lack of evidence does not support a recommendation for routine echocardiographic testing of all POPE patients.

CLINICAL MANAGEMENT

What Is the Usual Clinical Course of POPE?

Following relief of the acute upper airway obstruction, the onset of POPE is generally rapid, i.e., within minutes; however a minority of case reports document delayed onset of up to 4 to 6 hours,[5,38] suggesting that following an episode of acute, severe upper airway obstruction,[18] patients should be monitored for 6 to 12 hours. The same recommendation has been made for patients who have had surgical relief of chronic upper airway obstruction.[18]

In most cases, POPE runs a benign course, with symptoms, and clinical and radiologic signs clearing within 24 to 48 hours.[4–6,17,22,38,44,54]

How Is POPE Managed?

As the name implies, most cases of POPE present *after* the upper airway obstruction has been alleviated. After confirming airway patency, supplemental oxygen should be administered, and may be all that is required.[3,6,16,22] Continuous positive airway pressure (CPAP) by face mask has also been shown to be an effective intervention,[14,19] and the use of noninvasive ventilation has been reported.[26] Hypoxemia, or patient fatigue that is unresponsive to noninvasive methods may require reintubation and positive pressure ventilation. The larger case series report reintubation rates of between 66.5%[8] and 85%.[5,6,22] Of those patients reintubated, about half require mechanical ventilation[5] with[3,4,34] or without PEEP, usually for less than 24 hours.[6] In severe cases refractory to mechanical ventilation, venovenous ECMO may be of potential benefit.[55]

Although diuretics are often used in the setting of POPE[3,5,6,14,23,24,34,44] this practice has been questioned[5,24] based on the finding of normal central filling pressures, and the equally rapid resolution of symptoms when they are not used.[9,44] The use of steroids has been reported sporadically,[3,14,44] although as with the use of diuretics, their use is controversial[18] and without proven benefit. Other case reports make mention of fluid restriction[3,18] and the administration of medications such as morphine or digoxin.[22]

The available evidence would suggest that if the diagnosis of POPE is correct, drug therapy is unlikely to be of benefit, particularly in view of the self-limited and rapidly resolving course of the condition. With rare exceptions,[4,10] the same can be said of invasive hemodynamic monitoring.[16]

What Is the Differential Diagnosis of POPE?

The primary alternate diagnosis to POPE is aspiration pneumonitis, which may lead to pulmonary edema even when frank regurgitation has not been noted.[5] The initial management of this condition is identical to that of POPE, unless of course the aspirate is suspected to be particulate or contaminated by bacteria. It is more important to rule out other causes of pulmonary edema where management differs from that of POPE, including iatrogenic volume overload, primary cardiogenic causes, or drug reactions.

During the COVID-19 pandemic, POPE has the potential to be misdiagnosed as COVID-19 both radiologically and clinically. In addition to careful history-taking, imaging can be useful in the distinction of these two conditions. It has been shown that ground-glass opacities on chest computed tomography scanning is more centrally distributed in POPE and more peripherally distributed in COVID-19.[56]

What Are Risk Factors and Preventive Strategies for the Development of POPE?

A number of factors place the patient at higher risk for the development of POPE. Some are unavoidable, while some can be minimized by employing the principles of good airway management. The early recognition and management of acute, severe upper airway obstruction, and the conditions leading to it, are critical to the prevention of POPE:

- *Laryngospasm:* Most cases of POPE in adults, and many in children follow an episode of laryngospasm. Many case reports of POPE document laryngospasm following extubation during emergence from anesthesia, before the patient is fully awake.[44,57] Therefore, it is recommended that extubation be performed in patients who are either deeply anesthetized or fully awake. The prevention of intra-operative laryngospasm under mask or extraglottic device (EGD) anesthesia requires deep general anesthesia, particularly for highly stimulating surgical procedures. Prior to removing an ETT, suctioning of blood or secretions that may trigger laryngospasm is essential, particularly following upper airway surgery. Should laryngospasm occur, the initial treatment is to relieve any soft tissue obstruction together with gentle application of 10 to 20 cm H_2O CPAP by mask. However, the administration of succinylcholine 0.2 $mg \cdot kg^{-1}$ (or other appropriate neuromuscular blocking agent) may be indicated in patients making vigorous inspiratory efforts against a closed glottis, particularly if it persists for more than 30 seconds.[57]

- *Tube occlusion:* POPE has been described in patients who have "bitten down" to occlude ETTs[41,44] and EGDs (e.g., LMA).[11,12,58] Most reports have documented this occurring on emergence from anesthesia, although it has also been described during the positioning process.[11] Use of a rolled gauze bite block alongside the lumen of an endotracheal tube[9,41] or LMA (as recommended by its inventor[58]) ought to minimize this risk. Bite blocks, however, are not without their controversy. The use of oral airways as bite blocks can potentially increase the risk of dental damage at the level of the incisors as force tends to be concentrated in that area when patients reflexively bite down during emergence.[59] Gauze blocks have to be thick enough to prevent ETT occlusion, however not too bulky whereby they can potentially cause trauma to or impair the circulation of the tongue[60] especially during cervical surgeries which use motor-evoked potential (MEP) monitoring.[61] It is also important to fix the block in such a way to prevent accidental dislodgement.[62] Because of these factors, there might be a role for commercially available purpose-built bite blocks that fulfill these criteria. As with laryngospasm, the administration of a neuromuscular blocking agent may be indicated. Alternatively, deflation of the cuff of the ETT or EGD may permit sufficient alleviation of obstruction to prevent the marked negative intrathoracic pressure that leads to the development of POPE. Endotracheal tube clamping during intubation prior to connection to a ventilator circuit has also been described in the literature to mitigate the emission of aerosolized viral particles in COVID-19 patients. This technique is not recommended, as it may increase risk for POPE in already compromised patients from a respiratory perspective and may worsen overall hypoxemia and thus patient outcomes.[63]
- *Other soft tissue obstruction:* POPE has been described as a complication of obstructive sleep apnea, in patients with obesity and vocal cord paralysis, and in those with other risk factors for upper airway obstruction.[16,40] The preoperative identification of patients at risk for these conditions mandates full recovery of neuromuscular function and that they be fully awake prior to extubation.
- *Type of surgery:* A retrospective study by Deepika et al. showed that the majority of POPE cases (63%) occurred following surgery to the aerodigestive tract,[6] suggesting that vigilance be exercised in patients suffering from chronic tonsillar hypertrophy, goiter, and other conditions leading to chronic upper airway obstruction. In other published case series, none of the patients were undergoing aerodigestive tract surgery.[17]
- *Patient:* In adults, POPE occurs about twice as often in male patients,[4–6,8,17] and in those with an average age of 25 to 45 years.[4–6,8,17] The male preponderance may be related to well-developed musculature and their ability generate high negative intrathoracic pressures.[21] Early and aggressive treatment of airway obstruction should occur in this population.
- *Pharmacological agents:* There have been several case studies reporting POPE after utilizing sugammadex. The theory is that the rapid and dissociated reversal of muscular blockade in combination with upper airway obstruction or muscle rigidity (i.e., remifentanil-induced) can pose a potential risk for the development of POPE.[64–67]

What Is the Prognosis of POPE?

POPE is an important cause of morbidity in otherwise young, healthy patients that may lead to an unplanned hospital or ICU admission. With prompt recognition and appropriate therapy, the condition generally resolves inside 24 to 48 hours without long-term sequelae.[6,19] However, deaths can occur: a recent review of published adult case series of POPE reported 3 deaths in 146 patients—a mortality rate of 2%.[8]

PATIENT MANAGEMENT

Following extubation in the operating room, the patient exhibited clinical evidence of developing pulmonary edema and increasing respiratory distress. His oropharynx was suctioned and he was placed in a semi-sitting position. 100% oxygen was administered via a face mask through the anesthetic circuit and CPAP was applied. This failed to improve the SpO_2 above 90%, so assisted face-mask ventilation (FMV) was attempted. However, agitation and reduced lung compliance made assisted ventilation increasingly difficult, and the SpO_2 could not be maintained above 90%. Therefore, tracheal intubation was performed using a rapid sequence intubation technique. Following intubation, his SpO_2 returned to 97% with 2 minutes of mechanical ventilation using an FiO_2 of 100%; suctioning yielded copious quantities of pink, frothy fluid. Sedation was maintained with midazolam. An arterial line was placed, and the patient was admitted to the ICU. A chest X-ray showed signs of pulmonary edema. A 12-lead ECG was normal and troponins were negative. The patient remained sedated, intubated, and ventilated overnight. By the following day, his radiographic findings and arterial blood gases had improved, and extubation took place that evening. There were no further respiratory complications.

SUMMARY

Postobstructive pulmonary edema is an uncommon, yet potentially life-threatening condition. Occurring shortly after the relief of acute or chronic upper airway obstruction of varying cause, POPE presents with dyspnea, cough, progressive oxygen desaturation, tachypnea, and agitation. In most cases, POPE resolves within 24 to 48 hours. Sometimes, nothing more than supportive care with supplemental oxygen administration is required. Mask-delivered CPAP or noninvasive ventilation may also be effective. However, some patients with POPE may require tracheal intubation, mechanical ventilation with PEEP, or in severe cases venovenous ECMO to maintain adequate oxygenation. Although often used, the benefits of diuretics and steroids in managing POPE remain unproven.

Practitioners should be aware of this condition, be able to identify and where possible avoid the predisposing risk factors, and be able to manage it if it occurs. Prompt management of acute upper airway obstruction is crucial in reducing the incidence of POPE and improving outcome, particularly as deaths have been reported.

SELF-EVALUATION QUESTIONS

62.1. Which of the following situations would be **LEAST** likely to result in an episode of postobstructive pulmonary edema?

A. A 25-year-old male bites and occludes the endotracheal tube for a period of less than 60 seconds on emergence from a desflurane-based anesthetic. He never desaturates below a SpO_2 of 90%.

B. A 25-year-old male was scheduled for appendectomy. During RSI using fentanyl, propofol, and rocuronium, tracheal intubation was achieved with a Trachlight™ following three failed intubation attempts using a Macintosh blade; difficulty with BMV was experienced between intubation attempts.

C. A 25-year-old male has been extubated "deep" following surgery for a deviated nasal septum. At the time of extubation, end-tidal desflurane was 3%.

D. A 6-year-old child has presented to the ED with acute epiglottitis, is "tripoding" with stridor, drooling and respiratory distress. Intubation using an inhalational induction in the operating room is planned.

E. A 25-year-old male weighing 120 kg is having banding of hemorrhoids under general anesthesia with a laryngeal mask airway. Following a Propofol induction, he has been given a total of 100 μg of Fentanyl, is breathing a mixture of air and sevoflurane, with an end-tidal sevoflurane concentration of 1.7%.

62.2. Emerging from general anesthesia for shoulder acromioplasty and shortly after extubation, a 25-year-old man experiences an episode of laryngospasm and makes vigorous, yet futile inspiratory attempts against his closed glottis. Which of the following responses would be appropriate?

A. Suction the back of the throat with rigid tonsil suction, insert an oral airway, and perform an exaggerated jaw thrust.

B. Immediately give succinylcholine 100 mg as he is at high risk of postobstructive pulmonary edema.

C. As the laryngospasm is probably related to pain, give a dose of parenteral narcotic such as sufentanil 5.0 μg.

D. Give lidocaine 100 mg intravenously.

E. Perform an airway opening maneuver and apply CPAP by mask; if this does not break the laryngospasm within 30 seconds, give succinylcholine.

62.3. Which of the following patient conditions is considered a risk factor for the development of postoperative pulmonary edema?

A. The patient with an ASA of 3 or 4.

B. The patient emerging from surgery of the aerodigestive tract.

C. The patient with a history of difficult intubation.

D. The patient with a history of severe gastro-esophageal reflux.

E. The patient with a history of asthma.

62.4. Which of the following is **NOT** a characteristic of postobstructive pulmonary edema on imaging?

A. Peribronchial cuffing on CT scan

B. Airspace consolidation on chest radiographs

C. B-lines on ultrasound imaging

D. Peripherally distributed ground-glass opacities on CT scan

E. Interlobular septal thickening on CT scan

REFERENCES

1. Cormack RS, Lehane J. Difficult tracheal intubation in obstetrics. *Anaesthesia*. 1984;39:1105-1111.
2. Capitanio MA, Kirkpatrick JA. Obstructions of the upper airway in children as reflected on the chest radiograph. *Radiology*. 1973;107:159-161.
3. Oswalt CE, Gates GA, Holmstrom MG. Pulmonary edema as a complication of acute airway obstruction. *JAMA*. 1977 238:1833-1835
4. Goldenberg JD, Portugal LG, Wenig BL, Weingarten RT. Negative-pressure pulmonary edema in the otolaryngology patient. *Otolaryngol Head Neck Surg*. 1997;117:62-66.
5. Lang SA, Duncan PG, Shephard DA, Ha HC. Pulmonary oedema associated with airway obstruction. *Can J Anaesth*. 1990;37:210-218.
6. Deepika K, Kenaan CA, Barrocas AM, et al. Negative pressure pulmonary edema after acute upper airway obstruction. *J Clin Anesth*. 1997;9:403-408.
7. Cascade PN, Alexander GD, Mackie DS. Negative-pressure pulmonary edema after endotracheal intubation. *Radiology*. 1993;186:671-675.
8. Westreich R, Sampson I, Shaari CM, Lawson W. Negative-pressure pulmonary edema after routine septorhinoplasty: discussion of pathophysiology, treatment, and prevention. *Arch Facial Plast Surg*. 2006;8:8-15.
9. Koh MS, Hsu AA, Eng P. Negative pressure pulmonary oedema in the medical intensive care unit. *Intensive Care Med*. 2003;29:1601-1604.
10. Louis PJ, Fernandes R. Negative pressure pulmonary edema. *Oral Surg Oral Med Oral Pathol Oral Radiol Endod*. 2002;93:4-6.
11. Sullivan M. Unilateral negative pressure pulmonary edema during anesthesia with a laryngeal mask airway. *Can J Anaesth*. 1999;46:1053-1056.
12. Devys JM, Balleau C, Jayr C, Bourgain JL. Biting the laryngeal mask: an unusual cause of negative pressure pulmonary edema. *Can J Anaesth*. 2000;47:176-178.
13. Baltimore JJ. Postlaryngospasm pulmonary edema in adults. *AORN J*. 1999;70(3):468-479.
14. Jackson FN, Rowland V, Corssen G. Laryngospasm-induced pulmonary edema. *Chest*. 1980;78:819-821.
15. McConkey P. Airway bleeding in negative-pressure pulmonary edema. *Anesthesiology*. 2001;95:272.
16. Lorch DG, Sahn SA. Post-extubation pulmonary edema following anesthesia induced by upper airway obstruction. Are certain patients at increased risk? *Chest*. 1986;90:802-805.
17. Mulkey Z, Yarbrough S, Guerra D, et al. Postextubation pulmonary edema: a case series and review. *Respir Med*. 2008;102:1659-1662.

18. Guffin TN, Har-el G, Sanders A, et al. Acute postobstructive pulmonary edema. *Otolaryngol Head Neck Surg.* 1995;112:235-237.
19. McConkey PP. Postobstructive pulmonary oedema—a case series and review. *Anaesth Intensive Care.* 2000;28:72-76.
20. Galvis AG. Pulmonary edema complicating relief of upper airway obstruction. *Am J Emerg Med.* 1987; 5294-297.
21. Holmes JR, Hensinger RN, Wojtys EW. Postoperative pulmonary edema in young, athletic adults. *Am J Sports Med.* 1991;19:365-371.
22. Willms D, Shure D. Pulmonary edema due to upper airway obstruction in adults. *Chest.* 1988;94:1090-1092.
23. Sow Nam Y, Garewal D. Pulmonary hemorrhage in association with negative pressure edema in an intubated patient. *Acta Anaesthesiol Scand.* 2001;45:911-913.
24. Ringold S, Klein EJ, Del Beccaro MA. Postobstructive pulmonary edema in children. *Pediatr Emerg Care.* 2004;20:391-395.
25. Maniwa K, Tanaka E, Inoue T, et al. Interstitial pulmonary edema revealed by high-resolution CT after relief of acute upper airway obstruction. *Radiat Med.* 2005;23:139-141.
26. Ikeda H, Asato R, Chin K, et al. Negative-pressure pulmonary edema after resection of mediastinum thyroid goiter. *Acta Otolaryngol.* 2006;126:886-888.
27. Chaudhary BA, Nadimi M, Chaudhary TK, Speir WA. Pulmonary edema due to obstructive sleep apnea. *South Med J.* 1984;77:499-501.
28. Dohi S, Okubo N, Kondo Y. Pulmonary oedema after airway obstruction due to bilateral vocal cord paralysis. *Can J Anaesth.* 1991;38:492-495.
29. Pang WW, Chang DP, Lin CH, Huang MH. Negative pressure pulmonary oedema induced by direct suctioning of endotracheal tube adapter. *Can J Anaesth.* 1998;45:785-788.
30. Memtsoudis SG, Rosenberger P, Sadovnikoff N. Chest tube suction-associated unilateral negative pressure pulmonary edema in a lung transplant patient. *Anesth Analg.* 2005;101:38-40.
31. Goodman BT, Richardson MG. Case report: unilateral negative pressure pulmonary edema: a complication of endobronchial intubation. *Can J Anaesth.* 2008;55:691-695.
32. Ciavarro C, Kelly JP. Postobstructive pulmonary edema in an obese child after an oral surgery procedure under general anesthesia: a case report. *J Oral Maxillofac Surg.* 2002;60:1503-1505.
33. Thiagarajan RR, Laussen PC. Negative pressure pulmonary edema in children—pathogenesis and clinical management. *Paediatr Anaesth.* 2007;17:307-310.
34. Schwartz DR, Maroo A, Malhotra A, Kesselman H. Negative pressure pulmonary hemorrhage. *Chest.* 1999;115:1194-1197.
35. West JB, Tsukimoto K, Mathieu-Costello O, Prediletto R. Stress failure in pulmonary capillaries. *J Appl Physiol.* 1991;70:1731-1742.
36. Fremont RD, Kallet RH, Matthay MA, Ware LB. Postobstructive pulmonary edema: a case for hydrostatic mechanisms. *Chest.* 2007;131:1742-1746.
37. Kollef MH, Pluss J. Noncardiogenic pulmonary edema following upper airway obstruction. 7 cases and a review of the literature. *Medicine.* 1991;70:91-98.
38. Van Kooy MA, Gargiulo RF. Postobstructive pulmonary edema. *Am Fam Physician.* 2000;62:401-404.
39. Sofer S, Bar-Ziv J, Scharf SM. Pulmonary edema following relief of upper airway obstruction. *Chest.* 1984;86:401-403.
40. Brandom BW. Pulmonary edema after airway obstruction. *Int Anesthesiol Clin.* 1997;35:75-84.
41. Liu EH, Yih PS. Negative pressure pulmonary oedema caused by biting and endotracheal tube occlusion – a case for oropharyngeal airways. *Singapore Med J.* 1999;40:174-175.
42. Perez RO, Bresciani C, Jacob CE, et al. Negative pressure post-extubation pulmonary edema complicating appendectomy in a young patient: case report. *Curr Surg.* 2004;61:463-465.
43. Koch SM, Abramson DC, Ford M, et al. Bronchoscopic findings in post-obstructive pulmonary oedema. *Can J Anaesth.* 1996;43:73-76.
44. Herrick IA, Mahendran B, Penny FJ. Postobstructive pulmonary edema following anesthesia. *J Clin Anesth.* 1990;2:116-120.
45. Weissman C, Damask MC, Yang J. Noncardiogenic pulmonary edema following laryngeal obstruction. *Anesthesiology.* 1984;60:163-165.
46. Stradling JR, Bolton P. Upper airways obstruction as cause of pulmonary oedema. *Lancet.* 1982;1:1353-1354.
47. Picano, E, Pellikka, PA. Ultrasound of extravascular lung water: a new standard for pulmonary congestion. *Eur Heart J.* 2016;37(27):2097-2104.
48. Zhang, G, Huang, X, Wan, Q, Zhang, L. Ultrasound guiding the rapid diagnosis and treatment of negative pressure pulmonary edema: a case report. *Asian J Surg.* 2020;43(10):1047-1048.
49. Picano, E, Frassi, F, Agricola, E, Gligorova, S, Gargani, L, Mottola, G. Ultrasound lung comets: a clinically useful sign of extravascular lung water. *J Am Soc Echocardiogr.* 2006;19(3):356-363.
50. Lichtenstein, D, Meziére, G. Relevance of lung ultrasound in the diagnosis of acute respiratory failure: the BLUE protocol. *Chest.* 2008;134:117-125.
51. Weitzel, WF, Hamilton, J, Wang, X, et al. Quantitative lung ultrasound comet measurement: method and initial clinical results. *Blood Purif.* 2015;39(1-3):37-44.
52. Buda, N, Kosiak, W. Is a linear probe helpful in diagnosing diseases of pulmonary interstitial spaces? *J Ultrason.* 2017;17(69):136-141.
53. Silva PS, Monteiro Neto H, Andrade MM, Neves CV. Negative-pressure pulmonary edema: a rare complication of upper airway obstruction in children. *Pediatr Emerg Care.* 2005;21:751-754.
54. Mehta VM, Har-El G, Goldstein NA. Postobstructive pulmonary edema after laryngospasm in the otolaryngology patient. *Laryngoscope.* 2006;116:1693-1696.
55. Grant BM, Ferguson DH, Aziz JE, Aziz SM. Successful use of VV ECMO in managing negative pressure pulmonary edema. *J Card Surg.* 2020;35(4):930-933.
56. Karaman, I, Ozkaya, S. Differential diagnosis of negative pressure pulmonary edema during Covid-19 pandemic. *J Craniofac Surg.* 2021;32(5):e421-e423.
57. Lee KW, Downes JJ. Pulmonary edema secondary to laryngospasm in children. *Anesthesiology.* 1983;59:347-349.
58. Brain AI. The laryngeal mask–a new concept in airway management. *Br J Anaesth.* 1983;55:801-805.
59. Windsor J, Lockie J. Anaesthesia and dental trauma. *Anesth Intensive Care Med.* 2008;9(8):355-357.
60. Deiner SG, Osborn IP. Prevention of airway injury during spine surgery: rethinking bite blocks. *J Neurosurg Anesthesiol.* 2009;21(1):68-69.
61. Tamkus A, Rice K. The incidence of bite injuries associated with transcranial motor-evoked potential monitoring. *Anesth Analg.* 2012;115(3):663-667.
62. Difficult Airway Society Extubation Guidelines Group; Popat M, Mitchell V, et al. Difficult Airway Society guidelines for the management of tracheal extubation. *Anaesthesia.* 2012;67:318-340.
63. Savaie M. Does endotracheal tube clamping during intubation of COVID-19 patients increase the risk of negative pressure pulmonary edema? *Can J Anaesth.* 2021;68(1): 165.
64. Choi WK, Lee JM, Kim, JB, et al. Diffuse alveolar hemorrhage following sugammadex and remifentanil administration. *Medicine.* 2019; 8(8):e14626.
65. Kao CL, Kuo CY, Su YK, Hung KC. Incidence of negative-pressure pulmonary edema following sugammadex administration during anesthesia emergence: a pilot audit of 27,498 general anesthesia patients and literature review. *J Clin Anesth.* 2020;62:109728.
66. Lee JH, Lee JH, Lee MH, Cho HO, Park SE. Postoperative negative pressure pulmonary edema following repetitive laryngospasm even after reversal of neuromuscular blockade by sugammadex: a case report. *Korean J Anesthesiol.* 2017;70(1):95-99.
67. Suzuki M, Inagi T, Kikutani T, Mishima T, Bito H. Negative pressure pulmonary edema after reversing rocuronium-induced neuromuscular blockade by sugammadex. *Case Rep Anesthesiol.* 2014:135032.

SECTION 10

PRACTICAL CONSIDERATIONS IN AIRWAY MANAGEMENT

CHAPTER 63

Difficult Airway Carts

Saul Pytka and Michael F. Murphy

INTRODUCTION

Why Are Difficult Airway Carts Necessary?

The concept of difficult and failed airway carts is not a novel one. These carts usually serve two purposes:

- Managing the anticipated difficult airway. As such they contain special devices (e.g., atomizers, Jackson Crossover forceps) and medications (e.g., lidocaine 5% ointment, lidocaine 4% aqueous) used to perform an awake intubation (see Chapter 3);
- Managing the failed airway. To this end they have devices (e.g., extraglottic devices [EGDs]) and prepackaged kits (e.g., open cricothyrotomy) used to manage the failed airway in an emergency.

Ordinarily, a single "airway" cart serves both functions and the contents do not vary significantly from unit to unit, except perhaps in regard to pediatrics where size related variations must be accounted for. The equipment, supplies, devices, and medications that they contain ordinarily are not otherwise immediately available on the majority of clinical units. For example, the difficult airway cart for the operating room (OR) rarely contains endotracheal tubes (ETTs), laryngoscopes, and stylets, as they are in every OR. On the other hand, in the postanesthesia care unit (PACU), the intensive care unit (ICU) and the emergency department (ED), difficult airway carts may well have these devices in the cart.

It has long been acknowledged that having emergency equipment readily available in a reliable location is a standard of care. The "cardiac crash cart," for example, is a mandatory addition to ORs, EDs, and other patient care areas where they may be required. Many labor and delivery rooms have an "emergency cart" ready for unanticipated "crash" cesarean sections, while trauma units have an emergency surgical setup for occasions when a chest or abdomen must be rapidly opened.

Although the literature is relatively silent on the actual benefits of having a difficult airway cart available for an emergency, there is strong consensus among experts that the ready access to alternative devices for airway management has the potential for reducing risks and complications in the management of the unanticipated difficult airway.[1–5] In 1993, the American Society of Anesthesiologists Task Force on Management of the Difficult Airway published their Practice Guidelines for Management of the Difficult Airway.[1] This document, subsequently updated in 2003, 2013 and 2022, contained a clear statement that *at least one portable storage unit that contains specialized equipment for difficult airway management should be readily available.*[2–4] They followed with a suggested list of specialized equipment that this "storage unit," or cart, should contain (Table 63.1).

Beyond the scope of the original ASA guidelines, the Canadian Airway Focus Group reviewed the pertinent literature

TABLE 63.1. Suggested Contents of the Portable Storage Unit for Difficult Airway Management[3]

- Rigid laryngoscope blades of alternate design and size from those routinely used
- Video laryngoscope
- Tracheal tubes of assorted sizes
- Tracheal tube guides. Examples include (but are not limited to) semirigid stylets, ventilating tube-changer, lightwands, and forceps designed to manipulate the distal portion of the tracheal tube.
- extraglottic devices (e.g., LMA or ILMA of assorted sizes for noninvasive airway ventilation/intubation).
- Flexible bronchoscopic intubation equipment.
- Equipment suitable for emergency invasive airway access.
- An exhaled carbon dioxide detector.

ILMA, intubating LMA; LMA, laryngeal mask airway.
The items listed in this table represent suggestions. The contents of the portable storage unit should be customized to meet the specific needs, preferences, and skills of the practitioner and healthcare facility.
Reproduced with permission from Apfelbaum JL, Hagberg CA, Caplan RA, et al. Practice guidelines for management of the difficult airway: an updated report by the American Society of Anesthesiologists Task Force on Management of the Difficult Airway. *Anesthesiology*. 2013;118:251-270.

on airway management in Canada and published recommendations for the management of the unanticipated difficult airway.[5] This group recommended that a "difficult airway cart" be available for emergency airway interventions in addition to the standard airway equipment available in every OR. They also suggested a minimum equipment list for such a cart.

It is important to note that two significant changes to the cart content recommendations have been made since the last edition of this text:

1. The cricothyrotomy kit must contain equipment to perform an OPEN cricothyrotomy.[6]
2. The difficult airway cart must contain lidocaine 5% ointment and lidocaine 4% aqueous for atomization, in accordance with the three step topicalization procedure of the upper airway recommended in Chapter 3.

Is There Any Evidence That Difficult Airway Carts Are Beneficial in the Setting of Difficult or Failed Airway Management?

The literature is replete with the advantages of using alternative airway devices in situations where a difficult airway is encountered, both anticipated and unanticipated. Just as emergency drugs and the presence of a defibrillator on the "crash cart" are indispensable in the management of a cardiac emergency, the readily available rescue airway devices in an airway emergency clearly represent an improvement in patient care.

The increase in morbidity and mortality associated with difficulties in airway management is well recognized.[7,8] Both the ASA and Canadian Airway Focus groups recommend limiting the number of attempts at direct laryngoscopy to 3 and 2, respectively.[1–5,9,10] Mort has shown that the increasing numbers of attempts at intubation by direct laryngoscopy correlate with an increased incidence of respiratory and hemodynamic complications.[11] In this study, a database was created to record complications following emergency airway interventions outside the OR. When three or more attempts were made to secure an airway by direct laryngoscopy, the incidence of hypoxemia increased from 11% to 70%, regurgitation from 2% to 22%, aspiration from 0.8% to 13%, and cardiac arrest from 0.7% to 11% (Table 63.2). One could speculate that the presence of alternate airway devices would have prevented the need for repeated attempts at direct laryngoscopy.

Mort reviewed the incidence and etiology of out-of-OR cardiac arrests occurring during emergency intubation before and after the introduction of emergency airway carts.[12] In 1995, the institution, a level-one trauma center, introduced airway carts, or kits containing "advanced" airway equipment and tracheal tube verifying devices. A retrospective study compared the time periods of 1990–1995 and 1995–2002 for a number of variables, the primary comparator being cardiac arrest. The compelling results showed an overall reduction of 50% in airway-related cardiac arrests between the two time periods, attributable to the presence of the carts (Figure 63.1).[12]

TABLE 63.2. Complications by Intubation Attempts

Complication	2 or Fewer Attempts (90%)	>2 Attempts (10%)[a]	Relative Risk for >2 Attempts	95% CI for Risk Ratio
Hypoxemia	10.5%	70%	9×	4.20-15.92
Severe hypoxemia	1.9%	28%	14×	7.36-24.34
Esophageal intubation	4.8%	51.4%	6×	3.71-8.72
Regurgitation	1.9%	22%	7×	2.82-10.14
Aspiration	0.8%	13%	4×	1.89-7.18
Bradycardia	1.6%	18.5%	4×	1.71-6.74
Cardiac arrest	0.7%	11%	7×	2.39-9.87

[a]All categories $p < 0.001$ when comparing 2 or fewer attempts to > 2 attempts. Hypoxemia—$SpO_2 < 90\%$; severe hypoxemia—$SpO_2 < 70\%$.
Data from Mort TC. The incidence and risk factors for cardiac arrest during emergency tracheal intubation: a justification for incorporating the ASA Guidelines in the remote location. *J Clin Anesth*. 2004;16(7):508-516.

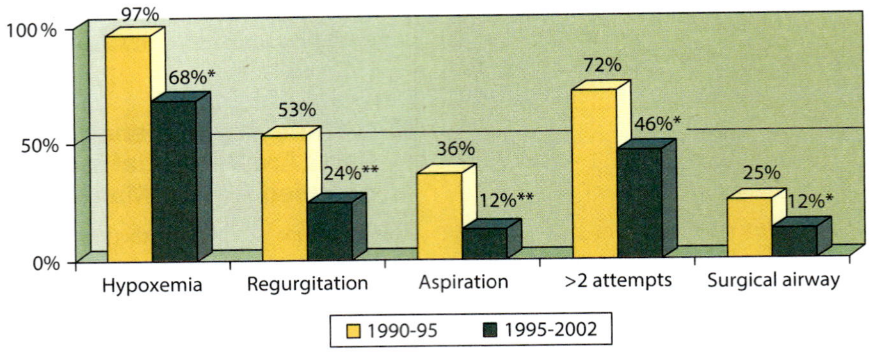

FIGURE 63.1. Complications associated with repeated attempts at laryngoscopic intubation. (Reproduced with permission from Mort TC. The incidence and risk factors for cardiac arrest during emergency tracheal intubation: a justification for incorporating the ASA Guidelines in the remote location. *J Clin Anesth*. 2004;16:508-516.)

Although the data compiled from these papers were gathered from non-OR locales, the conclusions are clearly applicable to all areas that airway management may be performed, including the OR. The ready accessibility of difficult airway carts is indispensable in reducing airway-related morbidity and mortality.

What Steps Should Be Taken to Ensure That the Carts Remain Well-Stocked and Contain Equipment in Good Working Order?

It is important that when an airway practitioner arrives at the scene of an airway emergency, or when the "Difficult Airway Cart" is summoned, all of the equipment that is needed must be present and functional. To achieve this, departmental and hospital policies or processes must be crafted, which should identify:

- The numbers and locations of such carts.
- A process of annual review of the cart locations and how they are equipped and updated.
- A qualified staff member must be responsible for the cart in each assigned area as the "keeper of the cart."
- How equipment is added to and deleted from the standard list of contents, and how such changes are suggested, vetted, implemented, and communicated to the relevant staff.
- How the drawers will be arranged and labeled.
- How equipment with schedules are to be maintained (e.g., flexible bronchoscopes [FBs]).
- Time frames and responsibilities regarding replenishment after equipment is used.
- Who will check the inventory and how often it will be checked. The checklist includes the functioning of essential equipment, such as bulbs and batteries, and time-sensitive supplies such as local anesthetic agents and vasoconstrictors.
- If cleaning is to be done, who will do it, how it will be done (e.g., bronchoscopes), and how long the "out of service for cleaning" interval will be.
- An inventory of replenishment supplies to be kept immediately on hand, particularly disposables (e.g., EGDs, open cricothyrotomy kit, etc.).
- Where equipment manufacturers' literature will be kept.

Routine airway management equipment that one expects to use in most, if not all, airway management emergencies, such as laryngoscopes, airways, ETTs, intubating tracheal introducers (e.g., Eschmann Introducer or Frova) and stylets, tonsil and catheter suction devices, etc., should be immediately available and not clutter the drawers of the cart. As mentioned above, this equipment need not be on an OR cart as each anesthetizing location ought to have them available. Carts should be located in each area of the hospital where airway management might reasonably be expected to occur, such as EDs, coronary care unit, cardiac catheterization units, labor and delivery suites, endoscopy suites, diagnostic imaging units, and other locations where sedatives will be administered. In locations where both children and adults are cared for, the pediatric cart should be distinctly separate from the adult cart (different style, and perhaps different color). An array of ETT sizes, masks, oral and nasal airways, etc., must be easily accessible in the event pediatric patients are cared for. Perhaps the best system currently available to meet this need is the Broselow-Luten System®.[13] Alternatively, canvas-pocketed systems that are rolled up for storage can easily and quickly be unrolled to access the equipment.

If at all possible, airway carts should be in a consistent location (e.g., with the cardiac crash cart). The cart should be secured with a plastic twist removable lock. The cart is secured after each check, signaling that the cart has been replenished and is ready for use. The absence of the lock signifies that the cart needs immediate inspection. A keyed lock may be required for drawers that contain medications. The locking mechanism for this drawer must be limited to this drawer only and should not impede access to the other drawers with airway devices.

DIFFICULT AIRWAY CART IN THE OPERATING ROOM

What Are the Guiding Principles for Establishing a Difficult Airway Cart for the OR Area?

Historically, the contents of the "difficult airway cart" in most anesthesia locations varied widely, as various practitioners demanded the addition of newer or their preferred devices. Unfortunately, items that nobody had ever used, or would ever use, were included. The contents would often be forgotten, and little or no maintenance would occur. Basically, they were difficult airway carts in name only.

Although a number of publications describe difficult airway cart setup, most are simply a description of the author's departmental cart.[14] However, such a list can be a good starting point for creating a useful cart, with the end-users customizing the contents according to departmental needs, preferences, and available resources. A designated individual or committee should be responsible for soliciting input from users in determining what should be on the cart. The decision about the contents ought to be reviewed quarterly or semiannually to ensure that carts have the most up-to-date and effective equipment. Deletions and additions need to be communicated to all users in a timely manner.

In principle, the cart should be one that is easily accessible and has equipment familiar to the users and other unit personnel. An assortment of well-arranged and quickly accessible devices should be available to handle most needs. Decisions about disposable versus reusable equipment should be made consistent with hospital policies and published evidence of equipment effectiveness (discussed later in this chapter).

In this all-inclusive difficult airway cart, all equipment needed for difficult airway situations (so-called Plan B and Plan C) should be present. As mentioned, equipment on the cart need not duplicate routine airway equipment otherwise available on anesthetic carts in the ORs. This may be where an OR difficult airway cart differs from airway carts in other locations: in ICU or ED settings, airway kits or carts may contain both routine and alternative airway equipment.

Familiarity with the difficult airway cart and its contents is crucial. Using "difficult airway" equipment for routine intubations will add to the skills in using alternative devices and will also help the anesthesia practitioner, and support personnel, gain needed familiarity with cart contents and location. This in turn will lead to more effective management of an emergency unanticipated difficult and failed airway, minimizing stress for all concerned. However, with regular use of the difficult airway cart, there must be a routine to ensure that it is properly maintained: disposables must be replenished and reusable equipment disinfected, and replaced as quickly as possible. This in turn implies that designated personnel familiar with the cart routinely check and replenish it. This is the same principle that applies to maintenance of the cardiac arrest "crash cart."

What Equipment Should Be Available on a Difficult Airway Cart for the OR?

The cart containing the equipment should be mobile, small enough to be safely and easily moved by one person, and should fit into the ORs through the doorways. It should be located in a central location that is familiar and visible to all. Smooth castors on the cart and the drawers are important to ensure that the cart does not become an obstacle in itself, and is safe from being overturned. Cables and cords should be neatly attached so that nothing can be snagged while the cart is being moved or people are working around it. Failure to pay attention to this could lead to damage to equipment or injury to staff. The drawers should be clearly labeled as per their contents.

In principle, the cart equipment should include all of the options that airway practitioners will require in a difficult airway scenario. The highly recommended use of algorithms on approaching anticipated and unanticipated difficult and failed airways, including the "cannot intubate, cannot oxygenate" (CICO) scenarios, will dictate what the local faculty are trained and familiar with. That should dictate what is on the carts and how they are organized. Well-labeled sections should be clearly visible to assist in locating what will be used. As an added resource, a large copy of the Difficult Airway Algorithm of the institution can be a valuable visual aid.

The equipment included on the cart should cover the range of options that might be needed in a difficult airway scenario. This will include categories such as:

- Equipment to facilitate mechanical (bag mask or EGD) ventilation
- High-flow nasal cannula to facilitate apneic oxygenation
- Adjuncts to direct and indirect laryngoscopy (e.g., tracheal introducers)
- Alternatives to direct laryngoscopy (e.g., video laryngoscopes, lightwands, etc.)
- Equipment to facilitate transtracheal access (e.g., cricothyrotomy kit or in house kits of scalpel, bougie, prep solutions)
- Light sources, cameras, and monitors for techniques requiring, or facilitated by, this equipment
- Equipment and drugs for application of topical airway anesthesia or airway blocks
- Miscellaneous equipment as determined by the location and facility

What Equipment to Facilitate Mechanical (Face Mask or EGD) Ventilation Should Be Included in the Difficult Airway Cart for the OR?

At least one face-mask device should be available for delivery of positive pressure ventilation. Nonstandard mask sizes (i.e., very large and very small) may belong on the cart. The group or individual responsible for the airway cart should decide which EGD to stock. If LMA®-Classic or disposable laryngeal mask airways (LMAs) are routinely stocked in an OR cart, then the cart may contain an LMA®-ProSeal™, and intubating LMA (LMA®-Fastrach™). Other EGDs such as the King LT® airway can be considered, but the devices should be the ones with which the department members have experience and have found useful. Second-generation EGDs (those with esophageal/gastric drainage tubes such as the King LTS-D®, LMA-ProSeal, LMA®-Supreme™, LMA®-Protector™, i-gel®, etc.) should be considered, especially in the wake of the findings of NAP4 where aspiration was the most common cause of death. Indeed, a much higher association of airway related deaths and serious brain injury was reported with the use of first-generation supraglottic devices than with second-generation devices, so the availability of these newer EGD is a strongly advised.[15,16]

What Adjuncts to Direct Laryngoscopy Should Be Included in a Difficult Airway Cart for the OR?

An assortment of alternate blades designed to fit standard laryngoscope handles used in the OR should be available. For example, Miller (straight) and Macintosh (curved) blades of various sizes, as well as levering tip (McCoy) laryngoscope blades,

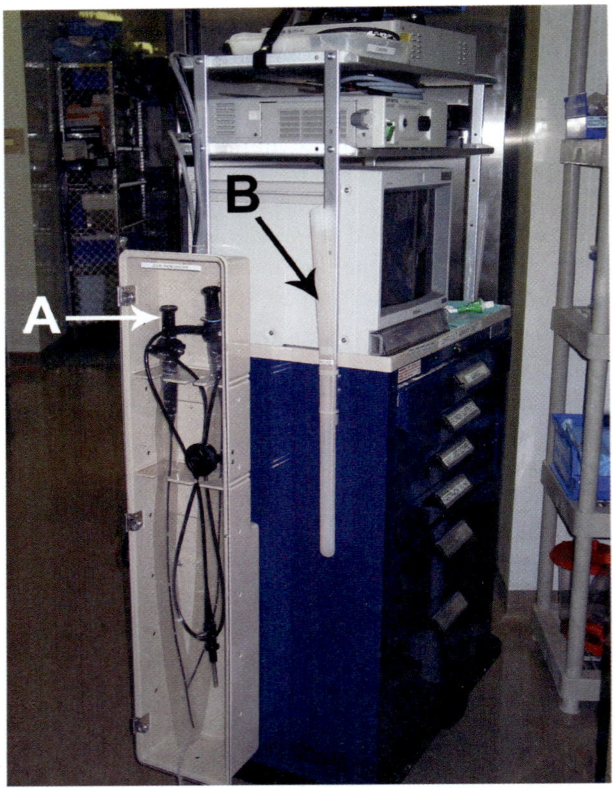

FIGURE 63.2. The proposed Difficult Airway Cart with different drawers for different airway equipment, video monitor, and flexible bronchoscope in a secure compartment **(A)**, and Eschmann Tracheal Introducer stored in its original shipping case **(B)**.

might be kept in this section. The presence of a variety of ETTs (e.g., Endotrol™, Microlaryngeal Tubes™, Parker FlexTip™) not routinely stocked in the OR, including a range of smaller sizes, is important.

The presence of a flexible, Coudé-tipped (distal 2.5 cm angled approximately 35 degrees) Eschmann Tracheal Introducer (also known the "gum-elastic bougie"), the SunMed Bougie™, Pocket Bougie or the single-use Cook Frova™ is an essential addition to an emergency cart. It can be guided below the epiglottis when a Mallampati class II or III view of the larynx is encountered, whereupon the ETT can be advanced over it (see Chapter 12). Because they should be kept straight (except the Pocket Bougie), rather than bent to fit into a drawer, some tracheal tube introducers (e.g., the Portex® Single-Use Bougie) may be stored in their original shipping case, secured to the side of the cart (Figure 63.2). As a simple, yet useful device, most would suggest that these introducers be an integral part of standard equipment found in every room or location where airways are routinely managed (e.g., anesthetizing locations, ED resuscitation rooms, etc.).

What Alternatives to Direct Laryngoscopy and Rescue Devices Should Be Included in a Difficult Airway Cart for the OR?

Here is where the list of objects becomes potentially extensive. Again, the principles are to not duplicate what already exists as routine airway management equipment in the OR, and to stock only those devices familiar to the anesthesia practitioner and support staff.

Options for inclusion in this section are as follows:

- Intubating LMA (LMA-Fastrach) in a variety of sizes (#3-#5), their dedicated silicone-ETTs (7-8 mm ID), and the tube stabilizer to aid with subsequent LMA-Fastrach removal.
- Intubating lighted stylet for light-guided intubation.
- Flexible bronchoscope (FB) devices. FB should be kept in a secure compartment, where it can be stored so that it is not tightly curled (Figure 63.2). This ensures maximum protection of the fragile shaft and the motion cable that controls the scope tip. FBs ought to be handled with great care as they are fragile devices and repairs may be expensive. Discussion often arises regarding the use of pediatric versus adult scopes. In a difficult intubation, particularly where failed attempts at direct laryngoscopy have traumatized the airway, the adult scope has the advantage of having a more functional suction lumen in addition to being a more rigid (and sturdy) scope. Ideally, a scope that will allow intubation with a 6 mm ID or larger ETT should be sought. Pediatric scopes are fragile and may not have the rigidity to facilitate the insertion of a large-diameter ETT tube around tight corners, and have smaller working channels compromising their suction capacity. They are, however, indispensable in performing an awake nasal intubation and confirming the position of devices when lung isolation is required. Included in the drawer where the FB equipment is kept should be devices to protect the scope from being bitten, such as a bite Williams Airway Intubator™ (see Figure 10.24), Ovassapian™ Fiberoptic Intubating Airway (see Figure 10.25), or Berman Intubating Pharyngeal Airways™ (see Figure 10.23) in an assortment of sizes.
- Most recently, single-use disposable FBs are commercially available from a number of manufacturers (Ambu®aScope™, Olympus, Storz, etc.). Because of the considerably lower cost than the reusable multiuse scopes, these could be deployed on multiple difficult airway carts in multiple locations. The cost of initial purchase, sterilization, as well as damage that can occur during the whole process of use to return needs to be factored in. Also, the loss of the reusable scope when it is sent for processing means that the cart is incomplete. Furthermore, the risks of infectious transmission from patients to handlers of the used scopes is eliminated. This is an important factor in the time of SARS-Cov-2 as well as other infectious processes.[17]

Rigid fiberoptic and video laryngoscopic devices. These devices provide indirect visualization of the larynx via fiberoptics, camera chips or alternative visual displays (e.g., Airtraq™ Optical Laryngoscope). Some devices such as the McGrath Mac™, GlideScope™, and C-MAC™ have a blade to aid with tongue control, while others, such as the Shikani SOS™, Clarus Video System™, Bonfils™, and Levitan FPS, are optical stylets, enabling visualization through an ensleeved ETT. Further details on these devices appear in Chapter 11. Many of these devices can be operated with batteries, making them portable.

A recent review of the literature revealed that, although visualization of the glottic opening is improved with many of these devices, insertion of the ETT may remain problematic.[18] Indeed, significant trauma to the pharyngeal and tracheal structures has been documented with some of these devices. Intubations, when confronted by distorted anatomy, are facilitated more by some video laryngoscopes than by others. In other words, none of the devices is a panacea. While video laryngoscopes are promising intubation devices, their precise role in difficult and failed airway management remains to be elucidated.

What Equipment to Facilitate Transtracheal Access Should Be Available in the Difficult Airway Cart for the OR?

In a failed airway situation, particularly when ventilation and intubation are not possible, quick direct transtracheal access to the airway must occur (see Chapter 14 for details). It is safe to say at this point in time that OPEN Cricothyrotomy is indicated in the CICO failed airway; and that trans-tracheal jet ventilation should be abandoned.[19] Commercial kits are available with equipment for one or both techniques. The Universal Cricothyrotomy Kit™ available from Cook Critical Care contains both open and Melker (needle cricothyrotomy) equipment. These cricothyrotomy kits now have cuffed cannulas, making them particularly useful when faced with the need for positive pressure ventilation. For those departments with members familiar with the technique, equipment for retrograde intubation can be considered an option in less urgent situations (e.g., "can't intubate, but can oxygenate" situation). The equipment for retrograde intubation is also available commercially in a Cook® Retrograde Intubation Set (Cook Medical, Bloomington, Indiana). As described in the NAP4 reports, a high degree of failure occurred with the use of percutaneous cricothyrotomy kits, and the recommendation for open access is strongly recommended by the NAP4 as well as numerous other papers. They are simple to do, and require a minimal amount of equipment, specifically a scalpel, bougie, and ETT. There should be a kit on every difficult airway cart. Anesthesiologists and surgeons should be experienced through simple courses or workshops in the provision of an emergency front-of-neck airway (eFONA) procedure.[15,16]

What Video Accessory Equipment Should Be Available in the Difficult Airway Cart for the OR?

Many of the newer flexible bronchoscopes can run on a battery-powered light source, while visualization occurs through a traditional eyepiece. Other FBs and the newer video bronchoscopes require a separate light source that attaches to the scope via a cable. This light source is generally brighter than the battery-powered light sources. A particularly useful device is a camera with an appropriate adaptor that attaches to a bronchoscope's eyepiece to give a video feed to a monitor (see Figure 63.2). This allows much better viewing of the airway, as the image is magnified and is brighter than that viewed through the eyepiece. It allows an assistant to visualize what is happening and in a teaching institution, it can be invaluable when explaining or directing a trainee what to do next. Still or video images can be recorded for documentation of the procedure as well as any pathology encountered.

What Other Miscellaneous Equipment Should Be Available in a Difficult Airway Cart?

Ancillary equipment, such as medication cups for holding and mixing solutions, tongue depressors, and tonsil forceps (e.g., the Kraus or Jackson forceps) for applying local anesthetic (e.g., lidocaine) containing gauze balls for superior laryngeal nerve blocks, as well as antifog agents for the FBs, are a few other additions to the cart. The need for awake intubation is always a possibility, so appropriate types and volumes of local anesthetic agents should also be kept on the cart (see Chapter 3). Water-soluble lubricants (e.g., AMG MedPro Lubricating Gel, AMG Medical Inc, Montreal, Canada), silicone fluid (Endoscopic Instrument Lubricant, ACMI, Norwalk, USA), or other anti-fog agents should also be available.

An array of airway exchange catheters is always appropriate, for use in changing tubes in difficult situations or for the extubation of the patient whose trachea was difficult to intubate.

Availability of pediatric equipment will be dictated by the practice pattern of the hospital, although very small-for-age adults, disaster preparedness, and airway pathology situations make it advisable for adult hospitals to carry some pediatric equipment. Other equipment for inclusion on the difficult airway cart will be dictated by the department's practice environment. For instance, some institutions include rigid bronchoscopes and anterior commissure scopes on their cart.

DIFFICULT AIRWAY CART OUTSIDE THE OR

How Might Equipment Requirements Differ for Out-of-OR Locations Such as the ICU or ED and Why?

The processes governing airway carts in non-OR areas are no different than those described above. A variety of policies and practices are essential in ensuring that vital life-saving equipment is available and in working order when required, including the following:

- Who should be involved in deciding what the cart contains?
- How are suggestions as to contents made and how are those decisions made?
- How are cart modifications communicated effectively to all staff that may be affected?
- How often is the cart checked for contents and equipment function, and by whom?
- Who is responsible to ensure that the carts are restocked routinely after use?
- How is this process documented?

Some areas are more "airway intervention prone" than others. EDs, ICUs, free-standing day-surgery operations, PACUs, pediatric dental clinics, nonhospital surgical facilities, and pediatric cancer care units are obvious examples. It is reasonable to expect that airway intervention may occur with some regularity in these environments, and that routine and difficult airway management equipment ought to be immediately available.

Others are less obvious. These include units where procedural sedation is undertaken, such as endoscopy suites, and angiography and cardiac catheterization units. While routine airway management equipment ought to be immediately available on these units, it may be financially prohibitive to create potentially expensive, fully equipped carts as described above. However, it is not unreasonable to expect that such units have relatively inexpensive, proven adjuncts, such as oral and nasal airways, and rescue devices such as disposable LMA® (LMA®-Unique™), LMA-Fastrach, and intubating stylets.

Some institutions designate staff from anesthesia, critical care, or emergency medicine, or hospitalists be a part of a team that responds to declared intrainstitutional airway emergencies. In response, some of these departments have created portable airway management bags to be taken to the site of the airway emergency. Policy considerations as to contents and their working order are no different for these kits than for the cart described above.

Furthermore, and crucially important from a medicolegal perspective, is the involvement of those departments tasked with emergency airway management in the design, equipping, and maintenance of unit resident carts in the units for which they are responsible. It is the duty of the hospitals and unit management, department leadership and airway practitioners to understand and embrace this accountability.

DISPOSABLE VERSUS REUSABLE DEVICES CONSIDERATIONS FOR DIFFICULT AIRWAY CARTS

What Is Transmissible Bovine Spongiform Encephalitis (BSE)? Should Airway Practitioners Be Concerned About It?

The widespread awareness of the possibility of transmission of infectious processes via the use of reusable medical equipment has led to adherence to standards for sterilization as a routine practice. Until recently, it was assumed that the adherence to these traditional sterilization measures would assure that prevention of iatrogenic disease transmission by this route would be effective.

Creutzfeldt-Jakob disease (CJD), Bovine Spongiform Encephalitis (BSE or mad cow disease), as well as variant CJD (vCJD) are examples of transmissible spongiform encephalopathies (TSE). All of these diseases are transmitted by malformed protein particles, referred to as prions. These infectious prion proteins attach themselves to native prion proteins in the recipient's brain, resulting in production of more of the distorted, abnormal prions, and the clinical specter of progressive neurological symptoms leading to death. Almost any symptom can present, from motor, to sensory, to cognitive dysfunction. This often makes the diagnosis difficult, as the symptoms can be confused with other neurological conditions. Definitive diagnosis is made histologically by biopsy or at autopsy. The term "Spongiform" refers to the spongy gross appearance of the brain caused by TSE.

The incidence of TSE in humans is extremely low. Sporadic (90% of CJD) and familial (10% of all CJD) forms of CJD occur at a frequency of 1:1,000,000 in the general population. Iatrogenic forms of CJD have occurred from transfer of infected neural tissues (pituitary extract, cornea, or dura mater) and represent <1% of all cases of CJD.

In 1986, the first case of BSE was reported in Britain. By 2001, it was estimated that 180,000 cattle were infected. One recalls the widespread control measures taken at that time, with the mass destruction of herds throughout the United Kingdom.

There appears to be a link between BSE and vCJD. This variant has some significant differences from the sporadic form of CJD. Among the differences between the two disease entities is the notable discovery of a prion specific to vCJD in lymphoid tissues (tonsil, spleen, appendix, and lymph nodes). Prior to this, the only location of the agents responsible for BSE was felt to be neural tissue involving brain, spinal cord, dura mater, or eye. The discovery of prions in lymphoid tissue occurs very early in the disease process, before the onset of clinical symptoms. Furthermore, the tissues are very highly infectious. A mass of 1 μg of infected lymphoid tissue has the same risk of infectivity as 1 g of neural tissue from sporadic CJD-infected subjects.[20,21] This makes the tissue infected with the vCJD prion particle 1000 times more infectious.

By the year 2002, a total of 134 cases of human TSE felt secondary to BSE had been reported worldwide.[20] The vast majority (126) were in the United Kingdom and Ireland, 6 in France, 1 in Italy, and 1 in the United States. The US (Florida) resident, however, was from the United Kingdom and it was felt the disease had been acquired there. Clearly, the transmission of TSE has been documented through the use of neural tissues, both dural grafts and pituitary growth hormone. It has also been reported to have passed from patient to patient via reusable neurosurgical instruments, despite employing standard cleaning and disinfection methods. While it is difficult to assess the risk of transmission via reusable airway instruments, either surgical or anesthetic, that have come in contact with lymphoid tissue in an infected patient, the infectivity of the vCJD prion from such tissue as mentioned above, is approximately 1000 times that of the material from neural tissue. In spite of the above data, there have been no reported cases, to date, of vCJD transmitted via contaminated airway equipment. Furthermore, projections of the future risks of deaths from vCJD show dramatic decreases, such that the incidence of deaths from the disease will be almost negligible over the next 70 years.[22]

How Effective Is Sterilization in Destroying the Prion Particle?

Discovery of prion transmission through the use of infected surgical instruments created an alarming realization that the usual methods of sterilization were not reliable in disinfecting medical equipment.[23,24] It has been shown that the prion particles associated with TSE are extremely resistant to accepted standard sterilization procedures; particles withstanding autoclaving (120°C), ultraviolet radiation, as well as ionizing radiation.[24] The discovery that protein residue is present in medical instruments used for airway manipulation after routine cleaning procedures creates even more concern. This is particularly worrisome in light of the presence of prions in lymphoid tissues in patients later diagnosed with vCJD. Miller et al. showed, in the assessment of 20 cleaned reusable LMAs, that all had residual protein deposits on them, ranging from mild (55%) to heavy staining (20%).[25] Similarly, of the 61 used laryngoscope blades that had been cleaned and returned for use, 50 were contaminated. This finding was confirmed by Clery and colleagues.[26]

The recognition that: (i) prions related to vCJD were present in tonsil tissue; (ii) the specific prion was much more virulent than the agent for vCJD; and (iii) material from patients was present on airway instruments in spite of adequate techniques of sterilization has led to the suggestion that single-use instruments be used in place of reusable varieties, where the risk of cross contamination with tonsil tissue can occur. Indeed, in 2001, the Department of Health in the United Kingdom mandated the use of disposable surgical and anesthetic instruments for use in tonsil surgery. However, within a year, the high incidence of surgical complications deemed to be secondary to the introduction of these disposable instruments led to the reversal of the directive. It was decided that the risk of complications from the disposable instruments outweighed the risk of transmission of vCJD from cross contamination of inadequately cleaned multiple use instruments. Although the ban on reusable anesthetic equipment was initially lifted, it was reimposed in 2002.

How Well Do Single-Use (Disposable) Airway Devices Work When Compared to the Reusable Instruments?

Following the concern that reusable airway equipment could cause the transmission of vCJD, a large number of single-use instruments were introduced into the market. These included, but were not limited to, laryngoscope blades, tracheal tube introducers (e.g., Eschmann Introducer), LMA®, and other EGDs, as well as disposable covers for laryngoscope blades. However, there are no strict testing or standards that must be met by any of these devices. Consequently, a great deal of controversy has arisen as to their effectiveness, when compared to the traditional equipment.

Twigg et al.[27] compared six single-use laryngoscope blades with the "standard" Macintosh blade in a simulator model. Twenty experienced anesthesiologists used each device, both in an "easy" scenario and a simulated difficult airway. Time to intubate, need for the use of an Eschmann Introducer, Cormack-Lehane (C-L) grading, and percentage of glottic opening visible (POGO) scores were recorded. Although considerable variability existed between the disposable devices, the best performer in both "normal" and "difficult" scenarios was the Macintosh blade. Not surprisingly, it was the difficult airway that brought out the greatest differences between the best and the worst performers. Some of the single-use blades performed reasonably well, the best being the Europa, which is a metal instrument. The results were so troubling that the investigators concluded, "We believe that intubation equipment that fails to match standard equipment should be avoided and is clinically unsafe. The unregulated use of single-use laryngoscopes must be questioned."[27]

Annamaneni et al.[28] demonstrated a difference between single-use and disposable tracheal introducers ("bougies") in simulated difficult intubations. Twenty anesthesiologists attempted intubation twice with both a reusable introducer and a single-use introducer, with success measured by tracheal as opposed to esophageal insertion. The success with first attempts was 85% versus 15% for the multiple use and disposable devices, respectively. The results were similar for the second attempt.

Evans et al.[29] compared disposable and nondisposable laryngoscopes by studying the time to intubate as well as measuring the force used to obtain an adequate laryngoscopic view, for both routine and difficult intubation in a manikin. They had 60 anesthesiologists performing intubations with five different laryngoscope blades, both routinely and with a cervical collar on the manikin. The blades included the standard Macintosh #3, a disposable metal, and three plastic blades. The time was significantly greater with the plastic blades when compared to the metal, for both the routine and "difficult" intubations. The increase ranged from 33% to 85%. Forces generated were statistically greater for the plastic blades when compared to those for the metal blades, by as much as 35%. The forces generated, even though they were not out of the range used clinically, were sufficient to cause three of the plastic blades to fracture during the study.

Anderson and Bhandal measured the effect on the illumination by placing a protective cover over a reusable Macintosh blade.[30] They showed that a predictable reduction in illumination occurred, with a mean reduction of 19%. Others have commented on their findings that disposable laryngoscope blades are inferior to reusable devices.[31,32]

One of the authors of this chapter (SP) had the experience of having been provided with a disposable plastic blade in the ICU when called to assist with a failed intubation. The blade fractured during the intubation attempt, causing a laceration on the patient's tongue and adding to an already stressful situation. Intubation was successful following the use of a reusable metal Macintosh blade.

Another area where the influx of single-use, disposable devices has flooded the market place is with the LMA. The reasons cited are again cost as well as infection control.

The significant increase in the marketing of these devices is unfortunately devoid of studies showing their safety and reliability. The materials used differ significantly from the ones used in the original LMA-Classic. In the LMA-Classic device, silicon was the chosen material. It produces a good seal, due to its pliability. It is, however, more expensive than the polyvinylchloride (PVC) material used in the single-use devices. Of note, Dr. Archie Brain rejected PVC as the materials for his LMA devices in the development stages. PVC, by its nature, is a rather rigid material, and therefore not very compliant. Plasticizers are needed to make PVC pliable and therefore produce a decent seal. These additives, however, potentially can make these products toxic, as phthalates—the most commonly used plasticizer—have been suggested as being potentially carcinogenic. Another concern regarding the use of single-use devices is the effects on the environment with the disposal of these nonbiodegradable plastic products.

Most importantly, there is a lack of standardized guidelines for the manufacturing of disposable devices, as well as the lack of studies comparing their efficacy to the original, reusable LMA devices. Just as with the disposable laryngoscopes and tracheal introducers, studies may reveal that the performance and safety of these devices may or may not meet expectations.

■ Should Reusable or Disposable Equipment Be Kept in the Difficult Airway Carts?

The only reliable ways to avoid the transmission of vCJD is to either use disposable instruments or not perform airway manipulation on patients infected with prion agent, and thus avoid contamination of reusable equipment. Clearly, the risk of contaminating equipment depends upon the probability of caring for an infected individual. The data from the World Health Organization (WHO) show that the incidence varies worldwide and is very low, even in countries at highest risk (i.e., the United Kingdom). Indeed, the risk of transmission through the use of contaminated instruments was felt to be less than the risk of complications posed by disposable surgical instruments used for tonsillectomy in 2001. Fortunately, the risks of anesthetic-related airway mishaps are lower than the risks posed by complications from our surgical colleagues. The numbers of failed intubations are too low to have adequate power to reveal what the increased risks posed are to patients by using disposable devices. Certainly, the risk posed by cross contamination of vCJD is unknown. However, as discussed earlier, there has not been a single reported case of transmission of vCJD via airway equipment at the time of this publication. In their editorial, Blunt and Burchett[20] discuss the hypothetical relative risks and come to the conclusion that the risk to the patient with poorly functioning airway equipment is likely greater than that of acquiring TSE through contaminated airway instruments.

The cost and reliability must be taken into account for all single-use instruments. Although Galinski et al.[33] felt that the disposable instruments were acceptable, they also state that, "it may be advisable to maintain conventional laryngoscopes in reserve for difficult intubations." More effective cleansing methods would also reduce risk, albeit not eliminate it. In the final analysis, it is important to weigh the relative risks of possible contamination with vCJD prions, negligible in most areas of the world and dropping, to those of risks created during airway management with what could, and has been shown to be, less than optimal equipment. The decision to keep reusable or disposable equipment in the difficult airway carts should be based on sound scientific evidence, relative risk, and cost-benefit assessments.

Unfortunately, a lack of studies supporting the efficacy and safety of the large number of disposable airway devices flooding the market is concerning, making informed decision difficult. Furthermore, many of the comparative studies have shown that these disposable devices are frequently substandard when compared to their reusable counterparts. The issue of cost, discussed by Cook in an editorial in the British Journal of Anesthesia suggests that this may not be the advantage as previously thought.[34]

Finally, when dealing with the most difficult airway situation, where the emergency airway cart is required, one could argue that the best, most reliable and proven equipment should be selected.

SAFETY OF ALL PERSONNEL PROVIDING CARE

Before concluding the discussions directed to the contents of the difficult airway cart, it is important to protect the health care providers known, and future unknown pathogens that are both airborne and transmitted through contaminated equipment and surfaces. Precautions should involve the need to limit the number of care providers exposed to the minimum required, to properly communicate using principles of Crisis Resource Management/simulation lessons, and to ensure adequate personal protective equipment (PPE) is readily available and properly applied and removed when dealing with patients requiring all airway interventions, but particularly in emergency situations where stress can lead to errors in protocols and judgment leading to mortality and morbidity of personnel following airborne generating medical procedures (AGMP), most recently with SARS-Cov-2. All difficult airway carts should be accompanied by a separate cart with a ready supply of PPE for all care providers.

SUMMARY

The use of alternative airway devices has clearly improved patient care. The ready availability of these devices is markedly facilitated by the creation of an airway cart. This cart should be easy to use, well laid out, and maintained to ensure optimal use. The contents should encompass a range of devices as described in various publications, and should be customized to the needs of a given department and its members. Although the decision to keep reusable or disposable equipment in these airway carts is not an easy one, it should be based on relative risk, scientific evidence, and the cost-benefit assessments.

The appendix itemizes how a difficult airway cart might be structured.

SELF-EVALUATION QUESTIONS

63.1. Which of the following is a known effective method of sterilization in destroying the prion particle?

A. Autoclaving (120°C)

B. Ultraviolet radiation

C. Ionizing radiation

D. Sterilization with ethylene oxide

E. none of the above

63.2. All of the following policy issues regarding a difficult airway cart are crucial EXCEPT:

A. Cart location.

B. Who is the cart "policy" manager?

C. Communications regarding contents.

D. Maintenance and replacement of contents.

E. Who is permitted to use the cart?

63.3. Since anesthesia practitioners are called to out-of-OR locations to manage airways:

A. They are liable for negative outcomes if the equipment they need is not available.

B. They must have input regarding contents of difficult airway carts in locations where they may be called to intervene.

C. They must ensure that policies regarding airway equipment maintenance in out-of-OR locations are in force and followed.

D. Noncompliance in any of the scenarios listed above (including the availability of essential equipment) would be grounds to refuse to participate in airway management in those locations.

E. All of the above.

REFERENCES

1. Practice guidelines for management of the difficult airway. A report by the American Society of Anesthesiologists Task Force on Management of the Difficult Airway. *Anesthesiology*. 1993;78:597-602.
2. American Society of Anesthesiologists Task Force on Management of the Difficult A. Practice guidelines for management of the difficult airway: an updated report by the American Society of Anesthesiologists Task Force on Management of the Difficult Airway. *Anesthesiology*. 2003;98:1269-1277.
3. Apfelbaum JL, Hagberg CA, Caplan RA, et al. Practice guidelines for management of the difficult airway: an updated report by the American Society of Anesthesiologists Task Force on Management of the Difficult Airway. *Anesthesiology*. 2013;118:251-270.
4. Apfelbaum JL, Hagberg CA, Connis RT, et al. 2022 American Society of Anesthesiologists Practice Guidelines for Management of the Difficult Airway. *Anesthesiology*. 2022;136:31-81.
5. Crosby ET, Cooper RM, Douglas MJ, et al. The unanticipated difficult airway with recommendations for management. *Can J Anaesth*. 1998;45:757-776.
6. Frerk C, Mitchell VS, McNarry AF, et al. Difficult Airway Society 2015 guidelines for management of unanticipated difficult intubation in adults. *Br J Anaesth*. 2015;115:827-848.
7. Rose DK, Cohen MM. The airway: problems and predictions in 18,500 patients. *Can J Anaesth*. 1994;41:372-383.
8. Schwartz DE, Matthay MA, Cohen NH. Death and other complications of emergency airway management in critically ill adults. A prospective investigation of 297 tracheal intubations. *Anesthesiology*. 1995;82:367-376.
9. Law JA, Broemling N, Cooper RM, et al. The difficult airway with recommendations for management. part 1. Difficult tracheal intubation encountered in an unconscious/induced patient. *Can J Anaesth*. 2013;60:1089-1118.
10. Law JA, Duggan LV, Asselin M, et al. Canadian Airway Focus Group updated consensus-based recommendations for management of the difficult airway: part 1. Difficult airway management encountered in an unconscious patient. *Can J Anaesth*. 2021;68:1373-1404.
11. Mort TC. Emergency tracheal intubation: complications associated with repeated laryngoscopic attempts. *Anesth Analg*. 2004;99:607-613.
12. Mort TC. The incidence and risk factors for cardiac arrest during emergency tracheal intubation: a justification for incorporating the ASA Guidelines in the remote location. *J Clin Anesth*. 2004;16:508-516.
13. Luten R, Broselow J. Rainbow care: the Broselow-Luten system. Implications for pediatric patient safety. *Ambul Outreach*. 1999:14-16.
14. McGuire GP, Wong DT. Airway management: contents of a difficult intubation cart. *Can J Anaesth*. 1999;46:190-191.
15. Cook TM, Woodall N, Frerk C, Fourth National Audit P. Major complications of airway management in the UK: results of the Fourth National Audit Project of the Royal College of Anaesthetists and the Difficult Airway Society. Part 1: Anaesthesia. *Br J Anaesth*. 2011;106:617-631.
16. Cook TM, Woodall N, Harper J, Benger J, Fourth National Audit P. Major complications of airway management in the UK: results of the Fourth National Audit Project of the Royal College of Anaesthetists and the Difficult Airway Society. Part 2: Intensive care and emergency departments. *Br J Anaesth*. 2011;106:632-642.
17. Barron SP, Kennedy MP. Single-use (disposable) flexible bronchoscopes: the future of bronchoscopy? *Adv Ther*. 2020;37:4538-4548.
18. Niforopoulou P, Pantazopoulos I, Demestiha T, Koudouna E, Xanthos T. Video-laryngoscopes in the adult airway management: a topical review of the literature. *Acta Anaesthesiol Scand*. 2010;54:1050-1061.
19. Duggan LV, Ballantyne Scott B, Law JA, Morris IR, Murphy MF, Griesdale DE. Transtracheal jet ventilation in the "can't intubate can't oxygenate" emergency: a systematic review. *Br J Anaesth*. 2016;117(Suppl 1):i28-i38.
20. Blunt MC, Burchett KR. Variant Creutzfeldt-Jakob disease and disposable anaesthetic equipment-balancing the risks. *Br J Anaesth*. 2003;90:1-3.
21. Bruce ME, McConnell I, Will RG, Ironside JW. Detection of variant Creutzfeldt-Jakob disease infectivity in extraneural tissues. *Lancet*. 2001;358:208-209.
22. Ghani AC, Donnelly CA, Ferguson NM, Anderson RM. Updated projections of future vCJD deaths in the UK. *BMC Infect Dis*. 2003;3:4.
23. Brown P, Preece M, Brandel JP, et al. Iatrogenic Creutzfeldt-Jakob disease at the millennium. *Neurology*. 2000;55:1075-1081.
24. Zobeley E, Flechsig E, Cozzio A, Enari M, Weissmann C. Infectivity of scrapie prions bound to a stainless steel surface. *Mol Med*. 1999;5:240-243.
25. Miller DM, Youkhana I, Karunaratne WU, Pearce A. Presence of protein deposits on "cleaned" re-usable anaesthetic equipment. *Anaesthesia*. 2001;56:1069-1072.
26. Clery G, Brimacombe J, Stone T, Keller C, Curtis S. Routine cleaning and autoclaving does not remove protein deposits from reusable laryngeal mask devices. *Anesth Analg*. 2003;97:1189-1191.
27. Twigg SJ, McCormick B, Cook TM. Randomized evaluation of the performance of single-use laryngoscopes in simulated easy and difficult intubation. *Br J Anaesth*. 2003;90:8-13.
28. Annamaneni R, Hodzovic I, Wilkes AR, Latto IP. A comparison of simulated difficult intubation with multiple-use and single-use bougies in a manikin. *Anaesthesia*. 2003;58:45-49.
29. Evans A, Vaughan RS, Hall JE, Mecklenburgh J, Wilkes AR. A comparison of the forces exerted during laryngoscopy using disposable and non-disposable laryngoscope blades. *Anaesthesia*. 2003;58:869-873.
30. Anderson KJ, Bhandal N. The effect of single use laryngoscopy equipment on illumination for tracheal intubation. *Anaesthesia*. 2002;57:773-777.
31. Babb M, Mann S. Disposable laryngoscope blades. *Anaesthesia*. 2002;57:286-288.
32. Jefferson P, Perkins V, Edwards VA, Ball DR. Problems with disposable laryngoscope blades. *Anaesthesia*. 2003;58:385-386.
33. Galinski M, Adnet F, Tran D, et al. Disposable laryngoscope blades do not interfere with ease of intubation in scheduled general anaesthesia patients. *Eur J Anaesthesiol*. 2003;20:731-735.
34. Cook TM. The classic laryngeal mask airway: a tried and tested airway. What now? *Br J Anaesth*. 2006;96:149-152.

APPENDIX: SAMPLE CONTENTS OF AN OPERATING ROOM DIFFICULT AIRWAY CART

Drawer #1: Awake intubation and topical anesthesia	• Endoscopic intubation guides such as Ovassapian™, Tudor Williams™, and/or Berman Intubating Pharyngeal (Breakaway) Airways™ • Mucosal Atomization Device (MAD™) • Anti-fog goggles. • Jackson Crossover Forceps. • Atomizer (e.g., single-use EZ-Spray™, Alcove Medical Corporation, Houston, Texas) with O_2 Tubing • Phenylephrine 0.5% (Neosynephrine®) nasal spray 15 mL • Lidocaine 4% aqueous 50-mL bottles. • Lidocaine 5% ointment (tube) with tongue depressors • Lidocaine 2% gel, Med Cups and cotton balls for use with Jackson forceps • Endoscopic light source replacement bulb • Portex flexible bronchoscope swivel adapter™ • Adult and Pediatric Magill forceps
Drawer #2	• Metered Dose Inhaler in-line administration adapters • Intravenous needle/catheters for transcricoid insertion (14- and 16-gauge × 2 of each) must be aspiration capable with 3-mL syringe with 7.0-mm ID ETT connector • ENK Oxygen Flow Modulator™ (Cook Critical Care). • 6.0-, 7.0-, and 8.0-mm ID Endotrol™ tubes: Mallinckrodt
Drawer #3	• King LTS-D of various sizes (Ambu) • Light wand
Drawer #4: LMAs	• LMA-Fastrach of various sizes • Second-generation EGDs of various sizes
Drawer #5: Surgical Airway	• Universal Cricothyrotomy Kit™ (Cook Critical Care) • Retrograde Intubation Kit™ (Cook Critical Care)
Drawer #6: Fiberoptics	• Cook Airway Exchange Catheters™ and Aintree catheter™ (Cook Critical Care)
Top of cart	• Bronchoscope Light Source • Spare Eschmann Tracheal Tube Introducer
Side cabinet	• 3.7-mm "pediatric" and 5.1-mm flexible bronchoscopes

CHAPTER 64

Point-of-Care Ultrasound (POCUS) of the Upper Airway in Airway Management

Eric You-Ten, Yeshith Rai, Michael S. Kristensen, Fabricio B. Zasso, and Naveed Siddiqui

CASE PRESENTATION

The following clinical scenario highlights the importance of upper airway point-of-care ultrasound (POCUS) in managing a patient in respiratory distress.

A 65-year-old male patient with a body mass index (BMI) 50 kg·m^{-2} presented to the emergency department in respiratory distress with associated fever, severe sore throat, and drooling. He reported progressive dysphagia and difficult phonating over the past couple of days. The patient's medical history was otherwise significant for hypertension, diabetes, and dyslipidemia. The patient was oxygenated with high-flow nasal cannula and immediately transferred to the operating room (OR) for an emergency intubation. Prior to airway management, neck landmarks were challenging to palpate on the thick neck, and ultrasonography of the upper airway was performed to identify swelling in the airway and to premark the cricothyroid membrane (CTM) location and its depth in preparation for a double set up with a front-of-neck airway (FONA). In the OR, the patient's airway was topicalized with lidocaine, and an awake intubation was attempted with a flexible bronchoscope, which revealed an inflamed and erythematous epiglottis. The intubation attempt was unsuccessful, and the patient experienced a complete airway obstruction, losing consciousness shortly after. Without delay, a front-of-neck cricothyrotomy using a scalpel-bougie-tube was successfully performed. The patient was subsequently transferred to the intensive care unit (ICU) and underwent an ultrasound-guided percutaneous tracheotomy (PCT) the next day.

INTRODUCTION

What Is the Role of POCUS in Surgical Cricothyrotomy?

The role of ultrasound for upper airway access has been described for a variety of procedures including endotracheal tube (ETT) placement, predicting difficult airways, and assessing airway anatomy and pathologies prior to surgical airway access.[1–3] During instances of "cannot intubate, cannot oxygenate" (CICO), difficult airway guidelines recommend establishing a surgical airway. In emergency settings, cricothyrotomies are preferred to tracheotomies as they are faster and easier to perform.[4,5] Successful cricothyrotomies are dependent on the rapid and accurate identification of the CTM. While POCUS has been described for assessment of the difficult airway, there is a relative paucity of literature regarding the use of ultrasound for CTM localization prior to cricothyrotomies. Location of the CTM by digital palpation (DP) has been shown to be challenging in emergency and nonemergency situations enhancing the risk of complications such as esophageal perforation, laryngeal trauma, and false passage cannulation.[6–8] Ultrasound plays an important preprocedure role when a surgical airway is a material possibility when managing a difficult airway.

Is the Use of Ultrasound Justified in Locating the CTM in an Emergency?

The utility of ultrasound in identifying the CTM becomes more apparent in individuals with difficult neck anatomy. Ultrasound is noninvasive, can accurately identify the CTM and can be performed relatively quickly. An early study compared CTM identification with ultrasound and conventional DP in higher BMI patients.[9] Investigators found that while increased BMI caused a significant increase in palpation difficulty, BMI did not impact CTM identification in the ultrasound group. Similar trends were seen comparing palpation accuracy of the CTM in obese and non-obese parturients. Palpation of the CTM in higher BMI parturients took longer, required a greater number of attempts, and was associated with lower accuracy rates.[10,11] In a study with cadavers exhibiting poorly defined neck anatomy, the preemptive use of ultrasound has been shown to improve cricothyrotomy success and decreased complications.[12] Specifically, the investigators found that while the ultrasound group was associated with longer total procedure times, their cricothyrotomies were associated with less severe injuries, fewer attempts, and higher CTM identification accuracy rates than the palpation group.

The use of ultrasound has its limitations; studies have shown that ultrasound takes significantly longer than palpation for initial identification of the CTM and subsequent airway device insertion.[9–13] This is a concerning finding given the time-sensitive nature of e-FONA. However, reduced CTM identification times by palpation is countervailed by its lower accuracy, lower success, and higher complication rates. Concerns that the use of ultrasound to locate the CTM may prolong the procedure time was investigated in a meta-analysis to determine whether the ultrasound-guided approach is superior to the palpation technique in terms of procedural-related accuracy and procedure time.[6] Although there was heterogeneity in the studies analyzed, no significant differences in time for the two procedures were identified. The marked enhancements in accuracy, success, and reduced complication rates related to the ultrasound location of the CTM reinforced its preemptive use in elucidating CTM and neck landmarks before airway management in patients with ill-defined airway anatomy.

Can Ultrasound Identification of the CTM Be Used as a Training Tool?

Employing ultrasound to identify CTM can be achieved with minimal ultrasound training, even when performed by relatively inexperienced trainees. A study involving 15 anesthesia practitioners with varying levels of training (junior residents, fellows, and anesthesia assistants) showed that ultrasound-guided palpation of neck landmarks improved the accuracy of CTM location. This improvement was brought about by a relatively short 1-hour training session with ultrasound.[13] Similarly, Oliveira and colleagues showed that ultrasound improves accuracy of CTM identification by anesthesia trainees following a 2-hour training session and these skills were retained 3 months after the initial training period.[14]

ULTRASOUND TECHNIQUES FOR IDENTIFICATION OF NECK LANDMARKS

What Are the Steps to Identify the CTM Using POCUS—Longitudinal and Transverse Techniques?

Accurate localization of the CTM is the first and most critical step when performing an emergency cricothyrotomy. Misidentification of the CTM is a major cause of tube misplacements, cricothyrotomy failures, and complications.[15] However, external palpation of the CTM by practitioners may be inaccurate, even under elective conditions.[16] Current evidence suggests that ultrasonography improves the accuracy of CTM localization and has been suggested before airway manipulation when a difficult airway is anticipated in nonemergency situations.[9–12]

Two techniques have been described for systematic, stepwise identification of the CTM:

1. The longitudinal "String of Pearls" (SOP) technique
2. The transverse "Thyroid-Airline-Cricoid-Airline" (TACA) technique

The "String of Pearls" (SOP) Technique

This technique is the most well published and has proven its superiority over palpation in a cadaveric study that demonstrated improved success and reduced tube misplacement in cricothyrotomy. Furthermore, this same technique can be used to identify the optimal interspace between tracheal rings for the placement of a tracheostomy tube. We recommend the longitudinal technique as the first to learn, and that every anesthesia department has the expertise and equipment to employ it.[17,18]

Performing the longitudinal SOP technique (*Figures 64.1A-D*)***:***

1. A right-handed operator stands on the patient's right side. The sternum is identified, and the transducer is placed transversely on the patient's neck just cephalad to the suprasternal notch to visualize the trachea—horseshoe-shaped dark structures with posterior white lines (Figure 64.1A).
2. The transducer is slid toward the patient's right side (towards the operator) such that the right border of the transducer is positioned midline of the trachea and the ultrasound image of the tracheal ring is thus truncated into half on the screen (Figure 64.1B).
3. The right end of the transducer is maintained over the midline of the trachea, while the left end is rotated 90° into the sagittal plane resulting in a longitudinal scan of the midline of the trachea. Several dark (hypoechoic) rings will be seen anterior to the white hyperechoic line (air-tissue border), akin to a "string of pearls." The dark hypoechoic "pearls" are the anterior part of the tracheal rings (Figure 64.1C).
4. The transducer is kept in the midline oriented longitudinally and slid cephalad until the cricoid cartilage comes into view (seen as a larger, more elongated, and anteriorly placed dark "pearl" compared with the other tracheal rings). Further cephalad, the distal thyroid cartilage can be seen as well. The longitudinal course of the midline of the airway can be marked with a pen.

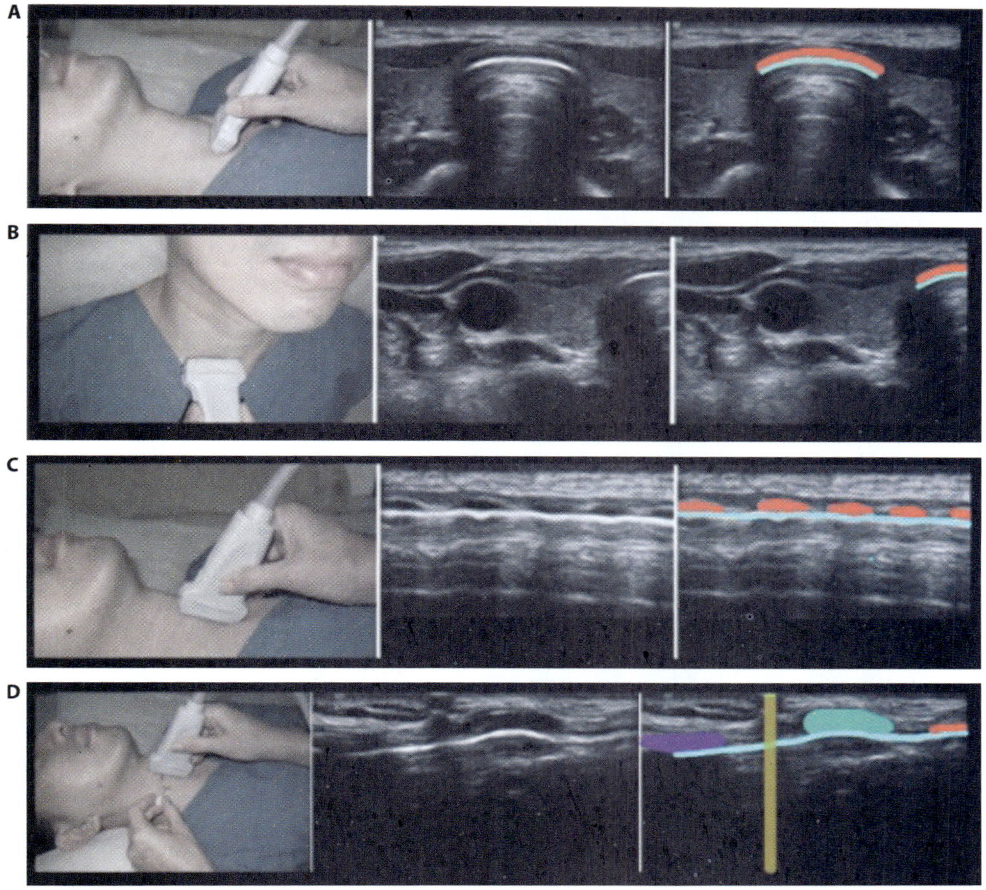

FIGURE 64.1. **(A)** The first step in performing the longitudinal "String of Pearls" technique is to place the transducer transversely on the patient's neck just cephalad to the suprasternal notch to visualize the trachea the horseshoe-shaped dark structures (highlighted in orange-red in the right panel) with posterior white lines. **(B)** The ultrasound view when the transducer is slid towards the patient's right side, the right border of the transducer is positioned midline of the trachea and the ultrasound image of the tracheal ring (in orange-red) is thus truncated into half on the screen. **(C)** The ultrasound view when the transducer is placed in a longitudinal position along the midline of the trachea. Several dark (hypoechoic) rings (also highlighted in orange-red in the right panel) will be seen anterior to the white hyperechoic line (air-tissue border), akin to a "string of pearls." **(D)** With the transducer oriented longitudinally and kept in the midline, slowly move the transducer cephalad until the cricoid cartilage comes into view (seen as a larger, more elongated, and anteriorly placed dark "pearl" (highlighted as green) compared with the other tracheal rings). The distal thyroid cartilage can also be seen (purple). The shadow from the needle (yellow) can be seen between the transducer and the skin.

5. While still holding the transducer, the other hand is used to slide a needle (as a marker, for its ability to cast a shadow in the ultrasound image) between the transducer and the patient's skin until the needle's shadow is seen midway between the caudal border of the thyroid cartilage and the cephalad border of the cricoid cartilage (Figure 64.1D).
6. Now the transducer is removed. The needle marks the center of the CTM in the transverse plane. This can be marked on the skin with a pen.

The TACA Technique

For patients with a very short neck, or flexion-deformity of the neck that leaves no space to place the ultrasound transducer in the longitudinal position, we recommend the transverse TACA technique to identify the CTM, as in these subsets of patients, this may be the only successful technique. Achieving a 100% success rate of identifying the CTM is possible when the longitudinal SOP technique is applied in tandem with the transverse TACA technique.[17,18]

Performing the transverse TACA technique (Figures 64.2A-D):

1. Estimate the thyroid cartilage's level on the neck and place the ultrasound transducer transversely over it, scanning to identify the thyroid cartilage as a hyperechoic triangular structure (Figure 64.2A).
2. Move the transducer caudally until the CTM is identified: this is recognizable as a hyperechoic white line resulting from the air-tissue border of the mucosal lining on the inside of the CTM, often with parallel white lines (reverberation artifacts) below (Figure 64.2B).
3. Move the transducer further caudally until the cricoid cartilage is identified—a black "lying C" with a white lining (Figure 64.2C).

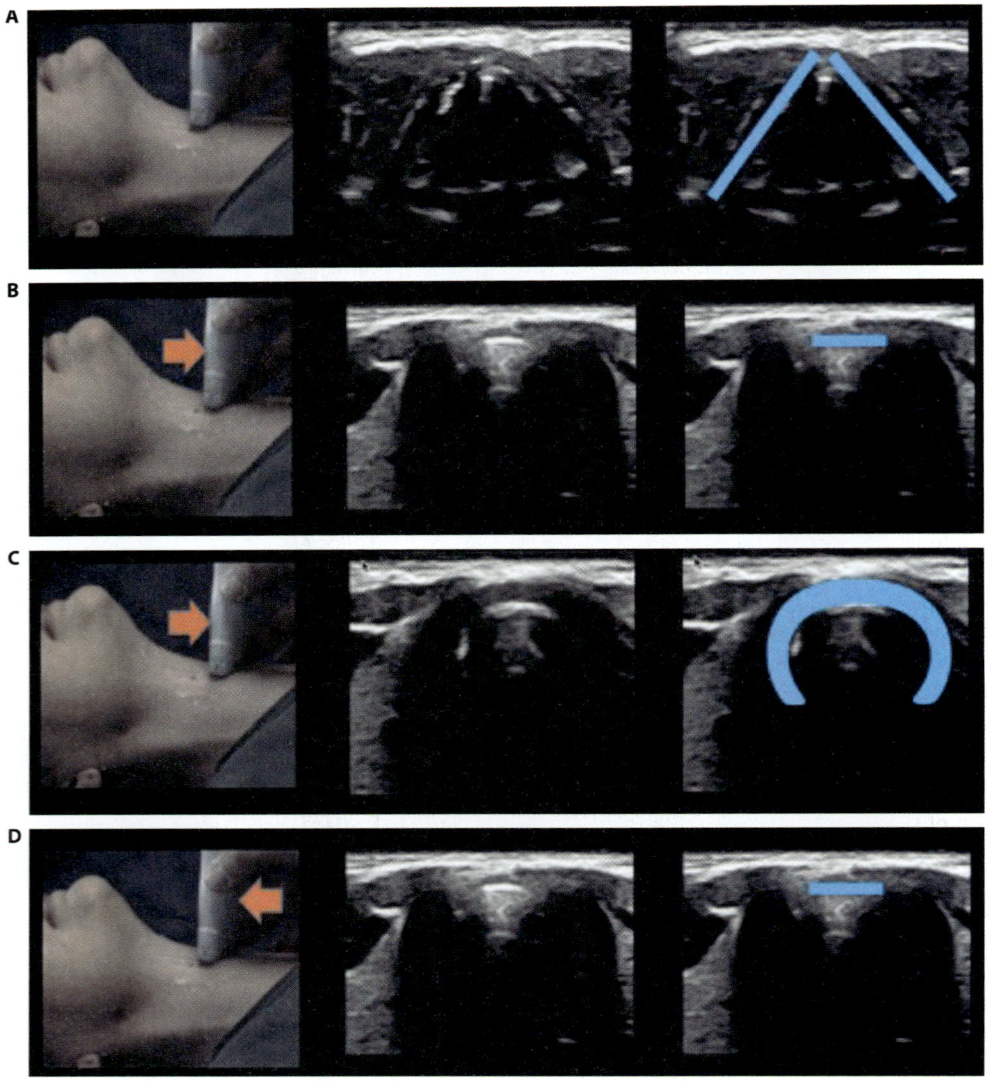

FIGURE 64.2. (A) The transverse "Thyroid cartilage, Airline, Cricoid cartilage, Airline" (TACA) technique: The ultrasound transducer is placed transversely over the thyroid cartilage, scanning to identify the thyroid cartilage as a hyperechoic triangular structure (the blue triangle). **(B)** The TACA technique: the cricothyroid membrane is identified as a hyperechoic white line (white line in the middle panel, highlighted blue in the right panel) resulting from the air-tissue border of the mucosal lining on the inside of the cricothyroid membrane, often with parallel white lines (reverberation artifacts). **(C)** The TACA technique: the cricoid cartilage is identified as the blue "lying C" when the transducer moves further caudally. **(D)** The last step of the TACA technique is to move the transducer slightly back cephalad until the center of the cricothyroid membrane (the blue horizontal line) is identified.

4. Finally, move the transducer slightly back cephalad until the center of the CTM is identified (Figure 64.2D).
5. The center can be marked both transversely and longitudinally on the skin with a pen. By identifying the highly characteristic shapes of both the thyroid and cricoid cartilages, both the cephalad and caudal borders of the CTM can be identified.

In summary, ultrasound-guided localization of the CTM fills the void of inaccurate localization by visualization or palpation. It is easily learned and should be used routinely, before embarking on the management of anticipated difficult airway situations.

What Are the Sonographic Characteristics of the CTM?

Knowing the likely depth and height of the CTM before emergency cricothyrotomy may improve success and decrease complications such as damage to posterior tracheal structures.

A cadaver study in Westerners demonstrated that the average width and height of the CTM membrane are 8.2 and 10.4 mm, respectively.[19] However, the dimensions of the CTM are variable among different racial populations. Investigators measured the dimensions of the CTM in adult South Indian populations to establish the association between these dimensions and select the appropriate sized ETT for the purpose of cricothyrotomy.[20]

These CTM dimensions in a neutral neck position, in men: width = 8.41 ± 2.11 mm, height = 6.57 ± 1.87 mm; in women: width = 6.30 ± 1.29 mm, height = 5.80 ± 1.56 mm. CTM dimensions are smaller in the Indian group compared with those published for western populations. ETTs ranging from size 3.0 to 6.0 mm internal diameter (ID) were found to be appropriate for cricothyrotomy in the adult South Indian population.[20]

CTM palpation is particularly challenging in obese patients, most likely due to the increased distance between the skin and the CTM (CTM depth). One study employing a CICO scenario coupled with CTM identification by DP recommended dissection of the neck down to the larynx in the event that surface DP CTM is impalpable. Measuring the CTM depth in a representative clinical sample having CT scans retrospectively quantified the relationship between BMI and CTM depth. The investigators found that CTM depth is strongly associated with BMI.[21] Another study in an obstetric population, using ultrasound compared the CTM depth between severely obese parturients and those with normal weight.[22] CTM depth was found to be significantly increased in severely obese versus normal-weight parturients independent of scanning plane, head and neck position, or transducer pressure. In a CICO failed airway, identification of the CTM and FONA cricothyrotomy should be anticipated to be challenging, particularly in the severely obese parturient, putting a finer point on preemptive ultrasound confirmation of CTM location in these patients.[22]

CONFIRMATION OF ENDOTRACHEAL TUBE

Can POCUS Be Used to Identify Endotracheal Tube or Esophageal Intubation?

There has been increasing evidence on the use of ultrasound for confirmation of ETT position as an adjunct to standard practices such as end-tidal CO_2, visualization of the ETT between cords, and endoscopic visualization of tracheal rings through the ETT. Ultrasound techniques of the lower airways have been used to visualize diaphragmatic movements, lung/pleura sliding, transtracheal identification of tube placement in the trachea, and whether the ETT is endobronchial.[23–26] Though current evidence regarding some of these findings is limited, ultrasound can be used to evaluate proper ETT placement in the trachea by indirectly ruling out an esophageal intubation.[27–29] A systematic review of over 2500 patients to determine the diagnostic accuracy of ultrasonography in confirmation of endotracheal intubation compared with standard confirmatory methods showed an estimated pooled sensitivity and specificity for ultrasonography of 0.98 (95% confidence interval [CI]: 0.97-0.99) and 0.96 (95% CI: 0.90-0.98), respectively.[27] Another systematic review and meta-analysis of a total of 12 eligible studies involving adult patients and cadavers found the diagnostic accuracy of using tracheal ultrasound to confirm ETT placement during emergency intubations (by indirectly excluding esophageal intubation) was determined to have a sensitivity of 0.93 (95% CI: 0.86-0.96) and specificity of 0.97 (95% CI: 0.95-0.98).[28] Similarly, a meta-analysis of 969 intubations performed in emergency and elective situations found that transtracheal ultrasonography used to rule out esophageal intubation, has pooled sensitivity and specificity of 0.98 (95% CI: 0.97-0.99) and 0.98 (95% CI: 0.95-0.99), respectively.[29] In emergency scenarios, transtracheal ultrasonography to rule out esophageal intubation showed an aggregate sensitivity and specificity of 0.98 (95% CI: 0.97-0.99) and 0.94 (95% CI: 0.86-0.98), respectively. In the absence of capnography and based on the findings of these studies with high sensitivity and specificity in the use of ultrasonography to confirm endotracheal intubation, transtracheal ultrasonography may play an important role in both elective and emergency intubations to evaluate proper ETT placement in the tracheal and indirectly rule out an esophageal intubation. However, end-tidal capnography remains to be the standard of care today in confirming correct tracheal placement.

Describe the Technique of Ultrasonographic Confirmation of Endotracheal Intubation

In this section, we explain the most consistently described ultrasound technique to suggest tracheal intubation by excluding esophageal placement of the ETT. A curved ultrasound probe may be used; however, tracheal rings are superficial and we recommend using a high-frequency linear probe. If time permits, one should visualize the patient's airway anatomy before placing the ETT, though clearly, this is not practical in an emergency.

1. The ultrasound probe should be placed above the suprasternal notch in a transverse direction.
2. Not to apply too much pressure as this may distort the airway anatomy.
3. On ultrasonography a tracheal ring is visualized as C-shaped hypoechoic (cartilage) and hyperechoic structures (the tissue-air border) with shadowing (Figure 64.3A).
4. The esophagus is usually seen on one side of the trachea as an oval structure with a hyperechoic wall and hypoechoic center.
5. Tracheal ultrasound can be performed in real-time as the ETT is passed. An esophageal intubation will reveal an adjacent hyperechoic structure with shadowing posterolateral to the trachea, consistent with the ETT location within the esophagus. This has been referred to as the "double tract sign" or "double trachea sign"[30] (Figure 64.3B).
6. If the esophagus is located directly posterior to the trachea, an esophageal intubation may be missed by ultrasound as this second hyperechoic structure will be obscured by the shadowing from the trachea.

TRACHEOTOMY

Can POCUS Be Used for Performing Tracheotomies?

Tracheotomy is a commonly performed procedure in ICUs for patients requiring long-term airway access. A body of evidence exists indicating that percutaneous tracheotomies (PCTs) are

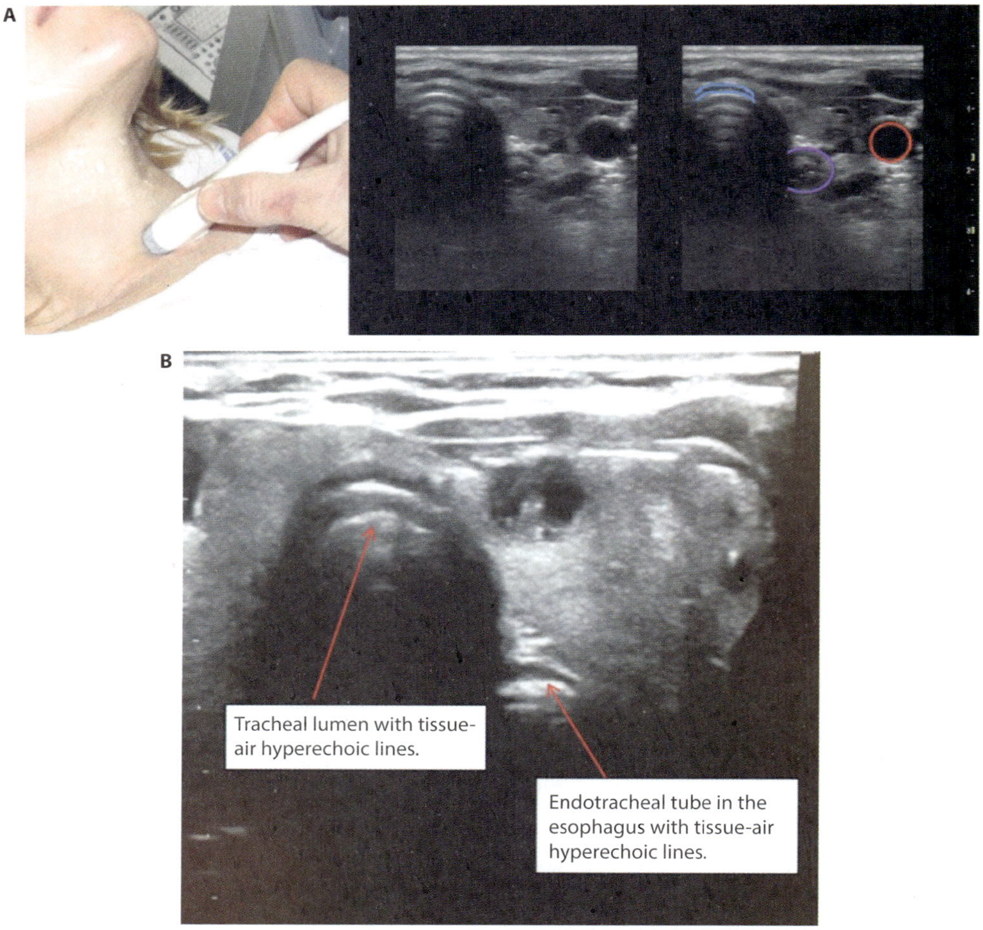

FIGURE 64.3. (A) With the ultrasound transducer placed above the suprasternal notch in a transverse direction, a tracheal ring is visualized as C-shaped (blue) hypoechoic (cartilage) and hyperechoic structures (the tissue-air border) with shadowing. The esophagus (purple) is usually seen on one side of the trachea as an oval structure with a hyperechoic wall and hypoechoic center. **(B)** An esophageal intubation is shown as an adjacent hyperechoic structure with shadowing posterolateral to the trachea, consistent with the endotracheal tube within the esophagus. The tissue-air hyperechoic lines are visualized in the trachea and esophagus (because of esophageal intubation); this has been referred to as the "double tract sign."

relatively safe compared to surgical tracheotomies.[31] Both surgical and percutaneous tracheotomies are associated with rare, but life-threatening complications including false-passage cannulation, esophageal or tracheal injury, and bleeding.[32]

Bronchoscopic-guided PCTs have been used by critical care teams to help reduce procedure-related complications. The use of bronchoscopy allows for indirect visualization of midline tracheal puncture, ETT depth, and tracheal wall injuries. However, among other complications, the use of bronchoscopic PCT is limited by its dependence on the operator, temporary hypoventilation, and risk of needle puncture of the bronchoscope.[33,34] Ultrasound guidance may be a useful adjunct in reducing complication rates and improving the accuracy of PCT. An earlier study in critically-ill patients in an ICU comparing PCT performed under ultrasound guidance (n = 166) and without ultrasound (n = 175), found that the use of ultrasound resulted in lower perioperative complication rates (7.8% vs. 15.0%, $p = .054$) and significantly lower number of multiple puncture attempts (3.9% vs. 13.6%, $p = .003$).[2] Not unexpectedly, total procedural time in the ultrasound-guided group took longer (24.09 minutes vs. 18.62 minutes, $p = .001$). More recently, a randomized controlled study compared outcomes between three techniques for PCT: traditional landmark, ultrasound-guided in-plane approach, and ultrasound-guided out-of-plane approach.[35] The ultrasound-guided out-of-plane approach had fewer punctures, lower complication rates, and higher first-entry success compared to the other groups. Investigators also noted that advanced patient age was negatively correlated with first-entry success, and more punctures resulted in increased complication rates.

There is a relative scarcity of literature directly comparing ultrasound-guided to bronchoscopy-assisted PCTs. The TRACHUS study found that ultrasound was at least equal to bronchoscope in primary and secondary outcomes.[36] Specifically, both groups had low procedure failure rates, with no major complications, similar rates of minor complications and procedure length.

To date, only a handful of single-center, relatively small randomized controlled trials have studied the utility of ultrasound-guided PCTs. While more studies are needed to firmly establish the advantages of ultrasound for PCTs, emerging evidence shows a clear trend toward improved safety and accuracy with ultrasound. Future studies should continue to explore the role of ultrasound as a useful bedside adjunct for PCTs while assessing long-term complication rates, the difference in techniques, patient profiles, and airway anatomy.

AIRWAY ASSESSMENT

Can POCUS Be Used to Predict a Difficult Airway?

The use of ultrasound has been described for various techniques in the context of airway management. Emerging research has been exploring the use of ultrasound parameters to predict difficult laryngoscopy and difficult tracheal intubation. Two recent meta-analyses compiled and examined data from more than 20 articles studying various ultrasound indicators of difficult intubation.[37,38] Of all the parameters studied, the hyomental distance (HMD)—distance from the hyoid bone to the tip of the chin—in the neutral position was found to be the most reliable parameter of difficult laryngoscopy and intubation. Specifically, difficult intubations were associated with a shorter HMD. Other parameters that were correlated with difficult laryngoscopy include tongue thickness, skin thickness at the epiglottis and hyoid levels, and HMD ratio (HMDR)—the ratio between HMD in the neutral and maximally extended neck positions. While numerous other ultrasound parameters were studied, they currently lack validation, and further research and large-scale randomized controlled trials are needed to substantiate these parameters as reliable predictors of difficult laryngoscopy and intubation.

SUMMARY

When confronted with a difficult airway, upper airway point of care ultrasound can be used at all stages, including prior to, during, and after the management of the airway. Prior to managing the airway, ultrasound can assess the ease of laryngoscopic intubation by measuring various anatomical parameters of the upper airway. Of all the parameters studied, the HMD—distance from the hyoid bone to the tip of the chin—in the neutral position was found to be the most reliable parameter of difficult laryngoscopy and intubation. Specifically, difficult intubations were associated with a shorter HMD. Thus, the role of ultrasound in assessing the anatomy parameters allows for better preparation in anticipation of difficult airways.

During airway management, ultrasound can be used to evaluate proper ETT placement in the trachea by indirectly ruling out an esophageal intubation since esophageal intubation can result in potentially serious complications of hypoxemia and aspiration pneumonitis. In both elective and emergency intubations, transtracheal ultrasonography to rule out esophageal intubation showed high aggregate sensitivity and specificity greater than 96%. However, end-tidal capnography remains to be the standard of care today in confirming correct tracheal placement.

The worst-case situation in managing a difficult airway can lead to a "CICO" scenario where the only life-saving procedure is a FONA. Airway ultrasound can be used to premark the CTM in anticipation of a potential FONA prior to airway management since palpation of the CTM is less accurate and can result in more complications and failed FONA.

Tracheotomy is a commonly performed procedure in ICUs for patients with prolonged intubation and requiring long-term airway access. A body of evidence exists indicating that PCTs are comparably safe compared to surgical tracheotomies. Ultrasound guidance may be a useful adjunct in reducing complication rates and improving the accuracy of PCTs.

SELF-EVALUATION QUESTIONS

64.1. Regarding the use of POCUS for airway management, which of the following statements is **NOT** true?

A. Ultrasound can be used as a preemptive tool to help delineate anatomical parameters in the neck.

B. Ultrasound can help reduce CTM identification and insertion times; however, this comes at the expense of decreased accuracy and precision.

C. Training with ultrasound helps users improve proficiency with identifying neck landmarks.

D. The transverse TACA technique is useful in identifying anatomical structures in those with very short neck, or neck-flexion deformities.

64.2. Which of the following is **NOT** true regarding the "String of Pearls" (SOP) technique?

A. It is the technique of choice for those with short necks or neck-flexion deformities.

B. The only vascular structure of note in the vicinity of the CTM is the superior thyroid arteries, which in 54% of people, courses along its lateral border.

C. The dark hypoechoic "pearls" represent the anterior part of the tracheal rings.

D. The cephalad border of the CTM is the distal thyroid cartilage, while the caudad border is formed by the proximal cricoid cartilage.

64.3. Which of the following is **TRUE** regarding the role of POCUS in the correct placement of the endotracheal tube in the trachea?

A. Correct placement of the endotracheal tube is confirmed using ultrasound by indirect visualization of the endotracheal tube in the trachea.

B. Hyperechoic signals in the endotracheal tube can be easily visualized using ultrasound.

C. Ultrasound confirms correct tube placement in the trachea indirectly by ruling out an esophageal intubation.

D. The diagnostic accuracy of ultrasound in esophageal intubation is low with sensitivity and specificity lower than 70%.

REFERENCES

1. Karacabey S, Sanri E, Gencer EG, Guneysel O. Tracheal ultrasonography and ultrasonographic lung sliding for confirming endotracheal tube placement: speed and reliability. *Am J Emerg Med.* 2016;34(6):953-956.
2. Yavuz A, Yilmaz M, Goya C, et al. Advantages of US in percutaneous dilatational tracheostomy: randomized controlled trial and review of the literature. *Radiology.* 2014;273(3):927-936.
3. Alansari M, Alotair H, Al Aseri Z, et al. Use of ultrasound guidance to improve the safety of percutaneous dilatational tracheostomy: a literature review. *Crit Care.* 2015;19(1):229.
4. Akulian JA, Yarmus L, Feller-Kopman D. The role of cricothyrotomy, tracheostomy, and percutaneous tracheostomy in airway management. *Anesthesiol Clin.* 2015;33(2):357-367.
5. Dillon JK, Christensen B, Fairbanks T, Jurkovich G, Moe KS. The emergent surgical airway: Cricothyrotomy vs tracheotomy. *Int J Oral Maxillofac Surg.* 2013;42(2):204-208.
6. Hung K-C, Chen I-W, Lin C-M, Sun C-K. Comparison between ultrasound-guided and digital palpation techniques for identification of the cricothyroid membrane: a meta-analysis. *Br J Anaesth.* 2021;126(1):e9-e11.
7. Zasso FB, You-Ten KE, Ryu M, Losyeva K, Tanwani J, Siddiqui N. Complications of cricothyroidotomy versus tracheostomy in emergency surgical airway management: a systematic review. *BMC Anesthesiol.* 2020;20(1):216.
8. Kristensen MS, Teoh WH. Ultrasound identification of the cricothyroid membrane: the new standard in preparing for front-of-neck airway access. *Br J Anaesth.* 2021;126(1):22-27.
9. Nicholls SE, Sweeney TW, Ferre RM, et al. Bedside sonography by emergency physicians for the rapid identification of landmarks relevant to cricothyrotomy. *Am J Emerg Med.* 2008;26(8):852-856.
10. You-Ten KE, Desai D, Postonogova T, Siddiqui N. Accuracy of conventional digital palpation and ultrasound of the cricothyroid membrane in obese women in labour. *Anaesthesia.* 2015;70(11):1230-1234.
11. Lavelle A, Drew T, Fennessy P, McCaul C, Shannon J. Accuracy of cricothyroid membrane identification using ultrasound and palpation techniques in obese obstetric patients: an observational study. *Int J Obstet Anesth.* 2021;48:103205.
12. Siddiqui N, Arzola C, Friedman Z, Guerina L, You-Ten KE. Ultrasound improves cricothyrotomy success in cadavers with poorly defined neck anatomy: a randomized control trial. *Anesthesiology.* 2015;123(5):1033-1041.
13. You-Ten KE, Wong DT, Ye XY, et al. Practice of ultrasound-guided palpation of neck landmarks improves accuracy of external palpation of the cricothyroid membrane. *Anesth Analg.* 2018;127(6):1377-1382.
14. Oliveira KF, Arzola C, Ye XY, et al. Determining the amount of training needed for competency of anesthesia trainees in ultrasonographic identification of the cricothyroid membrane. *BMC Anesthesiol.* 2017;17(1):74.
15. McGill J, Clinton JE, Ruiz E. Cricothyrotomy in the emergency department. *Ann Emerg Med.* 1982;11(7):361-364.
16. Lamb A, Zhang J, Hung O, Flemming B, Mullen T, Bissell MB, Arseneau I. Accuracy of identifying the cricothyroid membrane by anesthesia trainees and staff in a Canadian institution. *Can J Anaesth.* 2015 May;62(5):495-503.
17. Kristensen MS. Ultrasonography in the management of the airway. *Acta Anaesthesiol Scand.* 2011;55:1155-1173.
18. Kristensen MS, Teoh WH, Graumann O, Laursen CB. Ultrasonography for clinical decision-making and intervention in airway management: from the mouth to the lungs and pleurae. *Insights Imaging.* 2014;5:253-279.
19. Dover K, Howdieshell TR, Colborn GL. The dimensions and vascular anatomy of the cricothyroid membrane: relevance to emergent surgical airway access. *Clin Anat.* 1996;9(5):291-295.
20. Prithishkumar IJ, David SS. Morphometric analysis and clinical application of the working dimensions of cricothyroid membrane in south Indian adults: with special relevance to surgical cricothyroidotomy. *Emerg Med Australas.* 2010;22(1):13-20.
21. Ghaffar S, Blankenstein TN, Patel D, Theodosiou C, Griffith D. Quantification of the effect of body mass index on cricothyroid membrane depth: a cross-sectional analysis of clinical CT images. *Emerg Med J.* 2021;38(5):355-358.
22. Gadd K, Wills K, Harle R, Terblanche N. Relationship between severe obesity and depth to the cricothyroid membrane in third-trimester non-labouring parturients: a prospective observational study. *Br J Anaesth.* 2018;120(5):1033-1039.
23. Gottlieb M, Bailitz JM, Christian E, et al. Accuracy of a novel ultrasound technique for confirmation of endotracheal intubation by expert and novice emergency physicians. *West J Emerg Med.* 2014;15:834-849.
24. Chou HC, Chong KM, Sim SS, et al. Real-time tracheal ultrasonography for confirmation of endotracheal tube placement during cardiopulmonary resuscitation. *Resuscitation.* 2013;84:1708-1712.
25. Chou HC, Tseng WP, Wang CH, et al. Tracheal rapid ultrasound exam (T.R.U.E.) for confirming endotracheal tube placement during emergency intubation. *Resuscitation.* 2011;82:1279-1284.
26. Hosseini JS, Talebian MT, Ghafari MH, Eslami V. Secondary confirmation of endotracheal tube position by diaphragm motion in right subcostal ultrasound view. *Int J Crit Illn Inj Sci.* 2013;3:113-117.
27. Sahu AK, Bhoi S, Aggarwal P et al. Endotracheal tube placement confirmation by ultrasonography: a systematic review and meta-analysis of more than 2500 patients. *J Emerg Med.* 2020;59(2):254-264.
28. Chou EH, Dickman E, Tsou PY et al. Ultrasonography for confirmation of endotracheal tube placement: a systematic review and meta-analysis. *Resuscitation.* 2015;90:97-103.
29. Das SK, Choupoo NS, Haldar R, Lahkar A. Transtracheal ultrasound for verification of endotracheal tube placement: a systematic review and meta-analysis. *Can J Anaesth.* 2015;62:413-423.
30. Boretsky KR. Images in anesthesiology: point-of-care ultrasound to diagnose esophageal intubation: "the double trachea". *Anesthesiology.* 2018;129(1):190.
31. Al-Shathri Z, Susanto I. Percutaneous tracheostomy. *Semin Respir Crit Care Med.* 2018;39(6):720-730.
32. Dennis BM, Eckert MJ, Gunter OL, Morris JAJ, May AK. Safety of bedside percutaneous tracheostomy in the critically ill: evaluation of more than 3,000 procedures. *J Am Coll Surg.* 2013;216(4):857-858.
33. Iftikhar IH, Teng S, Schimmel M, Duran C, Sardi A, Islam S. A network comparative meta-analysis of percutaneous dilatational tracheostomies using anatomic landmarks, bronchoscopic, and ultrasound guidance versus open surgical tracheostomy. *Lung.* 2019;197(3):267-275.
34. Plata P, Gaszynski T. Ultrasound-guided percutaneous tracheostomy. *Anaesthesiol Intensive Ther.* 2019;51(2):126-132.
35. Kupeli I, Nalbant RA. Comparison of 3 techniques in percutaneous tracheostomy: Traditional landmark technique; ultrasonography-guided long-axis approach; and short-axis approach—Randomised controlled study. *Anaesth Crit Care Pain Med.* 2018;37(6):533-538.
36. Gobatto ALN, Besen BAMP, Tierno PFGMM, et al. Ultrasound-guided percutaneous dilational tracheostomy versus bronchoscopy-guided percutaneous dilational tracheostomy in critically ill patients (TRACHUS): a randomized noninferiority controlled trial. *Intensive Care Med.* 2016;42(3):342-351.
37. Gomes SH, Simões AM, Nunes AM, et al. Useful ultrasonographic parameters to predict difficult laryngoscopy and difficult tracheal intubation—a systematic review and meta-analysis. *Front Med.* 2021;8:671658.
38. Sotoodehnia M, Rafiemanesh H, Mirfazaelian H, Safaie A, Baratloo A. Ultrasonography indicators for predicting difficult intubation: a systematic review and meta-analysis. *BMC Emerg Med.* 2021;21(1):76.

CHAPTER 65

The Role of Robotics and Artificial Intelligence in Airway Management: Where Are We, and What Is the Future?

Janny Xue Chen Ke and Russell Taylor

CASE PRESENTATION

In 2035, a new class of highly infectious respiratory viruses plagues the world with severe multiorgan failure and high mortality. Scientists race against viral mutations with vaccines and boosters, but supplies are in dire shortage. Personal protective equipment (PPE) has been depleting rapidly due to overwhelming surge of patients and critical disruptions in the global supply and manufacturing chain.

As an anesthesiologist in a regional hospital a few hours away from the tertiary hospitals, you cover a wide area of rural and remote communities. On a stormy night, you receive a video call from the paramedics. They are in a remote area, in the home of Mr. A, a 40-year-old morbidly obese patient with a suspected respiratory infection. Due to weather constraints, the paramedics must rely on ground transport, and it will take a few hours to bring the patient by ambulance to the regional hospital due to poor visibility and road conditions. Since the paramedics arrived, the patient's condition has been deteriorating with increasing oxygen requirements and decreasing saturation, despite a trial of noninvasive ventilation, and the paramedics think it would be prudent to secure the airway prior to the drive.

The patient has multiple predictors of challenging intubation, usage of an extraglottic airway, and front-of-neck airway (FONA) access. He is extremely anxious and agitated due to his difficulty in breathing and has limited physiologic reserve. Moreover, while the paramedics have PPE, there remains concerns about viral transmission through aerosolization during tracheal intubation, especially if multiple attempts are needed. You assess the situation and ask the paramedics to prepare for robotic intubation using a flexible bronchoscope with the patient lightly sedated and spontaneously breathing. You also instruct them to set up backup airway equipment, optimize the position of the patient, denitrogenate, topicalize the airway, administer necessary medications, and deploy the remote-controllable intubation robot.

The intubation robot has some difficulty with automated movements initially due to the excessive airway tissues and secretions, but you guide it through properly from your regional hospital using a joystick. The robot navigates the rest of the way automatically. It identifies the vocal cords, sprays the vocal cords with local anesthetic, and inserts the tracheal tube. The paramedics secure the tracheal tube in place and connected the transport ventilator, and transport the patient sedated to your regional hospital. Along the way, you check in to provide any support they need.

INTRODUCTION

What Are Robotics and Artificial Intelligence, and What Are Their Potential Clinical Applications in Airway Management?

Robots are systems that process information into action in the physical world. Although robotic systems were first widely deployed in industrial applications[1], their potential for use is service applications (including health care) has been recognized since at least the 1980s.[2] Since then, robotic systems have been increasingly integrated into surgery and interventional medicine,[3,4] as a three-way partnership amongst medical practitioners, robotic technology, and information systems to improve the safety and scope of procedures while also reducing their invasiveness. Robots have been used successfully in applications such as preplanned tissue removal or stereotactic tasks with great accuracy,[5–8] or to provide surgeons the ability to perform high dexterity tissue manipulation tasks in endoscopic surgery.[9,10]

As these systems have become more capable physically, there has been increasing interest in expanding their control capabilities to enable the system to perform more sophisticated tasks "autonomously" or under the general supervision of the human medical practitioner. Although there have been several efforts to classify the "level" of autonomy in robotic systems,[11] there are fundamentally two questions: (1) how can the medical practitioner specify unequivocally what the robot is to do in a way that the robot controller can understand; and (2) how can the robot controller reliably and safely carry out the required tasks. For simple teleoperated systems such as the da Vinci surgical robot, this is straightforward. The surgeon observes the anatomy on a stereo video display and manipulates control handles to specify the desired surgical tool motions. The robot controller computes motor commands that move the tools to mimic the motion of the control handles. The remaining decisions are done by the surgeon, who must maintain complete situational awareness, based on the surgeon's understanding of the surgical task, patient anatomy, and what can be seen in the video display.

Increasing levels of task automation (such as automatic suturing or manipulating an endoscope to achieve a desired view) require that the robot controller have suitable representations of the patient anatomy and surgical task to be performed, along with suitable sensing and feedback mechanisms to relate these representations to the actual patient and to update them in real time. Advances in these areas thus depend heavily on advances in artificial intelligence (AI), which involves the "the theory and development of computer systems that are able to perform tasks that normally require human intelligence".[12] The synergistic development of extremely powerful and relatively inexpensive computer systems together with advances in "machine learning" methods over the past few years has greatly improved the ability of AI systems to perceive patient anatomy and to learn how to perform increasingly complex tasks without explicit direction and programming from a human.

There are many motivations for research in AI and robotics applied to airway management. Briefly, there are four broad categories discussed in the literature.[13–21] First, the most mentioned potential application is to assist those who do not have an expertise in airway management to improve the success rate. Second, AI could be used to enhance management in patients with difficult airways, particularly in the context of nonexperts. The third potential application would be deploying a robot in place of the health provider to reduce risks to humans, such as in the setting of infection, toxic gases, nuclear radiation, extreme temperatures, and battlefields. Finally, remote-controlled robotics could be integrated with telemedicine, where regional experts in airway management could support health providers in remote areas as in our case presentation. In this chapter, we will further assess the emerging literature on the use of robotics and AI in airway management.

What Areas in Airway Management Have Robotics and AI Research Been Performed?

So far, the literature on AI and robotics related to airway management addresses five domains, and its application in pediatrics has been reviewed in detail by Matava et al.[13] In assessing the literature in this area of research, it is important to consider whether the models have been validated and if so, in what populations, whether they can be extrapolated to the patient of interest, and how the models perform in more diverse populations.

Identification of Patients with Difficult Airways

The first domain of research involves the use of AI to enhance the identification of patients with anatomically difficult airway through photo images.[13,22–24] Existing physical examination findings have high specificity for identifying patients with difficult airways (specificity pooled point estimates range 0.84-0.98) but low sensitivity (pooled point estimates range 0.19-0.77).[25] Given the limited ability of existing predictors to rule out patients with potentially difficult airways, AI may identify new strategies by learning from large databases containing images from patients with a range of anatomically difficult airways. This may provide decision support for nonexperts. It may also aid planning during preoperative telemedicine consultations, commonly used during the COVID-19 pandemic, where the anesthesia practitioner may not be able to assess the patient's airway during a phone call. However, compared to existing physical examination predictors, the current machine learning models in the literature have only minimally improved sensitivity with worse specificity,[22] or showed high accuracy but did not report sensitivity nor specificity.

There are many issues associated with the use of AI algorithms to identify patients with a difficult airway. First is the possibility of bias, especially in ethnically and culturally diverse populations.[26] The bias may be compounded by the lack of interpretability in the algorithms, and users may not know when these algorithms should not be applied. In addition, the airway anatomy may change with time.[27] A classic example is the pregnant patient, whose airway becomes progressively more edematous during labor.[28] Moreover, the anatomical difficulty is only part of the difficult airway assessment. Physiological and contextual difficulties must also be considered.[29] Furthermore, policies for the confidentiality of patient images for the transmission and storage must be in place for real-time implementation.

Real-Time Image and Navigation Support

The second domain also involves image recognition but focuses on real-time decision support and automation for navigation from entry to the vocal cords. Research involves automatic labeling of key anatomic features (e.g., glottis) within airway images using techniques in AI.[13,17,30–32] This may be particularly helpful for novices or nonexperts. For example, a medical student during training could use a video laryngoscope that labels the vocal cords (in contrast to the esophagus) and correctly insert the endotracheal tube. However, these systems must be rigorously tested for reliability in a wide range of normal and abnormal anatomy. In situations of altered airway anatomy, such as upper airway obstruction after topicalization[33] or abnormal vocal cords, these systems may not be able to identify patterns that the algorithm did not train on. Also, the algorithms may be impaired by the poor image quality, such as in the presence of airway bleeding and secretions.

Monitoring and Risk Prediction

The third domain of research relates to monitoring and prediction of airway-related issues, such as airway obstruction and the need for reintubation.[13,34–42] Airway anatomy is dynamic in nature and a patient's airway difficulty and risk of complications evolve over time depending on surgical, patient, and anesthetic factors. Thus, airway reassessment should be done more often perioperatively in some patients, such as patients undergoing airway surgeries, or requiring prone or Trendelenburg positioning that is prolonged and/or coupled with significant fluid administration. Risk prediction models can help with planning for appropriate monitoring, disposition, and timely management of complications. Of note, an active area of research focuses on the identification of patients with obstructive sleep apnea (OSA).[38,43–45] This may be helpful due to the perioperative morbidity of patients with OSA, and the logistical barriers to diagnosis.

Training and Decision Support

The fourth domain centers around decision support and training. Example applications include airway and ventilator sensors, intelligent alarms, and virtual reality simulation.[46–51] It is paramount to maintain a high degree of situational awareness during airway management, and AI decision support may help the airway practitioner focus on the signal amongst the noise. However, these systems must be transparent with its underlying algorithm due to the catastrophic effects of potential errors (such as incorrect suppression of a critical alarm). Increased sophistication of simulation could also be helpful, particularly with nontechnical skills, but may not be sufficient for skills that require tactile feedback in real patients.

Robotic Techniques Related to Airway Management

The last domain of research is robotic techniques to assist with airway management, including automatic titration of inspired oxygen.[52] intubation,[15–20,53,54] and minimally-invasive tracheotomy.[55] Most of the literature centers on proof-of-concept studies in robotic tracheal intubation, which is the focus of the rest of this chapter. The sequence of steps during intubation by robots will be discussed (see Chapters 9, 10, and 11). For each step, specific considerations will be given to the roles of automation and robotic systems, and their limitations. Using robotic intubation as an example, this chapter will provide a multidisciplinary framework that can be applied to evaluate other novel airway technologies for the opportunity, feasibility, and limitations.

ROBOTIC INTUBATION

Overview

Several different designs of intubating robots have been published. The findings of these proof-of-concept studies are summarized in Table 65.1 and Figures 65.1 to 65.5. The approach to assessing a robotic product design includes determining the range of task(s) and patient population(s) where the robot can be used, the degree of autonomy, whether the robot can learn and respond to change, the durability of materials and construction, and logistical issues during clinical implementation. So far, all intubating robots incorporate equipment that is already central to airway management: the main intubating device is based on either the video laryngoscope or the flexible bronchoscope.

What Are the Critical Steps to Perform Tracheal Intubation, and Which Steps Can Potentially Be Performed by a Robot?

The process of intubation involves eight essential steps. The first step involves decision-making and situational awareness. One must correctly assess anatomic, physiological, and contextual factors to create a plan, including indication, urgency, equipment setup and personnel needed, medication, and the primary airway plan with backup plans.[29] This is perhaps the most complex step and is unlikely to be replaced by AI algorithms in the near future. However, decision support algorithms may play a role in helping nonexperts to identify patients with a difficult airway that could have been missed.

The second step of intubation involves preparation. Equipment setup should include the primary method of intubation and availability of backup plans and verification of the ventilator system. In particular, intubating robots based on a flexible bronchoscope would require lubrication and preloading of the endotracheal tube (ETT). Patient preparation includes denitrogenation, monitoring, positioning, medications, and reassessment. These consist of a wide range of distinct actions and will require a human expert.

The third step is the process of intubation. This first requires opening the mouth and positioning of the jaw, correct insertion of the scope without trauma, and/or suctioning. These tasks will likely require a human operator. This is followed by navigation and identification of relevant anatomy, in particular the glottic opening. This step could be manual, remote-controlled, machine-assisted, and/or automated in existing systems, though we caution against full automation due to potential variations in airway anatomy and the risk of airway trauma. Also, this step is particularly susceptible to poor image quality, such as due to fogging, secretions, bleeding, and/or a coughing or moving patient. The speed of successful intubation is paramount to reducing the risk of oxygen desaturation.

The next step involves accurately placing the ETT through the glottic opening into the trachea to the correct depth without trauma. Existing robot designs based on bronchoscopes may be able to automatically advance the ETT,[20,21] but the force must be carefully controlled to minimize the risk of vocal cord trauma and tracheal rupture. Importantly, bronchoscopic-based techniques do not allow for visualization of the ETT going through the vocal cords during insertion, since the camera is at the tip of the bronchoscope inside the trachea, and excessive force during advancement of the ETT into the trachea should be avoided. To avoid advancing the ETT into a false passage in

SECTION 10

TABLE 65.1. An Overview of Published Intubation Robot Designs and Studies

Study	Design and Main Components	Testing Population	Operator Population	Outcomes (Success Rate, Time for Intubation)
"REALITI" Biro 2020[15], Boehler 2020[21]	Manual or assisted endoscope steering, image recognition, and automated distal tip orientation in manikin.	Manikins	Anesthesia providers (4 physicians, 3 nurse anesthetists) vs. lay participants with no medical training (n = 7) Each performed 6 manual and 6 automated insertions.	Success rate (>95%) and time to glottic visualization without insertion (median 15-18s) were similar in experts and nonexperts, in either manual or automated insertions. Times improved with subsequent attempts.
"RRAIS" Wang 2018[16]	Intubation robot (self-made), control system (self-made), laptop (MSI GE62 6QC), and joystick (Cyborg V.1, MAD CATZ). The robot consisted of a tongue depressor, posture mechanism, and feeding mechanism for the ETT.	Pigs	10 medical students (with <10 prior intubations) inserted and fixed the robot between jaws, then 1 anesthetist operated the remote control. The medical students also performed direct laryngoscopy (DL) for comparison.	Time to intubation was 53.2(3.1)s for DL and 74.6(2.3)s, (23.4(0.7)s by medical students, and 51.2(1.6)s by anesthetist) for the robotic system. First-attempt and overall success rates, respectively, were 40% and 60% for DL, and 80 and 90% for the robot.
"Kepler intubation system" Hemmerling 2012[19,53]	ThrustMaster T. Flight Hotas X joystick (Guillemot Inc, New York, NY, USA), JACO robotic arm (Kinova Rehab, Montreal, QC, Canada), Pentax AWS video laryngoscope (Ambu A/S, Ballerup, Denmark), and software control system. Note that the Pentax AWS video laryngoscope was selected due to having two additional ports on the blade for suction and ETT loading, and a crosshair to indicate optimal scope positioning for ETT advancement. However, the blade is 2.5 cm wide and may not fit in small mouths.	12 patients (11 men and 1 woman), patients with difficult airways, and comorbidities were excluded. Neutral head positioning.	One operator (study team member), with previous experience in >90 intubations in manikins in a previous study[53]	First attempt success 91% (11/12). One failure due to fogging. Duration median (interquartile range, range) was 93 (87-109, 76-153)s.
Tighe 2010[54]	DaVinci Surgical System type S (DVS) (Intuitive Surgical, Sunnyvale, California): 4 separate robotic arms, 1 of which connected to a camera.	Manikin	A urologist steered the DVS for one nasal and one oral intubation. The bronchoscope was first manually placed into the respective pharynx.	Time from entry to carinal visualization was 75s and 67s for oral and nasal intubation, respectively.

TABLE 65.1. An Overview of Published Intubation Robot Designs and Studies (*Continued*)

Study	Design and Main Components	Testing Population	Operator Population	Outcomes (Success Rate, Time for Intubation)
"Intubot" Cheng 2018[20]	Separate motors to steer the stylet forward/ backward and bend the tip. Image-based navigation system can autonomously drive stylet to the glottis.	3D-printed silicone airway model, based on computed tomography images.	Manual initial insertion.	Steering capabilities were tested. The prototype was tested for its steering capabilities.

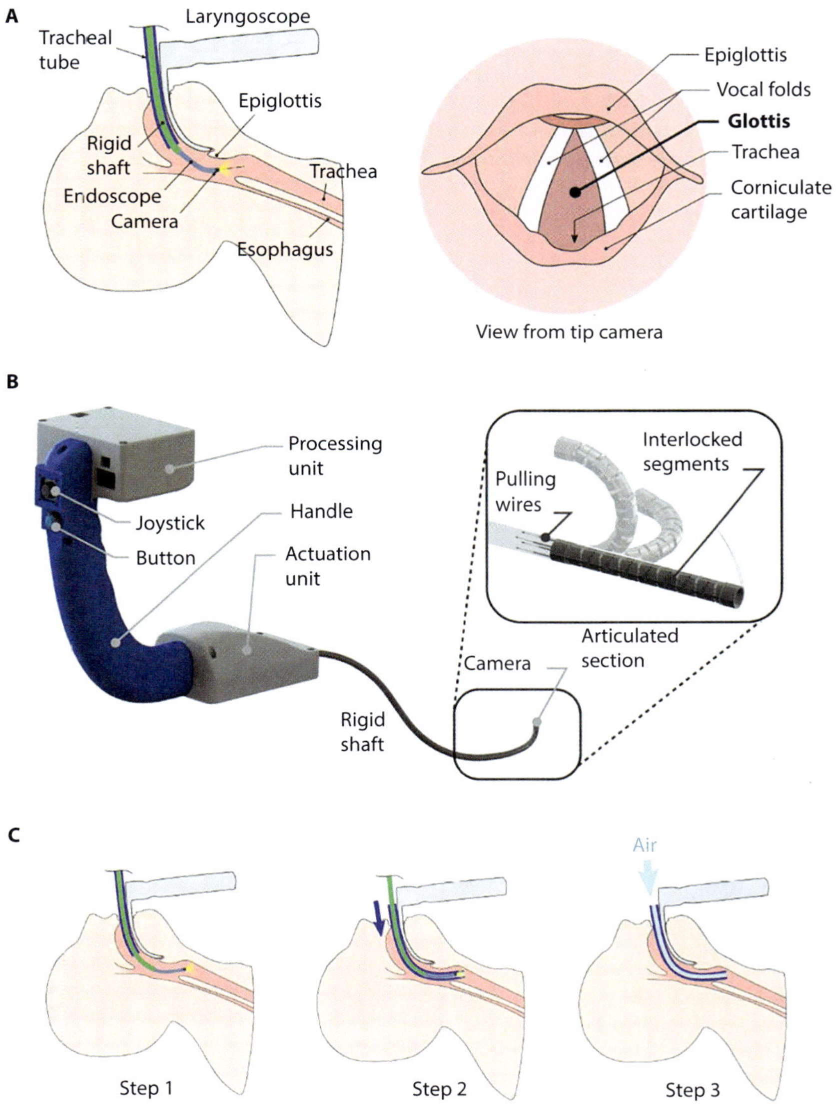

FIGURE 65.1. Tracheal intubation with **REALITI** robotic assistance. (**A**) Setup for the navigation in the larynx with a video endoscope, (**B**) **REALITI** device, and (**C**) intubation process with **REALITI**. (Reproduced with permission from Boehler Q, Gage DS, Hofmann P, et al. REALITI: A robotic endoscope automated via laryngeal imaging for tracheal intubation. *IEEE Trans. Med Robot Bionics*. 2020;2(2):157-164.)

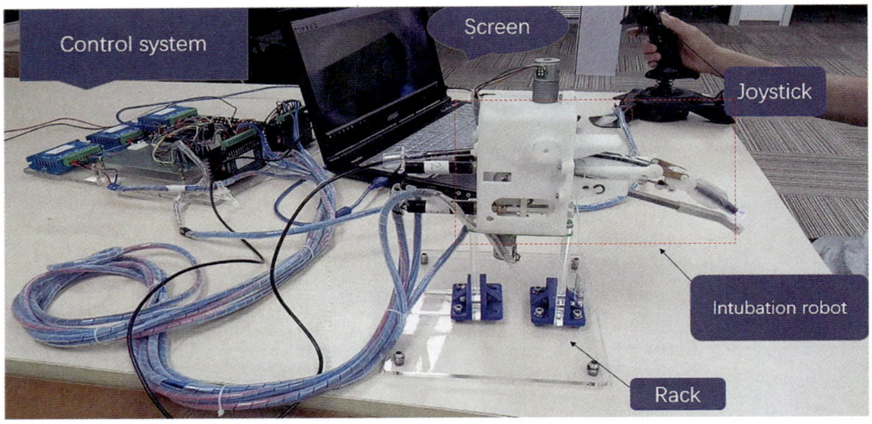

FIGURE 65.2. Four components of the remote robot-assisted intubation system (**RAAIS**): the intubation robot, the control system, the laptop, and the joystick. (Reproduced with permission from Wang X, Tao Y, Tao X, et al. An original design of remote robot-assisted intubation system. *Sci Rep.* 2018;8(1):13403.)

patients with an abnormal upper airway anatomy, it is necessary to use a combined technique, commonly with the addition of a hyperangulated video laryngoscope, to visualize the advancement of the ETT through the vocal cords. In addition, in current robot designs involving video laryngoscopes, a human operator is required to insert the ETT through a channel on the laryngoscope.[16,19] Due to these considerations, the actual insertion of the ETT will likely benefit from human presence.

The last steps involve multiple logistical tasks such as inflating the cuff of the ETT to the correct pressure, removal of the intubation device, securing the ETT, connecting to and starting the ventilator, confirmation of the correct ETT placement with capnography, reassessment of the situation, and adjustment of ventilation and medications. These steps also require a human operator.

In summary, intubation is a complex sequence involving multiple distinct steps. Most existing intubation robot research focuses on the third step: insertion of the intubation device and visualization of the vocal cords. This may be feasible in the

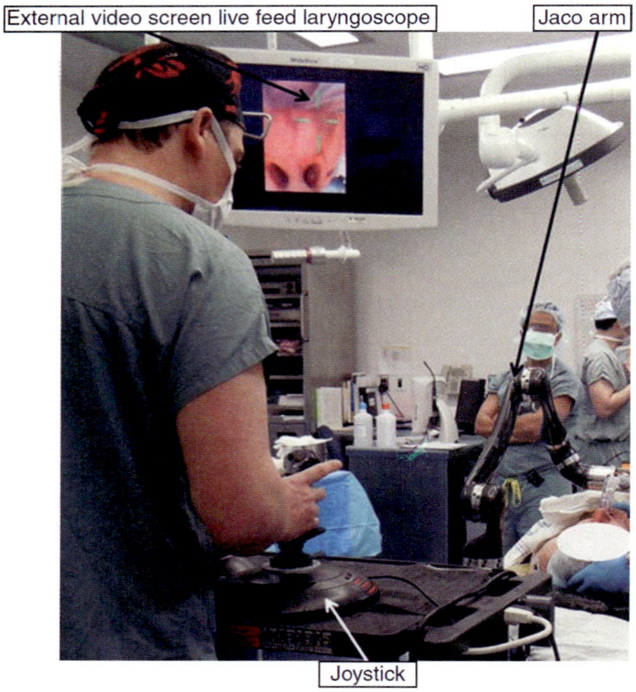

FIGURE 65.3. Illustration of the Kepler intubation system (KIS). The system consists of: a ThrustMaster T.Flight Hotas X joystick (Guillemot Inc), a JACO robotic arm (Kinova Rehab), a Pentax AWS video laryngoscope (Ambu A/S), and a software control system. An assistant is needed to open the mouth while performing robotic intubation. (Reproduced with permission from Hemmerling TM, Taddei R, Wehbe M, et al. First robotic tracheal intubations in humans using the Kepler intubation system. *Br J Anaesth.* 2012;108(6):1011-1016.)

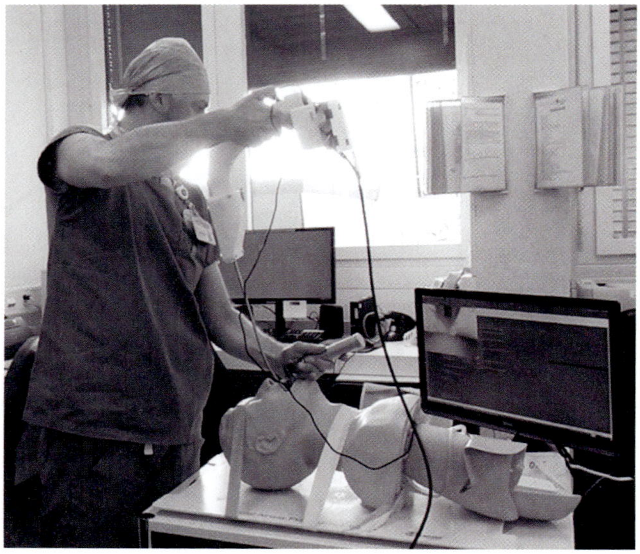

FIGURE 65.4. The setup of the automated tracheal intubation using a robotic endoscope: the intubation manikin and the video monitor displaying the tip camera view and steering information. (Reproduced with permission from Biro P, Hofmann P, Gage D, et al. Automated tracheal intubation in an airway manikin using a robotic endoscope: a proof of concept study. *Anaesthesia.* 2020;75(7):881-886.)

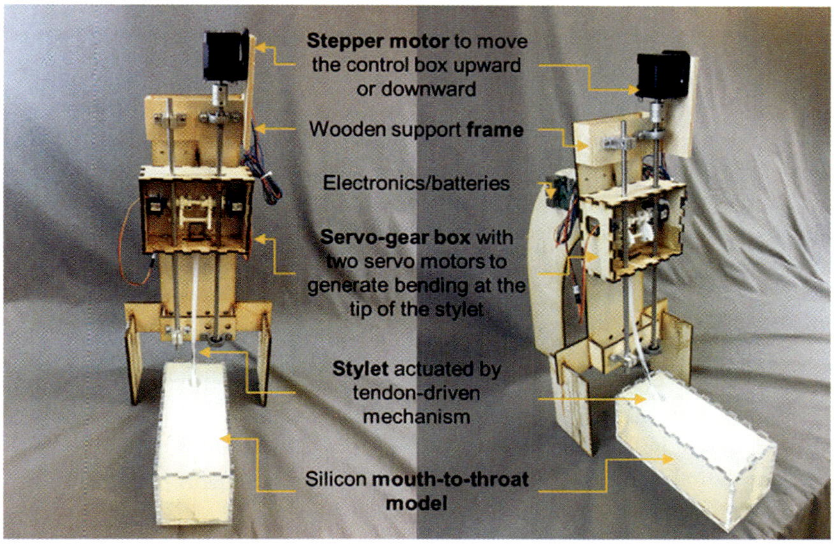

FIGURE 65.5. The prototype of IntuBot which consists of a stepper motor and two servo motors to generate linear and bending motions at the tip of the stylet to navigate through the airway. (Reproduced with permission from Cheng X, Jiang G, Lee K, et al. IntuBot: Design and Prototyping of a Robotic Intubation Device. 2018 IEEE International Conference on Robotics and Automation (ICRA) May 21-25, 2018, Brisbane, Australia.)

setting of remote expert support of a nonexpert intubator. If intubation robots are to be truly self-sufficient, the other steps in the intubation sequence need to be automated as much as possible. For use in areas of high occupational risk, a general-purpose robot that is able to do a variety of tasks may be more helpful than a specific robot that can only perform the insertion of the intubation device and ETT.

What Are the Limitations of Robotic Intubation, and What Should We Study About Them?

Airway management has significantly higher inherent risks than other applications of robotics, where delay or failure may lead to severe morbidity or death. Any robotic intubation system must have a high first-pass success rate and be time-efficient, due to the limited safe apnea period. The margin of safety is particularly small in situations where robotic intubation is purported to be particularly helpful, such as assisting paramedics in the field, use in a patient with respiratory failure with aerosolizing viruses, and deployment in patients with a difficult airway. Limitations to the use of robotics for intubation relate to issues of effectiveness, safety, resources and logistics, training and skill maintenance, and medical-legal regulations.

Robotic intubation needs to be reliably effective and efficient in a wide range of clinical situations. Whether the robot is remote-controlled or autonomous, it is still necessary to have the presence of a human operator to ensure that all steps of the intubation sequence proceed correctly and to provide a backup oxygenation plan if the system has failed. With AI image recognition becoming ever more sophisticated, it is anticipated that these systems will likely be able to identify key anatomic features correctly if given a sufficient variety of training images. However, the robot may struggle with correct navigation through soft tissue, particularly when image quality is impaired by fogging, secretions, blood, and movement of the patient. In the Kepler intubation system, there was one first-pass failure due to fogging during human testing.[19] Future designs may benefit from additional sensors to assist in situations of poor camera visualization. In addition, several studies mentioned potential difficulties in patients with a small mouth opening due to the size of the instruments.[19,20] Thus, prior to deployment, intubation robots must demonstrate success in patients with different types of anatomically difficult airways.

The next key issue is patient safety. First, the robotic intubation device must have force or pressure sensors or other design safeguards to avoid trauma, which can occur during the insertion of the intubation device or ETT. Second, potential contraindications for robotic intubation must be clearly defined to avoid serious adverse outcomes. One such situation involves patients with suspected traumatic airway disruption, where the advancement of the ETT must be clearly visualized to avoid the creation of false passages (see Chapter 10). Third, if there is a failure, the robot needs to be immediately removable to allow for a backup method of oxygenation to be applied. The current robotic designs often involve a mechanical arm installed directly over the patient and may limit access to the airway in an emergency. If the robot is to be deployed without human operators in the field (e.g., to a zone with high occupational risks), it must be designed to perform a variety of tasks including face-mask ventilation, insertion of an extraglottic airway, and a FONA access. Importantly, the robot needs to be able to rapidly make simple troubleshooting adjustments (e.g., for anatomical variations) and switch between tasks, and have a backup plan for failure. Remote human supervision is still required for situational awareness and decision-making.

In addition, since a key premise of the intubating robot is to support nonexperts, the robot needs to be simple enough for the health care provider to set up, operate, remove, and clean up even if the robot is controlled remotely. There needs to be a process to verify device functionality, similar to the checkout procedure in all modern ventilators. The operator should also be familiar with simple solutions to common potential mechanical and electronic failures. Also, the remote controller in current designs is often a joystick,[16,19] which represents different tactile motions and techniques from traditional motions that anesthesia practitioners are familiar with. Thus, when developing intubating robots, the learning curve and skill maintenance must be determined prior to implementation. Moreover, standardization of components and knobs is mandatory, to reduce increased setup and intubation times when different systems are in circulation.

Logistical issues must also be considered. A robotic system must be cost-effective and affordable for many health systems. For successful deployment, it needs to be built using durable material that is safe, lightweight, portable, and easy to sanitize for repeated use. The mechanical components must be simple for rapid troubleshooting, and replaceable using standardized components. The integration of manufacturing, software, and hardware must be seamless, to facilitate timely algorithm upgrades and repairs.

Lastly, ethical and medical-legal issues must be addressed. Who would be responsible for the mistakes, such as esophageal intubation or airway trauma, that are made by the autonomous robot? In addition, if the product is marketed to support nonexperts, supervision, and responsibility need to be clearly defined. For example, for a nonexpert who relies on the robotic system for support, a delayed call for urgent expert consultation when the robotic intubation has failed may lead to preventable morbidity and mortality in a critically ill patient. Furthermore, regulation needs to be in place for training, certification, and skill maintenance. With the availability of remote control, the geographic scope of licensure must be addressed. Given these considerations, robotic intubation systems may be most useful as remote-controllable, semiautonomous devices that could be deployed in the setting of dangerous exposures or remote expert support.

SUMMARY

In summary, this chapter provides a brief review of existing research involving robotics and AI in airway management. These include the identification of patients with difficult airways, real-time guided navigation, prediction and detection of airway complications, decision support, as well as robotic intubation systems. While there are significant opportunities in using these robotic and AI systems in different clinical settings, these systems have limitations that should be addressed prior to implementation. This chapter also discussed robotic intubation, to provide an example framework to evaluate the potential use of novel technologies in airway management. Intubation robots are promising technologies that may be particularly useful in settings of high occupational risk and remote expert support, though a human operator is still required in all existing designs. Future rigorous research is needed to validate the novel technologies in diverse populations and address potential limitations in effectiveness, harm, education, logistics, and legal issues.

SELF-EVALUATION QUESTIONS

65.1. What areas in airway management have robotics and AI research been performed?

A. Identification of patients with difficult airways
B. Real-time image and navigation support
C. Monitoring and risk prediction
D. Training and decision support
E. All of the above

65.2. What are the caveats to consider when assessing the feasibility for the implementation of a robotic and/or AI technology?

A. Reliability
B. Safeguards for patient safety
C. Learning and skill maintenance
D. Medical-legal issues
E. All of the above

65.3. Which of the following statements is **FALSE**?

A. Existing robotic intubation designs do not require human operators.
B. A robot that is autonomous means that it can perform tasks without specific human instruction.
C. AI algorithms for anatomical difficult airway prediction may not be adequate in situations of dynamic changes such as labor and postoperative airway edema.
D. One must correctly assess anatomic, physiological, and contextual factors to create a plan for airway management, which is unlikely to be replaced by AI in the near future.

REFERENCES

1. Engelberger J. *Robotics in Practice: Management and Applications of Industrial Robots*. Springer; 1980. Available at: https://link.springer.com/book/10.1007/978-1-4684-7120-5. Accessed December 28, 2021.
2. Engelberger JF. *Robotics in Service*. Cambridge, MA: MIT Press; 1989.
3. Lane T. A short history of robotic surgery. *Ann R Coll Surg Engl.* 2018;100 (6 sup):5-7.
4. Taylor RH. Computer-integrated interventional medicine: a 30-year perspective. In: Kevin Zhou S, Rueckert D, Fichtinger G, eds. *Handbook of Medical Image Computing and Computer Assisted Intervention*. Elsevier; 2019: 599-624.
5. Sefati S, Hegeman R, Iordachita I, Taylor RH, Armand M. A dexterous robotic system for autonomous debridement of osteolytic bone lesions in confined spaces: human cadaver studies. *IEEE Trans Robot.* 2022;38(2):1213-1229.
6. Kassamali RH, Ladak B. The role of robotics in interventional radiology: current status. *Quant Imaging Med Surg.* 2015;5(3):340-343.
7. Taylor RH, Mittelstadt BD, Paul HA, et al. An image-directed robotic system for precise orthopaedic surgery. *IEEE Trans Robot Autom.* 1994;10(3):261-275.
8. Solomon S, Patriciu A, Taylor R, Kavoussi L, Stoianvici D. CT guided robotic needle biopsy: a precise sampling method minimizing radiation exposure. *Radiology.* 2002;225:277-282.
9. Chen Y, Zhang S, Wu Z, Yang B, Luo Q, Xu K. Review of surgical robotic systems for keyhole and endoscopic procedures: state of the art and perspectives. *Front Med.* 2020;14(4):382-403.
10. Guthart GS, Salisbury JK. The Intuitive/sup TM/ telesurgery system: overview and application. In: *Proceedings 2000 ICRA Millennium Conference*

IEEE International Conference on Robotics and Automation Symposia Proceedings (Cat No00CH37065). 2000;1:618-621.
11. Yang G-Z, Cambias J, Cleary K, Daimler E, et al. Medical robotics—Regulatory, ethical, and legal considerations for increasing levels of autonomy. *Sci Robot*. 2017;2(4):eaam8638.
12. Joiner IA. Chapter 1: Artificial intelligence: AI is nearby. In: Joiner IA, ed. *Emerging Library Technologies*. Chandos Publishing; 2018:1-22. Available at: https://www.sciencedirect.com/science/article/pii/B9780081022535000022. Accessed December 28, 2021.
13. Matava C, Pankiv E, Ahumada L, Weingarten B, Simpao A. Artificial intelligence, machine learning and the pediatric airway. *Paediatr Anaesth*. 2020;30(3):264-268.
14. Zemmar A, Lozano AM, Nelson BJ. The rise of robots in surgical environments during COVID-19. *Nat Mach Intell*. 2020;2(10):566-572.
15. Biro P, Hofmann P, Gage D, et al. Automated tracheal intubation in an airway manikin using a robotic endoscope: a proof of concept study. *Anaesthesia*. 2020;75(7):881-886.
16. Wang X, Tao Y, Tao X, et al. An original design of remote robot-assisted intubation system. *Sci Rep*. 2018;8(1):13403.
17. Carlson JN, Das S, De la Torre F, et al. A Novel Artificial Intelligence System for endotracheal intubation. *Prehosp Emerg Care*. 2016 Oct;20(5):667-671.
18. Kurata S, Sanuki T, Okayasu I, Kawai M, Moromugi S, Ayuse T. A pilot study of upper airway management using a remote-controlled artificial muscle device during propofol anesthesia. *J Clin Anesth*. 2016;29:75-82.
19. Hemmerling TM, Taddei R, Wehbe M, Zaouter C, Cyr S, Morse J. First robotic tracheal intubations in humans using the Kepler intubation system. *Br J Anaesth*. 2012;108(6):1011-1016.
20. Cheng X, Jiang G, Lee K, Laker YN. IntuBot: Design and prototyping of a robotic intubation device. In: *2018 IEEE International Conference on Robotics and Automation (ICRA)*. IEEE; 2018:1482-1487.
21. Boehler Q, Gage DS, Hofmann P, et al. REALITI: a robotic endoscope automated via laryngeal imaging for tracheal intubation. *IEEE Trans Med Robot Bionics*. 2020;2(2):157-164.
22. Cuendet GL, Schoettker P, Yüce A, et al. Facial image analysis for fully automatic prediction of difficult endotracheal intubation. *IEEE Trans Biomed Eng*. 2016;63(2):328-339.
23. Yan H-M, Wei X-C, Zhang H, Chen X-F, Luo E-Q. Predicting Cormack classification based on neural network with multiple anthropometric features. In: *The 2010 International Conference on Apperceiving Computing and Intelligence Analysis Proceeding*. 2010:52-55.
24. Sreekantha DK, Rhea Carmel Glen R, Prajna MK, Mehandale SG, Saldanha RS, Krishnappa GJ. Prediction of difficulties in Intubation using an expert system. In: *2019 IEEE International Conference on Distributed Computing, VLSI, Electrical Circuits and Robotics (DISCOVER)*. 2019:1-7.
25. Detsky ME, Jivraj N, Adhikari NK, et al. Will this patient be difficult to intubate?: the rational clinical examination systematic review. *JAMA*. 2019;321(5):493-503.
26. Rauenzahn B, Chung J, Kaufman A. Facing bias in facial recognition technology. Available at: https://www.theregreview.org/2021/03/20/saturday-seminar-facing-bias-in-facial-recognition-technology/. Accessed December 28, 2021.
27. Hung OR, Morris I. Dynamic anatomy of upper airway: an essential paradigm. *Can J Anesth*. 2000;47(4):295-298.
28. Farcon EL, Kim MH, Marx GF. Changing Mallampati score during labour. *Can J Anaesth*. 1994;41(1):50–51.
29. Law JA, Duggan LV, Asselin M, et al. Canadian Airway Focus Group updated consensus-based recommendations for management of the difficult airway: part 2. Planning and implementing safe management of the patient with an anticipated difficult airway. *Can J Anaesth*. 2021;68(9):1405-1436.
30. Dunham ME, Kong KA, McWhorter AJ, Adkins LK. Optical biopsy: automated classification of airway endoscopic findings using a convolutional neural network. *Laryngoscope*. 2020;132(Suppl 4):S1-S8.
31. Siyambalapitiya SDMH, Wanigasekara RMR, Dissanayake SDSH, Jayaratne KL, Wickramasinghe MIE. Generate Navigations to Guide and Automate Nasotracheal Intubation Process. In: *2019 19th International Conference on Advances in ICT for Emerging Regions (ICTer)*. 2019:1-10.
32. Matava C, Pankiv E, Raisbeck S, Caldeira M, Alam F. A convolutional neural network for real time classification, identification, and labelling of vocal cord and tracheal using laryngoscopy and bronchoscopy video. *J Med Syst*. 2020;44(2):44.
33. Ho AMH, Chung DC, To EWH, Karmakar MK. Total airway obstruction during local anesthesia in a non-sedated patient with a compromised airway. *Can J Anaesth*. 2004;51(8):838-841.
34. Shashikumar SP, Wardi G, Paul P, et al. Development and prospective validation of a deep learning algorithm for predicting need for mechanical ventilation. *Chest*. 2021;159(6):2264-2273.
35. Siu BMK, Kwak GH, Ling L, Hui P. Predicting the need for intubation in the first 24 h after critical care admission using machine learning approaches. *Sci Rep*. 2020;10(1):20931.
36. Arvind V, Kim JS, Cho BH, Geng E, Cho SK. Development of a machine learning algorithm to predict intubation among hospitalized patients with COVID-19. *J Crit Care*. 2021;62:25-30.
37. Schwartz AR, Cohen-Zion M, Pham LV, et al. Brief digital sleep questionnaire powered by machine learning prediction models identifies common sleep disorders. *Sleep Med*. 2020;71:66-76.
38. Lim J, Alshaer H, Khan SS, Pandya A, et al. Diagnosis of obstructive sleep apnea during wakefulness using upper airway negative pressure and machine learning. *Annu Int Conf IEEE Eng Med Biol Soc*. 2019;2019:1605-1608.
39. Amaral JLM, Lopes AJ, Veiga J, Faria ACD, Melo PL. High-accuracy detection of airway obstruction in asthma using machine learning algorithms and forced oscillation measurements. *Comput Methods Programs Biomed*. 2017;144:113-125.
40. Knorr-Chung BR, McGrath SP, Blike GT. Identifying airway obstructions using photoplethysmography (PPG). *J Clin Monit Comput*. 2008;22(2):95-101.
41. Ren O, Johnson AEW, Lehman EP, et al. Predicting and understanding unexpected respiratory decompensation in critical care using sparse and heterogeneous clinical data. In: *2018 IEEE International Conference on Healthcare Informatics (ICHI)*. 2018:144-151.
42. Chen T, Xu J, Ying H, et al. Prediction of extubation failure for intensive care unit patients using light gradient boosting machine. *IEEE Access*. 2019;7:150960-150968.
43. Haidar R, Koprinska I, Jeffries B. Sleep apnea event prediction using convolutional neural networks and Markov chains. In: *2020 International Joint Conference on Neural Networks (IJCNN)*. 2020:1-8.
44. Hafezi M, Montazeri N, Saha S, et al. Sleep apnea severity estimation from tracheal movements using a deep learning model. *IEEE Access*. 2020;8:22641-22649.
45. Hurtado DE, Chávez JAP, Mansilla R, Lopez R, Abusleme A. Respiratory volume monitoring: a machine-learning approach to the non-invasive prediction of tidal volume and minute ventilation. *IEEE Access*. 2020;8: 227936-227944.
46. Das S, Carlson JN, De la Torre F, Phrampus PE, Hodgins J. Multimodal feature analysis for quantitative performance evaluation of endotracheal intubation (ETI). In: *2012 IEEE International Conference on Acoustics, Speech and Signal Processing (ICASSP)*. 2012:621-624.
47. Matsuoka Y, Bartolomeo L, Chihara T, et al. A novel approach to evaluate skills in endotracheal intubation using biomechanical measurement system. In: *2013 IEEE International Conference on Robotics and Biomimetics (ROBIO)*. 2013:1456-1461.
48. Noh Y, Shimomura A, Segawa M, et al. Development of Tension/Compression Detection Sensor System designed to acquire quantitative force information while training the airway management task. In: *2009 IEEE/ASME International Conference on Advanced Intelligent Mechatronics*. 2009:1264-1269.
49. Noh Y, Wang C, Tokumoto M, Matsuoka Y, et al. Development of the airway Management Training System WKA-5: Improvement of mechanical designs for high-fidelity patient simulation. In: *2012 IEEE International Conference on Robotics and Biomimetics (ROBIO)*. 2012:1224-1229.
50. Stegmaier PA, Brunner JX, Zollinger A. An intelligent airway sensor system to increase safety in computer controlled mechanical ventilation. In: *Proceedings of 17th International Conference of the Engineering in Medicine and Biology Society*. 1995;1:727-728.
51. Wang C, Noh Y, Ebihara K, et al. Development of a novel flow sensor to acquire quantitative information on BVM operation during airway management training. In: *2011 IEEE International Conference on Robotics and Biomimetics*. 2011:269-274.
52. Hansen EF, Hove JD, Bech CS, Jensen J-US, Kallemose T, Vestbo J. Automated oxygen control with O2matic® during admission with exacerbation of COPD. *Int J Chron Obstruct Pulmon Dis*. 2018;13:3997-4003.
53. Hemmerling TM, Wehbe M, Zaouter C, Taddei R, Morse J. The Kepler intubation system. *Anesth Analg*. 2012;114(3):590-594.
54. Tighe PJ, Badiyan SJ, Luria I, Lampotang S, Parekattil S. Robot-assisted airway support: a simulated case. *Anesth Analg*. 2010;111(4):929-931.
55. Botyrius M, Liu Q, Lim CM, Ren H. Design conceptualization of a flexible robotic drill system for minimally invasive tracheostomy. In: *2018 IEEE International Conference on Real-time Computing and Robotics (RCAR)*. 2018:584-588.

CHAPTER 66

Documentation of Difficult and Failed Airway Management

James Nielsen, George Zhong, Kar-Soon Lim, and Lucien Hackett

CASE PRESENTATION

A 39-year-old woman is booked for laparoscopic cholecystectomy. She takes no medications, has no allergies, and denies reflux. She is 5′4″ (163 cm) and 220 lb (100 kg), BMI 38.6 $kg{\cdot}m^{-2}$. On airway exam, she is Mallampati Class II, has 4 cm of mouth opening, good neck extension, and a thyromental distance of 5 cm. The anesthetic record from previous orthopedic surgery is requested but does not arrive before surgery.

After denitrogenation, anesthesia is induced with fentanyl 150 μg, propofol 200 mg, and rocuronium 60 mg. One-hand face-mask ventilation produces signs of airway obstruction and no capnograph. A two-hand technique with an oropharyngeal airway achieves a low-amplitude capnograph. Subsequent direct laryngoscopy reveals epiglottis only, with no improvement from external laryngeal manipulation. A tracheal introducer (commonly called "bougie") inserted blindly enters the esophagus so it is removed. Repeat face-mask ventilation remains difficult and the patient is becoming hypoxemic. A size 3 second-generation extraglottic device (EGD) insertion fails to produce a capnograph; a size 4 leaks but permits rescue oxygenation.

Help and the difficult airway cart are summoned. Video laryngoscopy with a hyperangulated blade reveals blood and swelling around the epiglottis. After suctioning, there is a partial view of the larynx with a head lift and external laryngeal manipulation. A bougie and size 7.0-mm internal diameter (ID) endotracheal tube (ETT) are inserted, and intubation is confirmed by the presence of end-tidal CO_2.

Surgery is routine. Extubation is smooth and the surgical recovery is uncomplicated, but the patient has a severe sore throat and hoarse voice for several weeks postoperatively. This significantly affects her work as a teacher.

INTRODUCTION

How Could Access to Documentation of Previous Airway Management Improve This?

Suppose the previous anesthetic record did arrive in time, and its airway section stated:

- Face-mask ventilation: difficult
- EGD: 2nd generation, size #4
- Laryngoscopy: grade 2 with video laryngoscope; bougie used

Would this have changed the approach to the patient's airway management?

What about this more detailed version, which documents both process and outcome?

- Face-mask ventilation: two-handed technique, oropharyngeal airway, muscle relaxation → minimal end-tidal CO_2
- EGD: second generation, size #3 → no capnograph; second generation, size #4 → low-amplitude capnograph, audible leak
- Direct Laryngoscopy: #3 Macintosh blade → Grade 3 view despite external laryngeal manipulation; bougie into

the esophagus. Video laryngoscope with hyperangulated blade → Grade 2 view; bougie inserted with external laryngeal manipulation and head lift.

Here is the same case managed with knowledge of this detailed previous anesthetic record.

A 39-year-old woman presents for laparoscopic cholecystectomy. A history of difficulty with face-mask ventilation and direct laryngoscopy is noted. The anesthetic team plan to avoid face-mask ventilation, give high-flow nasal oxygen before and during denitrogenation, tailor induction drugs to achieve intubating conditions sooner, and use a video laryngoscope with hyperangulated blade for their first laryngoscopy attempt.

The patient is meticulously positioned before denitrogenation. The difficult airway cart is brought into the operating room and a rescue size 4 second-generation EGD is prepared. Anesthesia is induced with alfentanil 1500 μg, propofol 200 mg, and rocuronium 100 mg. Video laryngoscopy 90 seconds later reveals a grade 2 laryngeal view and a bougie and a 7.0-mm ID ETT are inserted at the first pass. Surgery is routine, extubation smooth, and the recovery uneventful.

Afterward, the patient is grateful for her care and comments that "My voice is totally normal, unlike last time when it took weeks to recover!"

Why Should We Document the Difficult Airway?

The difficult airway is easier to manage when anticipated. The 4th National Audit Project (NAP4) on major complications of airway management in the United Kingdom found that failure to document and communicate airway difficulty was an important risk factor for subsequent airway complications.[1] Similarly, a Canadian case series examining airway-related medicolegal claims between 2007 and 2016 found that the most common contributing factor was inadequate airway assessment and planning.[2] Clinicians were often unaware of previous airway problems, especially when information was not readily available or was difficult to obtain.

Unfortunately, the prediction of difficulty based on clinical assessment alone is unreliable.[3,4] In large cohort studies from Denmark[4] (188,064 patients) and the United States[5] (176,679 patients), over 90% of cases of difficult intubation or difficult face-mask ventilation were unpredicted. In the US study, the positive predictive value of clinical assessment was only 3%,[6] even among patients with the most risk factors. Studies of the prediction of difficulty with extraglottic airway devices have also found low positive predictive values.[7,8]

Awareness of previous difficulty can improve both anesthesia planning and informed consent. It may prompt the anesthesia team to advise an awake airway technique or perhaps regional anesthesia to avoid any airway manipulation. It may also make the patient more amenable to that advice. NAP4 showed that awake flexible bronchoscopic intubation was frequently indicated but not used and this probably contributed to many of the ensuing complications. In some of these cases, airway practitioners were unaware of previous difficulties.[1]

If general anesthesia is unavoidable, the anticipation of risk enables airway practitioners to prepare. Assistance or special equipment can be readied before a hypoxemic crisis, not *during* one. Knowing what did and did not work previously also increases the chance of first-pass success by *not repeating previous failures*. First-pass success is a core objective when managing difficult airways[9] as trauma from multiple attempts increases morbidity (such as aspiration and cardiac arrest[10]) and it may make a difficult airway even harder.

AIRWAY MANAGEMENT DOCUMENTATION

What Should Be Documented?

Airway documentation should help future airway practitioners improve the anesthetic plan. To facilitate this, records should describe both the airway management *process* (techniques and equipment used) and its *outcome* (effects on the patient). Outcome measures can be defined as objective markers of the effectiveness of the procedure in the patient, distinct from techniques used by the airway practitioner.

Documentation of both process and outcome is a standard that should apply to all airway techniques, not just tracheal intubation. This includes face-mask ventilation, the use of extraglottic airway devices, and advanced techniques such as flexible bronchoscopic intubation and surgical airways.

Another important principle is that *all* attempts at airway management should be documented. To improve first-pass success, it is important to know the details of techniques that failed as well as those that succeeded. Comments on possible causes of failure may also be useful.

Finally, communication is better if it is concise and relevant and avoids information overload.[11] Some airway alerts include other information such as past medical and surgical histories, airway assessment, dentition, and planned operation, but excessive detail may add more distraction than value.

Face-Mask Ventilation (see Chapters 1 and 8)

Process: One or two hands, grip (C-E/V-E), airway adjuncts, head tilt, muscle relaxation, and operator comments on subjective difficulty

Outcome: Capnography waveform

Face-mask ventilation has been relatively neglected in anesthesia research. In a recent Cochrane difficult airway review, only 7 of 133 included studies that examined face-mask ventilation.[12] This neglect is reflected in clinical records. A single-center US audit of 23,011 anesthetic charts found almost 90% lacked data on face-mask ventilation.[13] Similarly, a 2016 editorial and survey of anesthetic records from 10 countries showed a near-exclusive focus on tracheal intubation.[14]

One likely cause for this is lack of consensus in *defining* difficult face-mask ventilation. The 2022 ASA Difficult Airway Guidelines offer a streamlined definition: failure to achieve adequate ventilation as measured by capnography.[9] End-tidal CO_2 ($ETCO_2$) has clear validity as an outcome measure: it is objective, immediate, and specific for alveolar ventilation. A 2019 Scandinavian survey found capnography to be the outcome most preferred by clinicians to assess face-mask ventilation.[15]

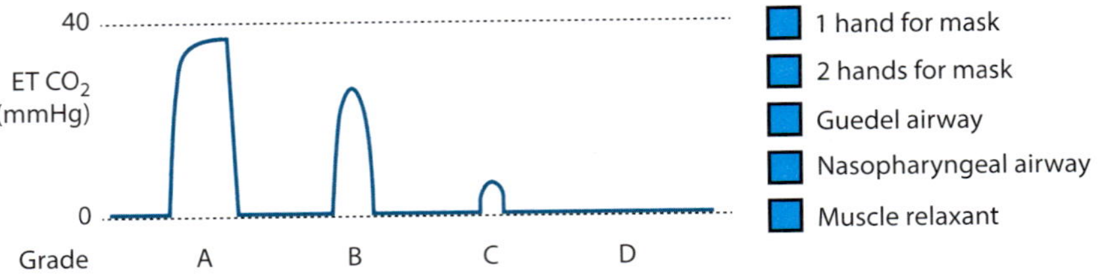

FIGURE 66.1. Objective grading scale for mask ventilation based on the capnograph. Grade A: plateau present. Grade B: no plateau, end-tidal $CO_2 \geq 10$ mmHg (≥ 1.3 kPa). Grade C: no plateau, end-tidal $CO_2 < 10$ mmHg (< 1.3 kPa). Grade D: no end-tidal CO_2/flatline.

Lim's scale (**Figure 66.1**) is a simple and pragmatic tool that uses capnography to grade face-mask ventilation objectively.[16] It helps airway practitioners assess face-mask ventilation in real-time and document it by both process and outcome afterward. This scale also provides an objective definition of difficult face-mask ventilation: when the best attempt results in a grade C or D capnograph.

Extraglottic Airway Device (EGD) Insertion

Process: Type and size of EGD, insertion maneuvers, airway positioning, airway cuff pressure, muscle relaxation, and number of attempts

Outcome: Capnography waveform, leak pressure, details of intubation through the EGD if applicable

EGDs are the most common airways used in general anesthesia,[1] but no scale is widely accepted to grade their outcome or difficulty. Records often describe only the type and size of EGD used. Airway cuff pressure and the number of insertion attempts both correlate with morbidity[17] and the risk of EGD failure,[18] but these are rarely documented.

The use of an EGD may also result in a spectrum of outcomes between success and failure. An optimally positioned EGD supports positive pressure ventilation with a good seal; a malpositioned EGD may leak at low pressure or require excessive pressure to achieve adequate tidal volumes; a failed EGD may result in complete airway obstruction. The airway practitioner's threshold to accept the outcome may also vary. An outcome considered inadequate for a long case might be "adequate" for a short one or even deemed a "success" for reoxygenation in a crisis (as in the case above). Documenting the details of these outcomes can improve future airway planning.

The 2022 ASA Guidelines on the Difficult Airway recommend $ETCO_2$ as the marker to assess ventilation through an EGD in the pediatric flowchart but do not specify an outcome measure in their adult one.[9] The authors of this chapter consider $ETCO_2$ to be a valid outcome measure for EGD insertion in both children and adults.

Laryngoscopy and Tracheal Intubation

Process: Type of laryngoscope and blade, patient positioning, maneuvers, adjuncts to aid tube delivery, number of attempts

Outcome: Laryngoscopic view, confirmation ($ETCO_2$ and auscultation), insertion depth

For the process, it is routine to report the type of laryngoscope and blade, use of adjuncts to aid tube delivery (e.g., bougies, stylets), and size and type of ETT. The number of attempts correlates with airway difficulty and morbidity and is simple to record, but it is subject to multiple confounders. The definition of "attempts" is unclear, and their invasiveness varies: compare one diagnostic look with a video laryngoscope to a direct laryngoscopy with multiple passes of a bougie. Thus, beyond the number of attempts, the inclusion of details associated with each attempt, its outcome, and the likely causes of difficulty is more clinically useful.

For outcome, the Cormack and Lehane grading scale[19] (in various versions) is widely used to describe the view of the larynx on direct laryngoscopy. Its advantages are simplicity, familiarity, objectivity, and reproducibility, although knowledge and interpretation of it may vary.[20] However, it was not designed for video laryngoscopy and describes only the view achieved, not tube delivery. With the increased use of video laryngoscopy, alternatives such as the percentage of glottic opening[21] and Fremantle[22] scales have been developed but are yet to gain widespread acceptance. The authors believe that for video laryngoscopy, it is important to document details on the process, outcome, and difficulty of tracheal intubation, not only the Cormack and Lehane grade.[23]

Awake Techniques

Process: Positioning of airway practitioner and patient, sedation, topicalization, oxygenation method, type and size of scope and ETT, adjuvant insertion maneuvers, number of attempts

Outcome: Ability to pass flexible bronchoscope through cords, ability to pass ETT through cords (type of ETT: Magill or Parker), patient cooperation and/or tolerance, anatomical abnormalities

Awake techniques include flexible bronchoscopic intubation and awake laryngoscopy (usually video laryngoscopy). There is limited guidance on how to document them.

A joint Australian and New Zealand guideline on awake flexible bronchoscopic intubation[24] notes that patients may have to undergo this procedure repeatedly. Clear documentation of what worked, what failed, and any suggestions for improvement are important for future care. This guideline also recommends performing conventional laryngoscopy after flexible bronchoscopic intubation and documenting the resulting Cormack-Lehane grade—while recognizing that the presence of an ETT may alter the view obtained.

Front-Of-Neck Airway (FONA) and Failed Airway Management

Process: Equipment and method used, positioning, use of ultrasound,

Outcome: Ability to oxygenate through cannula/bougie measured by oxygen saturations, presence of chest rise. Ability to ventilate measured by capnography. Immediate patient disposition (e.g., intensive care, death).

Failure of conventional airway management requiring FONA is a critical incident with a high risk of mortality. Records are important for quality assurance, morbidity and mortality reporting, and medicolegal reasons. Clear documentation of the details of failed attempts is essential to plan future care.

DISSEMINATION OF DIFFICULT AIRWAY INFORMATION

How Should Difficult Airway Records Be Disseminated?

As our case study illustrates, records are only useful to subsequent airway practitioners if they are readily accessible. This requirement becomes especially challenging when care occurs at different hospitals or locations.

The process to make airway information more accessible begins with a postoperative visit to explain the critical importance of airway difficulty to the patient. A letter or card for the patient and their family doctor helps to reinforce this.[25,26]

Although these are standard recommendations, they do not always occur in practice. A New Zealand survey of patients with a difficult airway found that only 12% recalled a postoperative visit, 11% received a letter or card, and only 10% of family doctors received a record of airway difficulty.[27] These findings highlight the need for a multimodal approach to communicating this information.

While the patient is in the hospital, useful methods include signs at the bedside, wristbands, and flags in the electronic medical record. After discharge, options include alert cards, medical alert bracelets, and information carried on the patient's smartphone. Finally, system-based resources include electronic health records and online airway databases.

Bedside Alerts

Difficult airway alerts can be placed at the patient's bedside—for example, signs which identify post-tracheotomy patients as having either a patent or closed upper airway. This method may restrict the warning to the bedside, however, and not cover situations where the airway management occurs elsewhere.

Wristbands

A colored wristband noting difficult intubation has been advocated, just as wristbands are used to warn of allergies.[28] As it is attached to the patient, this simple alert covers all locations in the hospital.

Permanently Worn Alerts

Patients can wear permanent alerts as a bracelet or necklace, or in a smartwatch. The medical alert bracelet may also be linked to online databases, although this may entail costs to create the tag and maintain a database subscription.

Electronic Medical Record (EMR) Alerts

Airway alerts can be added to a patient's EMR. However, these alerts may be difficult to access at the bedside or during a crisis, and they may not be accessible from other institutions.

Standardized coding may help identify patients with difficult airways on electronic health records. SNOMED-CT (systematized nomenclature of medicine–clinical terms) aims to standardize nomenclature for medical terminology.[29] It includes a code for difficulty with face-mask ventilation and tracheal intubation (718446005).

Smartphones

Airway alerts can be stored on patients' smartphones as an app[30] or simply as a photo of a difficult airway alert letter. This takes advantage of the fact that these devices are both widely available and routinely carried by the patient.

Online Difficult Airway Registries

Several online difficult airway databases exist. Two examples are the MedicAlert National Registry for Difficult Airway/Intubation in the United States[31] and the Difficult Airway Society database in the United Kingdom.[32] For the latter, an Airway Alert Card is issued to consenting patients and their anonymized data is entered into an online database. Patient information can be accessed by the NHS patient number or a unique code on the Airway Alert Card.[32]

Which Patients Should Receive an Alert?

In the United Kingdom, the Difficult Airway Society (DAS) offers a pragmatic recommendation: issue an alert "if an experienced clinician feels that the information provided will have a positive impact in the management of the patient's airway."[32]

Sample Difficult Airway Alert Forms

The Australian and New Zealand College of Anaesthetists (ANZCA) recently endorsed a Difficult Airway Alert form (Figure 66.2).[33] It is a comprehensive record of airway management in a concise and accessible format. The DAS alert form is another simpler example (Figure 66.3).[32]

SUMMARY

Airway documentation may seem a dry topic, but for the airway practitioner faced with a difficult airway, the previous airway record becomes acutely important.

A key part of managing a difficult airway is to document and disseminate information that will make future airway management safer. Both patients and future colleagues who look after them will benefit from this. To maximize that benefit, *all* airway attempts should be described by both process and outcome, and *multiple* methods used to share this information widely.

DO NOT WRITE IN THIS BINDING MARGIN

ANZCA FPM

Difficult Airway Alert

Facility: ....

(Affix identification label here)

URN:

Family name:

Given name(s):

Address:

Date of birth: Sex: ☐M ☐F ☐I

TO THE PATIENT:
- During your recent procedure your airway was found to be more difficult to manage than in most other people. This can make it more difficult to get oxygen to the lungs, heart, brain and other vital organs, which can potentially lead to serious and harmful outcomes, including death.
- Please keep this letter safe and show it to your doctor if you are admitted to hospital, and show it to the anaesthetic doctor if you need an operation.

TO THE GP: Please copy this letter with any future referral.

Summary of Airway Management

Date of intervention:		☐ Elective	☐ Emergency		Patient weight (kg):
Reason for airway intervention:					
Was difficulty predicted?	☐ Yes	☐ No			
Details:					
Bag mask ventilation Subjective	☐ Easy		☐ Difficult	☐ Impossible	☐ Not attempted
Capnography[§]	☐ A	☐ B	☐ C	☐ D	
Method	☐ 1 hand[†]	☐ 2 hands[†]	☐ OPA	☐ NPA	
Comments:					
Supraglottic airway ventilation	☐ Easy	☐ Difficult	☐ Impossible	☐ Not attempted	
Comments:					
Tracheal intubation	☐ Easy	☐ Difficult	☐ Impossible	☐ Not attempted	
Comments:					
Direct laryngoscopy C&L	☐ Grade 1	☐ Grade 2: ○A ○B	☐ Grade 3: ○A ○B	☐ Grade 4	
Comments:					
Video laryngoscopy	Type of VL:	Blade:	POGO score:		
Comments:					
Was a muscle relaxant used?	☐ BMV	☐ SGA	☐ Direct laryngoscopy	☐ Videolaryngoscopy	
Details:					
Was front of neck access attempted?	☐ Yes	☐ No			
Details:					

[§]See over for grading capnography reference image.
[†]1 or 2 hands for mask; OPA, oropharyngeal airway; NPA, nasopharyngeal airway; VL, videolaryngoscope; POGO, percentage of glottic opening.

Equipment and techniques used: *(Provide details of equipment/techniques used successfully or unsuccessfully. Where relevant, include comments on patient positioning and factors which may have contributed to difficulty).*

If you require further information, please contact the Anaesthetic Department

DIFFICULT AIRWAY ALERT

v3.00 - 09/2021

SW884

FIGURE 66.2. ANZCA Difficult Airway Alert, developed by Queensland Health. (©The State of Queensland (Queensland Health) 2023. Permission to reproduce should be sought from ip_officer@health.qld.gov.au.)